NORMAL RESPIRATION AND BLOOD PRESSURE READINGS FOR CHILDREN

AVERAGE RESPIRATORY RATES AT REST (BREATHS/MINUTE)

Age	Rate (breaths/minute)
Newborn	35
1-11 months	30
2 years	25
4 years	23
6 years	21
8 years	20
10 years	19
12 years	19
14 years	18
16 years	17
18 years	16-18

MEAN BLOOD PRESSURE AT WRIST AND ANKLE IN INFANTS (FLUSH TECHNIQUE)

Age	Blood pressure at wrist		Blood pressure at ankle	
	Mean	Range	Mean	Range
1-7 days	41	22-66	37	20-58
1-3 months	67	48-90	61	38-96
4-6 months	73	42-100	68	40-104
7-9 months	76	52-96	74	50-96
10-12 months	57	62-94	56	102

Data from Moss, A.J., and Adams, F.H.: Problems of blood pressure in childhood, Springfield, Ill., 1962, Charles C Thomas, Publisher; from Moss, A.J.: Indirect methods of blood pressure measurement, Pediatr. Clin. North Am. **25**:3-14, 1978.

Blood pressure percentiles (right arm, seated)

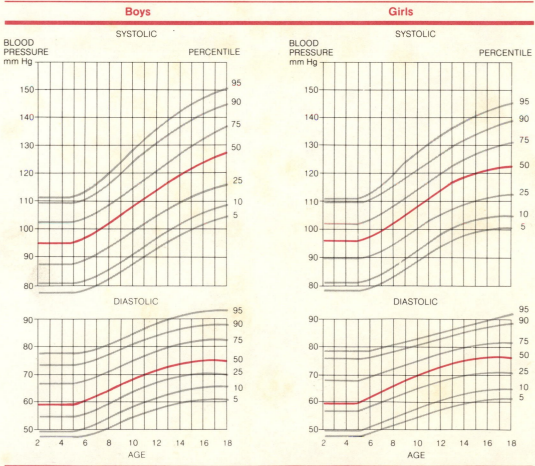

Redrawn from The National Heart, Lung, and Blood Institute's Task Force on Blood Pressure Control in Children: Report of the task force on blood pressure control in children, Pediatrics **59** (suppl. 5, pt. 2): 797-820, May 1977.

ESSENTIALS OF PEDIATRIC NURSING

SECOND EDITION
WITH 593 ILLUSTRATIONS

LUCILLE F. WHALEY, R.N., M.S.
Consultant, Parent-Child Nursing,
Formerly Professor of Nursing,
San Jose State University,
San Jose, California

DONNA L. WONG, R.N., M.N., P.N.P.
Nurse Counselor and Consultant in Private Practice,
Tulsa, Oklahoma

The C. V. Mosby Company

ST. LOUIS • TORONTO • PRINCETON 1985

A TRADITION OF PUBLISHING EXCELLENCE

Editor: David P. Carroll

Assistant editor: Bess Arends

Editing supervisor: Peggy Fagen

Manuscript editors: Jennifer Collins, Gayle May

Book design: Anne Canevari Green

Cover design: Kathleen A. Johnson

Production: Kathleen L. Teal, Teresa Breckwoldt

Cover photo of Nina Wong taken by Ting Wong

Second edition

Previous edition copyrighted 1981

Printed in the United States of America

The C.V. Mosby Company
11830 Westline Industrial Drive, St. Louis, Missouri 63146

Library of Congress Cataloging in Publication Data
Whaley, Lucille F., 1923-
 Essentials of pediatric nursing.

 Includes bibliographies and index.
 1. Pediatric nursing. I. Wong, Donna L., 1948-
II. Title.
RJ245.W46   1985   610.73'62   84-18976
ISBN 0-8016-5414-9

C/VH/VH   9 8 7 6 5 4 3 2 1   05/D/616

To my mother, Isabella Fillmore
To the memory of my father, Marvin Fillmore
L.F.W.

To my family,
Ting
Nina
Rudy
Who give me the loving support to continue
D.L.W.

PREFACE

The second edition of this book retains the major features that were so well received by our students and colleagues. The philosophy and purpose remain unchanged—the promotion of optimum health and development for children at any stage of health or illness. The emphasis is again on providing the reader with the basic information that is essential to the delivery of safe, comprehensive, and holistic care to children and their families.

The basic organization and presentation of content have been preserved from the first edition. The early chapters of the book emphasize normal development and common health problems encountered at various age levels and stress the role of the nurse in child health maintenance. The latter chapters focus on serious health problems of infants and children that frequently require hospitalization.

Unit 1 introduces the reader to child health promotion, including an overview of childhood mortality and morbidity, the role of pediatric nurses in health care delivery systems, and the needs of all children. It also presents an overview of the child in terms of his environment, especially the influence of the family, of ongoing developmental changes from birth through adolescence, and of the role of genetic and environmental influences in growth and maturation. Unit 2 provides an introduction to the principles and skills of nursing assessment, including communication, history taking, observation, physical and behavioral assessment, and developmental screening techniques.

Unit 3 is devoted to the stresses of the neonatal period, the time of greatest risk to survival. Units 4, 5, and 6 present detailed discussions of the major developmental stages that were introduced in Unit 1 and some of the health problems commonly associated with each age level. Unit 7 is concerned with the child who has special health or developmental problems but who has the same developmental needs as other children.

Units 8 through 12 describe the various types of serious health problems in children. Unit 8 sets the focus of the succeeding chapters through its discussion of the needs of the hospitalized child and his family and of the safe and competent implementation of hospital and home care procedures. In Units 9 through 12 the biologic-dysfunction framework allows for a conceptual approach to common symptoms and therapies as well as a discussion of the distinctive manifestations of specific disorders. Emphasis is placed on the special physiologic or emotional problems related to specific age-groups when appropriate. The reader is expected to apply the basic concepts of growth and development introduced in the early units when formulating individualized nursing care plans.

NEW FEATURES

The most notable features of the second edition are the inclusion of objectives for learning and identification of nursing diagnoses, both of which appear at the beginning of each chapter. Numerous new photographs and illustrations help clarify content and enhance the appearance of the book. An outstanding supplement that is available to instructors is an extensive resource manual with suggestions for learning activities, audiovisual materials, and a set of transparencies selected to augment the teaching process. A computerized test bank and booklet of test questions is also available.

The book has been updated to include current management and therapy, and new material has been added to increase the comprehensiveness and the usefulness of the book as a reference and a text. There is increased emphasis on the family in child health care, including expanded sections on fathers and siblings. The discussions of emotional care are highlighted whenever possible and are included in the numerous summaries of nursing care.

The sections on communication techniques, preparation of children for procedures (including parent teaching), pain assessment and management, and application of developmental principles have been expanded to facilitate the planning and implementation of nursing care to children of all ages and in a variety of settings, including the intensive care unit and the home environment. The discussions of normal growth and development now include segments that outline body image and moral and spiritual development. The section on mortality and morbidity includes a discussion of the evolution of child health care. The overview of the nursing process emphasizes the formulation of nursing diagnoses, a feature that is integrated throughout the text.

New material has been added to health problems of the neonate, such as birthmarks, hypotonia, neonatal seizures, intracranial lesions, and defects caused by maternal infection or chemicals. Supplemental information is included on health problems related to the adolescent reproductive system, shock in children, inhalation injury, and some of the newer health problems such as acquired immune deficiency syndrome and mucocutaneous lymph node syndrome. Accident prevention focuses on recent hazards to children, such as ingestion of button-size batteries, and includes a discussion of plant poisoning.

ACKNOWLEDGMENTS

We wish to express our appreciation to those persons who offered comments and suggestions for this revision. We again extend thanks to those institutions that have welcomed us to the units providing care to infants and children: Hillcrest Medical Center and St. Francis Hospital, Tulsa, Oklahoma; Santa Clara Valley Medical Center, San Jose, California; El Camino Hospital, Mt. View, California; and the library staffs at Santa Clara Valley Medical Center and Hillcrest Medical Center, especially Peggy Cook and Charlotte Wood.

In addition, a number of our colleagues provided reviews of specific content areas. Their criticisms and suggestions have been invaluable in ensuring accurate and up-to-date material that reflects current clinical practice. A very special thanks to Cathy Ayoub, clinical specialist, child psychiatry, Boston, Massachusetts; Linda Greenman, speech pathologist, Developmental Center, Tulsa County Schools; Mary Henley, clinic coordinator, Tulsa Cystic Fibrosis Center; Elizabeth Hiltunen, instructor, Boston College School of Nursing; Jacque Hodges, rehabilitation engineering technician, and Charles J. Laenger, rehabilitation engineer, Tulsa Rehabilitation Center; Christina Kasprisin, pediatric clinical specialist, and Marilyn Knoy, patient care supervisor of newborn nursery, St. Francis Hospital; Jim Keith, pharmacist, Eli Lilly and Company; Nannette Murrin, first president of Tulsa chapter of the National Federation of the Blind; Kristie Nix, assistant professor, University of Tulsa, and president of BELT (Buckle Every Little Tot); Donald Segal, executive director, Association for Brain Tumor Research; Marvin E. Spears, attorney-at-law, Tulsa, Oklahoma; and Patricia Thompson, associate professor, Northwestern State University of Louisiana.

We are especially indebted to all the children and families who have allowed us to take photographs. We also wish to thank the numerous persons who have generously contributed or otherwise provided photographs to this volume: Betty Stuart, Ogden, Utah; Ann Kunke, San Jose, California; Rick and Jackie Bender, Salt Lake City, Utah; Judy Dougherty, Danville, California; Roy Garibaldi, San Lorenzo, California; Kathleen Whaley and the San Lorenzo High School yearbook staff, San Lorenzo, California; Mike and Sue Riley and Dave and Mary Ann Bindbeutel, St. Louis, Missouri; Dave and Nan Carroll, Little Silver, New Jersey; and Joyce Bell, Loyal LaPlante Supply Company; Connie Morain, formerly child life specialist, Hillcrest Medical Center; the faculty and students of Holland Hall Primary School; Bo and Sherri Farmer; Mike and Karen Hess; Duke and Christina Kasprisin; and Mark and Kristie Nix, Tulsa, Oklahoma. Our collaboration with George Wassilchenko, Oral Roberts University, and with Kerri McGhee has generated additional illustrations for this volume and we are grateful for their efforts.

No book is ever a reality without the dedication and perseverance of the editorial staff. At The C.V. Mosby Company we are especially grateful to Bess Arends, Dave Carroll, and Mike Riley for their efforts in ensuring an excellent publication. This edition also marks the major transition to computerization of the manuscript process, a task made infinitely easier by Ann French, who patiently translated word processing into a usable language.

As always we wish to thank those members of our family whose substantial contributions as well as their devotion, patience, and forebearance are a constant source of support and encouragement. While it is never possible to adequately credit them with the numerous efforts and sacrifices each makes, we would like to thank Ting Kin Wong for the many long hours he spent taking and developing photographs, Bert Whaley and Rudolph Mitchko for assuming many of the tedious yet essential tasks associated with manuscript preparation, and Nina Wong for continuing to be a patient and precious child. Last of all, we thank each other for the shared excitement of exploration and the stimulation and mutual esteem that issue from this collaboration.

Lucille F. Whaley
Donna L. Wong

CONTENTS

UNIT 4
INFANCY

UNIT 5
EARLY CHILDHOOD

UNIT 6
MIDDLE CHILDHOOD AND ADOLESCENCE

UNIT 7
THE CHILD WITH LONG-TERM PHYSICAL OR DEVELOPMENTAL PROBLEMS

16 THE CHILD WHO IS HANDICAPPED, CHRONICALLY ILL, OR POTENTIALLY TERMINALLY ILL   440

UNIT 8
THE HOSPITALIZED CHILD

UNIT 9
THE CHILD WITH PROBLEMS RELATED TO THE TRANSFER OF OXYGEN AND NUTRIENTS

UNIT 11
THE CHILD WITH A DISTURBANCE OF REGULATORY MECHANISMS

24 THE CHILD WITH GENITOURINARY DYSFUNCTION 774

25 THE CHILD WITH CEREBRAL DYSFUNCTION 810

UNIT 12
THE CHILD WITH A PROBLEM THAT INTERFERES WITH LOCOMOTION

APPENDIXES

ESSENTIALS
OF
PEDIATRIC
NURSING

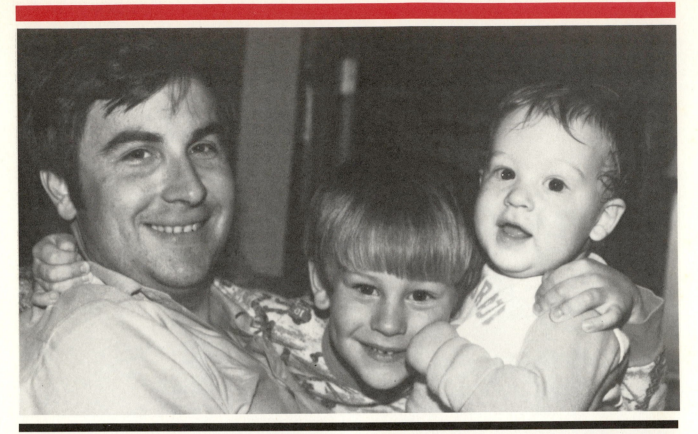

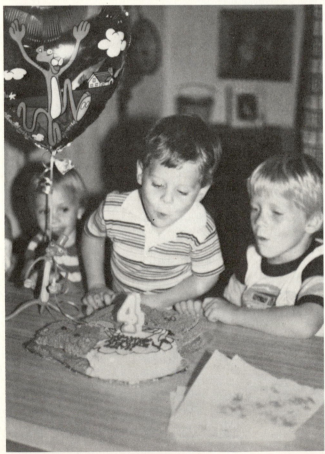

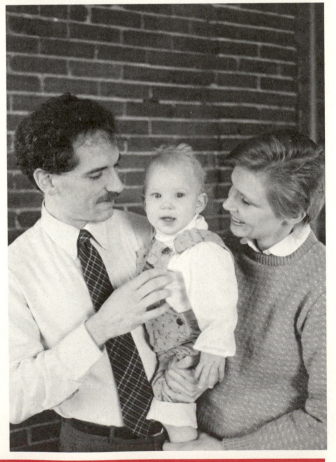

UNIT 1

CHILDREN, THEIR FAMILIES, AND THE NURSE

The ultimate goal of infant and child care is the promotion of optimum health and development for children at any stage of health or illness. To accomplish this purpose, nurses need an understanding of children and the way in which they grow and relate with significant persons in their environment, as well as an awareness of the multiple factors that contribute to the uniqueness of each child. To assess and evaluate the health and development of children, it is essential to be aware that the child is in the process of becoming.

Chapter 1, *Perspectives of Pediatric Nursing,* directs the focus for the remainder of the book, which emphasizes a child- and family-centered approach rather than a disease-centered approach to nursing of infants and children. Childhood health is viewed from the perspective of mortality and morbidity trends at various ages. An historical overview of child health care in the United States is given to serve as a basis for understanding the changes that have occurred in pediatrics. Nursing is viewed as a process and the nurse is viewed as a person who can work effectively with infants and children and who can help create the kind of conditions in which others, particularly the parents, can function more effectively in child care. The child is presented as a unique individual on a life-long developmental continuum, whose needs are the same as, yet different from, those of all other children.

Chapter 2, *Children: Their Environment and Development,* is concerned with children in their family setting.

It includes cultural, psychologic, and sociologic forces in the family situation that determine to some extent the way the family influences development. It examines various aspects of the family and the child's place within it, with emphasis on the role of parents in shaping the child's attitudes and behavior. This chapter also presents a vertical or longitudinal view of the alterations that take place during growth and development and serves as a preface to the horizontal view of the various age-related units that follow. The discussion focuses on general body changes, specific organ and system alterations, and a brief overview of the major theories of development.

Chapter 3, *Preconceptual and Prenatal Influences on Development and Health,* is concerned with genetic factors that affect the growth and health of children, maternal factors that may affect the outcome of the pregnancy, and the nurse's role in counseling parents of children with defects of hereditary origin.

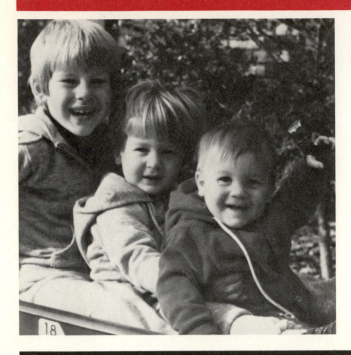

1

PERSPECTIVES OF PEDIATRIC NURSING

OBJECTIVES

On completion of this chapter the reader will be able to:

■ Define the terms *mortality* and *morbidity*

■ Identify two ways that knowledge of mortality and morbidity can improve child health

■ List three major causes of death during infancy, early childhood, later childhood, and adolescence

■ List two major causes of illness during childhood

■ Outline four events that were significant in the evolution of child health care in the United States

■ Define nursing diagnosis as a part of the nursing process

■ Describe five broad functions of the pediatric nurse in promoting the health of children

■ List three universal needs of children

NURSING DIAGNOSES

Because of the introductory nature of this chapter, nursing diagnoses are not identified. However, the concept of nursing diagnosis as part of the nursing process is discussed on p. 12 and a list of the diagnoses referred to throughout the text is presented on p. 13.

Health care of children has changed dramatically in the past century. It has paralleled society's change from a view of children as "miniature adults," whose value to the community was measured in productivity, to recognition and appreciation of children as unique individuals with special needs and qualities. There has been a shifting focus in their care from treatment of disease to prevention of illness and promotion of health. Nurses are no longer solely involved in the episodic care of children during an acute illness. They are increasingly responsible for providing comprehensive, distributive care that attempts to meet the needs of children and their families.

This chapter presents an overview of child health through discussion of past and present trends in childhood mortality and morbidity and the significant historical events that shaped present pediatric health care. It discusses the role of the pediatric nurse in both traditional and extended-role situations. The process of nursing children is briefly reviewed since it is the basis of all nursing action. Needs of children are presented because regardless of their immediate problem, these needs must be met for them to prosper and grow to the fullest.

HEALTH DURING CHILDHOOD

Health is a complex phenomenon. As defined by the World Health Organization (WHO), it is "a state of complete physical, mental, and social well-being and not merely the absence of disease." Despite this broad definition, however, health is traditionally assessed by observing *mortality* (death) and *morbidity* (illness) over a period of time. Therefore the *presence* of disease becomes a prime indicator of health.

Information concerning mortality and morbidity is of importance to nurses. Such data yield significant information about (1) the causes of death and illness, (2) high-risk age-groups for certain disorders or hazards, (3) advances in treatment and prevention, and (4) specific areas of health counseling. Statistics enumerating incidence according to race (color) demonstrate that health care is not equally benefiting all segments of society. Nurses who are aware of such information can better guide their planning and delivery of care.

Mortality

Figures describing rates of occurrence for events such as death in children are often referred to as *vital statistics*. *Mortality* statistics describe the incidence or number of individuals who have died over a specific period of time. They are usually presented as rates per hundred thousand because of their lower frequency of occurrence. Such rates are calculated from a sample of death certificates.

TABLE 1-1. INFANT MORTALITY FOR 20 COUNTRIES WITH POPULATION GREATER THAN 2 MILLION IN 1981

COUNTRY	RATE PER 1000 LIVE BIRTHS
Finland	6.5
Sweden	6.9
Japan	7.1
Norway	7.5
Switzerland	7.6
Denmark	7.9
Netherlands	8.3
France	9.6*
Canada	9.6
Hong Kong	9.8*
Australia	10.0
Spain	10.3
Ireland	10.6
Singapore	10.7*
United Kingdom	11.2*
German Federal Republic	11.6
United States	11.7*
Belgium	11.7
New Zealand	11.7
German Democratic Republic	12.3

From Wegman, M.E.: Annual summary of vital statistics—1982, Pediatrics **72**(6):755-756, 1983.
*Provisional data.

Infant mortality. *Infant mortality* is defined as the number of deaths per 1000 live births during the first year of life. It may further be divided into *neonatal* (first 28 days of life) and *postneonatal* (1 to 11 months) mortality. In the United States there has been a dramatic decrease in infant mortality during the 1900s. At the beginning of the twentieth century the rate was about 200 infant deaths per 1000 live births. In 1982 the number had dropped to an estimated 11.2 deaths per 1000 live births, the lowest rate ever recorded in the United States. This decrease has primarily resulted from infectious disease control and nutritional advances during the early twentieth century, the advent of antibiotic, antibacterial agents in the middle of the century, and recent improvements in perinatal care. However, from a worldwide perspective, the United States lags significantly behind other well-developed countries. In 1981 it ranked seventeenth among the 20 countries with the lowest infant death rates, with Finland having the lowest rate (Table 1-1). This is far behind neighboring countries such as Canada, which ranked ninth.

While there has been a steady and significant decline in infant mortality, the number of deaths occurring at this age is still proportionately high when compared with death

TABLE 1-2. DEATH RATES FOR CHILDREN, CANADA, 1981 (rates per 1000 population)

	RATE		
AGE (years)	TOTAL	MALE	FEMALE
Under 1	9.6	10.8	8.4
1-4	0.5	0.6	0.5
5-9	0.3	0.3	0.3
10-14	0.3	0.4	0.2
15-19	0.9	1.4	0.5
20-24	1.0	1.6	0.5

Data from Vital statistics, volume I, births and deaths: 1981, Statistics Canada, Minister of Supply and Services, 1983.

TABLE 1-3. DEATH RATES BY AGE, UNITED STATES, 1981 (rates per 100,000)

AGE (years)	RATE
Under 1	1143.7
1-4	55.5
5-14	27.8
15-24	104.7
25-34	126.9
35-44	207.9
45-54	556.4
55-59	1033.5
60-64	1574.6
65-69	2411.7
70-74	3516.7
75-79	5270.7
80-84	8107.1
85 and over	15,228.6

Data from National Center for Health Statistics: Annual summary of births, deaths, marriages, and divorces: United States, 1982. Monthly vital statistics report **31**(13):20, Public Health Service, Hyattsville, Md., 1983.

TABLE 1-4. LEADING CAUSES OF DEATH IN INFANTS UNDER 1 YEAR OF AGE, UNITED STATES, 1982 (estimated rates per 100,000 live births)

RANK	CAUSES OF DEATH	RATE
1	Other conditions originating in the perinatal period	295.1
2	Congenital anomalies	237.0
3	All other causes	177.1
4	Sudden infant death syndrome	127.2
5	Respiratory distress syndrome	107.2
6	Disorders relating to short gestation and unspecified low birth weight	98.8
7	Intrauterine hypoxia and birth asphyxia	39.7
8	Birth trauma	15.4
9	Pneumonia and influenza	20.0
10	Certain gastrointestinal diseases	7.3

Data from National Center for Health Statistics: Annual summary of births, deaths, marriages, and divorces: United States, 1982. Monthly vital statistics report **31**(13):8, Public Health Service, Hyattsville, Md., 1983.

rates at other ages. This is true of other countries, such as Canada (Table 1-2). As Table 1-3 shows, the death rate for infants under 1 year is greater than the rates for individuals ages 1 through 59 years. It is not until age 60 and over that the death rate begins to exceed the rate for infants.

During the first half of the 1900s, neonatal mortalities had not shown the remarkable reduction observed in infant mortality. In the early 1960s attention focused on perinatal health care in an effort to decrease the number of deaths.

As a result, neonatal mortality declined from 20.0 per 1000 in 1950 to 7.8 per 1000 in 1981. This has largely resulted from better treatment of perinatal illnesses, particularly asphyxia, immaturity, respiratory disorders, and gastrointestinal problems. As Table 1-4 demonstrates, most of the 10 leading causes of death during infancy continue to occur during the perinatal period. In fact almost three quarters of all infant deaths occur within the first 20 days of life.

While a number of perinatal problems have benefitted from improved treatment, congenital anomalies continue to be a leading cause of infant mortality, accounting for over 20% of those deaths. The incidence of the majority of birth defects has remained substantially the same. The relative stability of the incidence of congenital anomalies suggests the need for discovering and implementing improved prevention strategies (Kalter and Warkany, 1983).

When infant death rates are categorized according to race, an interesting paradox is seen. The infant mortality for whites is considerably lower than that for all other races in the United States, with blacks having almost double the rate for whites. One encouraging note is that the gap in death rates between whites and nonwhites has been narrowing. Since the Indian Health Service assumed responsibility for the health of American Indians in 1955, infant mortality has declined by 75%.

TABLE 1-5. FIVE LEADING CAUSES OF DEATH IN CHILDREN AT SELECTED AGE INTERVALS, UNITED STATES, 1980 (rates per 100,000)

AGES 1-4 YEARS	RATE	AGES 5-14 YEARS	RATE	AGES 15-24 YEARS	RATE
Accidents	25.9	Accidents	15.0	Accidents	61.7
Congenital anomalies	8.0	Cancer	4.3	Homicide	15.6
Cancer	4.5	Congenital anomalies	1.6	Suicide	12.3
Homicide	2.5	Homicide	1.2	Cancer	6.3
Heart disease	2.6	Heart disease	0.9	Heart disease	2.9

Data from National Center for Health Statistics: Advance report, final mortality statistics, 1980. Monthly vital statistics report **32**(4):17-18, Suppl., Public Health Service, Hyattsville, Md., Aug. 11, 1983.

Childhood mortality. After 1 year of age, there is a dramatic change in the causes of death in children. For all ages past 1 year the leading cause of death is accidents. As Table 1-5 illustrates, accidents account for nearly half of all childhood deaths from ages 1 to 24 years and claim more lives than all the next nine causes combined. In young adults ages 15 to 24, accidents, homicide, and suicide are responsible for more than 75% of all deaths. The pattern of deaths caused by accidents, especially from motor vehicles, drowning, and burns, is remarkably consistent in most Western societies, such as Canada.

Table 1-6 compares the six leading causes of accidental deaths for each age-group according to sex. The overwhelming majority of deaths at each age for both sexes is caused by motor vehicle fatalities. The group at highest risk includes infants less than 6 months of age. Factors that may be responsible are the greater frequency of their being held on an adult's lap or being placed on the front seat (Pless and Stulginskas, 1982).

From 1978 to 1982 nearly 3400 child passengers under 5 years of age were killed in traffic accidents and an additional 250,000 were injured. Tragically, up to 90% of the fatalities and 67% of the disabling injuries could have been prevented by the proper use of child safety restraints (National Transportation Safety Board, 1983). One encouraging note is that the incidence of vehicular accidents especially among young children has been declining, probably as a result of child passenger restraint laws. Currently, most of the states in the United States have enacted legislation requiring young children to be properly restrained in motor vehicles.

When accidental deaths are compared according to sex, it is obvious that the death rate is consistently higher for males than females and the causes of death may differ. Drowning and burns are the second and third leading causes of death in boys ages 1 to 14 years, but the order is reversed in girls. This probably reflects greater activity of boys outside the home and increased interest of girls in household activities, particularly in the kitchen. Also,

TABLE 1-6. MORTALITY FROM LEADING TYPES OF ACCIDENTS, UNITED STATES, 1978-1979 (rates per 100,000 population in specified group)

TYPE OF ACCIDENT	AGE (years)		
	1-4	5-9	10-14
Males			
Accidents (all types)	32.6	21.5	24.8
Motor vehicle	16.1(1)*	16.1(1)	14.2(1)
Drowning†	7.1(2)	4.2(2)	4.4(2)
Fires and flames	6.6(3)	2.3(3)	1.1(4)
Firearm missile	—	.8(4)	2.0(3)
Inhalation and ingestion of food or other object	1.6(4)	—	—
Falls	1.1(5)	.4(5)	.6(5)
Poisoning	.9(6)	—	—
Water transport	—	.3(6)	.4(6)
Accidents as a percent of all deaths	43%	54%	56%
Females			
Accidents (all types)	23.0	12.1	10.3
Motor vehicle	12.7(1)	9.8(1)	7.7(1)
Drowning†	3.4(3)	1.2(3)	1.1(2)
Fires and flames	5.0(2)	1.9(2)	1.1(2)
Firearm missile	—	.3(4)	.3(3)
Inhalation and ingestion of food or other object	1.0(4)	—	—
Falls	.7(6)	.2(5)	.1(4)
Poisoning	.9(5)	—	—
Water transport	—	.2(5)	.1(4)
Accidents as a percent of all death	39%	44%	41%

Data from Fatal accidents at the preschool ages, Stat. Bull. Metropol. Life. Insur. Co. **63**(4):12-15, 1982, and Fatal accidents among school-age children, Stat. Bull. Metropol. Life Insur. Co. **62**(3):10-12, 1981.
*Indicates rank among the leading types of accidents.
†Exclusive of deaths in water transportation.

while firearms are a major cause of death in males, they are not in females.

Analyzing deaths from specific types of accidents by age and sex is useful in identifying high-risk groups. It is also clear from a comparison of accidental deaths to other causes of childhood mortality that the greatest promise for improving childhood survival lies in preventing accidents. Certainly nurses play a major role in providing anticipatory guidance to parents and older children regarding hazards during each age period. In each succeeding chapter discussing growth and development, there is a lengthy discussion of accident prevention as part of health promotion.

The total number of deaths is also significant when each age-group is compared (Table 1-7). The school-age years have the lowest incidence of deaths. However, there is a sharp rise during later adolescence, when in addition to accidents, the next two leading causes of death, homicide and suicide, are also potentially preventable. Violent deaths have been steadily increasing among all groups of children. In the age-group 15 to 19, there has been a three to four times rate of increase since 1950 and the rate for those 10 to 14 is also increasing. Part of the reason for this in young children is more accurate identification of child abuse. Among adolescents, it may reflect an unhealthy preoccupation with violence and unresolved social tensions. Prevention lies in a better understanding of the social and psychologic factors that lead to the high rates of homicide and suicide. Nurses need to be especially aware of young people who are depressed, repeatedly in trouble with the criminal justice system, or associated with groups known to be violent. Prevention requires identification of these youngsters as well as therapeutic intervention by qualified professionals.

The general trend in racial differences that occurs in infant mortality is also apparent in childhood deaths. As Table 1-7 demonstrates, for all ages and for both sexes whites have fewer deaths. The accidental death rate for American Indian children ages 1 to 4 years is 3 times the average rate. For all ages and racial groups the number of male deaths outnumber female. This difference is particularly striking in the later adolescent years, when males have about a three times greater number of deaths than females.

The causes of death are also heavily influenced by race. For the white male between ages 15 and 19 years, the leading cause of death is motor vehicle accidents. For males in the ''all other'' category, the greatest number of deaths is from homicide. This same trend applies to females. However, for all groups the differences in suicide are comparatively small, with white males and females having a somewhat higher rate.

The absence of infectious diseases as a leading cause of death in the age-groups over 5 years is testimony to the role that antibiotic/antibacterial agents and immunizations

TABLE 1-7. NUMBER OF CHILDREN DYING AT SELECTED AGE INTERVALS ACCORDING TO SEX AND RACE, UNITED STATES, 1982 (rates per 100,000)				
AGE INTERVAL (years)	**WHITE**		**ALL OTHER**	
	MALE	**FEMALE**	**MALE**	**FEMALE**
Under 1	1129.2	906.2	1823.8	1440.4
1-4	55.5	44.3	95.0	62.9
5-14	32.1	20.2	45.4	23.7
15-24	148.2	52.3	186.8	60.9

Data from National Center for Health Statistics: Annual summary of births, deaths, marriages, and divorces: United States, 1982. Monthly vital statistics report **31**(13):20, Public Health Service, Hyattsville, Md., 1983.

have played in the declining death rates and the specific causes of death. More effective treatment of severe infections has resulted in other disorders becoming more prominent in the list of leading killers. Most notable among these are the neoplasms. Cancer is the leading cause of death from disease in children ages 3 to 14 years. It strikes some 6000 children annually. The most common form of cancer in the age-groups up to 9 years is leukemia. The lymphomas are most common in children 10 to 14 years. About 40% of all cancer occurs during the ages 4 and under. The school-age years have the lowest incidence, which may be attributable to the fact that this is a quiescent period of growth before puberty. The mortality for cancer in children has declined from 8.3 per 100,000 in 1950 to 4.4 in 1979. About 1600 deaths occur annually and about half of these are from leukemia (Cancer Facts and Figures, 1984).

Morbidity

Morbidity statistics describe the prevalence of a specific illness in the population at a particular time. These are generally presented as rates per 1000 population because of their greater frequency of occurrence. Unlike mortality statistics, morbidity is very difficult to define and measure. Morbidity may denote acute illness, chronic disease, or disability. The source of data also greatly influences the resulting statistics. Common sources include reasons for visits to physicians, diagnosis for hospital admission, or household interviews. The following discussion is intended to present an overview of illness in children from a variety of perspectives.

Childhood morbidity. Acute illness may be defined as symptoms severe enough to limit activity or require medical attention. According to the National Health Survey, children under 5 years of age have about 3.5 acute illnesses per year with 8.8 days of restricted activity. Children ages 5 to 14 years have 2.9 episodes and 9.4 days of disability. As a general rule, acute illness is less frequent in children under 6 months of age, increases thereafter until age 3 or 4 years, and then gradually decreases throughout middle and older childhood. There is a slight peak again during the first year or two of school, probably as a result of increased exposure to new contagions (Green and Haggerty, 1984).

Infections account for nearly 80% of all childhood illnesses, and respiratory infections lead the list, occurring two to three times as often as all other illnesses combined. The chief illness of childhood is the common cold. The average child has between one and two colds per year. One third of all children have at least one episode of some other infection annually as well. About 3% of all acute illnesses are caused by accidents, which generally require more medical care because they are more serious.

From the perspective of seeking medical care, more children from white families have acute illnesses than those from black families. However, the illnesses reported by black mothers are more likely to be severe. This is probably in part a result of different attitudes toward health care. For most American children in the middle and upper socioeconomic levels, serious physical illness is an uncommon event, but for those from underprivileged environments, critical physical disease still occurs.

Another area of morbidity is chronic disorders, which may be roughly defined as conditions that persist for more than 3 months. Statistics regarding the prevalence of chronic disorders are discussed in Chapter 16.

Probably the most important aspect of morbidity is the degree of disability it produces. Disability can be measured in days off from school or days confined to bed. It can be the result of acute or chronic disorders. On an average, a child loses 5.6 days of school per year. Boys miss somewhat more school than girls, chiefly because of injuries. Of all children under 17 years of age, over 95% are not disabled in any way. About 2% have mild disability, another 2% have moderate disability, and 0.2% are severely disabled (Pless, 1978).

While childhood is a time of relative health, it is the rare child who never becomes ill. Most children experience one or more episodes of acute illness annually and may be disabled for a short period of time. The rapidity with which children become ill is often a source of great anxiety for parents, who fear that the illness is serious. Part of nurses' intervention is education of parents regarding the usual types of childhood illness and recognition of those symptoms requiring treatment, such as signs of respiratory distress or dehydration. Certainly, nurses should also be aware of signs of potentially fatal illnesses. However, the future progress in decreasing childhood morbidity, as in childhood mortality, rests more on parent education than on miraculous discoveries such as the antibiotic. Nurses play a vital role in advancing child care through health promotion.

The new morbidity. In addition to disease and injury, children face other problems that can significantly alter their health. These include behavioral, social (family), and educational problems that are sometimes referred to as the new morbidity. Estimates on the incidence of these problems vary, but they represent at least 5% and as much as 25% to 30% in specific age-groups, social classes, and medical facilities (Starfield, 1980). These include children (1) from the lowest socioeconomic strata, (2) in the first and second grades, (3) with reading skills below grade level, and (4) with higher rates of school absenteeism (Nader and others, 1981). There is also some evidence that increasing maternal education is associated with decreasing numbers of children with "new morbidity" problems. However, these mothers are more likely to seek professional help and talk about the child's behavior, school problems, or social adjustment.

EVOLUTION OF CHILD HEALTH CARE IN THE UNITED STATES

Children in colonial America were born into a world with many hazards to their health and survival. Epidemics were common and no control or treatment was known. Physicians were few and only a small number had any formal training. Midwives also were untrained, usually practicing because of past experiences. Books providing information on child care and feeding were scarce and, when available, were useful only to a minority of literate parents.

Medical care by physicians was limited to wealthy European families who lived in or could travel to more developed cities. Children who lived on farms were cared for mainly by another family member or by a competent neighbor. Traveling medicine men, with their various forms of quackery, were common. Black children who were bought as slaves or born to slaves had only as much care as their owner was able or willing to provide. American Indian children were treated for disease according to the tradition of each tribe, which was often a mixture of medicine, magic, and religion. With the colonization of America the Indians were exposed to many new diseases.

Statistics on childhood mortality during the colonial period are largely unavailable. Epidemic diseases were prevalent, however, and included smallpox, measles, mumps, chickenpox, diphtheria, yellow fever, cholera, and whooping cough, but the disease that surpassed all others as a cause of childhood death was dysentery. Sometimes entire families succumbed to this illness. Other major contributors to childhood illness and death were tuberculosis, nutritional diseases, and accidents (Schmidt,

1976). Accidents included skull fractures from playing in the streets; burns from open fireplaces, candles, and gunpowder; scalds resulting from falling into open kettles of boiling milk, water, and chocolate; and drownings from falling into unprotected wells (Cone, 1976).

Although scientific knowledge was accumulating, especially from work done in Europe, there were no organized efforts in the United States to apply that knowledge to the care of the sick. It was not until the Industrial Revolution was well underway in the nineteenth century that the consequences of childhood illness and injury and the effects of poverty and neglect became more widely recognized. The end of the nineteenth century is often regarded as the dark age of pediatrics, and the first half of the twentieth century is regarded as the dawn of improved health care for children.

The study of pediatrics began in the last half of the 1800s, under the influence of a Prussian-born physician, Abraham Jacobi (1830-1919). Because of his many accomplishments, he is referred to as the Father of Pediatrics. With several other physicians he pioneered in the scientific and clinical investigation of childhood diseases. One achievement was the establishment of ''milk stations,'' where mothers could bring sick children for treatment and learn the importance of pure milk and its proper preparation. The crusade for pure milk helped bring the dairy industry under legal control and led to the establishment of infant welfare stations. The remarkable declines in infant mortality since 1900 have been achieved through prevention and health-promoting measures such as improved sanitation and pasteurization of milk. Before these regulations existed, the unsanitary milk supply was a chief source of infantile diarrhea and bovine tuberculosis. Cows were often kept in filthy stables and fed garbage and distillery wastes. Milk from cows fed distillery wastes was reported to make infants ''tipsy.'' Some of the cows were so diseased with tuberculosis that they had to be raised on cranes to be milked (Cone, 1976).

Arising about the same time as these developments was the increasing concern for the social welfare of children, especially those who were homeless or employed as factory laborers. The work of one such reformer, Lillian Wald (1867-1940), founder of the Henry Street Settlement in New York, led President Theodore Roosevelt to call the first White House Conference on Children in 1909. It focused on care of dependent children and attempted to address the deplorable working conditions of youngsters. As a result of this conference, the U.S. Children's Bureau was established under the jurisdiction of the Department of Labor, since at that time laws to regulate child labor were seen as the greatest need. Later, the Bureau was placed under the Department of Health, Education and Welfare (now the Department of Health and Human Services). White House conferences have been held approximately

every 10 years to address the welfare, health, education, social, economic, and psychologic needs of children.

Wald's work has had far-reaching effects on child health and nursing. She started visiting nurse services in New York City and was instrumental in establishing the role of the first full-time school nurse. An outgrowth of nursing involvement in school health was the development of pediatric courses and specialized clinical experience in schools of nursing.

As more causes of disease were identified, there was an emphasis on isolation and asepsis. In the early 1900s children with contagious diseases were isolated from adult patients. Parents were prohibited from visiting because they might transmit disease to and from the home. Even toys and personal articles of clothing were kept from the child. It was not until the 1940s and the famous work of Spitz and Robertson on institutionalized children that the effects of isolation and maternal deprivation were recognized. This brought forth a surge of interest in the psychologic health of children and resulted in changes for hospitalized children, such as rooming in, sibling visitations, child life (play) programs, prehospitalization preparation, parent education, and hospital schooling.

On a national level the establishment of the Children's Bureau in 1912 marked the beginning of a period of studies of economic and social factors related to infant mortality, maternal deaths, and maternal and infant care in rural areas, all of which created the basis for stimulating better standards of care for mothers and children. This helped lead to the first Maternity and Infancy Act (Sheppard-Towner Act) in 1921 and to a much broader Maternal and Child Health program under Title V of the Social Security Act in l935. The program consisted of three proposals: (1) aid to dependent children; (2) maternal and child health services, including Crippled Children's Services (CCS) (now the Special Child Health Services); and (3) child welfare services. The first programs provided by Title V were prenatal and postnatal clinics, child health clinics, and training of professional personnel. Since 1935 numerous other federal programs have been developed. Some of those that have had a major impact on maternal and child health include the following (Better Health for Our Children, 1981):

1. **Medicaid and EPSDT.** In 1965 Medicaid was created under Title XIX of the Social Security Act to reduce financial barriers to health care for the poor. In 1964 all states were required to provide early and periodic screening, diagnosis, and treatment (EPSDT) to children under Medicaid.
2. **WIC.** In 1966 the Special Supplemental Food Program for Women, Infants, and Children (WIC) was passed. It provides nutritious food and nutrition education to low-income, pregnant, postpartum, and lactating women, and to infants and children up to age 5.

3. **Education for All Handicapped Children Act (P.L. 94-142).** In 1975 P.L. 94-142 was passed to provide a free appropriate public education to all handicapped children from ages 3 to 21 and to provide for those supportive services (such as speech and counseling) that ensure the benefit of special education.
4. **CMHC and Service Systems.** This law, passed in 1980 and effective in 1982, replaces the 1963 Community Mental Health Centers (CMHC) Act and should provide a substantial increase in the availability of mental health centers to indigent and low-income families.

Nurses need to be aware of the types of programs available and the nature of the services rendered to individuals. Fragmentation of care can be prevented if professionals take the time to coordinate services and act as advocates for families.

UNITED NATIONS' DECLARATION OF THE RIGHTS OF THE CHILD
All children need:
To be free from discrimination
To develop physically and mentally in freedom and dignity
To have a name and nationality
To have adequate nutrition, housing, recreation and medical services
To receive special treatment if handicapped
To receive love, understanding, and material security
To receive an education and develop his/her abilities
To be the first to receive protection in disaster
To be protected from neglect, cruelty and exploitation
To be brought up in a spirit of friendship among people

THE PEDIATRIC NURSE

Nursing of infants and children is based on the premise that its purpose is to promote the highest possible state of health in each child. It consists of preventing disease or injury; assisting children, including those with a permanent handicap or health problem, to achieve and maintain an optimum level of health and development; and treating or rehabilitating children who have health deviations. This implies that nursing is involved in every aspect of a child's growth and development. Nursing functions vary according to regional job structures, individual education and experience, and personal expectations of their profession. Just as clients (children and their families) present a vast and unique background, so it is that each nurse will bring to the clients an individual set of variables that will affect their relationship. No matter where pediatric nurses practice, their primary concern is the welfare of the child and his family.

Family advocacy

Although the nurse is responsible to self, the profession, and the institution of employment, the primary responsibility is to the recipients of nursing services, the child and family. The nurse must work with members of the family, identifying their goals and needs, and plan interventions that best meet the defined problems. As a consumer advocate the nurse must strive to ensure that families are aware of all available health services, informed adequately of treatments and procedures, involved in the child's care when possible, and encouraged to change or support existing health-care practices. The pediatric nurse is aware of the United Nations Declaration of the Rights of the Child (see boxed material) and practices within these guidelines to ensure that every child receives optimum care. As child advocate the nurse utilizes this knowledge to adapt care for the child's optimum physical and emotional well-being. Examples of this may be fostering the parent-child relationship during hospitalization, preparing the child before any unfamiliar treatment or procedure, allowing the child privacy, providing play activities for expression of fear, aggression, or loss of control, and respecting cultural differences relating to feeding or childrearing practices.

The nurse is aware of the needs of children and works with all caregivers to ensure that these fundamental requirements are met. This often necessitates that the nurse expand the boundaries of practice to less traditional settings. As a child advocate the nurse may be involved in education, political/legislative change, rehabilitation, screening, administration, and even engineering and architecture. Regardless of how removed from direct patient care individual nurses become, they continue to foster health-care practices that promote the optimum well-being of children by incorporating knowledge of child growth and development into particular roles of practice.

Prevention

The emerging trends toward health care have been prevention of illness and maintenance of health, rather than treatment of disease or disability. Nursing has kept pace with this change, especially in the area of child care. In 1965 specialized programs for pediatric nurse associates/practitioners began to develop that have led to several specialized ambulatory or primary care roles for nurses. The thrust of these programs has been to educate nurses beyond the basic preparational stage in areas of child health maintenance in order for all children to receive high-quality care. An outgrowth of the practitioner programs has been expanded programs for school nurse practitioners.

Obviously, the thrust of these nurse practitioner programs is prevention. However, preventive care is not limited to them. Every nurse involved with child care must practice within the overall dimension of preventive health. Regardless of the identified problem, the role of the nurse is to plan care that fosters every aspect of growth and development. Based on a thorough assessment process, problems related to nutrition, immunizations, safety, dental care, development, socialization, discipline, or schooling frequently become obvious. Once the problem is identified, the nurse acts to intervene directly or to refer the family to other health persons or agencies.

The best approach to prevention is education and anticipatory guidance. In this book each chapter on growth and development includes sections on anticipatory guidance. With an appreciation of the hazards or conflicts of each developmental period, the nurse is able to guide parents regarding child-rearing practices aimed at preventing potential problems.

Prevention involves less obvious aspects of child care. Besides preventing physical disease or injury, the nurse's role is also to promote mental health. For example, it is not sufficient to administer immunizations without regard for the psychologic trauma associated with the procedure. Optimum health involves the practice of good medicine with a humane approach to health care; the nurse is often the one professional capable of ensuring ''humanity.''

Health teaching

Health teaching is inseparable from family advocacy and prevention. Health teaching may be a direct goal of the nurse, such as during parenting classes, or may be indirect, such as informing parents and children of a diagnosis or medical treatment, encouraging children to ask questions about their bodies, referring families to health-related professional or lay groups, supplying patients with appropriate literature, and providing anticipatory guidance.

Health teaching is often one area in which nurses feel competent because it involves translating information rather than receiving messages, translating them, and planning intervention. In other words, it is a concrete, structured, or incidental type of communication as opposed to other, emotionally laden, nondirected types of interaction. However, the nurse focuses on giving appropriate health teaching with generous feedback and evaluation to promote learning.

Support/counseling

Attention to emotional needs necessitates support and sometimes counseling. Frequently, the role of child advocate or health teacher is supportive by the very nature of the individualized approach. Support can be offered in many ways, the most common of which include listening, touching, and physical presence. The last two are most helpful with children because they facilitate nonverbal communication.

Counseling involves a mutual exchange of ideas and opinions that provides the basis for mutual problem solving. Although it is similar to health teaching, its focus is broader and more intense because it frequently implies some crisis or upsetting event that needs intervention. It involves support as well as teaching, techniques to foster expression of feelings or thoughts, and approaches to help the family cope with stress. Although counseling is often the role of more specialized nurses, counseling techniques are discussed in various sections of the text to help students and nurses cope with immediate crises about them and refer families for additional professional assistance.

Therapeutic role

The most basic of all nurses' roles is the restoration of health through care-giving activities. Nurses are intimately involved with meeting the physical and emotional needs of children, including feeding, bathing, toileting, dressing, security, and socialization. They are primarily responsible for instituting physicians' prescriptions; they are also held singularly accountable for their own actions and judgments regardless of written orders.

A significant aspect of the therapeutic role is continual assessment and evaluation of physical status. Only when aware of normal findings can the nurse intelligently identify and document deviations. In addition the pediatric nurse never loses sight of the emotional and developmental needs of the individual child, which can significantly influence the course of the disease process.

Restoration frequently implies habilitation and rehabilitation. Through expanding roles nurses are increasingly responsible for health care of handicapped children. For example, school nurses or pediatric nurse practitioners are involved in programs for severely developmentally disabled children in order to facilitate their attendance in regular classes.

Coordination/collaboration

The nurse as a member of the health team collaborates and coordinates nurses' services with other professionals' activities. Working in isolation does not serve the child's best interest. First, the concept of ''holistic care'' can only be realized through a unified interdisciplinary approach. Second, aware of individual contributions and limitations to the child's care, the nurse must collaborate with other specialists to provide for high-quality health services. Failure to recognize limitations can be nontherapeutic at best and destructive at worst. For example, the nurse who feels competent in counseling when really inadequate in this area may not only prevent the child from dealing with a crisis but may also retard his future success with a qualified professional.

Even nurses who practice in geographically isolated areas widely separated from other health professionals cannot be considered independent. Every nurse works interdependently with the child and family, collaborating on needs and interventions so that the final care plan is one that truly meets the child's needs. Unfortunately, this is one aspect of collaboration and coordination that is lacking in health care planning. Often numerous disciplines work together to formulate a comprehensive approach without consulting with clients regarding their ideas or preferences. The nurse is in a vital position to include consumers in their care, either directly or indirectly, by communicating their thoughts to the group.

Health care planning

So far, the nurse's role has been viewed through the nucleus of a family. However, the nursing role is far more extensive and includes the community or society as a whole. Traditionally nurses have been involved in public health care, either on a distributive or on an episodic basis. Rarely, however, have nurses been involved in health care planning, especially on a political or legislative level. Their role must also involve the decision-making body of government. Nursing, as the largest health profession, needs to have a voice, especially as family/consumer advocate. This does not mean that the nurse must hold public office. Rather it refers to knowledge and awareness of community needs, interest in government formulation of bills and support of politicians to assure passage (or rejection) of significant legislation, and active involvement in groups dedicated to the welfare of children, such as

---

AMERICAN NURSES' ASSOCIATION STANDARDS OF MATERNAL-CHILD HEALTH NURSING PRACTICE

Standard I
Maternal and child health nursing practice is characterized by the continual questioning of the assumptions upon which practice is based, retaining those which are valid and searching for and using new knowledge.

Standard II
Maternal and child health nursing practice is based upon knowledge of the biophysical and psychosocial development of individuals from conception through the childrearing phase of development and upon knowledge of the basic needs for optimum development.

Standard III
The collection of data about the health status of the client/patient is systematic and continuous. The data are accessible, communicated and recorded.

Standard IV
Nursing diagnoses are derived from data about the health status of the patient.

Standard V
Maternal and child health nursing practice recognizes deviations from expected patterns of physiologic activity and anatomic and psychosocial development.

Standard VI
The plan of nursing care includes goals derived from the nursing diagnoses.

Standard VII
The plan of nursing care includes priorities and the prescribed nursing approaches or measures to achieve the goals derived from the nursing diagnoses.

Standard VIII
Nursing actions provide for client/patient participation in health promotion, maintenance and restoration.

Standard IX
Maternal and child health nursing practice provides for the use and coordination of all services that assist individuals to prepare for responsible sex roles.

Standard X
Nursing actions assist the client/patient to maximize his health capabilities.

Standard XI
The client's/patient's progress or lack of progress toward goal achievement is determined by the client/patient and the nurse.

Standard XII
The client's/patient's progress or lack of progress toward goal achievement directs reassessment, reordering of priorities, new goal setting and revision of the plan of nursing care.

Standard XIII
Maternal and child health nursing practice evidences active participation with others in evaluating the availability, accessibility and acceptability of services for parents and children and cooperating and/or taking leadership in extending and developing needed services in the community.

From American Nurses' Association, *Standards of Maternal-Child Health Nursing Practice,* American Nurses' Association, Kansas City, 1973.

professional nursing societies, parent-teacher organizations, parent support groups, religious affiliations, and voluntary organizations.

Health care planning involves not only providing new services but also promoting the highest quality of existing ones. Nursing needs to ensure the excellence of its own profession through each individual member, who practices according to the Code of Ethics and Standards of Practice. Pediatric nurses are obligated to follow the Standards of Maternal and Child Health Nursing (see the boxed material, p. 11). Each standard is followed by rationale and pertinent assessment factors. Nurses should also help to make certain their colleagues implement the standards, through education, role modeling, and supervision.

Throughout the text the highest standards of nursing practice are continually reflected in the emphasis on thorough assessment, focus on scientific rationale as the basis for care, summary of nursing care goals and responsibilities, and comprehensive discussion of growth and development. Family-centered principles are continually evident in the consideration of dynamics affecting the child, parents, siblings, and extended members. The nurse is viewed as a vital component of the health care delivery system. Although nursing functions are clearly outlined, nursing responsibilities must be equally emphasized. It is hoped that the roles briefly described here will be studied, practiced, and implemented to the benefit of all children.

THE PROCESS OF NURSING CHILDREN

Planning and implementing nursing care to meet the needs of infants and children require a systematic approach to decision making. The problem-solving process consists of five operational phases: assessment, problem identification (nursing diagnosis), plan formulation, implementation, and evaluation. It involves both cognitive and operational skills. How successfully the process is carried out depends on such factors as the nurse's level of competence, the formation of the nurse-child-family relationship, and the goals and capabilities of the family members.

Summary of the nursing process

Assessment is a continuous process that is operative at all phases of problem solving and is the foundation for decision making. Derived through multiple nursing skills, it consists of the purposeful collection, classification, and analysis of data from a variety of sources. To ensure an accurate and comprehensive assessment, the nurse must consider information about the patient's biophysical, psychologic, sociocultural, and spiritual background.

Analysis and synthesis of the collected data results in *problem identification*. In order to solve a problem it is essential to acknowledge that it exists and to describe its nature. The problem may involve an unmet need, an unrealized expectation, an interrupted process, or a community crisis. In some instances no actual problem is identified but present health practices or coping mechanisms may need to be maintained. Potential problems may be recognized because of the identified risk, such as an infection or a skin problem. *Nursing diagnoses* are used to describe these problems or concerns.

One currently accepted definition of a nursing diagnosis states that it is "a clinical judgment about an individual, family, or community derived through the deliberate, systematic process of data collection and analysis which provides for the prescription of definitive therapy for which the nurse is accountable" (Shoemaker, 1984). Currently accepted nursing diagnoses are listed in the boxed material according to eleven functional health patterns (Gordon, 1982). The functional health patterns serve as a framework for organizing a nursing assessment and standardizing data collection. Additional research is needed to broaden the list, especially for specialty areas such as pediatrics. However, these nursing diagnoses are the beginning of a scientific basis for nursing practice. Throughout the text selected nursing diagnoses are listed at the beginning of the chapter to emphasize those nursing diagnoses that relate to specific conditions or disorders.

Plan formulation is the decision-making phase of the process. With a specific nursing diagnosis identified, the nurse designs a plan of action to meet a goal (objective or expected outcome). A design for action involves the selection of a plan that is based on scientific principles derived from a variety of disciplines. Interventions are chosen that are most likely to achieve the desired consequence with a minimum of risk to the persons involved.

The phase of *implementation* begins when the nurse puts the selected intervention into action and accumulates feedback regarding its effects. The feedback returns in the form of observation and communication and provides a data base on which to evaluate the outcome of the nursing intervention. Throughout the implementation stage, the patient's physical safety and psychologic comfort are the main concerns.

Evaluation is the last step in the decision-making process. The nurse gathers, sorts, and analyzes data to determine if (1) the goal has been met, (2) the plan requires modification, or (3) another alternative should be considered. This evaluation either completes the nursing process or serves as the basis for selection of other alternatives for intervention in solving the specific problem.

Primary nursing

Inherent in the decision-making process is accountability. Nurses are responsible for their actions, both in the legal

---

NURSING DIAGNOSES ACCORDING TO FUNCTIONAL HEALTH PATTERNS

Health perception-health management patterns
Health maintenance, alterations in
*Infection, potential for
Injury, potential for (specify: poisoning, suffocation, trauma)
Noncompliance (specify)

Nutritional-metabolic pattern
Fluid volume deficit, actual
Fluid volume deficit, potential
Fluid volume, alterations in: excess
Nutrition, alterations in: less than body requirements
Nutrition, alterations in: more than body requirements
Nutrition, alterations in: potential for more than body requirements
Oral mucous membranes, alterations in
Skin integrity, impairment of: actual
Skin integrity, impairment of: potential

Elimination pattern
Bowel elimination, alterations in: constipation
Bowel elimination, alterations in: diarrhea
Bowel elimination, alterations in: incontinence
Urinary elimination, alteration in patterns

Activity-exercise pattern
Activity intolerance
Airway clearance, ineffective
Breathing patterns, ineffective
Cardiac output, alterations in: decreased
Diversional activity deficit
Gas exchange, impaired
Home maintenance management, impaired
*Joint contractures, potential for
Mobility, impaired physical
Self-care deficit (specify level: feeding, bathing/hygiene, dressing/grooming, toileting)
Tissue perfusion, alteration in

Sleep-rest pattern
Sleep-pattern disturbance

Cognitive-perceptual pattern
Comfort, alterations in: pain
Knowledge deficit (specify)
Sensory-perceptual alterations
Thought processes, alterations in

Self-perception—self-concept pattern
Anxiety
Fear (specify)
Powerlessness
Self-concept, disturbance in

Role-relationship pattern
Communication, impaired verbal
Family process, alterations in
Grieving, anticipatory
Grieving, dysfunctional
Parenting, alterations in: actual
Parenting, alterations in: potential
Social isolation
Violence, potential for

Sexuality-reproductive pattern
Rape trauma syndrome
Sexual dysfunction

Coping-stress tolerance pattern
Coping, family: potential for growth
Coping, ineffective family: compromised
Coping, ineffective family: disabling
Coping, ineffective individual

Value-belief pattern
Spiritual distress

From Kim, M., McFarland, G., and McLane, A.: Classification of nursing diagnoses: proceedings of the fifth national conference, St. Louis, 1984, The C.V. Mosby Co.
*Additional diagnoses from Gordon, M.: Manual of nursing diagnosis, New York, 1982, McGraw-Hill Book Co.

---

and ethical senses. Part of the trend in nursing practice is a deeper commitment to accountability. One of the outgrowths of this has been the movement toward *primary nursing*. Primary nursing involves 24-hour responsibility and accountability by one nurse for the care of a small group of patients. The primary nurse becomes the bedside nurse, with few if any duties delegated to other staff. If responsibilities are shared, it is usually with an associate primary nurse who maintains continuity of care when the primary nurse is not on duty.

One of the traditional problems with primary nursing is providing consistency in scheduling the same nurse and associate. An approach that minimizes this difficulty is to designate one primary nurse and as many associates as are needed to ensure that the same group of nurses care for the child. This *primary core team* necessitates that at least one nurse is assigned to the patient for each shift and that additional nurses are assigned for these individuals' days off. By identifying the core team in advance for a specific period, all the nurses working with the child can plan care jointly, with the primary nurse maintaining overall responsibility.

The philosophy of primary care is supported throughout the discussion of nursing of children. In some instances the one-to-one relationship between child and nurse is emphasized because of its therapeutic benefit, such as in nonorganic failure to thrive. However, primary nursing is universally a supportive intervention in pediatric nursing because it provides a consistent caregiver for the child and focuses on the family unit as an integral component in the planning and implementation of care.

THE CHILD

All children are basically alike. They follow the same pattern of development and maturation, whereas, at the same time, their hereditary, cultural, and experiential backgrounds make each a distinct and unique individual. They differ in their rate of growth, their ultimate size and capabilities, and the way in which they respond to their environment. However, regardless of his stage of development, his state of health, or the situation in which he is encountered, *the child is first of all a child.*

In most instances parents assume the responsibility of child rearing with the intent to produce a well-adjusted member of society. Most succeed. The exceptional failures are usually attributed to faulty parenting in which the level of maturity, cultural background, and the quality of the parents' own upbringing influence their ability to provide for the care and nurture of their children. Parents and child can seldom be separated one from the other in child care. Anything that affects the parents will also affect the child. It is not uncommon for a child to develop physical symptoms as a response to intrafamily stress or disharmony. Nurses who assist parents to a successful relationship with their children will assure a healthier environment for the children.

Needs of infants and children

Every society and every generation has regulated child care practices and used children for its own purposes. Child rearing has been based on traditional beliefs and practices and dictated by cultural and religious values, political and economic requirements, and a variety of ideas and purposes that were often remote from the children themselves. Today the trend in the care and nurture of children is based on their developmental needs. Children need ample physical room in which to grow as well as support from the adults in their environment. Because they do not have the resources for coping with the world, children need to be surrounded by caring people who are willing to share their pleasures and help them through troubling times.

Although the emphasis and classification may vary according to the interpreter, the essential needs of children during all stages of development are physical, biologic, and emotional needs, including love, emotional security, discipline, independence, and self-esteem.

Physical and biologic needs. First of all, children's basic physical and biologic needs for food, water, air, warmth, elimination, and shelter must be met. Infants, except for limited reflex responses, are totally dependent on adults for satisfaction of even the most basic needs. As development proceeds, children begin to communicate their needs verbally and nonverbally and to assume increasing responsibility for their basic need gratification.

Those who care for children come to understand the physical changes that take place during the process of development and the special needs generated by these changes, for example, the nature and quantity of the food intake, the method and frequency of feeding, and the amount of sleep and activity that change during childhood. Health and safety hazards associated with every phase of development require implementation of measures to provide for the child's physical safety, including prevention of accidents and disease and education of children, families, and communities regarding these potential threats to health and well-being.

Love and affection. The single most important emotional need of children is to be loved and to feel secure in that love. Children strive above all else to gain the love and acceptance of those who are significant in their lives. When they feel secure in this love they are able to withstand the normal crises associated with growing up and those unexpected crises (such as illness or loss) that are superimposed on the anticipated course of development.

Children cannot receive too much love. However, this love must be communicated to them through words and actions that tell them that they are loved, not for their actions or achievement, but for what they are or simply *because they are.* Although love is closely associated with discipline, independence, and other factors that influence the child's self-concept, it is an undemanding, accepting love that is indispensable to the development of a healthy personality. Unconditional love, freely bestowed, helps establish a sense of security and a positive sense of self within children that will persist throughout their lifetime. It is important that children know they are loved and that whatever happens they can depend on this love. For many children spiritual love is a very significant source of complete undemanding love. Without the security of loving relationships, children may become tense and insecure and develop undesirable behavior patterns as they attempt to obtain that love or try to compensate for its loss.

The primary source of love, particularly during infancy, is the parent, usually the mother, or mothering person. The importance of establishing this early love attachment (or bonding) profoundly influences subsequent interpersonal relationships. With ever-widening relationships, children need the love and acceptance of others.

They need to feel they are wanted, accepted, and belong in whatever relationships are important to them at each stage of development.

Parents may truly love their children but be unable to communicate this love to them. Parents who are insecure in their parenting skills frequently seek advice and reassurance from health professionals. Nurses who are aware of indications of parental insecurity will be able to provide assistance and reassurance that can preserve and enhance the parent-child relationship and build a sense of confidence in the parent.

Security. Closely allied to the need for love is the need for a sense of security. As they grow and develop in a complex world, children encounter many threats to their sense of security. Indeed, most behavior problems of childhood are associated with an element of insecurity. Every change in themselves or their environment creates a feeling of uncertainty. Faced with confusing, conflicting adjustments, young children need the security provided by relatively stable situations and dependable human relationships. The degree to which they can cope with these stresses depends on the patience and support they receive from those most closely involved in their care.

There are a multitude of factors that generate a feeling of insecurity in children. Ordinarily the parents, who are sources of comfort, guidance, and encouragement, provide a measure of security in an insecure world. To achieve this security children need the warm acceptance of loving parents, a stable family unit, and judicious handling of stress-provoking situations such as sibling rivalry, relocation to a new neighborhood, and illness in themselves or other members of the family. A disturbed home environment caused by such factors as marital discord, illness of a parent or family member, or death of a family member can shatter their equilibrium.

Infants are disturbed by physical threats, such as hunger, cold, or discomfort. Small children are physiologically disturbed by emotions such as anger, fear, and grief, which they can release only in overt behavior. A measure of relief from these feelings can be obtained by the reassurance that their physical needs will be met, restraints will be placed on their behavior, and expectations that keep pace with their inner controls will be held. Rejection by significant persons, social ineptitude, and physical handicaps often produce insecurity in a child. The number and variety of factors originating within or outside the child are often difficult to determine; therefore, those responsible for the child's care must be alert for cues that reveal threats to this sense of security.

Discipline and authority. Because children live in an organized society, they must be prepared to accept restrictions on their behavior. Discipline is not punishment. Rather it is the teaching of desirable behavior. Children need to learn the rules governing behavior in the home, the neighborhood, the school, and the community at large. To learn acceptable behavior that permits them to live enjoyably with themselves and others, children need the steady, firm guidance of loving parents and others in authority roles. Good discipline provides children with protection from dangers (from within and without) and relieves them of the burden of decisions that they are not prepared to make, yet allows them to develop independence of thought and action within a secure framework.

Children who learn to live within reasonable rules are happier and more secure children. Without the stabilizing influence of controls, children feel uncertain and insecure. Too often, inexperienced and insecure parents fear the loss of a child's love, suffer feelings of guilt over disciplinary action, or may even relinquish their authority to the child. To discipline is to teach reality. Sensible, mature parents establish fair rules and regulations in the home and then see that they are carried out. Parents should never exploit children's love for them as a means to control their children. Children's anxiety lest they lose that love is already great. Discipline based on love of the child and carried out with conviction, confidence, and consistency will produce a self-reliant, buoyant, and self-controlled child.

Dependence and independence. As children grow and mature, they are increasingly able to direct their own activities and to make more independent decisions. However, there are great fluctuations in their ability to function independently. Even with a compelling inner drive to master and achieve, they are not always able to cope with difficult and frustrating problems or conflicts. All children feel the urge to grow up and move forward toward maturity, but they have at their disposal only those energies that are not being used to maintain their mastery over old conflicts. Independence should be permitted to grow at its own rate.

Periods of regression and dependence are not only normal but are often necessary and helpful. If children feel sufficiently comfortable and content in a situation or relationship and reasonably certain that they can return to this safety and security, they will venture into the untried and untested on their own. If they feel doubtful concerning their abilities to cope, regression to a more comfortable level of competence allows them to replenish their inner resources and prepare to move ahead once again. Independence grows out of dependence; one cannot be considered as distinct from the other.

Children will learn independence of thought and decision making provided the opportunity is not withheld from them. If they are pushed into acting independently before they feel themselves ready, they may withdraw from independence. When they choose not to relinquish the joys of independence and autonomy or move ahead to new worlds of independence, they will dawdle. Parents, teachers, nurses, and others responsible for child care must be able to adjust their expectations and support to meet the child's needs of the moment. It is important to recognize when to help and when not to help children to experiment with their immature and imperfect self-control, when to make demands that require children's utmost ability, and when to allow them to function temporarily on a more immature level. They need these freedoms and controls in the process of becoming mature, self-reliant adults.

Self-esteem. Self-esteem is children's personal, subjective judgment of their worthiness. It is the result of self-evaluation, principally in the areas of competence and social acceptance.

The content of self-esteem changes with children's development. Highly egocentric toddlers are unaware of any difference between competence and social approval. They are the center of their world and, to them, all positive experiences are evidence of their importance and value. Preschool and early school-age children, on the other hand, are increasingly aware of the discrepancy between their competencies and the abilities of more advanced children. They are expected to evaluate a situation and anticipate the consequences of their behavior before they act. The acceptance of adults and peers outside the family group become more important to them. Since these valued persons may not be as proud of their achievements or as understanding of their limitations as their families are, their recently acquired capacity for guilt may lead to anxiety over failure, and they will be more vulnerable to feelings of worthlessness and depression. As their competencies increase and they develop meaningful relationships, their self-esteem rises. Their self-esteem is again at risk during early adolescence when they are defining an identity and sense of self in the context of their peer group.

Unless children are continually made to feel incompetent and of little worth, a decrease in self-esteem during vulnerable periods is only temporary. It can be expected that there will be transitory periods of lowered self-esteem at the stages of development when they must set new goals or where there are very obvious discrepancies in competence. A constant source of anxiety arises from the endless number of separations that occur in the process of acquiring autonomy, independence, and individuality. As an expression of their own urgencies, parents often set overambitious goals for their children and expect them to perform beyond the limits of their capacity. Also, children's attempts at autonomy and achievement are often thwarted by parental overprotection, either because the parents fear that they will be hurt or because it is more convenient for the parents to do things for them.

In order to develop and preserve self-esteem, children need to feel that they are worthwhile individuals who are in some way different from, superior to, and more lovable than any other individual in the world. They need recognition for their achievements and the approval of parents and peers. Parents and other authority figures can foster a positive self-concept by providing appropriate encouragement and recognition for achievement and by discouraging inappropriate behaviors. However, when disapproval is being expressed, it is imperative to convey to a child that it is the *behavior* that is unacceptable, not the child.

Children who experience warm, affectionate relationships with parents, who are accepted by their parents, and who are aware of their parents' positive attitudes toward them are more accepting of themselves. Children who have a strong sense of their own worth are confident, able to initiate activities, explore their environment, and take risks in their behavior when confronted with new or novel situations. They approach tasks and relationships with the expectation that they will be well received and successful. Such is the focus of nursing—to allow children to grow and prosper from their experiences in health and illness.

REFERENCES

Better health for our children: a national strategy, The Report of the Select Panel for the Promotion of Child Health, vol. II, Analysis and recommendations for selected federal programs, Department of Health and Human Services (PHS) Pub. No. 79-55071, 1981.

Cancer facts and figures 1984, New York, 1983, American Cancer Society, Inc.

Cone, T.E., Jr.: Highlights of two centuries of American pediatrics, 1776–1976, Am. J. Dis. Child. **130:**762-775, July 1976.

Gordon, M.: Nursing diagnosis: process and application, New York, 1982, McGraw-Hill Book Co.

Green, M., and Haggerty, R.: Episodic problems. In Green, M., and Haggerty, R., editors: Ambulatory pediatrics III, Philadelphia, 1984, W.B. Saunders Co.

Kalter, H., and Warkany, J.: Congenital malformations: etiologic factors and their role in prevention, part I, N. Engl. J. Med. **308:**424-431, Feb. 1983; part II, **308:**491-497, Mar. 1983.

Nader, P., and others: The new morbidity: use of school and community health care resources for behavioral, educational and social-family problems, Pediatrics **67**(1):53-60, 1981.

National Transportation Safety Board: Safety study: child passenger protection against death, disability, and disfigurement in motor vehicle accidents, Washington, D.C., 1983, United States Government.

Pless, I.: Current morbidity and mortality among the young. In Hoekelman, R.A., and others: Principles of pediatrics: health care of the young, New York, 1978, McGraw-Hill Book Co.

Pless, I., and Stulginskas, J.: Accidents and violence as a cause of morbidity and mortality in childhood, Adv. Pediatr. **29:**471-495, 1982.

Schmidt, W.M.: Health and welfare of colonial American children, Am. J. Dis. Child. **130:**694-701, July 1976.

Shoemaker, J.: Essential features of nursing diagnoses. In Kim M., McFarland, G., and McLane, A.: Classification of nursing diagnoses: proceedings of the fifth national conference, St. Louis, 1984, the C.V. Mosby Co.

Starfield, B.: Psychosocial and psychosomatic diagnoses in primary care of children, Pediatrics **66:**159-163, Aug. 1980.

BIBLIOGRAPHY
Vital statistics/evolution of child health care

Better health for our children: a national strategy, The Report of the Select Panel for the Promotion of Child Health, vol. I, Major findings and recommendations, Department of Health and Human Services (PHS) Pub. No. 79-55071, 1981.

Bloch, H.: Jewish children in colonial times, Am. J. Dis. Child. **130:**711-713, July 1976.

Cone, T.E., Jr.: History of American pediatrics, Boston, 1980, Little, Brown & Co.

Holaday, B.: Changing views of infant care 1914-1980, Pediatr. Nurs. **7**(1):21-25, 1981.

National Center for Health Statistics: Health, United States, 1983, D.H.H.S. Pub. No. (PHS) 84-1232, Public Health Service, Washington, D.C., 1983.

Radbill, S.X.: Reared in adversity: institutional care of children in the 18th century, Am. J. Dis. Child. **130:**751-761, July 1976.

Rogers, D., and others: Some observations on pediatrics: its past, present, and future, Pediatrics (suppl.) **67**(5):776-784, 1981.

Sayre, J.W., and Sayre, R. F.: American children and the ''children of nature'', Am. J. Dis. Child **130:**716-723, July 1976.

Surgeon General's Report on Health Promotion and Disease Prevention: Healthy people, Department of Health, Education and Welfare (PHS) Pub. No. 79-55071, 1979.

The pediatric nurse and the child

Brown, B., and Chard, M.: Nurse practitioners: a review of the literature, 1965-1979, American Nursing Association Publication **I-VIII:**1-24, 1980.

Carpenito, J.L.: Nursing diagnosis: application to clinical practice, Philadelphia, 1983, J.B. Lippincott Co.

Chaisson, G.M.: Patient education: whose responsibility is it and who should be doing it? Nurs. Adm. Q. **4:**1-11, 1980.

Ciske, K.L.: Accountability—the essence of primary nursing, Am. J. Nurs. **79**(5):890-894, 1979.

Diers, D., and Molde, S.: Nurses in primary care: the new gatekeepers? Am. J. Nurs. **83**(5):742-745, 1983.

Fond, K.: Child advocacy: ideas for action, Pediatr. Nurs. **5:**18-19, 1979.

Griffith, J., and Christensen, P.: Nursing process: application of theories, frameworks, and models, St. Louis, l982, The C.V. Mosby Co.

Hymovitch, D.: How children, mothers, and nurses view primary and team nursing, Am. J. Nurs. **80**(11):2041-2045, 1980.

Kohnke, M.F.: The nurse as advocate, Am. J. Nurs. **80**(11):2038-2040, 1980.

Mullen, P.D.: Promoting child health: channels of socialization, Fam. Comm. Health J. **5**(5):52-68, 1983.

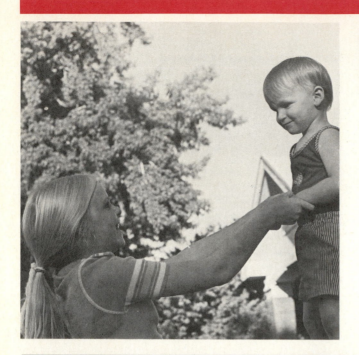

CHILDREN: THEIR ENVIRONMENT AND DEVELOPMENT

OBJECTIVES

On completion of this chapter the reader will be able to:

- Discuss cultural and subcultural influences on child growth and development

- Demonstrate an understanding of the factors within the family that influence the growth and development of the child

- Describe major trends in growth and development

- Explain the alterations in the major body systems that take place during the processes of growth and development

- Discuss the development and relationships of cognitive, personality, and moral development

- Demonstrate an understanding of the role of endogenous and exogenous factors in the physical and emotional development of children

- Describe the role of play in the growth and development of children

- Discuss the relationship between growth and development and childhood accidents

NURSING DIAGNOSES

Nursing diagnoses identified for developmental and environmental influences on the child and family include but are not restricted to the following:

Health perception-health management patterns

- Injury, potential for, related to developmental accomplishments

Activity-exercise pattern

- Self-care deficit, total or partial, related to developmental level

Self-perception—self-concept pattern

- Anxiety related to (1) previous experience(s); (2) perception of impending events; (3) knowledge deficit

- Self-concept, disturbance in, related to (1) interpersonal relationships; (2) environmental factors

Growth and development are complex processes involving numerous components that are subject to a wide variety of influences. All facets of the child's body, mind, and personality develop simultaneously, at varying rates and sequences, but not independently. Development of one part may be controlled or influenced by the activity of another part. Physical development proceeds at an orderly rate and sequence, but this development is strongly influenced by the environment in which the child grows and develops. A holistic view of any child requires that nurses acquire not only a knowledge of normal growth and development but also develop some understanding of the ways that culture contributes to the development of social and emotional relationships and attitudes toward health. This includes an awareness of the nurse's own cultural frame of reference.

THE INTERPERSONAL ENVIRONMENT OF THE CHILD

The manner and sequence of growth and development are universal and fundamental features of all children; however, the variations in behavioral responses that children display to similar events are believed to be determined by the culture in which they live and mature.

Culture and conformity

A culture is, essentially, the way of life of a group of people that incorporates experiences of the past, influences thought and action in the present, and transmits these traditions to future group members. People from one culture differ from those in other cultures in the way they think and solve problems and in the way they perceive and structure the world. The culture in which children are reared determines the type of food they will eat, the language they will speak, the ideals of behavior, and the way in which social roles should be conducted. To be acceptable members of the culture, children must learn how the culture expects them to behave toward others in the group. In turn, they learn how they can expect others to behave toward them. A set of values learned in childhood is apt to characterize children's attitudes and behavior for life— to guide their long-range strivings and to monitor their short-range, impulse-driven inclinations.

The culture into which children are born outlines the roles of their parents, structures their relationships with other people, and determines much of the behavior they acquire. The culture fosters and reinforces those behaviors deemed desirable and appropriate; it attempts to depress or extinguish those that are at conflict with cultural norms. Some cultures encourage aggressive behaviors in their children, others favor amiability and compliance; some

Role-relationship pattern

- Family process, alterations in, related to (1) loss or acquisition of family members; (2) situational crises (specify); (3) temporary family disorganization

- Grieving, anticipatory, related to (1) expected loss (specify); (2) expected change

- Parenting, alterations in: potential related to (1) skill deficit; (2) family stress

Coping-stress tolerance pattern

- Coping, family: potential for growth

cultures foster individual resourcefulness and competition, and others emphasize cooperation and submission to group interest. Since standards and norms vary from location to location, a practice that is accepted in one area may meet with disapproval or create tension in another. The extent to which cultures tolerate divergence from the established norm varies among cultures and subcultural groups. Although conformity provides a degree of security, it is a decided deterrent to change.

Subcultural influence

Except in rare situations, children grow in a blend of cultures and subcultures, those smaller groups within a culture that possess many characteristics of the larger culture while contributing their own particular values. In a large, complex society such as the United States, there are different groups that have their own set of standards, values, and expectations within the collective ways of the large culture. Most were formed when groups of people clustered together by preference, by external pressures from the majority culture, or by geographic isolation. Although many cultural differences are related to geographic boundaries, subcultures are not always restricted by location.

Children's membership in a cultural subgroup is, for the most part, involuntary. They are born into a family with a specific ethnic or racial heritage, socioeconomic level, and religious beliefs. Although in the complex society of the United States there are countless subcultures and considerable variation in the way of life between regions, ethnic groups, and social classes, those that seem to exert the greatest influence on child rearing are ethnicity, social class, and occupational role.

Ethnicity. Ethnic differences extend to many areas that include such manifestations as family structure, language, food preferences, moral codes, and expression of emotion. Children learn how to adhere to a mode of behavior that is in accordance with standards distinctive to their cultural group. They take cues for behavior from observing and imitating those to whom they are exposed. These perceptions are then incorporated into their own self-concept.

The religious orientation of the family dictates a code of morality and a meaning for life's mysteries as well as behavior standards. The religious affiliation influences the family's attitudes toward education, male and female role identity, and attitudes regarding their ultimate destiny. In many cultures the religious beliefs are such an integral part of the culture that it is difficult to distinguish one from the other. In a few instances religion is the basis of a common way of life that determines where the children are reared and a totally individualistic life-style.

Social class. Those who have made extensive studies conclude that probably the greatest influence on child-

rearing practices and their results is the social class of the family into which a child is born. Differences in child-rearing goals and practices as well as attitudes toward health have been found to be greater between social classes than between races or ethnic groups.

Upper and middle class children live in an enriched environment that provides material comforts and broader opportunities. The parents are usually educated, and other authority figures such as teachers with whom the children are routinely in contact are usually from a middle class background and have activities and expectations for the children that are similar to those of the parents. Parents have occupations that require judgment, creativity, and resourcefulness, and these attributes are fostered in their children.

Although differences in parental behavior in different social classes are less marked than they have been in the past, one of the distinctions that is observed in middle classes but not in lower classes is the willingness to delay gratification. The uncertainty of their life leads members of the lower classes to take advantage of gratifications when they are available. This characteristic has caused lower classes to be labeled as present oriented, whereas middle classes seem to be future oriented. Middle class parents have higher education and occupational aspirations for their children and use long-range planning to meet these goals.

There appear to be differences in intellectual skills and scholastic achievement between children in the upper and middle classes and those in the lower classes. There is a higher incidence of academic failure in children from the lower class with its attendant dropout rate. It has been found that lower class parents value the concrete and tangible rather than the abstract and are, therefore, less inclined to encourage these qualities in their children. Their own educational level discourages these parents from reading to their children and providing other means for learning in the home.

Middle class parents are positively oriented toward change, whereas working class parents remain tradition oriented. Consequently, the working class emphasizes conformity to parental values and external regulations, whereas middle class parents are more concerned with producing self-directed children. This may reflect the occupation orientation of the different classes. Middle class occupations tend to involve more self-direction and getting ahead; lower class occupations tend to be standardized with direct supervision.

With few exceptions, parents in all classes love their children and, in a broad sense, have similar goals regarding child rearing. Differences lie in the parental behavior toward the children in attempting to help them to reach these goals. Lower class parents are more restrictive and rely on coercive techniques in child training. They stress obedience and conformity, and the most frequently used form of discipline for undesirable behavior is physical punishment. Middle class parents are more apt to make use of manipulative techniques such as reasoning and drawing on the child's sense of guilt. They tend to scold and use isolation rather than physical punishment.

Occupational role. Some authorities believe that the occupational environment of the family head correlates more closely than does social class with the direction of child rearing and the values parents attempt to convey to their children. There appear to be differences in the way of life between "entrepreneurial" and "bureaucratic" parents.

Entrepreneurial occupations include the smaller and more traditional enterprises, such as small businessmen, salesmen, physicians, and so on, that require self-reliance and independence. Parents in these occupations rear their children in a more authoritarian manner. They emphasize self-control, self-denial, and responsible independence with a vigorous and control-oriented approach to life. They lean toward more rigid delineation of sex roles and a more traditional orientation to family life.

The term "bureaucrat" is applied to the "organization man," a person with a position in a large organizational structure where job security is high and risk taking is minimal; where there is more adjustment to and dependence on others. Bureaucratic parents tend to foster passivity, dependency, and some degree of impulse expression. They are more socially minded and usually allow their children more freedom. The general trend toward passivity and outer-directedness among young Americans may be rooted in this philosophy.

Cultural influence on health and health services

To begin to understand and to deal with families in a multicultural community, it is most important that nurses be aware of their own attitudes and values regarding a way of life, including health practices. Nurses, too, are products of their own cultural background and education. Those who are aware of their own culturally founded behavior are more sensitive to cultural behavior in others. To recognize that a behavior may be a characteristic of a culture rather than an "abnormal" behavior places nurses at an advantage in their relationships with families. When nurses respect the cultural differences of a family, they are able to postpone judgment until it is determined whether the behavior is distinctive to the individual or a characteristic of the culture.

Nurses continually encounter beliefs and practices that may facilitate or impede nursing interventions, including attitudes toward family planning, food habits, and folkways that are firmly entrenched in the culture. The language of the client may be different from that of the larger culture, or there may be regional or ethnic peculiarities in the use of basic English. Subcultural influences, such as some religious beliefs and practices, may be in conflict with standard health practices and therapeutic interventions.

The most overwhelming adverse influence on health is socioeconomic status. A higher percentage of individuals are suffering from some health problem at any one time in lower classes than in any other group. In the lower classes, children are less likely to be immunized against preventable diseases than they are in the upper and middle classes. Lack of funds or inaccessibility to health services inhibits treatment for any but severe illness or accident. Health care is sometimes inadequate because of ignorance. In some areas a disorder is so commonplace that it is looked on as unavoidable and is not recognized as something out of the ordinary that requires (or is amenable to) treatment.

Upper and middle class parents are likely to seek treatment for many more types of symptoms than are lower class parents, and they are more concerned with detecting and preventing illness in their children. The disinclination to use preventive health services by lower class parents is probably another symptom of the fatalistic approach to problems and a time orientation that is concentrated on the present rather than the future. Preventive dental care, immunization, and prenatal care are examples of such health services.

Nurses should make themselves aware of any specific attitudes regarding the manner of approach to a child in a given culture. Navajo Indians do not like a stranger near their infants. It is feared that the stranger may "witch" the child and produce harmful effects on his life. On the other hand, if a stranger, particularly a woman, lavishes attention on a Mexican-American infant but fails to touch him, he will develop symptoms of the "evil-eye," or *mal ojo,* that include restlessness, crying, diarrhea, vomiting, and fever. The concept of the "evil-eye" is common to many cultures throughout the world and serves to explain inexplicable onset of illness, particularly in infants and small children.

The person who represents the family regarding health matters differs among cultures. For example, in most cultural groups the mother assumes this responsibility. In others both parents are involved equally in relationships with health workers. A somewhat different approach is apparent in some of the oriental cultures. For example, the father in Vietnamese families is traditionally the family member who interacts with persons outside the family unit. Therefore, he is the one who represents the family in all health matters.

To aid their efforts to understand and respect the cultural beliefs of families, it is helpful for nurses to have an available resource file containing pertinent information about the cultural and subcultural characteristics of the community in which they practice. To bridge cultural gaps in delivery of health care to children requires the establishment of a close relationship with the influential persons in the community, such as the local health healer. In this way good health practice can be presented and carried out within the framework of the culture.

THE FAMILY

The family is an open system, and as such, it contains all the elements of a system—structure, purpose or function, and internal organization. It has definite boundaries and consists of components (a natural grouping of persons) mutually interacting among themselves and with their environment. As in any system, anything that affects one component (person) affects all other components. Any alteration, originating either inside or outside the system boundaries, has an impact on all others in the system. This concept has implications for health workers who are continually forming short- and long-term relationships with children and their families. In assessing and analyzing health problems the nurse must consider all members of the family and those factors outside as well as within the family system that might impinge on the health of the child and the family.

The family provides each newborn member of a society with legitimacy, that is, a family connection (usually symbolized by a family name), and an ascribed position in the societal strata. A family is traditionally conceptualized as consisting of more than one person, and the belief has been held that, ideally, both the mother and the father are needed to rear a child. During the long period of time required for human infants to reach a level of independence, families assume the responsibility for their rearing, although they differ considerably in form, complexity, and goals for socialization.

Functions of the family

Children bring very little predetermined behavior into the world with them; therefore, they depend on their parents to meet the primary requirements for growth and development and to establish for them an atmosphere of security. Although goals for socialization and child-rearing practices differ from one culture to another, in most societies the family appears to serve three principal functions in relation to children: (1) to provide physical care for children; (2) to educate and train children for adjustment to the culture; and (3) to accept responsibility for children's psychologic and emotional welfare.

Physical care. Human infants are totally helpless and require a long period of time to reach a level of inde-

pendence, which makes them dependent on adults for their survival. The family takes responsibility for providing the child's basic needs for food, clothing, shelter, protection from harm, and health care.

Education and training. One of the major functions of the family is to socialize children. It is through the family that infants receive their contact with culture directly. They learn the language, the appropriate role behavior, and the value system and ethical standards of the culture. Later, school, peers, and others will exert influence, but the family remains the primary socializing influence during childhood.

Psychologic and emotional welfare. Only recently has psychologic and emotional welfare been stressed as a major family function. Relatively recent studies have emphasized the importance of the early psychologic relationship between parents and child to later emotional adjustment of the child. Through relationships with family members children learn patterns of behavior that are extended to relationships with other persons and to other situations. It is these interactions with others that contribute most to formation of the self-concept, social competence, and the ability to form warm relationships with others during later years. The foundation of a healthy personality is laid within the family unit.

Family structure

A structure is a manner of organization or the arrangement of a number of parts that are interrelated in specified, recurring ways. The family structure consists of individuals with socially recognized statuses and positions who interact with one another on a regular, recurring basis and in socially sanctioned ways. Traditionally the family structure is referred to as either *nuclear* or *extended,* and the predominant pattern in any society depends to a large extent on the mobility of the families as they pursue economic goals.

Nuclear family. The nuclear or conjugal family structure consists of a man, his wife, and their children (natural or adopted) who live in a common household. This is the reproductive unit in which the marital tie (legally or otherwise sanctioned) is the chief binding force. In some instances one or more additional persons (such as a relative, friend, foster child, or others) may reside in the same household. The strongly functional nuclear family is the prototype of human relationships and the basic unit from which more complex familial forms are composed.

The nuclear family, the predominant structure in the United States, is characteristic of an urban mobile society. It is highly adaptable, with the ability to adjust and reshape its structure when needed. Although extended families residing in the same household are rapidly disappearing in American society, the isolated nuclear family without relatives within easy visiting distance is rare. This is most often seen where there has been extreme mobility of separate generations, such as wide geographic separations or marriages into different social classes, religions, or roles. Most consanguineous family members maintain contact through visits, telephone calls, letters, and gift exchanges.

Single-parent family. Variations on the traditional nuclear family have come about as a result of some recent social phenomena. For example, the *single-parent family* is now recognized as a family and has emerged partially as a consequence of women's rights movements wherein more women have established separate households as a result of divorce, death, desertion, or illegitimacy. Also the more liberal attitude of the courts has made it possible for divorced fathers to retain custody of children and for single persons to adopt children, whereas previously, rigid prerequisites specified that both a father and a mother must be present in the home.

Extended family. The extended, or consanguineous, family consists of the nuclear family plus lineal or collateral kinsmen. Traditionally it is composed of two or more nuclear families affiliated through extension of the parent-child relationship, that is, grandparents, parents, and grandchildren. Broader views recognize the affiliation of collateral kinsmen as an extended family—not necessarily organized into nuclear families. Rare in the United States today, the best examples of extended family units can be found in groups of individuals with great wealth, successful farmers, American Indians, certain recent immigrants, and single parents who reside with the grandparents or with whom a grandparent resides.

Alternative family structures. An alternative lifestyle, the *communal family,* has seemed to emerge, as have all previous experimental communities, from a disenchantment with most contemporary life choices. Although they may have divergent beliefs, practices, and organization, the basic impetus has been dissatisfaction with social systems and life goals of the larger communities and with the nuclear family structure as it exists—either from an ideologic or a practical perspective. Unlike the traditional family systems where the total responsibility for child rearing is left to the parents and the school, in the commune the parental role is deemphasized, and all children are the collective responsibility of the adult members.

There are other family forms that are relatively rare. Although it is not legally sanctioned, the conjugal unit can be extended by the addition of spouses in *polygamous* matings. Most often mothers and their children share a husband and father, usually with each mother and her children maintaining a separate household. Another form that has yet to be fully evaluated is the *homosexual* family, in which there is a marital or common-law tie between two persons of the same sex who have adopted children or in which one or both partners have natural children from a heterosexual mating.

Family relationships affecting children

Numerous familial factors can alter the childhood environment. No two children grow in exactly the same environment, although identical twins more nearly approximate this. For example, in a nuclear family with two children—even of the same sex—one will live in a family with an older sibling whereas the other will be reared in a family with a younger sibling. In a family where there is a 10-year age span between children, one may be born to a 20-year-old mother, the other to a 30-year-old mother. For the child in each situation the environment is different.

Family size. The size of the family of orientation has a decided impact on the child. In the small family more emphasis is placed on the individual development of the children. Parenting is intensive rather than extensive, and there is constant pressure to measure up to family expectations. Children in a large family are able to adjust to a variety of changes and crises. There is more emphasis on the group and less on the individual. Cooperation is essential, often because of economic necessity. The number of children reduces the intimate, one-to-one contact between the parent and any individual child. Consequently, children turn to each other for what they cannot get from their parents. The reduced parent-child contact encourages individual children to adopt specialized roles in an attempt at recognition in the family.

Discipline is often administered by older siblings in large families. Siblings are usually better attuned to what constitutes misbehavior, and sibling disapproval or ostracism is frequently a more meaningful disciplinary measure than parental spankings or scoldings. Large families seem to generate a sense of security in the children fostered by sibling support and cooperation.

Sibling position. Relationships between siblings in the family group duplicate, to some extent, many of the social interaction experiences of later years. Through relationships with siblings, children learn patterns of loyalty, competition, dominance, cooperation, sharing, and so on. Such factors as whether a child is the firstborn, a middle child, or the youngest child or whether there is 1 or 6 years separating him from his sibling affect his view of the world and his relationship with others inside and outside the family.

Firstborn children are more achievement oriented than children born later, and they exhibit strong drive and ambition. They usually receive more physical punishment than younger children and are allowed to show more aggression toward their younger siblings. They have stronger consciences and are usually more self-disciplined, inner-directed, and prone to feelings of guilt, which may account for a higher intellectual achievement. Firstborn children are better represented in college populations than are younger siblings.

Younger children reflect the decrease in the amount of parental attention and anxieties. On the whole, mothers are warmer toward the youngest child than the oldest and middle child, and the youngest child receives little physical punishment. The youngest child is less dependent than a firstborn and more apt to be left to manage things for himself. Younger children are usually more backward than the firstborn in language development and articulation. They appear to be less tense, more affectionate, and more good-natured than the firstborn, and they tend to identify more with the peer group than with parents.

The middle children appear to occupy the most difficult position. There are more demands on them for help with household tasks, they are praised less often for good behavior, and they receive less of the mother's time for pleasurable activities.

The age difference between siblings affects the childhood environment. The arrival of a sibling has the greatest impact on the older child, and a 2- to 4-year difference in age appears to be most threatening. When the older child is very young, his self-image is too immature to be threatened. At an older age he is better able to understand the situation and, therefore, less likely to see the newcomer as a threat, although he does feel the loss of his only-child status.

In general the narrower the spacing between siblings, the more the children influence one another, especially in emotional characteristics; the wider the spacing, the greater the influence of the parents. Also, younger children tend to identify with older siblings. Consequently they assume some of the personality characteristics of the older child.

The only child. Only children have been described as selfish, spoiled, dependent, and lonely. However, research indicates that there are no essential differences between a child reared alone and one who is reared with one or more siblings. They display no more evidence of maladjustment or self-centeredness than any other children and tend to strongly resemble firstborn children in such aspects as higher educational goals. Only children perform better on cognitive tests, are more mature and cultivated, are more socially sensitive, and demonstrate superiority in language facility.

Only children also enjoy the advantage of having parents who, without the distraction of other children, are able to devote more time to them, talk to them, and stimulate them in intellectual activities. However, parents also exert greater pressure for mature behavior at an early age and for achievement. Diminished contact with other children, such as siblings, encourages them to indulge in intellectual pursuits and encourages a rich fantasy life, independence, and originality.

Twins. It is well-known that twins are of two distinct types: *identical*, or *monozygotic*, and *fraternal*, or *dizygotic*. Dizygotic twins may be of the same or opposite sex, and they differ both physically and in genetic constitution. They are siblings who happen to be born at the same time. Monozygotic twins are always alike in their hereditary and physical characteristics, including sex.

A special kind of sibling relationship is observed in twins, although getting along with each other and quarreling is not too different from any other two siblings, especially if they are fraternal twins of opposite sex. Twins generally tend to work out a relationship that is reasonable and satisfactory to both and demonstrate early independence from parental attention. They develop a remarkable capacity for cooperative play and considerable loyalty and generosity toward each other. It is not uncommon for them to create a private language between themselves that may interfere with development of the family language.

In a twinship one member of the pair, to a greater or lesser extent, is more dominant, outgoing, and aggressive than the other; this often causes concern to their parents. However, the seemingly more passive twin is able to accomplish as much and get his way as frequently as the more aggressive twin.

Identical twins also differ in their response to the tendency of some parents to treat twins exactly alike. The present philosophy is to determine the degree to which the children demonstrate the inclination toward togetherness and to use this as a guide to relationships with them. Some twins thrive best when they are in the company of each other steadily; others prefer more individuality and separateness. Early years of togetherness are often the basis of the children's security. To separate them too early may produce unnecessary stresses. The trend among authorities is to recommend the fostering of individual differences in the children as they are evidenced in order to ease the process of separation when it becomes advisable.

The birth of twins can have a significant impact on the family—especially if the multiple birth was unexpected. There are few resources available for these families, and most have learned to deal with day to day problems as they arise. Because of this need "Mothers of Twins" clubs have been organized in many communities to provide support and information to families who are faced with this dilemma.

Working mothers. A great deal has been written and a variety of conclusions arrived at regarding the effects of mothers working outside the home. The number of women in the labor force has increased steadily during the past two decades and shows every indication of continuing. Mothers work for several reasons, but regardless of the mother's motivation, the consensus is that harmful effects on the children are related to the *quality* of the mother-child interaction rather then the *quantity* of time spent with the children. On the whole, children of working mothers are self-reliant, do better in school, and show relatively few ill effects of the separation.

The increasing numbers of working mothers and single parent families has given rise to a relatively recent phenomenon—*latch-key children*. Latch-key children are children who are expected to assume a greater amount of responsibility than children have in the past. They come home to an empty house after school (hence the name) and are often expected to do many of the more responsible household tasks such as tending younger children, cleaning, cooking, and other family needs. The effect on these children is variable. In some instances outside activities are curtailed and relationships with peers may be significantly diminished. In other cases the children benefit from the experience.

Absent father. Fathers have been referred to as "absentee fathers" because they are away from the home for the greater part of the day. Our concern here, however, is with the family without a father because of death, divorce, desertion, illegitimacy, or involuntary separation, such as military service, job demands, jail, and so on.

The primary effect of absence of either parent from the home is in the difficulty in adjustment and development of a sexual identity. This is more marked when the parental absence occurs early in the child's life and when it is the same sex parent. Girls from homes where fathers are absent are more dependent on their mothers and show some anxiety about relationships with males during adolescence. Boys from homes without fathers tend to be less aggressive, are more apt to have emotional and social problems, and demonstrate cognitive patterning more similar to that of girls. Overprotectiveness, extreme indulgence, and often prolonged physical contact with the mother over a period of years may contribute to serious sex identity problems in male children.

Divorce. Authorities agree that marital factors within the home contribute to children's development. Children from a happy, relaxed atmosphere in the home are less likely to have a negative outlook than are those from stressed homes. The child who becomes involved in divorce has feelings of terror and abandonment. As the parents become involved with their own feelings and concerns, they are less available and have less to give the children. The children see themselves apart from the family, feel alone and isolated, and long for consistency and order in their lives.

The impact of divorce on children depends on the age of the child and the quality of parental care during the years following the divorce. Although a child at any age is profoundly affected by divorce, the greatest amount of stress is suffered by preschool children; adolescents and school-age children are better able to cope with the separation.

Egocentric preschoolers, who see and understand things only in relation to themselves, assume themselves to be the cause of parental distress and interpret the separation as punishment. Moreover, they consciously fear that they may be abandoned by the remaining parent. Consequently it is essential that some kind of stability be established for these children; otherwise they will convert their energies to restabilization rather than to growth and development. They need frequent, repeated, and concrete explanations of what is going to happen to them and how they will be cared for and assurance that something new will take the place of the old and that they will not be deserted.

School-age children and adolescents are able to deal with parental separation better than younger children. They feel intense pain and loneliness, their ability to learn is affected since they are unable to focus on learning, and somatic complaints, especially in school-age children, and emotional disturbances in adolescents are observed. Often they must move to an unfamiliar environment and a new neighborhood and form new relationships in addition to coping with the alteration in their family structure. They almost invariably wish for the parents to reunite.

Adoption. Adoptive parents are those who, by whatever motivation, assume the sociologic and ethical responsibility of biologic parents. These ties of affection are just as strong as biologic ties. Persons are motivated to adopt a child for different reasons. However, in most instances it is a loving couple who find it impossible to have a child of their own or a single person who feels a responsibility to provide a home for a child who needs one (Fig. 2-1).

The major source of infants for adoption has been socially unsanctioned pregnancies, primarily unwed mothers. However, with the widespread use of contraception, more liberalized abortion laws, and more liberal attitudes toward out-of-wedlock parents, the number of these children available for adoption has significantly decreased.

Almost half the adoptable children in the United States are adopted by relatives. Nonrelative adoptions are primarily arranged through licensed social agencies. A small proportion are arranged independently by individuals such as physicians, nurses, clergymen, and lawyers. It is well recognized that the safest and most satisfactory adoptions are those conducted through a licensed social agency, either public or voluntary, and potential adoptive parents should be strongly urged to use this route for obtaining a wanted child. The welfare of the child should be the primary consideration in placement, and such motives as the need to strengthen an unstable marriage, to treat emotional

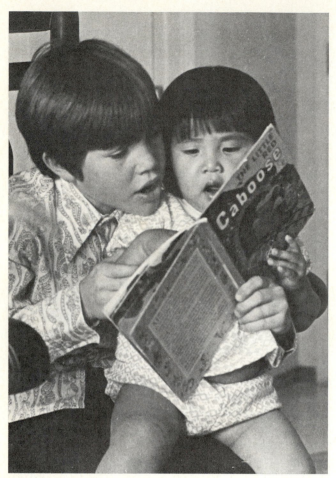

FIG. 2-1

A big brother is reading a story to his adopted sister.

problems (including grief over death of a child), or to treat psychogenic sterility should be carefully explored. When the adoption satisfies the needs of only one of the two parents, the outcome is questionable.

One of the major tasks in rearing adopted children is helping them to deal with the fact that they have had another set of parents. If the children are adopted after the age of 2 years, they maintain an image of the previous parenting persons that may cause the adopting parents some insecurity. The parents may not feel as close to these children as they would to those who are adopted in infancy. Also, the older child maintains the image of the natural parents. However, as they grow, the children are able to clearly distinguish between the parents who loved and cared for them and those who were merely responsible for their birth. Some of the early difficulties of adaptation are related to the change in surroundings, a change that is difficult for all children.

The task of telling children that they are adopted is a cause of deep concern and anxiety. Unfortunately there are no clear-cut guidelines for parents to follow in determining precisely when and at what age children are ready for the information, and parents are naturally reluctant to present the children with such unsettling news. However, it is an important aspect of their parental responsibilities, and, although they may be tempted to withhold the fact from a child, it is an essential component of the child's identity.

The timing seems to arise naturally as parents become aware of the child's readiness. Some authorities believe that the best time is between ages 7 and 10 years; others recommend an earlier age. The time must be right for both the parents and the child and is highly individual. One such time is when children ask where babies come from. At the same time children can be told the facts of their adoption. If they are told in such a way as to convey the idea that they were active participants in the selection process, they will be less apt to feel that they were abandoned victims in a helpless situation. Complete honesty between parents and child usually strengthens the relationship, and children should be encouraged to ask questions.

Influence of schools

When children enter school their radius of relationships extends to include a wider variety of peers and a new focus of authority. Although parents continue to exert the major influence on their children, in the school environment teachers have the most significant psychologic impact on the child's development. The function of teachers is primarily limited to teaching, but, like parents, they are concerned about the emotional welfare of the children. Both parents and teachers must constrain behavior, and both are in a position to enforce standards of conduct.

Classmates also have a significant impact on the socialization of individual children. For the first time children become members of a large group of individuals their same age, and peer relationships become increasingly important and influential as children proceed through school. It has a special impact during adolescence when the peer group plays such an important role in the transition from child to adult status. The kind of influence exerted by the peer group depends on the background, interests, and abilities of the individual child and on the degree to which the peer-group standards influence the child.

Influence of mass media of communication

There is no doubt that the communications media provide children with a means for extending their knowledge about the world in which they live and have contributed to narrowing the differences between classes.

Reading material. The oldest of the mass media— books, newspapers, and magazines—contribute to a child's competence in almost every direction, as well as provide enjoyment. Recognition of the impact that reading matter in the schools has on the value system and socialization processes has prompted reevaluation of the content of textbooks, for example, the biased presentation of male and female role models, the unrealistic, sugar-coated view of life situations, and an unrealistic, biased history of minority groups.

Fairy tales and comic books have acquired both critics and supporters as childhood reading material. Fairy tales that were previously believed to represent cruel and frightening themes have gained more acceptance in recent years, and comic books appear to have only a minor influence on acquisition of beliefs, values, and behaviors. Most seem to be relatively harmless to the majority of children, and in some ways they may even be beneficial.

Movies. Movies not closely bound to reality and often portraying an assortment of socially approved behaviors perhaps make a contribution to children's value systems, but they also provide opportunities for desirable social learning. On the other hand, children, especially adolescents, flock to the ''macho'' movies and those whose heroes resort to violent resolutions of problems, such as the use of karate techniques and wild automobile chases. It is also difficult to evaluate the effects of the recent proliferation of teenage horror and sex movies. The carry-over of these influences into daily life and relationships may account, in part, for the increase in violent behavior of young persons.

Television. The medium that has the most impact on children in the United States today is television, which has become one of the most significant socializing agents in the life of young children. Television is a solitary activity and, as such, increases passivity and decreases physical activity and peer group interaction. Controversy continues regarding the favorable vs harmful effects of television viewing. There is ample documentation to implicate television as a source for learning antisocial, aggressive behavior, but there is also evidence to indicate that television is a positive reinforcement for prosocial behavior. Most programs stress the triumph of good over evil with an unrealistically rapid resolution of problems, including moral dilemmas that are often accompanied by pain or violence.

GROWTH AND DEVELOPMENT OF THE CHILD

Growth and development, usually referred to as a unit, express the sum of the numerous changes that take place during a lifetime. The entire course is a dynamic process that encompasses several interrelated dimensions.

Growth implies a change in quantity. It results when cells divide and synthesize new proteins. This increase in the number and size of cells is reflected in an increase in the size and weight of the whole or any of its parts.

Maturation, which literally means to ripen, is described as aging or as an increase in competence and adaptability. It is usually used to describe a qualitative change, that is, a change in the complexity of a structure that makes it possible for that structure to begin functioning or to function at a higher level.

Differentiation is primarily a biologic description of the processes by which early cells and structures are systematically modified and altered to achieve specific and characteristic physical and chemical properties. It is sometimes used to describe one of the trends in development, that is, mass to specific.

Development is a gradual growth and expansion. It also involves a change, in this case from a lower to a more advanced stage of complexity. Development is the emerging and expanding of capacities of the individual to provide progressively greater facility in functioning. It is achieved through growth, maturation, and learning.

Stages of development

Most authorities in the field of child development conveniently categorize child growth and behavior into approximate age stages or in terms that describe the features of an age-group. The age ranges of these stages are admittedly arbitrary and, since they do not take into account individual differences, cannot be applied to all children with any degree of precision. However, this categorization affords a convenient means to describe the characteristics associated with the majority of children at periods when distinctive developmental changes appear and specific developmental tasks* must be accomplished. It is also significant for nurses to know that there are characteristic health problems peculiar to each major phase of development. The sequence of descriptive age periods and subperiods that are used here and elaborated in subsequent chapters include:

> **Prenatal period:** conception to birth
> EMBRYONIC: conception to 8 weeks
> FETAL: 8 to 40 weeks (birth)
> A rapid growth rate and total dependency make this one of the most crucial periods in the developmental process. The relationship between maternal health and certain manifestations in the newborn emphasizes the importance of adequate prenatal care to the health and well-being of the infant.

---

*A developmental task is a set of skills and competencies peculiar to each developmental stage that children must accomplish or master in order to deal effectively with their environment. (From Developmental tasks and education, ed. 3, by Robert J. Havighurst. Copyright © 1972 by Longman, Inc. Reprinted with permission of Longman, New York, and the author.)

Infancy period: birth to 12 or 18 months
NEONATAL: birth to 28 days
INFANCY: 1 to approximately 12 months
The infancy period is one of rapid motor, cognitive, and social development. Through mutuality with the caregiver (mother), the infant establishes a basic trust in the world and the foundation for future interpersonal relationships. The critical first month of life, although part of the infancy period, is often differentiated from the remainder because of the major physical adjustments to extrauterine existence and the psychologic adjustment of the mother.

Early childhood: 1 to 6 years
TODDLER: 1 to 3 years
PRESCHOOL: 3 to 6 years
This period, which extends from the time children attain upright locomotion until they enter school, is characterized by intense activity and discovery. It is a time of marked physical and personality development. Motor development advances steadily. Children at this age acquire language and wider social relationships, learn role standards, gain self-control and mastery, develop increasing awareness of dependence and independence, and begin to develop a self-concept.

Middle childhood: 6 to 11 or 12 years
Frequently referred to as the "school age," this period of development is one in which the child is directed away from the family group and is centered around the wider world of peer relationships. There is steady advancement in physical, mental, and social development with emphasis on developing skill competencies. Social cooperation and early moral development take on more importance with relevance for later life stages. This is a critical period in the development of a self-concept.

Later childhood: 11 to 18 years
PREPUBERTAL: 10 to 13 years
ADOLESCENCE: 13 to approximately 18 years
The tumultuous period of rapid maturation and change known as adolescence has been described in various ways. It is considered a transitional period that begins at the onset of puberty and extends to the point of entry into the adult world—usually high school graduation. Biologic and personality maturation are accompanied by physical and emotional turmoil, and there is redefining of the self-concept. In the late adolescent period the child begins to internalize all the previously learned values and to focus on an individual, rather than a group, identity.

Patterns of development

There are definite and predictable patterns in growth and development that are continuous, orderly, and progressive. These patterns, which are sometimes referred to as trends or principles, are universal and basic to all human beings. Although they are more apparent with respect to physical growth, most of these patterns apply to psychologic and social growth as well. Growth and development follow predetermined trends in direction, sequence, and pace, but each human being accomplishes these in a manner and time unique to that individual.

Directional trends. Growth and development proceed in regular, related directions or gradients and reflect the physical development and maturation of neuromuscular functions (Fig. 2-2). The first pattern is the *cephalocaudal*, or head-to-tail, direction. That is, the head end of the organism develops first and is very large and complex, whereas the lower end is small and simple and takes shape at a later period. The physical evidence of this trend is most apparent during the period before birth, but it also applies to postnatal behavior development. Infants achieve structural control of the head before the trunk and extremities, hold their back erect before they stand, use their eyes before their hands, and gain control of their hands before they have control of their feet.

Second, the *proximodistal*, or near-to-far, trend applies to the midline-to-peripheral concept. A conspicuous illustration is the early embryonic development of limb buds, which is followed by rudimentary fingers and toes. In the infant, shoulder control precedes mastery of the hands, the whole hand is used as a unit before the fingers can be manipulated, and the central nervous system develops more rapidly than the peripheral nervous system.

These trends or patterns are bilateral and appear symmetric—each side develops in the same direction and at the same rate as the other. For some of the neurologic functions, this symmetry is only external because of uni-

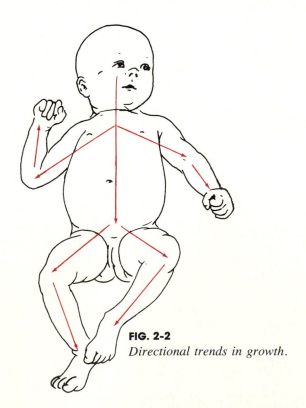

FIG. 2-2
Directional trends in growth.

lateral differentiation of function at an early stage of postnatal development. For example, by the age of approximately 5 years the child has demonstrated a decided preference for the use of one hand over the other, although previously he has used either one.

The third trend, the *mass to specific* trend (sometimes referred to as differentiation), describes development from simple operations to more complex activities and functions. From very broad, global patterns of behavior, more specific, refined patterns emerge. All areas of development (physical, mental, social, and emotional) proceed in this direction. Generalized development will precede specific or specialized development. Physically there are gross, random muscle movements before fine muscle control takes place. The child will at first run and jump for the sake of motion, but eventually these activities take the more complex form of a race or a game, for example, hopscotch. Infants will respond to people in general before they recognize and prefer their mothers.

Sequential trends. In all dimensions of growth and development there is a definite, predictable sequence. It is orderly and continuous, with each child normally passing through every stage. Children crawl before they creep, creep before they stand, and stand before they walk. Later facets of the personality are built on the early foundation of trust. The child babbles, then forms words and, finally, sentences; writing emerges from scribbling.

Developmental pace. Although there is a fixed, precise order to development, it does not progress at the same rate or pace. There are periods of accelerated growth and periods of decelerated growth. This includes both total body growth and the growth of subsystems. The very rapid growth rate before and after birth gradually levels off through early childhood. The rate is relatively slow during middle childhood, but there is a marked increase at the beginning of adolescence followed by a leveling off in early adulthood. Each child grows at his own pace. Marked individual differences are observed between children as they reach and surmount developmental milestones. Although the sequence remains unchanged, the rate varies with each child.

Sensitive periods. There are limited times during the process of growth when the organism will interact with a particular environment in a specific manner. The quality of interactions during these sensitive periods determines whether the effects on the organism will be beneficial or harmful. For example, physiologic maturation of the central nervous system is influenced by adequacy and timing of contributions from the environment, such as stimulation and nutrition. The first 3 months of prenatal life are sensitive periods for physical growth.

Psychologic development also appears to have sensitive periods when an environmental event has maximal influence on the developing personality. For example, primary socialization occurs during the first year when the infant makes the initial social attachments and establishes a basic trust in the world. A warm relationship with a mother figure is fundamental to a healthy personality. The same concept might be applied to readiness for learning skills such as toilet training or reading. In these instances there appears to be an opportune time when the skill is best learned.

PHYSICAL DEVELOPMENT

As children grow, their external dimensions change. These changes are accompanied by corresponding alterations in structure and function of internal organs and tissues that

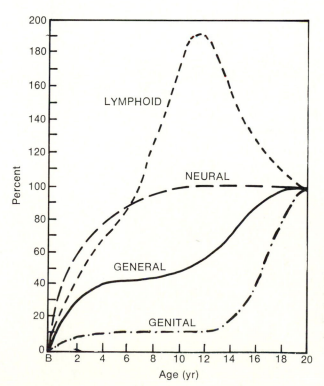

FIG. 2-3

Growth rates for the body as a whole and three types of tissues. Lymphoid type, *thymus, lymph nodes, and intestinal lymph masses;* neural type, *brain, dura, spinal cord, optic apparatus, and head dimensions;* general type, *body as a whole, external dimensions, and respiratory, digestive, renal, circulatory, and musculoskeletal systems. (Adapted from Harris, J.A., and others: The measurement of man, Minneapolis, 1930, University of Minnesota Press. Copyright 1930 by the University of Minnesota.)*

reflect the gradual acquisition of physiologic competence. Each part has its own rate of growth, which may be directly related to alterations in the size of the child (e.g., the heart rate). Skeletal muscle growth approximates whole body growth; brain, lymphoid, adrenal, and reproductive tissues follow distinct and individual patterns (Fig. 2-3).

External proportions

Variations in the growth rate of different tissues and organ systems produce significant changes in body proportions during childhood. The cephalocaudal trend of development is most evident in total body growth as indicated by these changes (Fig. 2-4). During fetal development the head is the fastest growing body part, and at 2 months of gestation the head comprises 50% of total body length. During infancy growth of the trunk predominates; the legs are the most rapidly growing part during childhood; in adolescence, the trunk once again elongates. In the newborn infant, the lower limbs are one third the total body length but only 15% of the total body weight; in the adult the lower limbs comprise one half the total body height and 30% or more of the total body weight. As growth proceeds, the midpoint in head-to-toe measurements gradually descends from a level even with the umbilicus at birth to the level of the symphysis pubis at maturity.

Growth in height and weight

Linear growth occurs almost entirely as a result of skeletal growth and is considered a stable measurement of general growth. Growth in height is not uniform throughout life but ceases when maturation of the skeleton is complete. The maximum growth in length occurs before birth, but the newborn continues to grow at a rapid, though slower, rate (Table 2-1).

Serial measurements of growth are plotted periodically on standard growth charts to determine the pattern of growth and to compare the individual child with the norm for that particular age-group (see Appendix B).

Weight at birth is more variable than height at birth and is, to a greater extent, a reflection of the intrauterine environment. The average newborn weighs 3175 to 3400 g (7 to 7.5 pounds). In general, the birth weight doubles by 5 to 6 months of age and triples by the end of the first year. By the end of the second year it usually quadruples. After this point the "normal" rate of weight gain, just as the growth in height, assumes a steady annual increase of approximately 2 to 2.75 kg (4.4 to 6 pounds) per year until the adolescent growth spurt (Table 2-1).

Alterations in water content

The changes in water content and distribution that occur with age reflect the changes that take place in the relative amounts of bone, muscle, and fat of which the body is composed. The percentage of total body water falls from 90% in the 1-month-old embryo to 75% or 80% of total body weight at birth. At 3 years of age body water comprises 63% of the total body weight and decreases slowly until age 12, when it reaches approximately 58%.

Another important aspect of growth changes in water distribution is related to the intracellular and extracellular fluid compartments. In the fetus and prematurely born infant, the largest proportion of body water is contained in the extracellular compartment. As growth and development proceed, the proportion within this fluid compartment decreases as the intracellular fluid and cell solids increase. The extracellular fluid decreases from approximately 40% of body weight at birth to 25% at 2 years of age and 20% at maturity (Fig. 2-5).

Temperature and metabolism

Body metabolism and its reflection in the temperature vary during development and according to circumstances that involve body activity or energy use.

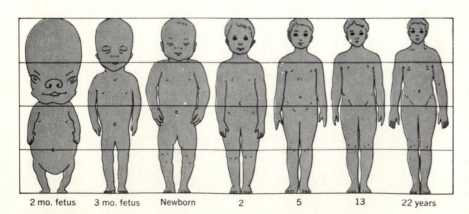

2 mo. fetus   3 mo. fetus   Newborn   2   5   13   22 years

FIG. 2-4

Changes in body proportions from before birth to adulthood. (From Crouch, J.E., and McClintoc, J.R.: Human anatomy and physiology, ed. 2, New York, 1976, John Wiley & Sons, Inc.)

TABLE 2-1. GENERAL TRENDS IN PHYSICAL GROWTH DURING CHILDHOOD

AGE	WEIGHT*	HEIGHT*
Infants		
Birth-6 months	Weekly gain: 140-200 g (5-7 ounces) Birth weight doubles by end of first 6 months	Monthly gain: 2.5 cm (1 inch)
6-12 months	Weekly gain: 85-140 g (3-5 ounces) Birth weight triples by end of first year	Monthly gain: 1.25 cm (0.5 inch) Birth length increases by approximately 50% by end of first year
Toddlers	Birth weight quadruples by age 2½ years Yearly gain: 2-3 kg (4.4-6.6 pounds)	Height at 2 years is approximately 50% of eventual adult height Gain during second year: about 12 cm (4.8 inches) Gain during third year: about 6-8 cm (2.4-3.2 inches)
Preschoolers	Yearly gain: 2-3 kg (4.4-6.6 pounds)	Birth length doubles by 4 years of age Yearly gain: 6-8 cm (2.4-3.2 inches)
School-age children	Yearly gain: 2-3 kg (4.4-6.6 pounds)	Yearly gain after age 7 years: 5.0 cm (2 inches) Birth length triples by about 13 years of age
Pubertal growth spurt		
Females—between 10 and 14 years	Weight gain: 7-25 kg (15-55 pounds) Mean: 17.5 kg (38.1 pounds)	Height gain: 5-25 cm (2-10 inches); approximately 95% of mature height achieved by onset of menarche or skeletal age of 13 years Mean: 20.5 cm (8.2 inches)
Males—between 11 and 16 years	Weight gain: 7-30 kg (15-65 pounds) Mean: 23.7 kg (52.1 pounds)	Height gain: 10-30 cm (4-12 inches); approximately 95% of mature height achieved by skeletal age of 15 years Mean: 27.5 cm (11 inches)

*Yearly height and weight gains for each age-group represent averaged estimates from a variety of sources.

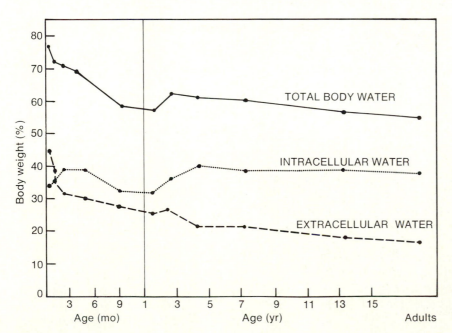

FIG. 2-5

Changes in total body water, extracellular water, and intracellular water, in percentages of body weight. (From Friis-Hansen, B.: Body water compartments in children, Pediatrics **28:***169, 1961. Copyright American Academy of Pediatrics 1961.)*

Metabolism. The rate of metabolism when the body is at rest (basal metabolic rate [BMR]) demonstrates a distinctive change throughout childhood. It is highest in the newborn infant and is closely related to the proportion of surface area to body mass, which changes as the body increases in size. In both sexes the proportion decreases progressively to maturity and determines the caloric requirements of the child. The basal requirement of infants is about 110 to 120 kcal/kg (50 to 55 kcal/pound) of body weight and decreases to 40 to 50 kcal/kg (18 to 25 kcal/pound) at maturity (see Appendix D). Children's energy needs vary considerably at different ages and with changing circumstances. The greatest proportion of calories in infancy is used for basal metabolic needs and growth. The energy requirement to build tissue steadily decreases with age, following the general growth curve; however, exercise needs vary with the individual child and may be considerably more.

Temperature. Body temperature, which reflects metabolism, displays the same decrement from infancy to maturity. Following the unstable regulatory ability in the neonatal periods, heat production (as reflected in body temperature) steadily declines as the infant grows into childhood. Individual differences of ½° to 1° are normal, and occasionally a child will normally display an unusually high or low temperature.

Even with improved temperature regulation, infants and young children are highly susceptible to temperature fluctuations. Body temperature responds to changes in environmental temperature and is increased with active exercise, crying, and emotional upset. Infections can cause a higher and more rapid temperature increase in infants and young children than in older children. In relation to body weight, an infant produces more heat per unit than children near maturity. Consequently, during active play or when heavily clothed, an infant or small child is likely to become overheated.

Growth of cartilage and bone

Growth of the skeleton follows a genetically programmed developmental plan that furnishes not only the best indicator of general growth progress but that also provides the best estimate of biologic age. The most accurate measurement of general development is the determination of osseous maturation by radiography. Skeletal age appears to correlate more closely with other measures of physiologic maturity (such as onset of menarche) than with chronologic age or height. This "bone age" is determined by comparing the mineralization of ossification centers and advancing bony form to age-related standards. Skeletal maturation begins with the appearance of centers of ossification in the embryo and ends when the last epiphysis is firmly fused to the shaft of its bone.

In long bones the ossification takes place in two centers. It begins in the *diaphysis* (the long central portion of the bone) from a "primary" center and continues in the *epiphysis* (the end portions of the bone) at "secondary" centers of ossification. These changes do not take place in all bones simultaneously but appear in a specific order and at a specific time. Although the speed of bone growth and the amount of maturity at specific ages vary from one child to another, the order of ossification is constant. New centers appear at regular intervals during the growth period and provide the basis for assessment of "bone age."

Skeletal development advances until maturity through growth of ossification centers and lengthening of long bones at the cartilage plate located between the diaphysis and the epiphysis. Linear growth can continue as long as the epiphysis is separated from the diaphysis by the cartilage plate; when the cartilage disappears, the epiphysis unites with the diaphysis and growth ceases. Epiphyseal fusion also follows an orderly sequence, thus the timing of epiphyseal closure furnishes another medium for measuring skeletal age.

Growth of muscle

As skeletal development is responsible for linear growth, muscle growth accounts for a significant portion of the increase in body weight. Differences in muscle size between individuals and differences in one person at various times during a lifetime are results of the ability of the separate muscle fibers to increase in size. This increase is most apparent during the adolescent growth spurt. The variability in size and strength of muscle is influenced by genetic constitution, nutrition, and exercise. At all ages muscles increase in size with use and shrink when inactive.

Lymphoid tissues

Lymphoid tissues, which are contained in the lymph nodes, thymus, spleen, tonsils, adenoids, and blood lymphocytes, follow a distinctive growth pattern unlike that of other body tissues. These tissues are small in relation to total body size, but they are well developed at birth. They increase rapidly to reach adult dimensions by 6 years of age and continue to grow. At about 10 to 12 years of age they reach a maximum development that is approximately twice their adult size. This is followed by a rapid decline to stable adult dimensions by the end of adolescence.

Adipose tissue

There is wide variation in the degree of fatness or thinness between individuals at all ages because of a multitude of factors. Normal fat distribution during childhood follows a definite pattern. There is a rapid accumulation from the seventh month of prenatal development through the first 6 postnatal months, and the amount of subcutaneous fat present in the newborn correlates with the weight of the infant.

After 6 months of age the rate of fat accumulation declines rapidly and then decreases steadily in both sexes until 6 to 8 years of age. From the ages of 6 to 8 years, fat again begins to accumulate slowly. It is during this period that obesity may begin to appear in some children. Many children also put on excess fat just before the adolescent growth spurt. Up to the time of the onset of puberty there is very little difference in fat accumulation and distribution in boys and girls. During the adolescent growth spurt the amount of fat in boys decreases sharply (especially in the limbs) and is not regained until early adulthood. In girls the fat accumulation continues but assumes a typical distribution pattern that produces the feminine curves of the mature female.

Dentition

Teeth are divided into quadrants of the lower (mandible) and upper (maxilla) jaws and are named for their location in each quadrant, such as central incisor, lateral incisor, and first and second molars. Teeth are also named for their specific function in the mastication of food. The knifelike shape of the incisors cuts the food. The two premolars, called bicuspids because of their two-pointed crown, crush the food. The permanent molars, with four or five cusps, grind the food.

About the middle of the first year the *primary (deciduous)* teeth begin to erupt, although calcification is not completed until sometime during the third year. The age of tooth eruption shows considerable variation among all children, but the order of their appearance is fairly regular and predictable (Fig. 2-6, *A* and *B*). The first primary teeth to erupt are the lower central incisors, which appear at approximately 6 to 8 months of age. This may vary from 4 months to 1 year in normal children, and infants may even be born with teeth. The total of 20 primary teeth is acquired in characteristic sequence by 30 months of age.

The first *secondary (permanent)* teeth erupt at about 6 years of age. Before their appearance they have been developing in the jaw beneath the primary teeth. Meanwhile, the roots of the latter are gradually being absorbed so that

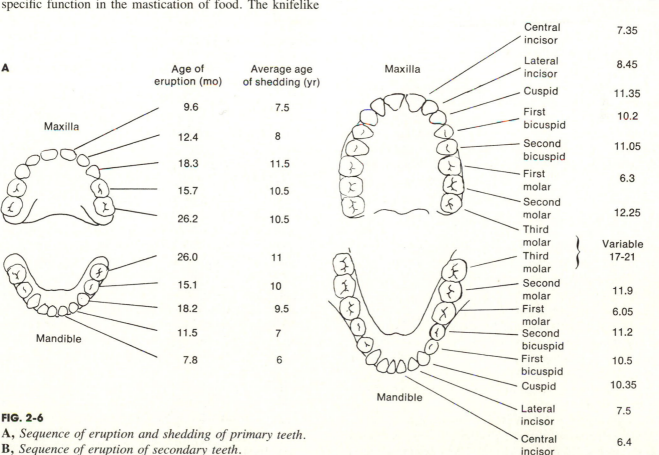

FIG. 2-6
A, *Sequence of eruption and shedding of primary teeth.*
B, *Sequence of eruption of secondary teeth.*

at the time a deciduous tooth is shed, only the crown remains. At 6 years of age all the primary teeth are present, and those of the secondary dentition are relatively well formed. At this time, eruption of the permanent teeth begins, usually starting with the 6-year molar, which erupts posterior to the deciduous molars. The others appear in approximately the same order as eruption of the primary teeth and follow shedding of the deciduous teeth. The pattern of shedding primary teeth and the eruption of secondary teeth are subject to wide variation among children. The eruption of teeth is sometimes used as a criterion for developmental assessment, especially the 6-year molar, which seems to be the most universally consistent in timing. However, dental maturation does not correlate well with bone age and is less reliable as an index of biologic age.

DEVELOPMENT OF MENTAL FUNCTION

Personality and cognitive skills develop in the same manner as biologic growth, and many aspects depend on physical growth and maturation for their accomplishment. This is not a comprehensive account of the multiple facets of personality and behavior development. Many aspects will be integrated with the child's emotional and social development in later discussions of the various age-groups.

Cognitive development

The term *cognition* refers to the process by which the developing individual becomes acquainted with the world and the objects it contains. Children are born with inherited potentialities for intellectual growth, but they must develop into that potential through interaction with the environment. By assimilating information through the senses, processing it, and acting on it, they come to understand relationships between objects and between themselves and their world. With cognitive development, individuals acquire the ability to reason abstractly, to think in a logical manner, and to organize intellectual functions or performances into higher-order structures. The best known and most comprehensive theory regarding children's thinking has been developed by the Swiss psychologist Jean Piaget. He believed that there are four major stages in the development of logical thinking. Each stage is derived from and builds on the accomplishments of the previous stage in a continuous, orderly process. The course of intellectual development is both maturational and invariant and is divided into the following stages (these ages are approximate).

Sensorimotor (birth to 2 years). The sensorimotor stage of intellectual development consists of six substages (see p. 223) that are governed by sensations in which simple learning takes place. Children progress from reflex activity through simple repetitive behaviors to imitative behavior. They develop a sense of ''cause-and-effect'' as they direct behavior toward objects. Problem solving is primarily trial and error. They display a high level of curiosity, experimentation, and enjoyment of novelty and begin to develop a sense of self as they are able to differentiate themselves from their environment. They become aware that objects have permanence—that an object exists even though it is no longer visible (see p. 223). Toward the end of the sensorimotor period children begin to use language and representational thought.

Preoperational (2 to 7 years). The predominant characteristic of the preoperational stage of intellectual development is *egocentricity*. Egocentricity in this sense does not mean selfishness or self-centeredness, but, rather, the inability to put oneself in the place of another. Children interpret objects and events, not in terms of general properties, but in terms of their relationships or their use to them. They are unable to see things from any perspective other than their own; they cannot see another's point of view, nor can they see any reason to do so.

Preoperational thinking is concrete and tangible. Children cannot reason beyond the observable, and they lack the ability to make deductions or generalizations. Thought is dominated by what they see, hear, or otherwise experience. However, they are increasingly able to use language and symbols to represent objects in their environment. Through imaginative play, questioning, and otherwise interacting, they begin to elaborate concepts more and to make simple associations between ideas. In the latter stage of this period their reasoning is *intuitive* (for example, the stars have to go to bed just as they do) and they are only beginning to deal with problems of weight, length, size, and time.

Concrete operations (7 to 11 years). At this age, thought becomes increasingly logical and coherent. Children are able to classify, sort, order, and otherwise organize facts about the world to use in problem solving. They develop a new concept of permanence—conservation. That is, they realize that volume, weight, number, etc. remain the same even though outward appearances are changed. They are able to deal with a number of different aspects of a situation simultaneously. They do not have the capacity to deal in abstraction; they solve problems in a concrete, systematic fashion based on that which they can perceive. Reasoning is inductive. Through progressive changes in thought processes and relationships with others, thought becomes decentered. They can consider points of view other than their own. Thinking has become socialized.

Formal operations (12 to 15 years). Formal operational thought is characterized by adaptability and flexibility. Adolescents can think in abstract terms, use abstract symbols, and draw logical conclusions from a set of observations. They can make hypotheses and test them; they can consider abstract, theoretic, and philosophic matters. Although they may confuse the ideal with the practical, most contradictions in the world can be dealt with and resolved.

Personality development

The personality evolves as children react to their changing bodies and to the environment. Personality development can be described by predictable age-related stages during which specific changes are assumed to take place. The most widely accepted and used is Erik Erikson's theory of personality development. Built on freudian theory, it emphasizes a healthy personality as opposed to a pathologic approach. In his theory, Erikson also uses the biologic concepts of sensitive or critical periods and epigenesis. Erikson describes key conflicts or core problems that the individual strives to master during critical periods in personality development. Successful completion or mastery of each of these core conflicts is built on the satisfactory completion or mastery of the previous core.

Each stage has two components, the favorable and un-

favorable aspects of the core conflict, and progression to the next stage depends on resolution of this conflict. No core problem is ever solved in its entirety; each new situation will present this conflict in a new form. For example, when children who have satisfactorily achieved a sense of trust and other tasks require hospitalization, they must again develop a sense of trust in those responsible for their care in order to master the situation.

Erikson's description of the core conflicts in the eight stages of personality development, which coincide with Freud's psychosexual stages, contains distinctive goals with lasting outcomes of their successful attainment. Also included are the processes by which these goals are attained and the psychosexual stages through which the individual is progressing (all ages are approximate) (Table 2-2).

Sense of trust (birth to 1 year). The first and most important attribute of a healthy personality to develop is a basic trust. Establishment of basic trust dominates the first year of life and describes all the child's satisfying experiences at this age. Corresponding to Freud's oral stage, it is a time of "getting" and "taking in" through all the senses. It exists only in relation to something or someone; therefore, consistent, loving care by a mothering person

TABLE 2-2. SUMMARY OF PERSONALITY DEVELOPMENT

	STAGE	AGE (years)	PSYCHOSEXUAL STAGES	PSYCHOSOCIAL STAGES	CENTRAL PROCESS	LASTING OUTCOMES
I	Infancy	Birth to 1	Oral sensory	Trust vs mistrust	Mutuality with caregiver	Drive and hope
II	Toddlerhood	1-3	Anal-urethral	Autonomy vs shame and doubt	Imitation	Self-control and will-power
III	Early childhood	3-6	Phallic-locomotion	Initiative vs guilt	Identification	Direction and purpose
IV	Middle childhood	6-12	Latency	Industry vs inferiority	Education	Method and competence
V	Adolescence	13-18	Puberty	Identity and repudiation vs identity confusion	Peer pressure Role experimentation	Devotion and fidelity
VI	Early adulthood		Genitality	Intimacy and solidarity vs isolation	Mutuality among peers	Affiliation and love
VII	Young and middle adulthood			Generativity vs self-absorption	Creativity	Production and care
VIII	Later adulthood			Ego integrity vs despair	Introspection	Renunciation and wisdom

Data from Erikson, E.H.: Childhood and society, ed. 2, New York, 1963, W.W. Norton & Co.; Newman, B.M., and Newman, P.R.: Development through life, rev. ed., Homewood, Ill., 1979, The Dorsey Press; Smart, M.S., and Smart, R.C.: Children: development and relationships, ed. 3, New York, 1977, Macmillan, Inc.

(the caregiver) is essential to development of trust. *Mistrust* develops when trust-promoting experiences are deficient or lacking or when basic needs are inconsistently or inadequately met. Although shreds of mistrust are sprinkled throughout the personality, from a basic trust in parents stems a basic trust in the world, other people, and oneself. The result is faith and optimism.

Sense of autonomy (1 to 3 years). Corresponding to Freud's anal stage, the problem of autonomy can be symbolized by the holding on and letting go of the sphincter muscles. The development of autonomy during the toddler period is centered around children's increasing ability to control their bodies, themselves, and their environment. They want to use their powers to do for themselves—these newly acquired motor skills of walking, climbing, and manipulating and mental powers of selection and decision making. Much of their learning is acquired through the process of imitating the activities and behavior of others. Negative feelings of *doubt* and *shame* arise when children are made to feel small and self-conscious, when their choices are disastrous, when others shame them, or when they are forced to be dependent in areas in which they are capable of assuming control. The favorable outcome of this stage is self-control and willpower.

Sense of initiative (3 to 6 years). This stage is characterized by vigorous, intrusive behavior, enterprise, and a strong imagination. Children explore the physical world with all their senses and powers. They develop a conscience. No longer guided only by outsiders, there is an inner voice that warns and threatens. Their circle of relationships extends beyond the family group and they begin to identify with role models both in and outside the family. Being made to feel that their activities or imaginings are bad produces a sense of *guilt*. This stage corresponds to Freud's infantile genital or phallic stage. An outstanding feature of this stage is the Oedipus complex—the child forms an attachment to the parent of the opposite sex. The favorable outcome of this stage is direction and purpose.

Sense of industry (6 to 12 years). Having achieved the more crucial stages in personality development, children are now ready to be workers and producers. They want to engage in tasks and activities that they can carry through to completion. They need and want real achievement. Through the process of education, they learn to compete with others and to cooperate, and they learn the rules. It is a decisive period in their social relationships with others. Feelings of inadequacy and *inferiority* may develop if too much is expected of them or if they believe that they cannot measure up to the standards set for them by others. This is the latency period of Freud. The favorable outcome of a sense of industry is method and competence.

Sense of identity (12 to 18 years). Corresponding to Freud's stage of puberty, this period of identity development is characterized by rapid and marked physical changes. Previous trust in their bodies is shaken, and children become overly preoccupied with the way they appear in the eyes of others as compared with their own self-concept. Adolescents struggle to fit the roles they have played and those they hope to play with the current style, to integrate their concepts and values with those of society, and to come to a decision regarding an occupation. Peer relationships become increasingly important forces in their development with pressure to conform to group standards. Inability to solve core conflicts results in *role diffusion*. The outcome of successful mastery is devotion and fidelity.

Sense of intimacy (early adulthood). A sense of intimacy is established on a firmly acquired sense of identity. It is the capacity to develop an intimate love relationship with another and intimate interpersonal relationships with friends, partners, and so on. This is Freud's stage of genitality. Without intimacy, the individual feels *isolated* and alone. The favorable outcome is affiliation and love.

Sense of generativity (young and middle adulthood). Central to this stage of development is the creation and care of the next generation. The essential element is to nourish and nurture that which has been produced. It may be directed toward one's own children, children of others, or products of creativity of other sorts. The individual who fails in this component of personality development becomes *self-absorbed* and stagnant. The favorable outcome of this stage is production and care.

Sense of ego integrity (old age). A sense of integrity results from satisfaction with life and acceptance of what has been; despair arises from remorse for that which might have been. The favorable outcome is renunciation and wisdom.

Moral development

Children also acquire moral reasoning in a development sequence. To understand the stages in the development of moral judgment, it is important to be aware of the relationship to cognitive development and the stages of logical thought as well as to moral behavior. According to Piaget there are three stages of reasoning: intuitive, concrete operational, and formal operational. When they enter the stage of concrete logical thought at about age 7 years, children are then able to make logical inferences, classify, and deal with quantitative relationships about concrete things. Not until adolescence are they able to reason abstractly with any degree of competence.

Moral development is based on cognitive developmental theory and consists of the following three major levels, each of which has two stages (Kohlberg, 1975).

Preconventional level. The preconventional level parallels the preconventional level of cognitive development and intuitive thought. Culturally oriented to the labels of good/bad and right/wrong, the child integrates these in terms of the physical or pleasurable consequences of his actions.

At first the child determines the goodness or badness of an action in terms of its consequences. He avoids punishment and obeys without question those who have the power to determine and enforce the rules and labels. He has no concept of the basic moral order that supports these consequences.

Later he determines that the right behavior consists of that which satisfies his own needs (and sometimes the needs of others) Although elements of fairness, give and take, and equal sharing are evident, they are interpreted in a very practical, concrete manner without loyalty, gratitude, or justice.

Conventional level. At this stage the child is concerned with conformity and loyalty. He values the maintenance of family, group, or national expectations regardless of consequences. Behavior that meets with approval and pleases or helps others is considered to be good. One earns approval by being ''nice.'' Obeying the rules, doing one's duty, showing respect for authority, and maintaining the social order is the correct behavior. This level is correlated with the stage of concrete operations in cognitive development.

Postconventional, autonomous, or principled level. At this level the individual has reached the cognitive stage of formal operations. Correct behavior tends to be defined in terms of general individual rights and standards that have been examined and agreed on by the entire society. Although procedural rules for reaching consensus become important with emphasis on the legal point of view, there is also emphasis on the possibility for changing law in terms of societal needs and rational considerations.

The most advanced level of moral development is one in which self-chosen ethical principles guide decisions of conscience. These are abstract and ethical but universal principles of justice and human rights with respect for the dignity of the persons as individuals. It is believed that few persons reach this stage of moral reasoning.

Spiritual development

Spiritual beliefs are closely related to the moral and ethical portion of the child's self-concept and, as such, must be considered as part of the child's basic needs assessment. Children need to have meaning, purpose, and hope in their lives, and the need for confession and forgiveness is present even in very young children. Fowler (1974) has identified stages in the development of faith that are closely associated with and that parallel cognitive and psychosocial development.

Stage 0: Undifferentiated. This stage of development encompasses the period of infancy during which time children have no concept of right or wrong, no beliefs, and no convictions to guide their behavior. However, the beginnings of a faith are established with the development of basic trust through their relationships with the primary caregiver.

Stage 1: Intuitive-projective. Toddlerhood is primarily a time of imitating the behavior of others. Children imitate the religious gestures and behaviors of others without comprehending any meaning or significance to the activities. During the preschool years the child assimilates some of the values and beliefs of his parents. Parental attitudes toward moral codes and religious beliefs convey to children what they consider to be good and bad. Children still imitate behavior at this age and follow parental beliefs as part of their daily lives rather than through an understanding of their basic concepts.

Stage 2: Mythical-literal. Through the school-age years, spiritual development parallels cognitive development and is closely related to children's experiences and social interaction. Most have a strong interest in religion during the school-age years. The existence of a deity is accepted and petitions to an omnipotent being are important and expected to be answered; good behavior is rewarded and bad behavior is punished. Their developing conscience bothers them when they disobey. They have a reverence for thoughts and matters and are able to articulate their faith. They may even question its validity.

Stage 3: Synthetic-convention. As the child approaches adolescence, however, he becomes increasingly aware of spiritual disappointments. He recognizes that prayers are not always answered (at least on his own terms) and may begin to abandon or modify some religious practices. He begins to reason, to question some of the established parental religious standards, and to drop or modify some religious practices.

Stage 4: Individuating-reflexive. Adolescents become more skeptical and begin to compare the religious standards of their parents with others. They attempt to determine which to adopt and incorporate into their own set of values. They also begin to compare religious standards with the scientific viewpoint. It is a time of searching rather than reaching. Adolescents are uncertain about many religious ideas but will not achieve profound insights until late adolescence or early adulthood.

Sex role identification

From the moment of birth a child is treated differently by the parents based on the biologic sex of the infant. Almost immediately the infant is placed in a male or female category with a given name that clearly indicates a sex, dressed in pink if a girl or blue if a boy, and referred to as either "he" or "she." Thus information regarding a sexual identity is conveyed to the child and to the world, and along with these overt messages a set of sex-related attitudes toward the child emerges. Parental attitudes and expectations regarding sex-appropriate behaviors, acquired from their own upbringing, influence the manner in which they react to the infant. These attitudes and expectations are transmitted to the infant first in subtle then in more obvious ways.

Four dimensions appear to be involved in the development of sex role identification. Children (1) learn to apply the appropriate gender label to themselves, (2) acquire sex-appropriate standards of behavior, (3) develop a preference for being the sex that they are, and (4) identify with their parent of the same sex.

The *gender label* is achieved early and subtly through imitation of the parents' expressions as they refer to the child's gender, for example, "That's a good girl," or "That's a good boy." Since it is such an important and basic component of the child's total identity, it is vital that the appropriate gender be assigned as soon as possible in rare cases where the sex of the infant is in doubt.

Beginning when a child is a toddler, *sex role standards* are differentiated and continuously developed throughout childhood. By the time children are 3 years old, they know whether they are boys or girls and they have acquired considerable knowledge of and a preference for sex-appropriate behaviors. They can differentiate one sex from the other even before they learn anatomic differences; a 2-year-old child can identify others as girls or boys based on external appearances. Toddlers are given sex-appropriate toys and objects and are encouraged in activities that are appropriate to their sex.

Preschool children have definite impressions of masculinity and femininity, which are reflected in overt play. Most children in this age-group engage in stereotyped sex-appropriate play activities. Little girls play at housekeeping, taking care of dolls, dressing up, and cooking; boys choose trucks, blocks, and more physically active play.

A *gender preference* for the sex into which the child is born is acquired over a long period of time and depends on several things. Children will prefer to be a member of their own sex when their own behaviors and competence closely approximate the sex role standards, when they like their parent of the same sex, and when they believe that their sex is valued. A deterrent to sex role preference by the child can exist in a family where the parents, at a specific birth, had hoped strongly for a child of the opposite sex. The environmental cues within the family will convey to this child that the opposite sex is a preferred one.

The process by which children come to style themselves after the parent of the same sex and to internalize their values and outlook is *identification*. Most children wish to be like their parent of the same sex, and, although the motivation for identification is still unsettled, children are more willing to share these parental attributes when they are able to see a degree of similarity between themselves and their parents. Once this identification is formed, it can be strengthened by the continued positive conception of the role model or weakened if the child does not perceive the model as desirable.

The formation of a sexual identity and role is influenced by a number of factors and is an enduring part of the personality that affects behavior, attitudes, and relationships in many aspects of daily life. The outcome of the identification process depends on the characteristics of the parents and other role models, the innate capacities and preferences of the child, and the value (cultural and familial) placed on his or her particular sex.

Development of body image

Body image is a complex phenomenon that evolves and changes during the process of growth and development. Children are continually bombarded by new data to be interpreted and accepted, revised, or rejected. They are strongly influenced by parental attitudes as values are conveyed to them that they interpret as desirable or undesirable. Some parts of the body appear to take on particular significance, and this varies with the individual child and with the stage of development. Any deviation from the "norm" (no matter how this is interpreted) is cause for concern. The extent to which a characteristic, defect, or disease affects children's body image is influenced by the attitudes and behavior of those around them.

The way children perceive their own bodies is basic to the establishment of an overall identity. Body image begins in infancy, first on a feeling level, then progresses to an interest in individual body parts, which they examine with the same impartial attention they direct toward toys or other objects. By the end of the first year they become aware of themselves as separate from their caregiver and separate from their environment. They can identify body parts and can recognize themselves in a mirror.

Toddlers continually modify the body image they have established as they become more mobile and imitate the behavior of other persons in their world. They learn that they are either a "boy" or a "girl" and gain impressions of themselves from the behavior and comments of other persons in their lives. For example, "Where did you get that curly hair (or dimples)?" They gain increased mastery over their body in performing basic motor skills, in language, and in control of body functions.

During the preschool period children begin to be concerned with what they will become. They continue imitation of parents and other persons in their world. They have no concept of their inner structure. Their awareness of internal organs comes from sensations and discomfort they feel and what they see entering and leaving their bodies. Sex typing and sex role identification are primary tasks during this time. Children are concerned with their genitals and discover pleasurable sensations by touching and manipulating the genital area. Masturbation is practiced to some extent by all preshool children. They compare their own genitals with those of parents, siblings, and playmates. This is a time when conflicts arise between the gratification received by these activities and the censure they often evoke from parents and society.

The school-age child compares his skills and abilities as well as his physical characteristics with those of his peers. The school-age child is highly concerned about how he looks to others as his social contacts expand. He is acutely aware of physical defects and other deviations from the normal in other persons. The school-age child has countless misconceptions about his inner structure but is interested to learn. Masturbation and sex play are still practiced.

Adolescence is probably the significant period of development for body image formation. The rapid changes of puberty cannot be ignored; they are apparent to the individual and to others. Consequently, an adolescent is forced to alter his body image to accommodate these physical changes. Adolescents focus a great deal of attention on their appearance and make frequent comparisons with their peers and the cultural norms of the society. Identity formation is the prime developmental task of adolescence and any event that alters the body at this time can have a crucial impact on body image construction.

FACTORS THAT INFLUENCE PHYSICAL AND EMOTIONAL DEVELOPMENT

Children are engaged in a continuous and ever-changing series of environmental and interpersonal interactions. It is impossible to include a discussion of all the complex and interrelated factors that influence the development of children as unique individuals. Children are affected by physical factors such as the climate in which they live, physiologic influences such as their innate characteristics and susceptibilities, the value system of their families and culture, and psychologic influences such as the quality of parenting and the number, sex, and personalities of the significant persons in their lives. Some factors that may be facilitated, modified, or otherwise influenced by nursing interventions will be mentioned, although specific activities and elaboration will be discussed elsewhere as appropriate.

Heredity

Inherited characteristics have a profound influence on development. The sex of the child, determined by random selection at the time of conception, directs both his pattern of growth and the behavior of others toward him. In all cultures, attitudes and expectations are different with respect to the sex of the child. Sex plus other hereditary determinants strongly affect the end result of growth and the rate of progress toward it. There is a high correlation between parent and child with regard to traits such as height, weight, and rate of growth. Most physical characteristics, including shape and form of features, body build, and physical peculiarities, are inherited and can influence the way in which children grow and interact with their environment. Many dimensions of personality, such as activity level, responsiveness, and a tendency toward shyness, are also inherited.

Differences in health and vigor of children may be attributed to hereditary traits. An inherited physical or mental defect or disorder will alter or modify a child's physical and/or emotional growth and interactions. The extent to which handicapping conditions interfere with the child's growth and well-being will be considered in relation to numerous disabilities throughout the remainder of the book.

Neuroendocrine

Probably all hormones affect growth in some fashion. Growth hormone (somatotropin), secreted by the anterior lobe of the pituitary gland, maintains the normal rate of protein synthesis in the body but produces its main effect on linear growth. An excess of growth hormone can produce a pituitary giant; a deficiency causes pituitary dwarfism. The thyroid hormones (thyroxine and triiodothyronine), secreted by the thyroid gland in response to the stimulation of thyrotrophic hormone, are essential for normal growth. They stimulate general metabolism and are especially important for growth of bones, teeth, and brain. A deficiency of thyroid hormone produces the stunted growth, mental retardation, and other manifestations of cretinism. The androgens produced and secreted by the adrenal cortex under the stimulation of adrenocorticotropin are responsible for many anabolic effects and for the adolescent growth spurt observed at puberty. These three hormones—somatotrophic hormone, thyroid hormone, and androgens—when given to persons in whom these hormones are deficient, stimulate protein anabolism and thereby produce retention of elements essential for building protoplasm and bony tissue. Other hormones that contribute effects on growth and development include insulin, cortisol, parathyroid hormone, and the sex hormones—testosterone and estrogen.

Nutrition

Nutrition is probably the single most important influence on growth. Dietary factors regulate growth at all stages of development, and their effects are exerted in numerous and complex ways. During the rapid prenatal growth period, faulty nutrition may influence development from the time of implantation of the ovum until birth. During infancy and childhood, the demand for calories is relatively great, as evidenced by the rapid increase in both height and weight. At this time, protein and caloric requirements are higher than at almost any period of postnatal development. As the growth rate slows with its concomitant decrease in metabolism, there is a corresponding reduction in caloric and protein requirement.

Growth is uneven during the periods of childhood between infancy and adolescence when there are plateaus and small growth spurts. The child's appetite will fluctuate in response to these variations until the turbulent growth spurt of adolescence, when adequate nutrition is extremely important but may be subject to numerous emotional influences. Adequate nutrition is closely related to good health throughout life, and an overall improvement in nourishment is evidenced by the gradual increase in size and early maturation of children in this century.

Malnutrition. The term *malnutrition* in its strictest sense is usually used to describe undernutrition, primarily that resulting from insufficient caloric intake. However, malnutrition may result from the following: (1) a dietary intake that is quantitatively or qualitatively inadequate, or both, including overnutrition; (2) disease that interferes with appetite, digestion, or absorption while increasing nutritional requirements; (3) excessive physical activity or inadequate rest; or (4) disturbed interpersonal relationships and other environmental or psychologic factors. Severe malnutrition during the sensitive periods of development, particularly the first 6 months of life, is positively correlated with diminished height, weight, and intelligence scores. Throughout this book, the importance of nutrition as a vital aspect of health promotion during all phases of the illness-wellness continuum is included as it relates to developmental phases and to specific health problems.

Socioeconomic level

There is evidence to indicate that socioeconomic level has a significant impact on development. At all age levels children from upper and middle class families are taller than children from the lower class and girls from the upper class attain menarche somewhat earlier than those in the lower class.

The cause of these discrepancies is not clear, although nutrition probably plays a prominent role. Poorer families are less likely to consistently provide the food the children need. This is especially critical during the sensitive periods in development. Related factors that might influence nutrition and growth in the lower socioeconomic levels are irregularity of eating, sleeping, and exercising, and, as a rule, these families have larger numbers of children who must compete with one another for available food supplies.

Disease

Altered growth and development is one of the clinical manifestations in a number of hereditary disorders. Growth impairment is particularly marked in skeletal disorders, such as the various forms of dwarfism and at least one of the chromosomal anomalies (Turner syndrome). Many of the disorders of metabolism, such as vitamin D–resistant rickets, the mucopolysaccharidoses, and the numerous endocrine disorders, interfere with the normal growth pattern. In other disorders the tendency is toward the upper percentile of height, for example, Klinefelter syndrome and Marfan syndrome.

Many chronic illnesses that are associated with varying degrees of growth failure are congenital cardiac anomalies and respiratory disorders such as cystic fibrosis. Any disorder characterized by the inability to digest and absorb body nutrients will have an adverse effect on growth and development. These include the malabsorption syndromes and defects in digestive enzyme systems. Almost any disorder or disease state that persists over an extended period, particularly during a critical period of development, may have a permanent effect on growth.

Interpersonal relationships

It is well established that relationships with significant others play an important role in development, particularly in emotional, intellectual, and personality development. Not only do the quality and quantity of contacts with other persons exert an influence on the growing child, but the widening range of contacts is essential to learning and the development of a healthy personality.

The mother or mothering person is unquestionably the single most influential person during early infancy. She is the one who meets the infant's basic needs of food, warmth, comfort, and love. She provides stimulation for his senses and facilitates his expanding capacities. Through her, the child learns to trust the world and feel secure to venture in increasingly wider relationships.

The sphere of persons from whom children seek approval widens to include other members of their family, their peers, and, to a lesser extent, other authority figures (for example, teachers). The increasing importance of the peer group in determining the behavior of school-age children and adolescents is well documented.

It is generally the parents who are most influential in assisting the child to assume sex role identification. Parents define and reinforce acceptable sex role behavior and provide sex-appropriate role models for the child. In the absence of a sex role model in the family setting, the child may adopt some characteristics of the opposite sex parent or sibling. Frequently, the child identifies with a teacher or other significant person of the same sex.

Siblings are the child's first peers, and the way in which he learns to relate to them affects later interactions with peers outside the family group. For example, a first-born child who is accustomed to a position of leadership with siblings will tend to assume the same position with peers; younger children are more often followers. Ease in relationships with peers of the same or opposite sex is frequently associated with similar associations in the home.

Emotional deprivation. The most prominent feature of emotional deprivation, particularly during the first year, is developmental retardation. Much of the information regarding the adverse effects of interpersonal influences on development has been acquired through retrospective studies of gross deprivation and trauma. The most notable instances involved homeless infants who were placed in institutions for care. These infants, who did not receive consistent mothering care, failed to gain weight even with an adequate diet; were pale, listless, and immobile; and were unresponsive to stimuli that usually elicits a response in the normal infant, such as smiling, cooing, and so on. It has been found that if the emotional deprivation continues for a sufficient length of time, the child may not survive infancy.

Although the most remarkable examples of emotional deprivation were first recognized among infants in institutions, the term ''masked deprivation'' has been used to describe children who are reared in homes where there is a distorted mother-child relationship or otherwise disordered home environment. Infants do not thrive if the mothering person is hostile, fearful of handling them, or indifferent to them and their needs. Such children exhibit poor growth even though apparently free of physical disease. Growth retardation in these children is believed to be caused by a psychologically induced endocrine imbalance that interferes with growth. These same infants and children display ''catch-up'' growth in a changed environment.

ROLE OF PLAY IN DEVELOPMENT

It is through the universal medium of play that children learn what no one can teach them. They learn about their world and how to deal with this environment of objects, time, space, structure, and people. They learn about themselves operating within that environment—what they can do, how to relate to things and situations, and how to adapt themselves to the demands society makes on them. It has been said that play is the *work* of the child. In play, children continually practice the complicated, stressful processes of living, communicating, and achieving satisfactory relationships with other people. In addition, while promoting and advancing development and relationships, play is its own reward.

Classification of play

From a developmental point of view, patterns of children's play can be categorized according to the *content* and the *social character* of play. In both there is an additive effect. Each builds on past accomplishments, and some element of each is maintained throughout life. At each stage in development the new predominates.

Content of play. Play begins with *social-affective* play, wherein the infant takes pleasure in relationships with people. As adults talk, fondle, nuzzle, and in various ways elicit a response from the infant, he soon learns to provoke parental emotions and responses with such behaviors as smiling, cooing, or initiating games and activities. The type and intensity of the adult behavior with children vary among cultures.

Sense-pleasure play is a nonsocial stimulating experience that originates from outside the individual. Objects in the environment—light and color, tastes and odors, textures and consistencies—attract a child's attention, stimulate his senses, and give pleasure. Pleasurable experiences are derived from handling raw materials (water, sand, food), from body motion (swinging, bouncing, rocking), and from other uses of senses and abilities, such as smelling and humming. Once infants have developed the ability to grasp and manipulate, they persistently demonstrate and exercise their newly acquired abilities through *skill play*, repeating an action over and over again.

One of the vital elements in the child's process of identification is *dramatic* play. It begins in toddlerhood and is the predominant form of play in the preschool child. Once children begin to invest situations and people with meanings and to attribute affective significance to the world, they can pretend and fantasize almost anything. By acting out events of daily life, children learn and practice the roles and identities modeled by the members of their family and society. Their small toys, replicas of the tools of the society in which they live, provide a medium for learning about these adult roles and activities that may be both puzzling and frustrating to them. Interacting with the world is one of the ways in which children get to know it. The simple, imitative, dramatic play of the toddler, such as using the telephone, driving a car, or rocking a doll, evolves into more complex, sustained dramas of the preschooler that extend beyond common domestic matters to the wider aspects of the world and the society, such as playing policeman, storekeeper, teacher, nurse, and so on. Older children work out elaborate themes, act out stories, and compose plays.

Very young children participate in simple, *imitative games* such as pat-a-cake and peekaboo. Preschool children learn and enjoy *formal games* that begin with ritualistic, self-sustaining games, such as ring-around-a-rosy and London Bridge, then progress to *competitive games,* such as cards, checkers, or baseball.

Social character of play. The play interactions of infancy are between the child and an adult. Children continue to enjoy the company of an adult but are increasingly able to play alone. As age advances, interaction with agemates increases in importance and becomes an essential part of the socialization process. Through it, the highly egocentric infant, unable to tolerate delay or interference, ultimately acquires concern for others and the ability to delay gratification or even to reject gratification at the expense of another. A pair of toddlers will engage in a good deal of combat since their personal needs cannot stand delay or compromise. By the time they reach age 5 or 6 years, children are able to arrive at a compromise or make use of arbitration—usually after each child has attempted but failed to gain his own way. Through continued interaction with peers and the growth of conceptual abilities and social skills, children are able to increase participation with others.

Social involvement during play can be categorized by the following:

Onlooker play

In onlooker play the child watches what other children are doing but makes no attempt to enter into the play activity. There is an active interest in observing the interaction of others but no movement toward participating. Watching television is a common example of the onlooker role.

Solitary play

In solitary play children play alone and independently with toys different from those used by other children within the same area. They enjoy the presence of other children but make no effort to get close to or speak to them. Their interest is centered on their own activity, which they pursue with no reference to the activities of the others.

Parallel play

In parallel play children play independently but among other children. They play with toys that are like those that the children around them are using, but as each sees fit, neither influencing nor being influenced by the other children. Each plays beside, but not with, other children. Parallel play is the characteristic play of the toddler, but it may also occur in other groups of any age. Individuals who are engaged in a creative craft with each person separately working on his own project are in parallel play.

Associative play

In associative play children play together and are engaged in a similar or even identical activity, but there is no organi-zation, division of labor, leadership assignment, or mutual goal. There is borrowing and lending of play materials, following one another with wagons and tricycles, and sometimes attempts to control who may or may not play in the group. Each child acts according to his own wishes; there is no group goal. An example of associative play is two children playing with dolls, each borrowing articles of clothing from the other, engaging in similar conversation, but neither directing the other's actions nor establishing rules regarding the limits of the play session. There is a great deal of behavioral contagion—when one child initiates an activity, the entire group follows the example.

Cooperative play

Cooperative play is organized, and the child plays in a group *with* other children. The children discuss and plan activities for the purposes of accomplishing an end—to make something, to attain a competitive goal, to dramatize situations of adult or group life, or to play formal games. The group is loosely formed, but there is a marked sense of belonging or not belonging to the group. The goal and its attainment require organization of activities, division of labor, and playing roles. The leader-follower relationship is definitely established, and the activity is controlled by one or two members who assign roles and direct the activities of the others. The activity is organized to allow one child to supplement another's function in order to complete the goal.

Functions of play

The specific values of play or the functions that it serves throughout childhood include sensorimotor development, intellectual development, socialization, creativity, self-awareness, and therapeutic and moral value.

Sensorimotor development. Sensorimotor activity is a major component of play at all ages and is the predominant form of play in infancy. Active play is essential for muscle development and serves a useful purpose as a release for surplus energy. Through sensorimotor play children explore the nature of the physical world. Infants gain impressions of themselves and their world through tactile, auditory, visual, and kinesthetic stimulation. Toddlers and preschoolers revel in body movement and exploration of things in space. Children continue to engage in sensorimotor play, although with increasing maturity the play becomes more differentiated and involved. Very young children run for the sheer joy of body movement, and older children incorporate or modify the motions into increasingly complex and coordinated activities such as races, games, roller skating, and bicycle riding.

Intellectual development. Through exploration and manipulation, children learn colors, shapes, sizes, textures, and the significance of objects. They learn the significance of numbers and how to use them, they learn to associate words with objects, and they develop an understanding of abstract concepts and spatial relationships, such as up, down, under, over, and so on. Activities such as puzzles and games help them to develop problem-solving skills. Books, stories, films, and collections expand knowledge and provide enjoyment as well. Play provides a means to practice and expand language skills. Through play, children continually rehearse past experiences to assimilate them into new perceptions and relationships. Play helps children to comprehend the world in which they live and to distinguish between fantasy and reality.

Socialization. From very early infancy, children show interest and pleasure in the company of others. Their initial social contact is with the mothering person, but through play with other children they learn to establish social relationships and solve the problems associated with these relationships. They learn to give and take, which is more readily learned from critical peers than from the more tolerant adults. They learn the sex role that society expects them to fulfill as well as approved patterns of behavior and deportment. Closely associated with socialization is development of moral values and ethics. Children learn right from wrong, the standards of the society, and to assume responsibility for their actions.

Creativity. In no other situation is there more opportunity to be creative than in play. Children can experiment and try out their ideas in play through every medium at their disposal, including raw materials, fantasy, and exploration. Creativity is stifled by pressure toward conformity; therefore, striving for peer approval may inhibit creative endeavors in the school-age or adolescent child. Creativity is primarily a product of solitary activity, as opposed to group activity. Once children feel the satisfaction of creating something new and different, they transfer this creative interest to situations outside the world of play.

Self-awareness. Beginning with active explorations of their bodies and awareness of themselves as separate from the mother, the process of self-identity is facilitated through play activities. Children learn who they are and what their place is in the world. They become increasingly able to regulate their own behavior, to learn what their abilities are, and to compare their abilities with those of others. Through play, children are able to test their abilities, to assume and try out various roles, and to learn the effect that their behavior has on others.

Therapeutic value. There is no doubt that play is therapeutic at any age. It provides a means for release from the tension and stress encountered in the environment. In play, children can express emotions and release unacceptable impulses in a socially acceptable fashion. Children are able to experiment and test fearful situations and can assume and vicariously master the roles and positions that they are unable to perform in the world of reality. Children reveal much about themselves in play. Through play, children are able to communicate to the alert observer the needs, fears, and desires that they are unable to express with their limited language skills.

Throughout their play, children need the acceptance of adults and their presence to help them control aggression and to channel their destructive tendencies.

Moral value. Although children learn at home and at school those behaviors that are considered right and wrong in the culture, the interaction with peers during play contributes significantly to their moral training. Nowhere is the enforcement of moral standards so rigid as in the play situation. If they are to be acceptable members of the group, children must adhere to the accepted codes of behavior of the culture—fairness, honesty, self-control, consideration for others, and so on. Children soon learn that their peers are less tolerant of violations than are adults and that to maintain a place in the play group they must conform to the standards of the group.

Toys

The type of toys chosen by and/or provided for children can facilitate their development in the areas just outlined. Toys that are small replicas of the culture and its tools help them assimilate their culture. Toys that require pushing, pulling, rolling, and manipulating teach them about physical properties of the items and help to develop muscles and coordination. Rules and the basic elements of cooperation and organization are learned through board games.

In providing toys for children it is well to keep in mind that raw materials with which they are able to use their own creativity and imaginations are sometimes superior to ready made items. For example, building blocks can be used to construct a variety of things, to count, and to learn shapes and sizes. Lewis and Block (1982) outline five ways in which parents can encourage their child's toy play:

1. Realize that play teaches skills and abilities that are the center of intelligence.
2. Play with your child, enroll the child in a play group that meets several times a week, or hire a babysitter who can act as a playmate.
3. Do not turn every play activity into an educational lesson.
4. Respect your child's likes and dislikes; remember that learning is best acquired in an enjoyable situation.
5. Observe your child at play so that you come to know favorite types of toys and activities.

ACCIDENTS IN CHILDHOOD

Accidents are the leading cause of death in children beyond 1 year of age, and the type of injury and the circumstances surrounding the accident are closely related to normal growth and development behavior. As the child develops, his innate curiosity impels him to investigate activities and to mimic the behavior of others. The developmental stage of the child partially determines the types of accidents that are most likely to occur at a specific age and thus helps provide clues to preventive measures that might be implemented. For example, small infants are helpless in any environment, and when they begin to roll over or otherwise propel themselves, they can fall from unprotected surfaces. The creeping infant with a natural tendency to place objects in the mouth is at risk of aspiration or poisoning. The mobile toddler with the instinct to explore and investigate and the ability to run and climb is subject to a variety of accidents, including falls, burns, and collision with objects. As children grow older their absorption with play often makes them oblivious to environmental hazards such as street traffic or water, and the need to conform and gain acceptance compels older children and adolescents to accept challenges and dares.

At all ages children are continually in contact with toys, tools, and an infinite variety of mechanical devices that are easily accessible and that they may explore without proper guidance or supervision. Although the highest incidence of accidental injury is in children less than 9 years of age (especially ages 2 and 3 years, with ages 5 and 6 years next), most fatal injuries occur in later childhood and adolescence. Older children have more accidents outside the home; younger children are more often injured in or around the home.

The personality of a child can be a factor in his susceptibility to accidents. The bright, alert, and adventuresome child is apt to have more accidents than the dull, passive, or less curious child. Boys, at all ages, have more accidents than girls, and this tendency increases as the child gets older. Because they are usually more closely supervised and have been taught to be more cautious, firstborn and only children seem to have fewer accidents than younger siblings.

Development and accidents

Accidents are amenable to control, and the preventive aspects of child care should be an ongoing part of health promotion throughout childhood. This necessitates protection, education, and legislation. To protect the child from accidental injury, persons who are responsible for children need to be aware of the normal behavior characteristics that render them vulnerable to accidents and to be alert to factors in the environment that create a hazard to their safety. Parents and others are often surprisingly out of tune with their child's developmental progress and seem unaware of their capabilities. Anticipatory guidance regarding developmental expectations serves to alert the parents to the type of accidents that are most likely to occur at any given age and to environmental circumstances that might precipitate an accident.

Toys. Selection of toys and play equipment is a joint effort between parents and children, but evaluation of their safety is the responsibility of the adult. Government agencies do not inspect and police all toys on the market. Therefore adults who purchase, supervise purchases, or allow the child to use play equipment need to evaluate such equipment for its safety. This often includes toys that are gifts or those that are purchased by the children themselves. Children need toys and activities that increase their sense of competence but that do not create a threat to their health and safety.

Accident prevention

Theoretically, all accidents are preventable, and one of the chief nursing responsibilities is to anticipate and recognize where safety measures are applicable. Safety should be an intrinsic element of nursing practice. Nurses who themselves practice safety, who are alert to safety needs in the environment, and who recognize the need for safety education contribute to accident reduction. Three major areas of focus for accident prevention in children are:

1. Improving the quality of child care
2. Instructing those concerned about measures to safeguard the environment so that *exogenous* factors are removed, such as attractive hazards
3. Being attentive and alert to the *endogenous* factors that are intrinsic in the behavioral characteristics of the developing child

To provide a safe environment for the child involves the combined efforts of family, nurses, and community. At each age level there are environmental attractions that are hazardous to the safety of the child. The specific hazards vary according to season (drowning, accidents related to winter heating devices), geographic area (water accidents in areas with swimming pools, rivers, and lakes; etc.; heater burns in cold climates), and socioeconomic level (lead poisoning and street injuries in slum areas, bicycle accidents in middle class areas). The special problems and preventive measures are discussed as appropriate throughout the book and are related to the various age levels and conditions that predispose to specific hazards.

REFERENCES

Fowler, J.W.: Toward a developmental perspective on faith, Relig. Educ. **69:**207-219, 1974.

Kohlberg, L.: The cognitive-developmental approach to moral education, Phi Delta Kappa **56:**670-677, 1975.

Lewis, M., and Block, J.R.: Toy play, IQ building. Mother's Manual Sept./Oct., 1982, pp. 31-32.

BIBLIOGRAPHY

Barnard, M.U.: Supportive care for the adoptive family, Issues Compr. Pediatr. Nurs. **2**(3):22-29, 1977.

Betz, C.L.: Faith development in children, Pediatr. Nurs. **7**(2):22-25, 1981.

Braff, A.M.: Telling children about their adoption: new alternatives for parents, Am. J. Maternal Child Nurs. **2:**254-259, 1977.

Briggs, E.: Transition to parenthood, Matern. Child Nurs. J. **8**(2):69-83, 1979.

Brockhaus, J.P.D., and Brockhaus, R.H.: Adopting an older child—the emotional process, Am. J. Nurs. **82:**289-291, 1982.

Brockhaus, J.P.D., and Brockhaus, R.H: Adopting an older child—the legal process, Am. J. Nurs. **82:**292-294, 1982.

Brown, V.: Providing a safe environment for children, Am. J. Maternal Child Nurs. **3**(1):53-55, 1978.

Clore, E.R., and Newberry, Y.S.G.: Nurse practitioner guidance for the adoptive family from birth to adolescence, Pediatr. Nurs. **7**(6):16-25, 1981.

Cronenwett, L.R.: Transition to parenthood. In McNall, L.K., and Galeener, J.T., editors: Current practice in obstetric and gynecologic nursing, St. Louis, 1976, The C.V. Mosby Co.

Coucouvanis, J.A., and Solomons, H.C.: Handling complicated visitation problems of hospitalized children, Am. J. Maternal Child Nurs. **8:**131-134, 1983.

Dresden, S.: The young adult: adjusting to single parenting, Am. J. Nurs. **76:**1286-1289, 1976.

Dudding, G.S.: Counseling children through their parents' divorce, Issues Compr. Pediatr. Nurs. **2**(3):40-51, 1977.

Engebretson, J.C.: Stepmothers as first-time parents: their needs and problems. Pediatr. Nurs. **8:**387-390, 1982.

Erikson, E.H.: Childhood and society, ed. 2, New York, 1963, W.W. Norton & Co., Inc.

Hammons, C.: The adoptive family, Am. J. Nurs. **76:**251-260, 1976.

Hollen, P.: Parents' perceptions of parenting support systems, Pediatr. Nurs. **8:**309-313, 1982.

Horowitz, J.A., and Perdue, B.J.: Single-parent families, Nurs. Clin. North Am. **12:**503-511, 1977.

Hrobsky, D.M.: Transition to parenthood: a balancing of needs, Nurs. Clin. North Am. **12:**457-468, 1977.

Jack, M.S.: The single-parent family: an issue in nursing, Issues Compr. Pediatr. Nurs. **2**(3):30-39, 1977.

Jackson, P.L.: Caring for children from divorced families, Am. J. Maternal Child Nurs. **8:**126-130, 1983.

Johnston, M.: Cultural variations in professional and parenting patterns. J. Obstet. Gynecol. Neonatal Nurs. **9**(7):9-13, 1980.

Johnston, M.: Folk beliefs and ethnocultural behavior in pediatrics, medicine or magic, Nurs. Clin. North Am. **12:**77-84, 1977.

Johnston, M.: Toward a culture of caring: children, their environment, and changing, Am. J. Maternal Child Nurs. **4:**210-214, 1979.

Johnston, M., Dayne, M., and Mittleider, K.: Putting more PEP in parenting, Am. J. Nurs. **77:**994-995, 1977.

Kaluger, G., and Kaluger, M.F.: Human development: the span of life, ed. 3, St. Louis, 1984, The C.V. Mosby Co.

Leninger, M.: Cultural diversities of health and nursing care, Nurs. Clin. North Am. **12:**5-18, 1977.

Lowrey, G.H.: Growth and development of children, ed. 7, Chicago, 1978, Year Book Medical Publishers, Inc.

Mussen, P.H., Conger, J.J., and Kagan, J.: Child development and personality, ed. 5, New York, 1979, Harper & Row, Publishers, Inc.

Newman, B.M., and Newman, P.R.: Development through life, revised, Homewood, Ill., 1979, The Dorsey Press.

Petrillo, M., and Sangay, S.: Emotional care of the hospitalized child, Philadelphia, 1980, J.B. Lippincott Co.

Phillips, J.L.: The origins of intellect: Piaget's theory, San Francisco, 1969, W.H. Freeman & Co. Publishers.

Reasoner, R.W.: Enhancement of self-esteem in children and adolescents, Fam. Comm. Health **6**(2):51-64, 1983.

Schilling, L.S.: The effects of divorce on children: a perspective for the pediatric health care provider, J. Assoc. Care Child. Health **11**(3):92-96, 1983.

Shelly, J.A.: Spiritual care. Planting seeds of hope, Crit. Care Update **9**(12):7-15, 1982.

Slevin, K.F.: Motherhood, culture, and change, Pediatr. Nurs. **8**(6):405-408, 1982.

Smart, M.S., and Smart, R.C.: Children: development and relationships, ed. 4, New York, 1982, Macmillan, Inc.

Stanwyck, D.J.: Self-esteem through the life span, Fam. Comm. Health **6**(2):11-28, 1983.

Stoll. R.I.: Guidelines for spiritual assessment, Am. J. Nurs. **79:**1575-1577, 1979.

Webster-Stratton, C., and Kogan, K.: Helping parents parent, Am. J. Nurs. **80:**240-244, 1980.

Women workers today, Nurs. Outlook **22:**191, 1974.

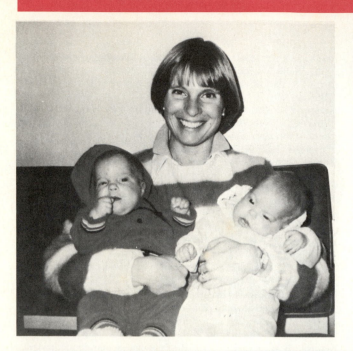

PRECONCEPTUAL AND PRENATAL INFLUENCES ON DEVELOPMENT AND HEALTH

OBJECTIVES

On completion of this chapter the reader will be able to:

- Differentiate between the classes of genetic disorders

- Describe the basic patterns of inheritance

- Determine the risk of recurrence of a disorder caused by a single gene

- Demonstrate an understanding of the processes responsible for abnormalities in chromosome number

- Explain the relationship between genes and environment in the causation of defects or disease

- Discuss the role of the nurse in genetic counseling

NURSING DIAGNOSES

Nursing diagnoses identified for preconceptual and conceptual influences on development include, but are not restricted to, the following:

Cognitive-perceptual pattern

- Knowledge deficit related to (1) lack of interest or motivation; (2) inability to use materials or information sources; (3) unfamiliarity with information resources

- Thought processes, alteration in, related to stress

Self-perception—self-concept pattern

- Anxiety related to (1) strange environment; (2) previous experience(s); (3) perception of impending events; (4) anticipated discomfort; (5) knowledge deficit

- Self-concept, disturbance in, related to (1) perception of hereditary disease; (2) nonintegration of physical changes

Role-relationship pattern

- Communication, impaired verbal, related to (1) language barrier; (2) cultural differences; (3) stress

- Family process, alterations in, related to (1) situational crisis (specify); (2) temporary family disorganization

Child development consists of both genetic components and environmental factors that interact to produce the physical, biochemical, and mental characteristics of the child. These include not only those traits that create the individuality of each child but also those characteristics that produce unpleasant symptoms or undesirable physical abnormalities that are interpreted as disease. Numerous defects and diseases are seen more frequently in the population and show an increased incidence in some families or under certain environmental conditions. Parents and health workers alike are concerned with the probability that a specific disease or disorder will recur in a family in which the condition has been known to occur. In order to be better able to counsel families and to anticipate probable problems, the nurse needs a fundamental understanding of the principles of heredity and the importance of heredity as an etiologic factor in diseases and disabilities.

BASIC CONCEPTS

To facilitate a discussion of the genetic influence on the health of children, it will be necessary to clarify some of the terms used to describe hereditary conditions.

congenital the condition is present at birth. The disorder may be brought about by genetic causes, nongenetic causes, or a combination of these.

familial a disorder that "runs in families" or is present in more members of a family than would be expected to occur by chance.

genetic the disorder is caused by a single harmful gene or by a deviation in chromosomal number or structure. A genetic disorder may or may not be apparent at birth.

inherited (heritable, hereditary) synonymous with genetic, although in the past was often used to describe a disorder that had appeared in parent and offspring over several generations.

Classification of genetic disorders

Genetic diseases can usually be classified into one of the following three broad categories according to the hereditary factors that produce the observed effect:

1. Chromosomal aberrations in which there is addition, loss, or structural alteration of a chromosome, for example, Down syndrome, Klinefelter syndrome, and Turner syndrome
2. Disorders that are caused by mutation of a gene or genes and that are distributed in families according to the basic mendelian inheritance patterns, for example, cystic fibrosis, hemophilia, muscular dystrophy, and phenylketonuria
3. The common diseases and disorders that are multifactorial, that is, result from a complex interaction of both genetic and environmental factors, for example, diabetes mellitus and congenital defects

■ Grieving, anticipatory, related to (1) expected loss (specify); (2) expected change

■ Social isolation related to body image disturbance

Sexuality-reproductive pattern

■ Sexual dysfunction related to fear of procreation of defective offspring

Coping-stress tolerance pattern

■ Coping, family: potential for growth

■ Coping, ineffective individual, related to (1) feelings of powerlessness; (2) situational crisis; (3) knowledge deficit; (4) problem-solving skills deficit

Value-belief pattern

■ Spiritual distress related to decisions regarding procreation

Biologic basis of heredity

All the traits possessed by an individual are contained in minute segments of deoxyribonucleic acid (DNA) called *genes* that are distributed on microscopic structures called *chromosomes.*

All somatic (body) cells in humans contain two sets of genes, one set derived from each parent during the process of reproduction. Each gene has a definite position, or locus, on a specific chromosome and may take one of several different forms. When corresponding genes at a locus produce the same effect they are said to be *homozygous.* If the genes of a pair produce different effects they are said to be *heterozygous.*

The entire set of genes is contained in 46 (23 pairs of) chromosomes—22 pairs of *autosomes* and 1 pair of *sex chromosomes.* The autosomes are alike in both male and female; the sex chromosomes are alike in the female (XX) but are structurally different in the male (XY).

Somatic cells divide by *mitosis,* the process whereby each chromosome with all its genes reproduces itself exactly (equational division). Thus each resulting cell possesses the same kind and number of chromosomes found in the original cell. Germ cells *(gametes)* containing the X and Y sex chromosomes divide by a different process, *meiosis,* whereby the total number of chromosomes is reduced by half (reduction division). Therefore, when the resulting cells are united with a similar germ cell at fertilization, the original number is restored. In this process the paired chromosomes split so that one chromosome of each pair is distributed to each of the resulting cells. This segregation and distribution of chromosomes during the process of meiosis form the basis of the mendelian ratios that constitute the principles of inheritance.

When a gene is altered in some way, it produces an effect different from its original effect. This change in a gene is termed a *mutation.* A mutant gene remains unchanged and is transmitted during reproduction.

DISORDERS CAUSED BY A SINGLE MUTANT GENE

The fundamental principles of mendelian genetics, which describe the activity of genes during gamete formation and fertilization, form the basis for understanding these inherited disorders. The statistically predictable results of combinations and recombinations of genes and their distribution in families can be summarized as follows:

> **principle of dominance** not all genes that determine a given trait operate with equal vigor. When two genes at a given locus produce a different effect (for example, the gene for eye color), they may compete for expression in the individual. As a result, one may mask or conceal the effect of the other. The characteristic that appears in the individual (and the gene that produces the effect) is referred to as *dominant;* that which is hidden and does not appear is *recessive.*
>
> **principle of segregation** the paired chromosomes, bearing genes derived from each parent, are separated when gametes are formed during meiosis. Each gene segregates in pure form, and chance alone determines which gene (paternally derived or maternally derived) will travel to which gamete.
>
> **principle of independent assortment** the members of one pair of genes are distributed in the gametes in random fashion independent of other pairs.

Autosomal inheritance patterns

Conditions that can be directly attributed to a single gene are distributed in families in characteristic patterns according to the basic principles just described. Genes are either dominant or recessive in their effect, and most disorders caused by a single gene can be recognized readily by the simple patterns that they display.

The major inheritance patterns are described with models indicating the mendelian ratios that can be predicted in each type. Since there are 44 autosomes and only two sex chromosomes, the majority of hereditary disorders are a result of defective genes located on an autosome.

Autosomal-dominant inheritance. Characteristics of a condition caused by a dominant gene on an autosome include the following (Fig. 3-1):

1. Males and females are affected with equal frequency.
2. Affected individuals will have an affected parent (unless the condition is caused by a fresh mutation).
3. Half the children of a heterozygous affected parent will be affected.
4. Normal children of affected parents will have normal children.

FIG. 3-1

Possible offspring of mating between normal parent, aa, and parent with an autosomal-dominant trait, Aa.

5. Traits can be traced vertically through previous generations—a positive family history.

Examples of an autosomal-dominant disorder include achondroplasia, osteogenesis imperfecta, and Marfan syndrome.

Autosomal-recessive inheritance. Characteristics of a condition caused by a recessive gene on an autosome include the following (Fig. 3-2):

1. Males and females are affected with equal frequency.
2. Affected individuals will have unaffected parents who are heterozygous for the trait.
3. One fourth of the children of two unaffected heterozygous parents will be affected.
4. Two affected parents will have affected children only.
5. Affected individuals married to unaffected individuals will have normal children, all of whom will be carriers.
6. There is usually no evidence of the trait in previous generations—a negative family history.

Children who display an autosomal-recessive disorder will always be homozygous for that trait. Examples of an autosomal-recessive disorder include cystic fibrosis, phenylketonuria, and galactosemia.

X-linked inheritance patterns

Genes on the X chromosome differ from those on the Y chromosome; therefore, the transmission of traits caused by these genes will vary according to the sex of the individual who carries the gene. Because the male possesses only one X chromosome, a characteristic determined by a gene on the X chromosome is *always* expressed in the male.

X-linked dominant inheritance. Characteristics of a condition caused by a dominant gene on an X chromosome include the following (Fig. 3-3):

1. Affected individuals will have an affected parent.
2. All the daughters but none of the sons of an affected male will be affected.
3. Half the sons and half the daughters of an affected female will be affected.
4. Normal children of an affected parent will have normal offspring.
5. The inheritance pattern shows a positive family history.

Superficially this pattern resembles an autosomal-dominant inheritance pattern. An example of an X-linked dominant disorder is hypophosphatemic vitamin D–resistant rickets.

X-linked recessive inheritance. Characteristics of a disorder caused by a recessive gene on the X chromosome include the following (Fig. 3-4):

1. Affected individuals are principally males.
2. Affected individuals will have unaffected parents (except in the rare possibility that the father is affected and the mother is a carrier).
3. Half of the female siblings of an affected male will be carriers of the trait.
4. Unaffected male siblings of an affected male cannot transmit the disorder.
5. Sons of an affected male are unaffected.
6. Daughters of an affected male are carriers.
7. The unaffected male children of a carrier female do not transmit the disorder.

	Heterozygous parent A/a	
Gametes	A	a
A	AA Normal	Aa Carrier
a	Aa Carrier	aa Affected

(Left column label: Heterozygous parent A/a)

FIG. 3-2
Possible offspring of mating between two parents with a recessive gene, a, on an autosome.

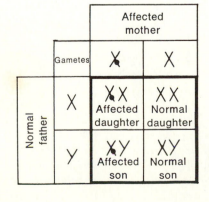

	Normal mother	
Gametes	X	X
X	XX Affected daughter	XX Affected daughter
Y	XY Normal son	XY Normal son

(Left column label: Affected father)

	Affected mother	
Gametes	X	X
X	XX Affected daughter	XX Normal daughter
Y	XY Affected son	XY Normal son

(Left column label: Normal father)

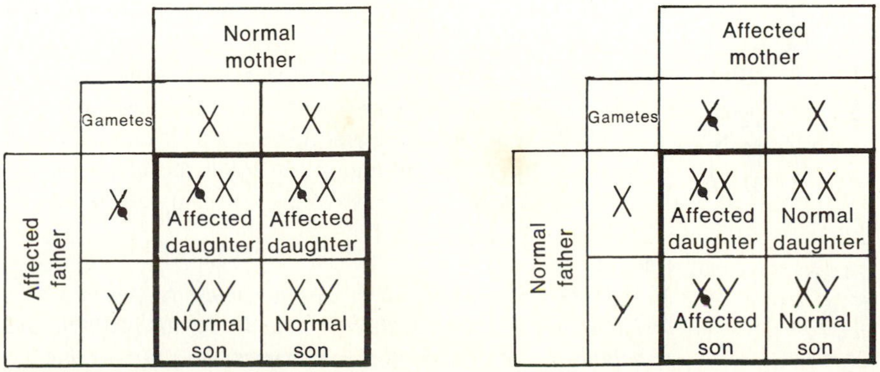

FIG. 3-3
Sex differences in offspring ratios in X-linked dominant inheritance. · = Dominant allele on X chromosome.

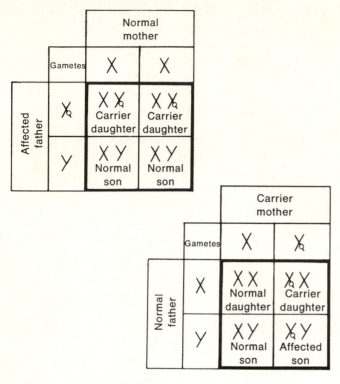

FIG. 3-4

Punnett square illustrating the sex differences in offspring ratios in X-linked recessive inheritance. ○ = Recessive allele on X chromosome.

The abnormal gene behaves as any recessive gene, that is, its effect will be hidden by a normal dominant gene. Examples of an X-linked recessive disorder include hemophilia and Duchenne type muscular dystrophy.

Codominance

In codominance both genes at the same point on a pair of chromosomes produce an effect—neither is recessive to the other. This is characteristic of the major blood groups, such as the ABO blood groups in which both the A and the B antigens are dominant traits. The O trait contains no antigens and therefore behaves as a recessive gene.

DISORDERS CAUSED BY CHROMOSOMAL ABERRATIONS

An aberration is defined as a deviation from that which is normal or typical. Chromosome aberrations are deviations in either structure or number of chromosomes, and the consequences in either situation can be readily observed in the affected individual.

A structural aberration involves loss, addition, rearrangement, or exchange of some of the genes of a chromosome. If there is sufficient remaining genetic material to render the organism capable of life, there can be an endless variety of clinical manifestations.

Deviations in chromosomal number involve the gain or loss of a chromosome and are designated with the suffix *-somy*. A cell that contains one less than the total number of chromosomes is called a *monosomy* because of the loss of one member of a chromosome pair; a cell containing one more than the total number of chromosomes that results from the addition of an extra member to a normal pair is called a *trisomy*. Trisomies are the chromosomal aberrations encountered most frequently by health workers.

Maldistribution of chromosomes

The mechanism that is considered to be responsible for maldistribution of chromosomes in the majority of cases occurs during meiosis. *Disjunction* refers to the normal separation of chromosomes during cell division; failure of this process is termed *nondisjunction*. The consequence of nondisjunction is an unequal distribution of chromosomes between the two resulting cells. When the cell with the extra chromosome is fertilized by a normal cell, the result

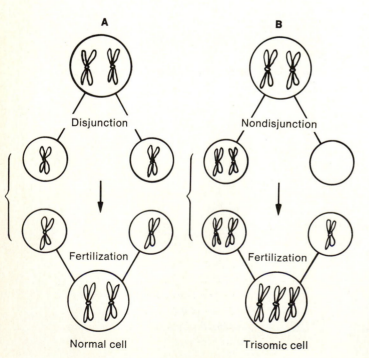

FIG. 3-5

*Mechanisms of distribution of chromosomes. **A,** Normal disjunction and balanced distribution. **B,** Nondisjunction and unbalanced distribution of chromosomes, resulting in one trisomic cell and one nonviable cell.*

is a trisomic cell (Fig. 3-5). The cell with the missing chromosome is nonviable. Nondisjunction can take place during ova formation or sperm formation and can involve autosomes or sex chromosomes.

Nondisjunction can occur in both maternal and paternal germ cell formation. The incidence of trisomic births strongly corresponds with increasing parental age, regardless of the number of pregnancies. The incidence is more frequently related to the age of the mother, however. There appears to be some factor that selects against fertilization by an abnormal sperm.

Chromosomes can be visualized under a microscope, photographed, and arranged in a *karyotype* according to size and shape. In this way the extra chromosome can be observed and classified to confirm a tentative diagnosis. A model of a normal karyotype is illustrated in Fig. 3-6; a trisomy of chromosome 21 is shown in Fig. 3-7.

Nondisjunction can also occur in somatic cells during the very early cell divisions following fertilization. This may or may not involve all the resulting cells. When the consequence is a mixture of both trisomic and normal cells, the result is termed *mosaicism*. The extent of clinical manifestations in the mosaic individual is determined by the type of tissues that contain cells with abnormal chromosomal numbers and may vary from near normal to a fully manifested syndrome.

Translocation. Translocation is a defect in chromosomal structure that occurs when one chromosome becomes attached to another to create one large chromosome. The translocations encountered most frequently are those between wishbone-shaped chromosomes, the best known being the fusion of a group D and a group G chromosome or two group G chromosomes. Because the cells of a person with a translocated chromosome have the normal amount of genetic material, there are no physical abnormalities associated with its possession, even though the total chromosome count is only 45. The attached chromosomes give the appearance of one large chromosome and,

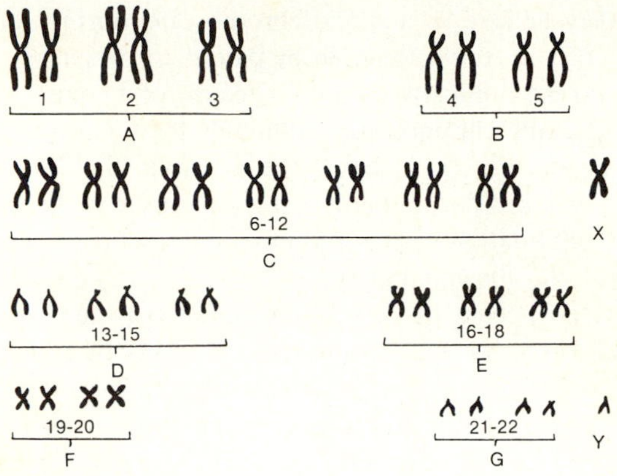

FIG. 3-6
Chromosomes arranged in a karyotype.

FIG. 3-7
Model of a female karyotype with trisomy of the 21 (G) chromosome group.

		Carrier parent D G (D G)							
		Balanced segregation			Unbalanced segregation				
	Gametes	D G	(D G)	or	G (D G)	D	or	G	D (D G)
Normal parent	D G	D G D G Normal	D G (D G) Carrier		D GG (D G) Down's	D D G Nonviable		D G G Nonviable	DD G (D G) Unknown

(D G) = translocated chromosomes D and G

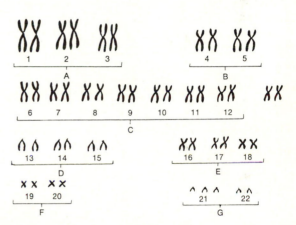

FIG. 3-8
Possible offspring from mating of a somatically normal carrier of a D/G translocation with a genetically and somatically normal individual.

since they behave as a single chromosome during cell division, can be transmitted from parent to offspring. Persons who are clinically affected because of a translocation have an extra chromosome, although their chromosomal count is 46. Fig. 3-8 shows the possible distribution of genetic material during germ cell formation and the results of the combination of these various cells with gametes of a normal chromosomal count.

There appears to be no correlation between parental age and a translocated chromosome. Parents of a child affected as a result of a translocated chromosome are generally in the younger age-group and have a history of spontaneous abortion of previous pregnancies or a family history of abortions. Often one parent is found to be a carrier with normal characteristics and a chromosomal count of 45 chromosomes.

Autosomal aberrations

Both numeric and structural abnormalities of autosomes account for a variety of disorders of infancy and childhood. A few are associated with a group of characteristics that clearly indicate the precise chromosomal anomaly. The first disorder in which an associated chromosomal abnormality was demonstrated is Down syndrome, in which there is an extra G group chromosome, usually number 21 (see Fig. 3-7). (See Chapter 17 for a further discussion of Down syndrome). The other known viable autosomal trisomies involve chromosomes 18 and 13. No known trisomies have been identified for the larger chromosomes, although abnormal chromosome counts have been detected in a large number of early aborted embryos. Table 3-1 describes the three autosomal trisomies encountered most frequently and cri du chat syndrome, which is caused by absence of a small segment of genetic material from a chromosome.

Abnormalities of sex chromosomes

Compared with most hereditary disorders, sex chromosomal aberrations are encountered with relatively high frequency. The possible mechanisms by which they may oc-

TABLE 3-1. COMMON AUTOSOMAL ABERRATIONS

SYNDROME	CHROMOSOMAL ABNORMALITY AND NOMENCLATURE	AVERAGE INCIDENCE	MAJOR CLINICAL MANIFESTATIONS
Cri du chat	Deletion of short arm of a B (No. 5) chromosome—46,XY,5p−		Distinctive weak, high-pitched mew-like cry resembling the cry of a cat; small head; hypertelorism; failure to thrive; severe mental retardation—profound with age
Trisomy 13 (Patau)	Trisomy of a group D (No. 13) chromosome—47,XY,13+	1/15,000	Multiple anomalies, including cleft lip and palate (frequently bilateral); ear malformations; microphthalmia; polydactyly; eye defects; mental retardation; early death
Trisomy 18 (Edwards)	Trisomy of a group E (No. 18) chromosome—47,XY,18+	1/5000	Deformed and low-set ears; micrognathia; rocker-bottom feet; overlapping (index over third) fingers; prominent occiput; hypertelorism; failure to thrive and early death; mental retardation
Trisomy 21 (Down)	Trisomy of a group G (No. 21) chromosome—47,XY,21+ (trisomy); 46,XY,D−,G−,(DqGq)+ (translocation); 46,XY/47,XY,21+ (mosaic)	1/500	Brachycephaly with flat occiput; inner epicanthal folds; small ears, nose, and mouth with protruding tongue; muscular hypotonia; broad, short hands with stubby fingers and transverse palmar crease; broad, stubby feet with wide space between big and second toes; mental retardation; variable life expectancy

cur are those previously described. Most are caused by an increase in sex chromosomal number as a result of nondisjunction during meiosis. An increase in the number of sex chromosomes does not produce the profound effects that are associated with the autosomal trisomies, although some degree of mental deficiency accompanies a large percentage of them.

This reduced disability in children with multiple sex chromosomes (when compared to the severe effects in children with additional autosomes) is attributed to an unusual characteristic of sex chromosomes—*X inactivation.* In all body cells only one X chromosome is biologically active; the other (or others) is in some way "switched off" or *inactivated* during the very early divisions of the zygote and remains so throughout life. This inactivated chromosome can be easily observed through a microscope as a condensed dark-staining mass lying on the periphery of the cell nucleus—the *sex chromatin* or *Barr body.* It is established that the maximum number of chromatin bodies is one less than the total number of X chromosomes in that cell nucleus (Fig. 3-9); therefore, female somatic cells are normally chromatin-positive (containing one active and one inactive X chromosome), and male cells are chroma-

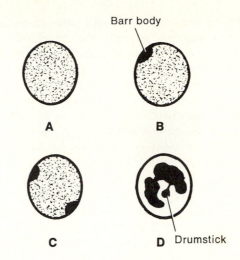

FIG. 3-9

Sex chromatin, or Barr body. **A,** *No sex chromatin is found in normal male somatic cells.* **B,** *One Barr body is normal in female somatic cells.* **C,** *Two Barr bodies are found in cells with three X chromosomes (XXX or XXXY).* **D,** *The drumstick is found in many polymorphonuclear leukocytes of the normal female.*

TABLE 3-2. COMMON SEX CHROMOSOMAL ABNORMALITIES

SYNDROME	CHROMOSOMAL NOMENCLATURE	PHENOTYPE	X CHROMOSOME	Y CHROMOSOME	CLINICAL MANIFESTATIONS
Turner	45,X	Female	0	0	Short stature; webbed neck; low posterior hairline; shield-shaped chest with widely spaced nipples; sterile
Triple X or superfemale	47,XXX (can also be 48,XXXX or 49,XXXXX)	Female	+1 or more	0	Normal female characteristics; usually mentally retarded; mental deficiency in others; fertile
XYY male	47,XYY (can also be 48,XYYY or mosaic)	Male	0	+1 or more	Usually normal sex development; tendency to be tall with long head; poor coordination; may demonstrate aberrant behavior
Klinefelter	47,XXY (48,XXYY, 48,XXXY, 49,XXXXY, etc. mosaics)	Male	+1 or more	+1 or more	Tall with long legs; hypogenitalism; sterile; male secondary sex characteristics may be deficient; may demonstrate aberrant behavior

tin-negative (containing only the one active chromosome). Visible in 20% to 50% of cells, the sex chromatin test provides a convenient means to determine the presence or absence of inactivated X chromosomes in somatic cells. Cells scraped from the buccal (cheek) mucosa are usually used for this test, which is often performed when a sex chromosomal abnormality is suspected in an infant. Sex chromatin can also be detected in polymorphonuclear leukocytes, where it appears as a drumstick-like mass attached to one of the nuclear lobes of the cell.

A number of sex chromosomal abnormalities have been described, and some are listed in Table 3-2. The more common of these, Klinefelter and Turner syndromes, are discussed further in relation to developmental problems of later childhood. Some general characteristics of sex chromosomal abnormalities are:

1. There is a direct relationship between the male or female phenotype and the presence or absence of a Y chromosome. It appears that the Y chromosome is essential for development of male characteristics.
2. The severity of defects is not related to the number of extra X chromosomes, except for mental retardation, which increases proportionately with each X chromosome.
3. The presence of more than one Y chromosome appears to have variable but as yet not well-defined effects on the phenotype.

DISORDERS CAUSED BY GENETIC AND ENVIRONMENTAL FACTORS

There are a number of diseases and defects that are frequently encountered in the population and that show an increased incidence in some families. Although this incidence is higher than would be expected by chance, no specific mode of inheritance can be identified—there is no clear-cut affected-unaffected classification. In some, environmental factors appear to play an important role. These are the conditions classified as *multifactorial*—disorders in which a genetic susceptibility combined with the appropriate environmental agents interact to produce a disease state.

Characteristics of multifactorial disorders are:

1. They are caused by a complex interaction of both hereditary and environmental factors, and the extent of the hereditary component varies from one condition to another.
2. They are multifactorial, that is, they involve a number of different hereditary and environmental influences.
3. The hereditary component is polygenic, that is, it consists of a number of minor genes, each of which makes a small contribution to produce a large effect.
4. The appearance of clinical manifestations requires strong genetic predisposition that places individuals at a point of risk at which environmental influences determine whether (and in some cases to what extent) they will be affected.
5. The closer the family relationship, the greater are the number of genes the members have in common; therefore, there is an increased likelihood that a combination of genes will be expressed more often when united with a similar combination of genes. The more distant the relationship, the fewer the shared genes. Disorders that are considered to be multifactorial include congenital defects (such as cleft lip and/or palate, pyloric stenosis, and meningomyelocele), and common diseases (such as diabetes, peptic ulcer, and schizophrenia).

When the laws of inheritance are applied to polygenic characteristics, it is expected that relatives will have more genes in common. Therefore, there is an increased likelihood that these genes will be expressed more often when united with a similar combination of genes. If the gene(s) is very common, relatives will receive it from different sources; if the gene is a rare one, they will seldom inherit it. Table 3-3 shows the difference in the likelihood of a disorder in a family when compared to the population as a whole.

Common diseases

There is evidence to indicate that heredity plays a role in the cause of numerous common diseases. It appears, for instance, that the genetic make-up of a person can have a decided effect upon the susceptibility and clinical course of some infectious diseases such as tuberculosis, rubeola, and paralytic poliomyelitis. In some diseases a genetic trait can be identified. For example, the development of peptic ulcer occurs more frequently in persons with type O blood;

TABLE 3-3. INHERITED COMPONENT IN SOME COMMON CONDITIONS

CONDITION	INCIDENCE	
	GENERAL POPULATION	FIRST-DEGREE RELATIVES
Cleft lip and palate	1/625	1/20
Clubfoot	1/1000	1/40
Congenital dislocated hip	1/500	1/20
Congenital heart disease	1/500	1/27
Juvenile diabetes mellitus	1/500	1/15
Pyloric stenosis	3/1000	1/15
Schizophrenia	1/100	1/10

however, environmental stresses are also important in the etiology.

The inherited histocompatibility antigens, similar to the blood group antigens, have been implicated in the development of many diseases. These antigens, termed the *human leukocyte antigen (HLA)* system, occur in linked pairs and are inherited in the same manner as the blood group antigens. A number of these antigens have been identified and a relationship between the HLA system has been shown for several disorders, for example, diabetes mellitus, hemochromatosis, and several forms of arthritis.

Congenital abnormalities

Congenital abnormalities, or birth defects, constitute a large group of defects and disorders that are so variable in type and causation that there is no satisfactory method for classifying them. A few are clearly caused by a single gene; others are associated with chromosomal abnormalities. There are some congenital malformations that are produced by known intrauterine environmental factors. However, many of the more common and severe defects (for example, central nervous system malformations, cataracts, and congenital heart disease) fit in no clearly defined category. There is a high correlation between the incidence of congenital abnormalities and the infant who is small for gestational age. The more severe the growth retardation, the more likely the chance for malformation.

Nongenetic factors can produce a congenital defect that imitates, or is indistinguishable from, one that is genetically determined. Such a condition is termed a *phenocopy*. For example, deafness, cretinism, and cataracts can all be caused by mutant genes, but they may also be caused by external agents. Deafness can be a result of a number of different agents, rubella virus can cause congenital cataracts, and lack of iodine in a child can produce cretinism.

Assigning a cause of mental retardation presents a particularly difficult problem. Mental retardation is a manifestation of a variety of syndromes, both single-gene and chromosomal, and numerous environmental agents are known to be damaging to brain tissue, for example, lack of oxygen as a result of anesthesia or drugs during labor and delivery. For this reason it is extremely important that such external factors be ruled out before any given congenital defect is labeled hereditary.

Before birth the maternal host determines the well-being of the fetus by the manner in which she protects, favors, or deprives it. An unfavorable maternally imposed environment may produce effects on the fetus that are of a transient nature with few, if any, harmful effects or can be serious enough to cause long-range health problems in the infant or child.

Parental age. There appears to be a relationship between the age of the mother at the time of birth and the outcome of pregnancy. Overall, mothers less than 20 years of age appear to encounter difficulties with greater frequency than do older mothers. Infants born to very young mothers are more apt to fall into the low birth weight category with an attendant increased risk of neonatal morbidity and mortality associated with these infants in general. However, there is not complete agreement regarding an increased incidence of malformations in infants of mothers less than 20 years of age.

Mothers who become pregnant in the later period of their biologic reproductive years (over age 35) seem to be less able to physically withstand the rigors of pregnancy and childbearing. A higher incidence of spontaneous abortion has been documented in this age-group, and the number of infants with chromosomal abnormalities, primarily Down syndrome, increases markedly when either parent is over age 35 years.

Chemicals. The relationship of the fetal and maternal circulations allows for the interchange of chemical substances across the placental membrane. During gestation, deficiencies in the fetal metabolism (such as hypothyroidism) are usually compensated by the maternal system to afford some measure of protection to the fetus. However, the limited metabolic capabilities of the fetal liver and its immature enzyme and transport systems render the unborn child ill equipped to absorb, distribute, detoxify, and excrete the substance. This includes both substances produced by the mother in response to a disease state (such as diabetes) and exogenous substances ingested or inhaled by the mother (such as drugs or gases).

Many drugs have been suspected of producing congenital malformations and some have been definitely implicated; however, none has created the impact of thalidomide, an efficient sleep-producing drug in the mother, that produced severe malformations in the fetus. When the drug was taken during the sensitive period, between the thirty-fourth and fiftieth days of gestation, the incidence of malformation reached 100% even with small doses. The drug was removed from the market as soon as the relationship between administration of the drug and defects in the infants was recognized.

It has been estimated that women take an average of four or five drugs—either prescription or over-the-counter preparations—during their pregnancy. Because they are frequently administered as drugs, hormones (such as insulin) are also classified as such. Hormones originate and circulate normally in all individuals; an exogenous source simply increases the amount already present in the body.

The extent to which chemical agents affect the unborn child depends on the interplay of several factors—the nature of the agent and its accessibility to the fetus, the time of its applications, the level and duration of the dosage, and the genetic makeup of the fetus. To help ensure that fewer women will inadvertently take some chemical that might be harmful to the fetus, labels on medications are now required to include information regarding the possible effects of the drug.

Infectious factors. The range of pathology produced by infectious agents is large, and the difference between the maternal and fetal effects of any one agent is also great. Severe maternal infections, especially during early pregnancy, can result in fetal loss or malformations caused by the debilitating effect on the health of the mother that may interfere with her ability to maintain the pregnancy, the infectious agent crossing the placental membrane to affect fetal development directly, or ascending inflammation crossing the fetal membranes by way of the cervix.

Because they are the smallest of the infectious organisms and cross the placenta more easily, viruses are important in the etiology of congenital defects. However, a great deal depends on the prevalence of these agents in the population. Some, such as respiratory and gastrointestinal viruses, tend to be present in almost all communities; others, such as smallpox and poliomyelitis, have been eliminated or reduced in most areas of the world. Data have implicated a number of viruses in health problems of infants. The most notable of these is rubella or German measles, a mild disease in adults but one that has been definitely shown to produce a high percentage of congenital malformation in the fetus when the mother is infected during the first 10 weeks of pregnancy. More frequent anomalies associated with rubella are congenital cataracts, deafness, mental retardation, and congenital heart disease. Other diseases that are known to cause defects or disease in the newborn are coxsackievirus, cytomegalic inclusion disease, toxoplasmosis, and syphilis.

Radiation. Ionizing radiation has been shown to be both mutagenic (capable of producing mutations) and teratogenic (capable of producing malformations) in humans. Pelvic irradiation of pregnant women—from natural background radiation that is present everywhere in varying degrees, from occupational exposure, and from diagnostic or therapeutic procedures—is believed to be hazardous to the embryo, although the extent of teratogenicity and the exact dosage required to induce tissue change are still under consideration. Radiation may damage the conceptus at any time during its prenatal existence, and it is known that rapidly dividing and differentiating cells, such as those of the embryo, have increased radiosensitivity. No amount of radiation can be considered absolutely safe; therefore, it is recommended that exposure to diagnostic or therapeutic radiation be carried out on women in the childbearing years only during the first half of their menstrual cycle

before fertilization and implantation are likely to have occurred.

Mechanical factors. The intrauterine environment minimizes the possibility of trauma to the fetus; however, during the later months of gestation the fetus may be subjected to a variety of positional abnormalities. As pregnancy advances, maintaining an attitude of complete flexion in the cramped quarters of the uterus predisposes the fetus to a number of deformities, for example, metatarsus varus, torticollis, and dislocation of the hip.

Defects sometimes occur as a result of amniotic bands or adhesions between the amnion and the fetus, such as the constriction of fetal limbs by bands of amniotic tissue that inhibit the growth of distal segments. Decrease in the production of amniotic fluid may create deformities of varying degrees as a result of the restriction of intrauterine space, for example, malformations of the jaw and ribs, asymmetry of the head, and compression marks on the body.

Temperature. There is increasing evidence to indicate that fetuses may be adversely affected by the high temperatures to which they are subjected when expectant mothers indulge in the hot environment of a hot tub or sauna. With the increasing popularity of these innovations, nurses should advise pregnant women to seek the advice of their physicians before extensive use of such items.

Nutritional factors. In recent years a great deal of attention has been centered on inadequate maternal nutrition and its long-term effects on organ growth and maturation. Current information indicates that the restriction of calories and protein during prenatal development profoundly affects the size, viability, postnatal growth, and behavior of children. The timing and duration of nutritional deprivation appear to be crucial. Of greatest concern are the consequences of dietary restriction at the time the brain is undergoing the most rapid growth and development. Insufficient nutrients to the fetus during the time of rapid brain cell division result in permanent deficiency in brain cell numbers. It appears that the critical period for increasing cell numbers in the brain takes place during the prenatal period and the first few months of life, with the greatest growth and development taking place during the third trimester of pregnancy. The long-term consequences of nutritional deficiency may be manifest as cognitive, behavioral, and language retardation.

Maternal health. Since the physiologic well-being of the fetus depends on the maternal environment in which it grows, any disorder that affects the maternal system will have some effect on the fetal system. Many of the specific disorders and related problems are discussed in Chapter 7 and elsewhere in the text.

Other factors. Other factors capable of adversely affecting the fetus include:

1. Physical factors such as high altitude, smoking, and excessive alcohol ingestion
2. Maternal disease such as toxemia of pregnancy, metabolic disorders such as diabetes and thyroid disease, and vascular diseases such as heart disease, lupus erythematosus, hypertension, and the hemoglobinopathies
3. Isoimmunization from maternal-fetal blood incompatibility
4. Prenatal diagnostic and therapeutic procedures

GENETIC COUNSELING

In recent years the significance of heredity as an etiologic agent in disease and disability has assumed a more prominent place in the nursing of infants and children. The clients, or persons who seek advice, may or may not be affected themselves but may request genetic counseling about the heritability of a trait that may be harmful, beneficial, or merely troublesome. Clients may be a young couple contemplating marriage or childbearing who are concerned about a disorder in one of their families, no matter how remote the relationship. They may seek advice because they are related. A couple who are both members of a population at risk for certain diseases may wish to determine whether they carry the harmful gene (for example, blacks and sickle cell anemia, Ashkenazic Jews and Tay-Sachs disease, or Italians and thalassemia). A couple planning adoption may seek counseling regarding a prospective child.

More often persons who inquire about the possibility of recurrence of a disease or disorder are parents of a child with a specific disease or defect that significantly impairs fitness who are concerned that they might produce another similarly affected child. This advice may be sought before the couple initiate another pregnancy, after the mother is already pregnant, or after the birth of another child. There may be concern regarding the risk to unaffected siblings of the affected child or to the affected child's future children.

Some families may need counseling in regard to the advisability of sterilization, artificial insemination, prenatal diagnosis, or termination of a pregnancy. Infertility or recurrent abortion in a family may indicate a need for counseling. Occasionally a counselor becomes involved in cases of disputed paternity, rape, and incestuous matings. Delayed or abnormal sexual development may be a reason to seek genetic advice.

The nurse and genetic counseling

Genetic counseling is a communication process that deals with the human problems associated with the occurrence, or risk of occurrence, of a genetic disorder in a family. Nurses in the field of infant and child care continually encounter genetic diseases and families in which there is a risk that a disorder may be transmitted to an offspring. It is a responsibility of nurses to be alert to situations in which persons could benefit from genetic counseling, to become familiar with facilities in their areas where genetic counseling is available, and to learn the basic principles of heredity. In this way they will be able to direct individuals and families to take advantage of needed services and to be active participants in the counseling process.

Counseling services. The most efficient counseling service consists of a group of specialists that may include physicians, geneticists, psychologists, biochemists, cytologists, nurses, social workers, and other auxiliary personnel. The services are most often under the leadership of a physician trained in medical genetics who assumes responsibility for the medical aspects of the group. The counseling service may serve only as a referral group, or it may conduct a regular clinic service. Most often it is associated with a large medical center. There are numerous specialty clinics that deal with specific genetic disorders (such as cystic fibrosis, muscular dystrophy, hemophilia, or diabetes) and provide their own genetic counseling services. Unfortunately these units are concentrated in and around large metropolitan areas. As a result, counseling is not always accessible to the large number of persons who would benefit from the service.

The nurse is frequently the family's initial contact with a counseling service. An intake interview is conducted before the primary counseling session or diagnostic workup to assess the needs of the family and attempt to reduce their anxiety; therefore, ample time should be allotted. In the process of the interview the nurse takes a family history for pertinent information and explains the clinic procedures carefully. Many families are concerned about such things as whether they will be required to undress, if blood is to be drawn, or if they can accompany the child during the visit. Families who have a relaxed and nonstressful initial discussion are able to gain more from a counseling session.

Follow-up care. The success of counseling is measured by the way in which the family utilizes the information presented to them. Maintaining contact with the family or referral to an agency that can provide a sustained relationship, usually the public health agency in their locality, is one of the most important aspects of the counseling process. Some families do not choose to have follow-up visits, but in most instances these visits make the family feel that they have not been abandoned and facilitate the process of adjustment to the problem.

Follow-up visits to the counseling service or in the home provide the family with the opportunity to ask questions that they did not ask on previous visits. Often the family have not really "heard" the information presented to them or have misinterpreted what they have heard so that it may be necessary to repeat and reinforce counseling. In some disorders a diagnosis of one family member places relatives at risk and is an indication for further screening. In a disorder such as phenylketonuria that requires conscientious diet management, it is important to make certain that the family understands and follows the advice. Children born later on must be carefully observed to assure early detection of symptoms in the event that they have also inherited the disorder.

Nurses should be prepared to help families arrive at tentative decisions regarding the future, including family planning, education or institutionalization of a handicapped child, plans for adoption, and many other problems related to their specific problems. Location of agencies and clinics specializing in the specific disorder that can provide services (such as equipment, medication, and rehabilitation), educational programs, and parent groups are all part of nurses' resources.

Psychologic aspects of genetic disease

It requires time and understanding to deal with the emotional tension and anxiety generated in families who are faced with the prospect of a genetic disorder. Knowledge of and the ability to deal with the range of psychologic responses and all their ramifications (such as the grief reaction, guilt, anger, and coping mechanisms) are essential components of the nursing role in genetic counseling.

It is important to stress that there is nothing shameful about an inherited or congenital defect and to emphasize any appropriate remedy. Families have a tendency to be more ashamed of a hereditary disorder than of one caused by self-indulgence, such as obesity or alcoholism. The threat of a hereditary "taint" often creates intrafamily strife, hostility, and marital disharmony, sometimes to the point of family disintegration. Relatives frequently cease reproduction after the diagnosis of a hereditary defect in a member, or the decision to marry may be postponed indefinitely on the basis of a disorder in a relative, even a remote one, in a prospective partner's family. While people may understand the situation on an intellectual level, this will not help them on an emotional level. A large and vital part of the nurse's role in genetic counseling is that of a sympathetic and supportive listener.

GENETICS AND SOCIETY

There is no doubt that genetic diseases constitute a significant portion of world health problems, and the advantages to improvement of the human race are seldom questioned. The controversy exists between those who advocate im-

provement in the species by selective breeding and those who recommend providing a better environment. Improvement of the human race through altering the genetic make-up of the individual is termed *eugenics;* improvement of the human race by modifying the environment is called *euthenics*.

Eugenics

Eugenics is essentially planned breeding designed to alter future generations. Such practice has been successfully used for many years by animal and plant breeders to develop superior food products. Eugenics can be further segregated into *positive eugenics* and *negative eugenics*.

Positive eugenics. Positive eugenics is the attempt to encourage reproduction among those individuals who are considered to possess superior or beneficial characteristics. Suggested means for accomplishing this purpose include selected mating of individuals with what are considered to be superior traits. Other methods are the establishment of sperm banks with sperm from a small, selected number of donors to be frozen and used to impregnate a large number of suitable women and the production of replicas of desirable persons by cloning (replacing the cell nucleus of a fertilized ovum with the nucleus of a cell from the desired individual; asexual reproduction). Some of the qualifications considered superior might be physical characteristics, socially desirable behavior, and superior intellect, as well as absence of genetically determined defects or disease.

Negative eugenics. Negative eugenics is the discouragement or prohibition of reproduction among individuals who are considered to be physically or mentally handicapped. Voluntary or legal prohibition of reproduction by persons with these characteristics might be accomplished with marriage laws, sterilization, and abortion.

Euthenics

An opposite point of view is taken by those who support euthenics, which advocates the modification of the environment to allow the genetically abnormal individual to live a relatively normal life. Examples of euthenic measures are prescription glasses for nearsighted persons and special schools for the deaf. Medical treatments such as special diets for children with inborn errors of metabolism, hormone replacement such as insulin for diabetic persons and thyroid for persons with cretinism, and special orthopedic appliances and prosthetic devices can be considered environmental manipulation. Providing better nutrition and home environment for children during the growing stages and educational and social stimulation are prime examples of euthenics.

BIBLIOGRAPHY

Afriat, C.I., and Schifrin, B.S.: Antepartum fetal evaluation. In McNall, L.K., and Galeener, J.T., editors: Current practice in obstetric and gynecologic nursing, vol. 2, St. Louis, 1978, The C.V. Mosby Co.

Brown, S.G.: The devastating effects of congenital rubella, Am. J. Maternal Child Nurs. **4:**171-173, 1979.

Claypool, J.M.: Rubella protection for maternal child health care providers, Am. J. Maternal Child Nurs. **6:**53-56, 1981.

Cohen, F.L.: Genetic knowledge possessed by American nurses and nursing students, J. Adv. Nurs. **4:**494-496, 1979.

Cowie, V.: Genetic causes of retardation, Nurs. Mirror **155:**29-34, Sept. 15, 1982.

Fitzsimmons, E.: Genetic counseling: learning to keep counsel, Nurs. Mirror. **153**(11):48-50, 1981.

Gullekson, D.J.K., and Temple, A.R.: Maternal drug use during the prenatal period, Fam. Comm. Health J. **1**(3):31-41, 1978.

Hopper, W.C., Jr.: A review of genetics in orthopaedics, Orthop. Nurs. **21:**37-38, 1983.

Iveson-Iveson, J.: Genetics. Part I, Nurs. Mirror, **154**(4):47, 1982.

Luke, B.: Maternal alcoholism and fetal alcohol syndrome, Am. J. Nurs. **77:**1924-1926, 1977.

McCance, K.L.: Genetics: implications for preventative nursing practice . . . identifying and evaluating susceptible families for cardiac risk, J. Adv. Nurs. **8:**359-364, 1983.

McKay, S.R.: Smoking during the childbearing years, Am. J. Maternal Child Nurs. **5:**46-50, 1980.

McNall, L.K., and Collea, J.V.: Environmental influences on embryonic and fetal development. In McNall, L.K., and Galeener, J.T., editors: Current practice in obstetric and gynecologic nursing, vol. 2, St. Louis, 1978, The C.V. Mosby Co.

Riccardi, V.M.: Health care and disease prevention through genetic counseling: a regional approach, Am. J. Public Health **66:**268-272, 1976.

Rozovky, L.E., and others: Genetic screening: public health and the law, Can. J. Public Health **72:**15-16, 1981.

Sahin, S.T.: The multifaceted role of the nurse as genetic counselor, Am. J. Maternal Child Nurs. **1**(4):211-216, 1976.

Sheffield, L.: Genetic counselling, Austr. Nurs. J. **11:**1-4, Mar. 1982.

Stagno, S.: Toxoplasmosis, Am. J. Nurs. **80:**720-722, 1980.

Summer, G.K., and Shoaf, C.R.: Developments in genetic and metabolic screening, Fam. Comm. Health, **4**(4):13-30, 1982.

Tishler, C.L.: The psychological aspects of genetic counseling, Am J. Nurs. **81:**733-734, 1981.

Weeks, H.F.: Perinatal pharmacology, Am. J. Maternal Child Nurs. **5:**143, 1980.

Whaley, L.F.: Genetic counseling in maternity nursing. In McNall, L.K., and Galeener, J.T., editors: Current practice in obstetric and gynecologic nursing, vol. 1. St. Louis, 1976, The C.V. Mosby Co.

Whaley, L.F.: Genetic counseling. In Curry, J.B., and Peppe, K.K., editors: Mental retardation: nursing approaches to care, St. Louis, 1978, The C.V. Mosby Co.

Wicklund, S.: Special report: drugs for two in pregnancy, Am. J. Nurs. **82:**980-981, 1982.

Williams, J.K.: Pediatric nurse practitioners' knowledge of genetic disease, Pediatr. Nurs. **9**(2):119-121, 1983.

Worthington, B.S.: Nutritional considerations during pregnancy and lactation, Fam. Comm. Health J. **1**(3):13-29, 1978.

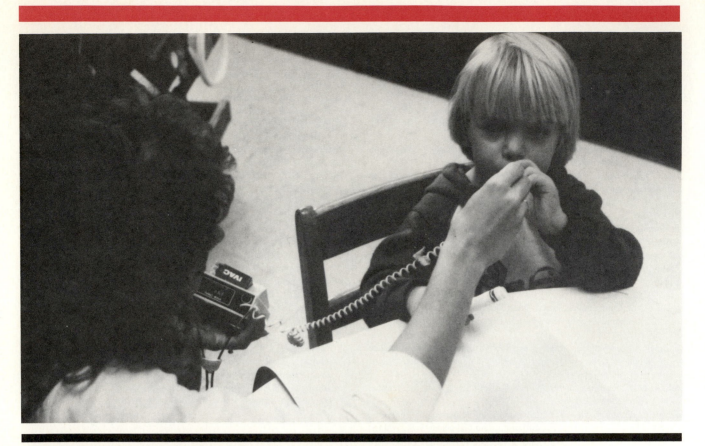

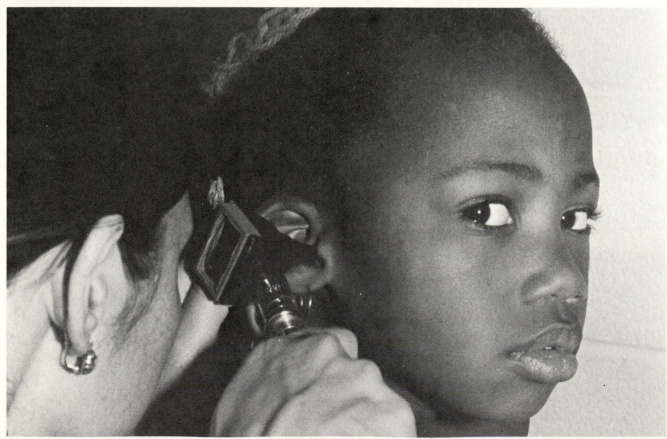

UNIT 2

ASSESSMENT OF THE CHILD AND FAMILY

Fundamental to the nursing process is assessment. Establishing a data base on which to formulate a nursing diagnosis, plan interventions, and evaluate outcomes of care is essential whether the nurse is involved with a healthy or ill child. Assessment facilitates identification of present problems and prevention of future ones. Although the assessment process focuses primarily on the child, it permits an exploration into the family dynamics and is often the first clue to cultural, environmental, socioeconomic, or religious traditions that influence the child's total well-being.

Assessment primarily involves some form of communication. Chapter 4, *Communication and the Health Interview,* is concerned with general aspects of communication as they relate to the nurse, parent, and child. It also discusses the interview process specifically in terms of history taking.

Chapter 5, *Physical Assessment of the Child,* deals with the procedures and skills required to perform a complete pediatric physical assessment, including sensory and developmental testing. Findings primarily related to normal structure and function are emphasized, with notation of those deviations that require further evaluation.

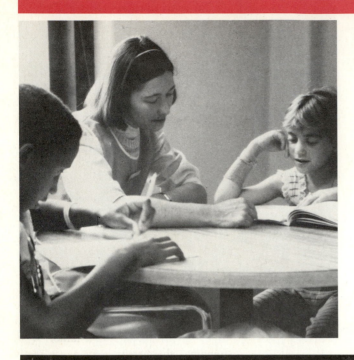

COMMUNICATION
AND THE HEALTH INTERVIEW

OBJECTIVES

On completion of this chapter the reader will be able to:

■ Describe guidelines for communication and interviewing

■ Identify communication strategies for interviewing parents

■ Formulate guidelines for using an interpreter

■ Identify communication strategies for communicating with children of different age-groups

■ Describe four communication techniques that are useful with children

■ State the components of a complete health history

NURSING DIAGNOSES

Nursing diagnoses identified for child and family communication include, but are not restricted to, the following:

Self-perception—self-concept pattern

■ Anxiety related to (1) strange environment; (2) previous experiences; (3) perception of impending events; (4) knowledge deficit

Role-relationship pattern

■ Communication, impaired verbal, related to (1) language barrier; (2) anxiety; (3) cultural factors

Essential to the nursing of children is communication. It is the most important skill used in assessment of children and their families and the most important feature in forming trusting relationships with them. Communication consists of all those behaviors by which one person, consciously or unconsciously, affects another. All behavior transmits a message: even the attempt not to communicate creates a particular impression. Inherent in communication are the power of observation, the use of all the senses, and the intangible influence of intuition.

This chapter is concerned with the communication process. In the first section guidelines for communication and interviewing are reviewed and specific suggestions for communicating with parents and children are presented. The second section deals with a particular type of interview, the health history. It is presented in some detail to give nurses the opportunity to learn to take a history, as well as to facilitate understanding those histories recorded by other members of the health team.

COMMUNICATION

The forms of communication may be verbal, nonverbal, or abstract. *Verbal* communication may involve language and its expression, vocalizations in the forms of laughs, moans, or squalls, or the implications of what is not said in light of what has been said. *Nonverbal* communication is often called body language and includes gestures, movements, facial expressions, postures, and reactions. *Abstract* communication takes the form of play, artistic expression, symbols, photographs, and choice of clothing. Because it is possible to exert greater conscious control over verbal communication, it becomes the least reliable indicator of true feelings. It is through the process of observation that one actively, consciously, and deliberately perceives messages communicated through nonverbal behavior.

There are many factors that influence the communication process. To be successful (gratifying), communication must be appropriate to the situation, properly timed, and clearly delivered. This implies that nurses understand and use techniques of effective communication, including listening. Verbal and nonverbal messages must be congruent, that is, two or more messages sent via different levels must not be contradictory.

Nurses need to recognize their own feelings and attempt to recognize those of the persons with whom the communicative interchange takes place. Biases and judgments interfere with all aspects of the process. The tendency to approve or disapprove another's statements inhibits positive reactions. In addition, the transmission and

reception of messages may be altered by influences of intimacy or distance, dependence and independence, trust and mistrust, security and insecurity, or caring and not caring on the part of the participants. The value of effective communication is increased understanding between the nurse, the child, and the family. Since nursing of infants and children always involves the inclusion of a caregiver, nurses must be able to communicate not only with children of all ages but with the adults in their lives as well.

VERBAL COMMUNICATION—THE POWER OF WORDS

Words are reality, and thus they hold tremendous power. One person can change another's perception of reality by the choice of words that are used. For example, if the diagnosis of cancer is always referred to as a tumor, cyst, malignancy, or carcinoma, the person may never really know that he has cancer. Consequently he may assume less responsibility for his care than if he were aware of his condition's seriousness. By learning to recognize how patients and health professionals use language to manipulate reality, one can also learn how to change one's perceptions and communicate more effectively.

Avoidance language. The most common way people try to alter reality is by avoiding words that truly describe it. For example, euphemisms such as ''passed on'' are used instead of the word ''death.'' Avoidance language indicates that a person wants to hide something, particularly his feelings. As a rule, accepting the person's use of euphemisms only serves to perpetuate his fears and never helps him to deal with them. In contrast, use of straightforward, precise, descriptive language lends perspective to the situation and allows the person to discuss his fears. Most often, imagined fears are much worse than the actual reality.

Distancing language. People may use impersonal words, such as ''it'' or ''others,'' to shield themselves from the painful reality of a situation. For example, parents may state that they know *someone* with a child who is slow, when they may actually be talking about personal fears regarding *their* child. By realizing that the parents may need to talk about this difficult subject, the nurse can provide sensitive statements that ease them into discussing their situation.

One of the dangers in supporting distancing language is that the person may effectively deny that a problem exists. To return to the previous example, if the issue of retardation is never approached directly but is allowed to be ''someone else's problem,'' the parents may not be able to make decisions for special schools or individualized training.

Sometimes distancing is desirable because the topic may be too painful to discuss directly. The use of the third-person technique (p. 72) may be very therapeutic in allowing an individual the opportunity to indirectly approach a subject and receive feedback but still remain in control.

NONVERBAL COMMUNICATION— PARALANGUAGE

In addition to the spoken word, messages are also relayed through nonverbal means, or paralanguage—the pitch, pause, intonation, rate, volume, and stress in speech. Young children become very adept at understanding paralanguage; long before they know the meaning of words, they sense anxiety or fear by the rise in pitch or the accelerated rate of the parent's voice. By careful observation of the spoken word, nurses can better understand the meaning of another's verbal message and more accurately control their own paralanguage.

Because most people do not exert conscious control over their paralanguage, it is a valuable clue to feelings and concerns. For example, pausing may signify a need to formulate thoughts, recall information, or fabricate a story. Frequent pauses often make the speaker sound unsure of himself. Long pauses may mean that the individual needs more information.

Rate is another characteristic that gives unspoken messages. Talking too fast usually makes the speaker sound glib and insensitive. Talking slowly with a firm tone and appropriate pauses conveys authority. Therefore, a person is much more likely to "hear" instructions if the latter approach is used. Children in particular respond attentively to a slow, even, steady voice.

GUIDELINES FOR COMMUNICATION AND INTERVIEWING

Since nurses' effectiveness in practice depends to a large extent on their ability to relate to others, they use the communication process to help children and their parents make use of the nurses' professional knowledge and skill. The most widely used method of communicating with parents on a professional basis is the interview process. Interviewing, unlike social conversation, is a specific form of goal-directed communication. As nurses converse with parents, they endeavor to focus on the parents to determine the kind of persons they are, their usual mode of handling problems, whether help is needed, and the way in which parents react to counseling. It requires time and patience to

develop interviewing skills. Some of the guiding principles and the obstacles that need to be avoided to facilitate this process are discussed here.

Establishing the setting

Part of the success in interviewing depends on the type of physical and psychologic setting the interviewer constructs. Appropriate introduction, role clarification, explanation of the reason for the interview, preliminary acquaintance with the family, and assurance of privacy and confidentiality are prerequisites for establishing a setting conducive to communication.

Appropriate introduction. Nurses introduce themselves to, and ask the name of, each family member who is present. During the interview, each person is addressed by name. If there is any question about using the person's first or last name, common courtesy should be the guiding rule. Asking individuals which name they wish to be called conveys respect and communicates a personal interest in them.

At the beginning of the visit, the nurse includes the child in the interaction by asking him his name, age, and other information. Nurses often direct all questions to the adult, even when the child is old enough to speak for himself. This serves to terminate one extremely valuable source of information, the patient himself. When including the child, the general rules for communicating with children are followed (p. 69).

Role clarification and explanation of the interview. During the introduction it is also necessary to clarify the nurse's particular role in the health setting. For example, nurses performing interviews may be pediatric nurse practitioners, inpatient staff nurses, clinic nurses, office nurses, visiting nurses, or school nurses. Since the format resembles a medical history, the nurse needs to clarify the reason for eliciting this information. A parent is much more likely to reveal personal information about the child and family if the relevance and importance of the interview are stressed. If this is not done, parents may refuse to elaborate on certain areas because they feel it has no bearing on the "problem." In addition, since more than one member of the health team may take a history during the course of a hospital admission, it is important to clarify the reason for each interview.

Another reason for role clarification is education of the health consumer. With expanded roles in nursing, it is not unusual for families to think that the examiner is a physician, not a nurse. Role clarification is especially important because some parents may feel deceived if they later are made aware of the nurse's identity. Since the general consumer acceptance of pediatric nurse practitioners has been very favorable, it is also important to acknowledge their expertise by emphasizing their role.

Preliminary acquaintance. In contemplating the personal and private nature of an in-depth interview, one may wonder at the human trust the person being interviewed needs to have to reveal such extensive information. It is best to commence the interview with some general conversation. The opening statements should be general but still informative. Comments such as, "How have things been since your last visit?" "Tell me about Johnny," or (to the child) "What do you think is going to happen today?" allow the parent or child to express his main concern in a casual, relaxed atmosphere.

The preliminary acquaintance conversation also reveals how responsive the informant may be to questions. For example, using open-ended statements, such as, "Tell me about the baby," may lead the parent into a lengthy detailed discussion. In this case it may be more beneficial to direct questions toward specific answers in order to avoid tangential remarks. At other times a parent may respond to open-ended questions with only minimal information, in which case the continued use of open-ended questions probably reveals more data than "yes" or "no" type questions.

Assurance of privacy and confidentiality. The place where the interview is conducted is almost as important as the interview itself. The physical environment should allow for as much privacy as possible. There should be minimal distractions during the interview, such as interruptions, ambient noise, or other visible activity. At times it may be necessary to turn off a television or radio. The environment should also have some play provision for young children to keep them occupied during the parent-nurse interview (Fig. 4-1). Parents who are constantly interrupted by their children are unable to concentrate fully on the questions asked of them. As a result they tend to give short, brief answers in order to terminate the interview as quickly as possible.

Confidentiality is another essential component of the initial phase of the interview. Since the interview is usually shared with other members of the health team or the teacher (as in the case of students), it is the interviewer's responsibility and obligation to inform the parents of the confidential limits of their conversation. Assuring privacy, communicating concern, and temporarily terminating questioning if interrupted signify confidentiality and therefore trust in the relationship.

COMMUNICATING WITH PARENTS

Although the parent and child are separate and distinct entities, relationships with the child are frequently mediated via the parent, particularly in the case of younger children. For the most part, information about the child is acquired by direct observation or is communicated to the nurse by

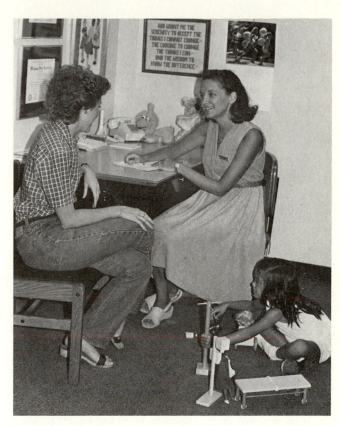

FIG. 4-1

A child is playing while the nurse interviews the parent.

the parents. Usually it can be assumed that because of the close contact with the child, the information imparted by the parent is reliable. To make an assessment of the child requires input from the child (verbal and nonverbal), information from the parent, and the nurse's own observations, including assessment of the child and interpretation of the relationship between the child and the parent. Counseling and guidance must be directed to the caregiver of infants and small children; when children are old enough to be active participants in their own health maintenance, the parent becomes a collaborator in health care. Usually mothers' communication concerning children will be used throughout most of this discussion. However, the communication might involve both parents, the father, or other caregivers.

Encouraging the parent to talk. Interviewing parents not only offers the opportunity to determine the health and developmental status of the child but also offers cues and guides to all those factors that influence the child's life. The mother is usually the most influential factor in the child's growth and adjustment; therefore anything that affects her will necessarily affect the child. Whatever the mother sees as a problem should be a concern of the nurse. These problems are not always easy to identify. Nurses will need to be alert for clues and signals by which a mother communicates worries and anxieties. Careful phrasing of inquiries is rewarded with the specific information needed and the feelings and attitudes of the parent. For example, one broad open-ended question such as "What is Jimmy eating now?" will provide more information than several single-answer questions such as "Is Jimmy eating what the rest of the family eats?" that can be answered with "yes" or "no."

Sometimes the parent will take the lead without prompting. At other times it may be necessary to direct another question based on an observation such as, "Connie seems unhappy today," or "Does it bother you when David cries?" If the mother appears to be tired or distraught, the nurse might ask, "What do you do to relax?" or "Do you get any help with the children?" A comment such as, "You handle the baby very well. Have you had a lot of experience with babies?" to a new mother who appears comfortable with her first child gives her positive reinforcement and provides an opening for any questions she might have regarding the care of her infant. Mothers who are relaxed and spontaneous are more likely to bring out useful information than are tense, defensive parents. Often all that is required to keep parents talking is a nod or saying "yes" or "uh-huh" to let them know the nurse is listening and interested.

When attempting to elicit feelings and covert problem areas, it is best to avoid beginning a question with "Does . . .," "Did . . .," or "It's . . .," which usually require only a single response. In addition, asking questions such as, "Do you have any problem with your son at school?" subtly implies a lack of parental skills and evokes defensiveness. Instead, it is helpful to say "What . . .," "How . . .," "Tell me about . . .," and to encourage elaboration with "You were saying . . .," "You say that . . .," or reflecting back a key word. Open-ended questions are nonthreatening and encourage description.

Directing the focus. The ability to direct the focus of the interview, while allowing for maximum freedom of expression, is one of the most difficult goals in effective communication. One approach is the use of open-ended or broad questions, followed with guiding statements. For example, if the parent proceeds to list the other children by name, the nurse can say, "Tell me their ages, too." If the parent continues on this theme by describing each child in-depth, which is not the purpose of the interview, the focus can be redirected by stating, "Let's talk about the other children later. You were beginning to tell me about Paul's activities at school." This approach conveys interest in the other children but focuses the data collection on the identified patient.

In the event that the parent has suggested that a problem exists with one of the other children, the nurse should reintroduce this subject at the end of the interview to assess the need for further family follow-up. Saying to the parent, "Before, you were mentioning that your older son is having trouble in school. Tell me what you see as the problem," reintroduces this subject but only in terms of the possible problem.

Listening. Listening is the most important ingredient for effective communication. When listening is truly aimed at understanding the client, it is an active process that requires concentration and attention to all aspects of the conversation—verbal, nonverbal, and abstract. Two of the greatest blocks to listening are environmental distraction and premature judgment.

The attitudes and feelings of the nurse are easily introduced into an interview. It is important that nurses understand and recognize their own reactions in order to minimize their potential impact on a parent. It is not uncommon for nurses (and parents) to react to emotions related to past experiences instead of to the circumstances of the present situation and then convey a false impression to the other person. Often nurses' perception of a parent's behavior is influenced by their own perceptions, prejudices, and assumptions, which may include racial, religious, and cultural stereotypes. What may be interpreted as passive hostility or disinterest in a parent may be shyness or an expression of anxiety.

For example, direct eye contact is frequently regarded as a sign of paying attention. However, in many American Indian tribes, looking into another's eyes is considered disrespectful. Therefore, judgments about "listening" need to be made with an appreciation of cultural differences.

Although it is necessary to make some preliminary judgments, the nurse must attempt to "hear" the parent with as much objectivity as possible by clarifying meanings and attempting to see the situation from the parent's point of view. Effective interviewers use conscious control over their reactions and responses and over the techniques they employ.

Use of minimum verbal activity with active listening facilitates parent involvement. Nurses are prone to become quite verbal when health education and advice are indicated. It is tempting to spend time explaining, describing, and interpreting health information when the opportunity presents itself. However, it is possible to provide effective health education by properly timing the information and presenting only as much as is necessary at the moment.

Careful listening facilitates the use of clues, verbal leads, or signals from the interviewee to move the interview along. Frequent references to an area, repetition of certain key words, or a special emphasis on something or someone serve as cues to the interviewer for the direction of inquiry. Concerns and anxieties are usually mentioned in a casual, offhand manner. Even though they are casual, they are of importance and deserve careful scrutiny. This serves to identify problem areas and to pursue the investigation and solution of a problem with systematic questioning. For example, a mother who is concerned about a child's habit of bed-wetting may casually mention that his bed was "wet this morning."

Because the interview is almost always triangular— that is, between the nurse, parent, and child—the parent may wish to convey information in such a way as to prevent the child from hearing it. This requires active listening on the part of the nurse to hear the unspoken message. The following example illustrates this point:

> During a routine health visit the nurse performed a complete history and physical examination on a 4-year-old girl. The child was accompanied by her mother, who appeared to be a reliable, well-informed, and talkative informant. During the child's birth history, the mother gave all the information asked. However, during the family history, the mother stated to the nurse, "I had a hysterectomy 6 years ago." Because the nurse gave no indication of acknowledging the significance of this statement, the mother repeated it, only this time she stressed the "6 years." The nurse, who had not been listening as attentively as she should have, realized that the mother was telling her something very important. The mother raised her eyebrows and gently shook her head "no," warning the nurse not to explore this area too openly. The nurse correctly read the cues and stated, "Let's return to your health history later."
> At the completion of the physical examination, the nurse brought the child to the health center's playroom and took the opportunity to investigate this contradictory information of a "4-year-old child born to a woman with a hysterectomy 6 years ago." The mother revealed that this child was adopted. The mother was greatly concerned about the fact that the child was unaware of this and requested the nurse's advice. Fortunately the nurse had "listened" carefully enough to realize the significance of this woman's concern and allowed her the opportunity to discuss it in private.

Listening is also helpful in assessing reliability. For example, the answers elicited at the beginning of the interview may differ from those at the end, when the parent feels more confident in revealing problems. It is important to identify any discrepancies and reintroduce those topics for further investigation.

Using silence. Silence as a response is often one of the most difficult interviewing techniques to learn. It requires a sense of confidence and comfort on the part of the interviewer to allow the interviewee space in which to think uninterrupted. Silence permits the interviewee to sort out thoughts and feelings or to search for responses to questions. It also allows for sharing of feelings in which two or more people absorb the emotion to its depth.

Sometimes it is necessary to break the silence and reopen communication. This should be done in such a way that the person is encouraged to continue talking about what is important to him. Breaking a silence by introducing a new topic or by prolonged talking essentially terminates the interviewee's opportunity to use the silence. Suggestions for breaking the silence include statements such as, "Is there anything else you wish to say?" "I see you find it difficult to continue; how may I help?" or "I don't know what this silence means. Perhaps there is something you would like to put into words but find difficult to say."

Providing reassurance. Most parents want to be "good" parents and have at least some anxiety about their ability to function in this role. Questionable behavior on the part of children tends to cast doubt on their success as parents. A mother's worries revolve around herself and her adequacy as a mother, as well as concern over the health and development of her children. When her feelings of maternal adequacy are threatened, her anxiety rises. She wants and needs reassurance that she is handling the task of parenthood, thus it is important to avoid communicating in a manner that is threatening to the client's self-esteem. For example, the statement, "Johnny is sleeping in his own room, of course," introduces the interviewer's values to the situation. The mother is most likely to respond affirmatively because she feels that the nurse wants to hear this or else will judge her as not behaving correctly as a parent.

Parents need to have the nurse show an interest in them as an individual as well as in their children. Questions such as, "How do you manage?" or "What do you do when things get difficult?" provide an opportunity for them to express those things that concern them but that are not directly related to the children. Being able to vent feelings to an accepting and impartial listener assists them in recouping their resources for problem solving and coping.

The expectations of parents are significant factors in determining the progress and outcome of an interview. They expect to receive guidance regarding health matters but are usually not prepared for the nurse's concern for their emotional needs. However, one objective of nursing is to help parents be better parents. In the process of assessing their capabilities and needs, nurses can provide them with reassurance that they are doing well when appropriate.

Concerned parents appreciate knowing that they have feelings and problems that are shared by other parents. All parents want to be reassured that their children are developing normally and most have some questions about feeding, sleep, behavior, and discipline. Occasionally parents do have negative feelings toward their children and need to know that such ambivalence is normal. If the nurse has determined that there is no physical or emotional problem underlying the reaction, parents can gain a measure of reassurance in knowing that this is a common feeling. The parent and nurse can work together to find possible avenues for coping with these feelings.

Defining the problem. In order to arrive at a solution to a problem, the nurse and the parent must agree that a problem exists. If neither believes that there is a problem, there is certainly no need to create one. Sometimes the parent may believe that there is a problem that the nurse is unable to see. For example, a mother was overly concerned about every small sniffle, sneeze, or cough in her infant who had been carefully examined and found to be healthy with no evidence of a respiratory problem. On careful questioning, the nurse discovered that a previous child had died of pneumonia in infancy. Consequently the nurse was able to better understand the mother's concern. Once the nurse acknowledges the mother's fear, she can help the mother deal with her special anxieties about her infant and teach her how to recognize when there is need for concern.

Occasionally the nurse identifies a problem that the parent denies exists. In this case the nurse should pursue the situation and either find a way to deal with the situation or enlist the aid of other health team members. For example, the parents of a child with Down syndrome may refuse to believe that their child is different from any other child of the same age. They may say, "He is just a little slow" and "All the child needs to do is to try harder." A child with an obvious behavior problem may be described by the parents as "stubborn" or "just behaving that way to spite us." Such statements may be clues that the parents have not progressed past the stage of denial in adjusting to the handicap.

Solving the problem. Once the problem is identified and agreed on by the parent and the nurse, they can begin to arrive at a solution. A parent who is included in the problem-solving process is more apt to follow through with a course of action. Such questions as "What have you tried so far?" or "What have you thought about doing?" provide leads for exploration and give the parents the feeling that their ideas and solutions are worthwhile. These can be followed by "What prevents you from trying that?" "That sounds like a good plan," and "You seem to be stumped. Have you considered trying this?" Such approaches reinforce rather than belittle parents' efforts to solve their problems and encourage active participation.

Sometimes the parents arrive at a solution that the nurse does not consider the best alternative. If it can be ascertained that it will do no harm and if the parents are convinced of its merits, it is usually best to allow them to continue with the plan. A course of action is more likely to be carried out when parents can reach their own conclusions. Parents believe, and rightly so, that they know what is best for their children. Decisions should be theirs with the nurse serving as a *facilitator* in problem solving.

Providing anticipatory guidance. The ideal way to handle a problem is to prevent it—to deal with it *before* it becomes a problem. The best preventive measure is anticipatory guidance. Parents who know what to expect will be prepared for a behavior when it appears. For example, a fussy, irritable infant will not worry parents who have been advised that the infant is at an age when he will normally cut a first tooth. Parents of a toddler will be prepared for his jealous behavior when he is confronted with a new brother or sister. Some developmental changes that may disturb unprepared parents are beginning locomotion, diminished appetite, negativism, altered sleeping patterns, toilet training, and anxiety toward strangers. Each of these is discussed in the chapters on growth and development to provide the nurse with knowledge to counsel parents.

Avoiding blocks to communication. There are a number of blocks to communication. Some of the more common blocks include:

Socializing
Giving unrestricted and sometimes unasked-for advice
Offering premature or inappropriate reassurance
Giving overready encouragement
Defending a situation or opinion
Using stereotyped comments or cliches
Cutting off expression of emotion by asking directed, close-ended questions
Interrupting and finishing the person's sentence
Talking more than the interviewee
Forming prejudged conclusions
Deliberately changing the focus

Each of these can be corrected by careful analysis of the interview process. One of the best methods for improving interviewing skills is audiotape and/or videotape feedback. With supervision and guidance, the interviewer can recognize the blocks and consciously avoid them.

Using an interpreter. Sometimes effective communication is blocked because two people speak different languages. In this case it is necessary to obtain information through a third party, the interpreter. When using an interpreter, the same guidelines for interviewing are employed, with the following modifications (Kohut, 1975).

Role clarification and explanation of the interview. The nurse introduces herself to the interpreter and explains the reason for the interview and the type of questions that will be asked. The interpreter should know whether a detailed or brief answer is required and whether the translated response can be general or literal.

Introduction and preliminary acquaintance. The nurse introduces the interpreter to each family member. Ideally the interpreter and parent are allowed some time together before the actual interview so that they can become acquainted.

Communicate directly with the parent. When asking questions, the nurse addresses the parent directly in order to reinforce interest in the parent. The nurse observes carefully for nonverbal expressions and mentally notes to ask the interpreter about these later. It is important to refrain from interrupting the parent and interpreter while they are conversing. If the parent answers statements with lengthy discussions, it may be necessary to use more direct questions, rather than open-ended ones. If the translation is shorter than the actual answer, the nurse should not assume that the interpreter is withholding information. He or she may have had difficulty in understanding the explanation and needed time for clarification.

The nurse should avoid commenting to the interpreter about the patient. It is best to presume that the parent understands some English.

Respect cultural differences. It is often necessary to pose questions about sex, marriage, or pregnancy indirectly. For example, it is best to ask about the child's "father" rather than the mother's "husband." The nurse must be aware of difficulty on the part of the interpreter in asking such questions.

Communicate directly with the interpreter. Following the interview, the nurse allows time to share information with the interpreter in private. This is the time to ask about nonverbal clues to communication, to ask for personal interpretations of the parent's reliability and ease in revealing information, and to allow the interpreter an opportunity to share something that he or she felt could not be said earlier.

Continuity. Whenever possible, the parent should speak with the same interpreter on subsequent visits. This helps all three parties feel more comfortable and facilitates effective translation of both words and feelings.

These guidelines apply primarily to the use of an adult interpreter. Often no one other than an older child is available to help translate. In this situation it is important to stress *literal* translation of parent responses. To maximize correct translations, it may be necessary to interrupt the parent and ask the child to translate every few sentences. When children are used as interpreters, the nurse needs to ask questions directed at specific answers and must assess the interpreted translation in terms of nonverbal expressions of communication.

COMMUNICATING WITH CHILDREN

Although the greatest amount of verbal communication is usually carried out with the parent, the child should not be excluded during the interview. Periodic attention to infants and younger children through play or by occasionally directing questions or remarks to them make children participants in the interview. Older children can be actively included as informants.

When relating with children of all ages it is the nonverbal components of the communication process that convey the most significant messages to them. It is difficult to disguise feelings, attitudes, and anxiety when relating to children. They are very alert to surroundings and attach meaning to every gesture and move that is made. This is particularly true with very young children. It is best to

avoid rushing in on a child with gestures or with words. The child should be allowed time to make the first move when possible. Sudden or rapid advances are frightening to a child, as are threatening gestures such as facial contortions, including very broad smiles. Although these are usually intended as friendly gestures, they frequently have the opposite effect.

Children are uncomfortable or even frightened when someone stares at them. It is best to refrain from extended eye contact with a child. Active attempts to make friends with children before they have had an opportunity to evaluate an unfamiliar person tend to increase their anxiety. A helpful tactic is to continue to talk to the child and parent but go about activities that do not involve the child directly, thus allowing him to carry out his observations from a safe position. If the child has a special toy or doll with him, it is helpful to "talk" to the doll first. Asking simple questions such as, "Does your teddy bear have a special name?" may ease the child into conversation.

Children are met on their own eye level since communicating down to children emphasizes their smallness. Adults in strange places may assume overwhelming proportions to children who believe themselves to be in helpless positions. Sitting on a low chair, kneeling, squatting, or even sitting on the floor, if appropriate, places the nurse in a more favorable and less threatening position (Fig. 4-2). With very young children every effort is made to pre-

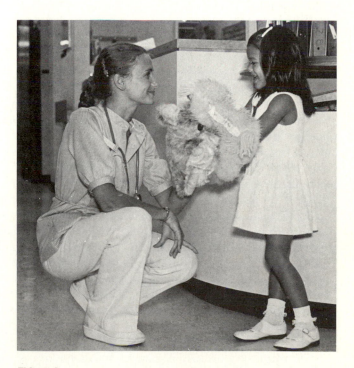

FIG. 4-2

A nurse talks to a child using puppets and assumes a position at the child's level.

serve physical closeness with the parent. Consequently the entire interview may be done with the child sitting on the parent's lap. Giving the child a toy, bottle, or pacifier helps to quiet him.

At any age children respond best to a quiet, unhurried, and confident voice. Children attend to softly spoken words; they tend to withdraw when a voice is raised. Even a crying, distressed child is more apt to "hear" a voice that speaks quietly than one that is attempting to compete with the child's own volume. This is the most successful approach to calming even an uncooperative child.

When giving directions to or seeking cooperation from a child, the nurse should speak clearly, be specific, and use as few words as possible. Simple language is more easily understood. In addition, children's language comprehension precedes their use of words. Although they may not yet talk, it does not mean that they do not understand. The same concept applies when nurses and parents discuss children in their presence. It is more effective to use a positive approach in relating with children. Directions and suggestions are best stated in a *positive* way. An easy way to do this is to avoid using the word "don't." There is more likelihood that a child's cooperation will be gained by saying, "The crayon is for writing" instead of "Don't eat the crayon."

The nurse should be honest with children and make no promises that are impossible to carry out. To assure them that a procedure, such as an injection, will not hurt is no measure of comfort to children who have either experienced the discomfort previously or who discover that indeed it *does* hurt. Any trust that has been built between the child and the nurse will be damaged by the deception, and the child will be justifiably angry.

Children should be told in advance what is going to happen to them. They are fearful of the unknown, and their active imaginations can fantasize images out of proportion to the actual event. The explanation or warning should immediately precede the action. Once the child has been told what to expect, the nurse should follow through without delay. Too much advance warning will be either nullified by intervening activities or will allow time for anxiety about the anticipated event to mount. When fearful procedures are being carried out, the child should be approached with confidence and the procedure executed swiftly and immediately following a brief warning. The child should be comforted with physical contact after a painful or stressful event. The parent who has always been the source of comfort to the child is an ideal person to provide consolation.

It is confusing to children when they are offered a choice when there actually is none. Again, a positive approach is most successful. For example, when clothes must be removed for an examination, the question "Would you like to take off your dress?" offers the child an alter-native she in fact does not have. The statement "We need the dress off so that I can listen to your chest. Shall I help you take it off?" gives the child an explanation, a choice, and some measure of control in the situation.

Communication related to development of thought processes

The normal development of language and thought offers a frame of reference in knowing how to communicate with children. Thought processes progress from concrete to functional and finally to abstract, formal operations.

Infancy. Because they are unable to use words, infants primarily use and understand nonverbal communication. Infants communicate their needs and feelings through nonverbal behaviors and vocalizations that can be interpreted by someone who is around them for a sufficient amount of time. Infants smile and coo when content and cry when distressed. Crying is provoked by unpleasant stimuli from inside or outside, such as hunger, pain, body restraint, or loneliness. Adults interpret this to mean that an infant needs something and consequently try to alleviate the discomfort and reduce tension. Crying (or the desire to cry) persists as a part of everyone's communication repertoire.

Infants respond to adults' nonverbal behaviors. They become quiet when they are cuddled, patted, or receive other forms of gentle, physical contact. They derive comfort from the sound of a voice even though they do not understand the words that are spoken. Until infants reach the age where they experience stranger anxiety, they readily respond to any firm, gentle handling and quiet, calm speech. Loud, harsh sounds and sudden movements are frightening.

Older infants' attentions are centered on themselves and their mothers; therefore, any stranger is a potential threat until proved otherwise. Holding out the hands and asking the child to "come" is seldom successful, especially if the infant is with the mother. If infants must be handled, the best approach is simply to pick them up firmly without gestures. It is helpful to observe the position in which the parent holds the infant. Most infants have learned to prefer a particular position and manner of handling. In general, infants are more at ease upright than horizontal. It is also best to hold infants in such a way that they can keep their parents in view. Until they have developed the understanding that an object (in this case the parent) removed from sight can still be present, they have no way of knowing that the object is still there.

Early childhood. Children less than 5 years of age are almost completely egocentric. They see things only in relation to themselves and from their point of view. Therefore, any communication to them should be focused on *them.* They need to be told what they can do or how they will feel. Experiences of others are of no interest to them. It is futile to use another child's experience as an attempt to gain the cooperation of very small children. They should be allowed to touch, examine, and familiarize themselves with articles that will come in contact with them. A stethoscope bell will feel cold; palpating a neck might tickle. Although they have not yet acquired sufficient language skills to express their feelings and wants, toddlers are able to communicate effectively with their hands to transmit ideas without words. They push an unwanted object away, pull another person to show them something, point, and cover the mouth that is saying something they do not wish to hear.

Everything is direct and concrete to small children. They are unable to work with abstractions and base all deductions on literal formulations. Analogies escape them because they are unable to separate fact from fantasy. For example, they attach literal meaning to such common phrases as "two-faced," "sticky fingers," or "coughing your head off." Children who are told they will get "a little stick in the arm" may not be able to envision an injection (Fig. 4-3). These literal interpretations are an appealing part of this phase of development, but nurses must be aware of inadvertently using a phrase that might be misinterpreted by a small child.

Language is used that is consistent with the child's developmental level. For example, in talking with a toddler, it is best to use simple, *short* sentences, repeat words that are *familiar* to the child, and limit descriptions to *concrete* explanations.

Children in this age category assign human attributes to inanimate objects. They endow mechanical devices and instruments with living characteristics. Consequently they fear that these objects may jump, bite, cut, or pinch all by themselves. Children do not know that these devices are unable to perform without human direction. Unfamiliar equipment needs to be simply explained without building the child's fantasies. Understanding comes slowly and is not usually achieved with one explanation, so things should be explained and described over and over again. If the child does understand, he may be seeking affirmation.

School-age years. Children ages 5 to 8 years rely less on what they see and more on what they know when faced with new problems. They want explanations and reasons for everything but require no verification beyond that. They are interested in the functional aspect of all procedures, objects, and activities. They want to know why an object exists, why it is used, how it works, and the intent and purpose of its user. They need to know what is going to take place and why it is being done to *them* specifically. For example, to explain a procedure such as taking a blood pressure, the nurse might show the child how squeezing the bulb pushes air into the cuff and makes the "silver" in the tube go up. The child should be permitted to operate

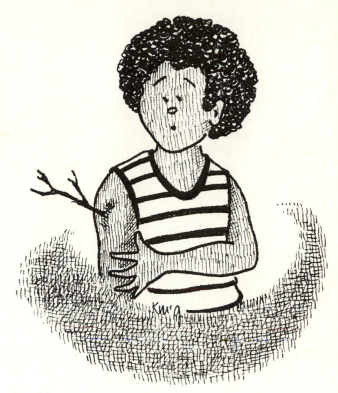

FIG. 4-3
To a young child the expression "a little stick in the arm" is taken literally.

the bulb. An explanation for the reason might be as simple as, "I want to see how far the silver goes up when the cuff squeezes your arm." Consequently the child becomes an enthusiastic participant. Allowing children to ask questions about what is happening to them and maintaining a permissive atmosphere is conducive to questioning.

Children at this age have a heightened concern about body integrity. Because of the special importance and value they place on their body, they are overly sensitive to anything that constitutes a threat or suggestion of injury to it. This concern extends to their possessions also, so that they may appear to overreact to loss or threatened loss of those objects that they treasure. Helping children to voice their concerns enables the nurse to provide reassurance and to implement activities that reduce their anxiety. For example, if a reticent child fears being the single object of probing inquiry, the nurse can ignore that particular child by talking and relating to other children in the family or group. When the child no longer feels like a single target, he will usually interject his ideas, feelings, and interpretations of events.

Older children have an adequate and satisfactory use of language. They still require relatively simple explanations, but their ability to think concretely can facilitate communication and explanation. Commonly they have sufficient experience with health and health workers to understand what is transpiring and generally what is expected of them.

Adolescence. As children move into adolescence, they fluctuate between child and adult thinking and behavior. They are riding a current that is moving them rapidly toward a maturity that may be beyond their coping ability. Therefore, when tensions rise, they may seek the security of the more familiar and comfortable expectations of childhood. Anticipating these shifts in identity allows the nurse to adjust the course of interaction to meet the needs of the moment. No single approach can be relied on consistently, and one can expect to encounter hostility, anger, bravado, and a variety of other behaviors and attitudes. It is as much a mistake to regard the adolescent as an adult with an adult's wisdom and control as it is to confine to him the concerns and expectations of a child.

Frequently adolescents are more willing to discuss their concerns with an adult outside the family, and they often welcome the opportunity to interact with a nurse. They are extremely susceptible to the advances of anyone who displays a genuine interest in them. However, adolescents are quick to reject persons who attempt to impose their values on them, whose interest is feigned, or who appear to have little respect for who they are and what they think or say.

As with all children, adolescents need to express their feelings. Generally they talk quite freely when given an opportunity. However, what adolescents say cannot always be taken at face value. When emotional factors are involved, the feelings that are interjected into words are as significant as the words that are used. The best way to give support is to be attentive, try not to interrupt, and avoid comments or expressions that convey disapproval or surprise. Prying and asking embarrassing questions should be avoided, and any impulse to give advice should be resisted. Frequently adolescents reveal their feelings or a source of concern or ask a question when they are involved in routine matters such as a physical assessment.

Teenagers characteristically have a language and culture all their own that further sets them apart from others. Since it is usually futile to attempt to keep abreast of the current vocabulary, frequent clarification of terms is advisable. Occasionally adolescents are reticent and answer only in monosyllables. Usually this happens when they are opposed to the contact with the nurse or do not yet feel safe enough to reveal themselves. In this instance the best approach is to confine discussions to irrelevant topics to reduce the element of threat until such time as they feel more secure. The nurse must be alert for signals that indicate they are ready to talk. The major sources of concern for adolescents are attitudes and feelings toward sex, relationships with parents, peer group acceptance, and developing a sense of identity.

Interviewing the adolescent presents some special situations to the interviewer. The first may be whether to talk to the adolescent alone, with the parents, or to each individually. Of course, if the adolescent is alone, there is no question, except that the nurse might want to suggest to the teenager that the nurse talk with the parents at another time. If parents and teenager are together, talking with the adolescent first has the advantage of immediately identifying with the young person, thus fostering the interpersonal relationship. However, talking with the parents initially may provide insight into the family relationship. Whichever decision is made, both parties need an opportunity to be included in the interview. If time constraints are important, such as during history taking, these need to be clarified at the onset to avoid appearing to ''take sides'' by talking more with one person than the other.

Confidentiality is of great importance when interviewing adolescents. The parents and the teenager need to know the limits of confidentiality, specifically that the young person's disclosures will be kept between him and the nurse. However, exceptions also must be clarified, such as breaking confidence if it is necessary for the welfare of the adolescent, as in the event of suicidal behavior.

Another dilemma in interviewing adolescents is that two views of a problem frequently exist—the teenager's and the parents'. Clarification of the problem is a major task. However, providing both parties with an opportunity to discuss their perceptions in an open and unbiased atmosphere can, by itself, be therapeutic. The nurse, by demonstrating positive communication skills, can help families communicate more effectively.

COMMUNICATION TECHNIQUES

Besides the conventional interviewing methods of reflection, open-ended questions, and leading statements, there are a number of techniques that encourage children, and sometimes other individuals, to express their thoughts and feelings in a less direct and confronting manner. The following is a discussion of several verbal and nonverbal approaches that can be helpful in a variety of instances. Throughout the book examples are given that use techniques described here.

Third-person technique. The third-person technique involves expressing a feeling in terms of a third person. This technique is less threatening than directly asking a child how he feels, because it gives him the opportunities to agree or disagree without being defensive. For example, the nurse may comment, ''Sometimes when a person is sick a lot he feels angry and sad because he cannot do what others can,'' and either wait silently for a response or encourage a reply with a statement such as, ''Did you ever feel that way?'' This approach allows the child three choices: (1) to agree and, hopefully, express how he feels,

(2) to disagree, or (3) to remain silent, in which case he probably has such feelings but is unable to express them at that time. Demonstrating to parents how useful such techniques are also helps them learn new ways of communicating with the child.

Storytelling. Storytelling uses the language of the child to probe into areas of his thinking while bypassing conscious inhibitions or fears. Children respond to a variety of storytelling techniques. The simplest is asking a child to relate a story about an event, such as "being in the hospital." Another approach involves showing him a picture of a particular event, such as a child in a hospital with other people in the room, and asking him to describe the scene. Comic strips cut from a newspaper with the words removed are excellent vehicles when the child ascribes his own statements to each comic scene (Epstein, 1975). If the child draws a family or hospital scene, he can fill in short verbal communication above each person, similar to a comic strip theme (Fig. 4-4).

Mutual storytelling involves a more therapeutic approach. It not only serves to uncover the child's thinking but also attempts to change the child's perceptions or fears by retelling a somewhat different story. It is a powerful tool and must be used wisely. It begins by asking the child to tell a story about something, followed by another story told by the nurse that is similar to the child's tale but that has differences that help the child in problem areas. A typical example is the child's story of going to the hospital and never seeing his parents again. The nurse's story is also of a child (using different names but similar circumstances) in a hospital whose parents visit everyday, but in the evening after coming home from work. In this way the child's fears of abandonment and separation are handled.

Sometimes children need help in beginning a story with encouragements, such as "Once upon a time . . . ," or the use of a tape recorder. For a less verbal child, having him draw pictures or write about an event may help him relate stories.

Bibliotherapy. Bibliotherapy involves the use of books in a therapeutic and supportive process. Its goal is to help the child express feelings and concerns through the familiar activity of being read to or reading to himself. Although it incorporates an educational component, it involves more than using a book for its preparatory value, such as familiarizing a child with hospitalization or a specific procedure. It provides the child with an opportunity to explore an event that is similar to his own but also sufficiently different to allow him to distance himself from it and remain in control. Since children tend to trust the characters in a book, they are able to feel familiar with the content even if they are suspicious of who reads the story. A book is essentially nonthreatening because the child can close it or stop reading it at any time.

Three wishes. Another simple device to engage children in conversation is the "three wishes" technique. The nurse asks, "If you could have any three things in the world, what would they be?" One child's answer to this was most revealing. He responded, "I don't want to be sick anymore." When asked about the other two wishes, he replied, "If that one came true, so would every other wish, so I don't have any more." Following this the nurse and boy were able to talk about what being sick meant to him. Although the nurse could not make him better, she was able to make some of the other "wishes" come true. One of them was to arrange for school friends to visit the child during his hospitalization and convalescence at home. Before this conversation the youngster's desire for peer companionship had never been revealed.

Rating scale. There are many applications of the rating scale. Some of them are particularly helpful in encouraging older children to talk. Instead of asking a youngster how he feels, the nurse asks him how his day has been "on a scale from 1 to 10, with 10 being the

FIG. 4-4

Filling in the blanks on a comic strip is an effective communication technique with older children.

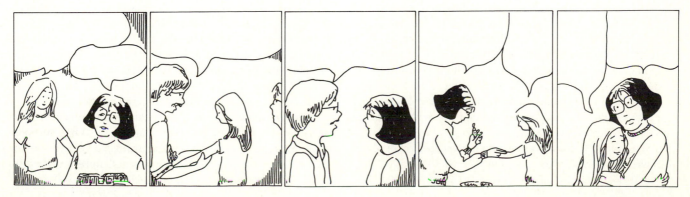

best.'' With a reply of ''Today is a 2,'' one can begin exploring why this day rates so poorly. An extension of this is to have the youngster keep a log of each day's rating and expand it into a diary. The use of a rating scale can be helpful in assessing the degree of pain or emotions such as sadness or happiness.

Word association game. Another approach is the word association game. The nurse can begin by having a list of key words and asking the child to say the first word that he thinks of when he hears the word. It is best to start with neutral words and then introduce more anxiety-producing words, such as illness, needles, hospitals, operation, and so on. The key words should be ones that relate to some significant event in the child's life.

Fill in the blanks. Without directly asking about feelings, one can probe into areas of concern by presenting a statement and having the child complete it. This is particularly useful with older school-age children and adolescents. Some sample statements are:

The thing I like best (least) about school is _____.
The best (worst) age to be is _____.
The most (least) fun thing I ever did was _____.
The thing I like most (least) about my parents is _____.
If I could change one thing about my family, it would be _____.
If I could be anything I wanted, I would be _____.
The thing I like most (least) about myself is _____.

Notice that the beginning statements are more neutral than the last ones, which center on feelings about oneself.

Pros and cons. A somewhat different approach to encouraging exploration of feelings is to select a topic, such as ''being in the hospital,'' and have the child list ''five good things and five bad things'' about it. This is an exceptionally valuable technique when applied to relationships. For example, family members can be asked to write down five things they like and dislike about each other. In reviewing the lists, each member has the opportunity to discuss his or her feelings in a nonjudgmental atmosphere. However, when this technique is used, the nurse must be able to handle feelings that can surface unexpectedly.

Writing. Many children and adults find talking about their feelings difficult. For them verbal communication may be more stressful than supportive. An alternative approach is writing. Some specific suggestions include (1) keeping a journal or diary, (2) writing down feelings or thoughts that are difficult to talk about, (3) writing ''letters'' that are never mailed (a variation is making up a ''pen pal'' and writing to him or her), or (4) keeping an account of the child's progress both from a physical and emotional viewpoint.

To initiate a conversation, the nurse can inquire about the writing, possibly even asking to read some of it. Fre-

quently, as a person writes down his ideas, thoughts, or feelings, there is also an urge to discuss them. Once they are written, they are more real and tangible but often less frightening than when kept locked inside the mind.

Drawing. Drawing is one of the most valuable forms of communication—both nonverbal, from looking at the drawing, and verbal, from the child's story of the picture. Children's drawings tell a great deal about them because they are projections of their personality. A child's drawing is usually of himself, his experience, or those who are significant to him. Besides communicating about himself, art also provides the child with a natural activity that helps him deal with conscious and unconscious feelings.

Drawing can be spontaneous or directed. *Spontaneous drawings* involve giving the child a variety of art supplies (older children like felt-tipped pens) and providing the opportunity to draw. The only encouragement may be the statement, ''Draw something for me.'' *Directed drawing* involves a more specific direction, such as ''Draw a person.'' In isolated figure drawings the child's response tends to be predominantly intellectual, in that he will produce a more complete picture with more parts than those he draws in a group picture.

If the child needs encouragement to draw, the ''three themes'' approach is helpful. It involves writing three statements about the child at the bottom of the paper, for example, ''I like playing the piano. I am in the hospital now. My dog's name is Poochie.'' The child chooses one theme to draw a picture (Fig. 4-5).

Group drawings are highly influenced by the child's feelings and the response is predominantly emotional. Consequently group drawings are highly valuable in disclosing what the child thinks about himself and others. The most valuable group drawing is of the family. A special type is the *kinetic family drawing* (Burns and Kaufman, 1970), in which the child is asked to, ''Draw your family doing something.'' In giving directions, the nurse must be careful to offer only a general statement of encouragement and refrain from suggesting themes. Drawing the family is appropriate for children over 4 years of age.

The basic assumption in interpreting drawings is that the child is revealing something about himself. However, interpretation must be undertaken with an understanding of normal development in art expression. For example, it is normal for a 4-year-old to draw arms attached to a head but highly questionable in a 6-year-old. Understanding how to ''read'' and use drawings takes considerable time, experience, study, and patience. It is just as dangerous to ''read'' too much into a drawing and mislabel a person as it is to disregard a drawing as meaningless. When studying a drawing, every detail must be evaluated, as well as relationships of one part to another. It is helpful to label the

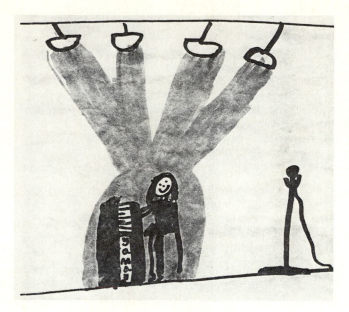

FIG. 4-5

Using the three themes approach, this child chooses to draw herself playing the piano; the spotlights focus on her as the center of attention, which was consistent with her position as an only child in the family.

characters (mother, father, and so on) and to denote the order in which each was drawn.

When evaluating a drawing the following features should be assessed:

1. The size of individual figures (expresses importance, power, authority)
2. The order in which figures are drawn (expresses priority in terms of importance)
3. The child's position to other family members (expresses feelings of status or alliance)
4. The exclusion of a member (may denote feeling of not belonging or desire to eliminate)
5. Accentuated parts (usually expresses concern for areas of special importance, for example, large hands may be sign of aggression)
6. Erasures, shadings, or cross-hatching (expresses ambivalence, concern, or anxiety with particular area)

These suggestions are by no means a complete inventory for analyzing drawing. However, they do provide initial guidelines that can offer much information about the child. One caution is that interpretation must be viewed in light of the child's particular circumstances. For example, while cross-hatching is generally a sign of anxiety, it can also be an attempt to reproduce a design in a particular artistic effect, in which case it has much less significance.

Play. Play is the universal language of children. It is one of the most important forms of communication and can be an effective technique in relating with them. Clues about physical, intellectual, and social developmental progress can often be derived from the form and complexity of a child's play behaviors. Therapeutic play requires little or no equipment and is often used to reduce the trauma of illness and hospitalization, as is discussed in Chapters 18 and 19.

Because their ability to perceive precedes their ability to transmit, small infants respond to activities that register on their senses. Patting, stroking, and other skin play convey messages. Repetitive actions such as stretching an infant's arms out to the side while he is lying on his back and then folding them across his chest or raising and revolving his legs in a bicycling motion will elicit pleasurable sounds. Colorful items to catch the eye or interesting sounds such as a ticking clock, chimes, bells, or singing can be used to attract the child's attention.

Older infants respond to simple games. The old game of peekaboo is an excellent means of initiating communication with infants while maintaining a "safe" nonthreatening distance. After this intermittent eye-to-eye contact, the nurse is no longer viewed as a stranger but as a friend. This can be followed by touch games. Clapping an infant's hands together for pat-a-cake or wiggling his toes for "this little piggy" delights an infant or small child. Much of the nursing assessment can be carried out with the use of games and simple play equipment while the infant remains in the safety of the parent's arms or lap. Talking to a foot or other part of the child's body is another effective tactic.

The nurse can capitalize on the natural curiosity of small children by playing games such as, "Which hand do you take?" and "Guess what I have in my hand" or by manipulating items such as a flashlight or stethoscope. Finger games are very useful. More elaborate materials, such as puppets and replicas of familiar or unfamiliar items, serve as excellent means to communicate with small children. The variety and extent are limited only by the nurse's imagination.

Through play children reveal their perceptions of interpersonal relationships with their family and friends or the hospital personnel. Children may also reveal the wide scope of knowledge they have acquired from listening to others around them. For example, through needle play children may disclose how carefully they have watched each procedure by precisely duplicating the technical skills.

Play sessions serve not only as assessment tools for determining children's awareness and perception of their illness but also as methods of intervention and evaluation. A change in the type of drawing or the theme of the play may indicate progression toward or away from an ability to deal with anxiety.

OUTLINE OF A PEDIATRIC HEALTH HISTORY

Identifying information

1. Name		6.	Sex
2. Address		7.	Religion
3. Telephone		8.	Nationality
4. Birth date and place		9.	Date of interview
5. Race		10.	Informant

Chief complaint (CC): to establish the major *specific* reason for the child's and parents' seeking professional health attention

Present illness (PI): to obtain *all* details related to the chief complaint

Past history (PH): to elicit a profile of the child's previous illnesses, injuries, or operations

1. Birth history (pregnancy, labor, and delivery; perinatal history)	4. Allergies
	5. Current medications
	6. Immunizations
2. Feeding history	7. Growth and development
3. Previous illnesses, injuries, or operations	8. Habits

Review of systems (ROS): to elicit information concerning any potential health problem

1. General	7. Mouth	13. Gastrointestinal
2. Integument	8. Throat	14. Genitourinary
3. Head	9. Neck	15. Gynecologic
4. Eyes	10. Chest	16. Musculoskeletal
5. Ears	11. Respiratory	17. Neurologic
6. Nose	12. Cardiovascular	18. Endocrine

Family history (FH): to identify the presence of genetic traits or diseases that have familial tendencies, to assess exposure to a communicable disease in a family member, to assess the individual's reactions to disease or death in the family, and to assess family relationships

1. Family pedigree
2. Familial diseases and congenital anomalies

Personal/social history (P/SH): to develop an understanding of the child as an individual and as a member of a family and a community

1. Home and community environment
2. Occupation and education of family members
3. Cultural and religious traditions
4. Geographic location
5. Marital and sexual history

Patient profile (P/P): to summarize the interviewer's overall impression of the child's physical, psychologic, and socioeconomic background

1. Health status
2. Psychologic status
3. Socioeconomic status

HISTORY TAKING

This section deals with interviewing as it relates to history taking. Each section of the history is discussed to allow the reader an opportunity to learn what constitutes a thorough assessment. The precise depth and extent of a nursing history vary with its intended purpose. The nurse uses judgment in deciding what data are necessary and relevant for the identification of problems.

The more complete the history is the more time consuming it is to take. A complete history can take an hour to complete. However, a thorough history at the beginning of the relationship is extremely helpful in planning care. For the healthy child, the nurse has background for identifying problems of a psychosocial nature and/or providing anticipatory guidance. For the ill child, there is the advantage of knowing the past and present health history, past experience with health care facilities, and the family constellation.

The format that is used resembles a medical history, but the objective of each assessment area is the identification of nursing diagnoses or patient problems. The value in following this well-established approach is that it is systematic and familiar in sequence and intent to members of the health team. The categories listed in the boxed material encompass the patient's current and past health status and information about his psychosocial environment.

PERFORMING A HEALTH HISTORY

The format used for history taking may be (1) *direct*—the nurse asks the information via direct interview with the informant, or (2) *indirect*—the informant supplies the information by completing some type of questionnaire. The direct method is superior to the indirect approach or a combination of both. However, in view of time constraints, the direct approach is not always practical. If the indirect method is used, it is important to review informants' written responses and question them regarding any unusual answers.

The direct method can lose its value if the nurse asks questions directly from a form. In essence, the parent is completing the form by listening to it rather than by reading it. Using a systematic approach does not imply rote memory of a specific outline. Rather, it denotes the use of categories to define what areas of information are required. If nurses use as a model the basic categories outlined above and understand the objective of each, they can then obtain the required information as it arises during the course of the interview. However, the history should be recorded using the specified format.

Identifying information

Much of the identifying information may already be available from other recorded sources. However, if the parent seems anxious, the nurse may ask about such information to help the parent feel more comfortable.

Informant. One of the important areas under identifying information concerns the informant, the person(s) who furnished the information. The following data about the informant are recorded: (1) who it is (child, parent, or other), (2) an impression of reliability and willingness to communicate, and (3) any special circumstances, such as the use of an interpreter or conflicting answers by more than one person.

Chief complaint

The chief complaint represents the specific reason for the child's visit to the clinic, office, or hospital. The chief complaint may be viewed as the theme with the present illness as the description of the problem. The chief complaint is elicited by asking open-ended neutral questions, such as, "Tell me what seems to be the matter," "How may I help you?" or "What brings you here?" Labeling-type questions, such as, "How are you sick?" are avoided, since it is possible that the reason for the visit is not because of illness.

Occasionally it is difficult to isolate one symptom or problem as the chief complaint because the parent may identify many. In this situation it is important to be as specific as possible when asking questions. For example, asking informants to state which *one* problem or symptom prompted them to seek help now may help them focus on the most immediate concern.

Present illness

The history of the present illness* is a narrative of the chief complaint from its earliest onset through its progres-

*The term *illness* is used in its broadest sense to denote any problem of a physical, emotional, or psychosocial nature. It is actually a history of the chief complaint.

sion to the present. Its four major components are: (1) the details of onset, (2) a complete *interval* history, (3) the *present* status, and (4) the reason for seeking help *now*. The focus of the present illness is on all factors relevant to the main problem, even if they have disappeared or changed during the onset, interval, and present.

Analyzing a symptom. Since pain is often the most characteristic symptom denoting onset of a physical problem, it is used as a prototype for analysis of a symptom. Assess pain for (1) type, (2) location, (3) severity, (4) duration, and (5) influencing factors. The *type* or character of pain should be as specific as possible. However, with young children, it is almost always impossible for them to describe the pain. Asking the parents how they know the child is in pain may help describe its type, location, and severity. For example, a parent may state, "My child must have a severe earache because she pulls at her ears, rolls her head on the floor, and screams. Nothing seems to help."

The nurse can help older children describe the pain by asking them if it is sharp, throbbing, dull, aching, stabbing, and so on. Whatever words they use are recorded in quotes.

The *location* of the pain must also be specific. "Stomach pains" is too general a description. Children can better localize the pain if they are asked to "point with one finger to where it hurts" or to "point to where mommy would put a bandaid." One can also determine if the pain radiates by asking, "Does the pain stay there or move? Show me where it goes with your finger."

The *severity* of pain is best determined by finding out how it affects the child's usual behavior. Pain that prevents a child from playing, interacting with others, sleeping, and eating is most often severe. It is preferable to record pain in terms of interference with activity, rather than to quote the parent's or child's adjectives.

Duration of pain should include the duration, onset, and frequency of attacks. It may be necessary to describe this in terms of activity and behavior, such as "pain lasted all night because child refused to sleep and cried intermittently."

Influencing factors are anything that causes a change in the type, location, severity, or duration of the pain. These include (1) precipitating events (those that cause or increase the pain), (2) relieving events (those that lessen the pain, such as medications), (3) temporal events (times when the pain is relieved or increased), (4) positional events (standing, sitting, and lying down), and (5) associated events (meals, stress, and coughing).

Past history

The past history contains information relating to all previous aspects of the child's health status and concentrates on several areas that are ordinarily deleted in the history of an adult, such as birth history, detailed feeding history, immunizations, and growth and development. Since a great deal of data is included in this section, it is more efficient to use a combination of open-ended and fact-finding questions. For example, the nurse may begin interviewing for each section with an open-ended statement, such as, ''Tell me about your child's birth,'' in order to provide the informant with the opportunity to relate what he or she thinks is most important. Fact-finding questions related to specific details are asked whenever necessary to focus the interview on certain topics.

Birth history. Birth history includes all data concerning (1) the mother's health during pregnancy, (2) the labor and delivery, and (3) the infant's condition immediately after birth. Since prenatal influences have significant effects on a child's physical and emotional development, a thorough investigation of birth history is essential. Since parents may question what relevance pregnancy and birth have on the child's present condition, particularly if the child is past infancy, it is best to explain why such questions are included. An appropriate statement may be: ''I will be asking you some questions about your pregnancy and . . . (refer to child by name) birth. Your answers will give me a more complete picture of his overall health.''

Because emotional factors also affect the outcome of pregnancy and the subsequent parent-child relationship, it is important to investigate (1) concurrent crises during pregnancy and (2) prenatal attitudes toward the fetus. It is best to approach the topic of parental acceptance of pregnancy through indirect questioning. Asking parents if the pregnancy was planned is a leading statement because they may respond affirmatively for fear of criticism if the pregnancy was unexpected. The nurse can encourage parents to disclose their true reactions by referring to specific facts relating to the pregnancy, such as the spacing between offspring, an extended or short interval between marriage and conception, or the concurrent experience of pregnancy and adolescence. The parent can choose to explore such statements with further explanations or, for the moment, may not be able to reveal such feelings. Silence should alert the nurse to the importance of refocusing on this topic later in the interview.

Feeding history. The exact questions needed to elicit a feeding history depend on the child's age. In general, the younger the child, the more specific and detailed the feeding history is. In regard to infant feeding, the following information is important:

1. Type of feeding (breast, commercial preparation, home preparation, special formulas)
2. Time and reason for changing feeding habits (breast to bottle, bottle to cup, one type of formula to another, formula to regular milk, introduction of solid foods)
3. Interval of feedings
4. Time required for one feeding
5. Apparent appetite
6. Quantity consumed
7. Addition of vitamins/minerals
8. Weight change
9. Any problems associated with feeding (vomiting, diarrhea, colic, ''spitting up,'' rumination, refusal to eat)
10. Remedies used for each problem

For older children it is best to use a ''diet diary'' approach for eliciting a feeding history by asking the parent to list what the child ate the previous day and ascertaining if that menu was typical. Specific questions are asked about snacks between meals, special likes and dislikes, changes in the appetite, and eating habits, such as time at the table. The daily food diary is then analyzed by comparing it to the four basic food groups. For example, if the list includes no vegetables, the nurse should ask the reason for this, rather than assume that the child dislikes vegetables, because it may be that none were served on that day. Based on the specific details of the nutrition history, appropriate counseling would be planned following completion of the assessment.

Because cultural practices are very prevalent in food preparation, it is important to consider carefully the kind of questions asked and the judgments made in regard to counseling. For example, some cultures, such as Hispanic, black, and American Indian, include many vegetables, legumes, and starches in their diet that together provide sufficient amounts of essential amino acids, even though the actual amount of meat or dairy protein may be low.

Previous illnesses, injuries, and operations. When inquiring about past medical illnesses, the nurse can begin with a general statement, such as, ''What other illnesses has your child had?'' Since parents are most likely to recall serious health problems, it is important to specifically ask about colds, earaches, and common childhood diseases, such as measles, rubella (German measles), chicken pox, mumps, pertussis (whooping cough), diphtheria, scarlet fever, strep throat, tonsillitis, or allergic manifestations.

In addition to illnesses, the parent is asked about injuries that required medical intervention, operations, and any other reason for hospitalization, including the dates of each incident. It is important to focus on injuries such as accidental falls, poisonings, chokings, or burns, since this may be a potential area for parental guidance.

Allergies. The nurse asks about commonly known allergic disorders, such as hay fever and asthma, as well as unusual reactions to foods, drugs, or contact agents, such as animals, household products, fabrics, or poisonous plants. It is especially important to have the parent describe the allergic reactions to drugs since a known side effect can be confused with an allergic reaction. If the child has a known allergy to antibiotics, it is important to inquire about reactions to specific immunizations, such as measles or rubella, which may contain neomycin.

Current medications. In addition to any drug allergies, the nurse asks about current drug regimens, including vitamins, aspirin, antibiotics, antihistamines, decongestants, or antitussives. All medications are listed, including name, dose, schedule, duration, and reason for administration.

Immunizations. A record of all immunizations or "baby shots" is essential. Since many parents are unaware of the exact name and date of each immunization, the most reliable source of information is a hospital, clinic, or private physician's record. All immunizations and "boosters" are listed, stating (1) the name of the specific disease, (2) the number of injections, (3) the dosage (sometimes lesser amounts are given if a reaction is anticipated), (4) the ages when administered, and (5) the occurrence of any reaction following the immunization. The nurse should also inquire about the previous administration of any horse or other foreign serum, recent administration of gamma globulin or blood transfusion, anaphylactoid reactions to neomycin or chicken eggs, and tuberculin testing. If testing was done, the child's positive or negative intradermal reaction is recorded.

Growth and development. The most important previous growth patterns to record are: (1) approximate weight at 6 months, 1 year, 2 years, and 5 years of age, (2) approximate length at ages 1 and 4 years, and (3) dentition, including age of onset, number of teeth, and symptoms during teething. Developmental milestones include: (1) age of holding up head steadily, (2) age of sitting alone without support, (3) age of walking without assistance, (4) age of saying first words with meaning, (5) present grade in school, (6) scholastic grades, and (7) interaction with other children, peers, and adults.

Specific and detailed questions are used when inquiring about each developmental milestone. For example "sitting up" can mean many different activities, such as sitting propped up, sitting in someone's lap, sitting with support, sitting up alone but in a hyperflexed position for assisted balance, or sitting up unsupported with the back slightly rounded. A clue to misunderstanding of the requested activity may be an unusually early age of achievement.

Habits. Habits are an important area to explore because numerous parental concerns may be discovered. They include:

1. Behavior patterns, such as nail-biting, thumb-sucking, pica, rituals ("security" blanket or toy), and unusual movements (head-banging, rocking, overt masturbation, and walking on toes)

2. Activities of daily living, such as hour of sleep and arising, duration of nighttime sleep and naps, type and duration of exercise, regularity of stools and urination, age of toilet training, and occurrences of daytime or nighttime bed-wetting

3. Usual disposition as well as response to frustration

4. Use or abuse of alcohol, drugs, coffee, and cigarettes

The last category is primarily applicable to adolescents, although nurses must be aware of the increasing juvenile experimentation and use of potentially harmful substances. If a youngster admits to smoking, drinking, or drug use, a specific average amount, such as one cigarette a week or two cans of beer on weekends, is recorded. A statement such as, "I pop pills once in awhile" has tremendously wide variations in meaning. Following this response with, "How many pills and when is once in a while?" may yield a measurable intake of drugs. If older children deny use of such substances, it is advisable to inquire about past experimentation. Asking, "You mean you never tried to smoke or drink?" implies that the nurse expects some such activity and consequently is likely to be nonjudgmental of an affirmative answer. One should also be aware of the confidential nature of such questioning and the adverse effect that the parents' presence may have on the adolescent's willingness to answer.

Review of systems

Review of systems is exactly what the title implies—a specific review of each body system, similar to the order of the physical examination. Often the history of the present illness provides a complete review of the system involved in the chief complaint. Since asking questions about other body systems may appear unrelated and irrelevant to the parents or child, it is important to precede the questioning with an explanation of why the data is needed (similar to the explanation concerning relevance of birth history) and reassurance that the child's main problem has not been forgotten.

The review of a specific system is begun with a broad statement, such as, "How has your child's general health been?" or "Has your child had any problems with his eyes?" If the parent states that there have been past problems with some body function, this is pursued with an encouraging statement, such as, "Tell me more about that." If the parent denies any problems, it is best to query for specific symptoms, such as, "No headaches, bumping into objects, or squinting?" If the parent reconfirms the absence of such symptoms, positive statements to this effect are recorded in the history, such as, "Mother denies headaches, bumping into objects, or squinting." In this way, anyone who reviews the health history is aware of exactly what symptoms were investigated.

The following is an outline of suggested areas for review of each body system. Although medical terminology may be used to record a symptom during the interview, only terms that are clearly understood by the parent or child are used.

general overall state of health, fatigue, recent and/or unexplained weight gain or loss, period of time for either, contributing factors (change of diet, illness, altered appetite), exercise tolerance, fevers (time of day), chills, night sweats (unrelated to climatic conditions), frequent infections, general ability to carry out activities of daily living

integument pruritus, pigment or other color changes, acne, eruptions, rashes (location), tendency to bruising, petechiae, excessive dryness, general texture, disorders or deformities of nails, hair growth or loss, hair color change (for adolescent, use of hair dyes or other potentially toxic substances, such as hair straighteners)

head headaches, dizziness, injury (specific details)

eyes visual problems (ask about behaviors indicative of blurred vision, such as bumping into objects, clumsiness, sitting very close to the television, holding a book close to the face, writing with head near desk, squinting, rubbing the eyes, bending the head in an awkward position), "cross-eye" (strabismus), eye infections, edema of lids, excessive tearing, use of glasses or contact lenses, date of last optic examination

nose nosebleeds (epistaxis), constant or frequent running or stuffy nose, nasal obstruction (difficulty in breathing), sense of smell

ears earaches, discharge, evidence of hearing loss (ask about behaviors, such as need to repeat requests, loud speech, inattentive behavior), results of any previous auditory testing

mouth mouth breathing, gum bleeding, toothaches, toothbrushing, use of fluoride, difficulty with teething (symptoms), last visit to dentist (especially if temporary dentition is complete), response to dentist

throat sore throats, difficulty in swallowing, choking (especially when chewing food—may be from poor chewing habits), hoarseness or other voice irregularities

neck pain, limitation of movement, stiffness, difficulty in holding head straight (torticollis), thyroid enlargement, enlarged nodes or other masses

chest breast enlargement, discharge, masses, enlarged axillary nodes (for adolescent female, ask about breast self-examination)

respiratory chronic cough, frequent colds (number per year), wheezing, shortness of breath at rest or on exertion, difficulty in breathing, sputum production, infections (pneumonia, tuberculosis), date of last chest x-ray examination

cardiovascular cyanosis or fatigue on exertion, history of heart murmur or rheumatic fever, anemia, date of last blood count, blood type, recent transfusion

gastrointestinal (much of this in regard to appetite, food tolerance, and elimination habits has been asked elsewhere), nausea, vomiting (not associated with eating may be indicative of brain tumor or increased intracranial pressure), jaundice or yellowing skin or sclera, belching, flatulence, recent change in bowel habits (blood in stools, change of color, diarrhea, or constipation)

genitourinary pain on urination, frequency, hesitancy, urgency, hematuria, nocturia, polyuria, unpleasant odor to urine, force of stream, discharge, change in size of scrotum, date of last urinalysis (for adolescent, venereal disease, type of treatment; for male adolescent, ask about testicular self-examination)

gynecologic menarche, date of last menstrual period, regularity or problems with menstruation, vaginal discharge, pruritus, date and result of last Pap smear (include obstetric history as discussed under birth history when applicable); if sexually active, type of contraception

musculoskeletal weakness, clumsiness, lack of coordination, unusual movements, back or joint stiffness, muscle pains or cramps, abnormal gait, deformity, fractures, serious sprains, activity level

neurologic seizures, tremors, dizziness, loss of memory, general affect, fears, nightmares, speech problems, any unusual habits

endocrine intolerance to weather changes, excessive thirst, excessive sweating, salty taste to skin, signs of early puberty

Family history

The medical family history is primarily for the purpose of discovering the potential existence of hereditary or familial diseases in the parents and child. However, it affords much more information in terms of status of the marital relationship, availability of support systems in extended relatives, and age relationships among siblings.

In general, information about the family is confined to first-degree relatives. In the case of children, this includes the maternal and paternal parents, siblings, and offspring. Information for each includes age, state of health if living, cause of death if deceased, and any evidence of the following conditions: heart disease, hypertension, cancer, diabetes mellitus, obesity, congenital anomalies, allergy, asthma, tuberculosis, sickle cell disease, mental retardation, convulsions, insanity or other emotional problems, syphilis, or rheumatic fever. The accuracy of the reported incidence is confirmed by inquiring as to the symptoms, course, treatment, and sequelae of each diagnosis.

The family history should also include a general overview of family interaction. Asking questions concerning with whom the child shares a room, the child's household chores, and activities the family does together gives some idea of how the family functions together. It is best to avoid direct questions such as, "How does your family get along with each other?" because the usual response is "Okay." An effective way of approaching this topic, especially with adolescents, is use of the third-person technique. The nurse may say, for example, "Teenagers and parents have a way of seeing things differently, especially when it comes to money, dating, clothes, using the car, and curfew. Have you and your parents ever disagreed about such things?" The young person is then allowed an opportunity to present his views because he is aware that the nurse expects such events and is therefore less likely to judge or criticize his response.

Personal/social history

This section of the history includes all the personal, sociocultural, spiritual, and economic factors that influence the child's and family's overall psychobiologic health. It focuses on (1) the home and community environment, (2) the occupation and education of family members, (3) the cultural and religious traditions, (4) the geographic location, and (5) the marital and sexual history of the parents and child (see below). Since the information elicited in this part of the history is often the most personal and confidential, it is left to the end of the interview, when the nurse-parent-child rapport should be well established.

1. Home and community environment
   a. Type of dwelling
   b. Number of rooms/occupants
   c. Sleeping arrangements
   d. Number of floors, accessibility of stairs, elevators
   e. Adequacy of utilities
   f. Safety features (fire escape, smoke detector, guardrails on windows, use of car restraint)
   g. Environmental hazards (chipped paint, insects, poor sanitation, no sunlight, industrial pollution, high incidence of crime, heavy street traffic)
   h. Availability of schools, play areas, health facilities
   i. Relationship with neighbors
   j. Recent crises or changes in home
2. Occupation and education of family members
   a. Type of employment
   b. Work schedule
   c. Work satisfaction
   d. Exposure to environmental/industrial hazards
   e. Source of income
   f. Adequacy of income
   g. Effect of illness on financial status
   h. Highest degree or grade attained
3. Cultural and religious traditions
   a. Adherence to cultural/religious practices
   b. Language spoken in home
4. Geographic location
   a. Recent travel
   b. Contact with foreign visitors
5. Marital and sexual history
   a. Marital status of parents
   b. Marital stability
   c. Sexual activity/concerns of adolescent

The degree of inquiry into the parents' sexual activity depends on many factors. For example, it may be limited to a brief discussion of their plans regarding future children and the methods used to ensure their wishes, such as the type of contraception. In instances where overt adult sexual activity may be having an adverse effect on the children, a more detailed exploration is warranted. This decision is based on facts learned during the interview, because this line of questioning should never be wanton prying. If parents ask the relevance of revealing such matters, the nurse must be prepared to offer a sound and logical explanation. It is every person's right to refuse to disclose personal information, especially if he or she is not informed of its importance.

A sexual history is an essential component of adolescent health assessments. It is warranted regardless of their degree of sexual activity since concerns about sexual matters may bear heavily on their physical and psychologic well-being.

One way of initiating a conversation about sexual concerns is to begin with a history of peer interactions. Open-ended statements such as, "Tell me about your social life," or "Who are your closest friends?" generally leads into a discussion of dating and sexual issues. Sometimes, to probe further, one can ask about the adolescent's attitudes on sex education, "going steady," "living together," and premarital sex.

Since homosexual experimentation may occur during adolescence and since it can be a great source of concern and anxiety for the teenager, it is important to investigate this area. One approach is to use nonspecific questions and to refer to all sexual partners as "partners," not as "girlfriends" or "boyfriends." This allows for a more open discussion because the interviewer has not biased the questioning with expected heterosexual relationships.

Occasionally a teenager may reveal very intimate details of a sexual relationship. One of the dangers in allowing this to occur is that the adolescent may later regret having revealed "too much" and consequently retreat from further contact with the nurse or limit subsequent interactions to superficial topics. Sometimes the elaboration of one topic is an attempt to prevent the interviewer from asking questions. In either situation it is best to limit the conversation with a statement such as, "It seems that this is something we should explore further. Right now, let's talk about your earlier concern with school."

In any conversation regarding sexual history, the nurse must be aware of the language that is used in either eliciting or conveying sexual information. For example, when asking if the adolescent is "sexually active" or "having sex," the exact meaning of either phrase is clarified to avoid misunderstanding. To some it may signify foreplay, self-stimulation, erotic visual stimulation, or intercourse. Adolescents' fantasies and strong sexual desires alone are sufficient to cause them concern. Therefore, the nurse not only wants to know the incidence of intimate sexual contacts but also areas of sexual concern.

Patient profile

The patient profile is a summary of one's impression of the child's health status and the psychologic-socioeconomic variables that influence his total well-being. It is sometimes written after completion of the physical examination and includes pertinent physical findings regarding the child's present state of health.

A well-written patient profile is actually the beginning of a problem list or nursing diagnoses (see p. 13) of both objective findings and subjective impressions. Frequently, physical findings during the examination yield supportive data of initial concerns identified during the history. Some of the more common health problems discovered during the interview include visual disturbances, delayed speech development, the need for dental hygiene, nutritional inadequacy, the impact of family problems on the child, such as divorce or separation, and discipline or behavioral concerns.

REFERENCES

Burns, R.C., and Kaufman, S.H.: Kinetic family drawings, New York, 1970, Brunner/Mazel, Inc.

Epstein, C.: Nursing the dying patient, Reston, Va., 1975, Reston Publishing Co., Inc.

Kohut, S.A.: Guidelines for using interpreters, Hosp. Prog. **56**(4):39-40, 1975.

BIBLIOGRAPHY

Adams, G.: The sexual history as an integral part of the patient history, Am. J. Maternal Child Nurs. **1**(3):170-175, 1976.

Adamson, L.S.: Strategies for nurse-patient communication, Superv. Nurse **11**:44-45, Dec. 1980.

Anderson, M.L.: Talking about sex—with less anxiety, J. Psychiatr. Nurs. **18**:10-15, June 1980.

Baer, E.D., McGowan, M.N., and McGivern, D.O.: Taking a health history, Am. J. Nurs. **77**(7):1190-1193, 1977.

Benjamin, A.: The helping interview, Boston, 1974, Houghton Mifflin Co.

Bentz, J.M.: Missed meanings in nurse/patient communication, Am. J. Maternal Child Nurs. **5**(1):55-57, 1980.

Berg, P.J., Devlin, M.K., and Gedaly-Duff, V.: Bibliotherapy with children experiencing loss, Issues Compr. Pediatr. Nurs. **4**:37-50, Aug. 1980.

Brown, M.S., and Murphy, M.A.: Ambulatory pediatrics for nurses, New York, 1979, McGraw-Hill Book Co.

Cameron, C., Juszczak, L., and Wallace, N.: Using creative arts to help children cope with altered body image, Child. Health Care **12**:108-112, l984.

Cassell, E.J.: Learning language skills: changing the words changes the world, Patient Care **14**:126-142, June 1980.

Cassell, E.J.: Learning language skills: hear what the patient means, say what you mean, Patient Care **14**:80-90, Jan. 1980.

Cassell, E.J.: Learning language skills: listen: "illogical" patients often make sense, Patient Care **14**:91-106, Jan. 1980.

Cassell, E.J.: Learning language skills: untwisting the fibers of "paralanguage," Patient Care **14**:186-204, Sept. 1980.

Crews, N.E.: Developing empathy for effective communication, AORN J. **30**:536, 540, 542, 544-546, Sept. 1979.

Edwards, B.J., and Brilhart, J.K.: Communication in nursing practice, St. Louis, 1981, The C.V. Mosby Co.

Elmassian, B.J.: A practical approach to communicating with children through play, Am. J. Maternal Child Nurs. **4**(4):238-240, 1979.

Farr, K.: Communication pitfalls in routine counseling, Pediatr. Nurs. **5**(1):55-57, 1979.

Gelhard, H.L.: Drawing and development, Pediatr. Nurs. **4**(6):23-25, 1978.

Heineken, J. and Roberts, F.: Confirming, not disconfirming: communicating in a more positive manner, Am. J. Maternal Child Nurs. **8**:78-80, 1983.

Henrich, A.P., and Bernheim, K.F.: Responding to patients' concerns, Nurs. Outlook **29**:428-433, July 1981.

How should patients be addressed? AORN J. **31**:1142-1146, 1980.

Johnson, S.H.: Avoiding communication blocks with high-risk parents, Issues Compr. Pediatr. Nurs. **4**:61-72, Aug. 1980.

Jolly, J.D.: Through a child's eyes: the problems of communicating with sick children, Nursing (Oxford) **1**:1012-1014, 1981.

McLeavey, K.A.: Children's art as an assessment tool, Pediatr. Nurs. **5**(2):9-14, 1979.

McNally Forsyth, D.: Looking good to communicate better with patients, Nursing 83, **13**(7):34-37, 1983.

Orndorf, R., and Deutch, J.A.: The power of positive suggestion: persuading patients to cooperate, Nursing 81 **11**(8):73, 1981.

O'Sullivan, A.L.: Privileged communication, Am. J. Nurs. **80**:947-950, May 1980.

Pidgeon, V.A.: Characteristics of children's thinking and implications for health teaching, Maternal Child Nurs. J. **6**:1-8, Spring 1977.

Pontious, S.L.: Practical Piaget: helping children understand, Am. J. Nurs. **82**(1):114-117, 1982.

Programmed instruction: patient assessment: taking a patient's history, Am. J. Nurs. **74**(2):293-324, 1974.

Ryberg, J.W., and Merrifield, E.B.: Tuning in to parents' concerns, Child. Nurs. **2**(2):1-4, 1984.

Roznoy, M.S.: How to take a sexual history, Am. J. Nurs. **76**(8):1279-1282, 1976.

Shufer, S.: Communicating with young children: teaching via the play-discussion group, Am. J. Nurs. **77**:1960-1962, 1977.

Smith, E.C.: Communicating with young children: are you really communicating? Am. J. Nurs. **77**:1966-1967, 1977.

Wong, D.: Providing experience in physical assessment for students in basic programs, Am. J. Nurs. **75**(6):974-975, 1975.

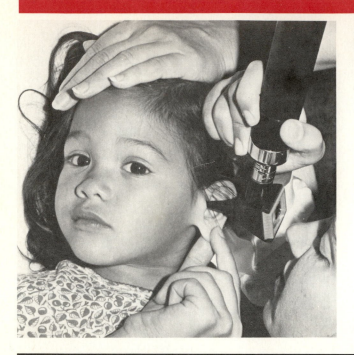

PHYSICAL ASSESSMENT OF THE CHILD

OBJECTIVES

On completion of this chapter the reader will be able to:

- Prepare a child for a physical examination based on his developmental needs

- Perform a physical examination in a sequence appropriate to the child's age

- Recognize expected normal findings for children at various ages

- Record the physical examination according to the traditional format

- Perform a developmental assessment using a standard screening test, such as the Denver Development Screening Test

NURSING DIAGNOSES

Nursing diagnoses identified for physical assessment of the child include, but are not restricted to, the following:

Health perception-health management pattern

- Infection, potential for, related to (1) improper handwashing; (2) improper care of instruments

- Injury, potential for, related to (1) incorrect use of instruments, (2) inattention to child's need for restraint

Cognitive-perceptual pattern

- Comfort, alterations in: pain related to (1) procedures; (2) positioning/restraint

- Thought processes, alteration in, related to sensory overload

Self-perception—self-concept pattern

- Anxiety related to (1) strange environment; (2) previous experiences; (3) perception of impending events; (4) anticipated discomfort; (5) knowledge deficit

Role-relationship pattern

- Communication, impaired verbal, related to (1) language barrier; (2) anxiety; (3) cultural factors

Coping-stress tolerance pattern

- Coping, ineffective individual, related to stress and/or anxiety

Physical assessment is a continuous process that begins during the interview, primarily by use of the tool of inspection or observation, and that continues to some degree through-out the professional relationship. While the format for organization of a systematic approach resembles that of a medical physical examination, the objective of each assessment area is to formulate nursing diagnoses and evaluate the effectiveness of interventions. Although the nurse may diagnose or assist in the establishment of a medical diagnosis, this is secondary to the primary goal of identifying patient problems.

This chapter discusses the influence of age in the preparation of children for physical examination, the performance of the examination, and the expected normal findings for children at various ages. It concludes with a discussion of developmental assessment and administration of the Denver Developmental Screening Test.

GENERAL APPROACHES TOWARD EXAMINING THE CHILD

Ordinarily the sequence for examining patients follows a head-to-toe direction. The main function of such a systematic approach is to provide a general guideline for assessment of each body area in order to minimize omitting segments of the examination. The standard recording of data also facilitates exchange of information among different professionals. The typical organization of a physical examination is listed here:

1. Growth measurements
   a. Height (length)
   b. Weight
   c. Head circumference
2. Physiologic measurements
   a. Temperature
   b. Pulse
   c. Respiration
   d. Blood pressure
3. General appearance
4. Skin
5. Lymph nodes
6. Head
7. Neck
8. Eyes
9. Ears
10. Nose
11. Mouth and throat
12. Chest
13. Lungs
14. Heart
15. Abdomen
16. Genitalia
17. Anus
18. Back and extremities
19. Neurologic assessment
   a. Cerebellar functioning
   b. Reflexes
   c. Cranial nerves
20. Developmental screening

In examining children, this orderly sequence is frequently altered to accommodate the child's developmental needs, although the examination is recorded following the traditional model. Using developmental and chronologic age as the main criteria for assessing each body system accomplishes several goals:

1. It minimizes stress and anxiety associated with assessment of various body parts.
2. It fosters a trusting nurse-child-parent relationship.
3. It allows for maximum preparation of the child.
4. It preserves the essential security of the parent-child relationship, especially with young children.
5. It maximizes the accuracy and reliability of assessment findings.

Certain behaviors signal readiness to cooperate, such as the child's willingness to talk to the nurse, make eye contact, accept the offered equipment, allow physical touching, smile, or choose to sit on the examining table rather than the parent's lap. Failure to observe these behaviors indicates a need to postpone the examination to allow the child to "warm up." Several approaches can be used to facilitate this:

1. Talk to the parent while essentially "ignoring" the child; gradually focus on him or a favorite object, such as a doll.
2. Make complimentary remarks about the child's dress and appearance.
3. Tell a funny story or play a simple trick.
4. Have a nonthreatening friend available, such as a hand puppet to "talk" for the nurse.
5. Allow choices whenever possible, such as, "Would you like to sit up on the table or in your mom's lap?"
6. Begin the examination with those activities that can be presented as games, such as tests for the cranial nerves (p. 127) or parts of the Denver Developmental Screening Test (DDST) (p. 126) and end with the more traumatic procedures, such as examining the ears and mouth.

Another approach that is effective in preparing the child for the examination is the "paper-doll technique." The child lies supine on the examining table and his length is measured by marking the end points of the head and heels on the paper. When he sits up, the nurse asks him to look at the two marks and suggests that the rest of him be filled in to see "how big" he is. Children are usually amazed to see their body outline and quickly become absorbed in drawing more parts. Consequently, before areas of the body are assessed, they can be drawn on the "paper doll" and "examined." For example, before auscultating the heart, the nurse can draw in the heart, "listen" to it on the paper, and then say to the child, "Let's listen to your heart and see what sound it makes" (Fig. 5-1). With older children the nurse can use a more detailed drawing to help them learn about their bodies. At the conclusion of the visit the child can bring the paper doll home as a memento of his experience.

Whatever approach is used, statements are made in a positive manner and in a tone of voice that says, "I expect you to cooperate." Suggestive statements, such as, "I am going to feel your belly but it won't hurt," are avoided, since the child immediately assumes it will hurt. Instead the nurse states what is going to be done and offers distractions, such as those suggested on p. 118.

Although the variations in the general approaches are numerous, some of them are elaborated here because they are more common. For example, the suggested sequence may change considerably when the child is in pain or when obvious physical defects are present. In either situation it is preferable to examine the affected area last to minimize distress early in the examination and to focus on normal, healthy, or functioning body parts rather than defective ones.

Positioning may also be altered because of physical distress. For example, the child who is having difficulty breathing may not be able to lie down, necessitating that as much of the physical examination as possible be performed in a sitting or slightly reclining position or that the examination be completed at another time.

Although parental presence is almost always conducive to a child's cooperation and sense of security, there are occasions when parents' anxiety increases the child's emotional distress or when older children prefer to be examined alone. In these instances it is best to request parents to leave the room before the examination begins. When the nurse and child are alone, the nurse can begin to establish rapport on a one-to-one basis by talking to or playing with the child and using appropriate preparatory measures rather than immediately initiating the examination. If the nurse judges that assistance may be needed, another person's help is enlisted.

Table 5-1 summarizes guidelines for positioning, preparing, and examining children at various ages. Since few children fit precisely into one category, it may be necessary to vary one's approach after a preliminary assessment of the child's development. For example, some preschoolers may require more of the "security measures" em-

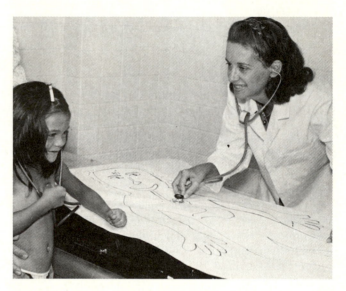

FIG. 5-1
Using paper-doll technique to prepare child.

TABLE 5-1. GENERAL APPROACHES TO PHYSICAL EXAMINATION DURING CHILDHOOD			
AGE	**POSITION**	**SEQUENCE**	**PREPARATION**
Infant	Before sits alone: supine or prone, preferably in parent's lap After sits alone: use this position whenever possible in parent's lap If on table, place with parent in full view	If quiet, auscultate heart, lungs, abdomen Record heart and respiratory rates Palpate and percuss same areas Proceed in usual head-toe direction Perform traumatic procedures last (eyes, ears, mouth [while crying], rectal temperature [if taken]) Elicit reflexes as body part examined Elicit Moro reflex last	Completely undress if room temperature permits Leave diaper on male Gain cooperation with distraction, bright objects, rattles, talking Smile at infant; use soft, gentle voice Pacify with bottle of sugar water or feeding Enlist parent's assistance for restraining to examine ears, mouth Avoid abrupt, jerky movements

TABLE 5-1. GENERAL APPROACHES TO PHYSICAL EXAMINATION DURING CHILDHOOD—cont'd

AGE	POSITION	SEQUENCE	PREPARATION
Toddler	Sitting or standing on/by parent Prone or supine in parent's lap	Inspect body area through play: "count fingers," "tickle toes" Use minimal physical contact initially Introduce equipment slowly Auscultate, percuss, palpate whenever quiet Perform traumatic procedures last (same as for infant)	Have parent remove outer clothing Remove underwear as body part examined Allow to inspect equipment; demonstrating use of equipment usually ineffective If uncooperative, perform procedures quickly Use restraint when appropriate; request parent's assistance Talk about examination if cooperative; use short phrases Praise for cooperative behavior
Preschool child	Prefer standing or sitting Usually cooperative prone/supine Prefer parent's closeness	If cooperative, proceed in head-toe direction If uncooperative, proceed as with toddler	Request self-undressing Allow to wear underpants if shy Offer equipment for inspection Briefly demonstrate use Make up "story" about procedure: "I'm taking blood pressure to see how strong muscles are" Use paper-doll technique Give choices when possible Expect cooperation; use positive statements: "Open your mouth"
School-age child	Prefer sitting Cooperative in most positions Younger age prefer parent's presence Older age may prefer privacy	Proceed in head-toe direction May examine genitalia last in older child Respect need for privacy	Request self-undressing Allow to wear underpants Give gown to wear Explain purpose of equipment and significance of procedure, such as otoscope to see eardrum, which is necessary for hearing Teach about body functioning and care
Adolescent	(Same as for school-age child) Offer option of parent's presence	(Same as older school-age child)	Allow to undress in private Give gown Expose only area to be examined Respect need for privacy Explain findings during examination: "Your muscles are firm and strong" Matter-of-factly comment about sexual development: "Your breasts are developing as they should be" Emphasize normalcy of development Examine genitalia quickly

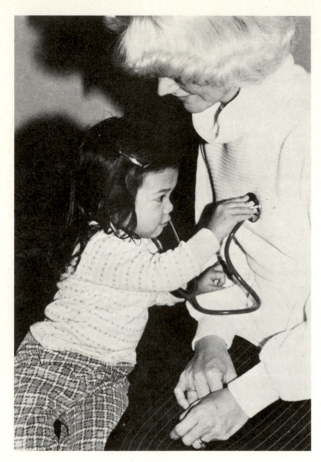

FIG. 5-2
Preparing the child for the physical examination.

ployed with younger children, such as performing the examination on the parent's lap, and less of the "preparatory measures," such as playing with the equipment (Fig. 5-2).

PHYSICAL EXAMINATION

Although the approach to and sequence of the physical examination differ according to the child's age, the following discussion outlines the traditional model for physical assessment. It emphasizes normal findings, indications for counseling, and general abnormalities that necessitate appropriate referral. While the focus includes all age-groups, the reader is referred to Chapter 6 for a discussion of newborn assessment.

Growth measurements

Measurement of physical growth in children is a key element in evaluation of the health status of children. Physical growth parameters include height (length), weight, and head circumference. Values are plotted on growth charts,

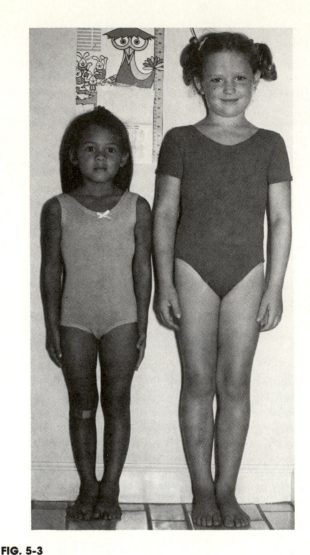

FIG. 5-3
These children of identical age (5¾ years) are markedly different in size. The child on the left, of part Oriental descent, is at 5th percentile for height and weight. The white child on the right is above 95th percentile for height and weight. However, both children demonstrate normal growth patterns.

and the child's measurements in percentiles are compared to those of the general population. Although some studies conclude that differences in height and weight among well-nourished children of different ethnic backgrounds are relatively small and that the present growth charts can be used for all racial or ethnic groups with a similar socioeconomic level, others demonstrate that ethnic differences are significant. For example, a comparison of the average growth of American and Chinese children demonstates that on the standard National Center for Health Statistics (NCHS) growth charts (see Appendix B), the average height and weight for Chinese children based on growth

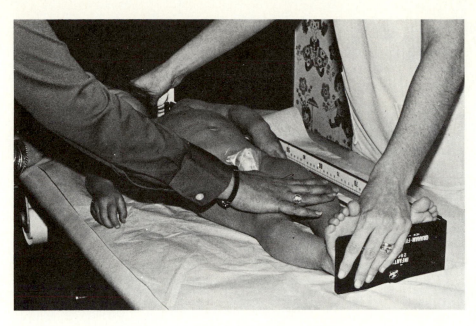

FIG. 5-4
Measurement of child's length.

standards from China (see Table B-1) falls on the 10th percentile, not the 50th percentile.

The growth charts listed in Appendix B use the 5th and 95th percentiles as criteria for determining which children fall outside the normal limits for growth. In general, those whose weight or height fall below the 5th percentile are considered underweight or small in stature; those whose height and weight fall above the 95th percentile are considered overweight or large in stature.

Overall evaluation of growth requires judgment in interpretation of growth percentiles. Children who fall above or below the standard deviation in both height and weight may not be abnormal but may reflect a genetically large or small frame (Fig. 5-3). Comparing their growth trends with those of their parents and siblings is essential in evaluating adequate growth. Children whose growth may be questionable include: (1) children whose height and weight percentiles are widely disparate, for example, height in the 10th percentile and weight in the 90th percentile may indicate that the child is overweight; (2) children who fail to show the expected gain in height and weight, especially during the rapid growth periods of infancy and adolescence; and (3) children who show a sudden increase or decrease in a previously steady growth pattern that is inappropriate for their age, such as puberty. Since growth is a continuous but uneven process, the most reliable evaluation lies in comparison of growth measurements over an extended period of time.

Length.   Until children are 24 months old, recumbent height or length is measured in the supine position. Because of their normally flexed position during infancy, measuring length requires full extension of the legs by (1) holding the head in midline, (2) grasping the knees to-

gether gently, and (3) pushing down on the knees until the legs are fully extended and flat against the table. If a measuring board is used, the head is placed firmly at the top of the board and the heels of the feet are placed firmly against the footboard (Fig. 5-4).

If such a measuring device is not available, the child's length is measured by placing him on a paper-covered surface, marking the end points of the top of the head and heels of the feet, and measuring between these two points. For accurate measurement the writing utensil is held at a right angle to the table when the cephalic point is marked and the feet are positioned with the toes pointing directly to the ceiling when the heel point is marked. Regardless of the method used, the parent's assistance in holding the child's head in midline should be enlisted while the nurse extends the legs and takes the measurements.

Height.   Recumbent or standing height may be taken in children who are over 24 months of age, although the latter is the usual procedure for those 3 years of age or older. Standing height is measured by having the child remove his shoes and stand as tall and straight as possible, with the head in midline and the line of vision parallel to the ceiling or floor. The child's back should be to the wall or other vertical flat surface, with the heels, buttocks, and back of the shoulders touching the wall. Any flexion of the knees, slumping of the shoulders, or raising of the heels of the feet are checked and corrected.

Height is measured by placing a firm, flat surface against the vertex or crown of the head. The movable measuring rod of platform scales is accurate only if it maintains a parallel position to the floor and rests securely on the topmost part of the head. One way of improvising a flat surface for measuring length is to attach a paper or

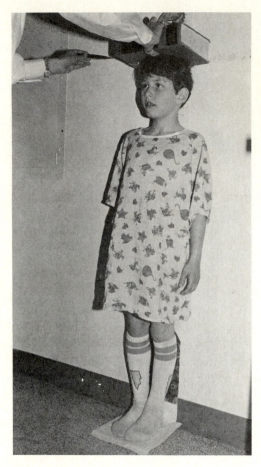

FIG. 5-5
Improvising for accurate measurement of height.

metal tape or yardstick to the wall, position the child adjacent to the tape, and place a thick book on the head, making sure that the end of the book rests firmly against the wall to form a right angle. The point of juncture of the underside of the book and the tape or yardstick is marked (Fig. 5-5). Length or stature should be measured to the nearest 1 mm or ⅛ inch.

Weight. Weight is measured using an appropriate-sized beam balance scale that measures weight to the nearest 10 g or ½ ounce for infants and 100 g or ¼ pound for children. Before weighing children, the scale is balanced by setting it at zero and noting if the balance registers exactly in the middle of the mark. If the end of the balance beam rises to the top or bottom of the mark, more or less weight, respectively, must be added. Some scales are designed to allow for self-correction, and others need to be recalibrated by the manufacturer.

Measurements should be made in a comfortably warm room. Infants are weighed nude; older children are usually weighed while wearing their underpants or a light gown in order to respect their need for privacy. If the child must be weighed wearing some article of clothing or some type of special device, such as a prosthesis, this is noted when the weight is recorded. Children who are measured for recumbent height are usually weighed on a large platform-type infant scale and placed in a lying-down or sitting position (Fig. 5-6, *A*). When weighing infants, the nurse places the hand slightly above the infant to prevent him from accidentally falling off the scale (Fig. 5-6, *B*). Once the standing height is taken, the weight can also be done on a standing-type upright platform scale. For maximum asepsis, scales are covered with a clean sheet of paper that is changed between each child's measurement.

Head circumference. Head circumference is usually taken in all children up to 36 months of age and in

FIG. 5-6
A, *Weighing a toddler on infant platform.* **B,** *Infant on scale.*

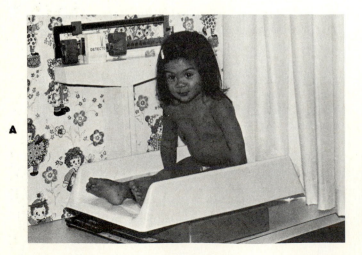

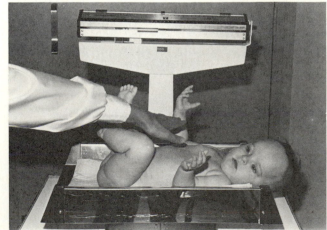

any child whose head size is questionable, such as a child with hydrocephalus. The head is measured at its greatest circumference, that is, slightly above the eyebrows and pinna of the ears and around the occipital prominence at the back of the skull (Fig. 5-7). A paper or metal tape is used since a cloth tape may stretch and give a false measurement. The head size is plotted on the growth chart under head circumference (see Appendix B). Generally head and chest circumference are equal at about 1 to 2 years of age. During childhood, chest circumference exceeds head size by about 5 to 7 cm (2 to 3 inches). (For head and chest circumference measurements of the newborn see p. 142.)

Physiologic measurements

Physiologic measurements include temperature, pulse, respiration, and blood pressure. Although not usually recorded on a graph similar to growth charts for determination of percentiles, each physiologic recording is compared with normal values for that age-group (see the inside front cover). In addition, values taken on preceding health visits should be compared with present recordings.

As in most procedures carried out with children, older children and adolescents are treated much the same as are adults. However, special consideration must be given to preschool children, whose fear of mutilation is intensified with any intrusive procedure (p. 313). Rectal temperatures are particularly threatening. When taking vital signs on infants, the usual order of approach is reversed for best results. That is, respirations are counted first, before the infant is disturbed, the pulse rate is measured next, and the rectal or axillary temperature is measured last. The tem-

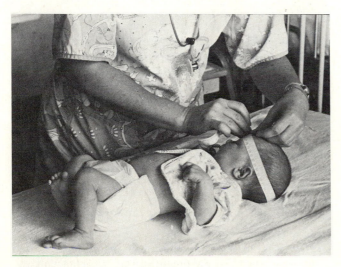

FIG. 5-7
Measuring head circumference.

perature, if taken first, is likely to initiate crying, which increases the respiratory rate and pulse. If the vital signs cannot be taken without disturbing the child, the child's behavior (e.g., crying) is recorded with the vital signs.

Temperature. Temperature can be taken by the oral, rectal, or axillary route. The only difference in selection of thermometers is that the rectal type has a rounded, blunt bulb as compared to the oral type, which has a slender, elongated tip. The newer electronic temperature-measuring equipment is ideally suited to pediatric use because the plastic sheath is unbreakable, because the child's mouth can remain open during an oral temperature reading, and because the temperature registers within seconds. Electronic thermometer measurement has been shown to be accurate for all three routes. When used to take an axillary temperature, it is an ideal substitute for intrusive rectal temperatures in young children.

Oral temperatures are taken in children who can be trusted to keep the thermometer under their tongue with their mouth closed without biting on the glass. Some institutions have set a specific age for permitting oral temperatures, such as after 5 or 6 years of age. In some instances even young preschoolers can cooperate.

When taking an oral temperature, the thermometer is placed under the tongue in the right or left posterior sublingual pocket, not in the area in front of the tongue. Contrary to traditional belief, the sublingual site indicates changes in core body temperature *better* than the rectum. The sublingual area has a rich blood supply derived from the carotid arteries, which are close to the temperature-regulating center in the brain and the central circulation at the heart.

Rectal temperatures may be indicated in infants and young children; in children whose mental age precludes understanding of instructions and cooperation; in unconscious, seriously ill, or agitated children; and in those children with oral injuries or surgery. To take a rectal temperature, children can be placed in a side-lying or prone position. A convenient position for infants is supine with the knees flexed toward the abdomen. This position is maintained with one hand while the other hand is used to insert the lubricated bulb of the thermometer (Fig. 5-8, *A*). The thermometer is inserted a maximum of 2.5 cm (1 inch). Further insertion increases the risk of perforation because the colon curves at a depth of about 3 cm (1¼ inches). It is advisable to cover the penis because this procedure often stimulates urination.

An alternative position that works very well, especially with toddlers because it preserves parental closeness and maintains an upright position, is to hold the child with his arms hugging the parent's neck and the legs wrapped around the parent's waist. With the child in this straddle position, the thermometer is gently inserted in the rectum.

Axillary temperatures are often recommended for chil-

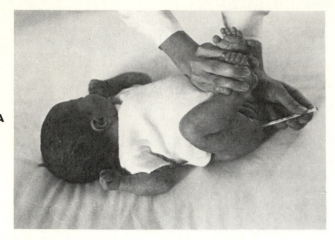
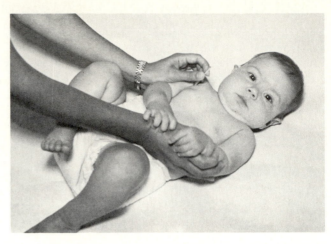

FIG. 5-8

A, *Position for taking rectal temperature in infant.* **B,** *Position for taking axillary temperature.*

dren who object strongly to a rectal temperature but on whom an oral temperature is not feasible. Axillary temperatures have the advantage of avoiding an intrusive procedure and eliminating the risk of rectal perforation and possible peritonitis. To take an axillary temperature, the thermometer is placed in the axilla with the arm kept close to the child's side (Fig. 5-8, *B*). Temperatures of newborn and premature infants are only taken by the axillary route.

There is no universal agreement regarding the length of time the thermometer should be kept in place; general recommendations are: 7 minutes for an oral reading; 4 minutes for a rectal reading; and 5 minutes for an axillary reading.

Normal body temperature registers 37.0° C (98.6° F) via the oral route. Traditionally it has been assumed that rectal temperatures are 1° F higher and axillary temperatures 1° F lower than oral temperatures. However, it has been demonstrated that this difference may be considerably less. Because of these variations, the route is charted along with the recorded temperature reading.

A characteristic of some small children is the tendency toward a rapid temperature elevation with the associated risk of precipitating seizures. Whenever a child feels extra warm to the touch, his temperature should be taken, even if it was found to be normal only a short time before. Children under 3 years of age are especially vulnerable to febrile seizures.

Pulse. A satisfactory pulse can be taken radially in children over 2 years of age. However, in infants and young children the apical pulse (heard through a stethoscope held to the chest at the apex of the heart) is more reliable. (See Fig. 5-34 for location of the apex and Fig. 5-35 for location of pulses.) The pulse is counted for 1 full minute in infants and young children because of pos-

sible irregularities in rhythm. (See the inside front cover for normal rates for pediatric age-groups.)

Respiration. The respiratory rate is counted in the same manner as it is in the adult patient except that, in infants, the movements are primarily diaphragmatic and, therefore, observed by abdominal movement. Since they are irregular, they should be counted for 1 full minute for accuracy (see also p. 111). (See the inside front cover for normal respiratory rates in children.)

Blood pressure. Blood pressure measurements are considered part of a routine vital sign determination in children 3 years of age and older. Blood pressure can be obtained by several techniques: palpation, auscultation, flush method, Doppler instrument, or an electronic monitoring device. Since the child should be quiet and relaxed during the procedure, the blood pressure is measured before any anxiety-producing procedures are performed. Infants and small children may be quiet if the reading is taken while they are sitting in the parent's lap. Children's cooperation can be enlisted if the equipment and each step of the procedure are explained and if they are told how it will feel to them.

There are no definite data to indicate that one position, sitting or supine, is superior to the other. However, the arm should be positioned at the level of the heart. If the arm is positioned below this point, gravity will add its pressure to the brachial artery pressure, producing falsely high readings.

Selection of cuff. Accurate measurement requires the use of an appropriately sized cuff. The width of the cuff should cover approximately two thirds of the upper arm (or thigh) or be 20% greater than the diameter of the extremity without causing pressure in the axilla or impinging on the antecubital fossa. In infants and young children

GUIDELINES FOR SELECTION OF BLOOD PRESSURE CUFFS		
	DIMENSIONS OF BLADDER (cm)	
AGE	WIDTH	LENGTH
Newborn	2.5-4	5-10
Infant	6-8	12-13.5
Child	9-10	17-22.5
Adult	12-13	22-23.5
Large adult arm	15.5	30
Adult thigh	18	36

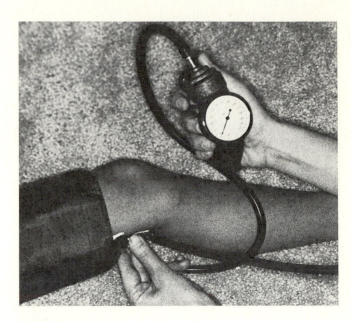

FIG. 5-9
Using the popliteal artery for blood pressure.

a cuff width greater than two-thirds the length of the upper arm is recommended. The length of the inflatable bladder inside the cuff should be long enough to sufficiently encircle the extremity without overlapping.

Ill-fitting cuffs are a common cause of incorrect blood pressure readings. A small cuff causes a falsely elevated reading. This may be a problem in the very obese child. Sometimes an adult thigh cuff may be needed for the severely obese adolescent, or the largest size arm cuff can be placed above the wrist and the radial artery used for auscultation or palpation. The systolic pressure in the radial artery is 10 mm Hg lower than in the brachial artery.

Generally a large cuff results in a falsely low reading. Compression of the brachial artery in the axilla by clothing pushed up the arm may also produce a falsely low reading. However, wide cuffs apparently do not cause the low readings observed in adults (Steinfeld and others, 1978). Therefore, when choosing cuff sizes, it is preferable to use an oversized cuff rather than an undersized one when the correct size is not available. Approximate guidelines for selection of cuff sizes are listed in the boxed material above, although the selection of a cuff must be individualized for each child. Guidelines are based on the range of cuff sizes sold by U.S. manufacturers. References to cuff size refer only to the inner inflatable bladder, not to the cloth covering, which can be considerably wider and longer than the bladder (Blumenthal and others, 1977).

Measurement. The technique of blood pressure measurement in children is generally the same as that used for adults. Thigh blood pressure can be taken on small children when only large cuffs are available. The cuff is wrapped around the thigh just above the knee and the popliteal artery is auscultated or palpated (Fig. 5-9). The pressure recorded in the thigh averages 10 mm Hg higher than the pressure recorded in the arm. A lower pressure in the lower extremities may indicate some interference with circulation such as coarctation of the aorta. The average blood pressure readings at various ages throughout childhood are listed on the inside back cover. For quick reference the following formula gives an approximate average systolic blood pressure for females ages 5 to 16 and males ages 5 to 18 years:

83 + (2.5 × Age in years) = Average systolic blood pressure

For children ages 2 to 4 years, the blood pressure is the same as that of the 5-year-old.

The blood pressure can be taken by the conventional *auscultation* method by listening for the sound at the brachial artery in the antecubital fossa. A systolic reading can be obtained by *palpation* and is measured as the point at which the pulse at the radial or brachial artery reappears as the cuff is deflated. A pediatric stethoscope with a small-diameter diaphragm and amplification is helpful for hearing blood pressure sounds in small children and infants. In some cases the *Doppler* instrument is used. This apparatus translates changes in ultrasound frequency caused by blood movement within the artery to audible sound by means of a transducer in the cuff.

In newborns (including premature infants) or in small infants whose pressure is difficult or impossible to obtain by other techniques, the *flush* method is employed. Although the flush blood pressure reflects the *mean* blood pressure (average of systolic and diastolic pressures), it has been found to correlate well with the mean aortic pressure in comparison tests. Although current standards for flush blood pressure readings have not been established for infants at all weights, a range of 30 to 60 mm Hg is considered normal for infants over 2500 g. The pressure of most larger infants is outlined on the inside back cover. A flush blood pressure determination is performed as follows:

1. Apply blood pressure cuff (usually 5 cm) to extremity.
2. Elevate extremity and wrap portion of extremity distal to cuff snugly with elastic bandage; wrap from fingers or toes toward cuff for complete capillary emptying.
3. Inflate cuff to 120 to 140 mm Hg.
4. Remove elastic bandage.
5. Gradually deflate cuff at the rate of approximately 5 mm/ second.
6. Read manometer at first full flush.

The point at which the earliest discernible flush is observed in the blanched extremity is considered the *flush end point* (Fig. 5-10). Although many nurses can blanch the extremity satisfactorily by applying compression with one hand while inflating the cuff with the other, greatest accuracy is achieved with the use of an elastic bandage.

General appearance

The general appearance of the child is a cumulative, subjective impression of the child's physical appearance, state of nutrition, behavior, and development. Although general appearance is recorded in the beginning of the physical examination, it encompasses all the observations of the child during the interview and physical assessment.

Physical appearance.   The description of physical appearance should make special note of *facies,* the facial expression and appearance of the child. For example, the facies may give clues to children who are in pain, have difficulty in breathing, or feel frightened. The child with low self-esteem or a feeling of rejection may assume a

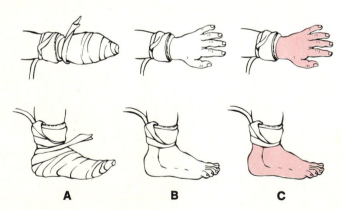

FIG. 5-10

*Indirect method of measuring blood pressure. **A,** Extremity wrapped with elastic bandage. **B,** Cuff inflated. **C,** Flush indicates return of circulation to extremity. (Color added.) (From Moss, A.J., and Adams, F.H.: Problems of blood pressure in childhood, Springfield, Ill., 1962, Charles C Thomas, Publisher.)*

slumped, careless, and apathetic type pose or posture. Likewise, a child with confidence, a feeling of self-worth, and a sense of security usually demonstrates a tall, straight, well-balanced posture. Although the nurse observes such ''body language,'' it must not be interpreted too freely but rather recorded objectively.

Posture, position, and types of body movement are also important in the overall assessment of physical appearance. The child with hearing or vision loss may characteristically tilt his head in an awkward position to facilitate perception of sound or sight. The child in pain may favor a body part.

Hygiene is noted in terms of cleanliness, unusual odor, the condition of the hair, neck, nails, teeth, and feet, and the condition of the clothing. Such observations give excellent clues to possible instances of neglect, inadequate financial resources, housing difficulties such as no running water, or lack of knowledge of children's needs.

Nutrition.   General appearance includes an overall impression of the child's state of nutrition. This impression is more than a statement describing body weight or stature, such as ''slender and tall.'' It is an estimation of the quality, as well as the quantity, of nutritional intake. For example, two children can be of the same height and weight, yet one can appear overweight because of flabby, loose skin, while the other child appears strong, robust, and well built because of firm, well-defined musculature.

The nurse's impression of nutritional state should be compared with the parents' history of feeding practices. Discrepancies between the two ''impressions'' may be a valuable area for nutritional counseling. For example, parents who believe that their child is too thin and eats too little, despite evidence of adequate growth and physical signs of proper nutrition, may find it helpful to keep a daily diary in order to calculate the child's cumulative food intake. When this is done, many parents are surprised at the quantity of food ingested, even though the amounts at each meal or snack are small.

Behavior.   Behavior includes the child's personality, level of activity, reaction to stress, requests, frustration, interactions with others (primarily the parent and nurse), degree of alertness, and response to stimuli. Some mental questions that serve as reminders for observing behavior include: What is the child's overall personality? Does he have a long attention span or is he easily distracted? Can he follow two or three commands in succession without the need for repetition? What is his response to delayed gratification or frustration? Does he use eye-to-eye contact during conversation? What is his reaction to the nurse and parents? Is he quick or slow to grasp explanations?

Development.   An overall estimate of the child's speech development, motor skills, degree of coordination, and recent area of achievement is recorded under general appearance. The impressions should be documented with screening tests, such as the Denver Developmental Screening Test (DDST) (see p. 126).

Skin

Skin is assessed for color, texture, temperature, moisture, and turgor. Examination of the skin and its accessory organs primarily involves inspection and palpation. The normal color in light-skinned children varies from a milky-white and rose color to a deep-hued pink color. Dark-skinned children, such as those from American Indian, Hispanic, or black descent, have inherited various brown, red, yellow, olive-green, and bluish tones in their skin. Oriental persons have skin that is normally of a yellow tone.

Normally the skin of young children is smooth, slightly dry to the touch, not oily or clammy, and of even exterior temperature. Skin temperature is evaluated by symmetrically feeling each part of the body and comparing upper areas with lower ones. Any distinct difference in temperature is noted.

Tissue turgor refers to the amount of elasticity in the skin. It is best determined by grasping the skin on the abdomen between the thumb and index finger, pulling it taut, and quickly releasing it. Elastic tissue immediately assumes its normal position without residual marks or creases. In children with poor skin turgor the skin remains suspended or tented for a few seconds before slowly falling back on the abdomen. Skin turgor is one of the best estimates of adequate hydration and nutrition.

Accessory organs. Inspection of the accessory organs of the skin, namely the hair, nails, and dermatoglyphics may be performed while the skin is being examined or when the scalp and extremities are being assessed.

Hair. The hair is inspected for color, texture, quality, distribution, and elasticity. Children's scalp hair is usually lustrous, silky, strong, and elastic. Genetic factors affect the appearance of hair. For example, the hair of black children is usually curlier and coarser than that of white children. Hair that is stringy, dull, brittle, dry, friable, and depigmented may suggest poor nutrition. Any bald or thinning spots are recorded. Loss of hair in infants may indicate lying in the same position and may be a clue for counseling parents concerning the child's stimulation needs.

The hair and scalp are inspected for general cleanliness. Various ethnic groups condition their hair with oils or lubricants, which, if not thoroughly washed from the scalp, clog the sebaceous glands, causing scalp infections. The hair and scalp are also examined for lesions, scaliness, evidence of infestation, such as lice or ticks, and signs of trauma, such as ecchymosis, masses, or scars.

In older children who are approaching puberty, growth of secondary hair is noted as signs of normally progressing pubertal changes (see p. 393). Precocious or delayed appearance of hair growth is noted because, although not always suggestive of hormonal dysfunction, it may be of great concern to the early- or late-maturing adolescent.

Nails. The nails are inspected for color, shape, texture, and quality. Normally the nails are pink, convex in shape, smooth, and hard but flexible (not brittle). The edges, which are usually white, should extend over the fingers. Dark-skinned individuals may have more deeply pigmented nail beds.

Dermatoglyphics. Each individual has a distinct set of handprints and footprints created by epidermal ridges and creases formed in the third month of prenatal life and cracks that develop subsequently throughout a lifetime. The patterns, or *dermatoglyphics,* are unique to the individual and vary a great deal in detail and complexity. The palm normally shows three flexion creases (Fig. 5-11, *A*). In some situations the two distal horizontal creases are fused to form a single horizontal crease called a *single palmar crease* or *simian crease* (Fig. 5-11, *B*), which is noted in almost all conditions that are caused by chromosomal abnormalities. If grossly abnormal lines or folds are observed, the nurse should sketch a picture to describe them and refer the finding to a specialist for further investigation.

Lymph nodes

Lymph nodes are usually assessed when the part of the body in which they are located is examined. Although the body's lymphatic drainage system is extensive, the usual sites for palpating accessible lymph nodes are shown in Fig. 5-12.

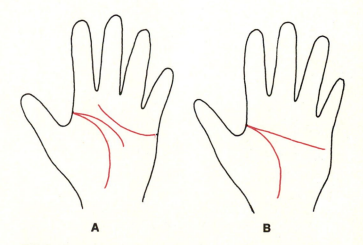

FIG. 5-11

Examples of flexion creases on the palm. **A,** *Normal.* **B,** *Simian line.*

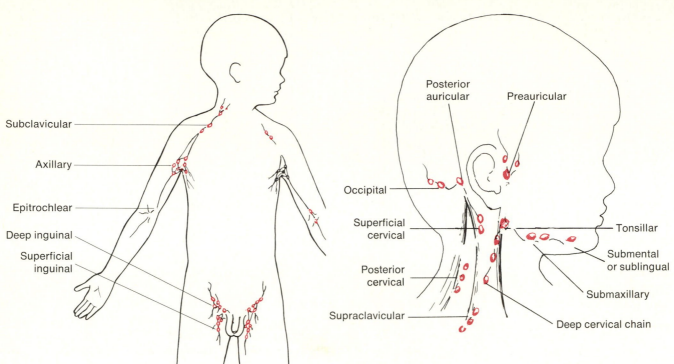

FIG. 5-12
Location of superficial lymph nodes.

Nodes are palpated by using the distal portion of the fingers and gently but firmly pressing in a circular motion along the regions where nodes are normally present. When assessing the nodes in the head and neck, the child's head is tilted upward slightly but without tensing the sternocleidomastoid or trapezius muscles. This position facilitates palpation of the *submental, submaxillary, tonsillar,* and *cervical* nodes. The *axillary* nodes are palpated with the arms relaxed at the side but slightly abducted. The *inguinal* nodes are best assessed with the child in the supine position. Size, mobility, temperature, and tenderness are noted, as well as reports by the parents regarding any visible change of enlarged nodes. In children small, nontender, movable nodes are usually normal. Tender, enlarged, warm lymph nodes generally indicate infection or inflammation proximal to their location. Such findings are reported for further investigation.

Head

The head is inspected for general *shape* and *symmetry*. It should be symmetrical with frontal, parietal, and occipital prominences. Oriental children have broader heads than children of other races.

Head control is noted in infants, and head posture is noted in older children. Most infants by 4 months of age should be able to hold the head erect and in midline when in a vertical position. Significant head lag after 6 months of age strongly suggests cerebral injury. Range of motion is evaluated by asking the older child to look in each direction (to either side, up, and down) or manually putting the younger child through each position.

The *skull* is palpated for patent sutures, fontanels, fractures, and swellings. The posterior fontanel normally closes by 2 months of age, and the anterior fontanel closes between 12 and 18 months of age (see Chapter 6).

Neck

Besides assessing motility of the head and neck, the neck is inspected for size and palpated for associated structures. The neck is normally short with skin folds between the head and shoulders during infancy; however, it lengthens during the next 3 to 4 years.

The *trachea* is palpated by placing the thumb and index finger on each side and sliding them back and forth to note any masses. Normally the trachea is in midline. Any shift from midline or questionable masses in the neck are recorded and reported for further investigation.

Eyes

Examination of the eyes involves inspection of all exterior structures for size, symmetry, color, and motility, and inspection of the interior surfaces for examination of retinal structures. The latter requires the use of an ophthalmoscope and is a highly skilled procedure. Discussion of the retinal examination includes the basic normal findings that the nurse should be able to discern with some practice in

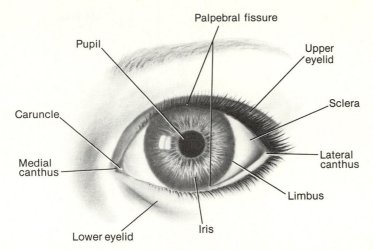

FIG. 5-13
External structures of the eye.

using the ophthalmoscope. The third part of the examination involves vision testing.

Inspection of external structures (Fig. 5-13). The *lids* are inspected for proper placement on the eye. When the eye is open, the upper lid should fall between the upper iris and the top portion of the pupil. When the eyes are closed, the lids should completely cover the cornea and sclera.

The general slant of the *palpebral fissures* or lids is inspected. The degree of slant is judged by drawing an imaginary line through the two points of the medial canthus and across the outer orbit of the eyes and aligning each eye on the line. Usually the palpebral fissures lie horizontally. However, in Oriental persons the slant is normally upward.

The lining of the lids, the *palpebral conjunctiva* is also inspected. Examining the lower conjunctival sac is easily accomplished by pulling the lid down while the patient looks up. To evert the upper lid, the child looks down while the nurse holds the upper lashes and gently pulls *down* and *forward*. Normally the conjunctiva appears pink and glossy. Vertical yellow striations along the edge are the meibomian or sebaceous glands near the hair follicle. Located in the inner or medial canthus and situated on the inner edge of the upper and lower lids is a tiny opening, called the lacrimal punctum. Any excessive tearing or inflammation of the lacrimal apparatus should be noted.

The *bulbar conjunctiva,* which covers the eye up to the limbus or junction of the cornea and sclera, should be transparent. The *sclera* or white covering of the eyeball should be clear. Tiny black marks in the sclera of heavily pigmented individuals are normal.

The *cornea,* or covering of the iris and pupil, should be clear and transparent. Any opacities are recorded since they can be signs of scarring or ulceration, which can interfere with vision. The best way to test for opacities is to illuminate the eyeball by shining a light at an angle (obliquely) toward the cornea.

The *pupils* are compared for size, shape, and movement. They should be round, clear, and equal. The nurse tests their *reaction to light* by quickly shining a source of light toward the eye and removing it. As the light approaches, the pupils should constrict; as the light fades, the pupils should dilate. *Accommodation,* or the focusing ability of the eyes to produce clear vision at different distances, is tested by having the child look at a bright, shiny object at a distance and quickly moving the object toward his face. The pupils should constrict as the object is brought near the eye. The normal findings when examining the pupils may be recorded as *PERRLA,* which means *pupils equal, round, react to light and accommodation.*

The *iris* is inspected for color, size, and clarity. Permanent eye color is usually established by 6 to 12 months of age. As the iris and pupil are inspected, the *lens* is also examined. Normally one should not see the lens while looking into the pupil.

Inspection of internal structures. The ophthalmoscope permits visualization of the interior of the eyeball with a system of lenses and a high-intensity light (Fig. 5-14). The lenses permit clear visualization of eye structures at different distances from the nurse's eye and correct visual acuity differences in the examiner and child. Use of the ophthalmoscope requires practice to know which lens setting produces the clearest image.

The ophthalmic and otic head are usually interchangeable on one "body" or handle, which encloses the power source, either disposable or rechargeable batteries. The nurse should practice changing the heads, which snap on and are secured with a quarter turn, and replacing the batteries and light bulbs. Nurses who are not directly involved in physical assessment are often responsible for assuring that the equipment functions properly.

Preparing the child. The child is prepared for the ophthalmic examination by showing him the instrument, demonstrating the light source and how it shines in the eye, explaining the reason for darkening the room, and

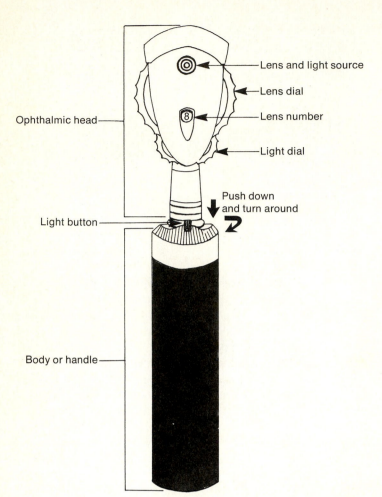

Lens and light source

Lens dial

Lens number

Light dial

Ophthalmic head

Push down
and turn around

Light button

Body or handle

FIG. 5-14
Ophthalmoscope.

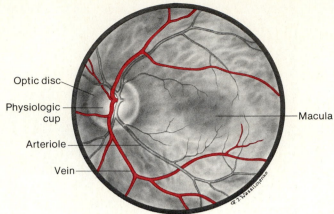

Optic disc

Physiologic
cup

Arteriole

Vein

Macula

FIG. 5-15
Structures of the fundus.

stressing that the procedure is not painful. For infants and young children who do not respond to such explanations, it is best to try and use distraction to encourage them to keep their eyes open. Forcibly parting the lids results in an uncooperative, watery-eyed child and a frustrated nurse. Usually, with some practice, the nurse can elicit a red reflex almost instantly while approaching the child and may also gain a momentary inspection of the blood vessels, macula, or optic disc.

The retinal examination. Fig. 5-15 illustrates the structures of the back of the eyeball or the *fundus*. In examining the interior of the eye, the nurse inspects the red reflex, the optic disc, the macula, and the blood vessels. It is important to remember that the ophthalmoscope permits only a small area of visualization. In order to perform an adequate examination, the nurse must move the ophthalmoscope systematically around the fundus to locate each structure.

The fundus derives its orange-red color from the inner two layers of the eye, the choroid and the retina, which are immediately apparent as the *red reflex*. The intensity

of the orange-red color increases in darkly pigmented individuals. A brilliant, uniform red reflex is an important sign, because it virtually rules out almost all serious defects of the cornea, aqueous chamber, lens, and vitreous chamber. Any dark shadows or opacities are recorded because they usually indicate some abnormality in any of these structures.

As the nurse approaches the child with the ophthalmoscope, the most conspicuous feature of the fundus is the *optic disc*, the area where the blood vessels and optic nerve fibers enter and exit from the eye. The color of the disc is creamy pink; it is lighter in color than the surrounding fundus. It derives its color from the rich capillary network. It is normally round or vertically oval. Its size is important because other structures of the fundus are measured in relationship to the disc's diameter (DD). Most discs have a small, pale depression in their center, called the *physiologic cup or depression,* which represents the blind spot of the retina. It is not always visible but, when large enough to be seen, should not extend to the disc margin.

After locating the optic disc, the area is inspected for *blood vessels*. The central retinal artery and vein appear in the depths of the disc and emanate outward with visible branching. The *veins* are darker in color and about one fourth larger in size than the *arteries*. Normally the branches of the arteries and veins cross each other.

About 2 DD temporal to the disc is the *macula,* the area of the fundus with the greatest concentration of visual receptors. It is about 1 DD in size and darker in color than the fundus (red reflex) or optic disc. The intensity of the color directly correlates with the individual's skin pigmentation, that is, the darker the skin, the darker the color of the macula. In the center of the macula is a minute glistening spot of reflected light called the *fovea centralis*. It is the area of most perfect vision. If locating the macula is difficult, the child should be asked to look directly at the

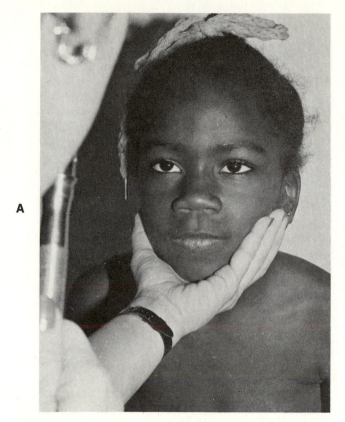 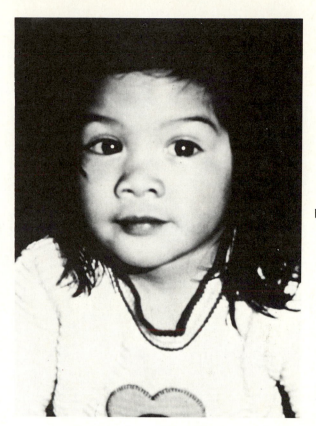

FIG. 5-16

A, *Corneal light reflex test demonstrating orthophoric eyes.* **B,** *Pseudostrabismus.*

light. However, since this is the most light-sensitive area of the retina, the nurse must be careful to focus on the macula only momentarily.

Vision testing. Several tests are available for assessing vision. This discussion focuses on four areas of vision testing: (1) binocularity, (2) visual acuity, (3) peripheral vision, and (4) color vision. The reader is referred to Chapter 17 for behavioral and physical signs that indicate visual impairment.

Binocularity. Normally, by the age of 3 to 4 months, children achieve the ability to fixate on one visual field with both eyes simultaneously (binocularity). One of the most important tests for binocularity is alignment of the eyes to detect nonbinocular vision or strabismus. In strabismus, or "cross-eye," one eye deviates from the point of fixation. If the malalignment is constant, the weak eye becomes "lazy," and the brain eventually suppresses the image produced by that eye (suppression scotoma). If strabismus is not detected and corrected by age 4 to 6 years, blindness, called *amblyopia,* may result.

Two tests commonly used to detect malalignment are the corneal light reflex test and the cover test. In the *corneal light reflex test* the nurse shines a flashlight or the light of the ophthalmoscope directly into the patient's eyes

from a distance of about 40.5 cm (16 inches). If the eyes are *orthophoric* or normal, the light falls perfectly symmetrically within each pupil (Fig. 5-16, *A*). If the light falls off center in one eye, the eyes are malaligned. *Epicanthal folds,* excess folds of skin that extend from the roof of the nose to the inner termination of the eyebrow and that partially or completely overlap the inner canthus of the eye, may give a false impression of malalignment (pseudostrabismus) (Fig. 5-16, *B*). Epicanthal folds are frequently found in Oriental children of Asiatic descent. When testing these children, one carefully observes the light reflection to rule out pseudostrabismus.

In the *cover test* one eye is covered and the movement of the *uncovered* eye is observed while the child fixes his gaze on a near (33 cm or 13 inches) or distant (50 cm or 20 inches) object. If the uncovered eye does not move, it is aligned. If the uncovered eye moves, a malalignment is present because when the stronger eye is temporarily covered, the weaker eye attempts to fixate on the object.

In the *alternate cover test* the nurse shifts occlusion back and forth from one eye to the other eye and observes movement of the *covered* eye while the child focuses on a point in front of him. If normal alignment is present, shifting the cover from one eye to the other eye will not cause

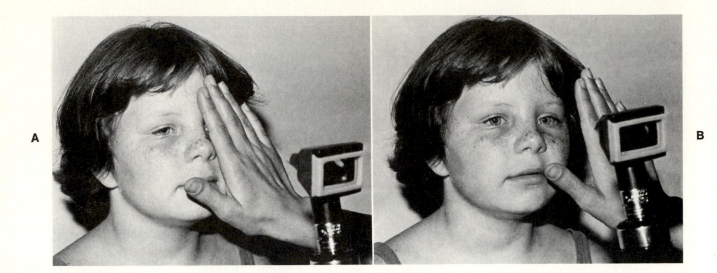

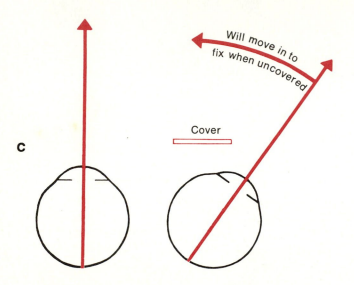

FIG. 5-17

*Alternate cover test for strabismus. **A,** Eye is occluded; child is fixating on a light source. **B,** If eye does not move when uncovered, eyes are aligned. **C,** Malalignment. As eye is uncovered it shifts to fixate on an object. (**C** adapted from Prior, J.A., Silberstein, J.S., and Stang, J.M.: Physical diagnosis: the history and examination of the patient, ed. 6, St. Louis, 1981, The C.V. Mosby Co.)*

movement of the covered eye. If malalignment is present, the covered eye will move from its position when covered to a straight position when uncovered. This test takes more practice than the other cover test because the nurse must move the occluder back and forth quickly and accurately in order to see the eye move. It is usually easier to perform this test by using one's hand rather than a card or other object as the occluder (Fig. 5-17). Since deviations can occur at different ranges it is important to perform the cover tests at both close and far distances.

Visual acuity. Visual acuity refers to the ability to see near and far objects clearly. The most common test for measuring visual acuity is the *Snellen alphabet chart* (see Appendix C). It consists of nine lines of letters in decreasing size. Each line is given a value, for example, line 8 is "20." The person to be tested stands 20 feet from the chart and reads each line. If he can read line 8, he has 20/20 vision, the accepted standard for normal acuity. If the person can only read line 2, he has 20/100 vision. That

means that what he is able to see at a distance of 20 feet, the person with 20/20 or normal eyesight can see at 100 feet. This test is suitable for most children above the third grade, who are familiar with the alphabet.

The 20-foot distance for measuring visual acuity is not a strict requirement and young children are often more attentive at closer range. If screening is done at a distance other than 20 feet with the appropriate chart an equivalent measurement is used. For example, in screening with the 10-foot chart the equivalent measurement for 20/40 is 10/20.

Another version of the Snellen chart is the *Snellen E Chart,* which uses the capital letter E pointing in four different directions. The child "reads" the chart by showing the direction of the letter E or the "legs of the table" either by pointing with his hand or by verbally identifying the direction, such as "toward the ceiling, floor, window, or wall." Preschoolers may have difficulty with this test because of confusion in identifying the direction rather than inability to see clearly. This can be corrected by giving them a large duplicate letter E and having them turn it to match the letter on the chart. The Snellen E Chart is available for home vision screening from the National Society to Prevent Blindness,* which recommends its use for children between preschool age and 6 years of age.

The National Society to Prevent Blindness (1982) recommends the following criteria for referring children when using the Snellen charts:

1. Three-year-old children with vision in either eye of 20/50 or less (inability to correctly identify one more than half the symbols on the 40-foot line) *or* a two-line difference in visual acuity between the eyes in the passing range; for example, 20/20 in one eye and 20/40 in the other
2. All other ages and grades with vision in either eye of 20/40 or less (inability to correctly identify one more than half the symbols on the 30-foot line)
3. All children who consistently show any of the signs of possible visual disturbances, regardless of visual acuity

Another test that is suitable for children age 2½ years and older is the *Denver Eye Screening Test* (DEST) (see Appendix C). It tests for visual acuity in children 3 years or older by using a single card for the letter E, and it tests from a distance of 15 feet, rather than 20 feet. The large E (20/100) is used primarily for explanation and demonstration of the procedure to the child. The small E (20/30) is used for testing. Failure to correctly identify the direction of the small E over three trials is considered abnormal. As with every other vision screening test, each eye is tested separately.

For children from 2½ to 2¹¹⁄₁₂ years of age or those who are untestable with the DEST letter E test, picture cards (or Allen cards) are used. Although the DEST is recommended for children beginning at age 30 months, the Allen cards can be used reliably with cooperative children from the age of 24 months. The pictures (a tree, birthday cake, horse and rider, telephone, car, house, and teddy bear) are shown to the child at close range to make certain that he can readily identify them and then are shown at a distance of 15 feet. If the child cannot correctly name three of the seven cards in three to five trials, his performance is considered abnormal.

The DEST also screens children from 6 to 30 months of age who may be at risk for visual problems by testing for (1) fixation (ability to follow a moving light source or spinning toy), (2) squinting (observation of the child's eyes or report by parent), and (3) strabismus (report by parent and performance on cover and pupillary light reflex tests). Abnormal findings include failure to fixate, pres-

ence of a squint, and/or failing two of the three procedures for strabismus.

In newborns, vision is tested mainly by checking for *light perception*; this done by shining a light into the eyes and noting responses such as blinking, following the light to midline, increased alertness, or refusing to open the eyes after exposure to the light. Vision can also be tested in an alert newborn by rotating a striped drum in front of his face and noting nystagmus, which indicates that vision is present. A more sophisticated and accurate test is the *visually evoked response (VER)*, which is determined by stimulating the eyes with a bright light and recording electrical activity through scalp electrodes placed on the head over the visual cortex.

Peripheral vision. In a child who is old enough to cooperate, peripheral vision, or the visual field of each eye, is estimated. The test is performed by having the child fixate on a specific point directly in front of him as an object, such as a finger or a pencil, is moved from beyond the field of vision into the range of peripheral vision. Each eye is checked separately and for each quadrant of vision. As soon as the child sees the object, he tells the nurse to stop moving it. At that point the angle from the anteroposterior axis of the eye (straight line of vision) to the peripheral axis (point at which the object is first seen) is measured. Normally the child sees about 50 degrees upward, 70 degrees downward, 60 degrees nasalward, and 90 degrees temporally. Limitations in peripheral vision may be indicative of blindness from damage to structures within the eye or to any of the visual pathways.

Color vision. Another important test is for color vision. It is estimated that from 6% to 8% of white males (1 in 17 to 1 in 13) and about half that percentage of black males have inherited the X-linked disorder known as *color blindness*. The two common types of impaired perception of color are confusion among browns, red, and black or among greens, browns, purples, and grays. Some of the difficulties encountered by these individuals in everyday life may be an inability to distinguish amber or red traffic lights, failure to see a red brake light on the rear of a car, difficulty in distinguishing green traffic lights from certain types of incandescent street lamps, and a poor sense of color coordination of clothing. For school-age children the greatest difficulty lies in performance of academic skills that use color as a visual aid. Adolescents who are color blind are ineligible for certain vocational opportunities, such as electrical careers, which use color coding of wires, and for several types of military service.

The tests available for color vision include the *Ishihara* test and the *Hardy-Rand-Rittler* (HRR) test. Each consists of a series of cards on which is printed a colored field composed of spots of a certain "confusion" color. Against the field is a letter or figure similarly printed in dots but of a color likely to be confused with the field

---

*The National Society to Prevent Blindness, 79 Madison Avenue, New York, NY 10016. Also available is an excellent book on vision screening for preschoolers and school age children entitled *Children's eye health guide*.

color by the color-blind person. As a result the figure or letter is invisible to an affected individual but is clearly seen by an unaffected person. Nurses administering the test must be familiar with the testing materials and should be able to inform the parents of the disorder's effects on practical areas of living, its genetic transmission, and its irreversibility.

Ears

Like the eyes, examination of the ears involves inspection of the external auditory structures, visualization of the internal landmarks using a special instrument called the otoscope, and screening for hearing ability.

Inspection of external structures.   The entire external earlobe is called the *pinna* or *auricle* and is located on each side of the head. The *height* alignment of the pinna is measured by drawing an imaginary line from the outer orbit of the eye to the occiput or most prominent protuberance of the skull. The top of the pinna should meet or cross this line. The *angle* of the pinna is measured by drawing a perpendicular line from the imaginary horizontal line and aligning the pinna next to this mark. Normally the pinna lies within a 10-degree angle of the vertical line (Fig. 5-18). If it falls outside this area, the deviation is recorded.

Normally the pinna extends slightly outward from the skull. Except in newborn infants, ears that are flat against the head or protruding away from the scalp may indicate problems. Flattened ears in infants may suggest a frequent side-lying position and, just as with isolated areas of hair loss, may be a clue to investigating parents' understanding of the child's stimulation needs.

The *skin* surface around the ear is inspected for small openings, extra tags of skin, or sinuses. If a sinus is found,

a special notation is made, since it may represent a fistula that drains into some area of the neck or ear. Cutaneous tags represent no pathologic process but may cause parents concern in terms of the child's appearance.

The ear is also assessed for general *hygiene*. An otoscope is not necessary for looking into the external canal to note the presence of cerumen, a waxy substance produced by the ceruminous glands in the outer portion of the canal. Cerumen is usually yellow-brown and soft. If an otoscope is used and any discharge is seen, its color and odor are noted. Care is taken to prevent transmitting potentially infectious material to the other ear or to another child. Handwashing and changing otic specula are essential preventive measures. Disposable specula are also available.

Inspection of internal structures.   The otic head permits visualization of the tympanic membrane by use of a bright light, a magnifying glass, and a speculum (Fig. 5-19). The speculum, which is inserted into the external canal, comes in a variety of sizes (2, 3, 4, and 5 mm) to accommodate different canal widths. The largest speculum that fits comfortably into the ear is used in order to achieve the greatest area of visualization. The lens or magnifying glass is movable, allowing the examiner to insert an object, such as a curette, into the ear canal through the speculum while still viewing the structures through the lens.

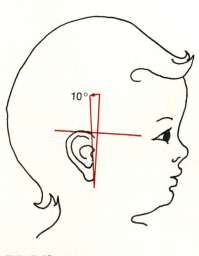

FIG. 5-18
Ear alignment.

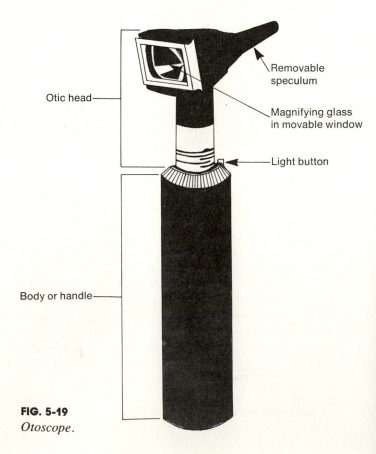

FIG. 5-19
Otoscope.

The handle is the same as for the ophthalmic head and operates similarly. The nurse should become familiar with the instrument and practice attaching the speculum securely to the head.

Positioning the child. Before beginning the otoscopic examination, the nurse positions the child. Older children are usually cooperative and need no type of restraint. They should, however, be prepared for the procedure by allowing them to play with the instrument, demonstrating how it works, and impressing upon them the need to remain still. It may be helpful to let them observe the nurse examine the parent's ear. The nurse can let older children view the inside of the ear. With younger children the nurse can explain that she is looking for a "big elephant" in the ear. This kind of "fairy tale" is an absorbing distraction and usually elicits ready cooperation. After examining the ear, it is important to clarify that "looking for elephants" was only pretending. As the speculum is inserted into the meatus, it should be moved around the outer rim to accustom the child to the feel of something entering the ear.

For their protection and safety infants and toddlers cannot be trusted to remain still, regardless of their former degree of cooperation. There are two general positions of restraint. In one the child is seated sideways in the parent's lap with one arm "hugging" the parent and the other arm at his side. The ear to be examined is toward the nurse. With one arm the parent holds the child's head firmly against his or her chest, and with the other arm "hugs" the child, thereby securing the child's free arm. The nurse

then examines the ear using the same procedure in holding the otoscope as described in the section that follows (Fig. 5-20, *A*).

The other position involves placing the child on his side or abdomen with his arms at his side and his head turned so that the ear to be examined points toward the ceiling. The nurse leans over the child and uses the upper part of the body to restrain his arms and upper trunk movements and the examining hand to stabilize his head. This position is practical for young infants or for older children who need minimal restraining, but it may not be feasible for other children who protest vigorously. For safety the nurse should enlist the parent's help in immobilizing the head by firmly placing one hand above the ear and the other on the child's back or side (Fig. 5-20, *B*).

Manipulating the otoscope. With the thumb and forefinger of the free hand, the nurse grasps the auricle. For either of the two positions of restraint, the otoscope is held upside down at the junction of its head and handle with the thumb and index finger. The other fingers are placed against the skull to allow the otoscope to move with the child in case he moves suddenly. In examining a cooperative child, the handle is held between the thumb and index finger with the otic head upright or upside down. The other fingers are still placed against the child's head to detect unexpected movement (see Fig. 5-20).

Entering the canal. Before entering the canal, one should imagine that the external ear and the tympanic membrane are superimposed on a clock (see Fig. 5-23). The numbers become important geographic landmarks.

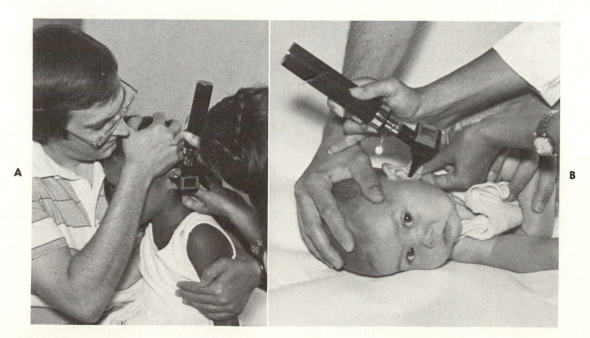

FIG. 5-20
Positions for restraining **A,** *child, and* **B,** *infant, during otoscopic examination.*

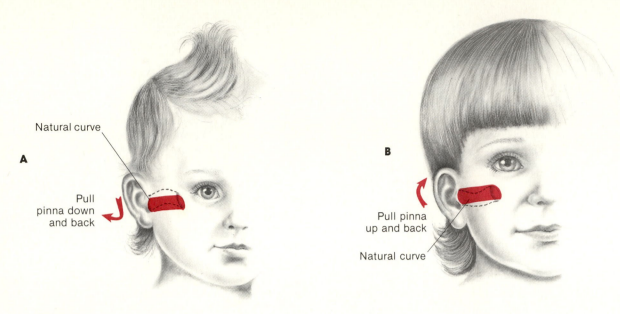

A Natural curve

Pull pinna down and back

B Pull pinna up and back

Natural curve

FIG. 5-21

Position of eardrum in **A**, *infant, and* **B**, *child over 3 years of age.*

The speculum is introduced into the meatus between the 3 and 9 o'clock positions in a downward and forward position. Because the canal is curved, the speculum does not permit a panoramic view of the tympanic membrane unless the canal is straightened. In infants the canal curves upward and the tympanic membrane lies almost horizontally along the upper wall of the canal. The pinna must be pulled *downward* and *backward* to the 6 to 9 o'clock range, which retracts the canal and the drum downward (Fig. 5-21, *A*).

With older children, usually those over 3 years of age, the canal curves downward and forward, and the drum, although more vertical, slopes inward and forward. Therefore the pinna is pulled *upward* and *backward* toward a 10 o'clock position (Fig. 5-21, *B*). The head is tilted slightly away from the nurse or toward the child's opposite shoulder to bring the drum into a 90-degree angle (Fig. 5-22). Proper positioning of the head is essential in achieving a full view of the membrane. If there is difficulty in visualizing the membrane, it can be brought into view by repositioning the head, introducing the speculum at a different angle, and pulling the pinna in a slightly different direction.

In neonates and young infants the walls of the canals are pliable and floppy because of the underdeveloped cartilaginous and bony structures. Therefore the very small 2 mm speculum usually needs to be inserted deeper into the canal than in older children. Great care must be exercised not to damage the walls or drum. For this reason, only an experienced examiner should insert an otoscope into the ears of very young infants.

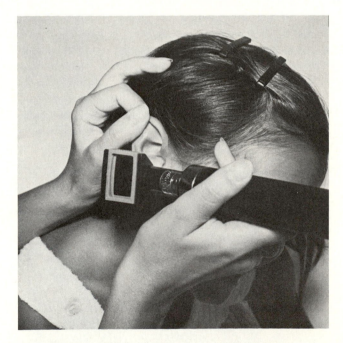

FIG. 5-22

Positioning head by tilting it toward opposite shoulder for full view of tympanic membrane.

Otoscopic examination. As the speculum is introduced into the external canal, the walls of the canal, the color of the tympanic membrane, the light reflex, and the usual landmarks of the bony prominences of the middle ear are noted. Fig. 5-23 illustrates the usual view of the tympanic membrane.

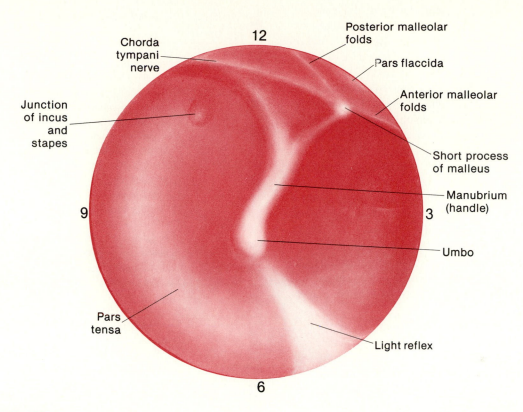

FIG. 5-23

Usual landmarks of right tympanic membrane with "clock" superimposed.

The *walls* of the external auditory canal are usually pink in color, although they are normally more pigmented in dark-skinned children. Minute hairs are evident in the outermost portion, where cerumen is produced.

The color of the *tympanic membrane* is normally a translucent light pearly pink or gray color. The characteristic tenseness and slope of the tympanic membrane causes the light of the otoscope to reflect at about the 5 or 7 o'clock position. The *light reflex* is a fairly well-defined cone-shaped reflection, which normally points away from the face.

The *bony landmarks* of the drum are formed by the *umbo,* or long arm of the malleus bone, which appears as a small, round, opaque concave spot near the center of the drum. The *manubrium,* the long process or handle of the malleus, appears as a whitish line extending from the umbo upward to the margin of the membrane. At the upper end of the long process near the 1 o'clock position is a sharp knoblike protuberance, representing the *short process* of the malleus. Absence of the light reflex or loss of any of these landmarks is always reported for further evaluation.

Auditory testing. Several types of hearing tests are available. Some of them, such as audiometric testing, use specialized equipment that measures the degree of hearing loss. Others, such as tests for the startle reflex in neonates, are rough estimations of perception of sound. The nurse must operate under a high index of suspicion for those children who may have conditions associated with hearing loss and who may have developed behaviors indicative of auditory impairment. Types, causes, clinical manifestations, and appropriate treatment of hearing loss are discussed in Chapter 17.

Audiometry. In audiometry an electrical instrument called an audiometer measures the threshold of hearing for pure-tone frequencies and loudness. A given sound is transmitted to the child's ear and is reduced until no longer heard. The child indicates when this point is reached and the intensity of the sound is recorded on graph paper (audiogram). This procedure is repeated for several sounds covering the range found in conversation. When an air conduction audiogram is being recorded, the sounds are transmitted through earphones. With bone conduction the sounds are passed through a plaque placed over the mastoid bone. Since the child is listening to very soft sounds, the audiogram is performed in a soundproof room.

The pure-tone audiogram provides valuable information regarding the severity of the hearing loss, the sound cycles involved, and the possible location of the defect. However, it requires specialized training of personnel, expensive equipment, and cooperation from the child in terms of confirming the perception of sound. Usually by preschool age audiometry can be performed.

Tympanometry. Another specialized test is *acoustic impedance* measurements or *tympanometry*. This technique measures tympanic membrane compliance (or mobility) and estimates middle ear air pressure. It is suitable for infants, young children, and those who are difficult to test by other methods because little cooperation is necessary, and the procedure is not painful. Like audiometry, this technique requires special equipment, although minimal training is necessary for the procedure. This test detects middle ear disease and abnormalities but does not indicate the degree of hearing loss or the interpretation of sound.

Clinical hearing tests. The following are tests that are more applicable for routine screening, that can be easily administered by the nurse, and that indicate the perception and interpretation of sound.

In newborns, hearing is best determined by eliciting the *startle reflex* (p. 150). Nurses also observe other neonatal responses to loud noises, such as facial grimaces, blinking, gross motor movements, quieting if crying or crying if quiet, opening the eyes, or ceasing sucking activity. An objective sign may be an increase in heart or respiratory rate following a loud noise. Absence of such alerting behaviors suggests a hearing loss.

During infancy the nurse can test hearing by making a noise and noting the child's specific reaction to *localization of sound*. The nurse stands about 18 inches away from the child, to the side, and out of his peripheral field of vision. With the room silent and the child sitting contentedly in his parent's lap, distracted by a toy or other object, the nurse makes a voice sound, such as PS or PHTH, which is high-pitched, or OO, which is low-pitched, rings a bell or a rattle, or rustles tissue paper. The child's response in terms of localizing the sound is compared to the expected age response (see the box on this page). This test is usually inadequate for toddlers and preschoolers because of less cooperation and the learned response to willingly inhibit sounds.

Brainstem-evoked response (BSER). In an attempt to objectively assess hearing in newborns and other hard-to-test children, a complex and expensive method called brainstem-evoked response audiometry has been developed. Through electrode wires attached to the infant's scalp, electrical or brain wave potentials generated within the auditory system are picked up and fed to a computer. Following repetitive acoustic stimulation, the average computer waveforms from a normal sleeping or quiet infant consist of several peaks and valleys that reflect activations of neural structures of the brain. This BSER audi-

MAJOR DEVELOPMENTAL CHARACTERISTICS OF HEARING

AGE (weeks)	DEVELOPMENT
Birth	Responds to loud noise by startle reflex
	Responds to sound of human voice more readily than to any other sound
	Low-pitched sounds, such as lullaby, metronome, or heartbeat, have quieting effect
8-12	Turns head to side when sound is made at level of ear
12-16	Locates sound by turning head to side and looking in same direction
16-24	Can localize sounds made below ear, which is followed by localization of sound made above ear; will turn head to the side and then look up or down
24-32	Locates sounds by turning head in a curving arc
	Responds to own name
32-40	Localizes sounds by turning head diagonally and directly toward sound
40-52	Learns to control and adjust own response to sound, such as listening for the sound to occur again

Adapted from Illingworth, R.S.: The development of the infant and young child, ed. 7, New York, 1980, Churchill Livingstone.

ogram is analyzed by a specially trained technician to determine the threshold of hearing response.

Crib-o-gram. The Crib-o-gram* is another neonatal screening tool. It analyzes hearing responses by comparing the infant's motor activity before, during, and after a sound is introduced. Both administration of the test and its scoring are totally automated. A motion-sensitive transducer is placed beneath the crib or Isolette mattress, and a microprocessor "reads" the infant's movement. A change in activity that coincides with the test sound is scored as a "pass." The sequence is repeated several times to assure reliability.

Conduction tests. Two tests are also used to distinguish between air and bone conduction—Rinne test and Weber's test. In air conduction sound is transmitted to the brain through the external, middle, and inner ear structures. In bone conduction the sound bypasses the external and middle ear and is transmitted to the brain through the mastoid bone to the inner ear structures and auditory nerve. Normally air conduction is considerably better than bone conduction.

In the *Rinne test* the stem of the tuning fork is placed

---

*Manufactured by Telesensory Systems, Inc., Palo Alto, CA 94304.

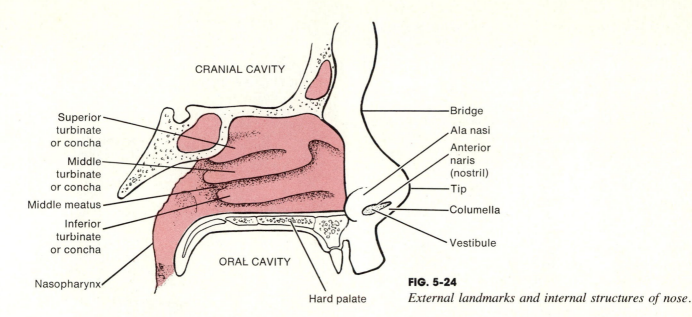

CRANIAL CAVITY

Superior turbinate or concha

Middle turbinate or concha

Middle meatus

Inferior turbinate or concha

Nasopharynx

ORAL CAVITY

Hard palate

Bridge

Ala nasi

Anterior naris (nostril)

Tip

Columella

Vestibule

FIG. 5-24

External landmarks and internal structures of nose.

against the mastoid bone until the sound ceases to be audible. It is then moved so that the prongs are held near, but not touching, the auditory meatus. The child should again hear the sound (Rinne positive). If the sound is not again audible (Rinne negative), some abnormality is interfering with the conduction of air through the external and middle ear chambers. This test requires the cooperation and ability of the child to signal when the sound is no longer audible and when it is again heard. It is not useful for most children before preschool age.

In *Weber's test* the stem of the tuning fork is held in the midline of the head. The child should hear the sound equally in both ears (Weber positive). With air conductive loss he will hear the sound better in the *affected* ear (Weber negative). This test is frequently not suitable for young children because of their difficulty in discriminating between "better, more, or less." Any child who is suspected of a hearing loss because of poor performance using any of these tests is referred for special audiometric testing.

Nose

The nose marks the beginning of the passageway through the respiratory tract. It is an important organ for filtration, temperature control, and humidification of inspired air, as well as a sensory organ for olfaction (smell). Each of these functions depends on the patency of the passageways and on the mucosal lining of the nasal cavity. Inspection is primarily used to assess the external and internal structures.

Inspection of external structures. The nose is located in the middle of the face just below the eyes and above the lips. Its placement and alignment can be compared by drawing an imaginary vertical line from the center point between the eyes down to the notch of the upper lip. The nose should lie exactly vertical to this line and each side should be symmetric. Its location, any deviation to one side, and asymmetry in overall size and in diameter of the nares (nostrils) are noted. The bridge of the nose is sometimes flat in black children or in children of Oriental descent. The alae nasi are observed for any sign of flaring, which may indicate respiratory difficulty. Fig. 5-24 illustrates the usual landmarks used in describing the external structures of the nose.

Inspection of internal structures. The anterior vestibule of the nose is inspected by pushing the tip upward, tilting the head backward, and illuminating the cavity with a flashlight or otoscope without the attached ear speculum.

The color of the *mucosal lining*, which is normally redder than the oral membranes, is noted. Any swelling, discharge, dryness, or bleeding are also noted. There should be no discharge from the nose.

On looking deeper into the nose, the *turbinates* or *concha,* plates of bone enveloped by mucous membrane that jut into the nasal cavity, are inspected. The turbinates greatly increase the surface area of the nasal cavity as air is inhaled. The spaces or channels between the turbinates are called *meatus* and correspond to each of the three turbinates. Normally the front end of the inferior and middle turbinate and the middle meatus are seen. They should be the same color as the lining of the vestibule.

Inside the nose, the *septum,* which should divide the vestibules equally, is also inspected. Any deviation is noted, especially if it causes an occlusion of one side of the nose. A perforation may be evident within the septum.

If this is suspected, the nurse can shine the light of the otoscope into one naris and look for admittance of light through the perforation to the other nostril.

Mouth and throat

With a cooperative child, almost the entire examination of the mouth and throat can be accomplished without the use of a tongue blade. The nurse asks the child to open his mouth wide, requests that he move his tongue in different directions for full visualization, and has him say "Ahh" in order to depress the tongue for full view of the back of the mouth (tonsils, uvula, and oropharynx). For a closer look at the buccal mucosa or lining of the cheeks, the nurse can ask the child to use his fingers to move the outer lip and cheek to one side. Performing the examination in front of a mirror is a great aid in enlisting children's cooperation. Another approach is using a puppet and letting the child examine its wide-open mouth (Fig. 5-25, *A*).

Infants and toddlers, however, usually resist attempts to keep the mouth open. Because it is an upsetting part of the examination, it is performed at the end of the physical examination (along with examination of the ears) or during episodes of crying. However, the use of a tongue blade to depress the tongue is necessary. The tongue blade is placed along the *side* of the tongue; it is not placed in the center back area where the gag reflex is elicited. Fig. 5-25, *B*, illustrates proper positioning of the child for the oral examination. If the child resists in opening his mouth, pinching the nostrils closed forces the child to open his mouth to breath.

The major structures that are visible within the oral cavity and oropharynx are the lips, the mucosal lining of the lips and cheeks, gums or gingiva, teeth, tongue, palate, uvula, tonsils, and posterior oropharynx (Fig. 5-26).

The major structure of the exterior of the mouth is the *lips*. The lips should be moist, soft, smooth, and pink, the color of a deeper hue than the surrounding skin. The lips should be symmetric when relaxed or tensed. Symmetry is easily assessed when the child talks or cries.

The nurse inspects all areas lined with *mucous membranes* (inside the lips and cheeks, gingiva, underside of tongue, palate, and back of pharynx), noting its color, any areas of white patches or ulceration, bleeding, sensitivity, and moisture. The membranes should be bright pink, smooth, glistening, uniform, and moist.

The *teeth* are inspected for number in each dental arch, for hygiene, and for occlusion or bite. The general rule for estimating the number of temporary teeth in children who are 2 years of age or younger is: *the child's age in months minus 6 months equals the number of teeth.* Discoloration of tooth enamel with obvious plaque (whitish coating on the surface of the teeth) is a sign of poor dental hygiene and indicates a need for dental counseling. Brown

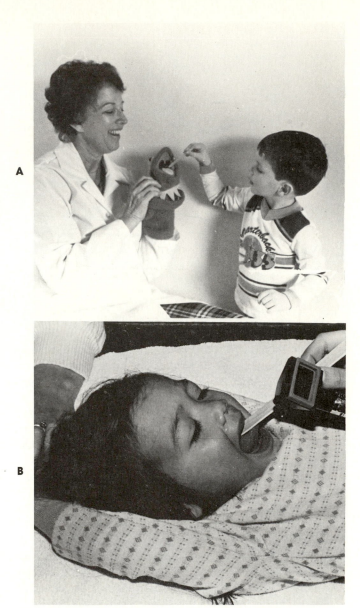

FIG. 5-25

A, *Encouraging child to cooperate.* **B,** *Positioning child for examination of mouth.*

spots in the crevices of the crown of the tooth or between the teeth may be caries. Teeth that appear greenish black may be stained from oral ingestion of supplemental iron. Although unsightly, this disappears after the iron is no longer given. Malocclusion or poor biting relationship of the teeth is also noted.

The *gums* (gingiva) surrounding the teeth are also examined. The color is normally coral pink, and the surface texture is stippled, similar to the appearance of orange peel. In dark-skinned children, the gums are more deeply colored, and a brownish area is often observed along the gum line.

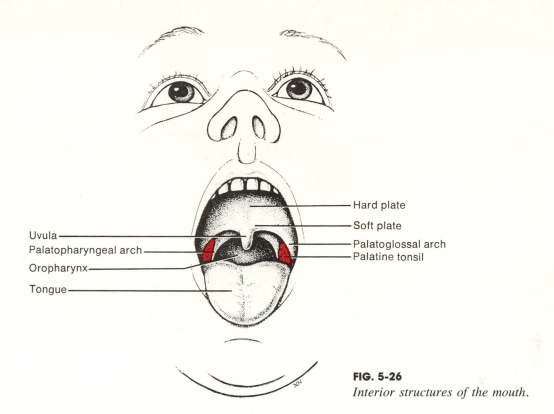

FIG. 5-26
Interior structures of the mouth.

Labels: Uvula, Palatopharyngeal arch, Oropharynx, Tongue, Hard plate, Soft plate, Palatoglossal arch, Palatine tonsil

The *tongue* is inspected for the presence of papillae, small projections that contain several taste buds each and give the tongue its characteristic rough appearance. The nurse also notes the size and mobility of the tongue. Normally the tip of the tongue should extend to the lips.

The roof of the mouth consists of the *hard palate,* which is located near the front of the oral cavity, and the *soft palate*, which is located toward the back of the pharynx and which has a small midline protrusion called the *uvula*. Both palates are carefully inspected to be sure that they are intact. The arch of the palate should be dome shaped. A narrow-flat roof or a high-arched palate affects the placement of the tongue and can cause feeding and speech problems. Movement of the uvula should be tested by eliciting a gag reflex. It should move upward to close off the nasopharynx from the oropharynx.

As the recesses of the oropharynx are examined, the size and color of the *palatine tonsils* are also noted. They are normally the same color as the surrounding mucosa, glandular, rather than smooth in appearance, and barely visible over the edge of the palatoglossal arches. The size of the tonsils varies considerably during childhood.

Chest

Although the thoracic cavity houses two vital organs, the heart and lungs, the anatomic structures of the chest wall are important sources of information concerning cardiac and pulmonary function, skeletal formation, and secondary

sexual development. The nurse inspects the chest for size, shape, symmetry, movement, breast development, and the presence of the bony landmarks formed by the ribs and sternum.

The *rib cage* consists of twelve ribs and the sternum, or breast bone, which is located in the midline of the trunk (Fig. 5-27). The *sternum* is composed of three main parts. The *manubrium,* the uppermost portion, can be felt at the base of the neck at the *suprasternal notch*. The largest segment of the sternum is the *body,* which forms the *sternal angle* as it articulates with the manubrium. At the end of the body is a small, movable process called the *xiphoid*. The angle of the costal margin as it attaches to the sternum is called the *costal angle* and is normally about 45 to 50 degrees. These bony structures are important landmarks in the location of ribs and intercostal spaces.

Intercostal spaces are the spaces between the ribs. They are numbered according to the rib directly *above* the space. For example, the space immediately below the second rib is the second intercostal space.

The *thoracic cavity* is also divided into segments by drawing imaginary lines on the chest and back. Fig. 5-28 illustrates the anterior, lateral, and posterior divisions. The nurse should become familiar with each imaginary landmark, as well as with the rib number and corresponding interspace because they are geographic landmarks for palpating, percussing, and auscultating underlying organs.

The *size* of the chest is measured by placing the measuring tape around the rib cage at the nipple line (Fig 5-

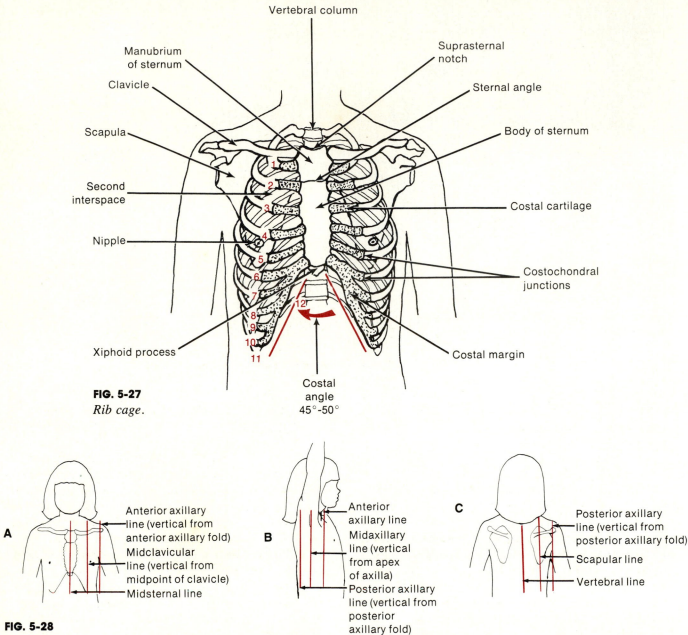

FIG. 5-27
Rib cage.

FIG. 5-28
Imaginary landmarks of chest. **A,** *Anterior;* **B,** *right lateral;* **C,** *posterior.*

29). For greatest accuracy two measurements are taken, one during inspiration and the other during expiration, and the average is recorded. Chest size is important mainly in comparison to its relationship with head circumference, which has been discussed on p. 91. Marked disproportions are always recorded. Most disproportions are caused by abnormal head growth, although some may be the result of altered chest shape, such as barrel chest or pigeon chest.

During infancy the *shape* of the chest is almost circular, with the anteroposterior (front-to-back) diameter equaling the transverse or lateral (side-to-side) diameter.

As the child grows the chest normally increases in the transverse direction, causing the anteroposterior diameter to be less than the lateral diameter. The nurse also notes the *angle* made by the lower costal margin and the sternum. As the nurse inspects the rib cage, the junction of the ribs to the costal cartilage (costochondral junction) and sternum is noted. Normally the points of attachment are fairly smooth.

Movement of the chest wall is noted. It should be symmetrical bilaterally and coordinated with breathing. During inspiration, the chest rises and expands, the dia-

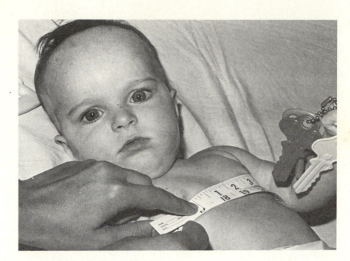

FIG. 5-29
Measuring chest circumference.

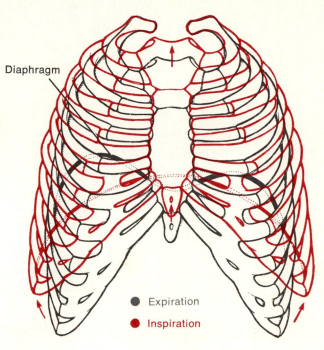

Diaphragm

● Expiration
● Inspiration

FIG. 5-30
Movement of the chest during respiration.

phragm descends, and the costal angle increases. During expiration, the chest falls and decreases in size, the diaphragm rises, and the costal angle narrows (Fig. 5-30). In children under 6 or 7 years of age, respiratory movement is principally abdominal or diaphragmatic. In older children, particularly females, respirations are chiefly thoracic. In either type, the chest and abdomen should rise and fall together. Any asymmetry of movement is an important pathologic sign and is reported.

On inspecting the skin surface of the chest, the position of the *nipples* is observed as well as any evidence of *breast* development. The nipples are normally located slightly lateral to the midclavicular line between the fourth and fifth ribs. The symmetry of nipple placement and the normal configuration of a darker pigmented areola surrounding a flat nipple in the prepubertal child are noted.

Any evidence of pubertal breast development, which usually begins in girls between 10 and 14 years of age, is noted. Precocious or delayed breast development is recorded, as well as evidence of any other secondary sexual characteristics. The nurse should investigate the child's feelings regarding breast development.

In adolescent females who have achieved sexual maturity, the breasts are palpated for evidence of any masses or hard nodules. This opportunity should also be taken to discuss the importance of routine breast self-examination. Although carcinoma of the breast is rare in women under 20 years of age, it is advisable to stress the value of routine breast self-examination so that it becomes a practiced habit during later years.

Lungs

Examination of the lungs involves the skills of inspection, palpation, percussion, and auscultation. The most impor-

tant of these are inspection and auscultation. Assessment of the lungs requires knowledge of their location and of their relationship to the rib cage (Fig. 5-31).

The lungs are situated inside the thoracic cavity, with one lung on each side of the sternum. Each lung is divided into an *apex,* which is slightly pointed and rises above the first rib, a *base,* which is wide and concave and rides on the dome-shaped diaphragm; and a body, which is divided into *lobes*. The right lung has three lobes: the upper, middle, and lower. The left lobe has only two lobes, the upper and lower, because of the space occupied by the heart.

Inspection. Inspection of the lungs primarily involves observation of respiratory movements, which are discussed on p. 92. Respirations are evaluated for rate (number per minute), rhythm (regular, irregular, or periodic), depth (deep or shallow), and quality (effortless, automatic, difficult, or labored). The character of breath sounds is noted, such as noisy, grunting, snoring, or heavy.

Palpation. Respiratory movements are felt by placing each hand flat against the back or chest with the thumbs in midline along the lower costal margin of the lungs. The child should be sitting during this procedure and, if cooperative, should take several deep breaths. During respiration the nurse's hands will move with the chest wall. The amount and speed of respiratory excursion is evaluated and any asymmetry of movement is noted.

Percussion. In percussing the chest, the anterior lung is percussed from apex to base, usually with the child

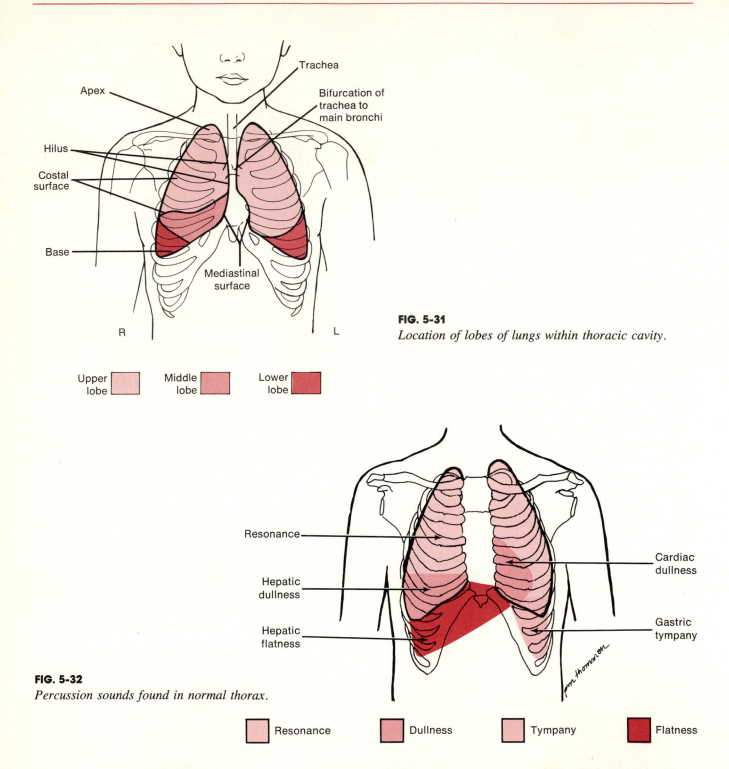

FIG. 5-31
Location of lobes of lungs within thoracic cavity.

Upper lobe ☐   Middle lobe ☐   Lower lobe ☐

FIG. 5-32
Percussion sounds found in normal thorax.

☐ Resonance   ☐ Dullness   ☐ Tympany   ☐ Flatness

in the supine or sitting position. Each side of the chest is percussed in sequence in order to compare the sounds. When percussing the posterior lung, the procedure and sequence are the same, although the child should be sitting.

Fig. 5-32 illustrates the usual percussion sounds within the anterior thorax. Resonance is heard over all the lobes of the lungs that are not adjacent to other organs.

Dullness is heard beginning at the fifth interspace in the right midclavicular line. Percussing downward to the end of the liver, the sound becomes flat, because the liver no longer overlies the air-filled lung. Cardiac dullness is normally felt over the left sternal border from the second to the fifth interspace medially to the midclavicular line. Below the fifth interspace on the left side, tympany results

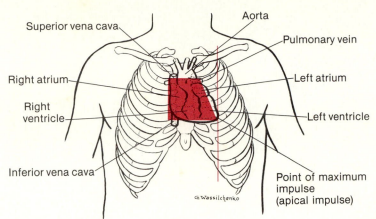

FIG. 5-33

Position of heart within thorax.

from the air-filled stomach. Normally, only resonance is heard when percussing the posterior thorax from the shoulder to the eighth or tenth rib. At the base of the lungs dullness is heard as the diaphragm is percussed. Deviations from expected sounds are always recorded and reported.

Auscultation. Auscultation involves using the stethoscope to evaluate breath sounds. In the normal lungs breath sounds are classified as vesicular or bronchovesicular. *Vesicular breath sounds* are heard over the entire surface of the lungs with the exception of the upper intrascapular area and the area beneath the manubrium. Inspiration is louder, longer, and higher-pitched than expiration. Sometimes the expiratory phase seems nearly absent in comparison to the long inspiratory phase. The sound is usually a soft swishing noise.

Bronchovesicular breath sounds are heard over the manubrium and in the upper intrascapular regions where there are bifurcations of large airways, such as the trachea and bronchi. Inspiration and expiration are of almost equal duration, quality, pitch, and intensity. Inspiration is normally louder and higher in pitch than that heard in vesicular breathing.

Another type of breathing that is normal only over the trachea near the suprasternal notch is *bronchial breath sounds*. They are almost the reverse of vesicular sounds; the inspiratory phase is short and the expiratory phase is longer, louder, and of higher pitch. They are usually louder than the normal breath sounds and have a hollow, blowing character. Bronchial breathing anywhere in the lung except over the trachea denotes some abnormality, such as consolidation or compression of lung tissue.

Absent or diminished breath sounds are always an abnormal finding warranting investigation. Fluid, air, or solid masses in the pleural space all interfere with the conduction of breath sounds. Diminished breath sounds in certain segments of the lung can alert the nurse to pulmonary areas that may benefit from postural drainage and percus-

sion. Increased breath sounds following pulmonary therapy indicate improved passage of air through the respiratory tract.

Various pulmonary abnormalities produce *adventitious sounds* that are not normally heard over the chest. These are not alterations of normal breath sounds but sounds that occur in addition to normal or abnormal breath sounds. They are classified into two main groups: rales (from the French word meaning "rattle") and rhonchi. Considerable practice with an experienced tutor is necessary to differentiate the various types of rales and rhonchi. Often it is best to describe the type of sound heard in the lungs rather than to try and label it correctly. Any abnormal sounds are always reported for further medical evaluation.

Heart

Examination of the heart involves the skills of inspection, palpation, percussion, and auscultation, although the last is the most significant. Knowledge of the location of the heart in relation to the rib cage is essential for evaluating and describing findings. Fig. 5-33 illustrates the usual position of the heart in the thorax.

The heart is situated like a trapezoid:

vertically along the right sternal border (RSB) from the second to the fifth rib

horizontally (long side) from the lower right sternum to the fifth rib at the left midclavicular line (LMCL)

diagonally from the left sternal border (LSB) at the second rib to the LMCL at the fifth rib

horizontally (short side) from the RSB and LSB at the second intercostal space

The *base* of the heart is actually the top of the trapezoid or the pulmonic and aortic areas. The *apex* is located at the left midclavicular line and fifth intercostal space or mitral area. The heart of the infant is more horizontally positioned; therefore, the apex is higher than (third to

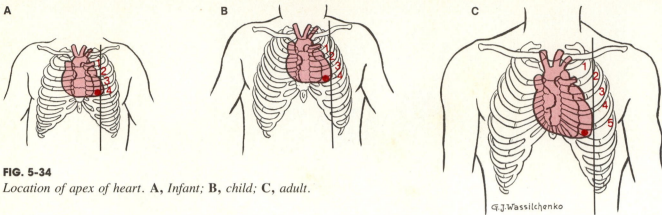

FIG. 5-34
Location of apex of heart. **A,** *Infant;* **B,** *child;* **C,** *adult.*

G.J.Wassilchenko

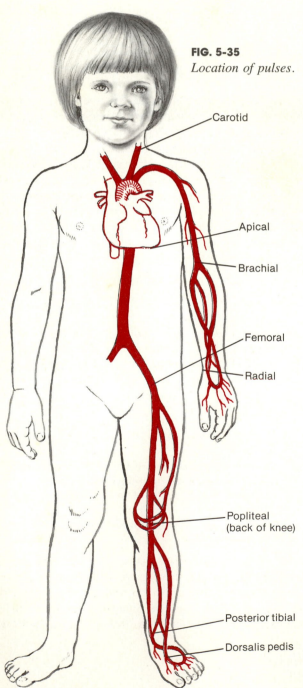

FIG. 5-35
Location of pulses.

Carotid

Apical

Brachial

Femoral

Radial

Popliteal
(back of knee)

Posterior tibial

Dorsalis pedis

fourth intercostal space) and to the left of the midclavicular line (Fig. 5-34). The apical impulse, or *point of maximum impulse* (PMI) (the area where the heartbeat is the loudest), is normally located at the apex.

Inspection. Inspection is best done by observing the child sitting in a semi-Fowler's position, looking at the anterior chest wall from an angle, and comparing both sides of the rib cage to each other. Normally they should be symmetric. In children with thin chest walls, the point of maximum impulse or apical pulse is sometimes apparent as a pulsation. Noting the location of the impulse gives some indication of the size and positioning of the heart.

Palpation. Palpation is useful in determining the size of the heart by feeling for the point of maximum impulse. It is felt by placing the fingertips or the palmar aspect of the fingers and hand at the fifth intercostal space and left midclavicular line. At this point in the examination other pulses may also be palpated, noting symmetry of pulsations (Fig. 5-35).

Percussion. Percussion is used mainly to determine the size of the heart by outlining its borders. Dullness is normally heard over the left area of the heart and partially over the right.

Auscultation. Auscultation involves listening for heart sounds with the stethoscope; it is similar to the procedure used in assessing breath sounds.

Origin of heart sounds. The heart sounds are produced by the opening and closing of the valves and the vibration of blood against the walls of the heart and vessels. Normally two sounds—S_1 and S_2—are heard, which correspond respectively to the familiar ''lub dub'' often used to describe the sounds. S_1 is caused by the closure of the *tricuspid* and *mitral valves* (sometimes called the atrioventricular valves). S_2 is the result of the closure of the *pulmonic* and *aortic* valves (sometimes called semilunar valves). Normally there is an audible pause or split between the two sounds that widens during inspiration.

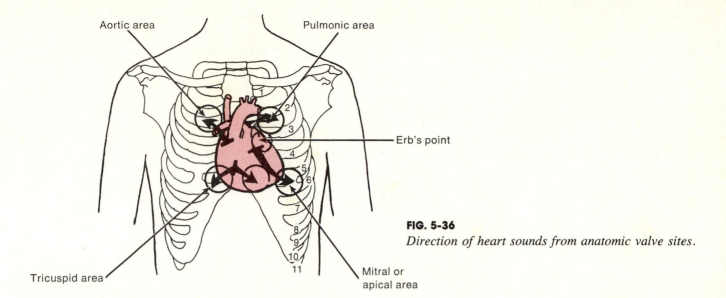

Aortic area

Pulmonic area

Erb's point

FIG. 5-36
Direction of heart sounds from anatomic valve sites.

Tricuspid area

Mitral or
apical area

"Physiologic splitting" is a significant normal finding that should be elicited. "Fixed splitting," in which the split in S_2 does not change during inspiration, is an important diagnostic sign of atrial septal defect and is always reported for further evaluation.

Two other heart sounds—S_3 and S_4—may be produced. S_3 is normally heard only in some children and young adults but is considered abnormal in older individuals. S_4 is rarely heard as a normal heart sound; usually it indicates the need for further cardiac evaluation.

Another important category of heart sounds is *murmurs*. Murmurs are produced by vibrations within the heart chambers or in the major arteries from the back and forth flow of blood. The description and classification of murmurs are skills that require considerable practice and training. The nurse should consult with a physician whenever a murmur is identified or suspected.

Differentiating normal heart sounds. Fig. 5-36 illustrates the approximate anatomic position of the valves within the heart chambers. It is important to note that the anatomic location of valves does not correspond to the area where the sounds are heard best. The auscultatory sites are located in the direction of the blood flow through the valves.

Normally S_1 is louder at the apex of the heart in the mitral and tricuspid area and S_2 is louder near the base of the heart in the pulmonic and aortic area. The nurse listens to each sound by inching down the chest in the sequence outlined in Table 5-2. If the nurse has difficulty in deciding which sound is S_1 or S_2, especially when the rate is rapid, the carotid pulse should be simultaneously palpated with the index and middle finger, while listening to the heart sounds. S_1 is synchronous with the carotid pulse. In addition to the areas listed in Table 5-2, the nurse should

also listen in the sternoclavicular area above the clavicles and manubrium, along the sternal border, along the left midaxillary line, and below the scapulae for sounds, such as murmurs, which may radiate to these areas.

The heart is auscultated with the child in at least two positions, sitting and reclining (Fig. 5-37). Both the diaphragm and bell chestpieces are used when listening to each auscultatory area. The diaphragm chestpiece is better for the detection of high-pitched sounds, such as S_1 and S_2. The bell chestpiece is used for low-pitched sounds, such as S_3, S_4, or murmurs.

Heart sounds are evaluated for:

1. **Quality,** which should be clear and distinct, not muffled, diffuse, or distant
2. **Intensity,** especially in relation to location or auscultatory site
3. **Rate,** which should be the same as the radial pulse
4. **Rhythm,** which should be regular and even

A particular arrhythmia that occurs normally in many children is *sinus arrhythmia,* in which the heart rate increases with inspiration and decreases with expiration. This can be differentiated from a truly abnormal arrhythmia by having the child hold his breath. In sinus arrhythmia cessation of breathing causes the heart rate to remain steady.

Abdomen

Examination of the abdomen involves the usual four skills, except that the order of their use is significantly changed. Inspection is followed by auscultation, percussion, and then palpation. Palpation is performed last because it may distort the normal abdominal sounds. The nurse must have

TABLE 5-2. SEQUENCE OF AUSCULTATING HEART SOUNDS*

AUSCULTATORY SITE	CHEST LOCATION	CHARACTERISTICS OF HEART SOUNDS
Aortic area	Second right intercostal space close to sternum	S_2 heard louder than S_1; aortic closure heard loudest
Pulmonic area	Second left intercostal space close to sternum	Splitting of S_2 heard best, normally widens on inspiration; pulmonic closure heard best
Erb's point	Second and third left intercostal space close to sternum	Frequent site of innocent murmurs and those of aortic or pulmonic origin
Tricuspid area	Fifth right and left intercostal space close to sternum	S_1 heard as louder sound preceding S_2 (S_1 synchronous with carotid pulse)
Mitral or apical area	Fifth intercostal space, left midclavicular line (third to fourth intercostal space and lateral to left midclavicular line in infants)	S_1 heard loudest; splitting of S_1 may be audible because mitral closure is louder than tricuspid closure S_3 heard best at beginning of expiration with child in recumbent or left side-lying position, occurs immediately after S_2, sounds like word "Ken-tuc-ky" $$S_1 \quad S_2 \quad S_3$$ S_4 heard best during expiration with child in recumbent position (left side-lying position decreases sound), occurs immediately before S_1, sounds like word "Ten-nes-see" $$S_4 \quad S_1 \quad S_2$$

*Use both diaphragm and bell chestpieces when auscultating heart sounds. Bell chestpiece is necessary for low-pitched sounds of murmurs, S_3, and S_4.

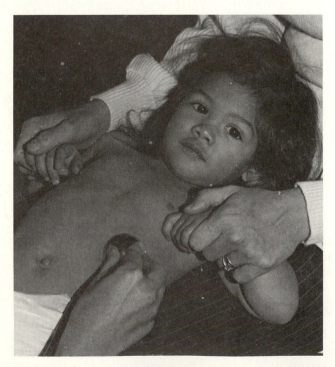

FIG. 5-37
Reclining position in parent's lap for auscultation of heart.

knowledge of the anatomic placement of the abdominal organs in order to differentiate normal, expected findings from abnormal ones (Fig. 5-38).

For descriptive purposes the abdominal cavity is divided into four quadrants by drawing a vertical line midway from the sternum to the pubic symphysis and a horizontal line across the abdomen through the umbilicus. Each section is named as follows: right upper quadrant (RUQ), right lower quadrant (RLQ), left upper quadrant (LUQ), and left lower quadrant (LLQ).

Inspection. The *contour* of the abdomen is inspected with the child erect and supine. Normally the abdomen of infants and young children is quite cylindric and, in the erect position, fairly prominent because of the physiologic lordosis of the spine. In the supine position the abdomen appears flat. A midline protrusion from the xiphoid to the umbilicus or pubic symphysis is usually *diastasis recti,* or failure of the rectus abdominis muscles to join in utero. In a healthy child a midline protrusion is usually a variation of normal muscular development. During adolescence the usual male and female contours of the pelvic cavity change the shape of the abdomen to form characteristic adult curves, especially in the female.

The condition of the *skin* covering the abdomen is noted. It should be uniformly taut, without wrinkles or

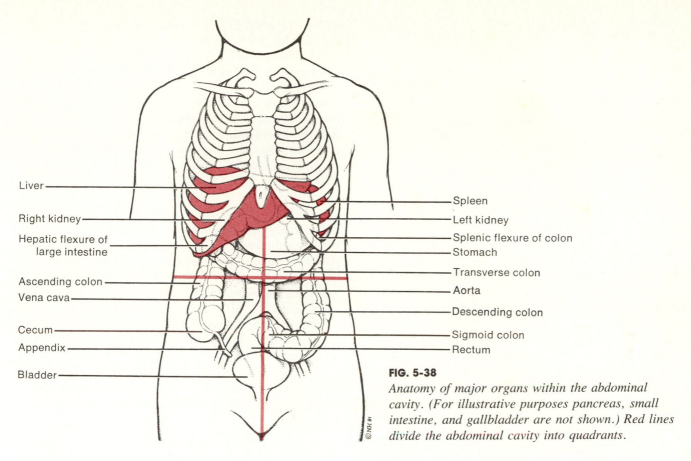

Liver
Right kidney
Hepatic flexure of
large intestine
Ascending colon
Vena cava
Cecum
Appendix
Bladder

Spleen
Left kidney
Splenic flexure of colon
Stomach
Transverse colon
Aorta
Descending colon
Sigmoid colon
Rectum

FIG. 5-38
Anatomy of major organs within the abdominal cavity. (For illustrative purposes pancreas, small intestine, and gallbladder are not shown.) Red lines divide the abdominal cavity into quadrants.

creases. Sometimes silvery, whitish striae are seen, especially if the skin has been stretched as in obesity.

Movement of the abdomen is observed. Normally chest and abdominal movements are synchronous. In infants and thin children, *peristaltic waves* may be visible through the abdominal wall; these always warrant careful evaluation. They are best observed by standing at eye level to and across from the abdomen.

The *umbilicus* is examined for size, hygiene, and evidence of any abnormalities, such as hernias. The umbilicus should be flat or only slightly protruding. If a herniation is present, the sac is palpated for abdominal contents and the approximate size of the opening is estimated. Umbilical hernias are common in infants, especially in black children.

Hernias are looked for elsewhere on the abdominal wall, such as in the inguinal or femoral region (Fig. 5-39). An *inguinal hernia* is a protrusion of peritoneum through the abdominal wall in the inguinal canal. It occurs most often in males, is frequently bilateral, and may be visible as a mass in the scrotum. It is palpated by sliding the little finger into the external inguinal ring at the base of the scrotum and asking the child to cough. If a hernia is present, it will hit the tip of the finger. If the child is too young to cough, he can be given a balloon to blow up. Just trying

to inflate the balloon raises the intra-abdominal sufficiently to demonstrate the presence of an inguinal hernia.

A *femoral hernia,* which occurs more frequently in girls, is felt or seen as a small mass on the anterior surface of the thigh just below the inguinal ligament in the femoral canal (a potential space medial to the femoral artery). Its location can be estimated by placing the index finger of the right hand on the child's right femoral pulse (left hand for left pulse) and the middle ring finger flat against the skin toward the midline. The ring finger lies over the femoral canal, where the herniation occurs. Palpation of hernias in the pelvic region, particularly inguinal ones, is often part of the examination of genitalia.

Auscultation.   The most important finding to listen for is *peristalsis* or *bowel sounds,* which sound like short metallic clicks and gurgles. Their frequency per minute should be recorded (for example, 15 bowel sounds/minute). Bowel sounds may be stimulated by stroking the abdominal surface with a fingernail. Absent bowel sounds or hyperperistalsis is recorded and reported, since either usually denotes an abdominal pathologic condition.

Percussion.   Percussion of the abdomen is performed in the same manner as percussion of the lungs and heart (see Fig. 5-32). Normally dullness or flatness is heard on the right side at the lower costal margin because

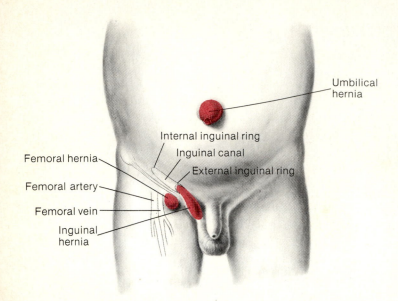

FIG. 5-39
Location of hernias.

of the location of the liver. Tympany is typically heard over the stomach on the left side and usually in the rest of the abdomen. An unusually tympanitic sound, like the beating of a tight drum, usually denotes air in the stomach, a common cause of which is mouth breathing.

Palpation. Two types of palpation are performed, superficial and deep. In *superficial palpation* the nurse lightly places the hand against the skin and feels each quadrant, noting any areas of tenderness, muscle tone, and superficial lesions, such as cysts.

Superficial palpation is often perceived as "tickling" by the child, which can interfere with its effectiveness. The nurse can avoid this problem in the older child by telling stories; by having him "help" with the palpation by placing his hand over the nurse's palpating hand, or with statements such as, "I am trying to feel what you had for lunch." Another approach is having the child place his hand on the abdomen with the fingers widely spaced and then palpating between the fingers. Admonishing the child to stop laughing only draws attention to the sensation and decreases cooperation. In a younger child, using the parent's lap as the examining surface, distracting him with toys or mobiles, or giving him a bottle or pacifier often increases relaxation and cooperation. A preferred position is lying supine with the legs flexed at the hips and knees.

Deep palpation is used for palpating organs and large blood vessels and for detecting masses and tenderness that were not discovered during superficial palpation. If the child complains of abdominal pain, that area of the abdomen is palpated last. Palpation usually begins in the lower quadrants and proceeds upward. In this way the edge of an enlarged liver or spleen is not missed. Except for palpating the liver, successful identification of other organs,

such as the spleen, kidney, and part of the colon, requires considerable practice with tutored supervision.

The lower edge of the *liver* is sometimes felt in infants and young children as a superficial mass 1 to 2 cm (0.4 to 0.8 inch) below the right costal margin (the distance is sometimes measured in fingerbreadths). If the liver is 3 cm (1.2 inches) or 2 fingerbreadths below the costal margin, it is considered enlarged, and this finding is referred to a physician. Normally the liver descends during inspiration as the diaphragm moves downward. This downward displacement should not be mistaken as a sign of liver enlargement.

The *spleen* is palpated by feeling it between the hand placed against the back and the other hand placed on the left upper quadrant. It is much smaller than the liver and positioned behind the fundus of the stomach. The tip of the spleen is normally felt during inspiration as it descends within the abdominal cavity. It is sometimes palpable 1 to 2 cm below the left costal margin in infants and young children. A spleen that is more than 2 cm below the right costal margin is enlarged and is always reported for further investigation.

The *bladder* may be palpated slightly above the pubic symphysis in infants and young children. It descends deeper into the pelvic cavity during adolescence, when it is not felt except if distended.

Other anatomic structures that are sometimes palpable in children include the kidney, cecum, and sigmoid colon. Although these structures are not routinely felt, the nurse should be aware of their relative location and characteristics in order not to mistake them for abnormal masses. Any questionable mass must be referred to a physician before it can be ruled out as benign.

During palpation of the abdomen the *femoral pulses* are felt by placing the tips of two or three fingers (index, middle, and/or ring) along the inguinal ligament about midway between the iliac crest and pubic symphysis. Both pulses are felt simultaneously to make certain that they are equal and strong (Fig. 5-40). Absence of femoral pulses is a significant sign of coarctation of the aorta.

Genitalia

Examination of genitalia conveniently follows assessment of the abdomen while the child is still supine. In adolescents inspection of the genitalia may be left to the end of the examination. The best approach is to examine the genitals quickly, placing no more emphasis on this part of the assessment than on any other segment. It helps to relieve children's and parents' anxiety by telling them the results of the findings as the nurse proceeds, for example, by stating, "Everything looks fine here." If the nurse finds it necessary to ask questions, such as about discharge, difficulty in urinating, and so on, consideration should be

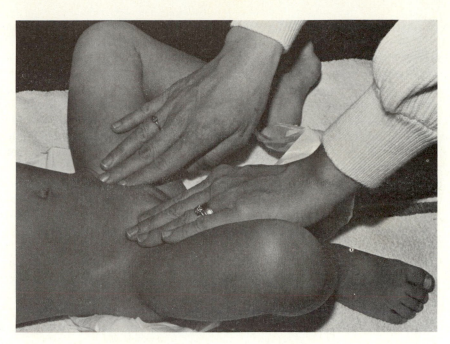

FIG. 5-40
Palpating for femoral pulses.

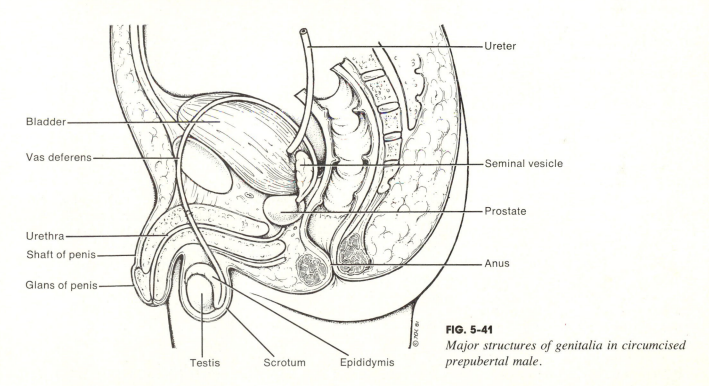

Bladder

Vas deferens

Urethra

Shaft of penis

Glans of penis

Testis   Scrotum   Epididymis

Ureter

Seminal vesicle

Prostate

Anus

FIG. 5-41
Major structures of genitalia in circumcised prepubertal male.

shown at all times, and the child's privacy should be observed by covering the lower abdomen with the gown or underpants.

Male genitalia. The external appearance of the genitalia is noted (Fig. 5-41). The size of the *penis* is generally small in infants and young boys, until puberty, when it begins to increase in both length and width. One should be familiar with normal pubertal growth of the external male genitalia in order to compare the findings with the expected sequence of maturation.

The *glans* (the head of the penis) and the *shaft* (the portion between the perineum and prepuce) are examined. If the child is uncircumcised, the *prepuce* or foreskin covers the glans or head of the penis. In infants the prepuce is normally tight for the first several months of life and should not be retracted for examination. In older infants and children the foreskin should be gently retracted for examination of the glans and the meatus.

The *urethral meatus* is carefully inspected for location and evidence of discharge. Normally it is centered at the tip of the glans.

The location and size of the *scrotum* are noted. They hang freely from the perineum behind the penis and the left scrotum normally hangs lower than the right. In infants the scrota appear large in relation to the rest of the genitalia. The skin of the scrotum is loose and highly rugated (wrinkled). During early adolescence the skin normally becomes redder and coarser. In dark-skinned children the scrota are usually more deeply pigmented.

Palpation of the scrotum includes identification of the testes, epididymis, and, if present, inguinal hernias. The two *testes* are felt as small ovoid bodies, about 1.5 to 2 cm (0.6 to 0.8 inch) long—one in each scrotal sac. They do not enlarge until puberty, when they approximately double in size.

Palpating for the presence of the testes requires an un-

derstanding of the normal anatomy and physiology of the coverings of the testes and scrotal sac. The scrotum and testes are surrounded by fascia called the cremaster muscle, which attaches to a point in the abdomen and extends downward along the inner surface of the thigh. The muscle or *cremasteric reflex* is stimulated by cold, touch, emotional excitement, or exercise. It causes the skin of the scrotum to shrink and pulls the testes higher into the pelvic cavity. Therefore the nurse must be careful not to elicit this reflex.

Several measures are useful in preventing the cremasteric reflex during palpation of the scrotum. First the hands should be warm, not cold. Second, if old enough, the child should be examined while sitting in a tailor or "Indian" position, which stretches the muscle, preventing its contraction. Third, the normal pathway of ascent of the testes can be blocked by placing the thumb and index finger over the upper part of the scrotal sac along the inguinal canal (Fig. 5-42). The site is the same as that described for locating the internal inguinal ring when palpating for her-

FIG. 5-42
A, *Preventing the cremasteric reflex by having the child sit in a "tailor" position.* **B,** *Blocking inguinal canal during palpation of scrotum for descended testicles.*

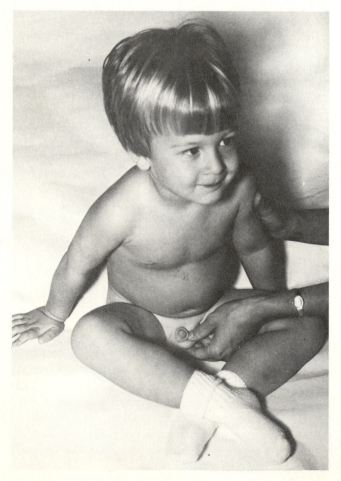

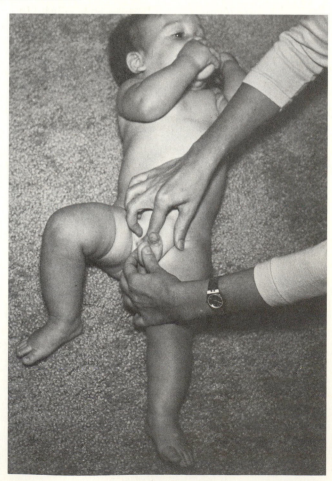

A

B

nias. The nurse should also place the index and middle finger in scissors fashion to separate the right and left scrotum if there is any question concerning the existence of two testes. If after each of these precautions the testes have not been palpated, the nurse feels along the inguinal canal and perineum to locate masses that may be incompletely descended testes. True undescended testes are reported and referred, although they may descend at any time during childhood and are therefore checked at each visit.

Hair distribution is also noted. Normally before puberty no pubic hair is present. Soft downy hair at the base of the penis is an early sign of pubertal maturation. In older adolescents the nurse notes the typical male pattern of hair distribution, which is usually triangular as it extends from the base of the penis along the midline to the umbilicus.

Female genitalia. A convenient position for examination of the genitalia involves placing the young child in a semireclining position on the parent's lap with the feet supported on the nurse's knees as the nurse sits facing the child. The child's attention is diverted from the examination by instructing her to try to keep the soles of her feet in apposition. The labia majora are held between the thumb and index finger and retracted outward in order to expose the labia minora, urethral meatus, and vaginal orifice.

The female genitalia are examined for size and location of the structures of the *vulva* or *pudendum* (Fig. 5-43). The *mons pubis* is a pad of adipose tissue over the

symphysis pubis. At puberty the mons is covered with hair, which extends along the labia. The usual pattern of female *hair distribution* is an inverted triangle. The appearance of soft downy hair along the labia majora is an early sign of sexual maturation.

The size and location of the *clitoris* are noted. It is a small erectile organ located at the anterior end of the labia minora. It is covered by a small flap of skin, the *prepuce*.

The *labia majora* are two thick folds of skin running posteriorly from the mons to the posterior commissure of the vagina. Internal to the labia majora are two folds of skin called the *labia minora*. Although the labia minora are usually prominent in the newborn, they gradually atrophy, which makes them almost invisible until their enlargement during puberty.

The inner surface of the labia should be pink and moist. The size of the labia and any evidence of fusion, which may suggest male scrota are noted. Normally no masses are palpable within the labia.

The *urethral meatus* is located posterior to the clitoris and is surrounded by Skene's glands and ducts. Although not a prominent structure, the meatus can be more readily identified by wiping downward along the vestibule toward the perineum. It will appear as a small V-shaped slit. The nurse notes its location, especially if it opens from the clitoris or inside the vagina. The glands, which are common sites of cysts and venereal lesions, are gently palpated.

The *vaginal orifice* is located posterior to the urethral meatus. Its appearance is variable depending on individual

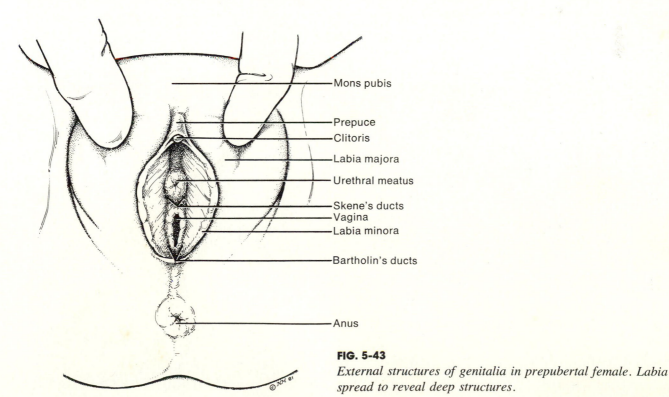

FIG. 5-43

External structures of genitalia in prepubertal female. Labia spread to reveal deep structures.

Mons pubis

Prepuce
Clitoris
Labia majora
Urethral meatus
Skene's ducts
Vagina
Labia minora
Bartholin's ducts

Anus

anatomy and sexual activity. Ordinarily examination of the vagina is limited to inspection. In virgins a thin crescent-shaped or circular membrane, called the *hymen,* may cover part of the vaginal opening. At times it completely occludes the orifice. After rupture, small rounded pieces of tissue called *carunculae* remain.

Surrounding the vaginal opening are *Bartholin's glands,* which secrete a clear, mucoid fluid into the vagina for lubrication during intercourse. The ducts are palpated for cysts. The discharge from the vagina, which is usually clear or white, is also noted.

Anus

Following examination of the genitalia, one can easily observe the anal area, although the child should be placed on the abdomen. The general firmness of the *buttocks* and symmetry of the gluteal folds are noted. The tone of the anal sphincter is assessed by eliciting the *anal reflex.* Scratching or gently pricking the anal area results in an obvious quick contraction of the external anal sphincter.

Back and extremities

While the child is prone, the back and spine are inspected. However, they are also observed with the child sitting and standing. The nurse notes the general *curvature* of the spine. Normally the back of a newborn is rounded or **C**-shaped from the thoracic and pelvic curves. The development of the cervical and lumbar curves approximates development of various motor skills, such as cervical curvature with head control, and gives the older child the typical double-**S** curve.

Marked curvatures in posture are noted. *Scoliosis,* lateral curvature of the spine, is an important childhood problem, especially in females. School-age children should be screened for the possibility of scoliosis. Screening procedures include: (1) having the child stand erect, clothed only in underpants (and bra if older girl), observing the child from behind, and noting asymmetry of the shoulders and hips, and (2) having the child bend forward so that the back is parallel to the floor, observing the child from the side, and noting asymmetry or prominence of the rib cage. A slight limp, a crooked hemline, or complaints of a sore back are other signs and symptoms of scoliosis.

The *back* is inspected especially along the spine for any tufts of hair, dimples, or discoloration. The spine is palpated to identify each spiny process of the vertebrae or lack of them. *Mobility* of the vertebral column is easily assessed in most children because of their propensity for constant motion during the examination. However, one can specifically test for mobility by asking the child to sit up from a prone position or to do a modified sit-up exercise.

Each extremity is inspected for symmetry of length and size; any deviation is referred for orthopedic evaluation. The fingers and toes are counted to be certain of the normal number. This is so often taken for granted that an extra digit (polydactyly) or fusion of digits (syndactyly) may go unnoticed.

The arms and legs are inspected for *temperature and color,* which should be equal in each extremity, although the feet may normally be colder than the hands.

The *shape* of bones is assessed. Several different variations of bone shape may be observed in children. *Bowleg* or *genu varum* is lateral bowing of the tibia. It is clinically present when the child stands with the medial malleoli (rounded prominence on either side of the ankle) in apposition and the space between the knees is greater than 1 inch (Fig. 5-44). Toddlers are usually bowlegged after beginning to walk until all their lower back and leg muscles are well developed. Persistence of genu varum may indicate rickets from a weakening of the bone.

Knock-knee or *genu valgum* appears as the opposite of bowleg in that the knees are close together but the feet are spread apart. It is determined clinically by using the same method as for genu varum but by measuring the distance between the malleoli, which normally should be less than 1 inch (Fig. 5-45). Knock-knee is normally present in children from about 2 to 7 years of age. Persistence of this leg posture can be a result of several disorders including rickets.

Tibial torsion is abnormal rotation or bowing of the tibia. The nurse tests for tibial torsion by laying the child on his back with his hips and knees flexed and his foot flat on the examining surface. An imaginary line drawn from the tibial tuberosity to the middle of the malleoli should parallel a straight tibial shaft (Fig. 5-46). If a bowing is

FIG. 5-44
Bowleg.

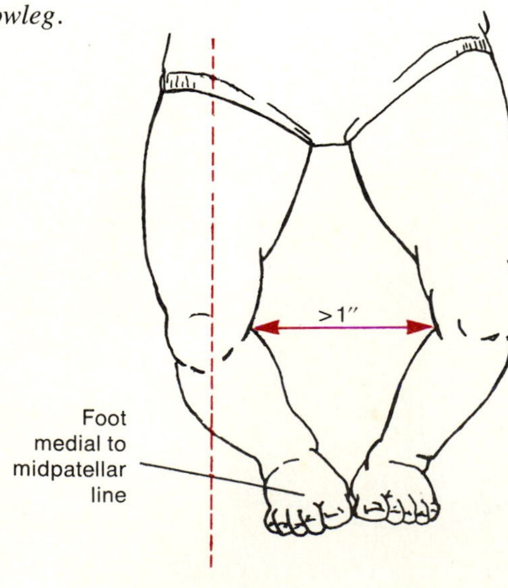

>1"

Foot medial to midpatellar line

present it will be evident as a nonparallel curved line to the imaginary line. This test is independent of associated foot anomalies. The nurse can also screen for this abnormality by placing the infant supine with the legs in a relaxed extended position or by having an older child stand naturally with both feet together. A straight line is drawn from the anterior superior iliac spine (felt externally as the "point" of the hip) through the center of the patella (knee cap). Normally this imaginary line intersects the second toe provided the foot is in normal alignment. If it intersects the fourth or fifth toe or bypasses the lateral aspect of the foot, the child is referred for orthopedic evaluation.

Next the *feet* are inspected. Infants' and toddlers' feet appear flat because the foot is normally wide and the arch is covered by a fat pad. Development of the arch occurs naturally from the action of walking. Normally at birth the feet are held in a valgus (outward) or varus (inward) position. To determine whether a foot deformity at birth is the result of intrauterine position or development, the outer, then inner, side of the sole is scratched. If the foot position is self-correctable, it will assume a right angle to the leg. As the child begins to walk, the feet should point straight ahead.

A common foot deformity is intoeing (pigeon toe, metatarsus varus), in which the forefoot or entire foot points inward. One cause of intoeing is tibial torsion. The opposite type deformity is toeing out (duck walk), in which the entire foot and leg turn outward. Both warrant further evaluation.

The *plantar* or *grasp reflex* is elicited by exerting firm but gentle pressure with the tip of the thumb against the lateral sole of the foot from the heel upward to the little toe and then across to the big toe. The normal response in children who are walking is flexion of the toes. *Babinski's sign,* dorsiflexion of the big toe and fanning of the other toes, is normal during infancy but abnormal after about 1 year of age or when locomotion begins (Fig. 5-47).

Inspection of the lower extremities also involves observing the child's *gait.* Normally toddlers have a "toddling" or broad-based gait, which facilitates walking by lowering the center of gravity. As the child reaches preschool age, the legs are brought closer together. By school age the walking posture is much more graceful and balanced.

Joints. The joints are evaluated for *range of motion.* Normally this requires no specific testing if the nurse has been observant of the child's movements during the examination. However, the hips should be routinely investigated in infants for congenital dislocation. Signs of congenital hip dislocation are discussed on p. 957. Any evidence of joint immobility or hyperflexibility is reported.

The joints are routinely palpated for *heat, tenderness,* and *swelling.* These signs, as well as redness over the joint, are referred to a physician for further investigation.

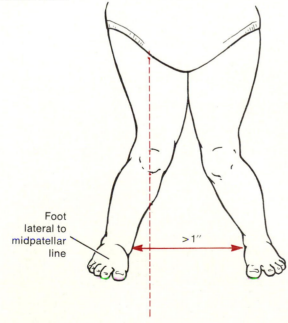

FIG. 5-45
Knock knee.

Foot
lateral to
midpatellar
line

>1"

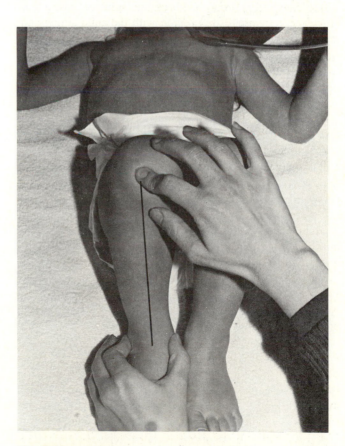

FIG. 5-46
Testing for tibial torsion.

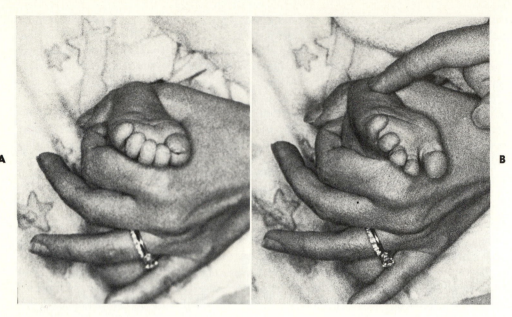

FIG. 5-47
A, *Plantar or grasp reflex.* **B**, *The Babinski reflex.*

Muscles.   Symmetry and quality of muscle development, tone, and strength are noted. *Development* is observed as one looks at the shape and contour of the body both in a relaxed and tensed state. *Tone* is estimated by grasping the muscle and feeling its firmness when it is relaxed and contracted. A common site for testing tone is the biceps muscle of the arm. Children are usually willing to "make a muscle" by clenching their fist.

Strength is estimated by having the child use an extremity to push or pull against resistance. For example, arm strength can be tested by having the child hold his arms outstretched in front of him. He is asked to raise his arms while the nurse applies downward pressure. Hand strength can be tested by using a "handshake," and finger strength can be tested by having the child squeeze one or two fingers of the nurse's hand. Leg strength can be tested by having the child sit on a table or chair with the legs dangling. The nurse holds the lower leg and while applying resistance asks the child to raise his legs. The symmetry of strength in each extremity, hands, and fingers is assessed, and any evidence of weakness is reported.

Neurologic assessment

The assessment of the nervous system is the broadest and most diverse since every human function, both physical and emotional, is controlled by neurologic impulses. This discussion will focus primarily on a general appraisal of cerebellar functioning, deep tendon reflexes, and the cranial nerves.

Assessment of neurologic function requires the use of a few additional tools. A reflex hammer, which has a small rounded rubber head, is used to test deep tendon reflexes. A pin and cotton are useful when testing sensory function. For the assessment of the cranial nerves, some flavors to taste and some odors to smell are necessary.

Cerebellar functioning.   The cerebellum controls balance and coordination. Much of the assessment of cerebellar functioning is included in observing the child's posture, body movements, gait, and development of fine and gross motor skills. Tests such as balancing on one foot and heel-to-toe walk on the Denver Developmental Screening Test assess *balance*. *Coordination* is tested by asking the child to reach for a toy, button his clothes, tie his shoes, or draw a straight line on a piece of paper, provided he is old enough to be expected to do each of these activities. Coordination can also be tested by any sequence of rapid successive movements, such as quickly touching each finger with the thumb of the same hand.

Several tests for cerebellar function that can be performed as games include:

1. **Finger-to-nose test:** with the child's arm extended, ask the child to touch his nose with the index finger both with his eyes open and then closed
2. **Heel-to-shin test:** with the child standing, have him run the heel of one foot down the shin or anterior aspect of the tibia of the other leg, both with his eyes opened and then closed
3. **Romberg test:** with the eyes closed, have the child stand with his heels together; falling or leaning to one side is abnormal and is called *Romberg's sign*

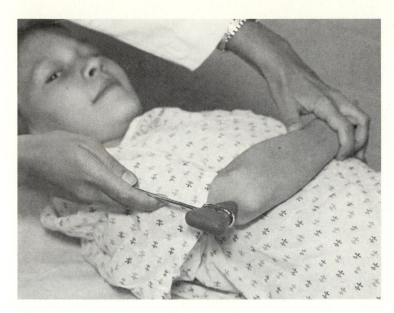

FIG. 5-48
Testing for triceps reflex. Child is placed supine, with his forearm resting over the chest, and triceps tendon is struck. Alternate procedure: Child's arm is abducted, with upper arm supported and forearm allowed to hang freely. Triceps tendon is struck. Normal response is partial extension of forearm.

School-age children should be able to perform these tests, although preschoolers normally can only bring the finger within 2 to 3 inches of their nose. Difficulty in performing these exercises indicates poor sense of position (especially with the eyes closed) and incoordination (especially with the eyes opened).

Reflexes. Testing reflexes is an important part of the neurologic examination. This discussion is primarily concerned with reflexes found in children past infancy. The primitive reflexes of the newborn are discussed in Chapter 6 under physical assessment of the neonate.

Reflexes can be elicited by using the rubber head of the reflex hammer, flat of the finger, or side of the hand. If the child is easily frightened by equipment, it is best for the nurse to use her hand or finger. Although testing reflexes is a simple procedure to perform, the child may inhibit the reflex by unconsciously tensing the muscle. The nurse should try to distract younger children with toys or by talking to them. Older children can concentrate on the exercise of grasping their two hands in front of them and trying to pull them apart. This diverts their attention away from the testing and causes involuntary relaxation of the muscles.

Deep tendon reflexes are stretch reflexes of a muscle. The most common deep tendon reflex is the *knee jerk,* or *patellar reflex* (this is sometimes called the *quadriceps reflex*). The reflexes normally elicited are described in Figs. 5-48 to 5-51. Any diminished or hyperreflexic response is reported for further evaluation.

Cranial nerves. Assessment of the cranial nerves is an important area of neurologic assessment (Table 5-3). With older children most of the tests can be made into games and, because no traumatic equipment is used, may

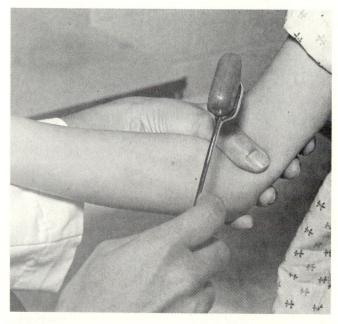

FIG. 5-49
Testing for biceps reflex. Child's arm is held by placing partially flexed elbow in examiner's hand with thumb over antecubital space. Examiner's thumbnail is struck with hammer. Normal response is partial flexion of forearm.

encourage trust and security at the beginning of the examination. However, if the nurse is familiar with the functions of each nerve, much of the testing can be included when each "system" is examined, such as tongue movement and strength, gag reflex, swallowing, and position of the uvula during examination of the mouth.

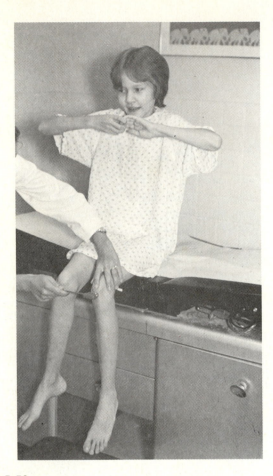

FIG. 5-50

Testing for patellar, or knee jerk, reflex, using distraction. Child sits on edge of examining table (or on parent's lap) with lower legs flexed at knee and dangling freely. Patellar tendon is tapped just below kneecap. Normal response is partial extension of lower leg.

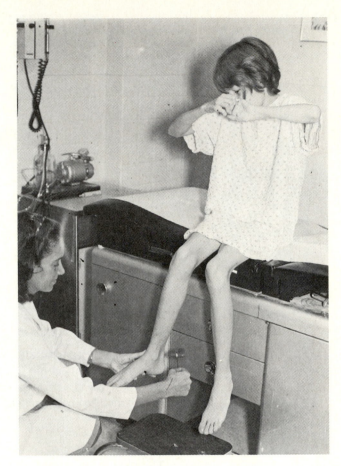

FIG. 5-51

Testing for Achilles reflex. Same position employed in eliciting knee jerk reflex is used. Foot is supported lightly in examiner's hand, and Achilles tendon is struck. Normal response is plantar flexion of foot (foot pointing downward).

DEVELOPMENTAL ASSESSMENT

One of the most essential components of a complete health appraisal is assessment of developmental functioning. *Screening procedures* are designed to identify quickly and reliably those children whose developmental level is below normal for their age and who, therefore, require further investigation. They also provide a means of recording objective measurements of present developmental functioning for future reference. In this discussion the nurse's role is viewed primarily in terms of screening.

Denver Developmental Screening Test

One of the most widely used screening tests for assessing a young child's development is the *Denver Developmental*

Screening Test (DDST) and the *Revised Denver Developmental Screening Test (DDST-R)* (see Appendix C). The tests are composed of four major categories: personal-social, fine motor-adaptive, language, and gross motor and are applicable for children from birth through 6 years of age. The age divisions are monthly until age 24 months and then every 6 months until 6 years of age. Allowances are made for infants who were born prematurely by subtracting the number of months missed gestation from their present age and testing them at the adjusted age. For example, a 9-month-old infant who was born 4 weeks before the expected date of confinement is tested at an 8-month level.

The results of the DDST and DDST-R compare favorably to other psychometric tests. However, one weakness

TABLE 5-3. ASSESSMENT OF CRANIAL NERVES

NERVE	DISTRIBUTION	TEST
I—Olfactory (S)*	Olfactory mucosa of nasal cavity	With his eyes closed, have child identify odors such as coffee, alcohol from a swab, or other smells. Test each nostril separately.
II—Optic (S)	Rods and cones of retina, optic nerve	Check for perception of light, visual acuity, peripheral vision, color vision, and normal optic disc.
III—Oculomotor (M)*	Muscles of eye	Have child follow an object such as a light or bright toy in all directions using only his eyes, not head movement. Perform PERRLA (p. 97).
IV—Trochlear (M)	Superior oblique muscle of eye	Have child look downward.
V—Trigeminal (M, S)	Muscles of mastication, skin of face, and two thirds of anterior scalp	Have child bite down hard and open his jaw; test symmetry and strength. With his eyes closed, see if child can detect light touch in the mandibular and maxillary regions. Test corneal and blink reflex by touching cornea lightly (approach child from the side so that he does not blink before cornea is touched).
VI—Abducens (M)	Lateral rectus muscle of eye	Have child look toward each side.
VII—Facial (M, S)	Nasal cavity and lacrimal gland, sublingual and submandibular salivary glands, muscles for facial expression, and anterior two thirds of tongue (taste)	Have child smile, make a funny face, or show his teeth to see symmetry of expression. Have child identify a sweet, sour, or bitter solution. Place each taste on anterior section and sides of protruding tongue; if child retracts tongue, solution will dissolve toward posterior part of tongue.
VIII—Auditory, acoustic, or vestibulocochlear (S)	Internal ear	Test hearing; note any loss of equilibrium or presence of vertigo.
IX—Glossopharyngeal (M, S)	Pharynx, tongue, and posterior one third of tongue for taste	Stimulate posterior pharynx with a tongue blade; child should gag. Test sense of taste on posterior segment of tongue.
X—Vagus (M, S)	Muscles of larynx, pharynx, some organs of gastrointestinal system, sensory fibers of root of tongue, heart, lung, and some organs of gastrointestinal system	Note hoarseness of voice, gag reflex, and ability to swallow. Check that uvula is in midline; when stimulated with a tongue blade, should deviate upward and to the stimulated side.
XI—Accessory (M)	Sternocleidomastoid and trapezius muscles of shoulder	Have child shrug shoulders while applying mild pressure. With the hands placed on his shoulders, have child turn his head against opposing pressure on either side. Note symmetry and strength.
XII—Hypoglossal (M)	Muscles of tongue	Have child move tongue in all directions. Have him protrude the tongue as far as possible; note any midline deviation. Test strength by placing tongue blade on one side of tongue and having child move it away.

*S—sensory; M—motor

is its possible limitation with minority ethnic groups. For example, there is a cultural bias in asking questions, such as "pedals tricycle," if the child has never had this opportunity. The nurse should evaluate cultural factors that may influence the child's performance on the test.

The major differences between the original DDST and the DDST-R are the arrangement of items on the form and the scoring. On the original form, items are scored as "P" for pass, "F" for fail, or "R" for refusal. On the DDST-R only the items passed are scored. The revised DDST-R has been found to have several advantages over the original form: (1) it is easier to use, especially for those not trained with DDST, (2) it facilitates using the short DDST (see p. 129), (3) it provides a more dynamic representation of the child's development because the form resembles a growth curve, and (4) subsequent testing of the child requires administering only those items not previously scored with a "P" that are to the left of the child's age line (Frankenburg and others, 1981).

The DDST-R is designed for administration by both professionals and paraprofessionals and takes about 15 to 20 minutes to complete. It is accompanied by a detailed instruction manual as well as by self-instructional units.* The kits for testing include a red wool "ball," raisins, a small clear bottle with a ⅝-inch opening, a rattle with a narrow handle, eight 1-inch square blocks in red, blue, yellow, and green colors, a small bell, a tennis ball, and a pencil.

Each item is designated by a bar that represents the ages at which 25%, 50%, 70%, and 90% of the tested population could perform the particular item. Scoring is based on the number of *delays*, which are defined as "failure to perform an item which is passed by 90% of the children who are of the same age or any item which falls completely to the *left* of the age line." *Abnormal* is determined by either:

1. Two or more sectors with two or more delays
2. One sector with two or more delays plus one or more sectors with one delay and, in that same sector, no passes through the age line

Questionable is determined by either:

1. One sector with two or more delays
2. One or more sectors with one delay and in that same sector no passes through the age line

If the child refuses to cooperate with testing so that a large number of items would be scored as failures, the child is evaluated as *untestable* and if possible retested at a future date. *Normal* is determined by any score that does not meet these three other criteria.

---

*The DDST-R and instruction manual can be purchased from LADOCA Publishing Foundation, East 51st Ave. and Lincoln St., Denver, CO 80216.

Although it is not the purpose of this discussion to detail the instruction manual, there are some points concerning preparation, administration, and interpretation of the DDST that necessitate emphasis. Before beginning the test, both the child and parent need an explanation. For parents this means clarifying that the DDST is *not* an intelligence test but a method of helping the nurse observe what the child can do at this age. It is best to deemphasize the word "test" while emphasizing that the child is *not* expected to perform each item on the sheet.

The parent is told before the testing begins that the results of the child's performance will be explained after all the items have been concluded. It is the nurse's responsibility to properly inform parents of any testing or screening procedure before its administration so that they are fully aware of its purpose and intent.

Toddlers and preschoolers are prepared for the test by presenting it as a game. Frequently the DDST is an excellent way to begin a health appraisal because it is nonthreatening, requires no painful or unfamiliar procedures, and capitalizes on the child's natural activity of play. Since children are easily distracted, it is best to perform the test quickly and to present only one toy from the kit at a time. After that toy's purpose is concluded, such as building a tower of blocks or identifying its color, the toy is replaced in the bag and another one is brought out for testing purposes. Other temporary factors that may interfere with the child's performance include fatigue, illness, fear, hospitalization, separation from the parent, or general unwillingness to perform activities asked of the child. In addition, undiagnosed mental retardation, hearing loss, vision loss, neurologic impairment, or a familial pattern of slow development greatly influences the child's performance.

Following completion of the DDST, the parent is asked if the child's performance was typical of his behavior at other times. If the parent replies affirmatively and if the child's cooperation was satisfactory, the nurse explains the results, emphasizing all successful items first, then those items failed but which the child was not expected to pass, and finally those items that were delays.

In explaining a normal score, the nurse should focus on how well the child performed and should reinforce the parents' efforts in satisfactorily stimulating their child. Although one does not wish to encourage parents to teach their child skills in order to pass the test, the DDST can be used to guide parents toward those activities that are appropriate, although not necessarily expected, for the child's age. For example, although not all 3-year-old children can button their clothes or dress with supervision, the nurse can inquire if the parent has presented such opportunities to the child. If the parent has not, the nurse can state that this is an activity that some 3-year-old children can perform, especially if encouraged and helped to do so.

In explaining delays, the nurse carefully notes the parent's response, especially casual acceptance, such as, "He'll catch up." Since all children with questionable or abnormal results should be rescreened before referral for diagnostic testing, some of the parents' more serious questions, such as, "Does this mean my child is retarded?" can be deferred until the next screening session. The nurse must be aware of personal anxieties during these situations and refrain from giving glib reassurances, such as, "I'm sure he will do better the next time." Rather, parents' questions should be answered honestly yet with appropriate flexibility and concern by stating, "I need to observe your child again before I can give you any answers or even make assumptions concerning his developmental progress. I will retest him next week, and then possibly I will know more. What are your thoughts about how he performed the items on the DDST?"

If the parents reply that the child's performance was not typical of his usual behavior, it is best to defer any scoring or discussion of the test results with the parents, especially if the refusals yield a questionable or abnormal rating. In this case the DDST is rescheduled for a time when the child is more likely to cooperate.

Short DDST

Several other screening tests are available. One is the short DDST. Using the DDST form, only the three items immediately to the left of the age line, but not intersecting the line, in each of the four sectors are administered. If all 12 items are passed, the child receives no further testing until the next scheduled visit. However, if one or more items are failed or refused, then the full DDST is administered while the child is in the test setting. The major advantages of the short DDST are that it takes less time and that the second stage testing can be done immediately if needed.

Denver Prescreening Developmental Questionnaire (PDQ)

Another prescreening test is the *Denver Prescreening Developmental Questionnaire (PDQ)*. It is designed to identify those children who require a more thorough screening with the DDST. It has the advantage of being very easy and rapid to administer (it takes parents about 5 minutes to answer the questions). It consists of a total of 97 questions that focus on a child's current behavior. Only 10 questions must be answered for any one child. The questions are arranged in chronologic order according to the age at which 90% of children passed the corresponding DDST item. Scores of 9 or 10 are considered nonsuspect. Children with scores of 8 or below are retested with the PDQ in 2 to 4 weeks. Children with rescreening scores of 6 or below should be referred for diagnostic testing.

Although screening tests are an effective method of applying the knowledge of children's expected rate of development to a large segment of the population, they are only as successful as the individuals' expertise in administering them. Since many of the screening tests are devised to be used by paraprofessionals, there are inherent risks in screening if such individuals are not properly trained or supervised. For example, false-positives can label the child as developmentally delayed and cause problems that otherwise might not have existed. It is the responsibility of the nurse to ensure that screening tests are properly administered and that the results are correctly interpreted. The complexity of mental and physical health can never be measured by any one index. Evaluation of the child's total well-being is the result of evaluating data from a comprehensive history, physical examination, and developmental screening.

REFERENCES

Blumenthal, S., and others: Report of the task force on blood pressure control in children, Pediatrics **59**(suppl.):797, 1977.

Frankenburg, W.K., and others: The newly abbreviated and revised Denver Developmental Screening Test, J. Pediatr. **99**(6):995-999, 1981.

National Society to Prevent Blindness: Children's eye health guide, New York, 1982, The Society.

Steinfeld, L., and others: Sphygmomanometry in the pediatric patient, J. Pediatr. **92**:934-938, June 1978.

BIBLIOGRAPHY

Adler, J.: Patient assessment: abnormalities of the heartbeat, Am. J. Nurs. **77**(4):647-673, 1977.

Alexander, M.M., and Brown, M.S.: Physical examination. Part 12. Examining the chest and lungs, Nursing 75 **5**(1):44-48, 1975.

Alexander, M.M., and Brown, M.S.: Physical examination. Part 13. Examining the abdomen, Nursing 76 **6**(1):65-70, 1976.

Alexander, M.M., and Brown, M.S.: Physical examination. Part 14. Male genitalia, Nursing 76 **6**(2):39-43, 1976.

Alexander, M.M., and Brown, M.S.: Physical examination. Part 16. The musculoskeletal system, Nursing 76 **6**(4):51-56, 1976.

Alexander, M.M., and Brown, M.S.: Physical examination. Part 17. Performing the neurological examination, Nursing 76 **6**(6):38-43, 1976.

Alexander, M.M., and Brown, M.S.: Physical examination. Part 18. Neurological examination, Nursing 76 **6**(7):50-55, 1976.

Barrus, D.H.: A comparison of rectal and axillary temperatures by electronic thermometer measurement in preschool children, Pediatr. Nurs. **9**(6):424-425, 1983.

Blackburn, N.A., and Cebenka, D.L.: Honing your respiratory assessment technique, RN **43**:28-33, May 1980.

Britton, C.V.: Blood pressure measurement and hypertension in children, Pediatr. Nurs. **7**(4):13-17, 1981.

Brown, J.: Child health maintenance, Nurse Pract. **5**:33-43, Jan./Feb. 1980.

Brown, M.S.: Vision tests for preschoolers, Nursing 75 **5**(5):72-74, 1975.

Brown, M.S., and Alexander, M.M.: Physical examination. Part 15. Female genitalia, Nursing 76 **6**(3):39-41, 1976.

Brown, M.S., and Murphy, M.A.: Ambulatory pediatrics for nurses, ed. 2, New York, 1979, McGraw-Hill Book Co.

Cannon, C.: Hands on guide to palpation and auscultation, RN **43:**20, 22-27, 76, March 1980.

Caufield, C.: A developmental approach to hearing screening in children, Pediatr. Nurs. **4**(2):39-42, 1978.

Chard, M.: An approach to examining the adolescent male, Am. J. Maternal Child Nurs. **1**(1):41-43, 1976.

Cohen, S.: Patient assessment: examination of the female pelvis. Part I, Am. J. Nurs. **78:**1717-1746, 1978.

Cohen, S.: Patient assessment: examination of the male genitalia, Am. J. Nurs. **79:**689-712, 1979.

Cohen, S.: Patient assessment: examining joints of the upper and lower extremities, Am. J. Nurs. **81:**763-786, 1981.

Delancy, V.L., and North, C.: Skin assessment, Topics Clin. Nurs. **5**(2):5-10, 1983.

Delaney, M.T.: Examining the chest. Part I. The lungs, Nursing 75 **5**(8):12-14, 1975.

Delaney, M.T.: Examining the chest. Part II. The heart, Nursing 75 **5**(9):41-44, 1975.

Dessertine, P.S.: Those neglected heart sounds, Pediatr. Nurs. **3**(1):18-20, 1977.

Dossey, B.: Perfecting your skills for systematic patient assessments, Nursing 79 **9**(2):42-45, 1979.

Eoff, M.J., and Joyce, B.: Temperature measurements in children, Am. J. Nurs. **81:**1010-1011, May 1981.

Erickson, R.: A source book for temperature taking, San Diego, 1980, The IVAC Corp.

Frankenburg, W.K., and others: The Denver Prescreening Developmental Questionnaire (PDQ), Pediatrics **57**(5):744-753, 1976.

Freis, P.C.: Sounds of a healthy heart, Issues Compr. Pediatr. Nurs. **3:**1-4, Dec. 1979.

Holland, S.H.: 20/20 vision screening, Pediatr. Nurs. **8**(2):81-87, 1982.

Holland, S.H.: Screening vision to detect eye disorders, Child. Nurs. **2**(1):1-3, 1984.

Hutchfield, K., and Crump, A.: Holding children for examination, Nursing (Oxford) **1:**1003-1005, March 1981.

King. R.C.: Examining the thorax and respiratory system, RN **45:**55-63, 1982.

Koeckeritz, J.L.: Assessing the heart: what's normal and what's not, RN **45:**59-63, l982.

Mechner, F.: Patient assessment: examination of the eye. Part I, Am. J. Nurs. **74**(11):1-24, 1974.

Mechner, F.: Patient assessment: examination of the ear, Am. J. Nurs. **75**(3):1-24, 1975.

Mechner, F.: Patient assessment: examination of the eye. Part II, Am. J. Nurs. **75**(1):1-24, 1975.

Mechner, F.: Patient assessment: examination of the head and neck, Am. J. Nurs. **75**(5):1-24, 1975.

Mechner, F.: Patient assessment: examination of the heart and great vessels. Part I, Am. J. Nurs. **76**(11):1807-1830, 1976.

Mechner, F.: Patient assessment: examination of the chest and lungs, Am. J. Nurs. **76**(9):1453-1475, 1976.

Mechner, F.: Patient assessment: neurological examination. Part III, Am. J. Nurs. **76**(4):608-633, 1976.

Mechner, F.: Patient assessment: auscultation of the heart. Part II, Am. J. Nurs. **77**(2):275-298, 1977.

Medenwald, N.A., and others: Is the DDST as good as you think it is? Pediatr. Nurs. **4**(5):53-55, 1978.

Mitchell, J.R.: Male adolescents' concern about a physical examination conducted by a female, Nurs. Res. **29**:165-169, May/June 1980.

Mizrahi, E.M., and Dorfman, L.J.: Sensory evoked potentials: clinical applications in pediatrics, J. Pediatr. **97**(1):1-10, 1980.

Moss, J.R.: Helping young children cope with the physical examination, Pediatr. Nurs. **7**:17-20, March/April 1981.

Moss, J.R.: Predicting young children's cooperation with the physical examination, Pediatr. Nurs. **9**(3):188-190, 1983.

Moss, M., and Schleutermann, J.: Assessment of the pediatric client. In Malasanos, L., and others: Health assessment, ed. 2, St. Louis, 1981, The C.V. Mosby Co.

O'Pray, M.: Developmental screening tools: using them effectively, Am. J. Maternal Child Nurs. **5**(2):126-130, 1980.

Peltzman, P., and Lipson, E.: Infant hearing assessment: a new approach, Pediatr. Basics **28**:11-14, 1981.

Performing palpation, Nursing 83 **13**(1):68-69, 1983.

Performing percussion, Nursing 83 **13**(2):63-64, 1983.

Roach, L.B.: Color changes in dark skin, Nursing 77 **7**(1):48-51, 1977.

Saul, L.: Heart sounds and common murmurs, Am. J. Nurs. **83**(12):1679-1689, 1983.

Schweiger, J., Lang, J., and Schweiger, J.: Oral assessment: how to do it, Am. J. Nurs. **80**(4):654-663, 1980.

Visich, M.A.: Knowing what you hear: a guide to assessing breath and heart sounds, Nursing 81 **11**(11):64-79, 1981.

Walleck, C.: A neurological assessment procedure that won't make you nervous, Nursing 82 **12**(12):50-56, 1982.

Wong, D.L.: The paper-doll technique, Pediatr. Nurs. **7** (6):39-40, 1981.

Yoos, L.: A developmental approach to physical assessment, Am. J. Maternal Child Nurs. **6**(3):168-170, 1981.

Younger, J.: Detecting visual problems in children, Pediatr. Nurs. **5**(6):50-51, 1979.

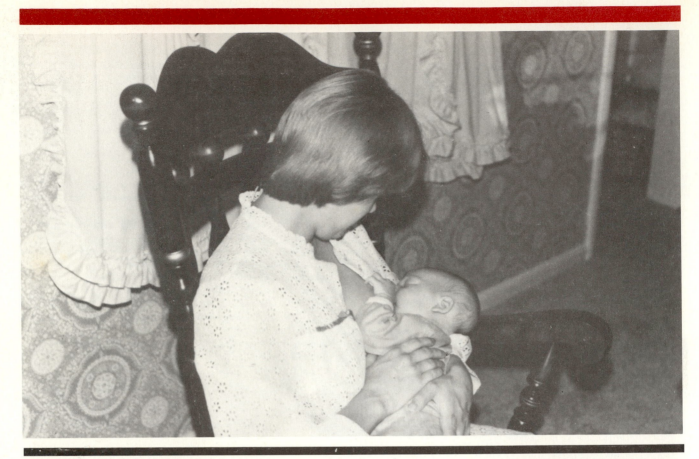

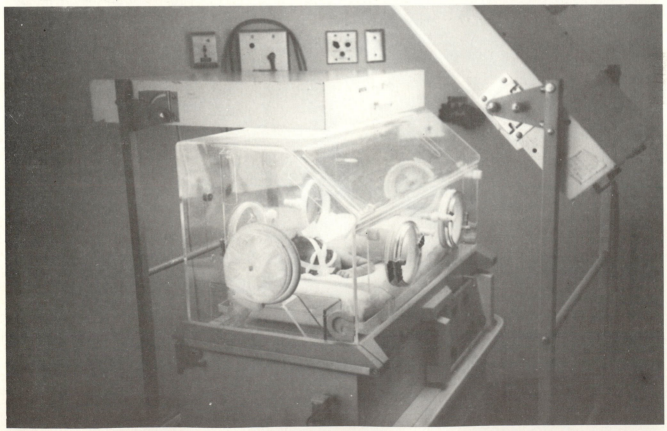

UNIT 3

THE NEONATE

Probably no event is more dramatic or miraculous than the birth of a child. It is the culmination of a 9-month gestation period during which the fetus prepares for extrauterine existence and the parents prepare for the addition of a totally dependent member to their lives. At the time of delivery, profound physiologic and psychologic reactions occur to initiate the child and parents' preparation for this experience.

In most instances the birth and perinatal period are uneventful, and the infant returns home with his parents to begin developing as a vital, healthy, and loved child. Chapter 6, *The Normal Neonate,* is concerned with the infant's normal adjustment to extrauterine life, his physiologic status at birth, and the nursing knowledge required to care for the infant at and immediately following delivery, to perform a physical assessment, and to promote the infant-parent attachment.

Chapter 7, *Health Problems of the Neonate,* is concerned with problems encountered during the neonatal period, including birth trauma, congenital defects, physiologic derangements, perinatal infection, and dysmaturity. The concept of high risk is introduced and focuses on identification and assessment of high-risk neonates, problems common to them because of their high-risk status, and supportive care of the child and family throughout his illness.

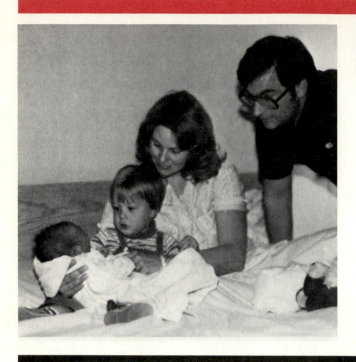

THE NORMAL NEONATE

OBJECTIVES

On completion of this chapter the reader will be able to:

- Identify the principle cardiorespiratory changes that occur during transition to extrauterine life

- Identify the immature physiologic functioning of each body system and its significance to nursing care of the neonate

- Perform an initial and transitional assessment of the newborn based on the Apgar score and periods of reactivity

- Perform a newborn physical assessment based on recognition of expected normal findings

- Administer safe care to the neonate in the nursery

- Assess and promote parent-infant attachment behaviors

NURSING DIAGNOSES

Nursing diagnoses identified for the normal neonate include, but are not restricted to, the following:

Health perception-health management pattern

- Infection, potential for, related to (1) immature immune defenses; (2) environmental hazards

- Injury, potential for (poisoning, suffocation, trauma), related to environmental hazards

Nutritional-metabolic pattern

- Fluid volume deficit, potential, related to (1) delayed feeding; (2) environmental hazards (overheating)

- Nutrition, alterations in: potential for more or less than body requirements, related to feeding problems

- Skin integrity, impairment of: potential, related to (1) birth injury; (2) environmental hazards

Activity-exercise pattern

- Airway clearance, ineffective, related to (1) excess mucus; (2) improper positioning

- Self-care deficit, total, related to developmental level

Role-relationship pattern

- Family process, alterations in, related to (1) gain of a new family member; (2) change in family roles

- Parenting, alterations in: potential, related to (1) skill deficit; (2) change in family unit

Coping-stress tolerance pattern

- Coping, family: potential for growth, related to (1) attachment to newborn; (2) complimentary family role change

Childbirth is an intense and exhausting physiologic and emotional experience for the mother and newborn. Even when this process progresses normally, the neonate is required to withstand extreme changes as he leaves a thermoconstant, aquatic, completely life-sustaining environment and enters a variable pressurized atmosphere that demands profound physiologic alteration for survival. The neonatal or perinatal period, the interval from viability until 28 days after birth, presents the greatest risk to the newborn. In fact, in the United States about three fourths of all deaths during the first year of life occur during these 4 weeks.

The nurse's role is one of supporting the mother and infant through the birth process, preventing physiologic complications in the neonate's adjustment to extrauterine life, and promoting the attachment process between child and parents. Expert technologic and psychologic nursing care during the immediate postpartum period lays a strong foundation for healthy parent-child development.

ADJUSTMENT TO EXTRAUTERINE LIFE

The most profound physiologic change required of the neonate is transition from fetal or placental circulation to independent respiration. The loss of the placental connection means the loss of complete metabolic support, the most important and essential function being the supply of oxygen and the removal of carbon dioxide. The normal stresses of labor and delivery produce alterations of placental gas exchange patterns, acid-base balance in the blood, and cardiovascular activity in the infant. Factors that interfere with this normal transition or that increase fetal asphyxia (a condition of hypoxemia, hypercapnia, and acidosis) will affect the fetus's adjustment to extrauterine life. Factors that influence neonatal adjustments are discussed in Chapter 3.

Immediate adjustments

The neonate's adjustment to extrauterine life is a complex physiologic process. The first 24 hours are the most critical since during this time respiratory distress and circulatory failure can occur rapidly and with little warning. There is a higher incidence of death during these initial 24 hours than during the entire succeeding perinatal period.

Respiratory changes. The most critical and immediate physiologic change required of the neonate is the onset of breathing. The stimuli that help initiate the first respiration are primarily chemical and thermal. The *chemical* changes in the blood—low oxygen, high carbon dioxide, and low pH—initiate impulses that excite the respiratory center in the medulla. The primary *thermal* stimulus is the sudden chilling of the infant as he leaves a warm environment and enters a relatively cooler atmosphere. This abrupt change in temperature excites sensory impulses in the skin that are transmitted to the respiratory center.

The significance of *tactile* stimulation is questionable. Probably descent through the birth canal and normal handling during delivery have some effect on initiation of respiration. Slapping the infant's heel or buttocks has no beneficial effect and usually does no harm, but it is an unnecessary maneuver that wastes precious time in the event of respiratory difficulty.

The initial entry of air into the lungs is opposed by the surface tension of the fluid that filled the fetal lungs and the alveoli. However, fetal lung fluid is removed by the lymphatic vessels and pulmonary capillaries. Some fluid is also removed during the normal forces of labor and delivery. As the chest emerges from the birth canal, fluid is squeezed from the lungs through the nose and mouth. Following complete delivery of the chest, a brisk recoil of the thorax occurs. Air enters the upper airway to replace the lost fluid.

In the alveoli the surface tension of the fluid is reduced by *surfactant,* a substance produced by the alveolar epithelium that coats the alveolar surface. Surfactant acts very much like a detergent in reducing the surface tension of the fluid. Its effect is greatest during expiration, when the alveoli are contracted, because the layer of surfactant becomes thicker. This is very fortunate because the enhanced effect of surfactant allows some air to remain in the alveoli at the end of expiration. Consequently, each respiration following the initial breath requires much less effort because the alveoli are already partially expanded. In the absence of surfactant, each respiration requires the same high pressure as the first breath, thus increasing the labor of breathing. This condition, known as *respiratory distress syndrome,* frequently develops in neonates born prematurely.

Circulatory changes. Equally as important as the initiation of respiration are the circulatory changes that allow blood to flow through the lungs. These changes occur more gradually and are the result of shifts in pressure in the heart and major vessels from increased pulmonary and systemic blood volume secondary to decreased pulmonary vascular resistance and increased systemic vascular resistance. The transition from fetal circulation to postnatal circulation involves the functional closure of the fetal shunts, the foramen ovale, the ductus arteriosus, and eventually the ductus venosus. (For a review of fetal circulation see p. 707.)

Once the lungs are expanded, the inspired oxygen dilates the pulmonary vessels, which causes a decrease in pulmonary vascular resistance and consequently, increased pulmonary blood flow. As the lungs receive blood, the pressure in the right atrium, right ventricle, and pulmonary

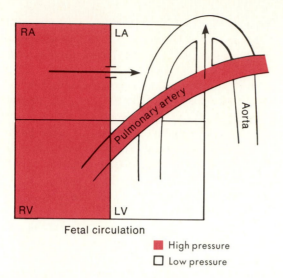
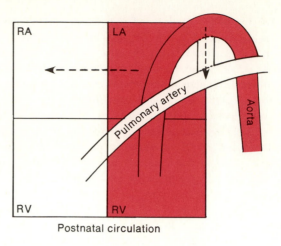

Fetal circulation

Postnatal circulation

■ High pressure
☐ Low pressure

FIG. 6-1

Changes in pressure at birth and their effect upon blood flow through the fetal shunts.

arteries decreases. At the same time there is a progressive rise in systemic vascular resistance from the increased volume of blood through the placenta at cord clamping. This increases the pressure in the left side of the heart. Since blood flows from an area of high pressure to one of low pressure, the circulation of blood through the fetal shunts is reversed (Fig. 6-1).

The most important factor controlling ductal closure is the oxygen concentration of the blood. Secondary factors are the fall in endogenous prostaglandins and acidosis. With the backward flow of blood through the fetal shunts, the high oxygen level of the blood causes the muscular walls of the ducts to constrict. The foramen ovale closes functionally at or soon after birth. The ductus arteriosus is closed functionally by the fourth day. Anatomic closure takes considerably longer. Failure of the ducts to close results in congenital heart defects (see Chapter 22).

Because of the reversible flow of blood through the openings during the early neonatal period, functional murmurs are occasionally heard. In conditions such as crying or straining the increased pressure shunts unoxygenated blood from the right side of the heart across the ductal opening, causing transient cyanosis.

PHYSIOLOGIC STATUS OF THE NEWBORN

The major life-dependent physiologic changes in the neonate have been discussed. All the systems undergo some change, and most are immature at birth. Each should be observed closely for proper functioning and adjustment to extrauterine life.

Hemopoietic system

The blood volume of the fetus at term is about 90 ml/kg. Immediately after birth the total blood volume averages 300 ml but varies depending on how long the infant is attached to the placenta. It is important that the delivery nurse take special note of the time interval between birth and cord clamping, since blood volume affects hematocrit values, initial blood pressure, and respiratory status.

The average red blood cell (RBC) count of the newborn is 5 million/mm^3. The mean hemoglobin value at birth is 16 to 18 g/100 ml of blood, the average hematocrit value is between 45 and 50 ml/100 ml, and the white blood cell (WBC) count is about 20,000/mm^3.

Fluid and electrolyte balance

Changes occur in the total body water volume, extracellular fluid volume, and intracellular fluid volume during the transition from fetal to postnatal life. At birth the total weight of the infant is 73% fluid, as compared to 58% in the adult. The infant has a proportionately higher ratio of extracellular fluid than the adult and consequently has a higher level of total body sodium and chloride and a lower level of potassium, magnesium, and phosphate.

Thermoregulation

The newborn's capacity for heat production is adequate. However, heat is not produced by shivering and voluntary muscular activity as in the older child and adult. Rather, heat production is from the oxidation of fat, particularly brown fat. Brown fat, which has a greater capacity for heat production, is located between the scapula, around the neck, and behind the sternum. Deeper layers surround the kidneys and adrenals. The location of the brown fat may explain why the nape of the neck frequently feels warmer than the rest of the infant's body. Heat generated in the brown fat is distributed to other parts of the body by the blood, which is warmed as it flows through the layers of this tissue. It is important to remember that heat production is through increased metabolic activity, which will affect calorie requirements and oxygen consumption.

Newborns can lose heat faster than they are able to produce it because their large surface area favors rapid heat loss, and the thin layer of subcutaneous fat provides poor insulation for conservation of heat. Fortunately, their normally flexed position decreases the surface area exposed to the environment. They also have difficulty dissipating heat because of the reduced ability of the eccrine glands to produce sweat. This increases the risk of hyperthermia.

Gastrointestinal system

The ability of the newborn to digest, absorb, and metabolize foodstuff is limited. Enzymes are adequate to handle the proteins and simple carbohydrates (monosaccharides and disaccharides), but deficient production of pancreatic amylase impairs utilization of complex carbohydrates (polysaccharides). Deficiency of pancreatic lipase limits absorption of fats, especially with ingestion of foods with high saturated fatty acid content, such as cow's milk.

The liver is the most immature of the gastrointestinal organs. The activity of the enzyme *glucuronyl transferase* is reduced, which affects the conjugation of bilirubin with glucuronic acid and contributes to the physiologic jaundice of the newborn. It is deficient in forming plasma proteins. The decreased plasma protein concentration probably plays a role in the edema usually seen at birth. Prothrombin and other coagulation factors are also low. The liver stores less glycogen at birth than later in life. Consequently the newborn is prone to hypoglycemia, which may be prevented by early feeding.

Some salivary glands are functioning at birth, but the majority do not begin to secrete saliva until about age 2 to 3 months, when drooling is frequent. The stomach capacity is limited to about 90 ml; thus the infant requires frequent small feedings. The emptying time is short, about 2½ to 3 hours, and peristalsis is rapid. These two factors increase the transit time of food passing through the stomach and colon. During the early weeks of life the newborn may have a bowel movement after each feeding.

The infant's intestine is longer in relation to body size than that in the adult. Therefore, there are a larger number of secretory glands and a larger surface area for absorption as compared to the adult's intestine. There are rapid peristaltic waves and simultaneous nonperistaltic waves along the entire esophagus. These waves, combined with an immature relaxed cardiac sphincter, make regurgitation a common occurrence.

Progressive changes in the stooling pattern indicate a properly functioning gastrointestinal tract. The infant's first stool is the sticky and greenish black *meconium,* which is composed of intrauterine debris, such as bile pigments, epithelial cells, fatty acids, mucus, blood, and amniotic fluid. Passage of meconium should occur within the first 36 hours.

Usually by the third day after the initiation of feedings, *transitional stools* appear. They are greenish brown to yellowish brown in color, less sticky than meconium, and may contain some milk curds. By the fourth day a typical *milk stool* is passed. In breast-fed infants the stools are yellow to golden in color and pasty in consistency. They have a peculiar odor, similar to that of sour milk. In infants fed cow's milk formula, the stools are pale yellow to light brown, are firmer in consistency, and have a more offensive odor.

Breast-fed infants usually have more stools than do bottle-fed infants. The stool pattern can vary widely; six stools a day may be normal for one infant, whereas a stool every other day may be normal for another.

Renal system

All structural components are present in the renal system, but there is a functional deficiency in the kidney's ability to concentrate urine and to cope with conditions of fluid and electrolyte stress, such as dehydration or a concentrated solute load.

Total volume of urine per 24 hours is about 200 to 300 ml by the end of the first week. However, the bladder voluntarily empties when stretched by a volume of 15 ml, resulting in as many as 20 voidings per day. The first voiding should occur within 24 hours. The neonate's urine is colorless and odorless and has a specific gravity of about 1.008.

Integumentary system

At birth all the structures within the skin are present, but many of the functions of the integument are immature. The two layers of the skin, the epidermis and dermis, are loosely bound to each other and are very thin. Slight friction across the epidermis causes separation of these layers and blister formation, such as from rapid removal of adhesive tape. The transitional zone between the cornified and living layers of the epidermis is effective in preventing fluid from reaching the skin surface.

The *sebaceous glands* are very active late in fetal life and in early infancy because of the high levels of maternal androgens. They are most densely located on the scalp, face, and genitalia and produce the greasy vernix caseosa that covers the infant at birth.

The *eccrine glands,* which produce sweat in response to heat or emotional stimuli, are nonfunctional at birth but become active during the next few days, beginning with sweating on the face, then on the palms. They produce sweat in response to higher temperatures than those required in adults and the retention of sweat may result in miliaria (minute vesicles and papules, sometimes called "prickly heat"). The *apocrine glands* remain small and nonfunctional until puberty.

The growth phases of hair follicles usually occur simultaneously at birth. During the first few months the synchrony between hair loss and regrowth is disrupted, and there may be overgrowth of hair or temporary alopecia. Boys' hair grows faster than girls' hair, and in both sexes scalp hair growth is slower at the crown.

Because melanin is low at birth, the newborn is lighter skinned than he will be as a child. This also means that the infant is more susceptible to the harmful effects of the sun.

Musculoskeletal system

At birth the skeletal system contains larger amounts of cartilage than ossified bone, although the process of ossification is fairly rapid during the first year. The nose, for example, is predominantly cartilage at birth and is frequently flattened by the force of delivery. The six skull bones are relatively soft and are separated only by membranous seams. The sinuses are incompletely formed in the newborn.

Unlike the skeletal system, the muscular system is almost completely formed at birth. Growth in the size of muscular tissue is caused by hypertrophy, rather than hyperplasia, of cells.

Defenses against infection

The infant is born with several defenses against infection. First, the *skin* and *mucous membranes* protect the body from invading organisms. Second, the *reticuloendothelial system* produces several types of cells capable of attacking a pathogen. The neutrophils and monocytes are phagocytes, which enables them to engulf, ingest, and destroy foreign agents. Eosinophils also probably have a phagocytic property, since in the presence of foreign protein they increase in number. The lymphocytes (T- and B-cells) are capable of being converted to other cell types, such as monocytes and antibodies. Although the phagocytic properties of the blood are present in the infant, the inflammatory response of the tissues to localize an infection is immature. The exact reason for this is unknown.

The third line of defense is the formation of specific *antibodies* to an antigen. This process requires exposure to various foreign agents for antibody production to occur. The infant is generally not capable of producing his own gamma globulins until the beginning of the second month of life but has received considerable passive immunity in the form of IgG from the maternal circulation. He is protected against most major childhood diseases, including diphtheria, measles, poliomyelitis, infectious hepatitis, and rubella, for about 3 months, provided the mother has developed antibodies to these illnesses.

In addition, breast-fed infants may acquire temporary immunity to such diseases as mumps, influenza, and chickenpox. Breast milk is rich in IgA and contains large numbers of macrophages, as well as a small number of lymphocytes, mainly B-lymphocytes with a minor T-lymphocyte component.

Endocrine system

Ordinarily the endocrine system of the newborn is adequately developed, but its functions are immature. For example, the posterior lobe of the pituitary gland produces limited quantities of antidiuretic hormone (ADH) or vasopressin, which inhibits diuresis. This renders the young infant highly susceptible to dehydration.

The effect of maternal sex hormones is particularly evident in the newborn because it causes a miniature puberty. The labia are hypertrophied and the breasts may be engorged and secrete milk during the first few days of life. Female newborns sometimes have pseudomenstruation from the sudden drop in the level of progesterone and estrogen.

Neurologic system

At birth the nervous system is incompletely integrated but sufficiently developed to sustain extrauterine life. Most neurologic functions are primitive reflexes. The autonomic nervous system is crucial during transition because it stimulates initial respirations, helps maintain acid-base balance, and partially regulates temperature control.

Myelination of the nervous system follows the cephalocaudal-proximodistal laws of development and is closely related to observed mastery of fine and gross motor skills. Myelin is necessary for rapid and efficient transmission of nerve impulses along the neural pathway. The tracts that develop myelin earliest are the sensory, cerebellar, and extrapyramidal. This accounts for the acute senses of taste, smell, and hearing in the newborn. All cranial nerves are present and myelinated except for the optic and olfactory nerves.

Sensory functions

The newborn's sensory functions are remarkably well developed and have a significant effect on growth and development, including the attachment process. Unfortunately, minimal research has been done on evaluating the senses, mainly because of the difficulty of accurately assessing them.

Vision. At birth the eye is structurally incomplete. The ciliary muscles are immature, limiting the ability of the eyes to accommodate and fixate on an object for any length of time. The infant can track and follow objects. The pupils react to light, the blink reflex is responsive to a minimal stimulus, and the corneal reflex is activated by a light touch. Tear glands usually do not begin to function until the neonate is 2 to 4 weeks of age.

The newborn has the ability to fixate momentarily on a bright or moving object that is within 20 cm (8 inches) and in the midline of the visual field. In fact the infant's ability to fixate on coordinated movement is greater during the first hour of life than during the succeeding several days. Although visual acuity is difficult to measure, it has been found that a newborn can respond to optokinetic stripes that are comparable to 20/50 vision.

The infant also demonstrates visual preferences: medium colors (yellow, green, pink) over bright (red, orange, blue) or dim colors; black and white contrasting patterns, especially geometric shapes and checkerboards; large objects with medium complexity rather than small, complex objects; and reflecting objects over dull ones.

Hearing. Once the amniotic fluid has drained from the ears, the infant probably has auditory acuity similar to that of an adult. The neonate is able to detect a loud sound of about 90 decibels and reacts with a startle reflex. The newborn's response to sounds of low frequency versus those of high frequency differs; the former, such as the sound of a heartbeat, metronome, or lullaby, tends to decrease an infant's motor activity and crying, whereas the latter elicits an alerting reaction. There also seems to be an early sensitivity to the sound of human voices, though not specifically speech sounds. For example, infants younger than 3 days of age can discriminate the mother's voice from that of other females. As early as age 2 weeks the infant may stop crying to listen to the sound of a voice.

At birth all the structural components of the ear are fully mature. However, the cortical activity associated with hearing or with any other sense is still incomplete because of the immature myelination of the various neural pathways beyond the midbrain. This lack of cortical integration is responsible for the infant's generalized response to sound.

Smell. Limited research has been done on the newborn's ability to smell. However, it is known that newborns will react to strong odors such as alcohol or vinegar by turning their heads away. Recent studies have demonstrated that breast-fed infants seem able to smell breast milk and will cry for their mothers when the breasts are engorged and leaking.

Taste. The newborn has the ability to distinguish between tastes. Various types of solutions elicit differing gustofacial reflexes. A tasteless solution elicits no facial expression, a sweet solution elicits an eager suck and a look of satisfaction, a sour solution causes the usual puckering of the lips, and a bitter liquid produces an angry, upset expression. During early childhood the taste buds are distributed mostly on the tip of the tongue.

Touch. At birth the infant is able to perceive tactile sensation in any part of the body, although the face (especially the mouth), hands, and soles of the feet seem to be most sensitive. There is increasing documentation that touch and motion are essential to normal growth and development. Gentle patting of the back or rubbing of the abdomen usually elicits a calming response from the infant. However, painful stimuli, such as a pinprick, will elicit an angry, upsetting response.

ASSESSMENT OF THE NEONATE

Once the infant is born, he requires thorough, skilled observation to ensure a satisfactory adjustment to extrauterine life. Assessment following delivery can be divided into three phases: (1) the initial assessment using the Apgar scoring system, (2) transitional assessment during the periods of reactivity, and (3) periodic assessment through systematic physical examination. Awareness of the expected normal findings during each assessment process helps the nurse recognize any deviation that may prevent the infant from progressing uneventfully through the early postnatal period.

Initial assessment: Apgar scoring

During the first seconds of the newborn's life, complex extensive physiologic changes occur. It is imperative that the nurse make astute observations during this time. One of the methods used to assess the newborn's immediate adjustment to extrauterine life is the Apgar scoring system. The score is based on observation of heart rate, respiratory effort, muscle tone, reflex irritability, and color (Table 6-1). Each item is given a score of 0, 1, or 2. Evaluations of all five categories are made at 1 and 5 minutes after birth and may be repeated until the infant's condition stabilizes. Total scores of 0 to 3 represent severe distress, scores of 4 to 6 signify moderate difficulty, and scores of 7 to 10 indicate absence of difficulty in adjusting to life.

The *heart rate* is the most evaluative of the five items. For accuracy, the heart rate should be counted for at least 30 seconds and correlated with the infant's activity.

TABLE 6-1. INFANT EVALUATION AT BIRTH—APGAR SCORING SYSTEM

	0	1	2
Heart rate	Absent	Slow (below 100 beats/minute)	Over 100 beats/minute
Respiratory effort	Absent	Slow or irregular	Good crying
Muscle tone	Limp	Some flexion of extremities	Active motion
Response to catheter in anterior nostril (tested after oropharynx is clear)	No response	Grimace	Cough or sneeze
Color	Blue or pale	Body pink, extremities blue	Completely pink

Respiratory effort is evaluated as an index of adequate ventilation. If the respirations are slow, shallow, irregular, or gasping, they indicate respiratory distress.

Muscle tone refers to the degree of flexion and resistance offered by the infant when the nurse attempts to extend his extremities. The normal infant's position is one of flexion—the extremities are flexed and close to the body, and the fist is tightly clenched. Any attempt to alter this flexed position should be met with resistance.

Reflex irritability is judged by the infant's response to passing a catheter into the tip of the nose after suctioning. It can also be evaluated by slapping the sole of the foot with the palm of the hand. The usual response from a healthy newborn is a loud, angry cry.

Color reflects peripheral tissue oxygenation. Few newborns are completely pink at 1 minute after birth. Most infants continue to have some blueness of the extremities, whereas the rest of the body is pink. In evaluating color of nonwhite newborns, it is important to inspect the color of the mucous membranes of mouth and conjunctiva as well as the color of the lips, palms of the hands, and soles of the feet.

Transitional assessment: periods of reactivity

The newborn exhibits behavioral and physiologic characteristics that can at first appear to be signs of stress. However, during the initial 24 hours, changes in heart rate, respiration, motor activity, color, mucus production, and bowel activity occur in an orderly, predictable sequence, which are normal and indicate lack of stress.

For 6 to 8 hours after birth, the newborn is in the *first period of reactivity*. During the first 30 minutes the infant is very alert, cries vigorously, may suck his fist greedily, and appears very interested in his environment. At this time his eyes are usually open, suggesting that this is an excellent opportunity for mother, father, and child to see each other. Because he has a vigorous suck, this is also an opportune time to begin breast-feeding. He will usually grasp the nipple quickly, satisfying both mother and infant. This is particularly important for nurses to remember, because after this initially highly active state the infant

may be quite sleepy and uninterested in sucking. Physiologically the respiratory rate during this period is as high as 82 breaths/minute, rales may be heard, heart rate reaches 180 beats/minute, bowel sounds are active, mucous secretions are increased, and temperature may decrease.

After this initial stage of alertness and activity, the infant's responsiveness diminishes. Heart and respiratory rates decrease, temperature continues to fall, mucus production decreases, and urine or stool is usually not passed. The infant is in a state of sleep and relative calm. Any attempt to stimulate him usually elicits a minimal response. This second stage of the first reactive period generally lasts 2 to 4 hours. Because of the continued decrease in body temperature, it is best to avoid undressing or bathing the infant during this time.

The *second period of reactivity* begins when the infant awakes from this deep sleep. The infant is again alert and responsive, heart and respiratory rates increase, the gag reflex is active, gastric and respiratory secretions are increased, and passage of meconium frequently occurs. This second period of reactivity lasts about 2 to 5 hours and provides another excellent opportunity for child and parents to interact. This period is usually over when the amount of respiratory mucus has decreased. Following this stage is a period of stabilization of physiologic systems and vacillating pattern of sleep and activity.

Physical assessment

An important aspect of the care of the newborn is a thorough physical examination that identifies normal characteristics and existing abnormalities and establishes a baseline for future physiologic changes. The physical assessment of the neonate should be one of the nurse's priorities in the plan of care. This discussion focuses on the newborn assessment with emphasis on normal findings (Table 6-2). In some facilities estimation of gestational age is also a routine procedure (see Chapter 7).

Examination of the newborn generally presents few problems in terms of gaining his acceptance or cooperation. However, a few comments may prove helpful. In

TABLE 6-2. SUMMARY OF PHYSICAL ASSESSMENT OF THE NEONATE

AREA	USUAL FINDINGS	COMMENTS
General measurements	Head circumference 33-35.5 cm (13-14 inches) Chest circumference 30.5-33 cm (12-13 inches) Head circumference should be about 2-3 cm (1 inch) larger than chest circumference Crown-to-rump length 31-35 cm (12½-14 inches) Crown-to-rump length approximately equal to head circumference Head-to-heel length 48-53 cm (19-21 inches) Birth weight 2700-4000 g (6-9 pounds)	Molding after birth may decrease head circumference Head and chest circumferences may be equal for first 1-2 days after birth
General appearance	Posture—flexion of head and extremities, which rest on chest and abdomen	In frank breech—extended legs, abducted and fully rotated thighs, flattened head, extended neck
Skin	At birth—bright red, puffy, smooth Second to third day—pink, flaky, dry Vernix caseosa Lanugo Edema around eyes, face, legs, dorsa of hands, feet, and scrotum or labia	Other common findings: Neonatal jaundice after first 24 hours Ecchymoses or petechiae caused by birth trauma Milia neonatorum Sudamina

Normal color changes:

Acrocyanosis—Cyanosis of hands and feet

Cutis marmorata—Transient mottling when infant is exposed to decreased temperature

Erythema toxicum—Pink papular rash with vesicles superimposed on thorax, back, buttocks, and abdomen; may appear in 24 to 48 hours and resolves after several days

Harlequin color change—Clearly outlined color change as infant lies on side; lower half of body becomes pink and upper half is pale

Mongolian spots—Irregular areas of deep blue pigmentation, usually in the sacral and gluteal regions; seen predominantly in newborns of African, Asian, or Hispanic descent

Telangiectatic nevi ("stork bites")—Flat, deep pink localized areas usually seen in back of neck

AREA	USUAL FINDINGS	COMMENTS
Head	Anterior fontanel—diamond-shaped 2.5-4.0 cm (1-1¾ inches) Posterior fontanel—triangular-shaped, 0.5-1 cm (¼-⅜ inch) Fontanels should be flat, soft, and firm	Molding usually follows vaginal delivery Fontanels may bulge because of crying or coughing
Eyes	Lids usually edematous Eyes usually closed Color—slate gray, dark blue, brown Absence of tears Presence of red reflex Corneal reflex in response to touch Pupillary reflex in response to light Blink reflex in response to light or touch Rudimentary fixation on objects and ability to follow to midline	Other common findings: Chemical conjunctivitis Searching nystagmus or strabismus
Ears	Position—top of pinna on horizontal line with outer canthus of eye Startle reflex elicited by a loud, sudden noise Pinna flexible, cartilage present	Inability to visualize tympanic membrane because of filled aural canals Pinna is flat against head

Continued.

TABLE 6-2. SUMMARY OF PHYSICAL ASSESSMENT OF THE NEONATE—cont'd

AREA	USUAL FINDINGS	COMMENTS
Nose	Nasal patency Nasal discharge—thin white mucus Sneezing	May be flattened and bruised
Mouth and throat	Intact, high-arched palate Uvula in midline Frenulum of tongue Frenum of upper lip Sucking reflex Rooting reflex Gag reflex Extrusion reflex Absent or minimal salivation	May see Epstein's pearls
Neck	Short, thick, usually surrounded by skin folds Tonic neck reflex	
Chest	Anteroposterior and lateral diameters equal Slight sternal retractions evident during inspiration Xiphoid process evident Breast enlargement	Secretion of milky substance from breasts is common in some female infants
Lungs	Rate—30-60 breaths/min Respirations chiefly abdominal Cough reflex absent at birth, present by 1-2 days Bilateral bronchial breath sounds	Rate and depth of respirations may be irregular, momentary apneic spells are common
Heart	Rate—120-140 beats/min and regular Apex—third to fourth intercostal space, lateral to midclavicular line S_2 slightly sharper and higher in pitch than S_1	Sinus arrhythmia is common Transient cyanosis is present on crying or straining
Abdomen	Cylindric in shape Liver—palpable 2-3 cm (about 1 inch) below right costal margin Spleen—tip palpable at end of first week of age Kidneys—palpable 1-2 cm (⅜ to ¾ inch) above umbilicus Equal bilateral femoral pulses	Umbilical hernia may be present

general it is best to proceed in an orderly head-to-toe progression. Since exposing an infant to the air when undressing him usually elicits crying, it is best to listen to the heart, lungs, and abdomen first. Head, chest, and length measurements are taken at the same time to mentally make a note of their relationship to each other. Weight is taken with the infant fully undressed. If clothing is not removed, the scale should be prebalanced to adjust for the excess weight by weighing similar articles of clothing first. If the newborn is irritable and crying during the examination, allowing him to suck on a nipple or on one's gloved finger usually pacifies him sufficiently to complete palpation and auscultation.

General measurements

There are several important measurements of the newborn that have significance when compared to each other as well as when recorded over time on a graph. For the full-term infant, average *head circumference* is between 33 and 35.5 cm (13 to 14 inches). Head circumference may be somewhat less immediately after birth because of the molding

TABLE 6-2. SUMMARY OF PHYSICAL ASSESSMENT OF THE NEONATE—cont'd

AREA	USUAL FINDINGS	COMMENTS
Female genitalia	Labia and clitoris usually edematous Labia minora larger than labia majora Urethral meatus behind clitoris Hymenal tag Vernix caseosa between labia	Blood-tinged discharge (pseudomenstruation) may be present in female infants
Male genitalia	Urethral opening at tip of glans penis Testes palpable in each scrotum Scrotum large, edematous, and pendulous; usually deeply pigmented in dark-skinned ethnic groups Smegma	Other common findings: Urethral opening covered by prepuce Inability to retract foreskin Epithelial pearls Erection or priapism Testes palpable in inguinal canal Scrotum small
Back and rectum	Spine intact, no openings, masses, or prominent curves Trunk incurvation reflex Patent anal opening	Mongolian spots
Extremities	10 fingers and toes Full range of motion Negative scarf sign—elbow does not reach midline Nail beds pink, with transient cyanosis immediately after birth Creases on anterior two thirds of sole Sole usually flat Symmetry of extremities Equal muscle tone bilaterally, especially resistance to opposing flexion	Other common findings: Partial syndactyly between second and third toes Clinodactyly of second toe with overlapping into third toe Wide gap between first and second toe Deep crease on plantar surface of foot between first and second toes Asymmetric length of toes Dorsiflexion and shortness of first toe
Neuromuscular system	Extremities usually maintain some degree of flexion Extension of an extremity followed by previous position of flexion Head lag while sitting, but momentary ability to hold head erect Able to turn head from side to side when prone Able to hold head in horizontal line with back when held prone	Quivering or momentary tremors are common

process that occurs during a normal vaginal delivery. Usually by the second or third day the normal size and contour of the skull have replaced the molded one.

Chest circumference is 30.5 to 33 cm (12 to 13 inches). The usual relationship between head and chest circumference is a difference of about 2 to 3 cm, or 1 inch. Because of the molding of the head during delivery, initially these measurements may appear equal.

Head circumference may also be compared with *crown-to-rump* length, or sitting height (Fig. 6-2). Crown-to-rump measurements are usually 31 to 35 cm (12.5 to 14 inches) and are approximately equal to head circumference. The relationship of the head and crown-to-rump measurements is more reliable than that of the head and chest.

Head-to-heel length is also measured in the newborn. Because of the usual flexed position of the infant, it is important to extend the leg completely when measuring total body length. The average length of the newborn is 48 to 53 cm (19 to 21 inches).

Body weight is taken in the delivery room because weight loss will occur fairly rapidly after birth. Normally

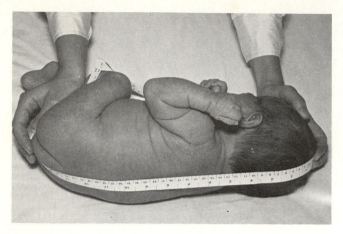

FIG. 6-2

Measurement of crown-to-rump length in appraisal of newborn.

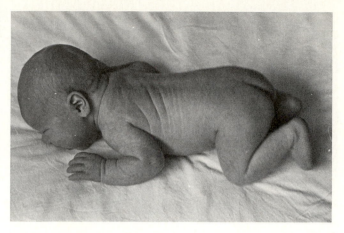

FIG. 6-3

Flexed position of neonate.

the neonate loses about 10% of the birth weight by 3 to 4 days of age because of loss of excessive extracellular fluid, meconium, and limited food intake. The birth weight is usually regained by the tenth day of life. Most newborns weigh 2700 to 4000 g (6 to 9 pounds), the average weight being about 3400 g (7.5 pounds). Newborns who weigh below 2500 g (5.5 pounds) are usually classified as low birth weight infants. (For additional information on this topic, see the discussion of weight related to gestational age located on p. 179.) Accurate birth weights and lengths are important because they provide a baseline for assessment of future growth.

Another category of measurements is *vital signs*. *Axillary temperatures* are taken because insertion of a thermometer into the rectum can cause perforation of the mucosa. Core (internal) body temperature varies according to the periods of reactivity but is usually 35.5° to 37.5° C (96° to 99.5° F). Skin temperature is slightly lower than core body temperature.

Pulse and *respirations* also vary according to the periods of reactivity and to the infant's behaviors but are usually in the range of 120 to 140 beats/minute and 30 to 60 breaths/minute, respectively. Both are counted for a full 60 seconds to detect irregularities in rate or rhythm. Heart rate is taken apically with a stethoscope. Although not a routine procedure in some nurseries, blood pressure should be taken in newborns to establish a baseline. The average systolic blood pressure is from 50 to 70 mm Hg and diastolic pressure is from 25 to 45 mm Hg.

General appearance

Before each body system is assessed, it is important to describe the general posture and behavior of the newborn.

The overall appearance yields valuable clues to the physical status of the infant.

Posture. In the full-term neonate the posture is one of flexion, a result of in utero position (Fig. 6-3). The infant born in a vertex position keeps the head flexed, with the chin resting on the upper chest. The arms are flexed at the elbows, and they rest, folded, on the chest. The hands are held in a clenched or fisted position. The legs are flexed at the knees, and the hips are flexed in such a position that the thighs rest on the abdomen. The feet are dorsiflexed and positioned on the anterior aspect of the legs. The vertebral column is also flexed. It is important to recognize any deviation from this very characteristic fetal position.

Behavior. The infant's behavior is carefully noted, especially the degree of alertness, drowsiness, and irritability, which are common signs of neurologic problems. Some questions to mentally ask when assessing behavior include is the infant awakened easily by a loud noise; is he comforted by rocking, sucking, or cuddling; do there seem to be periods of deep and light sleep; when he is awake, does he seem satisfied after a feeding; what stimuli elicit responses from him; and, when he is disturbed, how much does he protest? (See also pp. 149 and 160.)

Skin

The skin of the newborn is velvety smooth and puffy, especially about the eyes, the legs, the dorsal aspect of the hands and the feet, and the scrotum or labia.

Skin color depends on racial and familial background. The white infant is usually pink to red; the black newborn may appear a pinkish brown. Infants of Oriental descent may resemble a shade of tea rose; those of Hispanic de-

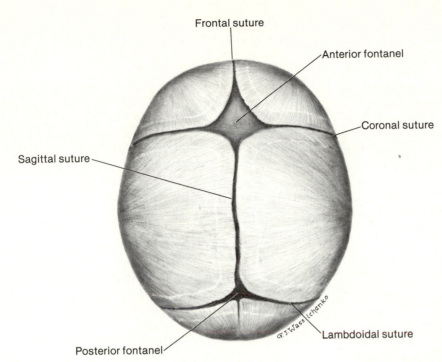

FIG. 6-4
Location of sutures and fontanels.

scent may have an olive tint or a slight yellow cast to the skin. By the second or third day the skin turns to its more natural tone and is more dry and flaky. Several color changes may be noted on the skin. These are summarized in Table 6-2.

At birth the skin is covered with a grayish-white, cheese-like substance called *vernix caseosa,* a mixture of sebum and desquamating cells. If it is not removed during the bath, it will dry and disappear by about 24 to 48 hours. A fine, downy hair called *lanugo* is present on the skin, especially on the forehead, cheeks, shoulders, and back. *Milia,* distended sebaceous glands, appear as tiny white papules on the cheeks, chin, and nose. They usually disappear spontaneously in a few weeks. *Sudamina* or *miliaria* are distended sweat (eccrine) glands that cause minute vesicles on the skin surface, especially on the face.

Head

General observation of the contour of the head is important since molding occurs in almost all vaginal deliveries. In a vertex delivery the head will usually be flattened at the forehead, with the apex elongated at the end of the parietal bones and the posterior skull or occiput dropping abruptly. The usual more oval contour of the head is apparent by 1 to 2 days after birth. The change in shape occurs because the bones of the cranium are not fused, allowing for overlapping of the edges of these bones to accommodate to the size of the birth canal during delivery.

Six bones—the frontal, occipital, two parietals, and two temporals—comprise the cranium. Between the junc-

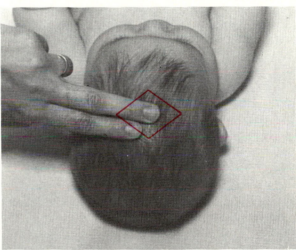

FIG. 6-5
Palpating anterior fontanel.

tion of these bones are bands of connective tissue called *sutures.* At the junction of the sutures are wider spaces of unossified membranous tissue called *fontanels.* The two most prominent fontanels in infants are the *anterior fontanel,* formed by the junction of the sagittal, coronal, and frontal sutures, and the *posterior fontanel,* formed by the junction of the sagittal and lambdoid sutures. One can easily remember the location of the sutures because the coronal suture "crowns" the head and the sagittal suture "separates" the head (Fig. 6-4).

The skull is palpated for all patent sutures and fontanels, noting size, shape, molding, or abnormal closure. The sutures feel like cracks between the skull bones, and the fontanels like wider ''soft spots'' at the junction of the sutures. These are palpated by using the tip of the index finger and running it along the ends of the bones (Fig. 6-5).

The *anterior fontanel* is diamond-shaped, measuring 2.5 cm (1 inch) along the coronal suture and 4.0 to 5.0 cm (about 2 inches) along the sagittal suture. The posterior fontanel is easily located by following the sagittal suture toward the occiput. The *posterior fontanel* is triangular-shaped, usually measuring between 0.5 and 1 cm (less than ½ inch) at its widest part. The fontanels should feel flat, firm, and well demarcated against the bony edges of the skull. Frequently pulsations are visible at the anterior fontanel. Coughing, crying, or lying down may temporarily cause the fontanels to bulge and become more taut. However, a widened, tense, bulging fontanel or a markedly sunken, depressed fontanel is always recorded and reported to the physician.

The degree of *head control* in the neonate is assessed. Although *head lag* is normal in the newborn, the degree of the ability to control the head in certain positions should be recognized. If the supine infant is pulled from the arms into a semi-Fowler's position, marked head lag and hyperextension are noted (Fig. 6-6, *A*). However, as one continues to bring the infant forward into a sitting position, the infant will attempt to control the head in an upright position. As the head falls forward onto the chest, many infants will attempt to right it into the erect position. Also, if the infant is held in ventral suspension, that is, held prone above and parallel to the examining surface, the infant will hold his head in a straight line with the spinal column (Fig. 6-6, *B*). When lying on the abdomen, the newborn has the ability to lift the head slightly, turning it from side to side.

Eyes

Usually the newborn will keep his eyes tightly closed. It is best to begin the examination of the eyes by observing the lids for edema, which is normally present for the first 2 days after delivery. The eyes are observed for symmetry.

In order to visualize the surface structures of the eye, the nurse holds the infant supine and gently lowers the head. The eyes will usually open, similar to the mechanism of dolls' eyes. The sclera should be white and clear.

The cornea is examined for the presence of any opacities or haziness. The *corneal reflex* is normally present at birth but is generally not elicited unless brain or eye damage is suspected. The pupil will usually respond to light by constricting. The pupils are normally malaligned. A searching *nystagmus* or *strabismus* is common. The color of the iris is noted. Most light-skinned newborns have slate gray or dark blue eyes, whereas dark-skinned infants have brown eyes.

A funduscopic examination is quite difficult to perform because of the infant's tendency to keep the eyes tightly closed. However, a red reflex should be elicited.

Ears

The ears are examined for position, structure, and auditory function. The top of the pinna should lie in a horizontal plane to the outer canthus of the eye. The pinna is often flattened against the side of the head from pressure in utero.

FIG. 6-6
Head control. **A,** *Inability to hold erect when pulled to sitting position.* **B,** *Ability to hold head erect when placed in ventral suspension.*

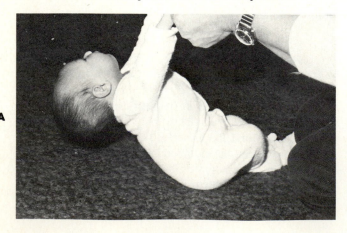
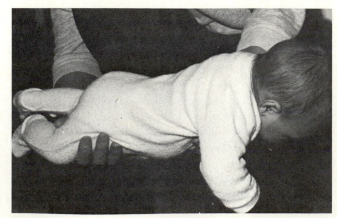

A

B

An otoscopic examination is ordinarily not performed because the *canals* are filled with vernix caseosa and amniotic fluid, making visualization of the drum difficult.

Auditory ability can be assessed by making a sharp, loud noise close to the infant's head. Normally the infant will respond with a *startle reflex* or twitching of the eyelids. Absence of any behavioral response to a sudden noise may indicate congenital deafness and is always reported.

Nose

The nose is usually flattened after birth, and bruises are common. Patency of the nasal canals can be assessed by holding the hand over the infant's mouth and one canal and noting the passage of air through the unobstructed opening. If nasal patency is questionable, it is reported because newborns are obligatory nose breathers.

Thin white mucus is very common in the newborn. Sneezing may be frequent and is normal.

Mouth and throat

The existing structures of the mouth are inspected. The palate is normally high arched and somewhat narrow. Rarely teeth may be present. A common finding is *Epstein's pearls,* small, white, epithelial cysts along both sides of the midline of the hard palate. They are insignificant and disappear in several weeks.

The frenum of the upper lip is a band of thick, pink

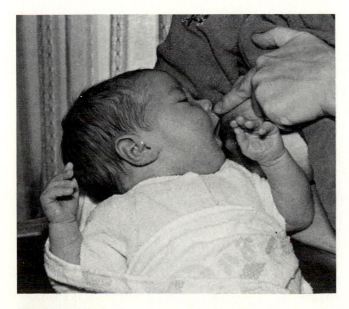

FIG. 6-7
Eliciting rooting reflex.

tissue that lies under the inner surface of the upper lip and extends to the maxillary alveolar ridge. It is particularly evident when the infant yawns or smiles. It disappears as the maxilla grows.

The *sucking reflex* is elicited by placing a nipple or tongue blade in the infant's mouth. The infant should exhibit a strong, vigorous suck. The *rooting reflex* is obtained by stroking the cheek and noting the infant's response of turning toward the stimulated side and sucking (Fig. 6-7).

It is difficult to examine the back of the throat. If the nurse attempts to depress the tongue, the infant will object with strong reflex protrusion of the tongue. Therefore it is best to visualize the uvula while the infant is crying and the chin is depressed. However, the uvula may be retracted upward and backward during crying. Tonsillar tissue is generally not seen in the newborn.

Neck

The newborn's neck is short and covered with folds of tissue. Adequate assessment of the neck requires allowing the head to fall gently backward in hyperextension while the back is supported in a slightly raised position. The nurse observes for range of motion, shape, and any abnormal masses.

Chest

The newborn's chest is almost circular because the anteroposterior and lateral diameters are equal. The ribs are very flexible, and slight intercostal retractions are normally seen on inspiration. The xiphoid process is commonly visible as a small protrusion at the end of the sternum. The sternum is generally raised and slightly curved.

Breast enlargement appears in many newborns of either sex by the second or third day and is caused by maternal hormones. Occasionally a milky substance sometimes called "witches' milk" is secreted by the infant's breasts by the end of the first week.

Lungs

The normal respirations of the newborn are irregular and abdominal, and the rate is between 30 and 60 breaths/minute. Periods of apnea less than 15 seconds are considered normal. After the initial forceful breaths required to initiate respiration, subsequent breaths should be easy and fairly regular in rhythm. Occasional irregularities occur in relation to crying, sleeping, and feeding.

It is important that the nurse learn to carefully assess the respiratory status of the newborn through observation, since auscultation is difficult because of the small size of the chest and the effective transmission of cardiac and bowel sounds to all parts of the pleural cavity.

Heart

Heart rate should always be auscultated and may range from 100 to 180 beats/minute shortly after birth and, when the infant has stabilized, from 120 to 140 beats/minute. The size and location of the heart should be determined. The *apex* of the heart is usually palpated or auscultated at the third or fourth intercostal space, lateral to the midclavicular line, because of its more horizontal position in the newborn (see Fig. 5-34).

Abdomen

The normal contour of the abdomen is cylindric and usually prominent with visible veins. Bowel sounds are heard a few hours after birth. Visible peristaltic waves may be observed in thin newborns, but should not be seen in well-nourished infants.

The umbilical cord is inspected to determine the presence of two arteries, which look like papular structures, and one vein, which has a larger lumen than the arteries and a thinner vessel wall. At birth the cord should appear bluish white and moist. After clamping it begins to dry and appears a dull, yellowish brown. It progressively shrivels in size and turns greenish black.

Palpation is done after inspection of the abdomen. The liver is usually located 2 to 3 cm (about 1 inch) below the right costal margin. The tip of the spleen can sometimes be felt in the newborn and usually by 1 week of age. Both kidneys should be palpated, especially soon after delivery when the intestines are still not filled with air. However, this requires considerable practice. When felt, the lower half of the right kidney and the tip of the left kidney are 1 to 2 cm above the umbilicus.

During examination of the lower abdomen, it is particularly important to palpate for femoral pulses, which should be strong and equal bilaterally.

Female genitalia

Normally the labia minora and clitoris are enlarged. Vernix caseosa may be present in large amounts between the labia. A hymenal tag is usually visible from the posterior opening of the vagina. It is comprised of tissue from the hymen and the labia minora. It usually disappears in several weeks. Generally the vaginal vault is not inspected.

Male genitalia

The penis is inspected for the location of the urethral opening, which is located at the tip. However, the opening may be totally covered by the prepuce, or foreskin, which covers the glans penis. A tight prepuce is a very common finding in the newborn. It should not be forcefully retracted, except to locate the urinary opening. *Smegma*, a white cheesy substance, is commonly found around the glans penis, under the foreskin. Small, white, firm lesions called *epithelial pearls* may be seen at the tip of the prepuce. An erection is common in the newborn.

The scrotum may be large, edematous and pendulous in the full-term neonate. The scrotal skin should be well rugated and more deeply pigmented than the surrounding area. Palpation of the scrotum is routinely performed for the presence of the testes, which should be descended in the full-term infant (see Fig. 5-42).

Back and rectum

With the infant prone, the spine is inspected. The shape of the spine should be gently rounded, with none of the characteristic S-shaped curves seen later in life. Stroking the back along one side of the vertebral column will cause the infant to move the hips toward the stimulated side *(trunk incurvation reflex)*.

With the infant still prone, symmetry of the gluteal folds is carefully noted. Any evidence of asymmetry is reported.

Passage of meconium indicates anal patency. If an imperforate anus is suspected, a rubber catheter should be inserted into the anal opening. In some institutions this is a routine procedure.

Extremities

The extremities are examined for symmetry, range of motion, and primitive reflexes. The fingers and toes are counted, and supernumerary digits *(polydactyly)* or fusion of digits *(syndactyly)* is noted. A partial syndactyly between the second and third toes is a common variation seen in otherwise normal infants. The nail beds should be pink, although slight blueness is evident in acrocyanosis.

The palms of the hands should have the usual creases (see Fig. 5-11). The full-term newborn usually has creases on the anterior two thirds of the *sole* of the foot. The soles of the feet are flat with prominent fat pads.

Range of motion of the extremities should be observed throughout the entire examination. The hips are rotated to identify a congenital dislocation. With the infant supine, the legs should be flexed at the hips and knees and abducted to almost 175 degrees. Limitation in abduction often indicates dislocation. Symmetry is noted when the infant moves, particularly when a Moro reflex is elicited.

Muscle tone should also be assessed. By attempting to extend a flexed extremity, the nurse determines if tone is equal bilaterally.

Two reflexes are elicited. The first is the *grasp*. Touching the palms of the hands or soles of the feet near the base of the digits causes flexion or grasping (see Fig. 5-47, *A*). The other is the *Babinski*. Stroking the outer sole of the foot upward from the heel across the ball of the foot causes the big toe to dorsiflex and the other toes to hyperextend (see Fig. 5-47, *B*).

Neurologic assessment

Assessing neurologic status is a critical part of the physical assessment of the newborn. Much of the neurologic examination takes place during examination of body systems, such as eliciting localized reflexes and observing posture, muscle tone, head control, and movement. However, several important mass (total body) reflexes also need to be elicited. They are usually left to the end of the examination because they may disturb the infant and interfere with auscultation. These reflexes are described in Table 6-3.

Behavioral assessment

Another important area of assessment is observation of behavior. It is becoming increasingly apparent that infants' behavior helps shape their environment. Their ability to react to various stimuli affects how others relate to them. The principal areas of behavior for newborns are sleep, wakefulness, and activity, such as crying. Besides the assessment below more advanced tools are available such as the Brazelton Neonatal Behavioral Assessment Scale (see p. 160).

Patterns of sleep and wakefulness. Newborns begin life with a systematic schedule of sleep and wakefulness that is initially evident during the periods of reactivity. For the first hour after birth the infant born of an unmedicated mother is intensely alert, the eyes are wide open, and sucking behavior is vigorous. The infant then becomes quiet and relatively unresponsive to either internal or external stimuli. He relaxes and falls asleep for a period of a few minutes to 2 to 4 hours. On awakening, the infant may be hyperresponsive to stimuli. This begins the second period of reactivity, which lasts from 2 to 5 hours. When the second period of reactivity is over, the infant's vital signs and patterns of sleep and activity stabilize. It is not unusual for the infant to sleep almost constantly for the next 2 to 3 days in order to recover from the exhausting birth process.

Five distinct states comprise the infant's sleep. During *regular sleep* the infant's eyes are closed, breathing is regular, and movement is absent, except for sudden generalized startles. Strong external or internal stimulation is absent or minimal, and mild stimuli, such as usual household noise, will not arouse the infant. During *irregular sleep* the eyes are still closed, but the breathing is irregular. Al-

though the body is still quiet, the muscles twitch occasionally. The external stimuli that were subliminal during regular sleep now cause the infant to smile, cry out, or groan.

The third state of sleep, *drowsiness,* occurs before or after regular and irregular sleep. The eyes may be open, breathing is irregular, and the body is actively moving. The infant is sensitive to such external stimuli as footsteps, voices, or the appearance of the mother. The occurrence of spontaneous discharges such as reflex smiles or startles, sucking movement, or erections are frequent. This period is followed by *alert inactivity,* provided that the infant's needs such as feeding and diapering have been satisfied. The infant responds to environmental stimuli by moving the head, limbs, and trunk and by staring at close-range objects, such as a swaying mobile or a smiling face. An interesting, stimulating environment can initiate or maintain a quiet, alert state.

The state that usually is most apparent to parents is *waking activity and crying.* Intense internal stimuli, such as hunger, pain, or cold, or intense external stimuli, such as removing the bottle while the infant is sucking or restraining the infant's extremities, will elicit such responses as a strong, angry cry and thrashing of the arms and legs in an uncoordinated manner. Attempts at quieting the infant may be ineffective unless the primary cause is removed.

The cycle of these sleep states is highly variable and is based on the number of hours an infant sleeps per day, which may range anywhere from 10½ to 23 hours, with an average of 16½ hours. Generally about 75% of the infant's sleep is in the irregular state.

States of sleep and periods of activity are highly influenced by environmental stimuli. Feeding usually terminates the crying when hunger is the cause. However, an awake infant exhibits more motor activity before feeding than after. Swaddling or wrapping an infant snugly in a blanket promotes sleep as well as maintains body temperature. Rocking the infant reduces crying and induces quiet alertness or sleep.

Cry. The newborn should begin extrauterine life with a strong, lusty cry. Variations in this initial cry can indicate abnormalities and are noted.

The sounds produced by crying can be classified into two groups, those of discomfort and those of comfort. Discomfort sounds initially consist of gasps and cries in which the consonant "H" is clearly distinguishable. Later the sounds of "W" and "L" are added. The almost universal "MAMA" sound is associated with much discomfort and is readily recognized by mothers.

The duration of crying is as highly variable in each infant as is the duration of sleep patterns. Some newborns may cry as little as 5 minutes or as much as 2 hours or more per day. Crying may continue to increase for the first

TABLE 6-3. ASSESSMENT OF REFLEXES IN THE NORMAL NEONATE

REFLEX	EXPECTED BEHAVIORAL RESPONSE	COMMENTS
Moro	Sudden jarring or change in equilibrium causes extension and abduction of extremities and fanning of fingers, with index finger and thumb forming a "C" shape, followed by flexion and adduction of extremities; legs may weakly flex; infant may cry (Fig. 6-8)	Should be elicited by holding the infant above the examining table in a supine position with one hand beneath the sacrum and the other supporting the upper back and head; the infant's head is then suddenly allowed to fall about 30 degrees. Should disappear after age 3-4 months, usually strongest during first 2 months
Startle	A sudden loud noise causes abduction of the arms with flexion of the elbows; the hands remain clenched	Should disappear by age 4 months
Tonic neck	When infant's head is quickly turned to one side, arm and leg will extend on that side, and opposite arm and leg will flex; posture resembles a fencing position (Fig. 6-9)	Should disappear by age 3-4 months, to be replaced by symmetric positioning of both sides of body
Dance or step	If infant is held so that sole of foot touches a hard surface, there will be a reciprocal flexion and extension of the leg, simulating walking (Fig. 6-10)	Should disappear after age 3-4 weeks, to be replaced by deliberate movement
Crawling	When infant is placed on abdomen, he will make crawling movements with the arms and legs (Fig. 6-11)	Should disappear at about age 6 weeks

several weeks of life but usually decreases at about 8 weeks when the infant is making other vocalizations, such as cooing.

NURSING CARE OF THE NEONATE

The main nursing goal for newborns is the promotion and maintenance of homeostasis or body equilibrium. Objectives of care for the newborn include: (1) establish and maintain a patent airway, (2) maintain a stable body temperature, (3) protect from infection and injury, (4) provide optimal nutrition, and (5) promote parent-infant attachment. Because of the importance of the last goal, promoting family relationships is discussed separately.

Establish and maintain a patent airway

Establishing a patent airway is a primary objective in the delivery room and is the responsibility of the attending physicians and obstetric nurses. Therefore, it is not discussed here.

Maintaining a patent airway continues to be a priority goal in the nursery with attention to proper positioning of the infant to facilitate drainage of secretions, especially after feeding (see Fig. 6-14). A bulb syringe should be available if suctioning of mucus is required. Any evidence of respiratory distress is reported immediately.

Vital signs. A minimal schedule for monitoring vital signs in normal neonates is every 15 minutes for at least 1 hour, every 2 hours for the next 8 hours, every 4 hours until 24 hours of age, and then twice a day until discharge. However, any change in the infant, such as in color, muscle tone, or behavior necessitates more frequent monitoring of vital signs.

Maintain stable body temperature

Conserving the newborn's body heat is an important nursing goal. It requires an understanding of the causes of heat loss: evaporation, radiation, conduction, and convection. Nursing care is based on preventing these from occurring.

At birth a major cause of heat loss is *evaporation*, the loss of heat through moisture. The amniotic fluid that bathes the infant's skin favors evaporation, especially when combined with the cool atmosphere of the delivery room. Heat loss through evaporation is minimized by rapidly drying the skin and hair with a warmed towel and placing the infant in a heated environment.

Another major cause of heat loss is *radiation*, the loss of heat to cooler solid objects in the environment that are not in direct contact with the infant. Loss of heat through radiation increases as these solid objects become colder and closer to the infant. The temperature of ambient or surrounding air in the Isolette or incubator essentially has

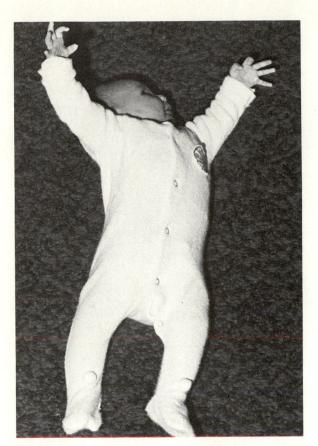

FIG. 6-8
Moro reflex.

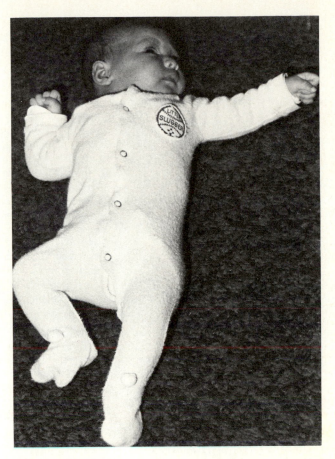

FIG. 6-9
Tonic neck reflex.

FIG. 6-10
Dance reflex.

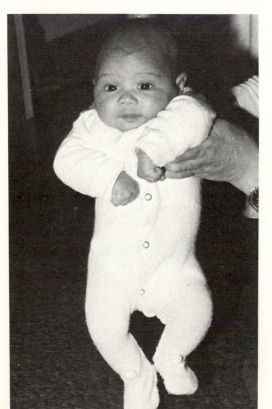

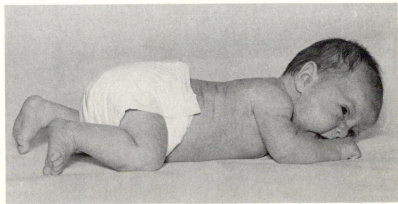

FIG. 6-11
Crawl reflex.

SUMMARY OF NURSING CARE OF THE NEONATE

GOALS	RESPONSIBILITIES
Establish and maintain patent airway	Perform as few procedures as possible on infant during first hour and have oxygen ready for use if respiratory distress should develop Take vital signs according to hospital policy Position infant on right side or abdomen after feeding to prevent aspiration Keep diapers, clothing, and blankets loose enough to allow maximum lung (abdominal) expansion Clean nares of any crusted secretions during bath or when necessary Keep bulb syringe near Isolette Check for patent nares
Maintain stable body temperature	Take infant's axillary temperature on arrival at nursery and, if stable, proceed according to hospital policy Maintain room temperature between 24° and 25.5° C (75° to 78° F) and humidity about 40% to 50% Monitor skin temperature and relate it to ambient air temperature; decreased skin temperature may indicate radiant heat loss Dress infant in a shirt and diaper and swaddle him in a blanket Postpone bath for first 4 to 6 hours until temperature stabilizes Postpone circumcision until after postnatal recovery period Prevent chilling of infant during daily bath If there is any question regarding stabilization of body temperature, postpone bath Keep infant's head covered if heat loss is a problem Warm all objects used to examine or cover infant, for example, place them under radiant warmer Uncover only one area of body for examination or procedures (for example, footprinting)
Protect infant from infection and trauma	Instill prophylactic eye medication into conjunctival sac of each eye from inner canthus outward; do not irrigate eyes with sterile saline Ideally, perform eye care after initial meeting of infant and parents, usually about 1 hour after birth (may be done in nursery) Check eyes daily for any discharge; explain to parents the reason for chemical conjunctivitis Administer vitamin K intramuscularly, using vastus lateralis muscle as site of injection Use plain warm water for daily bath; ideally, involve mother and father in bathing of infant Clean vulva in posterior direction to prevent fecal contamination of vagina or urethra; stress this to parents

SUMMARY OF NURSING CARE OF THE NEONATE—cont'd

GOALS	RESPONSIBILITIES
	While cleansing the penis, do not retract the foreskin; gently wipe away the smegma Maintain asepsis during circumcision If the infant has been circumcised, cover the area with a petrolatum jelly gauze (if ordered) for the first few hours, then remove the dressing Keep umbilical stump clean and dry; place diapers below umbilical stump
Protect infant from injury	Place identification bracelet(s) on infant immediately after birth; check often to ensure correct infant identity Never leave infant unsupervised on a raised surface without sides; newborns have been known to roll over, and the crawling reflex propels them short distances Always close diaper pins and place them away from infant's body Keep pointed or sharp objects out of infant's reach; grasp reflex can inadvertently be stimulated as hand approaches such an object and can cause damage to skin or, most importantly, to eyes Keep own fingernails short and trimmed; avoid jewelry that can scratch infant Collect blood specimens for required screening tests Discuss with parents the use of a suitable car restraint for transporting the infant home
Provide optimum nutrition	During first hour after delivery, put the infant to mother's breast when possible Postpone bottle-feeding of 5% glucose water until sucking and swallowing are well coordinated, usually after the second period of reactivity Do not offer water or supplementary feedings to breast-feeding infants, since this may satiate their hunger and interfere with lactation and breast feeding Bring breast-fed infants to their mothers on demand during day and night Offer bottle-fed infants 2 to 3 ounces of formula after they have retained their glucose feeding Support and assist breast-feeding mothers during initial feedings; encourage the father to remain with the mother to help her and the infant with positioning, relaxation, and reinforcement Encourage the father to participate in bottle-feeding Place infant on the right side after feeding to prevent regurgitation (see Fig. 6-14) Observe stool pattern

Continued.

SUMMARY OF NURSING CARE OF THE NEONATE—cont'd	
GOALS	**RESPONSIBILITIES**
Promote parent-infant attachment	As soon after delivery as possible, allow parents to see and hold their infant; place newborn close to face of parents so that visual contact can be established
	Identify for the parents specific behaviors manifested by the infant, for example, alertness, ability to see, vigorous suck, rooting behavior, and attention to the human voice
	Discuss with parents their expectations of fantasy child vs real child
	Encourage parents to "talk out" their labor and delivery experience; identify any events that signify loss of control to either parent, especially the mother
	Identify the behavioral steps in the attachment process and evaluate those aspects that could be considered positive and those that may represent inadequate or delayed parenting
	Observe and assess the reciprocity of cues between infant and parent
	Assist parents in recognizing attention-nonattention cycles and in understanding their significance
	Assess variables affecting the development of attachment through observing infant and parent and interviewing each parent or other significant caregiver
	If parent-infant attachment is at risk, refer to appropriate agencies (social services, family and child services, at-risk programs)

no effect on loss of heat through radiation. This is a critical point to remember when attempting to maintain a constant temperature for the infant because even though the temperature of the ambient air is optimal, the infant can be hypothermic.

An example of radiant heat loss is the placement of the incubator close to a cold window or air conditioning unit. The cold from either source will cool the walls of the incubator and, subsequently, the body of the neonate. To prevent this, the infant is placed as far away as possible from walls, windows, and ventilating units. If heat loss continues to be a problem, a radiant warmer may be placed over the infant or infant and mother.

Heat loss can also occur through conduction and convection. *Conduction* involves loss of heat from the body because of direct contact of skin with a cooler solid object. This can be minimized by placing the infant on a padded, covered surface and by providing insulation through clothes and blankets rather than by placing the infant directly on a hard table. Placing the newborn very close to his mother, such as in her arms or on her abdomen, is physically beneficial in terms of conserving heat as well as fostering maternal attachment.

Convection is similar to conduction, except that heat loss is aided by surrounding air currents. For example, placing the infant in the direct flow of air from a fan or air conditioner vent will cause rapid heat loss through convection. Transporting the neonate in a crib with solid sides reduces airflow around the infant.

Protect from infection and injury

The most important practice in preventing cross-infection is proper handwashing of all delivery and nursery room personnel. The nurse washes the hands before and after handling the infant.

In addition to handwashing, several procedures are done to prevent infection. These include eye care, bathing, and care of the circumcision and/or umbilical stump. To protect against injury vitamin K is administered, and several safety measures are practiced (see the summary on p. 153). In addition, screening tests such as for phenylketonuria, hypothyroidism, or galactosemia are performed to prevent serious consequences of undiagnosed disorders.

Eye care. Prophylactic eye treatment against *Neisseria gonorrhoeae,* which can cause blindness in infants born of mothers with gonorrhea, is done by instilling 2 drops of 1% silver nitrate solution into each eye. A separate ampule is used for each eye. Other local antibiotic preparations such as erythromycin (0.5%) or tetracycline (1%) can also be used for prophylaxis of chlamydial ophthalmia. Rinsing the eyes with sterile normal saline is *not* recommended. Proper instillation of silver nitrate into the conjunctival sac is essential because incorrect technique can cause a transient severe chemical conjunctivitis (see Fig. 19-27). It is very important for nurses to explain the reason for the instillation of silver nitrate, since the resultant conjunctivitis can be upsetting for new parents.

Traditionally antimicrobial preparations have been instilled in the newborn's eyes only minutes after birth. Studies on maternal attachment emphasize that in the first hour of life a newborn has a greater ability to focus on coordinated movement than at any other time during the next several days. This initial hour is very important in the development of maternal-infant bonding, one component of which is the establishment of eye-to-eye contact. Based on these findings, it is recommended that the routine administration of silver nitrate or antibiotics be postponed until after the parents and child have established such visual contact and bonding has begun (American Academy of Pediatrics, 1980). If the procedure is delayed, there must be some kind of checklist to ensure that the drug is given as soon as possible.

Bathing. The bath time can be an opportunity for the nurse to accomplish much more than general hygiene. It is an excellent time for observations of the infant's behavior, such as irritability, state of arousal, alertness, and muscular activity.

In hospitals where there is rooming-in of infant and mother, the bath time provides an opportunity for the nurse to involve the parents in the care of their child and to learn about his individual characteristics. Parents should be encouraged to examine every finger and toe of their infant. Frequently normal variations such as Epstein's pearls, mongolian spots, or stork bites cause parents undue concern because they are unaware of the insignificance of such findings. Minor birth injuries may appear as major defects to them. Explaining how these occurred and when they will disappear is reassuring to parents.

One of the most important considerations in skin cleansing is preservation of the skin's pH, which is about 5 soon after birth. The slightly acidic skin surface has bacteriostatic effects. Consequently, only plain warm water should be used for the bath. Alkaline soaps, such as Ivory, oils, powder, and lotions are not used because they alter the pH, thus providing a better environment for bacterial growth. Talcum has the added risk of aspiration if applied too close to the infant's face.

Bathing should be done in the nursery after the vital signs have stabilized. There is no need to immediately wash a newborn, except to remove the blood from the face and head. Cleansing proceeds in the cephalocaudal direction. A washcloth is used and turned so that a clean part touches the skin with each stroke. The eyes are carefully wiped from the inner to the outer aspect of the lid. The face is cleansed next. The nares are carefully inspected for any crusted secretions. The scalp is usually wiped, although it is sometimes necessary to shampoo the hair, which is best accomplished by positioning the infant's head over a small basin, lathering the scalp with a mild soap, and rinsing by pouring water from a small vessel over the head into the basin. The rest of the body should be covered during this procedure. The head is dried quickly in order to prevent evaporation heat loss.

The ears are cleaned with the twisted end of a washcloth or very carefully with a cotton-tipped swab. The swab is not inserted into the canal but is gently rotated around the pinna and immediate site of entry into the external canal.

The rest of the body is washed in a similar manner. Although the infant's skin requires little rubbing for adequate cleansing, certain areas such as the folds of the neck, the axillae, and creases at joints need special attention. The area around the neck is especially prone to a rash from regurgitation of feeding and should be thoroughly washed and dried.

The genitalia of both sexes require careful cleansing. In the female the labia are separated to remove the vernix caseosa, which is usually thick and adherent. Some of the vernix caseosa is removed at each diaper change, rather than at one time, in order to avoid irritation. Cleansing of the vulva is done in a front-to-back direction. The bath is a perfect opportunity to stress this part of hygiene to the mother, both for the infant's and for her own protection against urinary tract infection.

Cleansing the male genitalia involves washing the penis and scrotum. Sometimes smegma needs to be removed by wiping around the glans. The foreskin is not retracted because it is normally tight in newborns. If the infant is not to be circumcised, the parents are taught how to cleanse under and around the foreskin by retracting it gently *only* as far as it will go and returning it to its normal position. Leaving the prepuce retracted constricts the blood vessels supplying the glans penis, causing edema.

The buttocks and anal area are thoroughly cleansed of any fecal material. As with the rest of the body, the area is dried to prevent a warm, moist environment that fosters growth of bacteria.

Diapers are put on the infant after the bath. They should fit snugly around the thighs and abdomen to prevent urine from leaking. In males cloth diapers should be folded with extra thickness in the front to provide greater absorbency. In females the placement of the extra fold depends on whether the infant is prone or supine. Diapers are fastened with the back side overlapping the front side to allow full flexion of the hips.

The nurse should discuss the choice of cloth or disposable diapers with parents because of the cost difference. Using disposable diapers exclusively is the most expensive method, costing several times more than cloth diapers laundered at home. Diaper service costs vary but may be more than twice as much as the self-laundry method. Over 1 or 2 years the cost or savings can be considerable, particularly if more than one child is wearing diapers.

Care of the umbilicus and circumcision. The umbilical cord is clamped and cut after delivery. The stump deteriorates through the process of dry gangrene and falls off in 7 to 10 days. After the stump has fallen off, the cord base takes a few more weeks to heal completely.

The umbilical stump is an excellent medium for bacterial growth. To prevent infection, it is cleansed with mild soap and water during the bath and dried thoroughly. Wiping the base of the cord with an alcohol swab promotes drying. Some institutions may use additional drying and/or bacteriostatic agents. The diaper is placed below the cord to avoid irritation against the fabric.

The nurse instructs the parents regarding stump deterioration and proper umbilical care. Any signs of infection, such as presence of a malodorous, purulent discharge, are reported to the physician.

Circumcision is the surgical removal of the foreskin on the glans penis. In the Jewish culture circumcision is performed during a highly significant ceremony called a berith, or brit, which takes place on the eighth day of life. A rabbi skilled in the procedure usually performs the circumcision. However in most instances it is routinely done in the hospital by the physician.

There is much controversy regarding the benefits and risks of this widely practiced procedure. The American Academy of Pediatrics (1975) reaffirmed its position that there are no valid medical indications for circumcision of the newborn and that a program of good personal hygiene offers all the advantages of circumcision without the attendant surgical risks. Complications of circumcision include hemorrhage, infection, loss of penile skin, injury and/or laceration to the glans, penis, or scrotum, urethral fistula, and retained plastibell rings. In addition, the prepuce protects the glans from diapers and tight clothing.

Arguments for circumcision include prevention of penile cancer (a relatively rare form of cancer) and preservation of a male's body image with an appearance that is consistent with his peers, since circumcision is such a common practice in the United States. In light of these arguments, parents should be allowed an ''informed'' choice when considering circumcision.

Circumcision is usually performed in the nursery sometime after birth. It should not be performed immediately after delivery because of the neonate's unstabilized physiologic status and increased susceptibility to stress. Preoperative nursing care includes obtaining a signed informed consent from the parents, adequately restraining the infant, cleaning the penis with soap and water, and draping the infant with sterile towels to keep him warm and provide an aseptic field (Fig. 6-12). Even though no anesthesia is given, the infant is allowed nothing by mouth

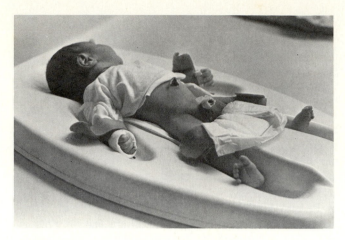

FIG. 6-12
Proper positioning of infant in Circumstraint.

before the procedure to prevent aspiration of vomitus. All the equipment used for the procedure, such as gloves, instruments, alcohol wipes, dressings, and draping towels, must be sterile.

The procedure involves freeing the foreskin from the glans penis by using a scalpel, a Yellen or Gomco clamp, or a Hollister plastibell. The clamp crushes the nerve endings and blood vessels, promoting hemostasis. After the procedure a petrolatum gauze dressing may be applied loosely for a few hours to prevent adherence to the diaper. If the dressing becomes dry, it is moistened with hydrogen peroxide before being removed.

As soon as the procedure is completed, the nurse releases the infant from the restraints and comforts him. Since parents are often concerned about the infant's well-being during this time, the nurse reassures them that the infant is recovering uneventfully. As soon as the infant is calmed and stabilized, he can be brought to the parents.

No special care following circumcision is required other than ordinary cleansing and observation for bleeding when the diaper is changed. Since the area is tender, the diaper is applied loosely to prevent friction against the penis. Normally on the second day a yellowish-white exudate forms as part of the granulating process. This is not a sign of infection and should not be forcibly removed. As healing progresses, the exudate disappears.

Vitamin K. Shortly after birth, vitamin K is administered intramuscularly to the newborn. Vitamin K is synthesized by the normal intestinal flora, but, since the infant's intestine is sterile at birth, the supply of vitamin K is inadequate for at least the first 3 to 4 days. The major function of vitamin K is to catalyze the synthesis of prothrombin in the liver, which is needed for blood clotting and coagulation and prevention of hemorrhagic disease of the newborn. It is important that the vastus lateralis muscle be used as the injection site because of the absence of other well-developed muscle masses.

Transportation after discharge. An important area of counseling is the safe transportation of the newborn home from the hospital. Ideally this counseling should occur *before* delivery to allow parents an opportunity to purchase a suitable infant car restraint. Parents are more likely to use a restraint if the proper use of one is demonstrated and its necessity is stressed, such as including this recommendation in discharge orders.

Provide optimal nutrition

Selection of a feeding method is one of the major decisions faced by parents. In general there are three acceptable choices: human milk, commercially prepared cow's milk formula, and modified cow's milk. There are significant nutritional, economic, and psychologic advantages and differences among each. Nurses need to be aware of the types of feeding to help parents choose the method that best meets their needs.

Comparison of human milk and cow's milk. There are significant nutritional differences between human milk and whole cow's milk. Cow's milk contains three times as much protein as human milk. Also, the type of protein differs. Human milk contains more lactalbumin, which is a more complete protein than casein because it contains a higher percentage of amino acids. The higher percentage of casein in cow's milk results in formation of large, hard curds. Human milk is more easily digested because of the presence of soft, flocculent curds. Therefore, stomach emptying time is more rapid with human milk, necessitating more frequent feedings.

Cow's milk and human milk both provide 20 kcal/ounce, but human milk contains a higher amount of lactose, a disaccharide that is converted into the monosaccharides glucose and galactose. Galactose is essential for the formation of galactolipids, which are necessary for the growth of the central nervous system.

Although the amount of fat in both types of milk is similar, the type of fat differs. Human milk contains more monounsaturated fatty acids, mainly oleic acid, whereas cow's milk has more polysaturated fatty acids. The unsaturated fatty acids in human milk enhance absorption of fat and calcium in the infant. In addition, the fat content of human milk varies during the feeding. It is higher toward the end of feeding and probably helps satisfy the infant longer as he completes breast-feeding.

The mineral content of cow's milk is considerably greater than that of human milk, with the exception of iron, fluoride, and copper. Although the amount of iron is low in both types of milk, the iron in human milk is much better absorbed by the infant. Another difference is the amount of calcium and phosphorus, minerals especially needed by the rapidly growing infant. Cow's milk contains more of these minerals but a lower calcium/phosphorus ratio (low calcium and high phosphorus). Because of the infant's immature regulatory mechanisms, calcium is excreted, resulting in tetany. Human milk contains a smaller but more balanced proportion of these minerals and a higher calcium/phosphorus ratio, which are adequate to meet the infant's needs. Both types of milk contain adequate amounts of zinc, a mineral identified as essential to the human. However, the zinc in human milk is more readily absorbed.

Both human and cow's milk provide adequate amounts of vitamins A and B complex. Vitamin C is low in cow's milk but higher in human milk provided the mother's intake is adequate. Vitamin D is low in human milk but adequate depending on the mother's intake and the infant's exposure to sunlight. Cow's milk and its preparations are usually fortified with vitamin D.

Evaporated milk and commercially modified formulas. The analysis of human and cow's milk shows that whole cow's milk is unsuitable for infant nutrition. It would have to be diluted to meet the protein requirement, but, when dilute, it does not meet the caloric or fat requirement. Therefore, evaporated whole milk is usually modified to meet the necessary nutritional demands. A common rule for preparing evaporated milk formula is diluting the 13-ounce can of milk with 17 ounces of water and adding 1 to 2 tablespoons of sugar or corn syrup.

Evaporated milk has many advantages over whole milk. It is readily available in cans, needs no refrigeration if unopened, provides a softer, more digestible curd, and contains more lactalbumin and higher calcium/phosphorus ratio. Evaporated milk must not be confused with condensed milk, which is a form of evaporated milk with 45% more sugar. Because of its high carbohydrate concentration and disproportionately low fat and protein content, condensed milk is not used for infant feeding. Likewise, skim milk should not be used because it is deficient in caloric concentration, significantly increases the renal solute load and water demands, and deprives the body of essential fatty acids.

Commercially prepared formulas (Similac, Enfamil, SMA) are milk-based formulas that have been modified to closely resemble human milk. Although they are not an exact substitute, they do provide an optimum source of nutrition. The formulas are available in three preparations: (1) a ready-to-use form in cans or bottles, (2) a concentrated liquid form that is diluted with an equal amount of water, and (3) a powdered form that must be prepared according to the manufacturer's directions. One consideration in the use of commercially prepared formulas is their cost. In general any of these preparations costs about twice as much as evaporated milk. It is wise to advise parents to do comparison shopping. For example, the concentrated liquid often costs less per ounce than the powdered form, which also requires more steps in its preparation.

Breast-feeding. Breast milk is the most perfect form of nutrition for the infant. In the United States about 60% of newborns in hospitals are breast-fed and there is a continuing trend for more mothers from all socioeconomic levels to breast-feed and to continue breast-feeding longer.

Probably the most outstanding benefit of breast-feeding besides the quality of the milk is the close maternal-child relationship. The infant is nestled very close to the mother's skin, can hear the rhythm of her heartbeat, feel the warmth of her body, and sense a peaceful security. The mother has a very close feeling of union with her child and feels a sense of accomplishment and satisfaction as the infant draws milk from her. Some mothers also experience a type of sensation similar to sexual excitement.

Breast-feeding is the most economical form of feeding, although it is not "free" milk because the lactating mother needs a high-protein, high-calorie diet. Breast milk is always available, ready to serve at room temperature, and free of contamination. In addition there is no need to sterilize bottles. There is also less chance of overfeeding and consequent obesity because the infant nurses until satisfied while bottle-fed infants are usually encouraged to finish all their formula. Consequently, bottle-fed infants gain weight faster than do breast-fed infants.

Breast-feeding offers some important physiologic advantages. Breast milk contains antibodies against such diseases as chickenpox, mumps, measles, and polio. The incidence of respiratory-related and gastrointestinal illnesses in breast-fed infants is lower during the first year. Colostrum and breast milk have a laxative effect; as a result, constipation is rare. Feeding difficulties such as colic, spitting up, and allergic reactions are much less common. There is a lower incidence of breast cancer in mothers who breast-feed their infants.

The few contraindications to breast-feeding include: any serious, debilitating illnesses (such as severe heart disease or advanced cancer) or infections (such as sputum-positive tuberculosis or hepatitis B) in the mother; mastitis if the discomfort is too great; and galactosemia in the infant. Breast milk may also produce hyperbilirubinemia (*breast-milk jaundice*) (see Chapter 7).

The birth of twins does not create a breast-feeding problem. If both twins are full-term, they can begin feedings immediately after birth (Fig. 6-13). Simultaneous feeding promotes the rapid production of milk needed for both infants and makes the milk that would normally be lost in the let-down reflex available to one of the twins. When only one infant is hungry, the mother should feed singly. She should also feed each infant on both breasts and avoid favoring one breast for one infant. The sucking patterns of infants vary and each infant needs the visual

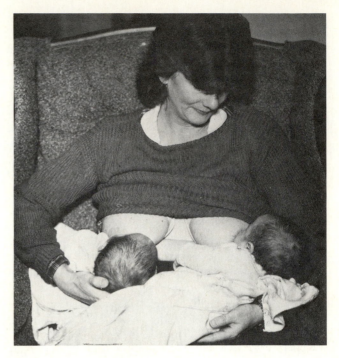

FIG. 6-13
Simultaneous breast-feeding of twins.

stimulation and exercise that alternating breasts provides.

Probably the greatest disadvantage of breast-feeding to most mothers is the inconvenience of having to be home more often. Many women resume their careers shortly after their pregnancy and prefer to use bottle-feeding. However, it is usually good to emphasize to new mothers that breast milk can be manually expressed for certain feedings and that formula can be substituted for one or two feedings during the mother's absence.

It is important to remember that successful breast-feeding probably depends more on the mother's desire to breast-feed than on any other factor. Contrary to popular belief, breast-feeding is not instinctive. Mothers need support, encouragement, and assistance during their postpartum hospital stay to enhance their opportunities for success and satisfaction. Frequent and early breast-feeding, especially during the first hour of life, increases the chances of success and mutual infant-mother satisfaction. Several excellent maternity texts (Jensen, Benson, and Bobak, 1981), books (Lawrence, 1980; Riordan, 1983), and organizations* are available as resources for the breast-feeding mother and professionals.

Bottle-feeding. Bottle-feeding is the most common method of feeding used in the United States. With commercial formulas that closely approximate human milk and

*La Leche League International, Inc., 9616 Minneapolis Ave., Franklin Park, IL 60131. A helpful book for breastfeeding twins is by Gromada, K.: Mothering multiples.

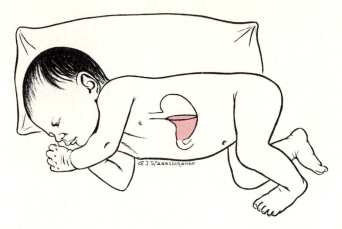

FIG. 6-14
Right side-lying position after feeding.

greatly improved conditions of sanitation, this is a perfectly acceptable method of feeding. Nurses should not assume that new mothers automatically know how to bottle-feed their infant. These mothers also need support and assistance in meeting their infant's needs. Providing the infant with nutrition is only part of feeding. Holding the infant close to the body and rocking or cuddling him help to assure the emotional component of feeding. There are a few important aspects of bottle-feeding that should be emphasized. The feeding should not be hurried. Even though the infant may suck vigorously for the first 5 minutes and seem to be satisfied, he should be allowed to continue sucking. Infants need at least 2 hours of sucking a day. If there are six feedings per day, then about 20 minutes of sucking should be allowed at each feeding for oral gratification.

Because infants do not have the motor control to voluntarily push the bottle away when finished, they may aspirate formula while sleeping. These infants also tend to contract more middle ear infections. As the infant lies flat and sucks, milk that has pooled in the pharynx becomes a suitable medium for bacterial growth. Bacteria then enter the eustachian tube, which leads to the middle ear, causing acute otitis media.

After feedings the infant is positioned on his right side to permit the feeding to flow toward the lower end of the stomach and to allow any swallowed air to rise above the fluid and through the esophagus (Fig. 6-14). This prevents regurgitation and distention. To maintain the side-lying position, a pillow can be propped behind the infant's back.

Propping the bottle should be discouraged. First of all, propping denies the infant the important component of close human contact. Feeding should be associated with socialization. Sucking on the bottle in a dark room is associated with separation of the mother.

Preparation of formula. The two traditional ways of preparing formula are the terminal heat method and the aseptic method. In the terminal heat method all the utensils and formula are boiled together for 25 minutes. In the aseptic method the equipment is boiled separately, after which the formula is poured into the bottles.

Because of improved sanitary conditions, in most instances it is not essential to do either of the above. The clean technique is satisfactory. However, new rubber nipples should be boiled 5 to 6 times, using fresh water for each boil, before the initial use to reduce the level of nitrosamines (Nitrosamines, 1984). The person preparing the formula washes his or her hands well and then washes all the equipment used to prepare the formula, including the cans of formula or evaporated milk. The formula is prepared and bottled immediately before each feeding. Warming the formula is optional, although many parents prefer to warm it before feeding. Any milk remaining in the bottle after the feeding is discarded because it is an excellent medium for bacterial growth. Opened cans of formula are covered and refrigerated.

Recent recommendations for labeling infant formulas require that the directions for preparation and use of the formula include pictures and symbols for nonreading individuals. In addition manufacturers are translating the directions into foreign languages, such as Spanish and Vietnamese, to prevent misunderstanding and errors in formula preparation.

Feeding schedules. Ideally feeding schedules should be determined by the infant's hunger. Feeding the infant when he signals his readiness is called *demand feeding*. More frequently, parents *schedule feedings* to meet their life-style. Most hospitals routinely feed infants every 4 hours. Although this is satisfactory for bottle-fed infants, it hinders the breast-feeding process. Breast-fed infants tend to be hungry every 2 to 3 hours, and, since lactation depends on breast stimulation, these infants should be on demand feedings.

Usually by 3 weeks of age lactation is well established and a feeding schedule has been formed. Bottle-fed infants retain about 2 to 3 ounces of formula at each feeding and are fed about six times a day. Larger infants are able to retain increased amounts because of greater stomach capacity; as a result they generally sleep through the night sooner than smaller infants or breast-fed infants.

PROMOTION OF PARENT-INFANT BONDING (ATTACHMENT)

The process of parenting is based on a mutual relationship between parent and infant. Much of past research on parent-child attachment has focused on the development of "mothering" or maternal attachment to the infant. Recently attention has focused on the infant's role in this process. Although the words "bonding" and "attachment" are sometimes referred to as separate phenomena with bonding as the development of emotional ties from parent to infant and attachment representing the emotional ties from infant to parent, in this discussion the words are used interchangeably to denote both processes.

As one learns of the complexity of the neonate and of his potential for influencing and shaping his environment, particularly his interaction with significant others, one cannot help but realize that promoting positive parent-child relationships necessitates an understanding of factors involved in identifying behavioral steps in attachment, variables that enhance or hinder this process, and methods of teaching parents ways to develop a stronger relationship with their child, especially by recognizing potential problems.

> ## HOW TO MAKE THE INFANT'S WORLD MORE EXCITING*
>
> Infant prefers animated and auditory objects.
> Infant enjoys novelty, quickly tires of seeing same objects; mobile should be changed frequently.
> Infant prefers to look at medium-intensity colors and contrasting colors, such as black and white.
> Infant likes geometric shapes and checkerboards; prefers patterns over straight lines.
> Contrasting lights and reflective surfaces such as mirrors are especially interesting.
> But most of all, nothing is as fascinating as the human face and voice!
>
> *Objects should be placed about 20 cm (8 inches) away from infant.

Infant behavior

Nurses must appreciate the individuality and uniqueness of each infant. According to the infant's temperament, he will change and shape his environment, which will undoubtedly influence his future development. Obviously an infant who sleeps 20 hours a day will be exposed to much fewer stimuli than the infant who sleeps 16 hours a day. In turn, each infant will likely effect a different response from his parents. The infant who is quiet, undemanding, and passive may receive much less attention than the infant who is responsive, alert, and active. Such behavioral characteristics have implications for parenting because forming a relationship is based on responding to reciprocal clues from each individual. The infant who responds to cuddling, smiling, and cooing invokes an attentive, pleasurable response from the parent, which will reinforce such behavior. An infant who stiffens when held, looks away when someone approaches too closely, or cries after feedings typically invokes feelings of rejection, dissatisfaction, and insecurity in the parent. This may very well be where child abuse or the maternal deprivation syndrome has its roots.

One method of systematically assessing the infant's behavior is the use of the *Brazelton Neonatal Behavioral Assessment Scale* (Brazelton, 1973). The scale is designed to assess the infant's response to 27 items, such as response to light or a bell, which are organized according to six categories, such as habituation or how soon the infant diminishes his response to stimuli.

Besides its use as an initial and ongoing tool to assess neurologic and behavioral responses, it can be used as a predictor of initial parent-child relationships, as a preventive instrument that identifies the caregiver as one who may benefit from a role model and as a guide for parents to help them focus on their infant's individuality and to develop a deeper attachment to their child. Studies have demonstrated that by showing parents the unique characteristics of their infant, there develops a more positive attitude toward the infant, less infant feeding and sleeping problems, and a consequently higher level of activity and alertness in the infant (Barnard, 1974).

Nurses can intervene and positively influence the attachment of parent and child. The first step is recognizing individual differences and explaining to parents that such characteristics are normal. For example, most people believe that infants sleep throughout the day, except for a half-hour feeding. For some newborns this may be true, but for many it is not. Understanding that the infant's wakefulness is part of his body rhythm and not a reflection of inadequate mothering can be crucial in promoting healthy parent-child relationships. Another aspect of helping parents concerns supplying guidelines on how to enhance the infant's development during awake periods. Placing the child in a crib to stare at the same mobile every day is not particularly exciting, but carrying him into each room as one does daily chores can be fascinating. A few simple suggestions can make life very stimulating for the infant and much more pleasurable and gratifying for the parents (see the boxed material).

Maternal attachment

During pregnancy, and in many cases even before conception occurs, parents develop an image of the ''ideal or fantasy infant.'' The unborn child has an imagined appearance, pattern of behavior, expected accomplishments, and predetermined effect on the life-style of the parents. At birth the fantasy infant becomes the real infant. How closely the dream child resembles the real child will influence the acceptance process. If the parents expected an alert, active infant who sleeps little and enjoys human contact and the real infant fulfills these expectations, the attachment process will be facilitated. If parents imagine that the newborn will sleep most of the time, will need little attention except feeding and diapering, and will not disturb their life-style significantly, the birth of a very active infant may cause considerable conflicts in the emotional bonding. Assessing such expectations during pregnancy and at the time of the infant's birth will allow nurses to identify discrepancies in the parents' view of the fantasy vs real child syndrome.

The labor process also significantly affects the immediate attachment of mothers to their newborn children. In general the mother's perception of maintaining control during the labor and birth process enhances the initial attachment, which, ideally, should take place during the first hour of life. A feeling of loss of control because of factors such as a long, difficult labor, excessive medication and sedation, or unwanted medical intervention will hinder the initial bonding process. Encouraging mothers to talk about their feelings of loss of control, particularly about the specific event that they perceive caused the lack of self-control, allows them to dissipate the emotional energy investigated in these feelings. It is not until such emotional tensions and anxieties are released that parents can attend to the emotional component of the attachment process.

It is believed that there is a *maternal sensitive period* immediately and for a short time after birth when parents have a unique ability to attach to their infants (Klaus and Kennell, 1982). Mothers demonstrate a predictable and orderly pattern of behavior during the development of the attachment process. When mothers are presented with their nude infants, they begin examining the infant with their fingertips, concentrating on touching the extremities, and then proceed to massage and encompass the trunk with their entire hands. Assuming the *en face* position, in which the mother's and the infant's eyes meet in visual contact in the same vertical plane, is significant in the formation of affectional ties (Klaus and others, 1972) (Fig. 6-15).

Observing such behavioral characteristics can assist nurses in identifying potential signs of inadequate or delayed mothering. For example, the mother who consistently feeds her infant while holding him at a distance from her body, who supports him with fingertips rather than encompassing him in her arm, who does not undress the infant for inspection, and who looks away from the infant most of the time is exhibiting behavior that needs to be assessed more carefully.

Recent studies have attempted to substantiate the long-term benefits of providing parents with opportunities to optimally bond with their infant during the initial postpartum period. There has been some evidence that increased parent-child contact at birth minimizes the risks of parenting disorders. However, not all studies support these findings and some authorities claim that the emphasis on bonding has been unjustified and may lead to guilt and fear in those parents who did not receive early contact with their infant.

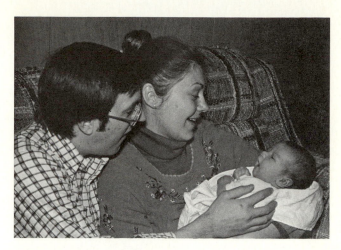

FIG. 6-15
En face position between parents and infant can be significant in attachment process.

Certainly, it should be stressed to parents that while early bonding may be valuable, it does not represent an "all or none" phenomenon. Throughout the child's life there will be multiple opportunities for the development of parent-child attachment. Bonding is a complex process that develops gradually and is influenced by numerous factors.

Another component of successful maternal attachment is the concept of *reciprocity*. As the mother responds to the infant, the infant must respond to the mother by some signal such as sucking, cooing, eye contact, grasping, or molding (conforming to the other's body during close physical contact). Five steps are described in positive mother-infant reciprocity (Brazelton, 1974). The first step is *initiation*, in which interaction between infant and parent begins. Next is *orientation*, which establishes the partners' expectation of each other during the interaction. Following orientation is *acceleration* of the attention cycle to a peak of excitement. The infant reaches out and coos, both arms jerk forward, the head moves backward, the eyes dilate, and the face brightens. After a short time *deceleration* of the excitement and *turning away* occur, in which the infant shifts his eyes away from his mother's and grasps his shirt. During this cycle of nonattention, repeated verbal or visual attempts to reinitiate his attention are ineffective. This deceleration and turning away probably prevent the infant from being overwhelmed by excessive stimuli. In a good interaction both partners have synchronized their attention-nonattention cycles. Parents or other caregivers who do not allow the infant to turn away and who continually attempt to maintain visual contact encourage the infant to turn off his attention cycles and thus prolong the nonattention phase.

Although this description of reciprocal interacting behavior is usually observable in the infant by 2 to 3 weeks of age, nurses can use this information to teach parents how to interact with their infant. Recognizing the attention cycle vs the nonattention cycle and understanding that the latter is not a rejection of the parent is one aspect in helping parents develop competence in parenting.

Monotropy is another component of attachment that has special meaning for health professionals. Monotropy refers to the principle that a person can become optimally attached to only one individual at a time (Klaus and Kennell, 1982). This is very significant in the attachment process that occurs in multiple births. If a parent can form only one attachment at a time, how then can all the siblings of a multiple birth receive optimum emotional care?

Even under the best circumstances mothers of twins may take months or even years to form individual attachments to each child and even longer if the twins are identical. The mother's separation from a sick twin during the perinatal period can have devastating results, since attachment to the well child occurs quickly but may impede attachment to the other twin. There are many practical suggestions for individualizing attachments to twins during the time of prenatal care to after delivery. However, the most important principle is to assist the parents in recognizing the individuality of the children. The mother should visit with each newborn as much as possible after birth. Rooming-in and breast-feeding are both feasible and should be encouraged. Any characteristics that are unique to each child are emphasized and each infant is called by his name, rather than ''the twins.'' Bonding behaviors are assessed and differences are noted, such as a parent's distinct preference for one twin over the other. In this situation the nurse can gently draw attention to these behaviors and encourage the parent to discuss feelings regarding a twin birth. The National Organization of Mothers of Twins Club, Inc.* has several local parents' groups that can be a source of support to new parents.

Paternal engrossment

Fathers also show specific behaviors during the attachment process, or what has been termed ''engrossment,'' forming a sense of absorption, preoccupation, and interest in the infant (Greenberg and Morris, 1974). The major characteristics of engrossment include (1) visual awareness of the newborn, especially focusing on the beauty of the child, (2) tactile awareness, often expressed in a desire to hold the infant, (3) awareness of distinct characteristics with emphasis on those features of the infant that resemble the father, (4) perception of the infant as perfect, (5) development of a strong feeling of attraction to the child that leads to intense focusing of attention on him, (6) experi-

encing a feeling of extreme elation, and (7) feeling a sense of deep self-esteem and satisfaction. These responses are greatest during the early contacts with the infant and are intensified by the neonate's normal reflex activity, especially the grasp reflex and visual alertness.

The development of engrossment has significant implications for nurses. Initially it is imperative that nurses recognize the importance of early father-infant contact in releasing these behaviors. Fathers need to be encouraged to express their positive feelings, especially if such emotions are contrary to the cultural belief that fathers should remain stoic. If this is not clarified, fathers may feel confused and attempt to suppress the natural sensations of absorption, preoccupation, and interest in order to conform with societal expectations.

Mothers also need to be aware of the responses of the father toward the newborn, especially since one of the consequences of paternal preoccupation with the infant is less overt attention toward the mother. If both parents are able to share their feelings, each can appreciate the process of attachment toward their child and will avoid the unfortunate conflict of being insensitive and unaware of the other's needs. In addition a father who is encouraged to form a relationship with his newborn is less likely to feel excluded and abandoned once the family returns home and the mother directs her attention toward caring for the infant.

Ideally the process of engrossment should be discussed with parents before the delivery, such as in prenatal classes, to reinforce the father's awareness of his natural feelings toward the expected child. Focusing on the future experience of seeing, touching, and holding one's newborn may also help expectant fathers become more comfortable in accepting their paternal feelings toward the unborn child. This in turn can assist them in being more supportive toward their wives, especially as the labor and delivery event draws near.

At the infant's birth the nurse can play a vital role in assisting the father in release or expression of engrossment by assessing the neonate in front of the couple, pointing out normal characteristics, especially the grasp reflex, encouraging identification through consistent referral to the child by using his name, encouraging the father to cuddle, hold, talk to, and/or feed the infant, and demonstrating whenever necessary the soothing powers of caressing, stroking, and rocking the child. The nurse observes for the same indication of affectional ties from the father as were discussed for the mother, such as visual contact in the *en face* position and embracing the infant close to the body. When present, such behaviors are reinforced. If such responses are not obvious, the nurse needs to assess the father's feelings regarding this birth, cultural beliefs that may prevent his emotional expression, and other factors in order to help him facilitate a positive attachment during this critical period.

---

*5402 Amberwood Lane, Rockville, MD 20853.

Siblings

Although the attachment process has been discussed almost exclusively in terms of the parents and infant, it is essential that nurses be aware of other family members, such as siblings and members of the extended family, who need preparation for the acceptance of this new child. Young children in particular need sensitive preparation for the birth to minimize sibling rivalry.

There is an increasing trend to allow siblings to visit the mother on the postpartum unit and in some instances to hold the newborn. Siblings have even been allowed to witness the birth, although they need preparation for and support during the event.

Assessment of attachment behavior

Unlike physical assessment of the neonate, which has concrete guidelines to follow, assessment of parent-child attachment requires much more skill in terms of observation and interviewing. The assessment process is even more challenging when one considers that postpartum hospital recovery is shorter and shorter. However, rooming-in of mother and infant and liberal visiting privileges for father, siblings, and grandparents facilitate recognition of behaviors that demonstrate positive or negative development of attachment.

What should the nurse observe when with the parents and the infant? Probably the most important activities to observe include feeding, bathing, and comforting. For example, when the infant is brought to the mother, does she reach out for him, call him by name, or involve the father in the greeting process? Do the parents speak about the child in terms of identification—who does he look like; what appears special about him over the other infants; how "smart" do they think he is? When the mother or father is holding the infant, what kind of body contact is there—do they feel at ease in changing the infant's position; are fingertips or whole hands used; are there parts of the body they avoid touching or parts of the body they investigate and scrutinize? When the infant is awake, what kinds of stimulation do the parents provide? Do they talk to the infant, to each other, or to no one? How do they look at the infant—direct visual contact, avoidance of eye contact, or looking at other people or objects?

Talking to the parents uncovers many variables that will affect the development of attachment and parenting. What expectations do they have for this child? In other words how similar are their predictions of the fantasy child and their realizations about the real child? They should be encouraged to talk about their relationship with their parents. Mothering and fathering of one's child are probably more dependent on the type of parenting that parents received as a child than on any other variable. Is this a planned birth, how do they see the addition of a dependent family member affecting their life-style, and what arrangements have they made in terms of such changes in life-style? What "support system" or significant others are available for assistance? What are their views regarding child rearing?

Professional support for parent-infant bonding should be continued from the hospital to the home through community services, such as visiting nurse agencies. Ideally the concept of family-centered care will be practiced when the family receives consistent comprehensive care from the same health team members, beginning with preventive prenatal care and continuing through child health maintenance.

REFERENCES

American Academy of Pediatrics, Committee on Drugs: Prophylaxis and treatment of neonatal gonococcal infections, Pediatrics **65:**1047-1048, May 1980.

American Academy of Pediatrics, Committee of Fetus and Newborn: Report of the Ad Hoc Task Force of Circumcision, Pediatrics **56:**610-611, Oct. 1975.

Barnard, K.: The acquaintance process. In Klaus, M., and others, editors: Maternal attachment and mothering disorders, New Brunswick, N.J., 1974, Johnson & Johnson Baby Products Co.

Brazelton, T.B.: Neonatal Behavioral Assessment Scale, Philadelphia, 1973, J.B. Lippincott Co.

Brazelton, T.B.: Mother-infant reciprocity. In Klaus, M., and others, editors: Maternal attachment and mothering disorders, New Brunswick, N.J., 1974, Johnson & Johnson Baby Products Co.

Greenberg, M., and Morris, N.: Engrossment: the newborn's impact upon the father, Am. J. Orthopsychiatry **44**(4):520-531, 1974.

Jensen, M.D., Benson, R.C., and Bobak, I.M.: Maternity care: the nurse and the family, ed. 2, St. Louis, 1981, The C.V. Mosby Co.

Klaus, M.H., and Kennell, J.H.: Parent-infant bonding, ed. 2, St. Louis, 1982, The C.V. Mosby Co.

Klaus, M., and others: Maternal attachment—importance of the first postpartum days, N. Engl. J. Med. **286:**460, 1972.

Lawrence, R.: Breast-feeding: a guide for the medical profession, St. Louis, 1980, The C.V. Mosby Co.

Nitrosamines in rubber baby bottle nipples, Pediatr. Alert **9**(1):2-3, 1984.

Riordan, J.: A practical guide to breastfeeding, St. Louis, 1983, The C.V. Mosby Co.

BIBLIOGRAPHY
Physiologic status of the newborn/assessment of the neonate

Arnold, H.W., and others: The newborn: transition to extra-uterine life, Am. J. Nurs. **65:**77, 1965.

Apgar, V.: The newborn (Apgar) scoring system, Pediatr. Clin. North Am. **13:**645, 1966.

Binzley, V.A.: State: an overlooked factor in newborn nursing, Am. J. Nurs. **77**(1):102-103, 1977.

Davis, V.: The structure and function of brown adipose tissue in the neonate, J. Obstet. Gynecol. Neonatal Nurs. **9**(6):368-372, 1980.

DeCasper, A.M., and Fifer, W.P.: Of human bonding: newborns prefer their mothers' voices, Science **208:**1174-1176, June 1980.

Fanaroff, A., and Martin, R., editors: Behrman's Neonatal-perinatal medicine: diseases of the fetus and infant, ed. 3, St. Louis, 1983, The C.V. Mosby Co.

The first six hours of life: assessment of risk in the newborn: evaluation during the transitional period, New York, 1980, March of Dimes/Birth Defects Foundation.

Graven, S.: Temperature control in newborn babies. In Neonatal thermoregulation, module 1, New York, 1976, The National Foundation—March of Dimes.

Johnson, T.R., and others: Children are different: developmental physiology, ed. 2, Columbus, Ohio, 1978, Ross Laboratories.

Ludington-Hoe, S.M.: What can newborns really see?, Am. J. Nurs. **83**(9):1286-1289, 1983.

Nursing care of the neonate

American Academy of Pediatrics, Committee on Fetus and Newborn: Statement: skin care of newborns, Pediatrics **54**:682, 1974.

American Academy of Pediatrics, Committee on Nutrition: Vitamin and mineral supplement needs in normal children in the United States, Pediatrics **66**:1015-1020, Dec. 1980.

Barness, L.A.: Nutritional requirements of the full-term neonate. In Suskind, R.M., editor: Textbook of pediatric nutrition, New York, 1981, Raven Press.

Boyer, K.B.: Routine circumcision of the newborn: reasonable precaution or unnecessary risk? J. Nurse Midwife. **25**:27- 31, Nov./Dec. 1980.

Callon, H.: Nursing responsibility in maintaining the body heat of the newborn infant. In Neonatal thermoregulation, module 1, New York, 1976, The National Foundation—March of Dimes.

Gibbons, M.B.: Circumcision: the controversy continues, Pediatr. Nurs. **10**(2):103-109, 1984.

Harris, C.C., and Stern, P.N.: Care of the prepuce in the uncircumcised child: reinforcing nature's laws of health, Issues Compr. Pediatr. Nurs. **5**:233-242, 1981.

Infant formula: labeling requirements, Federal Register **48**:31880-31887, July 1983.

Jeffries, R.D.: A short course in breastfeeding, Issues Compr. Pediatr. Nurs. **5**:243-251, 1981.

Kuller, J.M., Lund, C., and Tobin, C.: Improved skin care for premature infants, Am. J. Maternal Child Nurs. **8**(3):200-203, 1983.

La Leche League International: The womanly art of breastfeeding, Franklin Park, Ill., 1978, Interstate Printers Publishers.

Lum, B., and Lortz, R.: Reappraising newborn eye care, Am. J. Nurs. **80**(9):1602-1603, 1980.

National Society to Prevent Blindness, Committee on Ophthalmia Neonatorum: Prevention and treatment of ophthalmia neonatorum, New York, 1981, The Society.

Principles of infant skin care: A current guide for the pediatric health care professional, Skillman, N.J., Johnson & Johnson Baby Products Co., 1983.

Schlegel, A.M.: Observations on breast-feeding technique: facts and fallacies, Am. J. Maternal Child Nurs. **8**(3):204-208, 1983.

Shipman, S.C., and Robinson, D.B.: Normal newborn care. In Perez, R.H.: Protocols for perinatal nursing practice, St. Louis, 1981, The C.V. Mosby Co.

Strain, J.E.: First ride-safe ride, Pediatr. Nurs. **7**(4): 49, 1981.

Taylor, L.S.: Newborn feeding behaviors and attaching, Am. J. Maternal Child Nurs. **6**(3):201-202, 1981.

Wayland, J.R., and Higgins, P.G.: Newborn circumcision: father's involvement, Pediatr. Nurs. **9**(1):41-42, 1983.

Parent-infant attachment

Anderson, C.J.: Enhancing reciprocity between mother and neonate, Nurs. Res. **30**(2):89-93, 1981.

Buckner, E.B.: Use of Brazelton Neonatal Behavioral Assessment in planning care for parents and newborns, JOGN Nursing **12**:26-30, 1983.

Cannon, R.B.: The development of maternal touch during early mother-infant interaction, JOGN Nursing **6**(2):28-33, 1977.

Carter-Jessop, L.: Promoting maternal attachment through prenatal intervention, Am. J. Maternal Child Nurs. **6**(2):107-112, 1981.

Cropley, C.: Assessment of mothering behaviors. In Johnson, S.H., editor: High-risk parenting, Philadelphia, 1979, J.B. Lippincott Co., pp. 13-35.

The first six hours of life: early parent-infant relationships, New York, 1978, The National Foundation—March of Dimes.

Foley, K.L.: Caring for the parents of newborn twins, Am. J. Maternal Child Nurs. **4**(4):221-226, 1979.

Freeman, M.H.: Giving family life a good start in the hospital, Am. J. Maternal Child Nurs. **4**(1):51-54, 1979.

Gromada, K.: Maternal-infants attachment: the first step toward individualizing twins, Am. J. Maternal Child Nurs. **6**(2):129-134, 1981.

Jenkins, R.L., and Westhus, N.K.: The nurse role in parent-infant bonding: overview, assessment, intervention, JOGN Nursing **10**(2):114-118, 1981.

Mercer, R.T.: The nurse and maternal tasks of early postpartum, Am. J. Maternal Child Nurs. **6**(5):341-345, 1981.

Mitchell, K., and Mills, N.M.: Is the sensitive period in parent-infant bonding overrated?, Pediatr. Nurs. **9**(2):91-94, 1983.

Murphy, C.M.: Assessment of fathering behaviors. In Johnson, S.H., editor: High-risk parenting, Philadelphia, 1979, J.B. Lippincott Co., pp. 36-49.

Perez, P.: Nurturing children who attend the birth of a sibling, Am. J. Maternal Child Nurs. **4**(4):215-217, 1979.

Phillips, C.R., and Anzalone, J.T.: Fathering: participation in labor and birth, ed. 2, St. Louis, 1982, The C.V. Mosby Co.

Powell, M.: The Neonatal Behavioral Assessment Scale. In Powell, M.: Assessment and management of developmental changes and problems in children, ed. 2, St. Louis, 1981, The C.V. Mosby Co.

Rhone, M.: Six steps to better bonding, Can. Nurse **76**(10):38-41, 1980.

Weiser, M.A., and Castiglia, P.T.: Assessing early father-infant attachment, Am. J. Maternal Child Nurs. **9**(2):104-106, 1984.

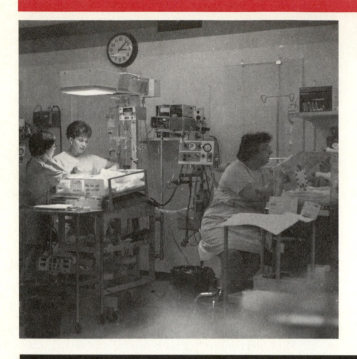

HEALTH PROBLEMS OF THE NEONATE

OBJECTIVES

On completion of this chapter the reader will be able to:

- Recognize common deviations from the normal expectations in the newborn infant

- Perform a systematic assessment of an ill newborn

- Determine the gestational age of a newborn infant

- Contrast the characteristics of a premature infant and a full-term infant

- Outline a general plan of care for a high-risk infant

- Modify a general care plan to meet the needs of an infant with a specific high risk health deviation

- Discuss the role of the nurse in facilitating positive parent-child relationships

NURSING DIAGNOSES

Nursing diagnoses identified for the neonate with health problems include, but are not restricted to, the following:

Health perception-health management pattern

- Infection, potential for, related to (1) presence of infective organisms; (2) impaired skin integrity; (3) denuded skin

- Injury, potential for, related to (1) use of specific therapies and appliances; (2) incapacity for self-protection; (3) immobility

Nutritional-metabolic pattern

- Fluid volume deficit, potential, related to (1) inability to regulate intake; (2) dehydrating effect of heat-producing devices and therapies

- Skin integrity, impairment of: potential related to (1) immature structure and function; (2) immobility

- Skin integrity, impairment of: actual related to (specific problem)

Activity-exercise pattern

- Airway clearance, ineffective, related to (1) accumulation of secretions; (2) immobility; (3) fatigue

- Diversional activity deficit related to lack of sensory stimulation

- Self-care deficit related to immaturity

Sleep-rest pattern

- Sleep pattern disturbance related to (1) frequent assessments; (2) therapies (specific)

Cognitive-perceptual pattern

- Sensory-perceptual alterations, visual, related to application of eye patches

- Sensory-perceptual alterations, tactile, related to protected environment

Role-relationship pattern

- Family process, alterations in, related to (1) situational crisis; (2) knowledge deficit; (3) temporary family disorganization; (4) inadequate support systems

- Grieving, anticipatory (parental), related to (1) expected loss (specify); (2) seriousness of infant's physical status

- Parenting, alterations in: potential related to (1) separation; (2) skill deficit; (3) family stress

Value-belief pattern

- Spiritual distress (parental), related to (1) inadequate support systems; (2) decisions regarding "right to life conflicts"

Factors that determine the degree to which the newborn adjusts to the extrauterine environment are numerous and varied. Certain factors determine the innate constitutional structure and function of the neonate. These include hereditary characteristics and environmental factors that influence development from the time of conception. The newborn's immature physiologic systems impose threats to his survival. Although infants are able to survive before the optimum level of maturity has been reached, there is a point at which extrauterine existence is impossible even with excellent, intensive prenatal, intrapartal, and postnatal care. In addition, there are all those factors that produce pathologic conditions in an otherwise normal, full-term infant. These pathologic conditions may be directly related to the birth process or may be postnatal hazards to the newborn. Some of the conditions require no intervention other than careful assessment and continued observation to distinguish them from potential pathologic situations. Others require immediate identification and intervention to prevent future problems. The nurse's ability to recognize such conditions and institute appropriate care significantly affects the neonate's immediate survival and later development.

BIRTH INJURIES

The forces of labor and delivery may result in trauma to the infant during the birth process, especially when the baby is large, when the presentation is breech, or when forceful extraction is used because of fetal distress. Many injuries are minor and spontaneously resolve in a few days; others, although minor, require some degree of intervention. Still others can be very serious, even fatal. Part of the nurse's responsibility is to identify such injuries in order that appropriate intervention can be initiated as soon as possible.

SOFT TISSUE INJURY

Various types of soft tissue injury may be sustained during the process of birth, primarily in the form of bruises and/or abrasions secondary to dystocia. Soft tissue injury usually occurs when there is some degree of disproportion between the presenting part and the maternal pelvis (cephalopelvic disproportion). Application of forceps to facilitate a difficult vertex delivery may produce discoloration or abrasion on the sides of the face with the same configuration as the forceps. Petechiae or ecchymoses may be observed on the presenting part following a breech or brow

delivery, and the sudden release of pressure on the head can produce scleral hemorrhages and/or generalized petechiae over the face and head following a difficult or too-rapid delivery, such as the ''precipitate'' delivery.

These traumatic lesions generally fade spontaneously within a few days without treatment. However, petechiae may be a manifestation of some underlying bleeding disorders and should be evaluated. Nursing care is primarily directed toward assessing the injury and providing an explanation and reassurance to the parents.

HEAD TRAUMA

Trauma to the head that occurs during the birth process is usually benign but occasionally results in more serious injury. The injuries that produce serious trauma such as intraventricular hemorrhage and subdural hematoma are discussed later in relation to neurologic disturbances (see Chapter 25). Skull fractures are discussed in association with other fractures sustained during the process of birth. The common injuries, caput succedaneum and cephalhematoma are discussed below and outlined in Table 7-1.

Caput succedaneum

The most commonly observed scalp lesion is caput succedaneum, a vaguely outlined area of edematous tissue situated over the portion of the scalp that presents in a vertex delivery (Fig. 7-1, *A*). The swelling consists of serum or blood, or both, accumulated in the tissues above the bone, and it often extends beyond the bone margins. The swelling may be associated with overlying petechiae or ecchymosis. No specific treatment is needed, and the swelling subsides within a few days.

Cephalhematoma

Infrequently, a cephalhematoma is formed when blood vessels rupture during a difficult labor or delivery to produce bleeding into the area between the bone and its periosteum. The boundaries of the cephalhematoma are sharply demarcated and do not extend beyond the limits of the bone (Fig. 7-1, *B*). The cephalhematoma may involve one or both parietal bones. Less frequently, the occipital and, rarely, the frontal bones are affected. The swelling is usually minimal at birth but increases in size on the second or third day.

No treatment is indicated for uncomplicated cephalhematoma, and most lesions are absorbed within 2 weeks to 3 months. Lesions that result in severe blood loss to the area or that involve an underlying fracture require further evaluation and appropriate therapy.

TABLE 7-1. COMPARISON OF CEPHALIC INJURIES CAUSED BY BIRTH TRAUMA

INJURY	TIME OF ONSET	PATHOLOGY	CLINICAL MANIFESTATIONS
Caput succedaneum	Within 24 hours after birth	Edema of soft scalp tissue	Outline is ill defined; mass is soft but not fluctuant; pressure causes pitting of edema
Cephalhematoma	After initial 24 to 48 hours after birth	Hematoma between periosteum and skull bone	Outline is well defined against edge of bone margin; mass is soft and fluctuant
Subdural hematoma	Variable—from a few hours to a few days after birth	Hematoma in space between dura and arachnoid linings of the brain	No mass is visible; signs are those of: Increased intracranial pressure: bulging and widened fontanels and sutures, high-pitched cry, vomiting, poor sucking reflex, irritability, lethargy, weak Moro reflex, flaccidity followed by spasticity, seizures, and coma Respiratory distress: cyanosis, apnea, and irregular respirations Progressive signs of hemorrhage and shock: pale, cold, clammy skin, weak pulse, and signs of jaundice and anemia

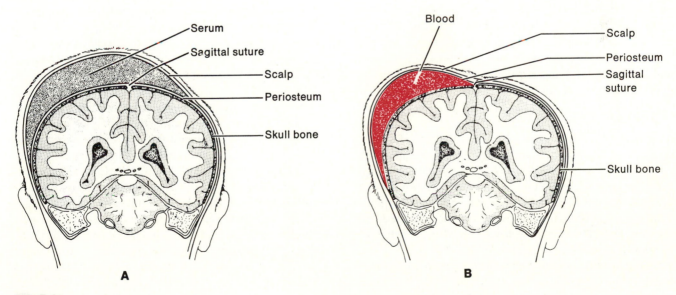

FIG. 7-1

Difference between caput succedaneum, **A,** *and cephalhematoma,* **B.** *See Table 7-1 for a further comparison of these injuries. (Modified from Jensen, M.D., Benson, R.C., and Bobak, I.M.: Maternity care: the nurse and the family, ed. 2, St. Louis, 1981, The C.V. Mosby Co.)*

Nursing considerations

Nursing care is directed toward assessment and observation of these two head injuries and vigilance in observing for possible associated complications such as subdural hematoma or intraventricular hemorrhage. Because both of these visible injuries resolve spontaneously, parents need reassurance of their usual benign nature.

FRACTURES

Fracture of the clavicle, or collarbone, is the most frequent birth injury. It is often associated with difficult vertex or breech birth and delivery of infants of above average weight. A fractured clavicle in a newborn may be asymptomatic but should be suspected if an infant demonstrates limited use of the affected arm, malposition of the arm, asymmetric Moro reflex, focal swelling or tenderness, or if he cries in pain when his arm is moved. Crepitus (the crackling sound produced by the rubbing together of fractured bone fragments) is often heard on further examination, and x-ray films usually reveal a complete fracture with overriding of the fragments.

Fractures of long bones, such as the femur or the humerus, are difficult to detect by radiologic examination. The epiphysis is mostly cartilage, which is usually not dense enough to show clearly on an x-ray film.

Fractures of the neonatal skull are uncommon. The bones, which are less mineralized and more compressible, are separated by membranous seams that allow sufficient alteration in the head contour so that it can adjust to the birth canal during delivery. Skull fractures usually follow prolonged, difficult delivery or forceps extraction. Most fractures are linear but some may be visible as depressed indentations resembling a ''ping-pong ball.''

Nursing considerations

Frequently, no intervention may be prescribed other than proper body alignment, careful dressing and undressing of the infant, and handling and carrying that support the affected bone. Occasionally, for immobilization and relief of pain, the arm on the side of the fractured clavicle may be fixed on the body by pinning the sleeve to the shirt or by application of a triangular sling or a figure-8 bandage.

Linear skull fractures usually require no treatment. A ''ping-pong'' fracture usually can be decompressed by nonsurgical methods. The infant is carefully observed for signs of cerebral complications. The parents of infants with a fracture of any bone should be involved in caring for the infant during hospitalization as part of discharge planning for care at home.

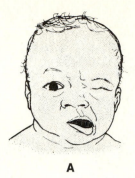 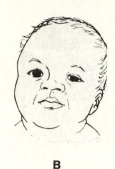

A   B

FIG. 7-2

A, *Paralysis of right side of face 15 minutes after forceps delivery. Absence of movement on affected side is especially noticeable when the infant cries.* **B,** *Same infant 24 hours later. Recovery was complete in another 24 hours. (From Jensen, M.D., Benson, R.C., and Bobak, I.M.: Maternity care: the nurse and the family, ed. 2, St. Louis, 1981, The C.V. Mosby Co.)*

PARALYSES

Pressure exerted on nerves during a difficult labor can cause injury and paralysis of muscles that they supply. The most frequently observed nerve injuries are those involving the brachial plexus and the facial nerve.

Facial paralysis

Pressure on the facial nerve during delivery may result in injury to cranial nerve VII. Clinical manifestations are primarily loss of movement on the affected side, such as inability to completely close the eye, drooping of the corner of the mouth, and absence of wrinkling of the forehead (Fig. 7-2). The paralysis is most noticeable when the infant cries. No medical intervention is necessary; the paralysis usually disappears spontaneously in a few days, but it may take as long as several months.

Nursing considerations. Nursing care involves aiding the infant to suck and assisting the mother with feeding techniques. If the lid of the eye on the affected side does not close completely, artificial tears can be instilled daily to prevent drying of the conjunctiva and injury to the sclera and cornea.

Brachial palsy

Plexus injury results from forces that alter the normal position and relationship of the arm, shoulder, and neck. *Erb palsy* (Erb-Duchenne paralysis), caused by damage to the upper plexus, is usually a result of stretching or pulling away of the shoulder from the head. The less common lower plexus palsy, or *Klumpke palsy,* results from severe

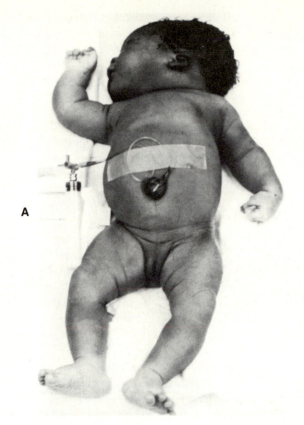

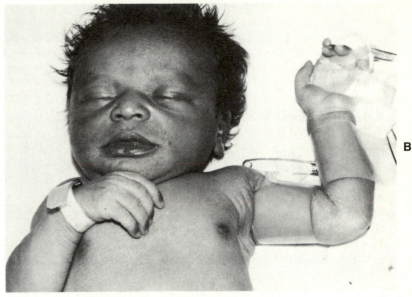

FIG. 7-3

A, *Brachial plexus (Erb) palsy, left sided. Note the extended, internally rotated arm and pronated wrist on the affected side.* **B,** *Recommended corrective positioning for treatment of Erb-Duchenne paralysis. Note abduction and external rotation at shoulder, flexion at elbow, supination of forearm, and slight dorsiflexion at wrist. (**A** from Korones, S.B.: High-risk newborn infant: the basis for intensive nursing care, ed. 3, St. Louis, 1981, The C.V. Mosby Co.; **B** from Behrman, R.E., and Mangurten, H.H.: Birth injuries. In Behrman, R.E., editor: Neonatology: diseases of the fetus and infant, St. Louis, 1973, The C.V. Mosby Co.)*

stretching of the upper extremity while the trunk is relatively immobile. The clinical manifestations of Erb palsy are related to the paralysis of the affected extremity and muscles. The arm hangs limp alongside the body, is internally rotated, and the wrist is pronated (Fig. 7-3, *A*). The muscles of the hand are paralyzed in lower plexus palsy, with absence of voluntary movements of the wrist. In severe forms of brachial palsy, the entire arm is paralyzed and hangs limp and motionless at the side.

Treatment of an affected arm is aimed at preventing contractures of the paralyzed muscles and maintaining correct placement of the humeral head within the glenoid fossa of the scapula. Complete recovery from stretched nerves usually takes about 3 months. Avulsion of the nerves may result in permanent damage, requiring surgical and orthopedic intervention.

Nursing considerations. Nursing care is primarily concerned with proper positioning of the affected arm. The arm is placed in an abducted, externally rotated position to relieve pressure on the stretched nerves. This is accomplished by means of casting or splinting, or the desired position is maintained by pinning the shirt sleeve to the mattress. A towel or diaper can be securely wrapped around the arm, in the manner of a sling, and attached to the mattress (Fig. 7-3, *B*).

The arm should also be put through complete passive range of motion exercises daily to maintain muscle tone and function. When dressing the infant, the nurse should always give special preference to the affected arm. Undressing should begin with the unaffected arm and redressing should begin with the affected arm to prevent unnecessary manipulation and stress on the paralyzed muscles.

Phrenic nerve paralysis

Phrenic nerve paralysis resulting in diaphragmatic paralysis sometimes occurs in conjunction with brachial palsy. Respiratory distress is the most common and important sign of injury. Because injury to this nerve is usually unilateral, the lung on the affected side does not expand and respiratory efforts are ineffectual. Breathing is primarily thoracic and cyanosis is a prominent sign. Pneumonia is a frequent complication.

Nursing care of the infant with phrenic nerve paralysis is the same as for any infant with respiratory distress.

COMMON PROBLEMS IN THE NEONATE

There are numerous problems encountered frequently in the newborn period. Many are innocuous conditions that are of concern only to the parents; others require intervention to prevent complications. Some are discussed elsewhere as appropriate throughout the book, for example, skin manifestations and color changes in the newborn (p. 141), diaper dermatitis, colic, and milk sensitivity (Chapter 9). One of the most common observations in the newborn period is jaundice but, since it can be a high-risk condition also, it is discussed at length under that category later in this chapter.

CANDIDIASIS

Candida infections, also known as *moniliasis*, are not uncommon in the newborn. *Candida albicans*, the usual organism responsible, may cause disease in any organ system. It is a yeastlike fungus (it produces yeast cells and spores) that can be acquired from a maternal vaginal infection during delivery, by person-to-person transmission (especially poor handwashing technique), or on contaminated hands, bottles, nipples, or other articles. Mucocutaneous, cutaneous, and disseminated candidiasis are all observed in this age-group. It is usually a benign disorder in the neonate, often confined to the oral and diaper regions.

Candidal diaper dermatitis

The warm, moist atmosphere created in the diaper area provides an optimal environment for candidal growth. The dermatitis appears in the perianal area, inguinal folds, and lower abdomen. The affected area is intensely erythematous with a sharply demarcated, scalloped edge, frequently with numerous satellite lesions that extend beyond the larger lesion. The usual source of infection is through the gastrointestinal tract when organisms are swallowed from the birth canal during delivery. It may also appear 2 to 3 days following an oral infection.

Therapy consists of applications of an anticandidal ointment, such as nystatin, with each diaper change. The caregiver is taught to keep the diaper area as clean and dry as possible and good hygienic care is essential to prevent spread. Sometimes the infant is given an oral antifungal preparation as well to eliminate any gastrointestinal source of infection (see the section on oral candidiasis).

Oral candidiasis (thrush)

Oral candidiasis is characterized by white adherent patches on the tongue, palate, and inner aspects of the cheeks. It is readily distinguished from coagulated milk when attempts to remove the patches are unsuccessful, usually resulting in bleeding from the scraped surfaces. The infant may refuse to suck because of pain in the mouth, but this is infrequent.

The condition tends to be acute in the newborn, chronic in infants and young children, and appear when the oral flora is altered as a result of antibiotic therapy. Although the disorder is usually self-limiting, spontaneous resolution may take as long as 2 months, during which time lesions may spread to the larynx, trachea, bronchi, and lungs and along the gastrointestinal tract. The disease should always be treated with good hygiene, application of a fungicide, and correction of any underlying disturbance. The source of infection should be identified to prevent reinfection.

Topical application of 1 ml nystatin (Mycostatin) over the surfaces of the oral cavity four times a day or every 6 hours is usually sufficient to prevent spread of the disease or prolong its course. Another effective therapy is application of 1% aqueous gentian violet three times a day.

Nursing considerations. Nursing care is directed toward preventing spread of the infection and correct application of the prescribed topical medication. Mycostatin is applied after feedings. The medication is distributed to the surface of the oral mucosa and tongue with an applicator and the remainder of the dose is deposited in the mouth to be swallowed in order to treat any gastrointestinal lesions. Therapy is continued for about 1 week, even when lesions have disappeared within a few days. The Mycostatin suspension is stable for only 1 week.

When gentian violet is used, the solution is applied directly to the patches. The infant should not be allowed to swallow any excess because the medication is irritating to trachea, larynx, and esophagus. After application of the solution, the infant should be placed prone for a short time to allow secretions to flow from the mouth. Special care should be taken when administering this preparation because gentian violet stains skin, clothing, bed linens, and other objects.

Other measures to control thrush, in addition to good hygienic care, include rinsing the infant's mouth with plain water after each feeding before applying the medication, boiling reusable nipples and bottles for at least 20 minutes after thorough washing (spores are heat resistant), and treating the source.

ERYTHEMA TOXICUM

Erythema toxicum, also known as ''flea bite dermatitis'' or newborn rash, is a benign, self-limiting eruption that usually appears within the first 2 days of life. The lesions vary in character and number. They may be firm pale yellow to white papules or pustules 1 to 3 mm in diameter on an erythematous base, erythematous macules, or simply blotchy erythema. The rash is most commonly located on the face, proximal extremities, trunk, and buttocks and is more obvious during crying episodes. There are no systemic manifestations and the cause is unknown. Although no treatment is necessary, parents are usually concerned about the rash and need to be reassured of its benign and transient nature.

''BIRTHMARKS''

Discolorations of the skin are very common findings in the newborn infant. (See skin assessment of the newborn, p. 141). Most, such as mongolian spots or telangiectatic nevi, involve no therapy other than reassurance to parents of their benign nature. Some can be a manifestation of a disease that suggests further examination of the child and other family members (for example, the multiple light brown *cafe au lait spots* that often characterize the autosomal-dominant hereditary disorder neurofibromatosis and are common findings in Albright syndrome).

Darker and/or more extensive lesions demand further scrutiny, and excision of the lesion is recommended when feasible or excisional biopsy is performed. These include the reddish-brown solitary nodule that appears on the face or upper arm that usually represents a spindle and epithelioid cell nevus (juvenile melanoma), a giant pigmented nevus (bathing trunk nevus), a dark brown to black irregular plaque that is at risk of transformation to malignant melanoma, and the dark brown or black macules that become more numerous with age (junctional or compound nevi).

Vascular birthmarks, those orange or light red (salmon patch) or dark red or bluish red (port wine stain) lesions, require no treatment but parents may need advice regarding the use of cosmetic coverings (such as Covermark) at a later time when they feel that the child may be adversely affected by the defect. Strawberry hemangiomas, those red, rubbery nodules with a rough surface, may not be present at birth but appear at 2 to 4 weeks of age. The parents can be reassured that they resolve spontaneously during childhood and usually require no treatment.

HYPOTONIA (FLOPPY INFANT SYNDROME)

Decreased muscle tone in an infant is not an unusual observation in the newborn nursery and is one of the most common presenting symptoms in neuromuscular disorders. It may also indicate a variety of systemic conditions. Probably the most frequent causes are cerebral trauma or hypoxia at birth and chromosome disorders, particularly Down syndrome.

Hypotonia, sometimes called the ''floppy infant syndrome,'' is marked by diminished muscle tone and weakness in response to both spontaneous and passive motion and to reflex testing. The infant, placed in a supine position, assumes a characteristic ''frog posture'' or lies in some other unusual position at rest. Normally, the young infant who is held in ventral suspension, that is, with the examiner's hand supporting the infant under the chest, will respond by slightly raising his head with his back relatively straight, arms flexed and slightly abducted, and knees partly flexed. The hypotonic infant droops over the supporting hand with head and extremities hanging loosely resembling an inverted ''U'' (Fig. 7-4). The muscles feel flabby when palpated and there is marked head lag when the infant is pulled to a sitting position. Poor sucking may be noted.

The management of these infants is determined by the cause of the hypotonia. It is a nursing responsibility to record and report findings that suggest hypotonia in an infant so that further evaluation can be carried out and therapeutic measures implemented if indicated.

THE HIGH-RISK INFANT

The high-risk neonate can be defined as the newborn, regardless of gestational age or birth weight, who has a greater than average chance of morbidity or mortality because of conditions or circumstances that are superimposed on the normal course of events associated with birth and the adjustment to extrauterine existence. The high-risk pe-

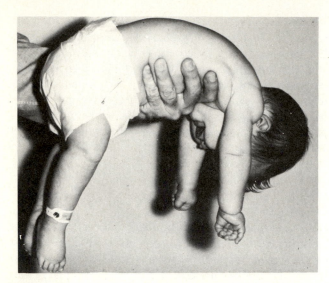

FIG. 7-4

Hypotonicity demonstrated by horizontal suspension in an infant with Werdnig-Hoffman disease. (From Swaiman, K.F., and Wright, F.S.: The practice of pediatric neurology, ed. 2, St. Louis, 1982, The C.V. Mosby Co.)

riod encompasses human growth and development from the time of viability until 28 days following birth and includes threats to life and health that occur during the prenatal, perinatal, and postnatal periods.

Congenital anomalies are often high-risk conditions, especially those involving the viscera and cranium, and are frequently complicated by prematurity. However, most of these are discussed elsewhere throughout the book and will be mentioned only briefly here. For a discussion of chromosome abnormalities that may also produce high-risk conditions, the reader is referred to Chapter 3.

CLASSIFICATION OF HIGH-RISK INFANTS

High-risk infants are most often classified according to size, gestational age, and the predominant pathophysiologic problems. The more common problems related to physiologic status are closely associated with the state of maturity of the infant; they usually involve chemical disturbances (hypoglycemia, hypocalcemia) and/or consequences of immaturely functioning organs and systems (hyperbilirubinemia, respiratory distress, hypothermia).

Classification according to size
Low birth weight (LBW) infant—an infant whose birth weight is less than 2500 g without regard to gestational age

Appropriate-for-gestational-age (AGA) infant—an infant whose intrauterine growth was normal at the moment of birth

Small-for-date (SFD) or small-for-gestational-age (SGA) infant—an infant whose rate of intrauterine growth was slowed and who was delivered at or later than term; these infants are usually two standard deviations below the mean for infants of appropriate weight at birth, and their birth weight falls below the 10th percentile on intrauterine growth curves

Intrauterine growth retardation (IUGR)—found in infants whose intrauterine growth is retarded (sometimes used as a more descriptive term for small-for-gestational-age infant)

Large-for-gestational-age (LGA) infant—an infant whose birth weight falls above the 90th percentile on intrauterine growth curves

Classification according to gestational age
Premature (preterm) infant—an infant born before completion of the thirty-seventh week of gestation, regardless of birth weight

Term infant—an infant born between the beginning of the thirty-eighth week and the completion of the forty-second week of gestation, regardless of birth weight

Postmature (postterm) infant—an infant born after completion of the forty-second week of gestational age, regardless of birth weight

Classification according to mortality
Fetal death—death of the fetus after 20 weeks of gestation and before delivery regardless of gestational age and with absence of any signs of life following birth

Neonatal death—death that occurs in the first 28 days of life; early neonatal or postnatal deaths occur in the first week of life

Perinatal mortality—describes the total number of fetal and early neonatal deaths per 1000 total births

Many problems can be anticipated before delivery. Prenatal testing and labor monitoring have reduced the incidence of perinatal mortality, and specialized care of the distressed newborn is increasing the survival rate of such infants. If an infant is likely to require special therapy at or soon after birth, plans should be made for delivery to take place at or near a hospital that has the facilities to provide such care. In this way there is no delay in initiating needed care, and some of the hazards associated with transporting the sick newborn are averted.

ASSESSMENT OF HIGH-RISK INFANTS

At birth the newborn is given a cursory assessment to determine any apparent problems and those that demand immediate attention. This examination is primarily concerned with evaluation of cardiopulmonary and neurologic function. The assessment includes assignment of an Apgar score (see p. 140) and evaluation for pallor, cyanosis, prematurity, any obvious congenital anomalies, or evidence of neonatal disease. If the infant displays any need for intensive care, he is taken immediately to the neonatal intensive care nursery for initiation of therapy and more extensive assessment.

Neonatal intensive care nursing is a highly specialized area of knowledge and practice that requires lengthy supervised experience to reach a level of competence that permits independent functioning. Neonatal intensive care nursing involves an understanding of neonatal physiology and characteristics, a knowledge of the function and management of a number of mechanical devices and apparatus, the ability to recognize very subtle deviations from the expected, and the ability to implement a judicious course of action.

Some major nursing observations and assessments apply to all high-risk infants, regardless of diagnosis. Therefore, the general aspects of assessment of the high-risk infant will be described briefly here. Many aspects were discussed in relation to the care of the newborn in Chapter 6. Others will be considered throughout the remainder of this chapter and summarized in relation to specific patient problems.

Maintaining detailed, ongoing records of all activities and observations is an important function of nurses in the intensive care setting. Knowledge and operation of complex pieces of equipment and mechanical devices are inherent in the care of the ill neonate. However, sophisticated monitoring and life-support systems cannot replace the vigilance and constant scrutiny of infants by experienced personnel. Subtle changes that are not apparent on mechanical devices can be detected by alert nurses. Some of the crucial factors in observation of ill newborns cannot be detected by monitors. These factors are as follows (Korones, 1981):

- Acceptance of feedings
- Course of weight gain
- Early detection of regurgitation
- Abdominal distention
- Frequency and character of stools
- Changes in behavior (lethargy, seizure activity, hyperactivity)
- Changes in color (jaundice, pallor, cyanosis)
- Skin lesions
- Deviations from prescribed volumes of intravenous infusions
- Edema
- Respiratory distress (tachypnea, retractions, flaring nares, grunting)
- Quality of breath sounds
- Character and location of heart sounds

Systematic assessment of the infant

Nurses are usually responsible for the same infant each day, which allows for more accurate determination of day-to-day progress. During the course of daily care the nurse makes frequent systematic assessments of physical status, since vital signs of small infants change several times in the period of a very few hours. It has been said that the newborn undergoes as many changes in 4 to 6 hours as an adult does in 24 hours.

In the course of an assessment the nurse ascertains whether the life-support apparatus is functioning properly—that the respiratory equipment is at the correct pressure and/or volume setting and no leaks are apparent, that the monitors are set at the desired limits and tracings are within normal limits, and that the infusion pump is delivering the correct volume and type of fluid. The assessment of the infant should proceed in a systematic manner. Each nurse develops an approach that is comfortable for him or her and follows the same pattern routinely. An observational assessment is usually performed hourly, or more frequently on very ill infants, and a synopsis is included in the charting. However, any assessment procedures that require that the infant be disturbed should be timed to allow for sufficient rest between assessments.

General assessment
- Weigh two or three times daily
- Describe general body shape and size, presence and location of edema, amount of body fat
- Describe any apparent deformities

Respiratory assessment
- Describe shape of chest (barrel, concave) symmetry, presence of incisions, chest tubes, and so on
- Describe use of accessory muscles—nasal flaring or substernal, intercostal, or subclavicular retractions
- Determine respiratory rate and regularity
- Describe breath sounds—rales, rhonchi, wheezing, grunts, areas of absence of sound, grunting, comparison among the four quadrants
- Determine whether suctioning is needed
- Describe cry
- Describe ambient oxygen and method of delivery—if intubated, describe size of tube, type of ventilator, and settings

Cardiovascular assessment
- Determine heart rate and rhythm
- Describe heart sounds, including any suspected murmurs
- Determine the point of maximum intensity (PMI), the point where the heartbeat sounds loudest (a change in the point of maximum intensity may indicate a mediastinal shift)
- Describe infant's color (may be of cardiac, respiratory, or hematopoietic origin)—cyanosis, pallor, plethora, jaundice

Determine blood pressure (indicate extremity used)

Describe peripheral pulses

Determine central venous pressure (if central venous pressure line is part of infant's apparatus)

Gastrointestinal assessment

Determine presence of any indication of abdominal distention—increase in circumference, shiny skin

Determine any signs of regurgitation, especially following feeding; character and amount of residual if gavage-fed; if nasogastric tube in place, describe type of suction, drainage (color, consistency, pH, guaiac)

Describe amount, color, consistency, and odor of any emesis

Describe amount, color, and consistency of stools; occult blood should be checked for, if indicated by physician's order or appearance of stool

Describe bowel sounds; presence or absence; visible peristalsis

Genitourinary assessment

Describe any abnormalities of genitalia

Describe amount (as determined by weight), color, and specific gravity (to determine adequacy of hydration) of urine

Neurologic-musculoskeletal assessment

Describe infant's movements—random, purposeful, jittery, twitching, spontaneous, elicited

Describe infant's position or attitude—flexed, extended

Describe reflexes observed—Moro, sucking, Babinski, and so on

Temperature

Determine axillary temperature

Determine relationship to environmental temperature

Skin assessment

Describe any discoloration, reddened area, or signs of irritation, especially where monitoring equipment, infusions, or other apparatus comes in contact with skin; note any discoloring preparation applied to the skin (such as povidone iodine)

Determine texture and turgor of skin—dry, smooth, flaky, peeling, and so on

Describe any rash or skin lesion

Determine whether intravenous infusion catheter or needle is in place, and observe for signs of infiltration

Describe parenteral infusion lines—location, type (arterial, venous, hyperalimentation, central venous pressure); type of infusion and relevant information; type of infusion pump and rate of flow; type of needle (butterfly, Quik-Cath); appearance of insertion site

The infant is weighed two or three times each day, and his position is changed every 1 to 2 hours. Any significant reaction to the changing or to a specific position is noted. To conserve the infant's energy, the position changing and periodic treatments should be timed to coincide with an assessment.

SUPPORTIVE CARE OF THE INFANT AND FAMILY

Professional health workers are often so absorbed in the life-saving physical aspects of care that the emotional needs of infants and their families are ignored. The significance of the early parent-child interaction and infant stimulation have been documented by reliable research, and nurses, aware of these infant and family needs, must incorporate activities that facilitate their development into the nursing care plan.

Neurologic impairment and serious sequelae appear to correlate with the size and gestational age of the infant at birth and with the degree of intensive care instituted. The greater the degree of immaturity, the greater the degree of handicap. Small-for-gestational-age infants appear to be less at a disadvantage than appropriate-for-gestational-age infants born early, although both are at a greater disadvantage than normal infants. There is an increase in the incidence of neurologic sequelae in preterm infants, such as cerebral palsy and the entity termed "attention deficit disorder," and intellectual functioning may be affected.

Infant stimulation

Recently, attention has been focused on the effects of early stimulation, or lack of it, on both normal and preterm infants. Findings indicate that infants are able to respond to a greater variety of stimuli than had been previously thought. Nurses who are aware of this need can incorporate a stimulation program into the nursing care plan, providing tactile, visual, and auditory stimuli whenever possible.

Touching is a vital part of any infant stimulation program. As soon as the infant's condition will allow, rocking in a specially designed sling inside the Isolette has been used in some areas to provide kinesthetic stimulation. Holding the infant in a rocking chair is a pleasant means for meeting this need in the infant who can tolerate room atmosphere.

Visual stimulation can be provided by hanging mobiles and placing colorful toys in the infant's line of vision. Nurses and others who care for the child should hold him in such a way that he can see the caregiver's face at close range, and they should attempt to get him to follow their head movements with his eyes. Talking to the infant is one of the best means of providing simultaneous auditory stimulation; many parents bring small music boxes or similar audio toys to place in the infant's crib or Isolette.

The effects of the intensive care environment on subsequent development has yet to be evaluated. Twenty-four-hour surveillance of sick infants implies maximum visibility. However, many units have instigated a program to help establish a night-day sleep pattern by either darkening the room, if the infant's condition allows, or placing patches over the infant's eyes at night. It has been found that the sound levels are significantly higher in the neonatal intensive care unit than in the regular nursery, but the long-term effects are not known.

Parental involvement

The birth of a premature infant is usually an unexpected and stressful event for which the family is emotionally unprepared. To compound the situation, the precarious nature of the infant's condition engenders an atmosphere of apprehension and uncertainty. The parents see the infant only briefly before he is removed to the intensive care unit or even to another hospital, leaving them with just the recollection of the infant's very small size and unusual appearance. The staff and physician are often guarded in discussing the infant's condition; the parents are continually expecting to hear that the infant has died.

If the infant is to be transported from the hospital in which he was born, the parents need information about the facility to which he is going, including the location, the care he is expected to receive, the name of his physician, and the telephone number of the nursery. Explanations should be simple, and parents should be given the opportunity to ask questions. Perhaps most important of all, the parents, especially the mother, should be allowed some contact with the infant before the transport.

When they visit the infant, the frightening array of equipment and activity is stressful to parents, and they need reassurance that the infant is receiving proper care. Once they understand that the infant needs this intensive care, they are content to be kept informed of his condition. It is not necessary to share too much information with the parents, such as very technical information that does not contribute to their understanding. Considering the parents' fears, the nurse can be truthful without being unduly candid regarding the more negative aspects of the child's condition.

There is increasing evidence to indicate that the emotional separation that accompanies the physical separation of mother and infant interferes with the normal maternal-infant attachment process (see p. 160). When the infant is sick, the necessary physical separation appears to be accompanied by an emotional estrangement on the part of the mother that may seriously damage her capacity for mothering the infant.

Facilitating parent-infant relationships. The current concept in the comprehensive management of the high-risk newborn is to encourage parental involvement rather than to isolate parents from the infant and his care. This is particularly important in relation to the mother. To reduce the effects of physical separation, the mother is united with her newborn at the earliest opportunity.

Preparing the parents to see their infant for the first time is a nursing responsibility. Before the first visit the parents should be prepared for the infant's appearance, the equipment that is attached to him, and some indication of the general atmosphere of the unit. At the bedside the nurse explains the function of each piece of equipment and the role it plays in facilitating recovery. When possible, some items related to therapy can be removed; for example, phototherapy can be temporarily discontinued and eye patches removed to permit eye-to-eye contact.

Parents will usually appreciate the support of a nurse during the initial visit with the infant, but they should be left alone with the infant for a short while. It is important during the early visits to emphasize positive aspects of the infant's behavior, to help the parents focus on the infant as an individual rather than on the equipment that surrounds him. Most institutions allow parents to visit their infants as often as they wish and encourage them to do so.

Most mothers feel very "shaky" and insecure about initiating interaction with the infant. Nurses can sense the mother's level of readiness and offer encouragement in these first efforts. Mothers of premature infants follow the same acquaintance process as do mothers of normal infants (Fig. 7-5). They may quickly proceed through the process, or they may require several days or even weeks to complete it. Throughout the maternal-infant acquaintance process, the nurse listens carefully to what the mother says, in order to assess her concerns and her progress toward incorporating the infant into her life.

Parents are encouraged to bring in clothes and toys for the infant, and the nurse helps the mother set goals both for herself and the infant. Feeding schedules are discussed, and the mother is encouraged to visit at times when she can become involved in the infant's care. Although the advisability of sibling visitation is still a matter of controversy in many neonatal units, the trend is toward allowing siblings into the unit as soon as the infant can be transferred to a transitional care unit (Fig. 7-6).

Preparation for discharge. Parents become very apprehensive as well as excited as time for discharge approaches. They have many concerns and insecurities regarding the care of the infant. Often all that the parent needs is reassurance that the behavior about which they are concerned is a normal reaction and that it will disappear as the infant matures (for example, the exaggerated Moro reflex or the inability to coordinate swallowing) or that they will have the support of the nurse during caregiving activities. Knowing that members of the staff are available for telephone or personal contact when they take the infant home provides a measure of security to insecure parents.

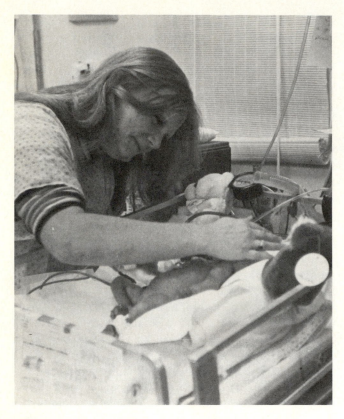

FIG. 7-5
Encouraging interaction of mother and premature infant facilitates maternal-infant attachment process.

Printed material is often a useful suggestion to offer parents of infants. Many units have such material to give to parents at the time of the birth or at the time of discharge. There are some excellent books that can be recommended, also.* Above all, encouragement and reinforcement for the parent during caregiving activities and interactions with the infant promote a healthy parent-child relationship.

Neonatal death

The precarious nature of many high-risk infants makes death a very real and ever-present possibility. Nurses in the intensive care unit are in an excellent position to prepare the parents for an inevitable death and to facilitate the family's grieving process after an expected or unexpected death. It is important that the staff allow the parents to hold and touch the infant before death and to be provided with an opportunity to see, touch, and hold the infant privately after death if they desire.

---

*Some suggestion for books for parents include: "Premature babies: a handbook for parents" by Sherri Nancy, Arbor House Publishing Co., Inc. and "The premature infant—a handbook for parents," available from The Hospital for Sick Children, Room 1218, 555 University Avenue, Toronto, Ontario, Canada MSG 1X8, for $3.00 a copy.

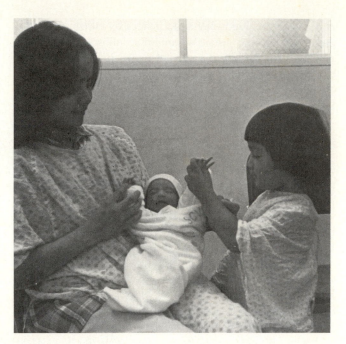

FIG. 7-6
Big sister gets acquainted with the new baby.

A photograph of the infant taken before or after his death is highly desirable. The parents may not wish to see the photograph at the time of death, but to be able to refer to it later will help make the infant seem more real, a part of the normal grief process (Wooten, 1981). Other tangible remembrances of the child can be provided, such as name tags, armbands, and locks of hair shaved for intravenous insertion or other procedures. If the parents have not done so, they should be encouraged to name the infant.

At least one nurse who is familiar to the family should be present during discussion of the dead or dying infant. Funeral arrangements should be discussed with parents openly and honestly, since few of them have had experience with this aspect of death. They need to be informed of options available, but it is preferable to encourage a funeral because the ritual provides an opportunity for parents to feel the support of friends and relatives. A clergyman of the appropriate faith should be offered if available.

Before the parents leave the hospital they should be given the telephone number of the unit (if they do not have it) and invited to call any time they have any further questions. Many intensive care units make it a point to contact the parents following a neonatal death to assess parents' coping mechanisms and provide support as needed.

Baptism. Since most Christian parents wish to have their children baptized if death is anticipated or a decided possibility, this becomes a nursing responsibility. Whenever possible, it is desirable that a representative of the parents' faith—that is, a Roman Catholic priest or a Protestant minister—perform the ritual. When death is imminent, however, a nurse or a physician can perform the baptism by simply pouring water on the infant's forehead (a medicine dropper is a convenient means) while saying, ''I baptize you in the name of the Father and of the Son and of the Holy Spirit.'' Such baptisms may need to be performed for newborns of any gestational age. Baptism is particularly important when the parents are of the Roman Catholic faith. When the faith of the parent is uncertain, a conditional baptism can be carried out by saying, ''If you are capable of receiving baptism, I baptize you in the name of the Father and of the Son and of the Holy Spirit.'' The fact of the baptism is recorded in the infant's chart, and a notice is placed on the crib or Isolette. Parents are informed at the first opportunity.

HIGH-RISK RELATED TO GESTATIONAL AGE

Since the majority of infants classified as high-risk are born before the estimated date of delivery, the major discussion of problems related to the high-risk neonate will be directed toward this group. The incidence of neonatal complications—for example, hyperbilirubinemia and hyaline membrane disease—is highest in the preterm infant, and other high-risk factors—for example, severe congenital defects often found in association with prematurity. Prematurity is generally accepted as the single largest factor contributing to infant mortality.

THE PREMATURE INFANT

The actual cause of prematurity is not known in most instances. The incidence of prematurity is lowest in the middle and high socioeconomic classes, in which pregnant women are generally in good health, are well-nourished, and receive prompt and comprehensive prenatal care. The incidence is highest in the low socioeconomic class, in which a combination of deleterious circumstances is present. Other factors, such as multiple pregnancies, toxemia, and placental accidents that interrupt the normal course of gestation before completion of fetal development, are responsible for a large number of premature births.

The outlook for a premature infant is largely, but not entirely, related to the state of physiologic and anatomic immaturity of the various organs and systems at the time of birth. The infant at term has advanced to a state of maturity sufficient to allow a successful transition to the extrauterine environment. The infant born prematurely must make the same adjustments but with functional immaturity that is directly related to the stage of development that has been reached at the time of birth. The degree to which the infant is prepared for extrauterine life can be predicted to some extent by weight and estimated gestational age.

Clinical characteristics

On inspection, the premature infant is very small and appears scrawny because of lack of or minimal subcutaneous fat deposits, with a proportionately large head in relation to the body, which reflects the cephalocaudal direction of growth. Of all the body measurements, the head is reduced least, and the sucking pads in the cheeks are strikingly prominent. The skin is bright pink, smooth, and shiny (may be edematous), with small blood vessels clearly visible underneath the thin, transparent epidermis. The fine lanugo hair is abundant over the body but is sparse, fine, and fuzzy on the head. The ear cartilage is soft and pliable, and the soles and palms have minimal creases, resulting in a smooth appearance. The bones of the skull and the ribs feel soft, and the prominent eyes are closed. Male premature infants have few scrotal rugae, and the testes are undescended; labia and clitoris are prominent in the female. (See Fig. 7-7 for a comparison of the features of normal and premature infants.)

In contrast to the full-term infant's overall attitude of flexion and continuous activity, the premature infant is inactive and motionless. The extremities maintain an attitude of extension and remain in any position in which they are placed. Reflex activity is only partially developed—sucking is absent, weak, or ineffectual; swallowing, gag, and cough reflexes are weak; and other neurologic signs are absent or diminished. Physiologically immature, the preterm infant is unable to maintain body temperature, has limited ability to excrete solutes in the urine, and has an increased susceptibility to infection. A pliable thorax and immature lung tissue and regulatory center lead to periodic breathing, hypoventilation, and frequent periods of apnea.

Weight related to gestational age

The weight of the infant at birth, which can be determined easily and reliably, correlates with the incidence of perinatal morbidity and mortality. Since many infants who weigh less than 2500 g are not premature by gestational age, there is often confusion in distinguishing between preterm and small-for-age infants. Fetal growth, gestational age, and fetal maturity are closely related but are not synonymous. Maturity implies functional capacity—the degree to which the neonate's organ systems are able to adapt to the requirements of extrauterine life. Therefore, gestational age is more closely related to fetal maturity than is birth weight (Fig. 7-8). Classification of infants at birth by both weight and gestational age provides the most

FIG. 7-7

The preterm infant lies in a "relaxed attitude," limbs more extended; his body size is small, and his head may appear somewhat larger in proportion to the body size. The term infant has more subcutaneous fat tissue and rests in a more flexed attitude.

The preterm infant's ear cartilages are poorly developed and the ear may fold easily; the hair is fine and feathery, and lanugo may cover the back and face. The mature infant's ear cartilages are well formed, and the hair is more likely to form firm separate strands.

The sole of the foot of the preterm infant appears more turgid and may have only fine wrinkles. The mature infant's sole (foot) is well and deeply creased.

The preterm female infant's clitoris is prominent, and labia majora are poorly developed and gaping. The mature female infant's labia majora are fully developed, and the clitoris is not as prominent.

The preterm male infant's scrotum is undeveloped and not pendulous; minimal rugae are present, and the testes may be in the inguinal canals or in the abdominal cavity. The term male infant's scrotum is well developed, pendulous, and rugated, and the testes are well down in the scrotal sac.

CLINICAL EVALUATION

PRETERM   TERM

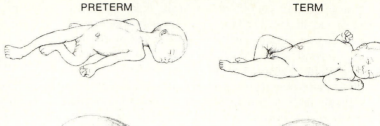
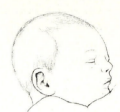
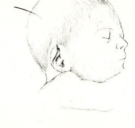
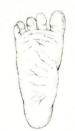
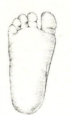
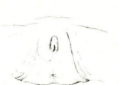

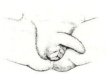
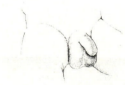

FIG. 7-7

Clinical and neurologic examinations comparing preterm and full-term infants. (From Pierog, S.H., and Ferrara, A.: Medical care of the sick newborn, ed. 2, St. Louis, 1976, The C.V. Mosby Co.)

NEUROLOGIC EVALUATION

PRETERM   TERM

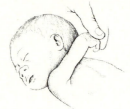
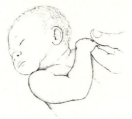

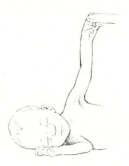
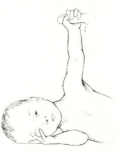

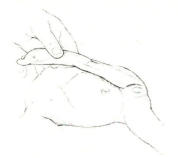
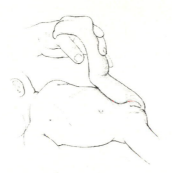

FIG. 7–7, cont'd

Scarf sign—The preterm infant's elbow may be easily brought across the chest with little or no resistance. The mature infant's elbow may be brought to the midline of the chest, resisting attempts to bring the elbow past the midline.

Grasp reflex—The preterm infant's grasp is weak; the term infant's grasp is strong, allowing the infant to be lifted up from the mattress.

Heel-to-ear maneuver—The preterm infant's heel is easily brought to the ear, meeting with no resistance. This maneuver is not possible in the term infant, since there is considerable resistance at the knee.

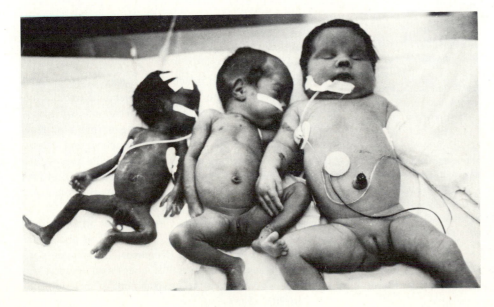

FIG. 7-8
Three babies, same gestational age, weight 600, 1400, and 2750 g, respectively from left to right. (From Korones, S.B.: High-risk newborn infants: the basis for intensive nursing care, ed. 3, St. Louis, 1981, The C.V. Mosby Co.)

satisfactory method for predicting mortality risks and providing guidelines for management of the high-risk neonate.

Assessment of gestational age

The preterm infant has a number of characteristics that are distinctive at various stages of development. Identification of these characteristics provides valuable clues to the gestational age and, hence, to the physiologic capabilities of the infant. The general outward physical appearance changes as the fetus progresses to maturity. Characteristics of skin, general attitude when supine, appearance of hair, and amount of subcutaneous fat provide clues to the newborn's physical development. Observation of spontaneous, active movements and responses to stimulation, as well as passive movement, contributes to the assessment of neurologic status. The appraisal is made as soon as possible after admission to the nursery, since much of the management of the infant depends on this information.

The physical neurologic features of the newborn at various stages of development are assessed according to the method presented in Fig. 7-9. The infant is observed first lying quietly in the supine position. The observer notes the attitude in which the child lies, including flexion, extension, and rotation of arms and legs. Muscle tone is assessed by simple testing of recoil. To facilitate the use of the assessment chart, the following tests and observations are described further:

resting posture with the infant lying in a supine position, the degrees of extension and flexion of arms and legs, knees and elbows, and adduction and abduction of hips are evaluated.

square window the examiner flexes the forearm, applying enough pressure to produce as full a flexion as possible, to measure the angle between the hypothenar eminence and the ventral aspect of the forearm.

recoil the arm is fully flexed for 5 seconds, then extended by means of traction on the hand; the maximum response is noted. Full flexion is a maximum response. A brisk return to full extension is characteristic of a full-term infant; a preterm infant displays sluggish return, only random movements, or no movement at all.

popliteal angle with the thigh in knee-chest position, the leg is extended by gentle pressure to measure the popliteal angle.

scarf sign the examiner attempts to move the infant's hand as far posteriorly around the neck as possible in the direction of the opposite shoulder.

heel-to-ear maneuver the infant's foot is drawn as near to the head as possible without the use of force. The degree of extension and the distance between the foot and the head are noted.

The sum of observations provides the examiner with a guide for management of the infant and special problems that might be anticipated in nursing care.

Nursing considerations

As a consequence of anatomic, physiologic, and biochemical inadequacies, the premature infant is prone to a variety of problems that must be anticipated and managed in the neonatal period. In addition to the regular assessment outlined earlier in the chapter, nurses must be aware of these special needs of the preterm infant and incorporate appropriate interventions to meet these needs.

Protection from infection is an integral part of all newborn care. Preterm and sick neonates are particularly susceptible; therefore, care must exercised to avoid their contact with contaminants. Thorough, meticulous handwashing is the foundation of a preventive program and includes all persons who come in contact with the infants and/or the equipment. Special clothing (scrub outfits, uniforms, cover gowns), furnished and laundered by the institution, is worn by everyone entering the unit. All linen and equipment used in the care of the infants are either sterile or scrupulously clean, and personnel with infectious disorders are either barred from the unit until they can no longer transmit the disease to the infants and other personnel or are required to wear suitable shields, such as masks or gloves, to reduce the likelihood of contamination.

Thermoregulation. After the establishment of respiration, the most crucial need of the premature infant is external warmth. To delay or prevent the effects of cold stress, preterm and other high-risk infants are placed in a heated environment immediately following birth; they remain there until they are able to maintain thermal stability (the capacity to balance heat production and conservation and heat dissipation).

The naked infant is placed in the controlled microenvironment of an Isolette or incubator. A Plexiglas top affords a clear view of the infant from all aspects. There is easy access through portholes that minimize temperature and oxygen loss and a large door that provides a more extensive approach (Fig. 7-10). Maximum accessibility is provided by an open unit with an overhead radiant warming system (Fig. 7-11).

Since overheating produces an increase in oxygen and calorie consumption, the infant is also jeopardized in a hyperthermic environment. A *neutral thermal environment* is one that permits the infant to maintain a normal core temperature with minimum oxygen consumption and calorie expenditure. The very small infant, especially one with a meager subcutaneous fat layer, can control body heat loss or gain only within a very limited range of environmental temperature.

Consumption of oxygen is minimum at an abdominal skin temperature of 36.5° C (97.7° F). When abdominal skin temperature increases or decreases, the oxygen consumption increases. The range of abdominal temperature resulting in a neutral thermal environment is 36.1° to 36.8° C (97° to 98.2° F).

CLINICAL ESTIMATION OF GESTATIONAL AGE

To calculate gestational age, place __X__ in each category in appropriate box. Derive gestation from total score.

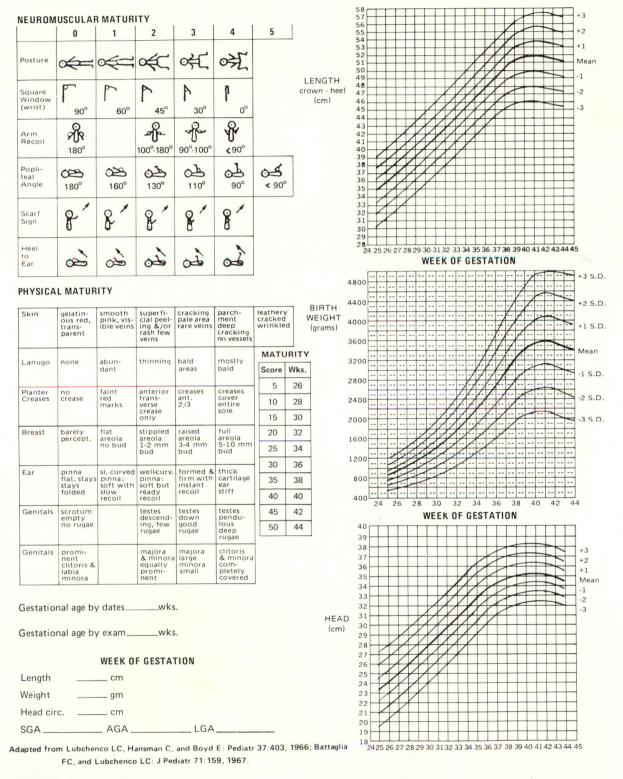

NEUROMUSCULAR MATURITY

	0	1	2	3	4	5
Posture						
Square Window (wrist)	90°	60°	45°	30°	0°	
Arm Recoil	180°		100°-180°	90°-100°	<90°	
Popliteal Angle	180°	160°	130°	110°	90°	< 90°
Scarf Sign						
Heel to Ear						

PHYSICAL MATURITY

Skin	gelatinous red, transparent	smooth pink, visible veins	superficial peeling &/or rash few veins	cracking pale area rare veins	parchment deep cracking no vessels	leathery cracked wrinkled
Lanugo	none	abundant	thinning	bald areas	mostly bald	
Planter Creases	no crease	faint red marks	anterior transverse crease only	creases ant. 2/3	creases cover entire sole	
Breast	barely percept.	flat areola no bud	stippled areola 1-2 mm bud	raised areola 3-4 mm bud	full areola 5-10 mm bud	
Ear	pinna flat. stays stays folded	sl. curved pinna; soft with slow recoil	well-curv. pinna; soft but ready recoil	formed & firm with instant recoil	thick cartilage ear stiff	
Genitals	scrotum empty no rugae		testes descending, few rugae	testes down good rugae	testes pendulous deep rugae	
Genitals	prominent clitoris & labia minora		majora & minora equally prominent	majora large minora small	clitoris & minora completely covered	

MATURITY

Score	Wks.
5	26
10	28
15	30
20	32
25	34
30	36
35	38
40	40
45	42
50	44

Gestational age by dates_____wks.

Gestational age by exam_____wks.

WEEK OF GESTATION

Length _____ cm

Weight _____ gm

Head circ. _____ cm

SGA_____ AGA_____ LGA_____

LENGTH crown - heel (cm) / WEEK OF GESTATION

BIRTH WEIGHT (grams) / WEEK OF GESTATION

HEAD (cm)

Adapted from Lubchenco LC, Hansman C, and Boyd E: Pediatr 37:403, 1966; Battaglia FC, and Lubchenco LC: J Pediatr 71:159, 1967.

FIG. 7-9

Scoring sheet for estimation of gestational age by maturity.

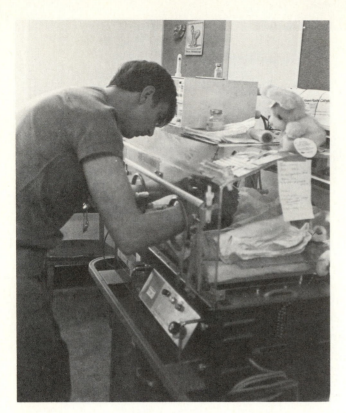

FIG. 7-10
Nurse caring for infant in Isolette.

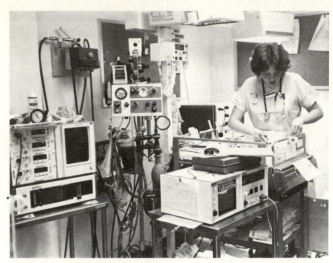

FIG. 7-11
Infant under overhead warming unit.

There are three methods for maintaining a neutral thermal environment: use of a radiant warming panel, use of an Isolette or incubator, and use of an open bassinet with cotton blankets. The dressed infant under blankets can maintain a temperature within a wider range of environmental temperatures; however, the close observations required by high-risk infants are best accomplished if the infants remain unclothed. When the infant is removed from the warm environment of the Isolette for feeding or cuddling, he is clothed and wrapped warmly in blankets.

The most effective means for maintaining the desired range of temperature in the naked infant is by way of a manually adjusted or automatically controlled (servocontrolled) heat panel or incubator, which adjusts automatically in response to signals from a thermal sensor attached to the abdominal skin. The mechanical temperature reading is periodically verified during routine assessments.

While loss of heat by convection is a constant problem in the open units, radiant heat loss is one of the greatest threats to temperature regulation in the Isolette, since the temperature of circulating air within has no influence on heat loss to cooler surfaces without, such as windows or walls, or on heat loss resulting from a lower nursery temperature. A high-humidity atmosphere provided from an external source such as humidified oxygen or air contributes to body temperature maintenance by reducing evapo-rative heat loss. Other methods of maintaining body temperature include use of plastic or rubber gloves filled with warm water, K-pads, and goose-necked lamps; however, extreme care must be exercised to avoid burning the infant's fragile skin. Lining the inside of the Isolette with aluminum foil may help prevent heat loss caused by radiation, and plastic bubble wrap, similar to that used as packing material, is sometimes used as a blanket to help preserve heat and prevent fluid loss, especially for infants under the radiant warmer.

Skin care. The skin of the premature infant is characteristically immature relative to that of the full-term infant. Because of the increased sensitivity and fragility of the premature skin it is recommended that no alkaline-base soap or detergent be used that might destroy the "acid mantle" of the skin. The skin is cleansed with plain clear water or mild nonalkaline cleanser (such as Aveeno, Neutrogena, Lowila)—usually only two to three times per week. Any topical preparation (including creams, lotions, or medicated ointments) should be carefully assessed for possible toxic effects before application. The increased permeability of the skin facilitates absorption of ingredients. Hexachlorophene has been discontinued as a cleansing agent because of its proven toxic effect.

The skin is easily excoriated and denuded; therefore, care must be exerted to avoid damage to the delicate structure. The total thickness of the skin is less than the full-term infant with fewer elastic fibers and there is less cohesion between the thinner skin layers. Adhesives used to secure monitoring equipment or intravenous infusions may adhere to the skin surface so well that the skin can be separated from understructures and pulled away with the tape. Paper tape is the only safe tape to apply directly to the skin of small infants. It is best to first apply a coating of a protective substance to which the adhesive tape is attached. The polyurethane elastic film, Op-Site, has been used with success in many units. The film forms a protective layer on which adhesive tape can be attached and serves as a protective layer over abrasions and excoriations. (Kuller, Lund, and Tobin, 1983).

Scissors are unsafe to use when removing dressings or tape because it is easy to snip off tiny extremities or nick the loosely attached skin.

Apnea. Characteristically, premature infants are periodic breathers—that is, they have periods of rapid respiration separated by periods of very slow breathing and, often, short periods during which there are no visible or audible respirations. Apnea is primarily an extension of this periodic breathing and can be defined as a lapse of spontaneous breathing for 20 or more seconds followed by bradycardia and color change. Apnea probably reflects the immature and poorly refined neurologic and chemical respiratory control mechanisms. As the gestational age increases, incidence of periodic breathing decreases.

Management of periodic apnea consists of monitoring respiration and/or heart rate routinely in all small preterm infants and prevention of conditions that might precipitate it. Since tactile stimulation decreases the incidence of neonatal apnea, many advocate routine cutaneous stimulation for 5 out of every 15 minutes to prevent apneic episodes. Mechanical apnea monitors provide a way to alert the staff to cessation of respiration, by means of a preset delay time (usually 10 to 15 seconds). However, these devices do not eliminate the need for alert nursing observation. Any mechanical device is subject to malfunction. Persistent and repeated periods of apnea are treated by mechanical ventilation, with the respirator set at low pressure and rate.

Nutrition. The initial feeding is not attempted until the infant has adapted to extrauterine existence, as evidenced by temperature neutrality, normal breathing, and good color, tone, and cry. The various mechanisms for ingestion and digestion of foods are not fully developed, and the younger the infant, the greater the problem. The infant's need for rapid growth and daily maintenance must be met in the presence of several anatomic and physiologic handicaps. Although sucking and swallowing are established before birth, coordination of these mechanisms does not occur until approximately 32 to 34 weeks of gestation and they are not fully developed until after birth. Consequently, the preterm infant is highly prone to aspiration, with its attendant dangers.

The nutritional needs vary with the size, age, and condition of the infant; therefore, the amount, interval, and method of feeding are individualized for each child. A vigorous infant can be fed with a soft nipple with little difficulty (Fig. 7-12), whereas a weaker infant will require an alternate method. It is important not to tire the infant or to overtax his capacity to retain the feedings.

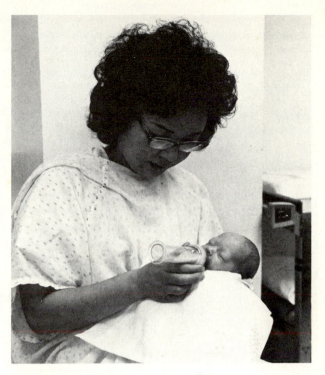

FIG. 7-12
Position for nipple-feeding the premature infant.

The preterm infant is often a slow feeder and requires periods of rest and frequent bubbling. When he is unable to tolerate bottle feedings, intermittent feedings by gavage are instituted until he gains enough strength and coordination to handle the nipple. Breast-feeding is almost universally impossible for the small preterm infant. However, breast milk obtained from the infant's mother or a milk bank is highly desirable and frequently used.

Sometimes, supplementary calories are needed in the form of dietary additives, such as Lipomul-Oral,* which provides vegetable fat and carbohydrate, and MCT oil,† which provides fat in the form of medium-chain triglycerides. Very small or ill infants are fed by the parenteral route until their condition is stabilized and their neurologic and physical states permit oral feedings. Often oral feedings are supplemented by parenteral infusions to assure an adequate intake of carbohydrate and water.

Gavage feeding. Intermittent gavage feeding is one of the safest means for meeting the nutritional requirements of the infant who is less than 32 weeks' gestation or who weighs less than 1650 g. Such infants are usually too weak to suck effectively and are unable to coordinate swallowing. In larger infants who become excessively tired, are listless, or become cyanotic, gavage feeding is used as an energy-conserving technique. A 15-inch size 5

*The Upjohn Co., Kalamazoo, MI.
†Mead Johnson & Co., Evansville, IN.

SUMMARY OF NURSING CARE OF THE PRETERM INFANT

GOALS	RESPONSIBILITIES
Determine gestational age	Weigh and measure infant Perform gestational age assessment based on external characteristics and neurologic signs
Ascertain infant's physiologic status	Perform routine systematic assessment Weigh daily
Prevent infection	Carry out meticulous hand washing before handling infant Place in protective environment Ensure that all equipment in contact with infant is scrupulously clean or sterile Prevent personnel with infections from coming into direct contact with infant Administer prophylactic antibiotics as ordered
Conserve energy	Maintain neutral thermal environment Concentrate activities to allow for longer periods of rest Administer gavage feeding when infant tires easily Ensure minimum handling of infant
Support respiratory efforts	Position for optimum air exchange (shoulder roll when on back or abdomen; head supported when on side) Observe for deviations from desired functioning; recognize signs of distress Suction as necessary to remove accumulated mucus from nasopharynx, trachea, and (where necessary) endotracheal tube Carry out percussion, vibration, and postural drainage to loosen secretions in respiratory tree Maintain ambient oxygen at level to assure satisfactory skin color with minimal respiratory effort and energy expenditure Prevent aspiration
Provide neutral thermal environment	Place infant in humidified Isolette, radiant warmer, or warmly clothed in open crib Monitor temperature hourly in unstable infants (take axillary temperature; check function of servocontrolled mechanism when used) Check temperature of infant in relation to temperature of heating unit and therapies, i.e., phototherapy Avoid situations that might predispose to chilling, such as exposure to cool air
Provide nutrition	Bottle-feed infant if strong sucking and swallowing reflexes are present Gavage feed if infant tires easily or has weak sucking, gag, or swallowing reflexes Measure specific gravity several times daily to help assess adequacy of hydration Maintain parenteral fluid or hyperalimentation therapy as ordered
Maintain hydration	Regulate parenteral fluids Monitor therapies that increase insensible water loss, e.g., phototherapy Assess hydration, e.g., skin turgor, temperature, urine specific gravity Avoid administering hypertonic substances, e.g., undiluted medications
Prevent skin breakdown	Cleanse with clear water or approved cleanser Avoid use of alkaline-based or hexachlorophene cleansing products or lotions Use paper tape only to secure items to the skin Apply protective covering to skin on which to attach tape or adhesive-backed items, e.g., electrodes Exert extreme care when performing activities involving skin, e.g., removing dressing, electrodes Place infant on water pillow or fleece Turn at least q 2 hrs

GOALS	RESPONSIBILITIES

Monitor physiologic data	Take vital signs as ordered (axillary temperature, apical pulse)
	Understand proper function and use of monitoring equipment and maintain at desired settings
	    Apnea monitor
	    Heart rate monitor, including oscilloscope and electrocardiograph printout units
	    Temperature monitor, usually with skin probe
	    Oxygen analyzers
	Collect specimens
	    Blood for glucose, bilirubin, electrolytes, and pH determinations
	    Blood for hemoglobin, hematocrit, microscopic examination, and culture
	    Urine for laboratory examination

Assist in specific therapies	Phototherapy—implement and maintain protective measures
	Administer medications as ordered
	    Antibiotics prophylactically or therapeutically
	    Vitamin K to prevent hemorrhage
	    Sedatives, etc., for withdrawal symptoms, seizures, irritability
	    Electrolyte replacement
	    Alkali therapy in acidosis
	Avoid use of substances known to be toxic to premature infants, e.g., benzyl alcohol or other preservatives
	Assisted ventilation
	Assist with other therapeutic measures as indicated

Encourage positive relationship with parents	Keep parents informed of infant's progress Answer questions; allow expression of concern regarding care and prognosis Encourage mother and father to visit and/or call unit Emphasize positive aspects of infant status Be honest but not overly candid or overly optimistic

Provide sensory stimulation	Tactile
	    Caress, fondle, and otherwise provide skin contact; hold and cuddle infant if condition permits
	Auditory
	    Talk to infant during care
	    Encourage parents and others to talk to infant
	    Allow parents to provide musical toys
	Visual
	    Place colorful mobiles and toys within visual field
	    Hold face within 9 to 12 inches of infant's face and stimulate to follow head movements

Facilitate parental-infant attachment process	Initiate parents' visit as soon as possible
	Encourage parents to
	    Visit infant frequently
	    Touch, fondle, and caress infant
	    Become actively involved in infant's care
	    Bring clothing to dress up infant as soon as condition permits
	Reinforce parents' endeavors
	Be alert to signs of tension in parents
	Allow parents to spend time alone with infant
	Help parents interpret infant responses; comment regarding any positive infant response
	Help parents by demonstrating techniques and offer support

Prepare for infant discharge	Assess readiness of parents (especially mother) to care for infant Teach necessary techniques and observations Arrange for public health referral if indicated Reinforce follow-up care Refer to appropriate agencies or services for needed assistance

or 8 French polyethylene feeding tube is used to instill the formula, and the usual methods for determining correct placement are employed (see p. 580 for technique). The procedure is best accomplished with the infant prone or lying on his right side and with the head slightly elevated. It is preferable to insert the tube through the mouth rather than the nares. Nose insertion interferes with obligatory nose breathing and may irritate the delicate nasal mucosa. Passage through the mouth also provides an opportunity to observe the sucking response. The formula is allowed to flow by gravity, and the length of time should approximate the time required for a nipple feeding.

The intermittent method of gavage feeding stimulates the infant to begin making attempts at sucking and swallowing. The nurse needs to observe the premature infant closely for behaviors that indicate readiness to handle bottle feedings. These include (1) a strong, vigorous suck, (2) coordination of sucking and swallowing, (3) sucking in response to the gavage tube or other objects placed near the mouth, and (4) wakefulness before and sleeping after feedings. When these behaviors are noted, the infant can be challenged with nipple feedings introduced slowly. It is often helpful to allow infants to suck on a pacifier during gavage feedings, so that their sucking ability can be assessed and so that they associate the sucking with the feeling of food in the stomach.

To determine how well the infant tolerates the feedings, the stomach contents are aspirated before each feeding and the residual fluid is recorded and replaced as part of the feeding. For example, if the feeding is 10 ml and 1 ml is aspirated, the 1 ml is returned to the stomach and the infant is given 9 ml of formula for a total of 10 ml.

THE POSTMATURE INFANT

Infants born of a gestation that extends beyond 42 weeks as calculated from the mother's last menstrual period are considered to be postmature or postterm, regardless of birth weight. This comprises approximately 12% of all births. The cause of delayed birth is unknown. Some infants are appropriate for gestational age, but many show the characteristics of progressive placental dysfunction. The appropriate-for-gestational-age infants are indistinguishable in appearance from term infants. Others—most often called postmature infants—display the characteristics of infants who are 1 to 3 weeks of age, such as absence of lanugo, little if any vernix caseosa, abundant scalp hair, long fingernails, and whiter skin than term newborns. Frequently the skin is cracked, parchmentlike, and desquamating. A common finding in postmature infants is a wasted physical appearance that reflects intrauterine impoverishment. There is a depletion of subcutaneous fat that gives them a thin, long appearance. The little vernix ca-

seosa that remains in the skin folds is usually stained a deep yellow or green.

There is a significant increase in fetal and neonatal mortality in postterm infants compared to those born at term. They are especially prone to intrauterine hypoxia associated with the decreasing efficiency of the placenta and to the meconium aspiration syndrome. The greatest risk occurs during the stresses of labor and delivery, particularly in infants of primigravidas (women delivering their first child). Cesarean section or induction of labor is usually recommended when the infant is significantly overdue.

HIGH RISK RELATED TO PHYSIOLOGIC COMPLICATIONS

There are a number of pathologic processes that interfere with the normal course of adjustment to extrauterine life. Some can be attributed directly to mechanical injuries during the birth process (intracranial hemorrhage, meconium aspiration), some are the result of postdelivery disturbances (hypoglycemia, hypocalcemia), and others are pathologic variations of certain physiologic peculiarities in some newborn infants (blood incompatibilities).

HYPERBILIRUBINEMIA

The term *hyperbilirubinemia* refers to an excessive accumulation of bilirubin in the blood and is characterized by *jaundice,* or *icterus,* a yellowish discoloration of the skin and other organs. Hyperbilirubinemia is a common finding in the newborn and, in most instances, relatively benign. However, it can also indicate a pathologic state. Following is a brief description of the pathophysiology of bilirubin production and excretion and a discussion of several disorders that cause hyperbilirubinemia in the newborn.

Pathophysiology

Bilirubin is one of the breakdown products of hemoglobin as a result of red blood cell destruction. When red blood cells are destroyed, the breakdown products are released into the circulation where the hemoglobin splits into two fractions, heme and globin. The globin (protein) portion is used by the body, while the heme portion is converted to unconjugated bilirubin, an insoluble substance bound to albumin. In the liver the bilirubin is detached from the plasma protein and in the presence of the enzyme *glucuronyl transferase* is conjugated with glucuronic acid to produce a highly soluble substance, bilirubin glucuronide, which is then excreted into the bile (Fig. 7-13).

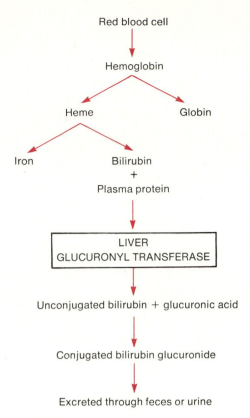

FIG. 7-13
Formation and excretion of bilirubin.

Normally the body is able to maintain a balance between the destruction of red blood cells and the utilization or excretion of by-products. When developmental limitations or a pathologic process interferes with this balance, bilirubin accumulates in the tissues to produce jaundice. In the newborn infant hyperbilirubinemia may be the result of (1) excess production of bilirubin, (2) disturbed capacity of the liver to conjugate bilirubin, or (3) bile duct obstruction resulting secondary to biliary atresia (see p. 694). The most common cause is the relatively mild and self-limited *physiologic jaundice.* However, it may be the result of a disease process such as hemolytic disease of the newborn or infection. As a rule, jaundice that appears within the first 24 hours is caused by hemolytic disease of the newborn, sepsis, or one of the maternally derived diseases (p. 190); jaundice that appears on the second or third day, peaks on the second to fourth days, and decreases between the fifth and seventh days is usually the result of physiologic jaundice; jaundice appearing after the third day but within the first week suggests sepsis.

Because unconjugated bilirubin is highly toxic to neurons, an infant with severe jaundice is at risk of developing *kernicterus,* severe brain damage resulting from the deposition of unconjugated bilirubin in brain cells when the serum concentration of bilirubin reaches toxic levels, regardless of the cause.

Physiologic jaundice (icterus neonatorum)

Physiologic jaundice is a result of immature bilirubin metabolism and transport in the newborn combined with an increased bilirubin load from pronounced hemolysis of red blood cells. Although almost all newborns experience elevated bilirubin levels (above the normal value of 0.2 to 1.4 mg/100 ml), only about half demonstrate observable signs of jaundice. In the newborn, bilirubin levels must exceed 5 mg/100 ml before jaundice or icterus is observable, principally in the sclera, nails, or skin.

The normal newborn produces an average of twice as much bilirubin as does an adult, because of higher concentrations of circulating erythrocytes (especially as a result of stripping of cord blood at delivery) and a shorter life span of red blood cells (only 60 to 80 days, in contrast to 120 days in the older child and the adult). In addition, the liver's ability to conjugate bilirubin is reduced because of diminished production of the enzyme glucuronyl transferase. The reabsorption of unconjugated bilirubin from the intestine is also a contributing factor.

Clinical manifestations. In full-term infants jaundice first appears after 24 hours. Bilirubin levels peak by the second to third day (mean bilirubin level, 6 mg/100 ml), rapidly decline by the fifth day, and slowly reach normal levels by the tenth day. In premature infants jaundice is initially evident by 48 hours. Bilirubin levels reach peak concentrations (10 to 12 mg/100 ml) by the fifth day and gradually return to normal by the end of the first month. Except for the icteric appearance, these infants are well. Postmature infants have little or no physiologic jaundice.

Infants of Oriental descent, including the American Indian, have mean bilirubin levels almost twice those seen in whites or blacks. In addition, individuals from certain geographic areas, particularly areas around Greece, demonstrate an increased incidence of hyperbilirubinemia in newborns.

Jaundice in breast-fed infants

Approximately 1 in 200 breast-fed infants with no evidence of disease develops elevated unconjugated bilirubin levels between the fourth and seventh days of life, which reach a peak during the third week, then gradually diminish but may persist for 3 to 10 weeks. This prolonged jaundice is thought to be caused by the presence of a factor in the breast milk of some women that reduces the bilirubin conjugation process by inhibiting the action of glucuronyl transferase in the infant liver.

Management consists of ceasing breast-feeding for 2 to 4 days. The serum bilirubin levels drop rapidly during this time and do not appear to return to the previous high levels after breast feeding is resumed.

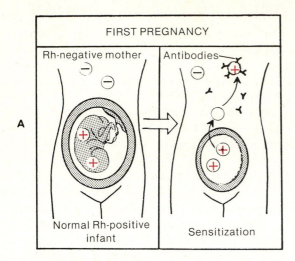

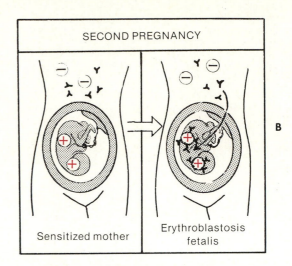

FIG. 7-14

Development of maternal sensitization to Rh antigens. **A,** *Fetal Rh-positive erythrocytes enter the maternal system. Maternal anti-Rh antibodies are formed.* **B,** *Anti-Rh antibodies cross the placental barrier and attack the fetal erythrocytes.*

Hemolytic disease of the newborn (erythroblastosis fetalis)

Hyperbilirubinemia in the first 24 hours of life is most often the result of an abnormally rapid rate of red cell destruction. Anemia caused by this destruction stimulates the production of red blood cells. which, in turn, provides increasing numbers of cells for hemolysis. Major causes of increased erythrocyte destruction are isoimmunization (primarily Rh) and ABO incompatibility.

The membranes of human blood cells contain a variety of antigens, also known as agglutinogens, substances capable of producing an immune response if recognized by the body as a foreign substance. It is the reciprocal relationship between the antigens on the red blood cells and the antibodies in the serum that causes agglutination to take place. In other words, antibodies in the serum of one group (except AB blood group, which contains no antibodies) will produce an agglutination or clumping reaction when mixed with antigens of a different blood group. In the ABO blood group system the antibodies occur naturally. In the Rh system the person must first be exposed to the Rh antigen before significant antibody formation takes place to cause a sensitivity response.

Rh incompatibility (isoimmunization). The Rh blood group consists of several antigens but, for simplicity, only the terms Rh-positive (presence of the antigen) and Rh-negative (absence of the antigen) are used in this discussion (see p. 49 for recessive inheritance). The presence or absence of the naturally occurring Rh factor determines the blood type. Ordinarily no problems are anticipated when the Rh blood types are the same in both mother and fetus or if the mother is Rh-positive and the infant Rh-negative. Difficulty may arise when the blood of the mother is Rh-negative and that of the infant is Rh-positive.

Although the maternal and fetal circulations are separate and distinct, sometimes fetal red blood cells (with antigens foreign to the mother) gain access to the maternal circulation through minute breaks in the placental vessels. The mother's natural defense mechanism responds to these alien cells by producing anti-Rh antibodies (isoimmunization).

Under normal circumstances, this process of isoimmunization has no effect on the fetus during the first pregnancy with an Rh-positive fetus because the initial sensitization to Rh antigens rarely occurs before the onset of labor. However, as larger amounts of fetal blood are transferred to the maternal circulation during placental separation, the maternal immune system is stimulated to form anti-Rh antibodies. During a subsequent pregnancy with an Rh-positive fetus, these previously formed maternal antibodies to Rh-positive blood cells enter the fetal circulation, where they attack and destroy fetal erythrocytes (Fig. 7-14). Since the disease begins in utero, the fetus attempts to compensate for the progressive hemolysis by accelerating the rate of erythropoiesis. As a result, immature red blood cells (erythroblasts) appear in the fetal circulation; hence the term *erythroblastosis fetalis.*

There is wide variability in the development of maternal sensitization to Rh-positive antigens. Sensitization may occur during the first pregnancy if the woman had previously received an Rh-positive blood transfusion. No sen-

TABLE 7-2. POTENTIAL MATERNAL-FETAL ABO INCOMPATIBILITIES

MATERNAL BLOOD GROUP	FETAL BLOOD GROUP
O	A or B
B	A or AB
A	B or AB

sitization may occur in situations where a strong placental barrier prevents transfer of fetal blood into the maternal circulation. In about 10% to 15% of sensitized mothers, there is no hemolytic reaction in the newborn.

In the most severe form of erythroblastosis fetalis, *hydrops fetalis,* the progressive hemolysis causes fetal hypoxia, cardiac failure, generalized edema (anasarca), and effusions of the pericardial, pleural, and peritoneal spaces. The fetus may be delivered stillborn or in severe respiratory distress. Even with immediate exchange transfusions, few hydropic infants survive.

Diagnostic evaluation. Diagnosis of the disease before delivery is confirmed through amniocentesis and analysis of bilirubin levels in amniotic fluid. Increasing bilirubin levels indicate progressive fetal hemolysis and may indicate the need for an intrauterine transfusion or immediate termination of the pregnancy.

Erythroblastosis fetalis can also be assessed by evaluating rising anti-Rh antibody titers in the maternal circulation (indirect Coombs' test). The disease can be confirmed postnatally by detecting antibodies attached to the circulating erythrocytes of affected infants (direct Coombs' test). The Coombs' test is routinely performed on cord blood samples from infants born to Rh-negative mothers.

Prevention. The administration of Rh_0 immune globulin (RhoGAM)* to all unsensitized Rh-negative mothers after delivery or abortion of an Rh-positive infant or fetus prevents the development of maternal sensitization to the Rh factor. When RhoGAM is given to unsensitized mothers within 48 hours after delivery or abortion, injected anti-Rh antibodies destroy the fetal erythrocytes passing into the maternal circulation before they are able to exert their immunogenic effect. To be effective, RhoGAM must be administered following the first delivery and repeated after subsequent ones. It is not effective against existing Rh-positive antibodies in the maternal circulation.

ABO incompatibility. Hemolytic disease can also occur when the major blood group antigens of the fetus are different from those of the mother. The most common blood group incompatibility occurs between an infant with A or B blood group and a mother with O blood group.

*Orthodiagnostics, Raritan, NJ.

(Other possible ABO incompatibilities are listed in Table 7-2.) The naturally occurring anti-A or anti-B antibodies already present in the maternal circulation cross the placenta and attack the fetal red blood cells, causing hemolysis. Usually, however, the hemolytic reaction is less severe than in Rh incompatibility. Since the anti-A or anti-B antibodies are naturally present in the serum, the number of pregnancies is insignificant in the development of ABO incompatibility and preventive measures such as those used in Rh incompatibility are not available.

Clinical manifestations. The clinical manifestations of blood incompatibility result from the hemolysis of large numbers of erythrocytes (anemia) and the liver's inability to conjugate and excrete the excess bilirubin (hyperbilirubinemia and jaundice). Most erythroblastotic newborns are not jaundiced at birth. However, shortly after birth (during the initial 24 hours), jaundice is evident and unconjugated bilirubin levels rise rapidly. Hepatosplenomegaly may be evident. If the fetus is severely affected, signs of anemia—notably, marked pallor—are seen in the newborn.

Therapeutic management

The aims of therapy for hyperbilirubinemia are to prevent kernicterus and, in any blood group incompatibility, to reverse the hemolytic process. The main forms of treatment involve phototherapy, exchange transfusion, and pharmacologic management.

Phototherapy. Phototherapy consists of the application of intense fluorescent light to the infant's exposed skin. Light in the blue range converts unconjugated bilirubin to a substance that is nontoxic to nervous tissue and excretable in the bile without conjugation—by the process of photoisomerization. Because blue light alters the appearance of the infant, the normal light of full-spectrum fluorescent bulbs is preferred so that the skin of the infant can be better observed for color, pallor, cyanosis, or other conditions. Although the value of phototherapy in effectively reducing or preventing rising bilirubin levels is well documented, its long-term effects are not.

Some institutions favor the use of phototherapy for all jaundiced infants (serum bilirubin levels of 5 mg/100 ml or more). However, such therapy does not follow recommended criteria for phototherapy. The suggested protocol involves carefully monitoring serum bilirubin levels, investigating possible pathologic causes for hyperbilirubinemia in which serum bilirubin levels exceed 5 mg/100 ml during the first 24 hours, and identifying high-risk infants who may develop kernicterus with bilirubin levels near 15 mg/100 ml such as premature neonates experiencing hypoxia and acidosis.

Phototherapy is not recommended for treatment of Rh

incompatibility, because the rate of hemolysis usually exceeds the rate of bilirubin diminution produced by photoisomerization. If used immediately following the initial exchange transfusion, phototherapy increases the rate of bilirubin removal from the tissues and may avert the need for repeated transfusions. It is indicated in ABO incompatibility when serum bilirubin levels are above 10 mg/100 ml but are below levels indicated for exchange transfusion and when anemia is absent or mild. Phototherapy is not effective for treatment of conjugated bilirubinemia.

Exchange transfusion. Exchange transfusion, in which the infant's blood is removed in small amounts (usually 10 to 20 ml at a time) and replaced with compatible blood (such as Rh-negative blood), is a standard mode of therapy for treatment of hyperbilirubinemia and the treatment of choice for hyperbilirubinemia caused by Rh incompatibility. Exchange transfusion removes the sensitized erythrocytes, lowers the serum bilirubin level to prevent kernicterus, corrects the anemia, and prevents cardiac failure. Indications for exchange transfusion include a positive direct Coombs' test, hemoglobin concentration of cord blood below 12 g/100 ml, and a bilirubin level of 20 mg/100 ml in the full-term infant or 15 mg/100 ml in the premature infant. An infant born with hydrops fetalis or signs of cardiac failure is a candidate for immediate exchange transfusion.

In exchange transfusion, fresh whole blood is used. It is typed and cross-matched to the mother's serum. The amount of donor blood used is usually double the blood volume of the infant, which is about 85 mg/kg, but no more than 500 ml is used. The two-volume exchange transfusion will replace approximately 85% of the neonate's blood.

An exchange transfusion is a sterile surgical procedure. The umbilicus is cut and a catheter is inserted into the umbilical vein and threaded into the inferior vena cava. Depending on the infant's weight 5 to 20 ml of blood is withdrawn within 15 to 20 seconds and the same volume of donor blood is infused over 60 to 90 seconds. If the blood has been citrated (addition of citrate phosphate dextrose adenine [CPDA] to prevent coagulation), calcium gluconate may be given after infusion of each 100 ml of donor's blood to prevent hypocalcemia.

Nursing considerations

The primary nursing consideration is recognition of jaundice and helping to distinguish the benign disorder from a threatening one. Part of the routine physical assessment includes observing for evidence of jaundice at regular intervals. Jaundice is most reliably assessed by observing the color of the sclera, nails, and skin, including palms, soles, and mucous membranes. Applying direct pressure to the skin, especially over bony prominences such as the tip of the nose or the sternum, causes blanching and allows the yellow stain to be more pronounced. For dark-skinned infants, the color of the sclera, conjunctiva, and oral mucosa is the most reliable indicator. The nurse observes the infant in natural daylight for a true assessment of color. Any neonate who becomes icteric during the first 24 hours of life and has rapidly rising bilirubin levels is referred to the physician for immediate evaluation.

The transcutaneous bilirubin meter has been shown to be a useful screening device and is used to detect neonatal jaundice in full-term infants. However, many institutions have found significant variations between bilirubinometry measurements and laboratory measurements. In addition, phototherapy reduces the accuracy of the instrument; therefore its value is limited to the initial assessment. Institutions in which the device is employed set up their own criteria based on their experience with the particular instrument used.

The lights should be turned off when blood samples are taken for bilirubin measurement to avoid a false reading from bilirubin destruction in the test tube.

Phototherapy. Several precautions are instituted to protect the infant during phototherapy. The infant's eyes are shielded by an opaque mask to prevent exposure to the light (Fig. 7-15). The eye shield should be properly sized and correctly positioned to prevent any occlusion of the nares. The infant's eyelids are closed before the mask is applied, since the corneas may become excoriated if they come in contact with the dressing. On each shift, the eyes are checked for evidence of discharge, excessive pressure on the lids, or corneal irritation.

The infant is placed nude under the fluorescent light and turned frequently to expose all areas to the light. To be effective, light must come in contact with the skin surface. Areas that are protected from the light retain their jaundiced appearance. There is evidence to indicate that a cap, fashioned from stockinette, worn by the infant during phototherapy prevents phototherapy-induced hypocalcemia (Blake, 1983).

At the present time the long-term risks from phototherapy are not known. However, minor side effects do occur and should be observed for and recorded. These include loose greenish stools, hyperthermia, increased metabolic rate, increased evaporative loss of water, and priapism. The temperature is closely monitored to detect early signs of hyperthermia and the skin observed for evidence of dehydration and drying, which can lead to excoriation and breakdown. Oily lubricants or lotions are not used on the skin in order to avoid increased tanning, or a so-called ''frying'' effect. Infants receiving phototherapy require up to 25% additional fluid volume to compensate for insensible and intestinal fluid loss.

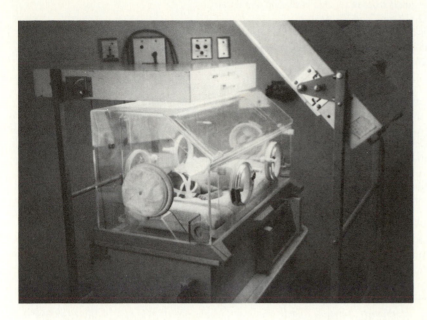

Fig. 7-15
Phototherapy unit combined with radiant heat warmer. Note that the bilirubin lights have been positioned laterally to increase the intensity of phototherapy.

Emotional support. Parents need constant reassurance concerning their infant's progress. All the procedures are explained to them so that they are aware of the benefits and risks. For example, they need to be reassured that the naked infant who is under the bilirubin light is warm and comfortable. Parents may be concerned about the blindfolds, since "blindness" is a frightening experience. Blindfolds are removed when the parents are visiting to facilitate the attachment process, and the parents can be reassured that the neonate is accustomed to darkness after months of intrauterine existence and benefits a great deal from auditory and tactile stimulation. They frequently feel guilty because they think they have caused the blood incompatibility. Parents should never be made to feel responsible or negligent. They should be encouraged to verbalize and express their thoughts. Actions they did to prevent any problems, such as frequent antepartum examinations and blood tests, should be referred to and praised.

Exchange transfusions. Besides assisting the physician during the initial stages of the procedure, the nurse keeps accurate records of blood volumes exchanged, including amount of blood withdrawn and infused, time of each procedure, and cumulative record of the total volume exchanged. Vital signs that are monitored electronically are evaluated frequently and correlated with removal and infusion of blood. If signs of restlessness or cardiac arrhythmias occur, the rate of infusion is slowed. Throughout the procedure the nurse attends to the infant's thermoregulation needs. He should be kept under a radiant warmer, and blankets should be available if he suddenly becomes chilled.

After the procedure is completed, the nurse inspects the umbilical site for evidence of bleeding. Usually, the catheter remains in place for use during repeated exchanges. A sterile dressing is applied and checked periodically for evidence of bleeding or infection.

HYPOGLYCEMIA

Hypoglycemia is said to be present when the infant's blood glucose concentration is significantly lower than that of the majority of infants of the same age and weight. In the newborn hypoglycemia is defined as plasma glucose concentrations of less than 35 mg/100 ml in the first 72 hours and 45 mg/100 ml thereafter in full-term infants; in low birth weight infants it is less than 25 mg/100 ml.

Following birth the infant must supply his own nutrients to meet his energy requirements for maintaining body temperature, respiration, muscular activity, and regulation of blood glucose. At birth he relies on the glycogen stores deposited in the liver, heart, and skeletal muscle during the last trimester of pregnancy, and the full-term infant, under normal circumstances, usually has sufficient sources for the first 2 or 3 days. However, any condition that causes increased energy requirements can rapidly deplete these stores. Four categories of neonatal hypoglycemia have been described:

Early transitional adaptive hypoglycemia These are the large- or normal-for-gestational-age infants including the infant of the mother with diabetes mellitus or gestational diabetes and erythroblastotic infants. These infants appear to be suffering from hyperinsulinism and are otherwise asymptomatic. The hypoglycemia responds readily to intravenous glucose infusions.

SUMMARY OF NURSING CARE OF THE NEONATE WITH HYPERBILIRUBINEMIA

GOALS	RESPONSIBILITIES
Prevent blood incompatibility	Encourage pregnant women to seek early antepartal care Determine blood group and Rh type Follow all Rh-negative pregnant women with possibility of Rh-positive fetus for rising bilirubin levels (amniocentesis, indirect Coombs' test) Administer RhoGAM to Rh-negative women at time of delivery or abortion
Identify infants at risk for hyperbilirubinemia and kernicterus	Observe color of amniotic fluid at time of rupture of membranes Observe for evidence of jaundice, anemia, and central nervous system irritability Refer infant with signs of jaundice and rising bilirubin levels during first 24 hours to physician Be aware of conditions (acidosis, hypoxia, hypothermia, and so on) that increase the risk of kernicterus at lower bilirubin levels Assess bilirubin levels and/or collect specimens for laboratory bilirubin determination
Assess general status	Perform routine assessments
Assist in medical therapies Phototherapy	Shield infant's eyes; check that lids are closed prior to applying shield; check eyes each shift for drainage or irritation Place infant under light nude Change position frequently Monitor body temperature; check axial temperature with reading on servocontrolled unit Ensure that protective Plexiglas shield separates infant from lights Chart duration of therapy, type of lights, distance of lights to infant, use of open or closed bassinet, and shielding of infant's eyes Avoid use of oily applications on the skin Observe for hyperthermia, signs of dehydration, loose stools, priapism Monitor hydration
Exchange transfusions Preprocedure	Give infant nothing by mouth prior to procedure (usually for 3 to 4 hours) Check donor blood with physician for correct blood group and Rh type Have resuscitative equipment (supplemental oxygen, airway, AMBU bag, endotracheal tube, and laryngoscope) at bedside
During procedure	Assist physician during procedure; ensure asepsis Keep accurate records of amounts of blood infused and withdrawn Monitor vital signs, especially following infusion of calcium gluconate Maintain optimum body temperature of infant during procedure (blankets, radiant warmer) Observe for signs of exchange transfusion reactions
Postprocedure	Apply sterile dressing to catheter site Monitor vital signs Observe for signs of kernicterus Check umbilical site for bleeding or infection Collect specimens for serum bilirubin levels
Observe for signs of kernicterus	Observe for signs of central nervous system depression (lethargy, diminished or absent reflexes, hypotonia, poor sucking reflex) or excitation (irritability, tremors, convulsions, high-pitched cry, opisthotonos)
Provide emotional support to parents	Explain reason for jaundice Discontinue phototherapy during parental visiting; remove infant's eye shields
Physiologic jaundice	Emphasize benign nature of condition Assure parents that skin will regain normal pigmentation Advise breast-feeding mothers of possibility of prolonged jaundice
Blood incompatibility	Explain therapies to parents Reassure parents during various procedures Allow parents to express any feelings regarding their "causing" the blood incompatibility Reinforce parents' previous attempts to provide optimum care for their infant, such as frequent antepartal checkups
Plan for follow-up, especially if bilirubin levels approached 20 mg/100 ml in full-term neonate	Encourage parents to report the perinatal history during subsequent infant assessments, especially when the child is seen by unfamiliar health personnel Plan for early developmental and hearing assessment Check blood during first 2 months for evidence of anemia and need for supplemental iron

Classical transient neonatal hypoglycemia This group consists of infants who have suffered intrauterine malnutrition that has reduced hepatic glycogen stores and body fat. In this category are the small-for-gestational-age infants, small twins, infants of toxemic mothers, and infants with abnormalities of the placenta. Males appear to be affected more frequently than females. Cardiomegaly and polycythemia may be present in addition to the hypoglycemia. The hypoglycemia may be more severe than other categories and is likely to recur.

Secondary hypoglycemia This type of hypoglycemia occurs as a response to a variety of perinatal stresses that have increased the metabolic needs relative to the glycogen stores available. Stresses include asphyxia, respiratory distress syndrome, pathologic conditions of the central nervous system, sepsis, hemorrhage, drug withdrawal, and iatrogenic events such as interruption of glucose infusions. This type of hypoglycemia responds to glucose administration and rarely recurs.

Recurrent, severe hypoglycemia This category consists of infants who have hypoglycemia secondary to an enzymatic or a metabolic-endocrine defect such as galactosemia, hypothyroidism, hypopituitarism, and any number of the inborn errors of metabolism. Diagnosis of the disorder determines the therapy.

Clinical manifestations

The signs of hypoglycemia are usually vague and often indistinguishable from those observed in other conditions, such as hypocalcemia, septicemia, central nervous system disorders, or cardiorespiratory problems. Because the brain depends on glucose for energy, cerebral signs such as jitteriness, tremors, twitching, weak or high-pitched cry, lethargy, limpness, apathy, convulsions, and coma are prominent. Other clinical manifestations include cyanosis, apnea, rapid and irregular respirations, sweating, eye rolling, and refusal to feed. Symptoms usually appear between 24 and 72 hours of age, but severely distressed infants may demonstrate signs of hypoglycemia within 6 hours after birth. Frequently, the symptoms are transient but recurrent.

Diagnostic evaluation

Diagnosis must be confirmed by direct analysis of blood glucose concentration. Two specimens of blood should be analyzed, because of the many factors that can affect correct readings. Proper handling of the specimen is essential, since storage at room temperature increases glycolysis. Accurate readings can be facilitated by storing the blood sample in ice or removing the red blood cells by centrifugation.

Blood sugar level may also be determined with a drop of blood placed on a reagent strip such as Dextrostix or Chemstrip-BG. Although a simple procedure, it is a very sensitive test and must be performed correctly to avoid false readings. For example, the blood must remain on the Dextrostix for exactly 1 minute and then be compared to the color chart. Inaccurate timing will produce varying stages of the reaction. Color changes that indicate a blood glucose level of less than 45 mg/100 ml should be confirmed by a laboratory analysis of whole blood.

Therapeutic management

Intravenous infusion of glucose is the therapy for hypoglycemia. Infants who are at increased risk for developing hypoglycemia should have their blood glucose measured within 1 hour after birth and repeated every 1 to 2 hours for the first 6 to 8 hours, then every 4 to 6 hours for 2 days.

Hypoglycemia can be prevented in most instances by the initiation of early feeding in normoglycemic newborns. Breast-fed infants should be put to breast as soon as possible after delivery. Bottle-fed infants should be offered 5% to 10% glucose and sterile water as early as 2 hours after birth, especially if the infant is at risk for hypoglycemia or if hypoglycemia is suspected. If feedings are poorly tolerated, intravenous glucose may be administered to these infants.

Nursing considerations

Much of the nursing responsibility for the hypoglycemic infant involves identification of the problem through careful observation of physical status. Another area of concern is to decrease those environmental factors that predispose the infant to the development of a decreased blood glucose level, such as cold stress and respiratory difficulty. Proper feeding technique of the breast-fed or bottle-fed infant promotes adequate ingestion of nutrients, particularly carbohydrates.

Preventing, anticipating, and recognizing potential dangers of concentrated dextrose infusion are also major nursing objectives. Too rapid infusion of the hypertonic solution can cause circulatory overload, hyperglycemia, and intracellular dehydration.

HYPOCALCEMIA

Hypocalcemia, like many conditions in the neonate, is difficult to differentiate from other disorders and the etiology is ill defined. There are two times during the neonatal period when the incidence is highest. *Early-onset hypocalcemia,* which appears within the first 48 hours, is the most common form and typically affects the premature or small-

---

SUMMARY OF NURSING CARE OF THE INFANT WITH HYPOCALCEMIA OR HYPOGLYCEMIA

GOALS	RESPONSIBILITIES
Recognize early signs of pathophysiologic state	Assess each system for signs and symptoms suggestive of each condition Correlate findings with general impression of progress of infant (feeding, weight gain, response to stimuli, and sleeping patterns)

Prevent or decrease potential side effects of medical intervention
Hypocalcemia
	Administer calcium gluconate slowly; if heart rate falls below 100 beats/minute, stop infusion
	Prevent extravasation of calcium gluconate into tissues:
	    Avoid scalp vein
	    Ensure placement of needle before administering drug
	    Tape needle securely at site of insertion
	    Apply pressure to puncture site after removal of needle
	Counsel mother regarding infant feeding (breast-feeding or appropriate formulas)

Hypoglycemia	Begin oral feeding as soon as possible after birth Administer glucose infusion carefully; avoid overloading the system by speeding up intravenous administration Observe for signs of hyperglycemia (acidosis) and possible need for insulin Decrease intravenous administration of glucose slowly to avoid hypoglycemia from physiologic hyperinsulinemia
Assess general status	Perform routine assessments
Monitor environment to decrease factors that will complicate recovery	Maintain thermoregulation, hydration, and oxygenation of infant Monitor vital signs and correlate with infant's progress
Hypocalcemia	Reduce environmental stimuli Organize care to ensure minimal handling of infant Discuss with parents reasons for minimal holding Institute seizure precautions
Observe for evidence of complications Hypocalcemia	Observe for tetany and convulsions
Hypoglycemia	Check heel blood with Dextrostix Check urine for glycosuria
Provide emotional support for parents	Allow parents the opportunity to express their feelings Keep parents informed of infant's progress Encourage frequent visiting and participation in care to foster parent-child attachment

for-date infant who has experienced perinatal hypoxia. Symptoms include apnea, cyanotic episodes, edema, a high-pitched cry, and abdominal distention.

Late-onset hypocalcemia, which is not apparent until after the first 3 to 4 days of life, is commonly referred to as cow's milk-induced hypocalcemia *or neonatal tetany*. It is observed in well-nourished infants who are fed unmodified cow's milk. Cow's milk with a high phosphorus-to-calcium ratio depresses parathyroid activity, resulting in diminished serum calcium levels. The manifestations of

neonatal tetany reflect neuromuscular irritation—twitching, tremors, and focal or generalized convulsive seizures that can be triggered by even minor stimuli and that vary from a few seconds to 10 minutes in duration.

Therapeutic management

Suspected hypocalcemia is confirmed by serum calcium determination. In most instances, early-onset hypocalcemia is temporary and reverses itself in 1 to 3 days. Restoration of a normal calcium concentration is facilitated by early feedings and oral administration of calcium supplements, usually calcium chloride, lactate, or gluconate. Calcium chloride, although effective, causes gastric irritation and should be given in concentrations of less than 2% and discontinued after 2 days.

Occasionally it may be necessary to administer calcium intravenously. Symptoms can be controlled by the administration of 10% calcium gluconate. It must be administered slowly, usually over a period of 5 minutes, to prevent nausea, vomiting, bradycardia, and circulatory collapse. If the heart rate falls below 100 beats/minute, the injection should be immediately discontinued. It is advisable to monitor the heart rate electronically. After the normal rate has resumed for at least 30 minutes, administration of the drug can be reinitiated. Care must be taken to ascertain that the needle is positioned within the vein, because extravasation into surrounding tissue causes local calcification and sloughing. Intramuscular administration of calcium gluconate is contraindicated because it precipitates in the tissue, causing necrosis. Phenobarbital may be necessary for seizures, especially if calcium cannot be administered.

Nursing considerations

Nursing care of the infant with hypocalcemia is directed toward identifying the cause of the manifestations observed and administration of calcium. Observation and management of neonatal seizures is discussed on p. 201 and will not be elaborated here.

The infant is monitored continuously during intravenous infusions. Calcium gluconate can cause tissue necrosis and scar formation; therefore, it is recommended that the scalp veins be avoided. To prevent tissue necrosis the infusion site should be changed frequently (ideally every 12 hours), the needle is firmly secured by tape to the skin, and during removal gentle pressure is applied at the puncture site for at least 1 minute.

The nurse also observes for signs of acute hypercalcemia (nausea, vomiting, bradycardia). If such symptoms occur, the injection or infusion is discontinued and the physician is notified. Since convulsions are common, seizure precautions are instituted. Minor stimuli, such as picking the infant up for a feeding or a sudden jarring of the crib, can provoke tremors or seizures. During the acute phase the environment is manipulated to allow for maximum rest and minimum activity around the infant to avoid tiring him.

If the infant is discharged on formula feedings supplemented with calcium salts, the parents are taught the correct procedure for diluting the mineral in the formula. Parents are advised to use only the prescribed formula, usually one with a low calcium/phosphorus ratio. Since oral calcium may result in more frequent bowel movements, the parents are also advised of this to prevent their associating this change with diarrhea or another gastrointestinal disorder.

RESPIRATORY DISTRESS SYNDROME

Respiratory distress is common in several neonatal disorders—for example, hypovolemia, hypoglycemia, congenital heart disease, and cerebral hemorrhage. However, the terms *respiratory distress syndrome* (RDS), *idiopathic respiratory distress syndrome* (IRDS), and *hyaline membrane disease* (HMD) are most often applied to the severe lung disorder that is not only responsible for more deaths in the pediatric age-group than any other disease but also carries the highest risk in terms of long-term neurologic complications. It is seen almost exclusively in the preterm infant, the infant of the diabetic mother, and the infant born by cesarean section.

Pathophysiology

The preterm infant is born before the lungs are fully prepared to serve as efficient organs for gas exchange. Most full-term infants successfully accomplish the respiratory adjustments to extrauterine life; the premature infant with respiratory distress is unable to do so. Although a number of factors is involved, most authorities believe that the central factor responsible for this adaptation is normal development of the surfactant system. Surfactant is a surface-active phospholipid secreted by the alveolar epithelium. Acting much like a detergent, this substance reduces the surface tension of fluids that line the alveoli and respiratory passages, resulting in uniform expansion and maintenance of lung expansion. Without surfactant, the infant is unable to keep the lungs inflated and, therefore, exerts a great deal of effort to reexpand the alveoli with each breath. This inability to maintain lung expansion produces widespread atelectasis, hypoxemia, and hypercapnia.

To compound this situation, increased amounts of lactic acid are formed to produce a metabolic acidosis and the inability of the atelectatic lungs to blow off excess carbon dioxide produces a respiratory acidosis. The acidosis causes vasoconstriction, which diminishes pulmonary circulation, and materials needed for surfactant production are not circulated to the alveoli.

The hyaline membrane, characteristic of the disorder, decreases the elasticity of the lungs, which become stiff and require far more pressure than do normal lungs to achieve an equal amount of expansion.

Clinical manifestations

The infant with respiratory distress syndrome can develop respiratory insufficiency either acutely or over a period of hours. Usually, the observable signs produced by the pulmonary changes begin to appear in an infant who apparently achieves normal breathing and color soon after birth. In 30 minutes to 2 hours, breathing gradually becomes more difficult and the infant displays substernal retractions. Retractions are a prominent feature of pulmonary difficulties in preterm infants (Fig. 7-16). Weak chest wall muscles and the highly cartilaginous nature of the rib structure produce an abnormally elastic rib cage. During this early period the infant's color remains satisfactory and auscultation reveals good air entry.

Within a few hours, respiratory distress becomes more obvious. The respiratory rate increases (to 80 to 120 breaths/minute), and breathing becomes more labored. It is significant to note that an infant will increase the *rate* of respiration rather than the *depth* of respiration when in distress. Substernal retractions become more pronounced, fine inspiratory rales can be heard over both lungs, and there is an audible expiratory grunt and flaring of the external nares. Cyanosis appears but can usually be abolished by administration of 40% to 50% oxygen.

As the disease progresses, the infant becomes flaccid, inert, and unresponsive and begins to display frequent apneic episodes. Auscultation of the chest reveals diminished breath sounds. Now the chances of recovery without assisted ventilation are very small. Severe respiratory distress is often associated with a shocklike state with diminished cardiac return and low arterial blood pressure. The lungs produce a typical ground-glass appearance on radiographic examination.

Therapeutic management

The treatment of respiratory distress syndrome is largely supportive; it includes all the general measures required of any premature infant. General supportive measures include minimal handling, maintaining a neutral thermal environment, and providing adequate caloric intake and hydration. Oral feedings are contraindicated in any situation that creates a marked increase in respiratory rate, because of the greater hazards of aspiration. Nutrition is provided by gavage and/or parenteral means.

The specific supportive measures that are most crucial to a favorable outcome are (1) correction of acidosis by intravenous administration of sodium bicarbonate or tromethamine (THAM), (2) maintenance of a neutral temperature environment to conserve utilization of oxygen, and (3) provision of oxygen by increasing the ambient oxygen concentration in the Isolette or via an oxygen hood or by instituting assisted ventilation.

The goals of oxygen therapy are to provide adequate oxygen to the tissues, prevent lactic acid accumulation resulting from hypoxia, and, at the same time, to avoid the toxic effects of oxygen—that is, retrolental fibroplasia and pulmonary oxygen toxicity. The most widely used method is assisted ventilation that supports the infant's own respiratory efforts. This method is known as continuous positive airway pressure (CPAP) or continuous positive pressure breathing (CPPB). The objective of continuous positive airway pressure is to apply just enough pressure to open and keep open (and yet avoid overdistending) the already expanded alveoli. If the oxygen saturation (Po_2) of the blood cannot be maintained at a satisfactory level and the carbon dioxide level (Pco_2) rises, the infant will require controlled ventilation, usually positive end-expiratory pressure (PEEP). The newer high-frequency ventilation (HFV), in which there is a very high respiratory rate with less tracheal pressure, is being used successfully with certain infants but is not uniformly accepted.

Prevention

The most successful approach to prevention of respiratory distress syndrome is prevention of premature delivery, especially in elective early delivery and cesarean section. Improved methods for assessing the maturity of the fetal lung by amniocentesis, although not a routine procedure, allow a reasonable prediction of whether the fetus of a high-risk pregnancy is likely to develop hyaline membrane disease. The principal test performed on amniotic fluid is determination of the lecithin/sphingomyelin (L/S) ratio.

In limited experiments, the administration of corticosteroids to mothers for 24 hours to 7 days prior to delivery has appeared to stimulate surfactant production in the fetus and to reduce the incidence of respiratory distress syndrome. No beneficial effects in the prevention of the disorder have resulted from administration of corticosteroids to infants after birth.

Nursing considerations

Care of the infant with respiratory distress syndrome includes all the nursing skills required for any high-risk infant, particularly those required for the premature infant. In addition, special skills and observations are required in relation to oxygen administration.

The most essential nursing function is to observe and assess the infant's response to therapy. Since oxygen concentration and continuous positive airway pressure are prescribed according to the infant's color and blood gas measurements and since the infant's status can change rapidly, frequent monitoring and close observation are mandatory. The amount of oxygen administered is based on these observations.

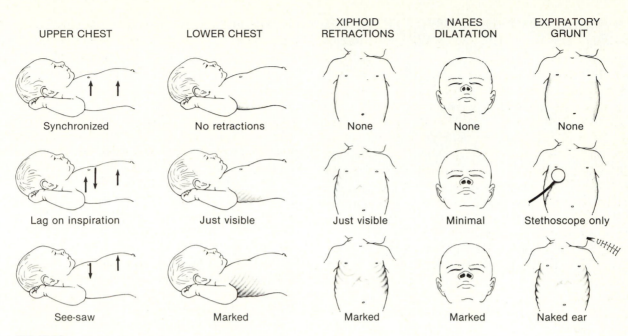

UPPER CHEST	LOWER CHEST	XIPHOID RETRACTIONS	NARES DILATATION	EXPIRATORY GRUNT
Synchronized	No retractions	None	None	None
Lag on inspiration	Just visible	Just visible	Minimal	Stethoscope only
See-saw	Marked	Marked	Marked	Naked ear

FIG. 7-16

Criteria for evaluating respiratory distress. (From Silverman, W.A., and Andersen, D.H.: Pediatrics **17:**1, *1956, Copyright American Academy of Pediatrics, 1956.)*

Arterial samples (PaO₂) are drawn from an umbilical artery catheter or from the radial or posterior tibial arteries by needle puncture. For capillary samples, blood is most often collected from the heel. In many instances the non-invasive technique of percutaneous blood gas analysis is employed. These nursing activities are frequently carried out at least every 4 hours on sick infants and as often as every 15 minutes on acutely ill infants.

Thick, tenacious mucus frequently forms in the respiratory tract, interfering with gas flow and predisposing the infant to obstruction of the air passages, including the endotracheal tube. Routine suctioning may be required every 2 hours or as needed based on assessment. Care must be exercised, since the procedure may cause bronchospasm or vagal nerve stimulation that can produce bradycardia. When the nasopharyngeal passages, trachea, or endotracheal tube is being suctioned, the catheter should be inserted gently but quickly; then intermittent suction should be applied as the catheter is withdrawn. It is imperative that the time the airway is obstructed by the catheter be limited to no more than 5 to 10 seconds. Also, continuous suction removes air from the lungs along with the mucus. One fourth to ½ ml of sterile normal saline instilled in the endotracheal tube before insertion of the suction catheter aids in loosening mucus and removing secretions.

Removal of secretions can be further facilitated by application of percussion and vibration to the thoracic wall. The technique and positioning for postural drainage, percussion, and vibration are outlined in Chapter 19. The principles are the same, but the cupped hand is much too

large to be used on the very small infant. An effective means to provide percussion is by the use of small plastic cups with padded rims or a small face mask with the airway opening occluded (Fig. 7-17). Vibration is even more difficult to accomplish on the infant whose respiratory rate is 60 to 80 breaths/minute. Some units have found a helpful aid in the electric toothbrush with foam padding placed over the handle. When applied to the chest, this provides effective vibrations. Percussion and vibration are performed every 2 hours, with rotation of segments of the lungs that are percussed. The preterm infant is usually unable to tolerate a full regimen each time. The length of time allotted to any given segment is also subject to the infant's tolerance and to the degree of lobar involvement, which is best determined by radiologic evaluation.

The most advantageous positions of the infant for facilitation of an open airway are on the side, with the head supported in alignment by a small folded blanket or towel, and on the back, with a small shoulder roll to keep the neck slightly extended. With the head in the "sniffing" position, the trachea is opened to its maximum; hyperextension reduces the tracheal diameter in the neonate.

Mouth care is especially important when the infant is receiving nothing by mouth, and the problem is often aggravated by the drying effect of oxygen therapy. Drying and cracking can be prevented by good oral hygiene using saline or glycerin swabs. The irritation to the nares or mouth that results from appliances used to administer oxygen may be reduced by the use of antibiotic ointment.

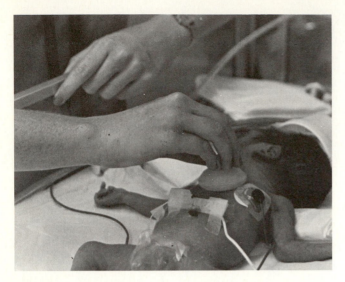

FIG. 7-17
Use of face mask for percussion of infant.

COMPLICATIONS OF OXYGEN THERAPY IN THE PREMATURE INFANT

Oxygen therapy, although lifesaving, is not without its hazards. Positive pressure introduced by mechanical apparatus has created an increase in the incidence of ruptured alveoli and subsequent *pneumothorax*. This complication can be suspected on the basis of absent or diminished breath sounds and a shift in location of maximum intensity of heart sounds; its presence is confirmed by radiographic examination. Treatment consists of monitoring and observation for increased respiratory distress, either aspiration of the accumulated air or insertion of the catheter into the pleural space, and use of water-seal drainage.

Retrolental fibroplasia (RLF)

Retrolental fibroplasia is a disease of the eyes related to elevated blood oxygen concentrations. It occurs almost exclusively in premature infants, and the incidence correlates with the degree of maturity—the shorter the gestational age, the greater the likelihood of its development. Vasoconstriction as a result of very high concentrations of oxygen in retinal capillaries causes a wild overgrowth of these developing blood vessels; veins become numerous and dilated. First the aqueous humor, followed by the vitreous humor, becomes turbid as new vessels proliferate toward the lens. The retina becomes edematous, and hemorrhages separate the retina from its attachment. Advanced scarring occurs from the retina to the lens, destroying the normal architecture of the eye. This extensive retinal detachment and scarring result in irreversible blindness. Unfortunately, there is no documented safety level of oxygen concentra-

tion or length of application. The best prophylaxis at present is to reduce the oxygen concentration to the minimum in terms of both amount and length of time required to relieve hypoxia. Therefore, careful monitoring of the infant and the arterial oxygen tension is essential.

Bronchopulmonary dysplasia (BPD)

Bronchopulmonary dysplasia, also known as *chronic* or *respirator lung disease,* is a pathologic process that may develop in the lungs of infants with respiratory distress syndrome who have required high concentrations of oxygen and assisted ventilation. The condition is characterized by epithelial damage, with thickening and fibrotic proliferation of the alveolar walls and squamous metaplasia of the bronchiolar epithelium.

The etiology and true incidence of bronchopulmonary dysplasia in survivors of respiratory distress syndrome is unknown. To date there is no evidence to indicate a relationship between the incidence of bronchopulmonary dysplasia and the increased survival of infants who received positive pressure ventilation for severe respiratory distress syndrome. The marked similarity between bronchopulmonary dysplasia and the *Wilson-Mikity syndrome* of alveolar thickening and cystlike patterns of hyperventilation seen in some premature infants has led some investigators to theorize that the two entities may be part of a continuous spectrum of the same lung disorder.

There is no specific treatment for bronchopulmonary dysplasia other than oxygen therapy and other supportive measures. Most infants recover by 6 months to 1 year of age, usually with normal pulmonary function, although some appear to have minimal obstructive and restrictive pulmonary deficiency that limits the tolerance of exercise.

MECONIUM ASPIRATION SYNDROME

Meconium aspiration is a serious condition occurring when the fetus has been subjected to some intrauterine insult that causes fetal distress, increasing peristalsis, relaxing of the anal sphincter, and passage of meconium into the amniotic fluid. Aspiration of meconium takes place either in utero or with the first breath. If sufficiently large amounts are aspirated, there is bronchial obstruction, alveolar overdistention, and atelectasis.

Meconium aspiration syndrome occurs primarily in full-term infants who are small for their gestational age or in the postmature infant. The infants are meconium stained, tachypneic, hypoxic, and depressed at birth and frequently require resuscitation. Respiratory distress may develop at once or may not appear until several hours later. There may be obvious cyanosis, but chest retractions are not usually prominent. Little can be done to remove meconium from deep in the respiratory tract, but the trachea is aspirated in all infants who emerge from stained amniotic fluid and evidence any respiratory difficulty. The care and management are the same as for any infant with respiratory distress.

HEMORRHAGIC DISEASE OF THE NEWBORN

Hemorrhagic disease of the newborn is a bleeding disorder that may appear within 1 to 5 days of life as a result of a severe transient deficiency of vitamin K-dependent factors II, VII, IX, and X. These blood factors normally decrease 2 to 3 days after birth then gradually return to normal levels by 7 to 10 days of age. This deficiency is probably related to (1) lack of free vitamin K in the mother, (2) the newborn's sterile intestinal tract being unable to synthesize the vitamin until feedings have begun, and (3) the immaturity of the infant liver where the blood factors are produced. Breast-fed infants are particularly at risk because human milk is a poor source of vitamin K. Hemorrhagic manifestations rarely occur in infants fed cow's milk on the first day of life because it is an adequate source of the vitamin.

Clinical manifestations

Signs and symptoms of hemorrhagic disease typically occur on the second or third day and include (1) oozing from the umbilicus or circumcision site, (2) bloody or black stools, (3) hematuria, (4) ecchymoses on skin and scalp, and (5) epistaxis.

Therapeutic management

The goal is prevention of hemorrhagic disease of the newborn with prophylactic administration of vitamin K. In most hospitals intramuscular administration of vitamin K (Aquamephyton, Mephyton) in a dose of 0.5 to 1 mg once during the first 24 hours of life is a standard practice.

In newborns with the disease, treatment is the same as the preventive measures, except that the vitamin may be given intravenously to prevent a hematoma at an intramuscular site. Bleeding usually ceases within 2 to 4 hours of vitamin K administration.

Nursing considerations

Nursing care is primarily directed toward prevention and involves careful administration of the vitamin into the vastus lateralis muscle because of absence of other well-developed muscle masses. In instances when this procedure is not routinely carried out (for example, home births or emergency deliveries), the nurse observes for signs of the disorder and notifies the physician for appropriate diagnosis and treatment.

NEONATAL SEIZURES

Seizures in the neonatal period are usually the clinical manifestation of a serious underlying disease. Therefore, seizures, although not life-threatening as an isolated entity, constitute a medical emergency because they signal a disease process that may produce irreversible brain damage. Consequently it is imperative to recognize a seizure and its significance so that the cause as well as the seizure can be treated.

The causes of neonatal seizures are many and varied including:

metabolic disorders such as hypoglycemia and hypocalcemia

toxic and electrolyte disturbances such as hypernatremia, hyponatremia, narcotic withdrawal, and bilirubin encephalopathy

infections such as bacterial meningitis, sepsis, herpes simplex, and cytomegalic inclusion disease

trauma at birth such as hypoxic encephalopathy and intracranial hemorrhage

congenital malformations such as hydrocephaly and central nervous system agenesis

miscellaneous disorders such as degenerative diseases

Clinical manifestations

The features of neonatal seizures are different from those observed in the older infant or child. The well-organized, generalized tonic-clonic seizures seen in older children are rare in the infant, especially the preterm infant. Seizures in the newborn may be subtle and barely discernible or grossly apparent. Neonatal seizures can be divided into five major types: subtle, generalized tonic, multifocal clonic, focal clonic, and myoclonic (Volpe, 1977).

Subtle seizures are often overlooked by the inexperienced observer. The manifestations include clonic horizontal eye deviation, repetitive blinking or fluttering of the eyelids, drooling, sucking or other oral-buccal-lingual movements, arm movements resembling rowing or swimming, leg movements described as pedaling or bicycling, and apnea. These signs may appear alone or in combination with other signs, especially apnea (a common phenomenon in the premature infant that in isolation almost always results from other causes).

Generalized tonic seizures usually manifest as extensions of all four limbs, similar to decerebrate rigidity, or occasionally the upper limbs are maintained in a stiffly flexed position resembling decorticate rigidity. Tonic seizures appear more frequently in premature infants.

Multifocal clonic seizures consist of rhythmic jerking movements, about 1 to 3 per second, which may migrate randomly from one part of the body to another. Simultaneous involvement of separate areas often occurs, and the convulsive movements may start at different times and at different rates.

Focal clonic seizures are usually well localized and frequently accompany other seizure types. *Myoclonic* seizures consist of single or multiple flexion jerks of the limbs. These last two types are relatively uncommon or rare in the newborn.

Jitteriness or tremulousness in the newborn is a repetitive shaking of an extremity or extremities that may be observed with crying, may occur with changes in sleeping state, or may be elicited with stimulation. Jitteriness is relatively common in the newborn and in a mild degree may be considered normal during the first 4 days of life. It can be distinguished from seizures by several characteristics: jitteriness is not accompanied by ocular movement as are seizures; the dominant movement in jitteriness is tremor, and seizure movement is clonic jerking that cannot be stopped by flexion of the affected limb; and jitteriness is highly sensitive to stimulation, whereas seizures are not. If jittery movements persist beyond the fourth day, if the movements are persistent and prolonged after a stimulus, or if they are easily elicited with minimal stimulus, further evaluation is indicated.

Diagnostic evaluation

Early evaluation and diagnosis of seizures are urgent. In addition to a careful physical examination, the pregnancy and family histories are investigated for familial and prenatal causes. Blood is drawn for glucose and electrolyte examination, and cerebrospinal fluid is obtained for examination for gross blood cell count, protein, glucose, and culture. Electroencephalography may help identify subtle seizures but is less helpful in establishing a diagnosis. Other diagnostic procedures such as computed tomography may be indicated.

Therapeutic management

Treatment is directed toward prevention of cerebral damage and involves correction of metabolic derangements, respiratory and cardiovascular support, and suppression of the seizure activity. The underlying cause is treated—for example, glucose infusion for hypoglycemia, calcium for hypocalcemia, and antibiotics for infection. If needed, re-

spiratory support is provided for hypoxia, and anticonvulsants may be administered, especially when the other measures fail to control the seizures. Phenobarbital is the drug of choice given orally or intramuscularly, but the intravenous route is used if seizures are severe and persistent. Other drugs that may be employed are diazepam (Valium), paraldehyde, and phenytoin (Dilantin).

Nursing considerations

The major nursing responsibilities in the care of the infant with seizures are to recognize when the infant is having a seizure so that therapy can be instituted, to carry out the therapeutic regimen, and to observe the response to the therapy and any further evidence of seizures or other symptomatology. Assessment and all other aspects of care are the same as for any high-risk infant. Parents need to be informed of the infant's status, with the nurse reinforcing and clarifying the explanations of the attending physician. The infant's behaviors need to be interpreted to the parents, and the significance of the infant's responses to the treatment must be anticipated and explained. Parents should be encouraged to visit the child and perform the parenting activities consistent with the plan of care. Seizures are a frightening phenomenon and generate a great deal of anxiety and fear, which is easily compounded by the justifiable concern of the staff. Providing support and guidance is an important nursing function.

PERINATAL HYPOXIC-ISCHEMIC BRAIN INJURY

Hypoxic-ischemic brain injury is the most common cause of neurologic impairment of a nonprogressive type observed in infants and children. Newborn infants are particularly vulnerable to ischemic injury caused by decreased cerebral blood flow following asphyxia. Most infants who have suffered intrauterine oxygen deprivation have low Apgar scores; thus a postnatal hypoxia is superimposed on an already existing problem.

The neurologic signs that indicate brain injury appear within the first hours after the hypoxic episode. The infant is stuporous or comatose, and seizures may begin after 6 to 12 hours and become more frequent and severe. Abnormal tone (usually hypotonia) and disturbances of sucking and swallowing are evident. Muscular weakness of the hips and shoulders is observed and apneic episodes are seen in approximately 50% of the affected infants.

Treatment involves vigorous supportive care directed toward adequate ventilation to prevent aggravating the existing hypoxia and measures to maintain cerebral perfusion and prevent cerebral edema. Seizures are managed as described in the previous section. Prevention is the most important therapy, however, and every effort should be expended to recognize the high-risk pregnancy, to monitor the fetus, and to initiate appropriate therapy early.

Nursing care is the same as for any high-risk infant—that is, careful assessment and observation for signs that might indicate cerebral hypoxia or ischemia, monitoring of ventilatory and intravenous therapy, observation and management of seizures, and general supportive care to the infant and parents.

INTRACRANIAL HEMORRHAGE

Intracranial hemorrhage is a common complication of premature birth as a result of either trauma or hypoxia. Fragility and increased permeability of capillaries and prolonged prothrombin time predispose the premature infant to trauma when delicate structures are subjected to the forces of labor. Traumatic bleeding in the newborn consists of four major types: subdural, primary subarachnoid, intracerebellar, and periventricular/intraventricular.

Subdural hematomas, life-threatening collections of blood in the subdural space, are most often produced by stretching and tearing of the large veins in the tentorium cerebelli (the dural membrane that separates the cerebrum from the cerebellum). Less frequently hemorrhage occurs when veins in the subdural space over the surface of the brain are torn.

Subarachnoid hemorrhage, although very common and a frequent cause of neonatal seizures, is of venous origin, usually self-limited, and seldom of major importance. *Intracerebellar hemorrhage* can be a primary hemorrhage in the cerebellum as a result of trauma, or it may occur secondary to extravasation of blood into the cerebellum from a ventricular hemorrhage. In the full-term infant the bleeding may follow a difficult delivery.

Periventricular/intraventricular hemorrhage is the most common type of intracranial hemorrhage and is responsible for a significant percentage of seriously ill infants and neonatal mortality. The disorder is extremely common in preterm infants, especially the very small infants who are subject to rupture in this heavily vascularized region.

Increase in intracranial pressure from hemorrhage is manifested by a tense, bulging anterior fontanel, separated sutures, and neurologic signs such as twitching, stupor, and convulsions. Consumption of clotting factors during periventricular hemorrhage may contribute to further bleeding and ventricular hemorrhage. Survivors of periventricular/intraventricular hemorrhage may develop hydrocephalus, a variety of motor deficits, and mental retardation.

Nursing care is the same as for high-risk infants and those with intracranial inflammation, intracranial pressure, and seizures.

HIGH RISK RELATED TO ENVIRONMENTAL FACTORS

The newborn infant is subject to environmental factors that cause injury or illness. His immature immune system and inability to localize infection renders him especially vulnerable to infectious organisms. Prevention of infection in the newborn, especially the infant who is already compromised by physiologic or structural disorders, is a primary nursing concern.

SEPSIS

Sepsis, or septicemia, refers to a generalized bacterial infection in the bloodstream. Neonates are susceptible to infection because they have diminished nonspecific (inflammatory) and specific (humoral) immunity. Because of the poor response to infectious agents, there is usually no local inflammatory reaction at the portal of entry to signal an infection and the resulting symptoms tend to be vague and nonspecific. Consequently, diagnosis and treatment may be delayed.

Sepsis in the neonatal period can be acquired prenatally or during labor from infected amniotic fluid, across the placenta from the maternal bloodstream, or by direct contact with maternal tissues during passage through the birth canal. Postnatal infection is acquired by cross-contamination from other infants, personnel, or objects in the environment, primarily life saving apparatus such as mechanical ventilators and indwelling venous and arterial catheters used for infusions, blood sampling, and monitoring vital signs. Neonatal sepsis is most common in the infant at risk, particularly the preterm infant and the infant born following a difficult or traumatic labor and delivery.

Clinical manifestations

A few neonatal infections (for example, pyoderma, conjunctivitis, omphalitis, and mastitis) are easily recognized. However, systemic infections are characterized by very subtle, vague, nonspecific, and almost imperceptible physical signs. Frequently the only complaint concerning the infant's progress is "failure to do well," "not looking right," or nonspecific respiratory distress. Rarely is there any indication of a local inflammatory response, which would suggest the portal of entry into the bloodstream.

All bodily systems tend to show some indication of sepsis. Respiratory distress is usually noticed because of periods of apnea, irregular, grunting respirations, and retractions. Gastric distress is evidenced by signs such as vomiting (vomitus may be bile stained), diarrhea, abdominal distention and absent stools as a result of paralytic ileus, and poor sucking and feeding. Skin manifestations may include cyanosis, pallor, mottling, or signs of jaundice, as well as the lesions associated with specific organisms. Signs of central nervous system involvement are similar to those seen in hypocalcemia or hypoglycemia, notably irritability, apathy, tremors, convulsions, and coma. Since meningitis is a frequent sequela of sepsis, signs of increased intracranial pressure may also be evident. Fever, which is usually characteristic of any infection, is frequently absent in neonatal sepsis. Body temperature is commonly normal or suboptimal.

Diagnostic evaluation

Isolation of the specific organism is always attempted through repeated blood cultures and analysis of potential primary sources of infection, such as the umbilicus, naso-oral-pharyngeal cavity, ear canals, skin lesions, cerebrospinal fluid, stool, and urine. Direct (conjugated) hyperbilirubinemia is frequently seen in infants with sepsis, particularly of gram-negative origin. Blood studies may show signs of anemia, leukocytosis, or leukopenia. Leukopenia is usually an ominous sign because it is frequently associated with high mortality.

Therapeutic management

Early recognition and diagnosis and institution of vigorous therapeutic measures are essential to increasing the chance for survival and reducing the likelihood of permanent neurologic damage. Treatment consists of aggressive administration of appropriate antibiotics and supportive therapy, careful regulation of fluids and electrolytes, and temporary discontinuation of oral feedings.

Supportive therapy usually involves administration of oxygen if respiratory distress or cyanosis is evident, adequate hydration with intravenous fluid and electrolytes, and isolation of the infant in an Isolette or incubator. Blood transfusions may be needed to correct anemia and/or shock, and electronic monitoring of vital signs and regulation of the thermal environment are mandatory.

Nursing considerations

Nursing care of the infant with sepsis is similar to the care of any high-risk infant. Recognition of the existing problem is of paramount importance; it is usually the nurse who frequently observes and assesses the infant who recognizes that "something is wrong" with the child. Awareness of the potential modes of transmission allows the nurse to identify those infants more at risk for developing sepsis.

Much of the care of the infant involves the medical treatment of illness. Knowledge of the side effects of the specific antibiotic and proper regulation and administration of the drug via the intravenous route is mandatory.

Part of the total care of the infant with sepsis is to decrease any additional physiologic or environmental stress. This includes providing an optimum, thermoregulated environment and anticipating potential problems such as dehydration or anoxia. Isolation of the infant prevents spread of infection to other newborns, but, in order to be effective, isolation must be carried out by all caregivers. Proper handwashing, use of disposable equipment (such as linens, catheters, feeding utensils, and intravenous equipment), disposing of excretions (such as vomitus and stool), and adequate housekeeping of the environment and equipment are essential. Since nurses are the most consistent caregivers involved with the sick infant, it is usually their responsibility to oversee that all aspects of isolation are maintained.

Another aspect of caring for the infant with sepsis involves observation for signs of meningitis, a frequent sequela of septicemia. The most common indication of meningitis is a full or bulging anterior fontanel.

A severe complication of sepsis is shock, which is caused by the release of toxins within the bloodstream. Signs of shock are often difficult to distinguish from those of sepsis, such as rapid, irregular respirations and pulse. However, blood pressure usually falls in shock, and, therefore, this measurement should be a part of the infant's routine vital signs. The nurse needs to be especially aware of the importance of blood pressure; this is one measurement that is frequently neglected in the assessment of children.

The newborn with sepsis is usually quite ill. The prognosis varies from patient to patient, but with immediate and vigorous antibiotic therapy, mortality is quite low.

STAPHYLOCOCCAL INFECTIONS

Skin eruptions in the newborn infant are less common than they are in children. However, because of their depressed immune system, infants are more vulnerable to bacterial invasion, which tends to be more serious and less likely to remain localized.

Bullous impetigo (Impetigo neonatorum)

Bullous impetigo is a superficial skin infection most often produced by group 2 phage type *Staphylococcus aureus*. It is characterized by the eruption of bullous vesicular lesions on previously untraumatized skin. The lesions may appear

SUMMARY OF NURSING CARE OF THE INFANT WITH BACTERIAL INFECTION

GOALS	NURSING RESPONSIBILITIES
Recognize signs of infection	Maintain high level of suspicion in infants with vague or nonspecific signs of illness Monitor suspicious cases Assist with diagnostic procedures and tests
Assess status	Perform routine assessments
Prevent spread of infection	Institute appropriate isolation measures Carry out meticulous handwashing technique Use cohort nursing for care of infant
Eradicate organism Skin lesions	Administer antibiotics as prescribed Perform skin care as indicated Apply appropriate topical medication or other substance

Maintain nutrition
 	
   Necrotizing enterocolitis
   (NEC)
	Regulate and monitor intravenous infusions
	Provide oral feedings as appropriate
	
	Discontinue oral feedings

Anticipate possible
   complications
   Skin lesions
 	
   Sepsis
   NEC
	Observe for signs of shock
	Observe for side effects or sensitivity to antibiotics
	Observe for signs of spread of infection to other areas or generalized sepsis
	Observe for signs of meningitis (especially bulging anterior fontanel)
	Observe for signs of perforation or peritonitis, acidosis

Support parents	Explain purpose of isolation Teach appropriate isolation precautions Explain tests and therapies Provide opportunity for visiting infant Provide opportunity to express feelings and concerns Keep informed of infant's progress

on any body surface, but the usual distribution involves the buttocks, perineum, trunk, and face but sometimes becomes widespread. They vary in size from a few millimeters to several centimeters in diameter, contain turbid fluid, and are easily ruptured. The bullae rupture in 1 to 2 days, leaving a superficial red, moist, denuded area with very little crusting.

Cultures are obtained from the lesion and, if the infant appears ill, blood cultures are indicated. Warm saline compresses are applied to the lesions followed by gentle cleansing and application of a topical antibiotic several times a day. Systemic antibiotics are also administered to small infants and those with widespread lesions. Recovery is usually rapid and uneventful.

Nursing considerations. The affected infant is isolated from other infants and other appropriate precautionary measures are instituted to prevent spread of the infection to other infants. Persons who have come in contact with the infant are investigated to determine a possible source of the infecting organism. Other infants in the nursery should be scrutinized for early detection of any signs of infection. Even though the affected infant is isolated, he should be held during feeding and rocked and cuddled as much as possible. Parents and other visitors are instructed regarding precautions for prevention of infection.

Staphylococcal scalded skin syndrome (SSSS)

The scalded skin syndrome is a severe bullous eruption caused by group 2 *Staphylococcus aureus*. The disorder appears first as a macular erythema with a ''sandpaper'' texture of the involved skin. The most common initial sites are the face, neck, axilla, and groin, but the infection frequently spreads rapidly to other areas. Within a short time (2 days or less) the upper layer of the affected areas becomes wrinkled and may separate after gentle stroking (Nikolsky sign). Soon large, flaccid bullae filled with clear fluid appear and the epidermis separates in large sheets, leaving a moist, glistening, denuded surface. The denuded areas quickly dry and heal rapidly without scarring.

Unlike bullous impetigo, the intact bullae of SSSS are sterile; therefore, cultures are obtained from suspected ports of entry such as from the blood, the skin of a preceding impetiginous infection, the nasopharynx, or the conjunctival sac. Treatment consists of prompt systemic administration of antibiotic and gentle cleansing of skin with compresses of saline, Burow solution, or 0.25% silver nitrate.

Nursing considerations. The nursing care of infants with SSSS is similar to nursing care of the infant with bullous impetigo. Because of the large areas involved the infant is subject to excessive fluid loss, difficulty regulating body temperature, and infection such as pneumonia, cellulitis, and septicemia. The nurse is continually observant for signs of these complications.

NECROTIZING ENTEROCOLITIS (NEC)

This serious condition in a premature infant may go undetected for some time because of the ambiguity of symptoms in the preterm infant and preoccupation with other life-threatening problems by members of the staff. Three factors appear to play an important role in its development: intestinal ischemia, bacterial colonization, and early enteric feeding.

Pathophysiology

The precise cause of the disorder is still speculative, although it appears to occur in an infant whose gastrointestinal tract has suffered a vascular compromise somehow related to an episode of hypoxia or sepsis or after an exchange transfusion. The reduced blood supply to the intestines causes damage and death to mucosal cells lining the bowel wall. They are unable to secrete protective mucus; therefore, the unprotected bowel wall is invaded by gas-forming bacteria producing pneumatosis intestinalis (presence of air in the submucosal or subserosal surfaces of the colon), a consistent and diagnostic finding.

There is a consistent relationship between the development of NEC and feedings of hypertonic formula, but it is unclear whether this is a result of the formula imposing a stress on an ischemic bowel or serving as a medium for bacterial growth.

Clinical manifestations

The nonspecific clinical signs of necrotizing enterocolitis include lethargy, poor feeding, hypotension, vomiting, apnea, decreased urine output, and unstable temperature. Specific signs are distended (often shiny) abdomen, blood in the stools or gastric contents, and gastric retention. Necrotizing enterocolitis has been found to be absent in breast-fed animals but the significance of these experiments is unclear.

Diagnostic evaluation

Radiographic studies show a sausage-shaped dilation of the intestine that progresses to marked distention and the characteristic pneumatosis intestinalis. Organisms are often cultured from blood, although bacteremia may not be prominent early in the course of the disease.

Therapeutic management

Treatment of necrotizing enterocolitis consists of discontinuation of all oral feedings and starting intravenous fluids, correction of fluid and electrolyte imbalances, institution of abdominal decompression via nasogastric suction, and administration of systemic antibiotics. If there is progressive deterioration under medical management or evidence of perforation, surgical resection and anastomosis are carried out. Extensive involvement may necessitate establishment of an ileostomy or a colostomy.

Nursing considerations

Nursing responsibilities begin with early recognition of the disease. Because the signs are similar to those observed in many other disorders of the newborn, nurses must be constantly aware of the possibility of this disease and alert to indications of its early development. Checking the abdomen frequently for distention, measuring for residual gastric contents before feedings, and listening for presence of bowel sounds are especially important in detecting the early signs of NEC.

When the disease is suspected, the nurse assists with diagnostic procedures and implements the therapeutic regimen. Vital signs, including blood pressure, are monitored for changes that indicate impending sepsis or cardiovascular shock. It is especially important to avoid taking rectal temperatures because of the increased danger of perforation. To avoid pressure on the distended abdomen, the infant is not diapered or positioned on the abdomen.

Confirmed cases are isolated from other infants and strict handwashing and other isolation precautions are instituted, such as wearing of long-sleeved gown and gloves and use of separate diapers with careful disposal and laundry handling. When possible the same nurses are designated to care for the infant and no person with gastrointestinal symptoms should be assigned to his care.

Conscientious attention to nutritional and hydration needs is essential, and antibiotics are administered as prescribed. The time at which oral feedings are reinstituted varies considerably but is usually at least 7 days following diagnosis. Plain water or electrolyte solution is given for two feedings, followed by dilute human milk formula. The concentration is gradually increased over 2 to 3 weeks until the infant is again taking full-strength feedings.

The infant who requires surgery requires the same careful care and observation as any infant with abdominal surgery, including colostomy care. Throughout the management of the infant with NEC the nurse is continually alert to signs of complications such as sepsis, disseminated intravascular coagulation, hypoglycemia, and other metabolic derangements.

HIGH RISK RELATED TO MATERNAL FACTORS

Some newborn infants are at risk because of adverse influences present before birth. These factors may be diseases of the mother that are transmitted to the infant (rubella), diseases or deficiencies of the mother that cause chemical or physiologic imbalances in the infant (diabetes mellitus), or chemicals that produce an undesirable effect in the infant (narcotics).

INFANT OF THE DIABETIC MOTHER (IDM)

Before the introduction of insulin therapy, few diabetic women were able to conceive, and, for those who did, the mortality rate for both mother and infant was extremely high. As a result of effective control of diabetes, more infants of diabetic mothers (IDMs) experience an uneventful perinatal course. However, where special care is not available, the infant death rate may be as high as 50%. As the incidence of diabetes rises in the population as a whole, increasing numbers of infants of diabetic mothers are admitted to intensive care nurseries.

The severity of the maternal disease affects infant and fetal survival, and there is a relationship between length of gestation and neonatal mortality. There is a higher incidence of stillborn infants in the more severely insulin-dependent diabetic women, and their live-born infants appear to be more at risk than those of mothers with less severe diabetic involvement.

It has been found that the gestational age most favorable to survival of infants of diabetic mothers is between 36 and 37 weeks. Delivery at an earlier age is associated with increased neonatal mortality, but the incidence of stillborn infants is higher in later deliveries, probably because of failing placental competence. The favored approach is to induce labor or to deliver the infant by cesarean section at approximately 37 weeks.

Pathophysiology

Hypoglycemia appears within a short period after birth and is associated with increased insulin activity in the blood. It is generally agreed that during fetal life high maternal blood sugar levels provide a continual stimulus to the fetal islet cells for insulin production. This sustained state of hyperglycemia promotes fetal insulin secretion, which ultimately leads to excessive growth and deposition of fat, which probably accounts for the infants who are large for gestational age. When this glucose supply is removed abruptly at the time of birth, the continued production of insulin soon depletes the blood of circulating glucose, creating a state of hypoglycemia within 2 to 4 hours. Sudden drops in blood glucose levels can cause serious neurologic abnormality or death.

Clinical manifestations

All infants of diabetic mothers have a characteristic appearance. They are oversized for their gestational age, very plump and full-faced, liberally coated with vernix caseosa, and plethoric. They are listless and lethargic. Although they are large, these infants are often prematurely born—either because of an elective early delivery or for other reasons. Their appearance has been described as that of a premature infant seen through a magnifying glass (Fig. 7-18).

There is an increase in congenital anomalies in this group as well as a high susceptibility to hypoglycemia, hypocalcemia, hyperbilirubinemia, and hyaline membrane disease. No satisfactory explanation has been accepted for all the abnormalities in these infants, although complications may be related to the prematurity factor in a number of complications.

Therapeutic management

If hypoglycemia is left untreated, it can cause rapid, irreversible central nervous system damage. The most effective management appears to be careful observation of all infants of diabetic mothers in the special-care nursery, with early feeding of 5% to 10% glucose followed by formula, if tolerated. Critically ill infants require intravenous infusions. Frequent determinations of blood glucose levels are needed for the first 2 days of life, to assess the degree of hypoglycemia present at any given time.

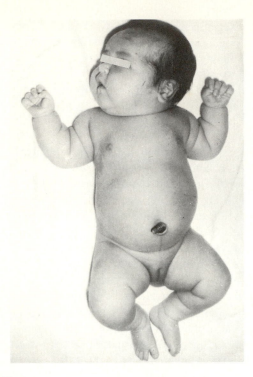

FIG. 7-18

*Infant of gestational diabetic mother born at 40 weeks'
gestation. Birth weight, 4.7 kg; postnatal age, 1 week.
(From Fanaroff, A.A., and Martin, R.J., editors: Behrman's neonatal-perinatal medicine, ed. 3, St. Louis, 1983,
The C.V. Mosby Co.)*

Nursing considerations

Nursing care of IDMs requires observation for signs of
complications to which they are more susceptible than
other neonates. Hypoglycemia is the most immediate and
consistent threat to these infants; therefore, feedings are
initiated early and the infant is observed for central nervous system signs such as hyperirritability, tremors, and
jitteriness during the early hours of life. Other complications that occur with increased frequency in the IDM are
polycythemia, hyperbilirubinemia, sepsis, and respiratory
distress syndrome. Vigilance is needed to detect signs that
indicate development of any of these neonatal problems.
(See p. 193 for care of the infant with hypoglycemia.)

NARCOTIC-ADDICTED INFANTS

Narcotics, which have a low molecular weight, readily
cross the placental membrane and enter the fetal system.
When the mother is a habitual user of narcotics, in particular heroin or methadone, the unborn child becomes passively addicted to the drug, which places such infants at
risk during the early neonatal period.

Clinical manifestations

Most passively addicted infants of drug-dependent mothers
appear normal at birth but begin to exhibit signs of drug
withdrawal within 12 to 24 hours if the mother has been
taking heroin alone. If she has been taking methadone, the
signs appear somewhat later, anywhere from 1 or 2 days
to a week or more after birth. The manifestations become
most pronounced between 48 and 72 hours of age and may
last anywhere from 6 days to 8 weeks, depending on the
severity of the withdrawal.

The clinical manifestations of withdrawal in the neonate, which are predominantly those of autonomic nervous
system hyperirritability, may persist for 3 or 4 months.
The most common acute signs are tremors, restlessness,
hyperactive reflexes, increased muscle tone, sneezing,
tachypnea, and a high-pitched, shrill cry. Although infants
undergoing withdrawal suck avidly on fists and display an
exaggerated rooting reflex, they are poor feeders, with uncoordinated and ineffectual sucking and swallowing reflexes. Regurgitation and vomiting after feedings are common, and diarrhea is a later manifestation. An unusual
observation in a large percentage of these infants is generalized sweating, the incidence of which is double that in
normal newborns who display sweating.

Not all infants of heroin-addicted mothers show signs
of withdrawal. Because of irregular and varying degrees of
drug use, varying quality of drug, and mixed drug usage
by the mother, some infants display mild or variable manifestations.

It is significant to note that, although passively addicted infants have some tachypnea, cyanosis, and/or apnea, they rarely develop respiratory distress syndrome.
Apparently, the heroin or related factors in the intrauterine
environment cause accelerated lung maturation in these infants, even in the face of a high incidence of prematurity.

Therapeutic management

The treatment of the infant consists of intramuscular administration of chlorpromazine or phenobarbital in four divided doses over 2 to 4 days and then orally in decreasing
doses for an additional 7 to 10 days. If there are gastrointestinal symptoms such as diarrhea, paregoric may be the
drug of choice.

Nursing considerations

The management of the infant of the drug-addicted mother
begins with recognizing manifestations that indicate withdrawal. Once the presence of withdrawal is identified in
an infant, nursing care is directed toward reducing the
stimuli that might trigger hyperactivity and irritability,
providing adequate nutrition and hydration, and promoting

maternal-infant relationships. Irritable and hyperactive infants have been found to respond to comforting, movement, and close contact. Wrapping the infant snugly to limit his ability to self-stimulate and holding him tightly and arranging nursing activities to reduce the amount of disturbance help to decrease external stimulation.

Loose stools together with poor intake and regurgitation following feeding predispose the infants to malnutrition, dehydration, and electrolyte imbalance that can progress to shock and coma. Frequent weights, careful monitoring of intake and output, and supplemental parenteral fluids may be necessary in addition to the care ordinarily afforded high-risk newborn infants. Monitoring and recording activity levels, and their relationship to other activities such as feeding and preventing complications are important nursing functions.

A valuable aid to anticipating problems in the newborn is recognizing drug addiction in the mother. Unless the mother is enrolled in a methadone rehabilitation program, she seldom risks calling attention to her habit by seeking prenatal care. Consequently, the infant and mother are exposed to the additional hazards of obstetric and medical complications. In addition, the nature of heroin addiction predisposes the user to disorders such as infection, hepatitis, and foreign body reaction, as well as the hazards of inadequate nutrition and premature birth. Methadone treatment does not prevent withdrawal reaction in the neonate, but the clinical course may be modified.

DISORDERS CAUSED BY MATERNAL FACTORS

A variety of disorders have been attributed to maternal infections during a sensitive period of fetal development. The clinical picture of disorders caused by transplacental transfer of infectious agents is not always well defined. One group of microbial agents can cause remarkably similar manifestations, and it is not uncommon to test for all when a prenatal infection is suspected. This is the so-called TORCH complex, an acronym that represents the following infections:

> **T**—toxoplasmosis
> **O**—other
> **R**—rubella
> **C**—cytomegalovirus infection
> **H**—herpes simplex

To determine the causative agent in a symptomatic infant, tests are carried out to rule out each of these infections. The ''O'' category may involve testing for several viral infections as well as testing for syphilis and listeriosis. Bacterial infections are not included in the TORCH workup because they are usually identified by clinical manifestations and readily available laboratory tests. Gonococcal conjunctivitis (ophthalmia neonatorum) has been virtually eliminated by prophylactic measures and is not discussed in this section. The major maternal infections, their possible teratogenic effects, and specific nursing considerations are outlined in Table 7-3. The two most common chemical agents are also included. For additional discussion of maternal influences on fetal development see Chapter 3.

Nursing considerations

One of the major goals in the care of infants suspected of a maternally derived infectious disease is identification of the causative agent. Until diagnosis is established, the infant is isolated from contact with other infants. In suspected cytomegalovirus and rubella infections, pregnant personnel are cautioned to avoid contact with the infant. Herpes simplex is easily transmitted from one infant to another; therefore, risk of cross-contamination should be eliminated.

Special feeding techniques may need to be implemented for infants with feeding difficulties, and infants subject to seizures should be protected from adverse environmental stimuli. Specimens need to be obtained for laboratory examinations, and the infant and parents need to be prepared for diagnostic procedures. When possible, long-term disabilities are prevented by early evaluation and implementation of therapy. If sequelae are inevitable, the family will need assistance in determining how they can best cope with the problems, such as assistance with home care, referral to appropriate agencies, or placement in an institution for care.

INBORN ERRORS OF METABOLISM

Inborn errors of metabolism is a term applied to a large number of inherited diseases caused by the absence or deficiency of a substance essential to cellular metabolism, usually an enzyme. When a normal metabolic process is interrupted as a result of the missing enzyme, the consequence is disease.

PHENYLKETONURIA (PKU)

Phenylketonuria is a genetic disease, inherited as an autosomal-recessive trait, caused by the absence of an enzyme that is necessary for the metabolism of the essential amino acid phenylalanine. It is not a common inborn error of

TABLE 7-3. CONGENITAL DISORDERS ACQUIRED FROM THE MOTHER

MATERNAL EXPOSURE	FETAL OR NEWBORN EFFECT	COMMENTS AND NURSING CONSIDERATIONS
Maternal infections Rubella virus (congenital rubella)	Eye defects: cataracts (unilateral or bilateral) microphthalmia, retinitis, glaucoma Central nervous system signs: microcephaly, seizures, severe mental retardation Congenital heart defects: patent ductus arteriosus Auditory: high incidence of delayed hearing loss Intrauterine growth retardation Hyperbilirubinemia, spinal fluid abnormalities, thrombocytopenia, hepatomegaly	Transmitted: first trimester; early second trimester Pregnant women should avoid contact with all affected persons, including infants with rubella syndrome Emphasize vaccination of all unimmunized prepubertal children, susceptible adolescents, and adult females of childbearing age Caution women against pregnancy for at least 3 months following vaccination Isolate affected infant
Cytomegalovirus (CMV) (cytomegalic inclusion disease—CMD)	Microcephaly, cerebral calcifications, chorioretinitis Jaundice, hepatosplenomegaly Petechial or purpuric rash Neurologic sequelae: seizure disorders, sensorimotor deafness, mental retardation	Transmitted: throughout pregnancy Affected individuals excrete the virus Pregnant women should avoid close contact with those who have known cases
Toxoplasma gondii (toxoplasmosis)	Microcephaly, hydrocephaly, cerebral calcifications, chorioretinitis Encephalitis, myocarditis, hepatosplenomegaly, anemia, jaundice, diarrhea, vomiting, seizures	Transmitted: throughout pregnancy Predominant host for organism is cats May be transmitted through cat feces, poorly cooked or raw infected meat Caution pregnant women to avoid contact with cat feces, e.g., emptying cat litter boxes Isolate infant
Herpes simplex virus (neonatal herpes)	Cutaneous lesions: vesicles at 6 to 10 days of age Disseminated disease: resembles sepsis Visceral involvement: granulomas Early nonspecific signs: fever, lethargy, poor feeding, irritability, vomiting May include hyperbilirubinemia, seizures, flaccid or spastic paralysis, apneic episodes, respiratory distress, lethargy, or coma	Transmitted: Intrapartum either ascending and/or direct contact Incubation period 6 to 10 days Rarely acquired as intrauterine infection during first trimester and intrapartum Cesarean section a frequent preventive measure Isolate infant until disease determined by blood cultures

TABLE 7-3. CONGENITAL DISORDERS ACQUIRED FROM THE MOTHER—cont'd

MATERNAL EXPOSURE	FETAL OR NEWBORN EFFECT	COMMENTS AND NURSING CONSIDERATIONS
Varicella virus (varicella) (chickenpox)	Skin lesions, microcephaly, limb deformities, encephalomyocarditis, visceral involvement	Transmitted: first trimester or intrapartum Isolate infant
Group B coxsackie virus	Poor feeding, vomiting, diarrhea, fever; cardiac enlargement, arrhythmias, congestive heart failure; lethargy, seizures, meningeal involvement	Transmitted: first trimester or late in pregnancy
Treponema pallidum (congenital)	Copper-colored maculopapular cutaneous lesions (after 7th day), mucous membrane patches, hair loss, nail exfoliation, snuffles (syphilitic rhinitis), profound anemia, poor feeding, pseudoparalysis of one or more limbs	Transmitted: transplacental, usually after 18th week of pregnancy Penicillin is treatment of choice Isolate infant
Neisseria gonorrhoeae (gonococcal disease)	Ophthalmitis Neonatal gonococcal arthritis, septicemia, meningitis	Transmitted: last trimester or intrapartum Apply prophylactic medication to eyes at time of birth Isolate suspected cases; obtain smears for culture Administer penicillin as ordered
Chlamydia trachomatis	Conjunctivitis, pneumonia	Transmitted: last trimester or intrapartum Apply prophylactic medication to eyes at time of birth
Chemical agents Alcohol (fetal alcohol syndrome)	Facial features: hypoplastic maxilla, micrognathia, hypoplastic philtrum, short palpebral fissures Neurologic: mental retardation, motor retardation, microcephaly, hypotonia Growth: prenatal growth retardation, persistent postnatal growth lag	Exact quantity of alcohol needed to produce teratogenic effects in fetus is not known Women with histories of heavy drinking should be counseled regarding risks to fetus
Tobacco smoking	Fetal growth retardation Increased perinatal deaths Increased spontaneous abortions	Women should be counseled regarding the risk to fetus

metabolism—it affects 1 in every 10,000 to 20,000 live births—but it accounts for about 1% of institutionalized mentally defective individuals. Phenylketonuria primarily affects whites, with the incidence being highest in people living in the United States or Northern Europe. It is very rare in the African, Jewish, or Japanese populations.

Pathophysiology

In PKU the hepatic enzyme *phenylalanine hydroxylase,* which normally controls the conversion of phenylalanine to tyrosine, is absent, resulting in the accumulation of phenylalanine in the bloodstream and urinary excretion of its abnormal metabolites, the phenyl acids (Fig. 7-19). One of these metabolites, phenylpyruvic acid, gives urine the characteristic musty odor associated with this disease, and is responsible for the term *phenylketonuria.* In addition to the accumulating phenylalanine, there is an absence of the amino acid tyrosine, which is needed for the formation of the pigment melanin and the hormones epinephrine and thyroxin.

Clinical manifestations

Decreased melanin production is responsible for the physical appearance of most phenylketonuric children. Typically they have blonde hair, blue eyes, and fair skin, which is particularly susceptible to eczema and other dermatologic problems.

Other clinical manifestations of untreated PKU include failure to thrive, frequent vomiting, irritability, hyperactivity, and unpredictable, erratic behavior. Bizarre or schizoid-like behavior patterns are common, such as fright reactions, screaming episodes, disorientation, failure to respond to strong stimuli, and catatonic-like positions. Many of the severely retarded children have convulsions, and about 80% of untreated persons with phenylketonuria demonstrate abnormal electroencephalograms, regardless of whether they have overt seizures.

Diagnostic evaluation

The objective in diagnosing or treating PKU is to prevent mental retardation. All the tests for PKU are based on the detection of increasing phenylalanine levels in the blood or

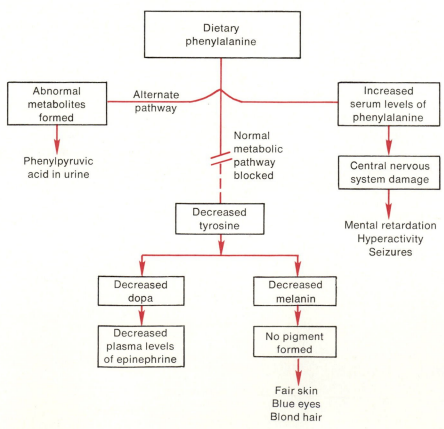

FIG. 7-19

Metabolic error and consequences in phenylketonuria.

characteristic metabolites in the urine. The most reliable test for screening newborns for phenylketonuria is the *Guthrie blood test,* which measures blood phenylalanine levels. The test is unreliable until the infant has ingested dietary protein (cow's milk or human milk) for 24 to 48 hours. Therefore, the test should not be performed before the third to sixth day of life. Retesting is recommended in 2 weeks for infants tested in the first 24 hours, those whose phenylalanine levels were greater than 20 mg/dl, and those with phenylketonuric siblings. At the present time the Guthrie blood test is mandatory for all newborns in most states.

Several tests exist for detecting phenylpyruvic acid in urine. All of them utilize the reagent ferric chloride, which turns green when in contact with phenylpyruvic acid. The Phenistix test* employs a dipstick that has a ferric salt impregnated in the filter paper. When it is dipped in urine or pressed against a wet diaper, the dipstick will turn green if abnormal phenylalanine levels are present. Fading of the color occurs within 1 minute. For reliable results, fresh urine and new filter paper must be used. False-positive results can occur if large amounts of ketones are present (diabetic acidosis). Aspirin and other salicylate-containing compounds will turn the paper a nonfading bluish purple.

Therapeutic management

Treatment of phenylketonuria is dietary. Since the genetic enzyme is intracellular, systemic administration of phenylalanine hydroxylase is of no value. Phenylalanine cannot be eliminated from the diet, because it is an essential amino acid, necessary for tissue growth. Therefore, dietary management must meet two criteria:

1. It must meet the child's nutritional need for optimum growth.
2. It must maintain phenylalanine levels within a safe range.

Since all natural food proteins contain about 5% phenylalanine, a specially prepared milk substitute (Lofenalac†) is usually given to the infant. It is usually well accepted by infants, although older children may not find it palatable. At present, most authorities suggest continuing the diet until the child is 6 to 8 years old, when at least 90% of brain growth has occurred.

If dietary management is begun after brain damage has occurred, it will not reverse the process but will limit its progress. Restricting phenylalanine in older children with phenylketonuria has proved to be of some benefit in improving behavior and motor ability and in decreasing exacerbations of eczema.

Nursing considerations

Although the treatment for phenylketonuria may sound simple, the task of maintaining such a strict dietary regimen is very demanding. Foods with low phenylalanine levels, such as vegetables, fruits, juices, and some cereals, breads, and starches, must be measured in order to provide the prescribed amount of phenylalanine. Most high-protein foods, such as meat or dairy products, are either eliminated or restricted to small amounts. Unfortunately, special formulas are quite expensive, adding financial burdens. However, it is essential that the formula be used in place of milk products. Milk can be used in the event that the formula is not available, but this must be a temporary exception. Families should be cautioned against giving the sweetening agent aspartame (NutraSweet) to children with PKU because the drug is converted to phenylalanine in the gut.

To evaluate the effectiveness of dietary treatment, frequent monitoring of urinary phenylpyruvic acid levels is necessary. Since suboptimal phenylalanine levels will retard the rate of growth, a careful record should be kept of weight and height. In addition, frequent urine and blood assays of phenylalanine should be performed.

GALACTOSEMIA

Galactosemia is an inborn error of carbohydrate metabolism, inherited as an autosomal-recessive trait, in which the hepatic enzyme *galactose-1-phosphate uridyl transferase* is absent, preventing the conversion of galactose to glucose. As galactose accumulates in the blood, several organs are affected. Hepatic dysfunction leads to cirrhosis, resulting in jaundice in the infant by the second week of life. The spleen subsequently becomes enlarged as a result of portal hypertension. Cataracts are usually recognizable by 1 or 2 months of age; cerebral damage is evident soon afterward, manifested by the symptoms of lethargy and hypotonia. Infants with galactosemia appear normal at birth, but within a few days after ingesting milk, which has a high lactose content, they begin to vomit and lose weight. Drowsiness, nausea, and diarrhea also occur. Death during the first month of life is not infrequent in untreated galactosemic infants.

Diagnosis of this rare disorder is made on the basis of galactosuria, increased levels of galactose in the blood, or decreased enzyme levels in erythrocytes. Screening tests are available and mandatory in several states.

Treatment of galactosemia is dietary; it consists of eliminating all milk and galactose-containing foods. This

---

*Ames Co., Elkhart, IN.
†Meade-Johnson & Co., Evansville, IN.

involves reading food labels very carefully for the addition of any form of dairy product, such as cream, yogurt, cheese, or butter. During infancy, soybean-based formulas are used. Many drugs, such as penicillin, contain lactose as fillers and must also be avoided.

Nursing considerations are similar to those for phenylketonuria.

REFERENCES

Blake, S.: The bright side of phototherapy, Am. J. Maternal Child Nurs. **8**:23, 1983.

Korones, S.B.: High-risk newborn infants: the basis for intensive nursing care, ed. 3, St. Louis, 1981, The C.V. Mosby Co.

Kuller, J.M., Lund, C., and Tobin, C.: Improved skin care for premature infants, Am. J. Maternal Child Nurs. **8**:200-203, 1983.

Volpe, J.J.: Neonatal seizures, Clin. Perinatol. **4**:43-63, 1977.

Wooten, B.: Death of an infant, Am. J. Maternal Child Nurs. **6**:257-260, 1981.

BIBLIOGRAPHY
General

Abbey, B.L., and others: Nursing responsibility in referring the convalescent newborn, Am. J. Maternal Child Nurs. **2**:295-297, 1977.

Blackburn, S.: The neonatal ICU: a high-risk environment, Am. J. Nurs. **82**:1708-1712, 1982.

Bresadola, C.: One infant/one nurse/one objective: quality care, Am. J. Maternal Child Nurs. **2**:287-290, 1977.

Buxton, A.E.: Nosocomial infection in the intensive care unit, Crit. Care Update **9**:32-37, 1982.

Chaze, B.A., and Ludington-Hoe, S.M.: Sensory stimulation in the ICU, Am. J. Nurs. **84**:68-71, 1984.

Gutrecht, N.M.V., and Khoury, G.: Cardiopulmonary emergencies in the newborn: diagnosis and management, Heart Lung **2**:878-883, 1973.

Guy, M.: Neonatal transport, Nurs. Clin. North Am. 3-12, 1978.

Korones, S.B.: High-risk newborn infants: the basis for intensive nursing care, ed. 3, St. Louis, 1981, The C.V. Mosby Co.

Kress, L.M.: Transporting the sick neonate, Issues Compr. Pediatr. Nurs. **2**(1):8-19, 1977.

Oelerich, W.J., and Dombrowski, J.M.: Mini IV patients ... maximum precautions, RN **44**(9):43-47, 1982.

Perez, R.H.: Protocols for perinatal nursing practice, St Louis, 1981, The C.V. Mosby Co.

Reid, T.J.: Newborn cyanosis, Am. J. Nurs. **83**:1230-1234, 1983.

Seaman, C.K.: Monitoring the neonate, Crit. Care Update **10**:23-29, 1983.

Thornton, J., Berry, J., and Dal Santo, J.: Neonatal intensive care: the nurse's role in supporting the family, Nurs. Clin. North Am. **19**:125-137, 1984.

Weeks, H.: Bioinstrumentation in the care of the neonate, Nurs. Clin. North Am. **13**:597-609, 1978.

Zamansky, H., and Strobel, K.: Care of the critically ill newborn, Am. J. Nurs. **76**:566-569, 1976.

Assessment of high-risk neonates

Black, M.: Assessment of weight and gestational age, Nurs. Clin. North Am. **13**:13-22, 1978.

Gunn, S.: Critical care concepts related to maturational problems, Crit. Care Q. **4**(1):1-7, 1981.

Luchner, K.R.: Stress in neonatal intensive care units, Issues Compr. Pediatr. Nurs. **2**(1):20-35, 1977.

Parental involvement

Aab, C.A.: Assessment of maternal behavior during early mother-infant interaction. In Brandt, P.A., Chinn, P.L., and Smith, M.E., editors: Current practice in pediatric nursing, vol. 1, St. Louis, 1976, The C.V. Mosby Co.

Barnard, M.U.: Supportive nursing care for the mother and newborn who are separated from each other, Am. J. Maternal Child Nurs. **1**(2):107-110, 1976.

Chitwood, L.: A lesson in living, Nursing 84 **14**(1):55-56, 1984.

Christensen, A.Z.: Coping with the crisis of a premature birth—one couple's story, Am. J. Maternal Child Nurs. **2**(1):33-37, 1977.

Clark, A.L., and Affonso, D.D.: Infant behavior and maternal attachment: two sides to the coin, Am. J. Maternal Child Nurs. **1**(2):94-99, 1976.

Cordell, A.S., and Apolito, R.: Family support in infant death, J. Obstet. Gynecol. Neonatal Nurs. **10**:281-285, July/Aug. 1981.

Donnelly, G.F., and Conroy, N.: Parent-neonate communication in the care-giving system, Top. Clin. Nurs. **1**(3):1-9, 1979.

Dubois, D.R.: Indications of an unhealthy relationship between parents and premature infant, J. Obstet. Gynecol. Neonatal Nurs. **4**:21, 1975.

Eager, M.: Long-distance nurturing of the family bond, Am. J. Maternal Child Nurs. **2**:293-294, 1977.

Erdman, D.: Parent-to-parent support: the best for those with sick newborns, Am. J. Maternal Child Nurs. **2**:291-292, 1977.

Houser, J.: Therapeutic groups for parents of high risk infants. Issues Compr. Pediatr. Nurs. **4**(4):31-35, 1979.

Mahan, C.K.: Care of the family of the critically ill neonate, Crit. Care Q. **4**:89-103, 1981.

Miller, C.: Working with parents of high-risk infants, Am. J. Nurs. **78**:1228-1230, 1978.

Slade, C.L.: Working with parents of high risk newborns, J. Obstet. Gynecol. Neonatal Nurs. **6**:21, March/April 1977.

Thomas, N., and Cordell, A.S.: The dying infant: aiding parents in the detachment process, Pediatr. Nurs. **9**(5):355-357, 1983.

Work, R.B.: When we cannot cure, care, (Letters to the editor), Am. J. Maternal Child Nurs. **8**:111-112, 1983.

The premature infant

Boggs, K.R., and Rau, P.K.: Breastfeeding the premature infant, Am. J. Nurs. **83**:1437-1439, 1983.

Brown, J., and Hepler, R.: Stimulation—a corollary to physical care, Am. J. Nurs. **76**:578-581, 1976.

Choi, M.W.: Breast milk for infants who can't breast-feed, Am. J. Nurs. **78**:852-855, 1978.

Conway, A., and Williams, T.: Parenteral alimentation, Am. J. Nurs. **76**:574-577, 1976.

Johnson, S.H., and Grubbs, J.P.: The premature infant's reflex behaviors: effects on the maternal-child relationships, J. Obstet. Gynecol. Neonatal Nurs. **4**:15-21, May/June 1975.

LaRossa, M.M., and Brown, J.V.: Foster grandmothers in the premature nursery, Am. J. Nurs. **82**:1834-1835, 1982.

Miner, H.: Problems and prognosis for the small-for-gestational-age and the premature infant, Am. J. Maternal Child Nurs. **3**:221-226, 1978.

Reid, T.J.: Newborn cyanosis, Am. J. Nurs. **82**:1230-1234, 1982.

Rothfeder, B., and Tiedeman, M.: Feeding the low-birth-weight neonate, Nursing 77 **7**(10):58-59, 1977.

Shalm, B., and Messerly, A.M.: Apnea in the premature infant. An overview of causes and treatment, Nurs. Clin. North Am. **13**:29-37, 1978.

Hyperbilirubinemia, hypoglycemia, and hypocalcemia

The first six hours of life: hypoglycemia in the newborn, module 2, New York, 1977, The National Foundation/March of Dimes.

Gannon, R.G., and Pickett, K.: Jaundice, Am. J. Nurs. **83:**404-407, 1983.

Matulich, N.: Jaundice in the neonate: theory and practice, Curr. Pract. Pediatr. Nurs. **3:**85-97, 1980.

McFadden, E.A., Zaloga, G.P., and Chernow, B.: Hypocalcemia: a medical emergency, Am. J. Nurs. **83:**227-230, 1983.

Taur, K.M.: Physiologic mechanisms in childhood hypoglycemia, Pediatr. Nurs. **9**(5):341-344, 1983.

Tripp, A.: Hyper- and hypocalcemia, Am. J. Nurs. **76**(7):1142, 1145, 1976.

Tufts, F., and Johnson, F.: Neonatal jaundice and phototherapy, Can. Nurse **75:**45-47, 1979.

Respiratory distress syndrome

Affonso, D., and Harris, T.: Continuous positive airway pressure, Am. J. Nurs. **76:**570-575, 1976.

Ennis, S., and Harris, T.R.: Positioning infants with hyaline membrane disease, Am. J. Nurs. **78:**398-401, 1978.

Fowler, M.D.: Idiopathic respiratory distress syndrome of the newborn. In McNall, L.K., and Galeener, J.T., editors: Current practice in obstetric and gynecologic nursing, vol. 1, St. Louis, 1976, The C.V. Mosby Co.

Mason, T.N.: A hand ventilation technique for neonates, Am. J. Maternal Child Nurs.**7:**366-369, 1982.

Sham, B., and Messerly, A.M.: Apnea in the premature infant, Nurs. Clin. North Am. **13:**29-38, 1978.

High-risk related to environmental factors

Bliss, V.J.: Nursing care for infants with neonatal necrotizing enterocolitis, Am. J. Maternal Child Nurs. **1:**37-40, 1976.

Flores, R.N.: Necrotizing enterocolitis, Nurs. Clin. North Am. **13:**39-46, 1978.

Gennaro, S.: Necrotizing enterocolitis: detecting it and treating it, Nursing '80 **80**(1):52-56, 1980.

Strodtbeck, F: Critical care concepts related to neonatal septicemia and septic shock, Crit. Care Q. **4**(1):71-77, 1981.

Infant of the diabetic mother

Dunn, P.: The infant of the diabetic mother, Issues Compr. Pediatr. Nurs. **2**(1):36-48, 1977.

Guthrie, D.W., and Guthrie, R.A.: The infant of the diabetic mother, Am. J. Nurs. **74:**2008-2009, 1974.

Jasper, M.L.: Pregnancy complicated by diabetes—a case study, Am. J. Maternal Child Nurs. **1:**307-312, 1976.

Narcotic addicted infant

Finnegan, L.P., and MacNew, B.A.: Care of the addicted infant, Am. J. Nurs. **74:**685-693, 1974.

Lemons, P.M.: Prenatal addiction: a dual tragedy, Crit. Care Quarterly **4**(1):79-88, 1981.

Lemons, P.K.M.: Victims of addiction. Crit. Care Update **10**(5):12-17, 1983.

Disorders caused by maternal factors

Bahr, J.: Herpesvirus Hominis Type 2 in women and newborns, Am. J. Maternal Child Nurs. **3:**16, 1978.

Brown, S.G.: The devastating effects of congenital rubella, Am. J. Maternal Child Nurs. **4:**171-173, 1979.

Enloe, C.F.: How alcohol affects the developing fetus, Nutr. Today, Sept./Oct. 1980, pp.12-15.

Jemison-Smith, P., and Hamm, P.: Rubella, Crit. Care Update **9**(12):34-36, 1982.

Luke, B.: Maternal alcoholism and fetal alcohol syndrome, Am. J. Nurs. **77:**1924-1926, 1977.

Lynch, J.M.: Helping patients through the recurring nightmare of herpes, Nursing 82, **12:**52-57, 1982.

Powell, J.J.: The tragedy of fetal alcohol syndrome, RN **44**(12):33-35, 92, 94, 96, 1981.

Stagno, S.: Toxoplasmosis, Am. J. Nurs. **80:**720-722, 1980.

Stephens, C.J.: The fetal alcohol syndrome: cause for concern, Am. J. Maternal Child Nurs. **6:**251-256, 1981.

Inborn errors of metabolism

Justice, P., and Smith, G.F.: PKU: phenylketonuria, Am. J. Nurs. **75:**1303-1305, 1975.

Reyzer, N.: Diagnosis: PKU, Am. J. Nurs. **78:**1895-1898, 1978.

Smith, E.J.: Galactosemia: an inborn error of metabolism, Nurse Pract. **5:**8-9, Mar./April 1980.

Wyatt, D.S.: Phenylketonuria: the problems vary during different developmental stages, Am. J. Maternal Child Nurs. **3**(5): 296-302, 1978.

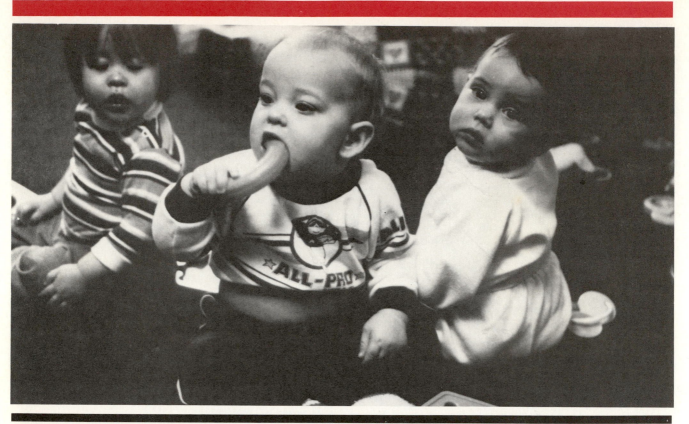

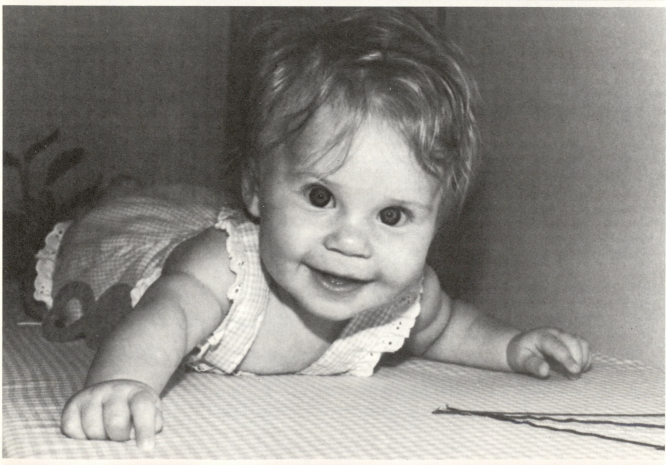

UNIT 4

INFANCY

The first 12 months of childhood is the period of most rapid gain in physical size and most dramatic achievement in developmental milestones of an individual's entire life. It is marked by an orderly progression of physical, intellectual, and social maturation. It is also a highly vulnerable period for both positive and negative influences governing optimum growth and development.

Chapter 8, *The First Year: Laying the Foundation,* investigates the infant's psychosocial, intellectual, biologic, and adaptive development. It is concerned with fostering optimum health through anticipatory guidance regarding nutrition, prevention of disease and accidental injury, and promotion of parent-child attachment. Chapter 9, *Health Problems During the First Year,* deals with health problems that commonly occur during the first year, usually as a result of environmental, rather than pathologic, processes and that therefore are amenable to prevention. It is also concerned with conditions of unknown cause, such as sudden infant death syndrome, which has profound emotional consequences on the developing family.

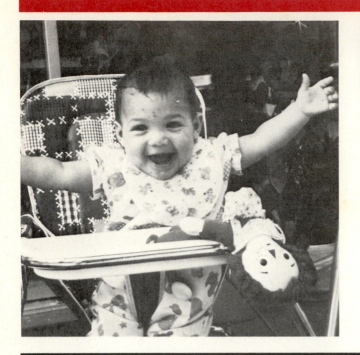

THE FIRST YEAR: LAYING THE FOUNDATION

OBJECTIVES

On completion of this chapter the reader will be able to:

- Identify the major biologic, psychosocial, cognitive, and adaptive developments during the first year

- Relate parent-child attachment, separation anxiety, and stranger fear to developmental achievements during infancy

- Define ''temperament'' and recognize its influence on parenting children of different temperament patterns

- Provide parents with feeding recommendations for infants during the first and second half of infancy

- Outline immunization requirements during infancy

- Administer immunizations safely

- List general contraindications to immunizations

- Provide anticipatory guidance to parents regarding accident prevention based on the infant's developmental achievements

- Provide anticipatory guidance to parents regarding common parental concerns during infancy

NURSING DIAGNOSES

Nursing diagnoses identified for the infant include, but are not restricted to, the following:

Health perception-health management pattern

- Infection, potential for, related to inadequate immunization

- Injury, potential for (poisoning, suffocation, trauma), related to environmental hazards

Nutritional-metabolic pattern

- Nutrition, alterations in: potential for more or less than body requirements, related to (1) knowledge deficit (parental); (2) cultural factors

Activity-exercise pattern

- Self-care deficit, total, related to developmental level

The miracle of birth is surpassed only by the wonder of unfolding in the succeeding months and years. The biologic growth and developmental maturation of the infant are a study of perfection in nature. The nurse's understanding of these processes is essential to the optimum care of the child and family. In order to present relevant data for appreciation of growth and development, it is necessary to systematize and categorize the facts into various levels of maturation and age-groups. However, one must always bear in mind that no child will be represented in any one table or chart, for each child is as much an individual as the number of variables that influence his existence.

GROWTH AND DEVELOPMENT

General concepts of growth and development, such as stages and patterns of development and individual differences, have been discussed in Chapter 2. This chapter is primarily concerned with biologic, psychosocial, cognitive, and adaptive development of the infant from 1 to 12 months of age.

Biologic development

During the first year growth is very rapid, especially during the initial 6 months. Infants gain 680 g (1.5 pounds) a month until age 6 months, when the birth weight has at least doubled. An average weight for a 6-month-old child is 7.26 kg (16 pounds). Weight gain decreases by half that amount during the second 6 months. By 1 year of age the infant's birth weight has tripled for an average weight of 9.75 kg (21.5 pounds).

Height increases by 2.5 cm (1 inch) a month during the first 6 months and half that amount during each of the second 6 months. Average height is 65 cm (25½ inches) at 6 months and 74 cm (29 inches) at 12 months. By 1 year the birth length has increased by almost 50%. The increase in length occurs mainly in the trunk, rather than in the legs, and contributes to the characteristic physique of the infant (see Fig. 8-6, *E*).

Head growth is also rapid. During the first 6 months head circumference increases approximately 1.5 cm (0.6 inch) a month but decreases to only 0.5 cm (0.2 inch) during the second 6 months. The average size is 43 cm (17 inches) at 6 months and 46 cm (18 inches) at 12 months. By 1 year head size has increased by almost 33%.

Another change is closure of the cranial sutures. The posterior fontanel is fused by 6 to 8 weeks of age, and the anterior fontanel closes by 12 to 18 months of age.

Expanding head size reflects the growth and differentiation of the nervous system. By the end of the first year the brain has increased in weight about two and one half

---

Sleep-rest pattern

■ Sleep-pattern disturbance related to fear of separation from parents

Cognitive-perceptual pattern

■ Comfort, alteration in: pain related to teething

Self-perception—self-concept pattern

■ Anxiety related to (1) stranger fear; (2) separation

Role-relationship pattern

■ Parenting, alteration in: potential, related to knowledge deficit (childrearing)

Coping-stress tolerance pattern

■ Coping, family: potential for growth, related to (1) attachment to infant; (2) successful parenting

NEUROLOGIC REFLEXES THAT APPEAR DURING INFANCY

Reflex	Expected Behavioral Response	Age of Appearance (months)
Labyrinth-righting	When infant is in prone or supine position, he is able to raise head	2, strongest at 10
Neck-righting	While infant is supine, head is turned to one side; shoulder, trunk, and finally pelvis will turn toward that side	3, until 24-36
Body-righting	A modification of the neck-righting reflex in which turning hips and shoulders to one side causes all other body parts to follow	6, until 24-36
Otolith-righting	When body of an erect infant is tilted, head is returned to upright, erect position	7-12, persists indefinitely
Landau	When infant is suspended in a horizontal prone position, the head is raised, legs and spine are extended	6-8, until 12-24
Parachute	When infant is suspended in a horizontal prone position and suddenly thrust downward, hands and fingers extend forward as if to protect himself from falling (Fig. 8-1)	7-9, persists indefinitely

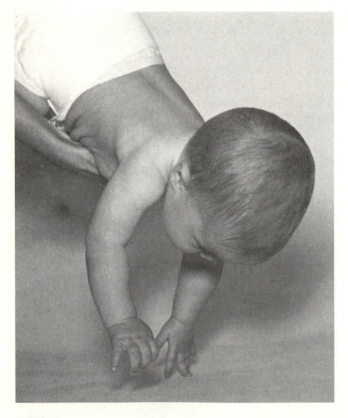

FIG. 8-1
Parachute reflex.

times. The maturation of the brain is exhibited in the dramatic developmental achievements of infancy (see Table 8-1). The primitive reflexes are replaced by voluntary, purposeful movement. New reflexes appear that influence motor development (see boxed material above).

Visual acuity gradually improves and binocular fixation is established. *Binocularity,* or the fixation of two ocular images into one cerebral picture (fusion), begins to develop by 6 weeks of age and should be well established by age 12 months. *Depth perception* (stereopsis) begins to develop by age 7 to 9 months but may exist earlier as an innate safety mechanism against accidental falling.

Other organ systems also change and grow during infancy. The respiratory rate slows somewhat (see inside front cover) and is relatively stable. Respiratory movements continue to be abdominal. Growth of the respiratory tract is gradual. The lumen of the trachea and bronchi enlarges but remains small in comparison to the total size of the lung. Also the ability of the entire respiratory tract to produce mucus is diminished, decreasing the humidification of the large volume of inspired air. In addition, the volume of dead space, that amount of air needed to fill the respiratory passages with each breath, is large, requiring the infant to breath about twice as fast as the adult to provide the body with the needed amount of oxygen.

The chest assumes a more adultlike contour, with the lateral diameter becoming larger than the anteroposterior diameter. The chest circumference approximately equals head circumference by the end of the first year.

The heart rate slows (inside front cover), and the rhythm is frequently *sinus arrhythmia,* in which the rate increases with inspiration and decreases with expiration. The regularity of the rhythm correlates with the respiratory rate: the faster the respiratory rate, the more regular the heartbeat, and the slower the respiratory rate, the more irregular the heartbeat. Consequently, sinus arrhythmia is most obvious during sleep.

The heart grows less rapidly than does the rest of the body. Its weight is usually doubled by 1 year of age in comparison to body weight, which triples during the same period of time. The size of the heart is still large in relation to the chest cavity; its width is about 55% of the width of the chest.

Blood pressure also changes during infancy (inside front cover). The rising systolic pressure is a result of the increasing ability of the left ventricle to pump blood into the systemic circulation. Fluctuations in blood pressure occur during varying states of activity and emotion.

Significant hemopoietic changes occur during the first year (Appendix A). Fetal hemoglobin is present for the first 5 months, with adult hemoglobin forming at about 13 weeks of age. Maternal iron stores are present for the first 5 to 6 months and then gradually diminish, which partially accounts for lowered hemoglobin levels toward the end of the first 6 months. *Physiologic anemia* is seen at 2 to 3 months of age because of the decreasing number of red blood cells. This phenomenon is thought to be caused by the suppression of the hemopoietic system from the high level of fetal hemoglobin, which suppresses the production of erythropoietin, a hormone released by the kidney. The occurrence of physiologic anemia is not affected by an adequate supply of iron. However, when erythropoiesis is stimulated, iron supplies are then necessary for formation of hemoglobin.

The majority of the digestive processes do not begin functioning until age 3 months, when drooling is common because of the poorly coordinated swallowing reflex. The enzyme ptyalin (also called amylase) is present in small amounts but usually has little effect on the foodstuff because of the limited amount of time the food stays in the mouth. Gastric digestion in the stomach consists primarily of the action of hydrochloric acid and rennin, an enzyme that acts specifically on the casein in milk to cause the formation of curds. A curd is a coagulated semisolid particle of milk. Curds cause the milk to be retained in the stomach long enough for digestion to occur.

Digestion also takes place in the duodenum, where pancreatic enzymes and bile begin to break down protein and fat. Secretion of the pancreatic enzyme amylase, which is needed for digestion of complex carbohydrates, is deficient until about the fourth month of life. Lipase is also somewhat limited, especially for highly saturated fats. Trypsin is secreted in sufficient quantities to catabolize protein into polypeptides and some amino acids.

The immaturity of the digestive processes is evident in the appearance of stools. During infancy solid foods, such as peas, carrots, corn, and raisins, are passed incompletely broken down in the feces. Not until the second year are fibrous foods more completely digested. An excess quantity of roughage easily disposes the child to loose, bulky stools.

The rapid peristaltic activity of the gastrointestinal tract slows down throughout infancy, and the stomach enlarges to accommodate a greater volume of food. By the end of the first year the infant is able to tolerate three meals a day and a before-bedtime bottle, and he may have one or two bowel movements daily. Bowel evacuation remains under involuntary, reflexive control until myelination of the spinal cord is complete, usually by 14 to 18 months of age.

Paralleling the ability of the gastrointestinal system to digest and absorb more complex foodstuff is the process of tooth eruption. Tooth eruption occurs in a fairly orderly sequence, although the rate may vary in different children (Fig. 2-6). The first teeth to erupt are the lower central incisors. One incisor will erupt, followed closely by the homologous incisor. These teeth usually are present by 6 to 7 months of age. The upper central incisors erupt by 7 or 8 months of age. The upper lateral incisors erupt at about ages 10 to 12 months, followed by the lower lateral incisors at ages 12 to 14 months. Primary dentition is usually complete by 2½ years of age.

The immunologic system undergoes numerous changes during the first year. The newborn receives significant amounts of maternal IgG, which confers immunity for about 3 months against antigens to which the mother was exposed. During this time the infant begins to synthesize his own IgG, and about 40% of adult levels are reached by 1 year of age. Significant amounts of IgM are produced at birth, and adult levels are reached by 9 months of age. The production of IgA, IgD, and IgE is much more gradual, and maximum levels are not attained until early childhood.

During infancy the ability of the skin to contract and shiver in response to cold increases and serves to regulate body temperature. In response to cold, the capillaries constrict, conserving core body temperature and decreasing potential evaporative heat loss from the skin surface. In response to heat the capillaries dilate, decreasing internal body temperature through evaporation, conduction, and convection. Shivering causes the muscles and muscle fibers to contract, generating metabolic heat, which is distributed throughout the body. Accumulation of adipose tissue serves to insulate the body against heat loss.

Adipose tissue, which is laid down during the last trimester of pregnancy, continues to accumulate during the next 6 months of life. The amount of adipose tissue laid down during infancy probably influences the predisposition to fat accumulation later in life and is an important fact to stress during nutritional counseling.

At birth there is a shift in the total body fluid of the neonate, resulting in a higher level of intracellular fluid to extracellular fluid, probably because of the progressive growth of cells at the expense of extracellular fluid. However, the proportion of extracellular fluid, which is composed of blood plasma, interstitial fluid, and lymph, still remains high in comparison to adult levels and predisposes the infant to a more rapid loss of total body fluid and consequently dehydration.

The immaturity of the renal structures also predisposes the infant to dehydration. Complete maturity of the kidney occurs during the latter half of the second year. Prior to this time the filtration capacity of the glomeruli is reduced.

Psychosocial development

Infants are born with the basic abilities needed for extra-uterine survival, such as respiration, thermoregulation, and digestion. However, they cannot survive without a caregiver to provide for their essential needs, such as food, warmth, and security. In addition to their basic needs, which must be supplied for them, infants have certain tasks that they must achieve for themselves during the first year of life. How their needs are met by others greatly determines to what degree they accomplish their tasks.

Developing a sense of trust. Erikson's phase I (birth to 1 year) is concerned with acquiring a sense of basic *trust* while overcoming a sense of mistrust. The trust acquired in infancy is foundational for all the succeeding phases. It allows the infant a feeling of physical comfort and security, which assists him in experiencing unfamiliar, unknown situations with a minimum of fear. The crucial element for the achievement of this task is the *quality* of the mother (caregiver)-child relationship. The provision of food, warmth, and shelter are alone inadequate for the development of a strong ego. The infant and mother must jointly learn to satisfactorily meet their needs in order for mutual regulation of frustration to occur. When this synchrony fails to develop, mistrust is the eventual outcome.

The acquisition of trust involves the libidinal or psychologic energy of the erotic centers of the body, especially the mouth. Erikson has described particular stages in the oral phase. The first social modality is primarily *oral*. During the first 3 to 4 months, food intake is the most important social activity the infant engages in. The newborn can tolerate little frustration or delay of gratification. Primary *narcissism* (total concern for oneself) is at its height.

However, as bodily processes such as vision, motor movements, and vocalization are better controlled, the infant realizes that the environment requires some adaptation from him in order to mutually meet the needs of all the individuals. For example, crying lessens as the infant uses other means to attract attention. Once he hears his mother's voice, he is able to wait for his needs to be met because he knows that she will be coming to him.

Failure to learn "delayed gratification" leads to mistrust. It can result from too much or too little frustration. If the mother always meets the child's needs before he signals his readiness, the infant will never learn to test his ability to control the environment. If the delay is prolonged, the infant will experience constant frustration and eventually mistrust others in their efforts to satisfy him.

The next social modality involves an incorporative mode of reaching out to others through *grasping*. Initially grasping is reflexive, but even as a reflex it has a powerful social meaning to the parents. The reciprocal response to the infant's grasping is the parents' holding on and touching. There is pleasurable tactile stimulation for both the child and parents.

Tactile stimulation is extremely important in the total process of acquiring trust. In fact, the degree of mothering skill, the quantity of food, or the length of sucking does not determine the quality of the experience. Rather, it is the total nature of the quality of the interpersonal relationship that influences the infant's formulation of trust.

During the second incorporative stage, the more active and aggressive modality of *biting* occurs. The infant learns that he can hold on to what is his own and can more fully control his environment. During this stage the infant may be confronted with one of his first conflicts. If he is breast-feeding, he quickly learns that biting causes withdrawal of the nipple and anxiety in the mother. Yet biting also brings internal relief from teething discomfort and a sense of power or control.

This conflict may be solved in a variety of ways. The mother may wean the infant from the breast and begin bottle-feeding. The infant may learn to bite substitute "nipples," such as a pacifier, and retain pleasurable breast-feeding. The successful resolution of this conflict strengthens the mother-child relationship because it occurs at a time when the infant is recognizing her as the most significant person in his life.

Cognitive development

Intellectual development is concurrent with biologic, adaptive, and psychosocial achievement. In fact, many of these must occur before learning can take place. For example, visual ability must be sufficient for the infant to see objects clearly before associations about the object can be made. As motor function progresses, learning occurs through the infant's more active participation in the environment.

The theory frequently quoted to explain *cognition,* or the ability to know, is by Jean Piaget, who referred to the period of birth to 24 months as the *sensorimotor phase*. During this phase the infant progresses from reflex behavior to simple repetitive acts to imitative activity.

Three crucial events take place during this phase. First, the infant learns to separate himself from other objects in the environment. In Freudian terms, the infant progresses from the id stage to ego development. He realizes that others besides himself control the environment and that certain readjustments must take place for mutual satisfaction to occur. This coincides with Erikson's concept of the formation of trust and mutual regulation of frustration.

The second major achievement is perceiving the concept of *permanency,* or the realization that objects that leave one's visual field still exist. A typical example of the development of object permanency is the infant's ability to separate from his parents at bedtime because of his realization that they will be present when he awakens. Eventually he broadens this concept to tolerate brief periods of separation with a different caregiver.

The last major intellectual development of this period is the ability to use symbols or "mental representation." The use of symbols allows the infant to think of an object or situation without actually experiencing it. The recognition of symbols is the beginning of understanding of time and space.

The sensorimotor phase is composed of six stages. The first stage, from birth to 1 month, is identified by the *use of reflexes.* At birth the infant's individuality and temperament are expressed through the physiologic reflexes of sucking, rooting, grasping, and crying. The repetitious nature of the reflexes is the beginning of associations between an act and a sequential response. When the infant cries because he is hungry, a nipple is put in his mouth, and he sucks, feels satisfaction, and sleeps.

The next stage, *primary circular reactions,* marks the beginning of the replacement of reflexive behavior with voluntary acts. During this period from 1 to 4 months, activities such as sucking or grasping become deliberate acts that elicit certain responses. The infant incorporates and adapts his reactions to the environment and recognizes the stimulus that produced a response. Previously the infant would cry until the nipple was brought to his mouth. Now he will associate the nipple with the sound of the mother's voice. He accommodates this new piece of information and adapts by ceasing to cry when he hears her voice, before he receives the nipple.

The next stage, *secondary circular reactions,* is a continuation of the previous one and lasts until 8 months of age. In this stage the circular primary reactions are repeated and prolonged for the response that results. Grasping and holding now become shaking, banging, and pulling. Shaking is performed to hear a noise, not solely for the pleasure of shaking. Quality and quantity of an act become evident. "More" or "less" shaking produces different responses. Causality, time, deliberate intention, and one's separateness from the environment begin to develop.

Three new processes of human behavior—imitation, play, and affect—occur. *Imitation* requires the differentiation of selected acts from several events. By the second half of the first year, the infant can imitate sounds and simple gestures. *Play* becomes evident as the infant takes pleasure in performing an act after he has mastered it. Much of the infant's waking hours are absorbed in sensorimotor play. *Affect* is seen as the infant begins to develop a sense of permanency. During the first 6 months the in-

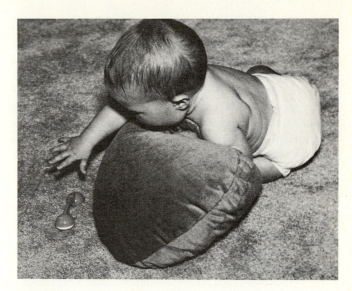

FIG. 8-2

Nine-month-old infant actively searches for object hidden behind pillow.

fant believes that an object exists only for as long as he can visually perceive it. In other words, out of sight—out of mind. When the object continues to be present or remembered even though it is beyond the range of perception, affect to external objects is evident. Object permanence is a critical component of parent-child attachment and is seen in the development of stranger anxiety at 6 to 8 months of age (p. 237).

During the fourth sensorimotor stage, *coordination of secondary schemata and its application to new situations,* the infant uses previous behavioral achievements primarily as the foundation for adding new intellectual skills to his expanding repertoire. This stage from 9 to 12 months is largely transitional. Increasing motor skills allow for greater exploration of the environment. The child begins to discover that hiding an object does not mean that it is gone and that removing an obstacle will reveal the object (Fig. 8-2). This marks the beginning of intellectual reasoning. Furthermore, he can experience an event by *observing* it, and he begins to associate symbols with events, such as "bye-bye" with "Daddy goes to work," but the classification is purely his own. Unlike the second stage, where the infant learned from the type of interaction between objects or individuals, in this stage the child learns from the object itself. Intentionality is further developed in that now the infant will actively attempt to remove a barrier to his desired (or undesired) action. If something is in his way, he will attempt to climb over it or push it away. Previously an obstacle would cause him to give up any further attempt to achieve his desired goal.

The last two stages occur during the toddler period of 12 to 24 months. These are discussed in Chapter 10.

Adaptive behaviors

As biologic maturation progresses, there is a concurrent development of behaviors that increasingly allow the infant to respond to and cope with the environment. These adaptive behaviors can be classified into various categories: (1) gross motor, (2) fine motor, (3) language, and (4) personal-social. The acquisition of skill in each area occurs in an orderly sequence, following the usual cephalocaudal-proximodistal laws.

Knowledge of the developmental sequence allows the nurse to assess normal growth as well as minor or abnormal deviations. Knowledge of developmental milestones helps parents gain realistic expectations of their child's ability and provides guidelines for suitable play and stimulation. Emphasizing the child's *developmental age* rather than chronologic age strengthens the parent-child relationship by fostering trust and lessening frustration. Therefore, one cannot overemphasize the importance of a thorough understanding and appreciation of the growth and developmental process of children. A summary of growth and development is presented in Table 8-1.

Gross motor behavior. Gross motor behavior includes developmental maturation in posture, head balance, sitting, creeping, standing, and walking.

Head control. The full-term newborn can momentarily hold the head in midline and parallel when the body is suspended ventrally and can lift and turn the head from side to side when prone. However, marked head lag is evident when the infant is pulled from a lying to a sitting position. By 3 months of age the infant can hold his head well beyond the plane of his body, and by 4 months of age he can lift the head and front portion of the chest about 90 degrees above the table, bearing his weight on the forearms. Only slight head lag is evident when the infant is pulled from a lying to a sitting position and by 4 to 6 months head control is well established (Figs. 8-3 and 8-4).

TABLE 8-1. SUMMARY OF GROWTH AND DEVELOPMENT DURING INFANCY*

AGE (months)	PHYSICAL	GROSS MOTOR	FINE MOTOR
Birth-1	Weight gain of 150 to 210 g (5 to 7 ounces) weekly for first 6 months Height gain of 2.5 cm (1 inch) monthly for first 6 months Head circumference increased by 1.5 cm monthly for first 6 months Primitive reflexes present and strong Obligatory nose breather	• Assumes flexed position with pelvis high, but knees not under abdomen when prone (at birth, knees are flexed under abdomen) • Can turn head from side to side when prone, lifts head momentarily from bed Marked head lag, especially when pulled from lying to sitting position Holds head momentarily parallel and in midline when suspended in prone position Assumes asymmetric tonic neck reflex position when supine	Hands predominantly closed Grasp reflex strong Hand clenches on contact with rattle
2	Posterior fontanel closed Crawling reflex disappears	• Assumes less flexed position when prone—hips flat, legs extended, arms flexed, head to side Less head lag when pulled to sitting position Can maintain head in same plane as rest of body when held in ventral suspension When prone, can lift head almost 45 degrees off table When held in sitting position, head is held up but bobs forward	Hands frequently open Grasp reflex fading

*Milestones that represent essential integrative aspects of development that lay the foundation for the achievement of more advanced skills are indicated by a bullet.

Rolling over. The newborn may roll over accidentally because of his rounded back. The ability to willfully turn from the abdomen to the back occurs at 5 months and from the back to the abdomen at 6 months. It is noteworthy that the parachute reflex, which elicits a protective response to falling, appears at 7 months.

Sitting. The ability to sit follows progressive head control and straightening of the back as shown in Fig. 8-5. For the first 2 to 3 months the back is uniformly rounded. The convex cervical curve forms at about 3 to 4 months when head control is established. The convex lumbar curve appears when the child begins to sit, about age 4 months. As the spinal column straightens, the infant is able to be propped in a sitting position. By ages 6 to 7 months he can sit alone, leaning forward on his hands for support. By ages 7 to 8 months he can sit well unsupported and begins to explore his surroundings in this position rather than in a lying position.

Locomotion. Locomotion involves acquiring the ability to bear weight, propel forward on all four extremities, stand upright with support, and finally walk alone (Fig. 8-6). By 6 to 7 months the infant is able to bear all his weight. By 9 months he stands holding on to furniture and can pull himself to the standing position but is unable to maneuver himself back down, except by falling. He also can crawl on all fours with his belly on the floor. At first crawling is often in reverse direction because the flexor muscles are stronger than the extensors. At 10 months he steps with one foot and crawls well. By 11 months he creeps (belly off the floor) and walks while holding onto furniture or with both hands held. By 1 year he may be able to walk with one hand held.

Fine motor behavior. Fine motor behavior includes the use of the hands and fingers in the prehension (grasp) of an object. Grasping occurs during the first 2 to 3 months as a reflex and gradually becomes voluntary. At

SENSORY	SPEECH/LANGUAGE	SOCIALIZATION/COGNITION
• Able to fixate on moving object Follows light to midline Quiets when hears a voice Visual acuity 20/50	Cries to express displeasure Makes small throaty sounds Makes comfort sounds during feeding	Watches parent's face intently as she or he talks to infant Totally autistic (self-centered)
Binocular fixation and convergence to near objects beginning When supine, follows dangling toy from side to point beyond midline Visually searches to locate sounds Turns head to side when sound is made at level of ear	• Vocalizes, distinct from crying Crying becomes differentiated Coos Vocalizes to familiar voice	• Social smile in response to various stimuli Visually prefers people to objects Excites in anticipation of objects

Continued.

TABLE 8-1. SUMMARY OF GROWTH AND DEVELOPMENT DURING INFANCY—cont'd

AGE (months)	PHYSICAL	GROSS MOTOR	FINE MOTOR
3	Primitive reflexes fading Landau reflex appears	Able to hold head more erect when sitting, but still bobs forward Only slight head lag when pulled to sitting Assumes symmetric body positioning Able to raise head and shoulders from prone position to a 45- to 90-degree angle from table; bears weight on forearms When held in standing position, able to bear slight fraction of weight on legs Regards own hand	Grasp reflex absent Hands kept loosely open • Actively holds rattle, but will not reach for it Clutches own hand, pulls at blankets and clothes
4	Drooling begins • Moro, tonic neck, and rooting reflexes have disappeared	• Almost no head lag when pulled to sitting position • Balances head well in sitting position Able to raise head and chest off couch to angle of 90 degrees Assumes predominantly symmetric position Rolls from back to side Able to sit erect if propped up	• Inspects and plays with hands, pulls clothing or blanket over face in play Tries to reach objects with hand but overshoots it Grasps object with both hands Plays with rattle placed in hand, shakes it, but cannot pick it up if dropped Can carry objects to mouth
5	Growth rate may begin to decline Beginning signs of tooth eruption Able to breathe when nose is obstructed	No head lag when pulled to sitting position When sitting, able to hold head erect and steady Able to sit for longer periods when back is well supported Back straight When prone, assumes symmetric positioning with arms extended When held in standing position, able to bear most of weight Can turn over from abdomen to back When supine, puts feet to mouth	• Able to grasp objects voluntarily Uses palmar grasp, bidexterous approach Plays with toes Holds one cube while regarding a second
6	Birth weight doubled Weight gain of 90 to 150 g (3 to 5 ounces) weekly for next 6 months Height gain of 1.25 cm (½ inch) monthly for next 6 months Teething may begin with eruption of two lower central incisors • Chewing and biting occur	When prone, can lift chest and upper abdomen off table, bearing weight on hands Sits in high chair with back straight Rolls from back to abdomen When held in standing position, bears almost all of weight	Resecures a dropped object Drops one cube when another is given Grasps and manipulates small objects Holds bottle Grasps feet and pulls to mouth

SENSORY	SPEECH/LANGUAGE	SOCIALIZATION/COGNITION
• Follows object to periphery (180 degrees) Locates sound by turning head to side and looking in same direction Begins to have ability to coordinate stimuli from various sense organs	• Squeals aloud to show pleasure Coos, babbles, and chuckles Vocalizes when smiling "Talks" a great deal when spoken to Less crying during periods of wakefulness	Much interest in surroundings Ceases crying when parent enters room Can recognize familiar faces and objects, such as feeding bottle
Able to accommodate to near objects Binocular vision fairly well established Can focus on a ½-inch block Beginning eye-hand coordination	Makes consonant sounds n, k, g, p, b Laughs aloud Vocalization changes according to mood	Demands attention by fussing; becomes bored if left alone Enjoys social interaction with people Anticipates feeding when sees bottle Shows excitement with whole body, squeals, breathes heavily Shows interest in strange stimuli Begins to show memory; aware of strange surroundings
Visually pursues a dropped object Able to sustain visual inspection of an object Can localize sounds made below the ear	• Squeals Vowel-like cooing sounds interspersed with consonantal sounds (for example, ah-goo)	Smiles at mirror image Pats bottle with both hands More enthusiastically playful, but may have rapid mood swings Able to discriminate strangers from family Vocalizes displeasure when an object is taken away Discovers parts of body
Adjusts posture to see an object Prefers more complex visual stimuli Can localize sounds made above the ear Will turn head to the side, then look up or down	• Begins to imitate sounds Babbling resembles one-syllable utterances—ma, mu, da, di, hi Laughs aloud Takes pleasure in hearing own sounds (self-reinforcement)	Recognizes parents; begins to fear strangers Holds arms out to be picked up Has definite likes and dislikes Beginning of imitation (cough, protrusion of tongue) Excites on hearing footsteps Briefly searches for a dropped object (object permanence beginning) Frequent mood swings—from crying to laughing with little or no provocation

Continued.

TABLE 8-1. SUMMARY OF GROWTH AND DEVELOPMENT DURING INFANCY—cont'd

AGE (months)	PHYSICAL	GROSS MOTOR	FINE MOTOR
7	Eruption of upper central incisors	• When supine, spontaneously lifts head off table • Sits, leaning forward on both hands Sits erect momentarily Bears full weight on feet When held in standing position, bounces actively	• Transfers objects from one hand to the other Bangs cube on table Rakes at a small object
8	Begins to show regular patterns in bladder and bowel elimination Parachute reflex appears	Sits steadily unsupported Readily bears weight on legs when supported, may stand holding on	Beginning pincer grasp using the index, fourth, and fifth fingers against the lower part of the thumb Releases objects at will Secures an object by pulling on a string Reaches persistently for toys out of reach
9	Eruption of upper lateral incisor may begin	Crawls, may progress backward at first Sits steadily on floor for prolonged time (10 minutes) Recovers balance when leans forward but cannot do so when leaning sideways Stands holding onto furniture Pulls self to standing position	• Ability to use thumb and index finger in crude pincer grasp Preference for use of dominant hand now evident
10		Crawls by pulling self forward with hands Can change from prone to sitting position Pulls self to sitting position Stands while holding onto furniture, sits by falling down While standing, lifts one foot to take a step	Crude release of an object beginning
11	Eruption of lower lateral incisors may begin	• Creeps with abdomen off floor Cruises or walks holding onto furniture	Can hold crayon to make a mark on paper Explores objects more thoroughly (for example, clapper inside bell)
12	Birth weight tripled Birth length increased by 50% Has total of six to eight deciduous teeth Anterior fontanel almost closed Landau reflex fading Babinski reflex disappears Lumbar curve develops, lordosis evident during walking	May attempt to stand alone momentarily Can sit down from standing position without help Walks with one hand held	• Neat pincer grasp Drops object deliberately for it to be picked up Puts one object after another into a container (sequential play) Releases cube in cup Attempts to build two-block tower but fails Tries to insert a pellet into a narrow-neck bottle but fails Can turn pages in a book, many at a time

SENSORY	SPEECH/LANGUAGE	SOCIALIZATION/COGNITION
• Can fixate on very small objects Responds to own name Localizes sound by turning head in a curving arch Beginning awareness of depth and space Has taste preferences	• Produces vowel sounds and chained syllables—baba, dada, kaka Vocalizes four distinct vowel sounds "Talks" when others are talking	• Increasing fear of strangers; shows signs of fretfulness when mother disappears Imitates simple acts and noises Tries to attract attention by coughing and snorting Plays peekaboo Demonstrates dislike of food by keeping lips closed Exhibits oral aggressiveness in biting and mouthing • Looks briefly for toy that disappears
	Makes consonant sounds t, d, and w Listens selectively to familiar words Combines syllables, such as dada, but does not ascribe meaning to them	Increasing anxiety over loss of parent, particularly mother, and fear of strangers Responds to word "no" Dislikes dressing, diaper change
Localizes sound by turning head diagonally and directly toward sound Depth perception increasing	Responds to simple verbal commands Comprehends "no-no"	Parent (mother) is increasingly important for own sake Increasing interest in pleasing mother Begins to show fears of going to bed and being left alone • Searches for an object if he sees it hidden
	• Says dada, mama with meaning Comprehends bye-bye May say one word (for example, "hi, bye, what, no")	Inhibits behavior to verbal command of "no-no" or own name Imitates facial expressions, waves bye-bye Extends toy to another person but will not release it Looks around a corner or under a pillow for an object Repeats actions that attract attention and are laughed at Pulls clothes of another to attract attention Plays interactive games such as pat-a-cake Reacts to adult anger, cries when scolded Demonstrates independence in dressing, feeding, locomotive skills, and testing of parents Looks at and follows pictures in a book
	Imitates definite speech sounds Uses jargon	Experiences joy and satisfaction when a task is mastered Reacts to restrictions with frustration
Discriminates simple geometric forms (for example, circle) Amblyopia may develop with lack of binocularity Can follow rapidly moving object Controls and adjusts response to sound; will listen for sound to recur	• Says two or more words besides dada, mama Comprehends meaning of several words (comprehension always precedes verbalization) Recognizes objects by name Imitates animal sounds Understands simple verbal commands (for example, "Give it to me," "Show me your eyes")	Shows emotions such as jealousy, affection (may give hug or kiss on request), anger, fear Shakes head for "no" Enjoys familiar surroundings and will explore away from mother Fearful in strange situation, clings to mother May develop habit of "security blanket" or favorite toy Unceasing determination to practice locomotor skills • Searches for an object even if he hasn't seen it hidden, but only where it was last seen

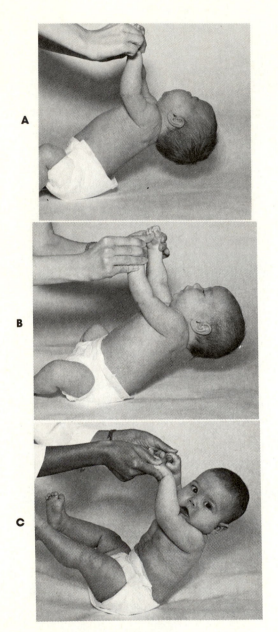

FIG. 8-3
Head control while pulled to sitting. **A,** *Complete head lag at 1 month.* **B,** *Partial head lag at 2 months.* **C,** *Almost no head lag at 4 months.*

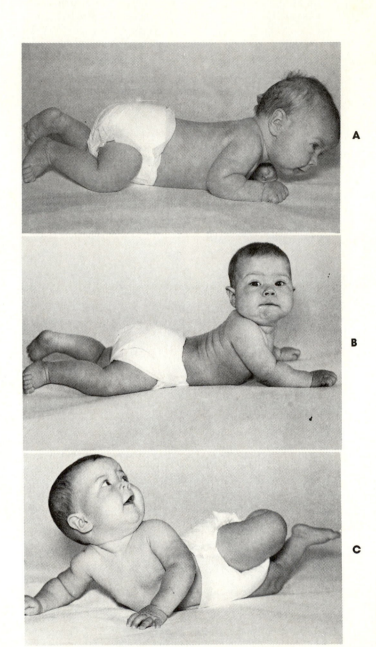

FIG. 8-4
Head control while prone. **A,** *Momentarily lifts head at 1 month.* **B,** *Lifts head and chest 90 degrees and bears weight on forearms at 4 months.* **C,** *Lifts head, chest and upper abdomen and can bear weight on hands at 6 months. Note how this position facilitates turning from abdomen to back.*

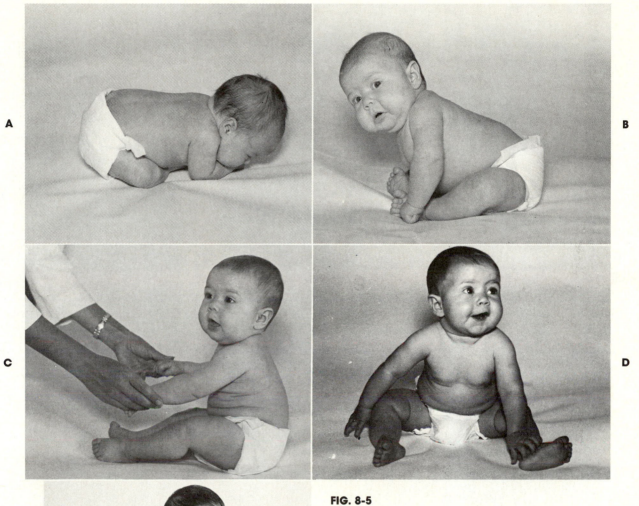

FIG. 8-5

Development of sitting. **A,** *Back is completely rounded, and infant has no ability to sit upright at 1 month.* **B,** *Back is still rounded, but infant can sit up momentarily with some head control at 2 months.* **C,** *Back is rounded only in lumbar area, and infant is able to sit erect with good head control at 4 months.* **D,** *Infant can sit alone, leaning on hands for support at 7 months.* **E,** *Infant sits without support at 8 months. Note transferring of objects that occurs at 7 months.*

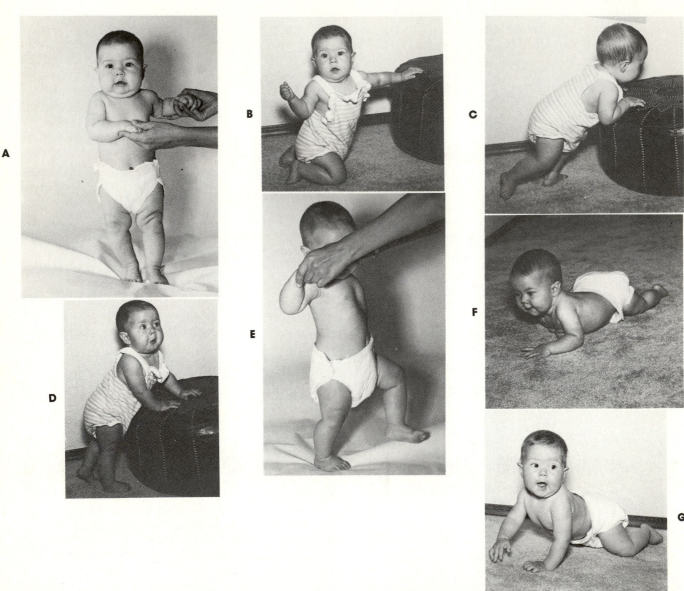

FIG. 8-6

Development of locomotion. **A,** *Infant bears full weight on feet by 7 months.* **B,** *Infant can maneuver from sitting to kneeling position.* **C,** *Infant can pull self to standing position, and* **D,** *infant can stand holding onto furniture at 9 months.* **E,** *While standing, infant takes deliberate step at 10 months.* **F,** *Infant crawls with abdomen on floor and pulls self forward with hands at 10 months.* **G,** *Infant creeps on hands and knees at 11 months.*

1 month the hands are predominantly closed and by 3 months are mostly open. By this time the infant demonstrates a desire to grasp an object, but he "grasps" it more with the eyes than with the hands. If a rattle is placed in his hand, he will actively hold onto it. By 4 months he regards both a small pellet and his hands then will look from the object to his hands and back again. Hand regard is common at this age because of the limitation of symmetric positioning that prevents the infant from exploring the periphery. Hand regard occurs in children who are blind because it is a developmental process that occurs without visual stimulation. By 5 months the infant is able to voluntarily grasp an object.

Gradually the palmar grasp (using the whole hand) is replaced with a pincer grasp (using the thumb and index finger). By 8 to 9 months the infant uses a crude pincer grasp but by 11 months has progressed to a neat pincer grasp (Fig. 8-7).

By 6 months the infant has increased manipulative skill. He holds his bottle, grasps his feet and pulls them to his mouth, and feeds himself a cracker. By 7 months he transfers objects from one hand to the other, employs one hand for grasping, and holds a cube in each hand simultaneously. He enjoys banging objects and will explore movable parts in a toy.

By 10 months pincer grasp is sufficiently established to enable the infant to pick up a raisin and other finger foods. He can deliberately let go of an object and will offer it to someone.

By 11 months he puts objects into a container and likes to remove them. By 1 year the infant tries to build a tower of two blocks but fails.

Language behavior. The infant is a very verbal being. His first means of verbal communication is crying and he learns to signal displeasure before pleasure. Vocalizations heard during crying eventually become the syllables and the words of the child. A classic example is the "mama" heard during vigorous crying. The infant vocalizes as early as 5 to 6 weeks of age by making small throaty sounds. By 2 months he makes single vowel sounds, such as ah, eh, and uh. By 3 to 4 months the consonants n, k, g, p, and b are added, and the infant coos, gurgles, and laughs aloud. By 8 months he adds the consonants t, d, and w and combines syllables, such as "dada," but does not ascribe meaning to the word until ages 10 to 11 months. By 9 to 10 months he comprehends the meaning of the word "no," obeys simple commands, and responds to his name. By age 1 year he can say two to three words with meaning.

During the acquisition of new language skills the child temporarily may give up other recently learned sounds or words. This is often distressing for parents after waiting in anticipation for the words "dada" or "mama." However, these sounds are frequently given up for other vocalizations and may not be repeated for several weeks. It is reassuring for parents to know that the child will again say these words, probably with meaning.

Personal-social behavior. Personal-social behavior includes the child's personal responses to his environment. It is the area most influenced by external stimuli but,

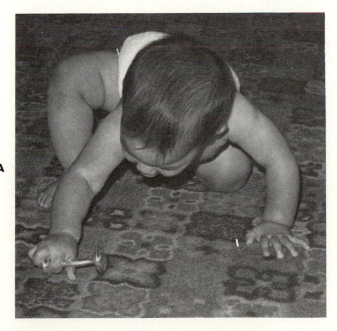
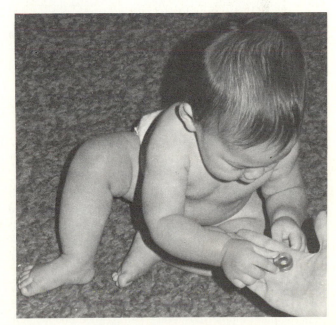

FIG. 8-7

A, *Crude pincer grasp.* **B,** *Neat pincer grasp.*

as in the other fields of behavior, follows certain developmental laws. Personal-social behavior implies communication with one's self and with others. It is foundational for the successful mastery of skills such as feeding, control of bodily functions, independence, and cooperativeness in play.

Recently research has confirmed what parents knew all along—that infants are responsive, social beings. They have the ability to shape their environment and to elicit certain responses. The newborn shows visual preference for the human face and, as early as 1 week of age, begins to watch his mother intently as she speaks to him. By ages 6 to 8 weeks a social smile in response to pleasurable stimuli is present. This has a profound effect on family members and is a tremendous stimulus for evoking continued responses from others. By 3 months he shows considerable interest in the environment: excitement when a toy is presented, refusal to be left alone, recognition of mother, and demonstration of pleasure by squealing. By 4 months he laughs aloud and enjoys strange, novel stimuli.

By age 6 months the infant is a very personable child. He plays games such as peekaboo when his head is hidden in a towel, he signals his desire to be picked up by extending his arms, and he shows displeasure when a toy is removed or his face is washed. There is increasing demonstration of his ability to control his environment. The acquisition of fine and gross motor skills allows him much more independence in movement.

By the second half of the first year the infant understands simple discipline, such as the meaning of the word "no" or a scolding remark. He comprehends different facial expressions and is sensitive to emotional changes in others. Imitation and independence are developing during this time. He is learning to feed himself and use a spoon and cup. He can help with dressing by putting his foot out for a shoe or pushing his arm through the sleeve. He not only comprehends the meaning of "no" but also shakes his head to signal his understanding. He can follow simple directions and will gladly perform for others to attract and prolong their attention.

Play

Play mirrors all of the developmental tasks and allows children to experiment safely with their newly learned skills. Play during infancy is representative of the various social modalities proposed by Erikson. The infant's activity is primarily narcissistic, revolving around his own body. At 2 months of age the infant will look at his extended hand as if it were an unfamiliar object. At about age 6 months the infant plays with his feet and finds fingers excellent nipple substitutes. During this time the ability to grasp is well under voluntary control, and everything is reached for and brought to the mouth for inquisitive ex-

ploration. When the pincer grasp is mastered, the infant is absorbed with growing independence, refusing to allow others to feed him.

At the same time, locomotion skills are developing rapidly, bringing previously unattainable areas within easy access. The infant is thus facing another conflict by learning the meaning of the word "no." His new independence in gross motor skills necessitates his learning and adapting to limits within his environment. This is another important time for child and parents since it represents the beginning of discipline and further delayed gratification.

Play reflects the infant's social development and his increasing awareness of the environment. From birth to age 3 months the infant's response to the environment is global and largely undifferentiated. Play is dependent; pleasure is demonstrated by a quieting attitude (age 1 month), later by a smile (age 2 months), and then by a squeal (age 3 months). From ages 3 to 6 months the infant shows more discriminate interest in the stimuli presented to him and begins to play alone with a rattle or soft stuffed toy or to play with someone else. There is much more interaction during play. By 4 months of age he laughs aloud, shows preference for certain toys, and is excited when food or a favorite object is brought to him.

By 6 months to 1 year of age, play is much more sophisticated and involves sensorimotor skills. Actual games are played, such as peekaboo, pat-a-cake, verbal repetition, and imitation of simple gestures in response to demonstration. Play is much more selective, not only in terms of specific toys but also in terms of "playmates." Although play is solitary or one-sided, the infant chooses with whom he will interact. At 6 to 8 months of age he usually refuses to play with strangers until he begins to know them. Parents are definite favorites, and he knows how to attract their attention. At 6 months he extends his arms to be picked up, at 7 months he coughs to make his presence known, at age 10 months he pulls the parent's clothing, and at 1 year he calls them by name. This represents a tremendous advance from the newborn who signaled biologic needs by crying to express displeasure.

Stimulation is as important for developmental growth as food is for biologic growth. Knowledge of developmental milestones allows nurses to guide parents regarding proper play for infants. It is not sufficient to place a mobile over a crib and toys in a playpen for a child's optimum social, emotional, and intellectual development. Play must provide interpersonal contact, as well as recreational and educational stimulation. Infants need to be *played with*, not merely allowed *to play*. Although the type of play infants engage in is called *solitary*, this is only a figurative, not literal, term to denote one-sided play. The kind of toys given to the child is much less important than the quality of personal interaction that occurs.

Table 8-2 lists play activities that are appropriate for

the developmental level of the infant in view of motor, language, and personal-social achievements. Although the activities are grouped according to the major mode of stimulation provided, there is overlap in many instances. In addition play activities suggested for one age-group may be appropriate for an older age-group but are generally inappropriate for a younger age-group.

PROMOTING OPTIMUM DEVELOPMENT

Although growth and development proceed in an orderly, predetermined sequence, environment does influence optimum development. No aspect of the environment is more important than the quality of emotional care that the infant receives, and the importance of human physical contact cannot be overemphasized. Parenting is not an instinctual

TABLE 8-2. PLAY DURING INFANCY

AGE (months)	VISUAL STIMULATION	AUDITORY STIMULATION	TACTILE STIMULATION	KINETIC STIMULATION
Suggested activities				
Birth-1	Look at infant within close range Hang bright, shiny object within 20-25 cm (8-10 inches) of infant's face and in midline	Talk to infant, sing in soft voice Play music box, radio, television Have ticking clock or metronome nearby	Hold, caress, cuddle Keep infant warm May like to be swaddled	Rock infant, place in cradle Use carriage for walks
2-3	Provide bright objects Make room bright with pictures or mirrors on walls Take infant to various rooms while doing chores Place him in infant seat for vertical view of environment	Talk to infant Include in family gatherings Expose to various environmental noises other than those of home Use rattles, wind chimes	Caress infant while bathing, at diaper change Comb hair with a soft brush	Use cradle gym or swing Take in car for rides Exercise body by moving extremities in swimming motion
4-6	Place infant so that he can look in mirror Place in front of television with family Give brightly colored toys to hold (small enough to grasp)	Talk to infant, repeat sounds he makes Laugh when he laughs Call him by name Crinkle different papers by his ear Place rattle or bell in hand, show him how to shake them	Give infant soft squeeze toys of various textures Allow to splash in bath Place nude on soft furry rug and move extremities	Use swing or stroller Bounce infant in lap while holding him in standing position Help him roll over Support him in sitting position, let him lean forward to balance himself Put him in an open box and tilt gently
Suggested toys				
	Nursery mobiles Unbreakable mirrors See-through crib bumpers Contrasting-colored sheets *Tracking tube *Visual panels	Music boxes Musical mobiles Crib dangle bells Small-handled clear rattle *Spin-a-round	Stuffed animals Soft clothes Soft or furry quilt Soft mobiles	Crib exerciser Crib gym Rocking crib/cradle Weighted or suction toy

*These toys are from a specially designed series called Playpath Playthings produced as part of the Johnson & Johnson Baby Products Child Development Program. They are available for purchase; information can be obtained by writing to Johnson & Johnson, Grandview Rd., Skillman, NJ 08558.

Continued.

TABLE 8-2. PLAY DURING INFANCY—cont'd

AGE (months)	VISUAL STIMULATION	AUDITORY STIMULATION	TACTILE STIMULATION	KINETIC STIMULATION
Suggested activities				
6-9	Give infant large toys with bright colors, movable parts, and noisemakers Infant enjoys mirror, pats it, talks to image Infant enjoys peekaboo, especially hiding his face in a towel Make funny faces to encourage imitation Give him paper to tear, crumble Give him ball of yarn or string to pull apart	Call infant by name Repeat simple words such as "dada, mama, bye-bye" Speak clearly Name parts of body, people, and foods Tell him what you are doing Use word "no" only when necessary Give simple commands Show him how to clap hands, bang a drum	Let infant play with various textures of fabric Have bowl with foods of different size and textures to feel Let him "catch" running water Encourage "swimming" in large bathtub or shallow pool Give wad of sticky tape to manipulate	Use walker Place infant on floor to crawl, roll over, sit Hold upright to bear weight and bounce Pick up—say "up" Put down—say "down" Place toys out of reach; encourage him to get them Play pat-a-cake
9-12	Show infant large pictures in books Take him to places where there are animals, many people, different objects (shopping center) Play ball by rolling it to child, demonstrate "throwing" it back Demonstrate building a two-block tower	Read infant simple nursery rhymes Point to body parts and name each one Imitate sounds of animals	Give infant finger foods of different textures Let him mess and squash food Let him feel cold (ice cube) or warm objects, say what temperature each is Let him feel a breeze (fan blowing)	Use walker Give large push-pull toys to encourage walking Place furniture in a circle to encourage cruising Encourage "roughhouse" play, turn in different positions
Suggested toys				
	Various colored blocks Nested boxes or cups Books with rhymes and bright pictures Strings of big beads and snap beads Simple take-apart toys Large ball Cup and spoon *Fitting forms Large puzzles	Rattles of different sizes, shapes, tones, and bright colors Squeaky animals and dolls Records with light, rhythmic music *Balls in a bowl	Soft, different textured animals and dolls Sponge toys, floating toys Squeeze toys Teething toys Books with textures/objects, such as fur and zipper	Exercise crib toy Activity box for crib Push-pull toys Walker Swing

*These toys are from a specially designed series called Playpath Playthings produced as part of the Johnson & Johnson Baby Products Child Development Program. They are available for purchase; information can be obtained by writing to Johnson & Johnson, Grandview Rd., Skillman, NJ 08558.

ability but a learned, acquired process. The attachment of parent and child probably begins before birth. Recently the importance of the first few hours of life has been studied and recognized. It is the nurse's responsibility to promote parent-child bonding through each stage of development, especially during infancy when the foundation of trust is being formed.

Attachment

Several components are crucial in the process of attachment. Some of them, such as the maternal sensitive period and paternal engrossment, have been discussed in Chapter 6 and emphasize the importance of the first hour and days of life. The following is a discussion of attachment after the neonatal period. Although the word "mother" is frequently used, it does not refer exclusively to the biologic mother but to the consistent caregiver with whom the child relates more than anyone else. In society's changing social climate and sex role stereotypes, this may very well be the father.

During infancy attachment progresses with the child assuming an increasingly significant role. Two components of cognitive development are required for attachment: (1) the ability to discriminate the mother from other individuals and (2) the achievement of object permanence. Both of these processes prepare the infant for an equally important aspect of attachment—separation from the parent.

During the formation of attachment to the parent the infant progresses through four distinct but overlapping stages. For the first few weeks the infant responds indiscriminately to anyone. Beginning at about 8 to 12 weeks of age, the infant cries, smiles, and vocalizes more to the mother than to anyone else but continues to respond to others, whether familiar or not. At about age 6 months the infant shows a distinct preference for the mother. He follows her more, cries when she leaves, enjoys playing with her more, and feels most secure in her arms. About 1 month after showing attachment to the mother, many infants begin attaching to other members of the family, most often the father.

Infants acquire other developmental behaviors that influence the attachment process. These include (1) differential crying, smiling, and vocalization (more to mother than to anyone else), (2) visual-motor orientation (looking more at mother even if she is not close), (3) crying when mother leaves the room, (4) approach through locomotion (crawling, creeping, or walking), (5) clinging (especially in presence of a stranger), and (6) exploring away from mother while using her as a secure base.

Separation anxiety. Between 4 and 8 months the infant begins to have some awareness of self and mother as separate individuals. At this same time object permanence is developing and the infant is aware that the parent can be absent. Consequently, separation anxiety develops and is manifest through a predictable sequence of behaviors.

During the early second half of the first year the infant protests when placed in his crib, and a short time later objects when his mother leaves the room. Subsequently the infant may not notice the mother's absence if he is absorbed in an activity. However, when he realizes her absence, he protests. From this point onward he becomes very alert to her activities and whereabouts. By 11 to 12 months he is able to anticipate her imminent departure by watching her behaviors and begins to protest *before* she leaves. At this point many parents learn to postpone alerting the child to their departure until just before leaving.

Stranger fear. As the infant demonstrates attachment to one person, he correspondingly exhibits less friendliness to others. Between ages 6 and 8 months fear of strangers and stranger anxiety become prominent and are related to the infant's ability to discriminate between familiar and nonfamiliar people. Such behaviors as clinging to the parent, crying, and turning away from the stranger are common (Fig. 8-8).

Parental guidance. Although interpreted by some individuals as a sign of undesirable, antisocial behavior, stranger fear and separation anxiety are important components of a strong, healthy parent-child attachment. However, this period can also be a most difficult time for parent and child. Parents may be more confined to the home because the infant protests to baby-sitters. Parents should be encouraged to have close friends or relatives visit often. This provides at least one other person with whom the child is comfortable and who can give parents time alone.

Infants also need opportunities to experience strangers safely. Usually toward the end of the first year infants are beginning to venture away from the parent and demonstrate curiosity in strangers. If allowed to explore at their own rate, many infants will eventually "warm up." If the parent holds the child away from her face, the infant can observe while maintaining close physical contact. The best approach for the stranger (who may be the nurse) is to talk to the parent, maintain a safe distance from the infant, and avoid gestures such as holding the arms out and smiling broadly.

Parents also may wonder whether they should encourage the child's clinging, dependent behavior, especially if there is pressure from others who view this as "spoiling." Parents need to be reassured that such behavior is healthy, desirable, and necessary for the child's optimum emotional development. If parents can reassure the infant of their presence, the infant will learn to realize that they are still there even if not present physically. Talking to infants when leaving the room, allowing them to hear the parent's voice on the telephone, and using transitional objects, such as a favorite blanket or "mommy's purse," reassures them of the parent's continued presence.

Infant temperament

The infant's behavior has a significant influence on the development of attachment or bonding. A highly responsive infant is more likely to evoke satisfaction and pleasure from a parent than is a passive, apathetic infant. Because of the importance of behavior in the attachment process, nurses need knowledge of how it is assessed and its relevance to childrearing.

Temperament is defined as *behavioral style* or the *how* rather than the what or why of behavior. Based on maternal interviews Thomas and Chess (1977) identified nine

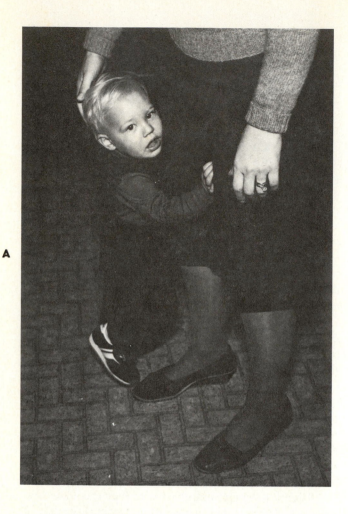

A

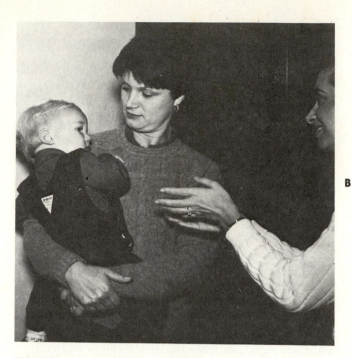

B

FIG. 8-8
*Stranger fear behaviors include **A,** clinging to the parent and **B,** turning away from a stranger.*

temperament variables and three common patterns of child temperament: the easy child, the difficult child, and the slow-to-warm-up child. However, not all children were characterized by one of these patterns.

The Infant Temperament Questionnaire (ITQ), (Carey and McDevitt, 1978) provides the nurse with a useful tool for parental guidance. It focuses on the nine temperament variables, but the questions relate specifically to activities such as sleep, feeding, play, diapering, dressing, and so on. There is no attempt to rate the behaviors as "good" or "bad." Rather, it is the degree of *fit* between the child and his environment, specifically his parents, that determines the degree of risk. The more dissonance between the child's temperament and the parent's ability to accept and deal with the behavior, the more chance of subsequent behavior problems.

Appropriate childrearing techniques for different temperament patterns include the following. The "difficult" child may respond better to scheduled feedings and structured care-giving routines than demand feedings and frequent changes in daily routines. Parents also benefit from knowing that this child sleeps about 2 hours less a night and 1 hour less during the day than the easy child.

The "highly distractible child" may require additional soothing measures such as swings, rocking, or being carried in a pack that the parent wears across the chest or back. The "high activity" child requires vigilant watching because he is prone to accidents. Parents need to take extra precautions in safeguarding the home. This child benefits from increased opportunities for gross motor activity to help channel his boundless energy.

Even the "easy child" can present problems because the parents may have to retrain him. For example, they may allow behaviors that they later regret, such as staying up late or frequent watching of television.

HEALTH PROMOTION DURING FIRST YEAR

The infant's first year is a time of monumental change and achievement. Each month and phase of development have implications for care of the child. Some of the general areas that are especially affected by the infant's development are feeding and safety. Physical care is fairly constant because the infant depends on others for bathing and diapering, and the degree of the child's independence usually is less influential than during the toddler years, when the achievement of autonomy and tasks such as toilet training are important goals.

Health promotion involves nutritional guidance, prevention of disease through immunization, provision of a safe environment, and counseling regarding common parental concerns. The recommended schedule for health supervision is monthly for the first 6 months and bimonthly for the second 6 months.

Nutrition

Ideally nutrition guidance should begin prenatally with the decision to breast- or bottle-feed the infant. During the 12 months following birth, growth needs and developmental milestones ready the child for introduction of solid foods. Frequently the nurse is asked when to begin feeding solid foods, how to introduce new foods, and what foods are best. A thorough understanding of each of these areas prepares the nurse to answer these questions in order to meet the nutritional needs of each child.

The first 6 months.   Human milk is the most desirable and complete diet for the infant for the first 6 months. The normal infant receiving breast milk from a well-nourished mother needs no specific vitamin and mineral supplements, with the exception of fluoride in a dose of 0.25 mg (regardless of the fluoride content of the local water supply) and iron by 6 months of age when fetal iron stores are depleted. Supplements of 400 IU of vitamin D daily may be indicated if the mother's vitamin D intake is inadequate or if the infant does not benefit from adequate ultraviolet light because of dark skin color or little exposure to light (American Academy of Pediatrics, 1980).

An acceptable alternative to breast-feeding is commercial iron-fortified formula. Like human milk, it supplies all the nutrients needed by the infant for the first 6 months. The only supplementation required is 0.25 mg of fluoride if the local water supply is not fluoridated or if the infant is given ready-to-feed formula that eliminates the use of fluoridated tap water.

If evaporated milk formula is given, supplemental iron, vitamin C, and fluoride (depending on local water supply) are required. Commercially prepared vitamin and iron preparations with or without fluoride are available to meet the specific needs of the infant. Obviously, the nurse needs to assess the type of formula given and the fluoride content of local water before advising the parent.

The addition of solid foods before 5 to 6 months is not recommended. During the early months solid foods are not compatible with the gastrointestinal ability and nutritional needs of the infant. For example, feeding solids to the infant exposes him to food antigens that may produce food-protein allergy. Developmentally, the infant is not ready. The extrusion (protrusion) reflex is strong and pushes food out of the mouth. The infant instinctively sucks when given food.

The second 6 months.   During the second half of the first year human milk or formula continues to be the primary source of nutrition. If breast-feeding is discontinued, commercial iron-fortified formula should be substituted. Whole cow's milk can be given if the infant is consuming one third of the calories as supplemental foods consisting of a balanced mixture of cereal, vegetables, fruits, and other foods to ensure adequate sources of iron and vitamin C (American Academy of Pediatrics, 1983).

The major change in feeding habits is the addition of solid foods to the infant's diet. Physiologically and developmentally 5 to 6 months is a transition period. By this time the gastrointestinal tract has matured sufficiently to handle more complex nutrients and is less sensitive to potentially allergenic foods. Tooth eruption is beginning and facilitates biting and chewing. The extrusion reflex has disappeared and swallowing is more coordinated to allow the infant to easily accept solids. Head control is well developed, permitting the infant to sit with support and purposely turn his head away to communicate disinterest in food. Voluntary grasping and improved eye-hand coordination gradually allow the infant to pick up ''finger'' foods and feed himself. His increasing sense of independence is evident in his desire to hold his own bottle and try to ''help'' during feeding.

The sequence of introducing solid foods is highly variable. The one generally accepted rule is the introduction of infant cereal as the first food because of its high iron content. Rice cereal is the preferred grain because it is least allergenic. Cereal should be mixed with formula or breast milk until whole milk is given. If fruit juices have been started, they can be mixed with the dry cereal. The vitamin C content of the juice enhances the absorption of iron in the cereal. Because of its benefit as a source of iron, infant cereal should be continued until the infant is 18 months of age.

The addition of other foods is arbitrary. A common sequence is strained fruits, followed by vegetables, and finally meats. At 6 months foods such as a cracker or zwieback can be offered as a type of finger and teething food. By 8 to 9 months junior foods and nutritious finger foods, such as firmly cooked vegetables, raw pieces of fruit, or cheese, can be given. By 1 year well-cooked table foods are served.

Introduction of solid foods.   When the spoon is first introduced to the infant, the likelihood is that he will push it away and appear dissatisfied. Some patience and skill are required to overcome this initial response. A small-bowled, straight, and long-handled spoon, similar to a demitasse spoon, allows a small portion of food to be placed toward the back of the tongue. If food is placed on the front of the tongue, it will be pushed out. It should simply be scooped up and tried again. As the child becomes accustomed to the spoon, he will more eagerly accept the food and will eventually open his mouth in anticipation (or keep it closed in dislike). Since the first introduction of food is a new experience, the spoon feeding should be attempted before or after ingestion of a small amount of breast milk or formula to associate this new experience with a pleasurable and satisfying experience. Trying to introduce a new food *after* the entire milk feeding is usually useless, since the infant is satiated and has no inclination to try something new.

After several spoon feedings, new food can be introduced at the beginning of a meal. It is best to introduce many new foods during the first year when the infant is more likely to eat them because of a hearty appetite resulting from a rapid growth rate.

Each new food is introduced at intervals of 4 to 7 days to allow for identification of food allergies. New foods are offered in small amounts, from 1 teaspoon to 1 to 2 tablespoons. As the amount of solid food increases, the quantity of milk is decreased to less than a liter a day to prevent overfeeding.

Food should not be mixed in the bottle and fed through a nipple with a large hole. This deprives the child of the pleasure of learning new tastes and developing a discriminating palate. It can also cause problems with poor chewing of food later in life since this experience would be lacking.

At the same time solid foods are introduced, fruit juice can be offered for its rich source of vitamin C and as a substitute for milk. Because vitamin C is naturally destroyed by heat, juice is not warmed. Containers of juice are always kept covered and refrigerated to prevent further vitamin loss. Fruit juice is offered only from a cup, rather than a bottle, to prevent the development of ''nursing bottle'' caries.

Weaning. Weaning, the process of giving up one method of feeding for another, usually refers to relinquishing the breast or bottle for a cup. In Western societies this is generally regarded as a major task for infants and is frequently seen as a potentially traumatic experience. It is psychologically significant because the infant is required to give up a major source of oral pleasure and gratification.

There is no one time for weaning that is best for every child, but generally most infants show signs of readiness during the second half of the first year. They have learned that good things come from a spoon. Their increasing desire for freedom of movement may lessen their desire to be held close for feedings. They are acquiring more control over their actions and can easily manipulate a cup to their lips (even if it is held upside down!). Since imitation becomes a powerful motivator by age 8 or 9 months, they enjoy using a cup or glass like others do.

Weaning should be gradual by replacing one bottle- or breast-feeding at a time. The last feeding to be discontinued is usually the nighttime one. If breast-feeding must be terminated before 5 or 6 months of age, weaning should

be to a bottle to provide for the infant's continued sucking needs. If discontinued later, weaning can be directly to a cup.

Nutritional counseling. The relatively simple feeding plan for infants, especially during the first 6 months, allows the nurse ample opportunity to educate parents regarding the nutritional needs of their child and to prepare them for the addition of solid foods. A prime consideration of counseling is provision of optimum nutrition. This includes education concerning what infants need and do not need. It may necessitate an introduction to the basic four food groups in order for the parents to wisely select foods for the infant's diet.

Another consideration in infant nutrition is home preparation of food. The choice to use commercial infant food or home preparation is an individual one. Both can supply adequate nutrition. In preparing the food moderate use of salt or sugar is recommended, since diets that avoid extremes are safest for children (American Academy of Pediatrics, 1983). If sweetening is needed, refined sugar or corn syrup can be used, but honey should be avoided because of the risk of infant botulism. Preferably, foods prepared for the infant should be fresh or frozen, since canned foods other than those prepared for infants may have excessive sodium or sugar or be a source of lead.

Preventing obesity. Besides selection of foods, the nurse must also consider amount of food. The most prevalent nutritional disorder in the United States is overeating, and prevention begins early. From the infant's first feeding parents should allow the child to regulate the amount of formula he desires. No attempt should be made to encourage the infant to finish the last drop or, later, to clean his plate.

Often eating habits are controlled by the sociocultural background of the family, rather than by their knowledge of well-balanced nutrition. Common myths such as ''a fat baby is a healthy baby'' are difficult to dispel. In some cultures overweight infants are regarded as a sign of good mothering, and any suggestion regarding altering the child's weight is threatening to the parent. Understanding cultural values is important in effecting change through counseling.

A thorough nutritional history is also a prerequisite for counseling. Asking questions such as, ''Does your child drink too much milk?'' may yield little reliable information. Phrasing the question by saying, ''Your child certainly looks well nourished (or well fed); how many bottles of milk a day does he drink?'' lessens parents' defensiveness and offers an objective number of ounces.

If too much formula or milk is the problem, the solution may be to dilute the feeding to decrease the calorie content, substitute water for a bottle of formula, or use a smaller-hole nipple to prolong sucking with less intake. A commercial formula, Advance,* is also available that provides 20% fewer calories than regular formula or whole cow's milk.

Dietary fat should not be restricted. For example, substituting skim or low-fat milk is unacceptable because the essential fatty acids are inadequate and the solute concentration of protein and electrolytes, such as sodium, is too high. Overall, the objective is not for the infant to lose weight but for his weight gain to slow until it is appropriate for his age and height.

The selection of solid foods is also an important aspect of controlling obesity. Approximately 20% of commercial baby foods contain less than 50 kcal/100 g, whereas another 20% contain more than 100 kcal/100 g. Choosing low-caloric foods can significantly lower the daily calorie intake without actually decreasing the total quantity of food. Table 8-3 lists calorie contents of various commercial baby foods. The selection of sweet foods should be kept to a minimum. This includes not adding additional sugar to the formula or cereal and avoiding finger foods such as cookies. Other foods rich in calories that should be restricted in serving size rather than eliminated include butter, cream, ice cream, pudding, and chocolate.

Immunizations

One of the most dramatic advances in pediatrics has been the decline of infectious diseases over the past 30 years because of the widespread use of immunization for preventable diseases. Although many of the presently available immunizations can be given to individuals of any age, the recommended primary schedule begins during infancy and, with the exception of boosters, is completed during early childhood. Therefore, the discussion of childhood immunizations for diphtheria, tetanus, pertussis, polio, measles, mumps, and rubella is included under health promotion during the first year.

The recommended age for beginning primary immunizations of normal infants is 2 months (Table 8-4). Recommended schedules for children not immunized during infancy are included in Table 8-5. Children who began primary immunization at the recommended age but for some reason did not receive all the doses do not have to begin the series again. They receive only those doses that were missed.

Certain combinations of simultaneously administered vaccines have been shown to be satisfactory. These include diphtheria-tetanus-pertussis (DTP) and oral poliovirus (OPV), DTP and measles-mumps-rubella (MMR), and MMR and the third or fourth dose of OPV. Although all possible combinations have not been tested, the American Academy of Pediatrics (1982) recommends that in situ-

ations when there is doubt that the child will return for immunization according to the optimum schedule, DTP, OPV, and MMR can be administered simultaneously. DTP and MMR are given in separate syringes in different injection sites.

One major change in the immunization schedule is the routine discontinuation of smallpox vaccination in the United States. This occurred because over a period of years, the risks from receiving the vaccination were greater

*Ross Laboratories, Columbus, OH.

TABLE 8-3. CALORIC CONTENT OF COMMERCIAL BABY FOOD

FOOD	CALORIC CONTENT
Juice (4.2 ounces)	
Apple, orange	70
Orange-apricot	80
Apple-grape	90
Orange-apple-banana	100
Meats (3.5 ounces)	
Veal	90
Beef, lamb	100
Ham	110
Pork	120
Chicken, turkey	130
Vegetables (4.5 ounces)	
Green beans	35
Squash, carrots	40
Beets	50
Peas	60
Sweet potatoes	90
Fruits (4.7 ounces)	
Pears	90
Applesauce	100
Peaches	110
Plums with tapioca	140
Dairy products	
Egg yolks (3.3 ounces)	180
Creamed cottage cheese with pineapple (4.5 ounces)	160
High meat-content dinners (4.5 ounces)	
Ham or veal with vegetables	90
Chicken or beef with vegetables	100
Turkey with vegetables	120
Vegetable and meat—combination dinners	
Vegetables and turkey or chicken	50
Macaroni and cheese	80
Vegetables and bacon	100

than the chance of contracting the actual disease. In 1980 the World Health Organization announced the worldwide eradication of smallpox.

Recommendations. In addition to the schedule for immunizations, the nurse needs to be aware of the latest recommendations regarding their use. It is the health professional's responsibility to be aware of these changes, which can differ from the following discussion.

Diphtheria. Diphtheria vaccine is commonly administered in three different ways: (1) in combination with tetanus and pertussis vaccines (DTP) for normal children under 7 years of age, (2) in a combined vaccine with tetanus (DT) for children under 7 years of age who have some contraindication to receiving pertussis vaccine, and (3) in smaller doses (15% to 20% of that in DTP or DT) with tetanus vaccine (Td) for use in children 7 years of age and over. Although the diphtheria vaccine does not produce absolute immunity, when given according to the recommended schedule, protective levels of antitoxin persist for 10 years or more.

Tetanus. Three forms of tetanus vaccine—tetanus toxoid (TT), tetanus immune globulin (TIG) (human), and tetanus antitoxin (TAT) (usually horse serum)—are available. Tetanus toxoid is generally used for routine primary immunization, usually in one of the combinations listed above, and provides protective antitoxin levels for 10 years or more.

Pertussis. Pertussis vaccine is recommended for all children under 7 years of age who have no neurologic contraindications to its use. It is not given to children 7 years or older because the risk of receiving the vaccine increases, while the incidence, severity, and fatality of the disease decrease.

Polio. The trivalent oral form of poliovirus (TOPV) (developed by Sabin) is recommended for all children under 18 years of age who have no specific contraindications, regardless of the number of administrations of inactivated poliovirus vaccine (IPV) (developed by Salk) they may already have received. For infants and children with immune deficiency diseases and for their siblings, the inactivated poliovirus vaccine is the vaccine of choice. Inactivated poliovirus vaccine has the disadvantage of being given by subcutaneous injection but has no reported history of ever causing a case of vaccine-associated paralysis.

Measles. Because of the presence of maternal antibodies, measles virus vaccine should be delayed until 15 months of age for infants who live in communities where the disease is not prevalent. However, during the course of measles outbreaks, the vaccine can be given any time after 6 months of age, followed by a second inoculation after age 15 months.

Mumps. Mumps virus vaccine may be given at any time to children between 15 months and 12 years of age who have not had the disease.

Rubella. Rubella is a relatively mild infection in

TABLE 8-4. RECOMMENDED SCHEDULE FOR ACTIVE IMMUNIZATION OF NORMAL INFANTS AND CHILDREN

AGE	IMMUNIZATION RECOMMENDED
2 months	DTP,* TOPV†
4 months	DTP, TOPV
6 months	DTP‡
1 year	Tuberculin tests§
15 months	Measles, rubella, mumps‖
18 months	DTP, TOPV
4-6 years	DTP, TOPV
14-16 years	Td¶—repeat every 10 years

Adapted from American Academy of Pediatrics: Report of the Committee on Infectious Diseases, III., ed. 19, 1982. Copyright American Academy of Pediatrics, 1982.
*DTP—diphtheria and tetanus toxoids combined with pertussis vaccine.
†TOPV—trivalent oral poliovirus vaccine. This recommendation is suitable for breast-fed as well as bottle-fed infants.
‡A third dose of TOPV is optional but may be given in area of high endemicity of poliomyelitis.
§Frequency of tuberculin testing depends on risk of exposure of the child and on the prevalence of tuberculosis in the population group. The initial test should be at or preceding the measles vaccine.
‖May be given at 15 months as measles-rubella or measles-mumps-rubella combined vaccines.
¶Td—combined tetanus and diphtheria toxoids (adult type) for those more than 6 years of age, in contrast to diphtheria and tetanus (DT) toxoids, which contain a larger amount of diphtheria antigen.

children. However, in a pregnant woman it presents serious risks to the developing fetus. The aim of rubella immunization is actually for protection of the unborn child rather than the recipient of the immunization. Because the live attenuated virus may cross the placenta and present a risk to the developing fetus, rubella vaccine should not be given to any pregnant woman or to any woman who may become pregnant in the 3 months following the immunization. The nurse must explain the necessity for adequate contraception for at least this 3-month period following the vaccine. There is no reported danger of giving a rubella immunization to a child if the mother is pregnant.

Rubella immunization is recommended for all children at 12 months of age or older. If administered in a combined form with measles vaccine, it should be given to children at about 15 months of age. Increased emphasis should be placed on vaccinating all postpubertal females of childbearing age.

Tuberculin test. Tuberculin testing is included as part of the immunization schedule to permit a systematic screening of the population for exposure to tuberculosis. It is not an immunization.

Two types of tuberculin preparations are used for skin tests: old tuberculin (OT) and purified protein derivative (PPD) of tuberculin. The PPD is used most widely, and the standard dose is 5 tuberculin units (TU) in 0.1 ml of solution, injected intracutaneously. The techniques for in-

TABLE 8-5. RECOMMENDED IMMUNIZATION SCHEDULES FOR INFANTS AND CHILDREN NOT INITIALLY IMMUNIZED AT USUAL RECOMMENDED TIMES IN EARLY INFANCY

TIMING	PREFERRED SCHEDULE	ALTERNATIVES* #1	#2	#3
First visit	DTP #1, OPV #1, tuberculin test (PPD)	MMR,† PPD	DTP #1, OPV #1, PPD	DTP #1, OPV #1, MMR, PPD
1 month later	MMR	DTP #1, OPV #1	MMR, DTP #2	DTP #2
2 months later	DTP #2, OPV #2	—	DTP #3, OPV #2	DTP #3, OPV #2
3 months later	DTP #3‡	DTP #2, OPV #2	—	—
4 months later	DTP #3 (OPV #3)§	—	(OPV #3)	(OPV #3)
5 months later	—	DTP #3 (OPV #3)	—	—
10-16 months after last dose	DTP #4, OPV #3, or OPV #4	DTP #4, OPV #3, or OPV #4	DTP #4, OPV #3, or OPV #4	DTP #4, OPV #3, or OPV #4
Preschool‖	DTP #5, OPV #4, or OPV #5	DTP #5, OPV #4, or OPV #5	DTP #5, OPV #4, or OPV #5	DTP #5, OPV #4, or OPV #5
Age 14-16	Td¶	Td	Td	Td

Adapted from American Academy of Pediatrics: Report of the Committee on Infectious Diseases, III., ed. 19, 1982. Copyright American Academy of Pediatrics, 1982.

*Alternative #1 can be used in children more than 15 months old if measles is occuring in the community.
Alternative #2 allows for more rapid DTP immunization.
Alternative #3 should be reserved for those whose access to medical care is compromised by poor compliance.
†MMR should be given to children no younger than 15 months.
‡Can be given if OPV #3 not administered until 10-16 months.
§OPV #3 optional for areas likely to import polio (some southwestern states).
‖Not necessary if DTP #4 administered after fourth birthday.
¶Repeat every 10 years.

jection are (1) the Mantoux test, in which 0.1 ml of PPD is injected directly into the dermis and (2) the multiple-puncture test (for example, the tine, Heaf, Sterneedle, or Mono-Vac test).

A positive reaction indicates that the person has been infected and developed a sensitivity to the protein of the tubercle bacillus. Once the individual reacts positively, he will continue to react positively. If a child who previously has reacted negatively shows a positive reaction, he has been infected since the last test. Tests are read according to instructions provided by the manufacturer.

Reactions. Vaccines for routine immunizations are among the safest and most reliable drugs available. However, minor side effects do occur following many of the immunizations, and, rarely, a serious reaction may result.

In general with inactivated antigens, such as DTP, side effects are most likely to occur within a few hours or days of administration. The common reactions are fever and soreness, redness, and swelling at the site of injection. Pertussis may be associated with more severe reactions such as loss of consciousness, convulsions, and thrombocytopenia.

With the live attenuated virus vaccines such as measles, mumps, rubella, and oral poliovirus possible unfavorable reactions and ''vaccine-associated'' disorders can occur for a period of 30 to 60 days. Poliovirus and mumps immunization have essentially no side effects, although a vaccine-associated paralysis rarely occurs from TOPV. Measles is occasionally associated with anorexia, malaise, rash, and fever 7 to 10 days after immunization. Rarely, a subsequent encephalitis may occur. In some children rubella vaccine causes mild rash, arthralgia, and/or paresthesia. However, in adults the reactions can be much more severe and prolonged. This is an additional reason for ensuring that individuals receive this immunization during childhood.

No specific treatment is required for the expected reactions. Acetaminophen given as soon as side effects occur is adequate. However, the nurse should advise parents to notify the physician immediately if any unusual symptoms or neurologic sequelae peculiar to pertussis occur.

Contraindications. The general contraindication for all immunizations is a severe febrile illness. This precaution is to avoid adding the risk of adverse side effects from the vaccine on an already ill child or mistakenly identifying a symptom of the disease as having been caused by the vaccine. The presence of minor illnesses, such as the common cold, are *not* contraindications.

Pertussis immunization is contraindicated for infants and children who have any of the following reactions after receiving a pertussis-containing vaccine: (1) a severe neurologic reaction; (2) persistent, unconsolable screaming for 3 hours or more; (3) a hyporesponsive, shock-like state; (4) a temperature of 40.5° C (105° F) or greater, unexplained by another cause within 24 hours following immunization; (5) a convulsion within 48 hours following immunization; or (6) an allergic reaction to the vaccine (American Academy of Pediatrics, 1984).

Live-virus vaccines are not given to anyone with an altered immune system because multiplication of the virus may be enhanced, causing a severe vaccine-induced illness. Such children include (1) those with immunologic-deficiency disease or diseases that suppress the immune system, such as leukemia, lymphoma, or generalized malignancy, and (2) those receiving immunosuppressive therapy, such as steroids, chemotherapy, or radiation. In addition household contacts of such children should not receive oral poliovirus vaccine because the excreted virus can be communicable to the immunosuppressed child. Another contraindication to live-virus vaccines is the presence of recently acquired passive immunity, including blood transfusions, immunoglobulin, or maternal antibodies. Administration of such vaccines should be postponed until 3 months after passive immunization with immune serum globulin.

Pregnancy is a known contraindication to immunization against mumps, measles, and rubella. In addition these vaccines should not be given to women who are likely to become pregnant within 3 months after vaccination. However, if rubella vaccination is given during pregnancy, it should not be a routine reason for therapeutic abortion. Oral poliovirus vaccine should also be withheld unless there is risk of exposure during an outbreak of polio.

A final contraindication is a known allergic response to a previously administered vaccine, such as pertussis, or a substance in the vaccine, such as preservatives or trace amounts of antibiotics, for example, neomycin. Although measles, mumps, and rubella virus vaccines contain minute amounts of neomycin, only a history of anaphylactoid reaction is considered a contraindication to their use. The nurse identifies this situation by carefully reading all package inserts and taking a detailed history regarding allergies to isolate the rare child who may not be able to receive the vaccine. A history of allergy to eggs, chickens, or chicken feathers is not a contraindication for receiving the live virus vaccines of rubella, mumps, or measles (American Academy of Pediatrics, 1982). However, if the child has a history of egg anaphylaxis, this is reported to the physician before administering the vaccine.

Administration/precautions. The principal precautions in administering immunizations include proper storage of the vaccine to protect its potency and following recommended procedure for injection. All the virus vaccines except oral polio are administered subcutaneously; DTP is given intramuscularly. Since the total series requires a number of injections, every attempt is made to administer them as painlessly as possible (see Chapter 19).

The DTP vaccines contain an adjuvant aluminum compound that can cause local irritation, inflammation, or abscess formation if given by subcutaneous or intracutaneous injection. These vaccines should be administered by deep intramuscular injection using an air bubble to avoid tracking the adjuvant through the superficial layers of the skin.

The manufacturer's package insert specifies proper storage and reconstitution techniques. Nurses are often responsible for the handling of immunizations. For example, if the vaccine is to be refrigerated, it should be stored on a center shelf, not on the door, where frequent temperature increases from opening the refrigerator can alter the vaccine's potency.

Accident prevention

Accidents are a major cause of death during infancy, especially for children 6 to 12 months old. Constant vigilance, awareness, and supervision are essential as the child gains increased locomotor and manipulative skills that are coupled with an insatiable curiosity about the environment. Accidents can be grouped into the following categories: aspiration of foreign objects, suffocation, falls, poisoning, burns, motor vehicle accidents, and bodily damage.

Table 8-6 lists the major developmental achievements of each period during infancy and the appropriate accident prevention plan.

Aspiration of foreign objects. Asphyxiation by foreign material in the respiratory tract is the leading cause of fatal injury in children under 1 year of age. As soon as the infant has the ability to find his mouth, he is vulnerable to aspiration of small objects, such as those left within his reach or removable parts of objects that may on initial in-

TABLE 8-6. ACCIDENT PREVENTION DURING INFANCY

AGE (months)	MAJOR DEVELOPMENTAL TASK	ACCIDENT PREVENTION
Birth-4	Crawling or Moro reflex may propel infant forward May roll over Increasing eye-hand coordination and voluntary grasp reflex	**Aspiration** Not as great a danger to this age-group but should begin practicing safe guarding early (see under 4-7 months) Inform parents of dangers from baby powder; encourage its proper use and storage if used **Suffocation** Keep all plastic bags stored away from infant's reach; discard large plastic garment bags after tying in a knot Do not cover mattress or pillows with plastic Use a firm mattress, no pillows, and loose blankets Make sure crib design follows federal regulations and mattress fits snugly Position crib away from other furniture Avoid sleeping in bed with infant Do not tie pacifier on a string around infant's neck Remove bibs at bedtime Drowning—never leave infant alone in bath **Falls** Always raise crib rails; tie them to crib if malfunctioning Never leave infant on a raised, unguarded surface When in doubt where to place child, use the floor Restrain child in the infant seat and never leave him unattended while the seat is resting on a raised surface Avoid using a high chair until child is old enough to sit well **Poisoning** Not as great a danger to this age-group but should begin practicing safeguarding early (see under 4-7 months) **Burns** Install smoke detectors in home Check bath water and warmed formula and food Do not pour hot liquids when infant is close by, such as sitting on lap Beware of cigarette ashes that may fall on the infant Do not leave infant in the sun for more than a few minutes Wash flame-retardant clothes according to label directions Use cool mist vaporizers Do not keep child in parked car Check surface heat of car restraint **Motor vehicles** Transport infant in a specially constructed, rearward-facing car seat with shoulder and waist restraints Do not place infant on the seat or in your lap Do not place a carriage or stroller behind a parked car **Bodily damage** Avoid sharp, jagged-edged objects Keep diaper pins closed and away from infant

Continued.

TABLE 8-6. ACCIDENT PREVENTION DURING INFANCY—cont'd

AGE (months)	MAJOR DEVELOPMENTAL TASK	ACCIDENT PREVENTION
4-7	Rolls over Sits momentarily Grasps and manipulates small objects Resecures a dropped object Has well-developed eye-hand coordination Can fixate and locate very small objects Mouthing very prominent	**Aspiration** Keep buttons, beads, and other small objects out of infant's reach Use pacifier with one-piece construction and loop handle Keep floor free of any small objects Do not feed infant hard candy, nuts, food with pits or seeds, or whole hot dogs Inspect toys for removable parts ·Avoid balloons as playthings Discard used button-size batteries; store new batteries in safe area **Suffocation** May begin to teach swimming as part of water safety **Falls** Restrain in a high chair Keep crib rails raised to full height **Poisoning** Make sure that paint for furniture or toys does not contain lead Place toxic substances on a high shelf and/or locked cabinet Hang plants or place on high surface rather than on floor Avoid storing large quantities of cleaning fluid, paints, pesticides, and other toxic substances Discard used containers of poisonous substances Do not store toxic substances in food containers Know telephone number of local poison control center **Burns** Keep faucets out of reach Place hot objects (cigarettes, candles, incense) on high surface **Motor vehicles** (See under Birth-4 months) **Bodily damage** Give toys that are smooth and rounded, preferably made of wood or plastic Avoid long, pointed objects as toys

spection appear safe. Rattles, for example, have small beads in them to produce noise. A broken or cracked rattle can be dangerous because the beads can easily be swallowed while the infant has the toy in his mouth. Stuffed animals are another potentially dangerous toy if any of the parts, such as the eyes or nose, are removable buttons or plastic pieces.

A previously unrecognized danger is ingestion of button-size batteries that are used in calculators and watches. Because they are bright and shiny they are attractive to children. However, they can cause severe morbidity, even death, if lodged in the esophagus.

When infant clothes are being purchased, the type of closure used should be considered. A front button can eas-

TABLE 8-6. ACCIDENT PREVENTION DURING INFANCY—cont'd

AGE (months)	MAJOR DEVELOPMENTAL TASK	ACCIDENT PREVENTION
8-12	Crawls Stands, holding onto furniture Stands alone Cruises around furniture Walks Climbs Pulls on objects Throws objects Uses pincer grasp for small articles Mouthing very prominent Dislikes being restrained Explores away from mother Increasing understanding of simple commands and phrases	**Aspiration** (See under 4-7 months) **Suffocation** Keep doors of ovens, dishwashers, refrigerators, and front-loading clothes washers and dryers closed at all times If storing an unused appliance, such as a refrigerator, remove the door Fence swimming pools; always supervise when near any source of water, such as cleaning buckets Keep bathroom doors closed **Falls** Fence stairways at top and bottom if child has access to either end Dress in safe shoes and clothing **Poisoning** Administer medications as a drug, not as a candy Do not administer medications unless so prescribed by a physician Replace medications and poisons immediately after use; replace caps properly if a child protector cap is used Advise parents regarding proper use of syrup of ipecac **Burns** Place guards in front of or around any heating appliance, fireplace, or furnace Keep electrical wires hidden or out of reach Place plastic guards over electrical outlets; place furniture in front of outlets Keep hanging tablecloths out of reach Do not allow infant to play with electrical appliance Apply a sunscreen when infant is exposed to sunlight **Motor vehicles** Do not use adult seat or shoulder belt without infant car seat Do not allow to crawl behind a parked car If infant plays in a yard, have the yard fenced or use a playpen **Bodily damage** Do not allow infant to use a fork for self-feeding Use plastic cups or dishes Check safety of toys and toy box Protect from young children and animals, especially dogs

ily be pulled off and swallowed. Safety pins for diapers should be kept closed and away from the dressing table. Even though a young infant may not search for them, practicing this good habit from the beginning prevents future accidents.

All toys must be carefully inspected for potential danger. An active infant can grab a low-hanging mobile and quickly chew off a small piece. As soon as the infant crawls or plays on the floor, one must be certain that the floor is free of any small articles that can be picked up and swallowed. Balloons, whether partially inflated, uninflated, or popped, cause more deaths in children than any other kind of small object and should be kept from infants and young children.

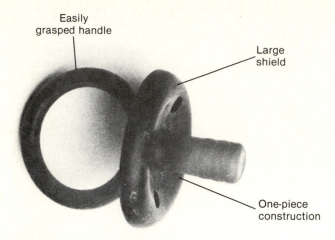

Easily grasped handle

Large shield

One-piece construction

FIG. 8-9
Design of a safe pacifier.

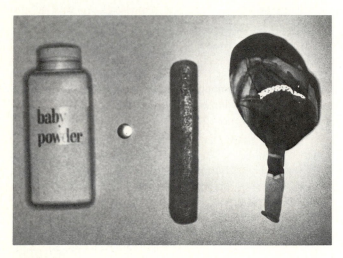

FIG. 8-10
Four common household objects that can be deadly to infants (from left to right): baby powder, button-size battery, whole hot dog, and balloon.

When new foods are given to the child, nuts, hard candies, or fruits such as grapes or those with pits or seeds should be avoided. A food that has caused several deaths is the hot dog, since its size (diameter), shape, and consistency allows for complete occlusion of the airway. If given to small children, it should be cut up into small noncircular pieces rather than served whole.

Pacifiers can also be dangerous because the entire object may be aspirated if it is small or the nipple and shield may become detached from the handle and become lodged in the pharynx. Safe pacifiers should be of one-piece construction, have a shield or flange that is large enough to prevent entry into the mouth, and have a handle that can be grasped (Fig. 8-9).

Another common source of aspiration is baby powder, which is usually a mixture of talc (hydrous magnesium silicate) and other silicates. Talc preparations can cause severe and often fatal inhalation episodes. One of the factors involved in talc aspiration is the similar appearance of baby powder containers and nursing bottles. Talc containers often become favorite playthings and are placed in the mouth. Parents should be advised of the danger of baby powder and encouraged to avoid it or use it properly (Fig. 8-10).

Suffocation. Mechanical suffocation is another important cause of death by asphyxiation and includes accidental asphyxiation by covering the mouth and nose, by pressure on the throat and chest, and by exclusion of air, such as refrigerator entrapment.

An infant who is placed in a bed under blankets and sheets that are tucked in can be caught under them and be unable to wriggle free. There are potential dangers in adults sleeping with a small infant because of the possibility of their rolling over and smothering the child. Even though this is a slight possibility, if it happens the consequent parental guilt can be devastating.

Another more common cause of suffocation is plastic bags. Large plastic bags used over garments are very lightweight and can easily and quickly be wrapped around the head of an active infant or pressed against his face. Pillows and mattresses should not be covered with plastic for this reason. Older infants may play peekaboo with a plastic bag and accidentally pull it over their heads. Since plastic is nonporous, suffocation takes place in a matter of minutes.

Anything tied around the infant's neck can potentially cause strangulation. Bibs should be removed at bedtime, and objects such as pacifiers should never be hung on a string around the infant's neck. This is a common practice in some cultures and can be remedied by pinning a short string tied to a pacifier on the child's shirt.

Toys that have strings attached, such as a telephone, or toys that are tied to cribs or playpens can be hazards, since the string can become wrapped around the child's neck. As a precaution all cords should be less than 30 cm (12 inches) long. Cradle gyms should be hung high enough so that the infant cannot become entangled in them.

Restraining straps, if applied too loosely or left unfastened, can be a hazard. For example, a child may slide off a high chair beneath the tray and strangle himself on the loose strap. All straps should be fastened securely.

Infant strangulation may occur if the infant's head becomes caught between the crib slats and mattress or objects close to the crib. According to federal regulation the distance between crib slats should not be more than 2⅜ inches (about 6 cm), roughly the width of three adult fingers. Mattresses and bumper pads should fit snugly against the slats. A general rule is that if two adult fingers can be placed between the mattress and crib side, the mattress is too small. A temporary solution is to place large, rolled towels in the space to create a snug fit. Ideally information regarding correct crib design should be given prenatally before parents have purchased or borrowed a crib.*

Toy box injuries can cause strangulation when the lid closes on the child's head or neck. Parents need to be warned of this danger and should supervise the child's exploring of toy chests in relatives' or neighbors' homes.

Mesh-sided playpens and cribs can result in death if the sides are left in the lowered position. Infants have suffocated when they fell off the edge of the mattress and the head or chest were compressed between the floorboard and mesh side. Parents should be advised of this danger and encouraged to *always* keep the sides locked securely in the up position whenever the child is in the playpen or crib.

The crib should be positioned away from large furniture because children who crawl out of the crib may become caught between the two objects. Cribs should also be located away from windows, where drape cords can become wrapped around the infant's neck.

Drowning is another cause of asphyxiation. Infants should never be left unsupervised in a bathtub or near a source of water, such as a swimming pool, toilet, or bucket. One way to stress water safety is to teach infants to swim. Infants under 6 months of age have two reflexes that enhance swimming. The crawl reflex causes a swimming motion strong enough to propel the infant through water for a short distance. The dive reflex inhibits breathing when the infant is submerged. Most infants, if introduced to the water properly, will not be afraid and can be taught to float and to swim underwater for a few feet. Not until they are 3 or 4 years old can they swim above water for longer distances because of the proportionately heavy weight of the head. Regardless of swimming instructions, no infant can be expected to learn the elements of water safety or to react appropriately in an emergency. Therefore, all young children need to be considered at risk when near water.

Falls. Falls are most common after 4 months of age when the infant has learned to roll over, but they can occur at any age. Newborns are normally active, assume a flexed position, and have crawling and Moro reflexes that can propel them forward. The best advice is never to place a child unattended on a raised surface that has no type of guardrails. When in doubt, the safest place is the floor. Even though young infants cannot climb over a partially raised crib rail, it is best to form a habit of raising the side rail all the way because some day that infant will be able to climb out. Crib sides should have a latching device that

cannot be easily released. Ideally cribs should be placed on carpeted, not hard, floors.

Another danger area for falling is a changing table, which is usually high and narrow. Although these tables have a restraining belt, it is unwise to leave the child unattended even when he is so restrained. The best way to avoid having to leave is to arrange the area with all necessary articles within easy reach so the child is always in full eyesight of the caregiver. It only takes a fraction of a second for the infant to fall off. During the latter half of the first year, infants usually resist dressing and diapering and may be difficult to manage. If there is danger that the child is strong enough to resist restraining, he should be changed on the floor.

Infant seats, high chairs, walkers, and swings present additional opportunities for accidental falls. If the infant seat is placed on a table where the child has an excellent panorama of his environment, he should never be left unrestrained or unattended. The same rule is essential for other baby equipment, particularly when the child has learned to crawl and stand up. Small infants can slip through a high chair if a protective harness is not used. High chairs are designed for older infants who can sit well and who are tall enough to have the tray at the level of their chest or abdomen. Walkers are responsible for a number of different types of injuries that occur because the walker tipped over or fell downstairs. Parents need to be warned of these dangers and encouraged to keep a constant vigil on their child's activities.

Although the infant begins to develop depth perception by age 9 months, that is no guarantee of his ability to perceive danger. His curiosity may still propel him forward and over, or his immature locomotor skills may be inadequate to keep him from falling even though he is aware of the danger. Infants should not be allowed to crawl unsupervised on any raised surface, near stairs, or near any water reservoir. Gates should be used at the bottom and top of stairs, since both present dangers to the crawling and climbing infant.

Sometimes, even when the environment is made safe, infants may literally trip over their own feet. Slippery socks, hard, slick soles on shoes or rubber soles that can catch, especially on a carpet, and long pants or pajama bottoms can easily upset a child's balance. Such dangers need to be pointed out to parents, especially when the infant is taking his first steps.

Poisoning. Accidental poisoning is one of the major causes of death in children under 5 years of age. The highest incidence occurs in those in the 2-year-old age-group, with the second highest incidence in 1-year-old children. The infant who has not learned to crawl is relatively free from danger of poisonous agents by virtue of his confinement. However, once locomotion begins, danger from poisoning is present almost everywhere. There are over 500

---

*A booklet, *It hurts when they cry,* gives basic information on hazards, safety features, and proper use of nursery furniture and equipment. It is available at no charge from the U.S. Consumer Product Safety Commission, Washington, DC 20207.

toxic substances in the average home, and about 34% of all poisonings occur in the kitchen.

The major reason for ingestion of poisons is improper storage. To protect the infant, avoid placing toxic agents on a low shelf, table, or floor. Drugs that are kept in a purse pose additional dangers; if the purse is given to the infant to play with, he may open it and ingest the contents. Another unrecognized hazard is during diaper changes when infants are near many toxic substances, such as ointments, creams, oils, and talc. Parents may even hand the infant a potentially poisonous object to quiet him. Such dangers need to be stressed to parents and toys kept at diapering areas to minimize these risks.

Poisoning is almost always the result of inadequate supervision, but it may not represent neglect. Children are very fast, and it takes only seconds to eat a bar of soap, cleanser from an open can, or a handful of detergent. Although infants usually do not possess the manipulative skill to open closed jars, they are amazingly persistent and inventive. For example, an ant trap placed in an out-of-the-way corner is easy for a crawling infant to find.

Plants are another source of poisoning for infants. Plants are frequently placed on the floor, where the leaves or flowers are attractive and easy to pull off. There are over 700 species of plants that are known to have caused illness or death.

The only sure way to prevent poisoning is to remove toxic agents, which means placing them high out of the infant's reach. However, since crawling infants soon become climbing toddlers, it is best to keep all toxic agents, especially drugs, in a locked cabinet. Special plastic hooks can be attached to the inside of cabinet doors to keep them securely closed (Fig. 8-11). Since it requires firm thumb pressure to unlatch the hook, small children are usually unable to manipulate them. Locks are best, but for cleaning agents frequently used, such as under a kitchen sink, hooks are a practical alternative. Impractical suggestions are usually ignored, and some protection is better than none.

With several hundred toxic substances in each house, locking all potentially toxic substances could present a problem; however, careful planning can help. A large surplus of cleaning agents, furniture polishes, laundry additives, paints, insecticides, and solvents should be avoided. Used poison containers should be promptly discarded and not used to store another poison without adequately marking the package. Since young children cannot read, any potentially hazardous substance should not be stored in any type of food container. A popular container that is used to store toxic liquids is a soda bottle. A child who is unaware of the dangerous contents is a vulnerable victim for poisoning. Parents should know the location of the local poison control centers and call them in the event of a sus-

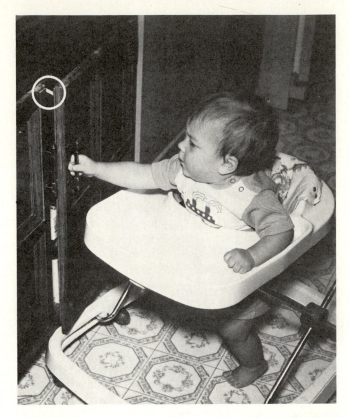

FIG. 8-11
Special plastic hooks as shown above prevent a young child from opening a cabinet door.

pected poisoning. Emergency measures for accidental poisoning are discussed in Chapter 12.

Burns. Burns are generally not thought of as a particular danger to infants, but several important hazards exist, such as scalding from water that is too hot, excessive sunburn, and burns from electrical wires, sockets, and heating elements such as radiators, registers, and floor furnaces. The infant's skin is particularly sensitive to irritation, and the mechanisms for temperature perception are not completely developed.

The bath water should be checked before the infant is immersed. Any food or formula warmed in a microwave oven must be checked before feeding since the container may remain cool while the contents are hot. The handles of cooking utensils should be turned toward the back of the stove. When the infant is underfoot, pouring hot liquids and cooking with hot oil should be avoided. Hanging tablecloths should be placed out of the infant's reach.

Sunburn can be a source of a first- or second-degree burn. Exposure to direct sunlight or filtered light through a window should be gradual, about 5 minutes initially. The infant's head should be covered, since it represents a large proportion of body surface. Sunscreen agents may be help-

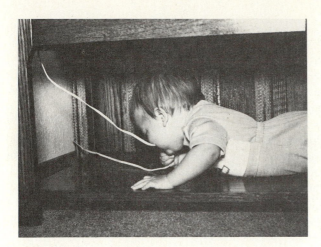

FIG. 8-12
Crawling infants can find hazardous electric wires even in "hidden" areas.

ful and should be applied 20 to 30 minutes before swimming. Although black-skinned infants burn less readily, their thin skin can become sunburned also.

Electrical outlets should be covered with protective plastic caps that prevent the child from sucking on the outlet or putting objects such as hairpins into it. Live wires are placed out of reach, since curious infants can chew on them and potentially break the rubber coating. Infants should not be allowed to play near televisions, stereo units, or other appliances, whether these units are on or off, since infants cannot determine when the appliance is safe (Fig. 8-12).

Any heat-producing element should have a guard placed in front of it. Fireplaces should be well screened because they are very appealing and within easy access. Small portable heaters should only be used when placed on a high surface. Floor furnaces should have barrier gates to prevent children from crawling or walking over them. Cigarettes, candles, and incense are kept out of reach.

Vaporizers are a hazard, particularly if they produce heated mist. Parents should be advised to purchase cool-mist vaporizers. If a heat-mist vaporizer is used, it is placed on a high surface, away from the crib. By law all infants' sleepwear must be flame retardant. Unfortunately this does not apply to all infants' clothes. Flame-retardant fabric must never be viewed as the ultimate protection against burns. Repeated washing reduces the flame-retardant properties, and the use of soap or bleach destroys the protection. Since only detergent should be used for washing flame-retardant clothing, infants who are sensitive to such wash agents are unprotected when their clothing is washed with a mild soap. If sleepwear is home sewn, mothers should be advised to look for specially treated flame-retardant fabric.

Another type of thermal injury occurs when children are exposed to excessive heat during confinement in poorly ventilated cars. The practice of leaving the windows open 2 to 3 inches does not appear to be protective. The nurse should caution parents never to leave children in parked cars, especially when the automobile is in direct sunlight.

Children can also be burned by overheated metal hardware and vinyl seats in cars parked in the sun. As a precaution the surface heat of car restraints should be determined before putting children in them. Covering the restraints and hardware (such as metal latch on seat belt) may be necessary to prevent skin burns. An additional safeguard is buying a light-colored restraint, which absorbs less heat.

In addition to these precautions parents are advised to have smoke and/or heat detectors in the home. This passive protection is considered one of the best burn safety measures.

Motor vehicle accidents. Automobile accidents are the leading cause of accidental deaths in children over 1 year of age. The major danger to the infant is improper restraint within the vehicle. It is recommended that all infants, newborns included, be secured in a special car restraint rather than held or placed on the car seat.

A variety of car seats are available for young children. For infants up to 9 kg (20 pounds) the recommended type is a rearward-facing, molded plastic shell seat or convertible infant-toddler seat that includes a shoulder restraint and uses the car seat belt (Fig. 8-13). In this position the most dangerous forces in a crash are absorbed by the infant's back.

Generally the middle of the back seat is considered the safest area of the car. However, with an infant restraint it is preferable to position the child in the front seat, where the driver can observe the infant without having to turn around.

For restraints to be effective, they must be used properly. Dressing the infant in an outfit with sleeves and legs allows the harness to be placed correctly. A small blanket or towel rolled tightly can be placed on either side of the head to minimize movement and increase comfort. Although many infant restraints can be recliners, they should only be used in the car in the position specified by the manufacturer. Many of the infant car restraints also serve as baby carriers, a point that should be stressed to parents to encourage their purchasing a suitable restraint. (For further discussion of restraints see Chapter 10.)

Another potential vehicular accident is placing a carriage or stroller behind a car, particularly a car parked in a garage or driveway. It is possible that the driver may not see the small stroller and, while driving in reverse, run over the child. Once the child crawls, he should not be allowed to play in areas where vehicles can be a hazard.

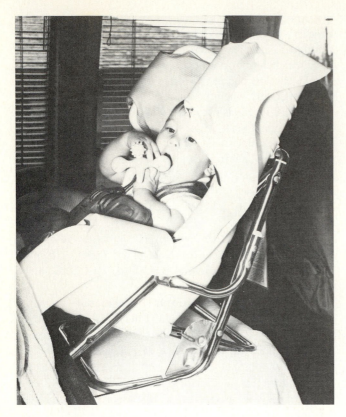

FIG. 8-13
Rearward facing shell car seat.

Bodily damage. Accidents can occur in other ways. Constricting clothing such as tight socks or loose yarn or thread can wrap around a toe or finger. Sharp, jagged-edged objects can cause wounds in the skin. Long, pointed articles can be poked into the eye, causing serious visual loss. The latter is particularly important to remember because infants have less well-developed fine motor control. For this reason forks should be avoided for self-feeding until the child has mastered the spoon, usually by age 18 months.

Another frequently unrecognized danger to infants is attacks by young siblings and pets, especially dogs and cats. Helpless infants, as newcomers to the home, can provoke jealousy in siblings or animals. Parents must be constantly vigilant of protecting the child from such dangers.

Nursing considerations: accident prevention and discipline

When one considers the potential environmental dangers to which infants are vulnerable, the task of preventing these accidents only begins to be appreciated. Nurses must be aware of the possible causes of injury in each age-group in order for *anticipatory* preventive teaching to occur. For example, the guidelines for accident prevention during in-

fancy presented in Table 8-6 should be discussed before the child reaches the susceptible age-group. Therefore, preventive teaching ideally occurs during pregnancy. Since two thirds of all accidents involving children occur in the home, the importance of safety cannot be overemphasized.

Accident prevention requires protection and education. For infants, this translates into protection of the child and education of the parents or caregiver. Nurses in ambulatory care settings, health maintenance centers, or visiting nurse agencies are in a most favorable position for accident education. This does not exclude nurses in inpatient facilities, who could utilize visiting times as an excellent opportunity for discussing this topic. One approach to teaching accident prevention is to relate why children in various age-groups are prone to special types of accidents. Stressing the prevention is just as important as emphasizing the *why* of the accident. However, accident prevention must also be practical. For example, suggesting that *all* potentially toxic substances be locked in a cabinet or placed on a high shelf is ideal but may be so impractical that no change will occur. Asking parents for their ideas will lead to realistic suggestions that can be followed. For instance, bathroom cleaning agents, cosmetics, and personal care items can be placed on a top shelf in the linen closet, and towels or sheets can be stored on the lower shelves and floor.

If an accident has occurred, the nurse should not be too quick to admonish the parent. Accidents do not always indicate neglect. It is a difficult task to watch children carefully without overprotecting or unnecessarily confining them. Small falls help children learn the dangers of heights. Touching a hot object once can emphasize to the child the pain of a burn. Allowing children to explore while maintaining *consistent, age-appropriate limit setting* is sound advice.

Parents need to remember that infants and young children cannot anticipate danger or understand when it is or is not present. A dead electrical wire may present no actual harm, but if the child is allowed to play with it, a poor habit is being practiced for when the child comes across live wires. Although it is always wise to explain why something is dangerous, one must remember that small children will need to be physically removed from the situation.

It is not easy to teach safety, supervise closely, and refrain from saying "no" a hundred times a day. Parents become acutely aware of this triangle as soon as the infant learns to crawl. Preventing accidents is usually the first reason for discipline because accidents not only can cause harm to children but may also damage valuable household objects. Small children must have dangerous objects removed or guarded and valuable articles placed out of reach. Children, even the youngest crawling infant, will almost always test their parents. It is better to learn a les-

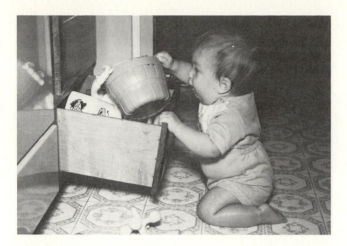

FIG. 8-14
A drawer filled with playthings can be a safe and fun area in the kitchen.

son from breaking an inexpensive ashtray than a valuable crystal decanter, or by falling off a step stool rather than down a flight of stairs. In either case the lesson is similar, but the price is different.

When children are taught the meaning of ''no,'' they should also be taught what ''yes'' means. Children should be praised for playing with suitable toys, their efforts at behaving or listening should be reinforced, and recreational toys that are innovative and creative should be provided for them. Infants love to tear paper and avidly pursue books, magazines, or newspapers left on the floor. Instead of always scolding them for destroying a valued book, old, discarded reading material should be kept available for them to play with. If they enjoy pots and pans, a cabinet can be arranged with safe utensils for them to explore (Fig. 8-14). These actions will result in much less frustration for everyone, and in time the infants will learn to distinguish between what is theirs and what belongs to others.

One additional factor must be stressed concerning accident prevention and discipline. Children are imitators; they copy what they see and hear. Practicing safety teaches safety, which applies to parents and their children as well as to nurses and their clients. Saying one thing but doing another confuses children and can lead to discipline problems as the child grows older.

PARENTAL CONCERNS

For new parents, as well as for some experienced parents, there are many concerns about childrearing during the first year. Should he suck his thumb? When will he sleep through the night? Why he is so irritable with each new tooth? Should we discipline him so soon? These are just a sampling of questions that parents ask. Nurses must be aware of these concerns and provide answers that give guidance and help decrease anxiety.

Thumb-sucking

Sucking is the infant's chief pleasure, and it may not be satisfied by breast- or bottle-feeding. It is such a strong need that infants who are deprived of sucking, such as those with a cleft lip repair, will suck on their tongue. Some newborns are born with sucking pads on their fingers from in utero sucking activity. Problems arise when parents are concerned about finger- or thumb-sucking and attempt to restrain this natural tendency. Before giving advice nurses should investigate the parents' feelings and base guidance on this information. For example, some parents may see no problem with the use of a pacifier but may find the use of a finger repulsive.

In general there is no need to restrain either. Malocclusion may occur if thumb-sucking persists past 4 years of age or when the permanent teeth erupt. There is probably less dental displacement with the use of pacifier than with the use of a hard, rigid finger. Pacifiers are usually relinquished earlier than thumbs because they are not so readily available.

Sucking pleasure can be increased by prolonging feeding time. A small-holed, firm nipple on the bottle causes stronger sucking and slower feeding.

Thumb-sucking reaches its peak at ages 18 to 20 months and is most prevalent when the child is hungry or tired. Persistent thumb-sucking in a listless, apathetic child always warrants investigation. It may be a sign of an emotional problem between parent and child or of boredom, isolation, and lack of stimulation.

Teething

One of the more difficult periods in the infant's (and parents') life is the eruption of the deciduous teeth, often referred to as teething. Teething is a physiologic process, and as the crown of the tooth breaks through the peridontal membrane considerable discomfort may be present. Some children show minimal evidence of teething, such as drooling or biting on hard objects. Others are very irritable, have difficulty in sleeping, and refuse to eat. Generally signs of illness such as fever, vomiting, or diarrhea are not symptoms of teething but of illness.

Since teething pain is a result of inflammation, cold is usually soothing. Giving the child a cold metal spoon, a frozen teething ring, or an ice cube wrapped in a washcloth helps relieve the inflammation. Analgesics, preferably nonaspirin compounds such as acetaminophen, can be given judiciously. The use of teething powders or procedures such as cutting the gums are discouraged, since ingestion of the powder or infection of the tissue can occur.

Sleep

Most infants have developed a nocturnal pattern of sleep by 3 months of age. By age 6 months the majority of infants sleep through the night, with naps during the day. An 8- or 9-month-old infant may take one or two naps during the day and sleeps about 12 hours during the night. However, there is no set schedule for any child. If parents question the infant's need for sleep, it is best to investigate the reason for their concern, stressing the individual needs of each child. Infants who are active during wakeful periods and who are growing normally are sleeping a sufficient amount of time. If waking during the night persists, the diet should be investigated, since hunger will cause infants to waken. Breast-fed or small infants usually sleep less prolonged periods than do bottle-fed or larger infants because of the more rapid digestion of human milk and lesser stomach capacity of smaller infants. Tooth eruption and sleeping in the parents' room are also associated with night waking.

Infant shoes

Many parents are unaware of the type of shoes that are appropriate for the older infant and succumb to buying expensive infant shoes because of misleading advertising claims. Inflexible shoes that have hard soles can be detrimental by delaying walking, aggravating intoeing and outtoeing, and impeding the development of supportive foot muscles. Therefore, counseling the parents regarding proper footwear should begin when the infant is about 5 to 6 months old.

When children begin walking, the main reason for shoes is *protection*. To provide protection, the shoe should retain its fit, be made of durable material with smooth interiors and few construction seams to irritate the skin, and be soft and flexible, especially in the toe area. A high-top shoe is not necessary for support but may be helpful in keeping the foot in the shoe. The shape of the shoe should conform to the anatomic shape of the foot. In particular the toe area should be rounded and have sufficient room. When bearing weight, there should be at least the space of half the width of the thumbnail, or 1.25 cm (½ inch), between the end of the longest toe and the shoe. Socks should also be roomy and square-toed to allow for proper growth and alignment. Inexpensive but well-constructed sneakers are suggested as adequate footgear for walking infants.

Anticipatory guidance—care of parents

Childrearing is no easy task; it presents challenges to new parents as well as to "seasoned" parents. With society's changing roles and mores, combined with a highly mobile population, there is little stability for traditional role models and time-honored methods of raising children. As a result, parents look more to professionals for guidance. Nurses are in an advantageous position for rendering assistance and suggestions. Every phase of a child's life has its particular traumas, whether it is toilet training for toddlers, unexplained fears for preschoolers, or identity crises for adolescents. For parents of an infant some challenges center around dependency, discipline, increased mobility, and safety. The major areas for parental guidance during the first year are listed in the boxed material above.

PARENTAL GUIDANCE DURING INFANT'S FIRST YEAR

First 6 months

Understand each parent's adjustment to newborn, especially mother's postpartal emotional needs

Teach care of infant and assist parents to understand his individual needs and temperament and that he expresses his wants through crying

Reassure that infant cannot be spoiled by too much attention during the first 4 to 6 months

Encourage parents to establish a schedule that meets needs of child and themselves

Help parents understand infant's need for stimulation in environment

Support parents' pleasure in seeing child's growing friendliness and social response, especially smiling

Plan anticipatory guidance for safety

Stress need for artificial immunization

Prepare for introduction of solid foods

Second 6 months

Prepare parents for child's "stranger anxiety"

Encourage parents to allow child to cling to mother or father and avoid long separation from either

Guide parents concerning discipline because of infant's increasing mobility

Encourage use of negative voice and eye contact rather than physical punishment as a means of discipline; if unsuccessful, use one slap on the hand

Encourage showing most attention when infant is behaving well, rather than when crying

Teach accident prevention because of child's advancing motor skills and curiosity

Encourage parents to leave child with suitable mother substitute to allow some free time

Discuss readiness for weaning

Explore parents' feelings regarding infant's sleep patterns

REFERENCES

American Academy of Pediatrics, Committee on Nutrition: The use of whole cow's milk in infancy, Pediatrics **72**(2):253-255, 1983.

American Academy of Pediatrics, Committee on Nutrition: Toward a prudent diet for children, Pediatrics **71**(1):78-80, 1983.

American Academy of Pediatrics, Committee on Nutrition: Vitamin and mineral supplement needs in normal children in the United States, Pediatrics **66**(6):1015-1020, 1980.

American Academy of Pediatrics, Report of the Committee on Infectious Diseases, Evanston, Ill., 1982, The Academy.

Baker, S.P., and Fisher, R.S.: Childhood asphyxiation by choking or suffocation, JAMA **244**(12):1343-1346, 1980.

Carey, W.B., and McDevitt, S.C.: Revision of the infant temperament questionnaire, Pediatrics **61**(5):735-739, 1978.

Thomas, A., and Chess, S.: Temperament and development, New York, 1977, Brunner/Mazel, Inc.

BIBLIOGRAPHY
Growth and development

Brown, M., and Murphy, M.: A child grows, Pediatr. Nurs. **1**:9, Jan./Feb. 1975.

Brown, M., and Murphy, M.: A child grows. Part II. How the child grows and develops psychologically, socially, and culturally, Pediatr. Nurs. **1**:22-30, March/April 1975.

Brown, M., and Murphy, M.: A child grows. Part III. The child's cognitive development, Pediatr. Nurs. **1**:7-12, May/June 1975.

Brown, M., and Murphy, M.: A child grows. Part IV. The child's perceptual and linguistic development, Pediatr. Nurs. **9**:15, July/Aug. 1975.

Chance, P.: Learning through play, Skillman, N.J., 1979, Johnson & Johnson Baby Products Co.

Chase, R.A., and Rubin, R.R.: The first wondrous year, New York, 1979, Macmillan, Inc.

Fraiberg, S.: The magic years, New York, 1968, Charles Scribner's Sons.

Illingworth, R.S.: Development of the infant and young child, ed. 7, New York, 1980, Churchill Livingstone, Inc.

Kaluger, G., and Kaluger, M.F.: Human development: the span of life, ed. 3, St. Louis, 1984, The C.V. Mosby Co.

Knobloch, H., and Pasamanick, B.: Gesell and Amatruda's developmental diagnosis, New York, 1974, Harper & Row, Publishers, Inc.

Maier, H.: Three theories of child development, ed. 3, New York, 1978, Harper & Row, Publishers, Inc.

Reilly, A.P., editor: The communication game, Skillman, N.J., 1980, Johnson & Johnson Baby Products Co.

Stern, D.: Play and learning in the first year: new insights, Pediatr. Nurs. **5**(5):37, 1979.

Thoman, E.B., and Trotter, S.: Social responsiveness of infants, Skillman, N.J., 1978, Johnson & Johnson Baby Products Co.

Attachment/infant temperament/stranger anxiety

Als, H.: Assessing infant individuality. In Brown, C.C., editor: Infants at risk, Skillman, N.J., 1981, Johnson & Johnson Baby Products Co.

Blosser, C.: Avoiding potential behavior problems in children, Pediatr. Nurs. **5**(3):11-15, 1979.

Harris, C.H.: Assessment of children's behavior. In Johnson, S.M.: High-risk parenting, New York, 1979, J.B. Lippincott Co.

Harris, F.G.: Strategies for parenting during the early stages of a child's life, Issues Ment. Health Nurs. **2**(3):71-84, 1980.

Klaus, M., and Kennel, J.: Parent-infant bonding, ed. 2, St. Louis, 1982, The C.V. Mosby Co.

Nelms, B.C.: Attachment versus spoiling, Pediatr. Nurs. **9**(1):49-51, 1983.

Powell, M.L.: Assessment of infant temperament. In Powell, M.L.: Assessment and management of developmental changes and problems in children, ed. 2, St. Louis, 1981, The C.V. Mosby Co.

Sherwen, L.N.: Separation: the forgotten phenomenon of child development, Topic Clin. Nurs. **5**(1):1-11, 1983.

Snyder, C., Eyres, S.J., and Barnard, K.: New findings about mothers' antenatal expectations and their relationship to infant development, Am. J. Maternal Child Nurs. **4**(6):354-357, 1979.

Nutritional guidance

American Academy of Pediatrics, Committee on Nutrition: On the feeding of supplemental foods to infants, Pediatrics **65**(6):1178-1181, 1980.

Crummette, B., and Munton, M.: Mothers' decisions about infant nutrition, Pediatr. Nurs. **6**(6):16-19, 1980.

Gulick, E.: Infant health and breast-feeding, Pediatr. Nurs. **9**(5):359-362, 1983.

Owens, A.L.: Feeding guide: a nutritional guide for the maturing infant. In Infant nutrition: a foundation for lasting health? Bloomfield, N.J., 1979, Health Learning Systems, Inc.

Pipes, P.L.: Nutrition in infancy and childhood, ed. 2, St. Louis, 1981, The C.V. Mosby Co.

Ross, L.: Weaning practices, J. Nurse Midwife. **26**(1):9-14, 1981.

Immunizations

American Academy of Pediatrics, Committee on Infectious Diseases: Pertussis vaccine, Pediatrics **74**(2):303-305, 1984.

Bindler, R.M.: Truths and trends in immunization, Child. Nurs. **2**(1):1-4, 1984.

Claypool, J.M.: Rubella protection for maternal child health care providers, Am. J. Maternal Child Nurs. **6**(1):53-56, 1981.

Infectious diseases update: it's not fun to be sticked by a needle! Emergency Medicine **14**:29-32, Aug. 1982.

Krugman, S., and Katz, S.: Infectious diseases of children, ed. 7, St. Louis, 1981, The C.V. Mosby Co.

Pajares, K., Parks, B.R., and Fischer, R.G.: Rubella vaccination, Pediatr. Nurse **10**(1):72, 1984.

Selekman, J.: Immunization: what's it all about? Am. J. Nurs. **80**(8):1440-1442, 1980.

Accident prevention

American Academy of Pediatrics, Committee on Pediatric Aspects of Physical Fitness, Recreation, and Sports: Swimming instruction for infants, Pediatrics **65**(4):847, 1980.

Feldman, K.W.: Prevention of childhood accidents: recent progress, Pediatr. Rev. **2**(3):75-82, 1980.

Johnson, N.: Pacifiers: safety and security, Pediatr. Nurs. **4**(6):58-60, 1978.

Marcus, D.F.: Child car seats: a must for safety, Pediatr. Nurs. **7**(3):13-17, 1981.

Post, C., and Robinson, J.: A "good beginning" for families, Pediatr. Nurs. **6**(4):32-36, 1980.

Reinhard, S.C.: Nursing responsibility in infant car safety, Am. J. Maternal Child Nurs. **5**(1):26, 1980.

Surveyer, J.A., and Halpern, J.: Age-related burn injuries and their prevention, Pediatr. Nurs. **7**(5):29-34, 1981.

Parental concerns

Bradshaw, T.W.: Teething, Pediatr. Nurs. **7**(3):41-42, 1981.

Osterholm, P., Lindeke, L.L., and Amidon, D.: Sleep disturbance in infants aged 6 to 12 months, Pediatr. Nurs. **9**(4):269-721, 1983.

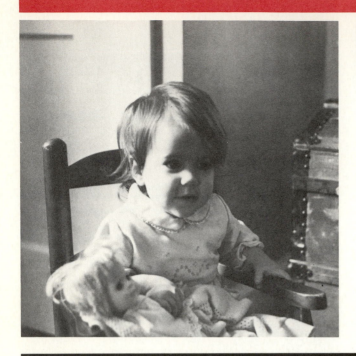

HEALTH PROBLEMS DURING THE FIRST YEAR

OBJECTIVES

On completion of this chapter the reader will be able to:

- Identify children at increased risk of developing nutritional disturbances

- Outline a nutritional counseling plan for vitamin deficiency and excess

- List measures that may prevent or minimize the development of allergies in children

- Outline a dietary plan for parents when the infant is sensitive to milk

- Differentiate ''spitting up'' and regurgitation from rumination and other types of vomiting

- Outline a feeding plan for the child with rumination

- List measures that can be used to alleviate colic

- Identify characteristics of failure-to-thrive children and their families

- Plan nursing care that meets the physical and emotional needs of the failure-to-thrive child and parent

- Provide nursing care that meets the immediate and long-term needs of the family who have lost a child from sudden infant death syndrome

NURSING DIAGNOSES

Nursing diagnoses identified for the infant with health problems include, but are not restricted to, the following:

Health perception-health management pattern

- Infection, potential for, related to nutritional disturbances

Nutritional-metabolic pattern

- Fluid volume deficit, potential, related to nutritional disturbances

- Nutrition, alterations in: less than body requirements related to (1) nutritional disturbances; (2) rumination; (3) failure to thrive

- Oral mucous membranes, alterations in, related to specific nutritional deficiencies (for example, vitamin C)

- Skin integrity, impairment of: actual, related to malnutrition

Activity-exercise pattern

- Activity intolerance related to malnutrition

- Diversional activity deficit related to developmental deprivation (failure to thrive)

- Home maintenance management, impaired, related to (1) knowledge deficit; (2) inadequate support system or overwhelming demands (autism)

- Mobility, impaired physical, related to specific nutritional deficiencies (for example, vitamin D)

- Self-care deficit, total, related to developmental level

Sleep-rest pattern

- Sleep-pattern disturbance related to excessive crying (colic)

Cognitive-perceptual pattern

- Comfort, alterations in: pain, related to specific nutritional deficiencies (for example, vitamin C)

- Knowledge deficit related to parenting skills

Self-perception—self-concept pattern

- Anxiety related to (1) colic; (2) death

Role-relationship pattern

- Communication, impaired verbal, related to autism

- Family process, alterations in, related to disruption in life style (colic, SIDS, autism)

- Grieving, dysfunctional, potential for, related to loss of child (SIDS)

- Parenting, alteration in: actual, related to disturbed parent-child relationship (failure to thrive)

- Parenting, alterations in: potential, related to (1) stress (colic, autism); (2) grief

Coping-stress tolerance pattern

- Coping, family: potential for growth, related to successful coping with loss

The infant's immature physiologic system predisposes him to several potential health problems during the first year. This chapter deals primarily with health problems that are influenced by environmental factors affecting the physical or psychologic development of the child. Some of the problems, such as the nutritional disturbances, have special implications for nurses because they are preventable. Others, such as sudden infant death syndrome, are uncontrollable and unpredictable; however, the intervention needed after the death of the child is crucial for the reintegration of the family. Although several topics discussed here can occur in other age-groups, the greatest significance of these disorders is evident during the early months of life. Prompt awareness and identification of health problems will avert complications in later life. Prevention rather than treatment whenever possible should be every health professional's goal in the care of children.

NUTRITIONAL DISTURBANCES

Malnutrition is a general term that refers to poor or inadequate nutrition. Although it is generally thought of in terms of undernutrition, it also includes overnutrition, which may be manifested as obesity or hypervitaminosis. Inadequate nutrition is most commonly seen as iron-deficiency anemia (Chapter 23) or vitamin deficiencies. The most severe states of malnutrition involve the protein and caloric deficiencies, kwashiorkor and marasmus.

Another category of nutritional disturbances is nutritional allergy, which is the result of the body's altered response to substance rather than an excess or deficiency of the nutrient. Nutritional allergy is discussed separately under the topic of allergy.

Vitamin disturbances

True vitamin disturbances are rare in the United States. Subclinical deficiencies are commonly seen, however, especially in lower socioeconomic groups where dietary intake may be unbalanced. Vitamin deficiencies of the fat-soluble vitamins A and D may occur in malabsorptive disorders. Recently, there has been an increase in vitamin D–deficient rickets. Populations at risk include (1) children born of mothers who are vitamin D deficient, (2) individuals who are exposed to minimal sunlight because of dis-

TABLE 9-1. SUMMARY OF VITAMINS AND THEIR NUTRITIONAL SIGNIFICANCE

VITAMINS*	PHYSIOLOGIC FUNCTION	SOURCES
A (retinol)	Necessary component in formation of pigment rhodopsin (visual purple)	Natural form—liver, kidney, fish oils, milk and nonskimmed milk products, egg yolk
	Formation and maintenance of epithelial tissue	
Provitamin A (carotene)	Normal bone growth and tooth development	Carrots, sweet potatoes, squash, apricots, spinach, collards, broccoli, cabbage, artichokes
	Needed for growth and spermatogenesis	
	Involved in thyroxine formation	

*For RDA (recommended daily dietary allowance) see Appendix D.

tinctive clothing, housing in areas of high pollution, or dark skin pigmentation, and (3) adherence to vegetarian diets that are low in sources of vitamin D.

With the addition of vitamins and minerals to commercially packaged foods, the potential for hypervitaminosis has escalated, especially when combined with the injudicious use of vitamin supplements. Hypervitaminosis can also occur from overfeeding of certain foods, such as liver, which has a large vitamin A content.

Deficiencies of vitamins A, B complex, C, D, E, and K and excesses of vitamins A, D, E, and K are summarized in Table 9-1. Excesses of the water-soluble vitamins B complex and C are known to occur but are less frequent. Therefore, they are not included in the table. The recommended daily dietary allowances (RDA) are listed in Appendix D. The main nursing goal for each excess and deficiency is prevention through appropriate nutritional counseling as outlined in Table 9-1.

Protein and calorie malnutrition (PCM)

Hunger is one of the world's gravest and most prevalent health problems. Three fourths of the world population suffers some form of malnutrition. Mortality and morbidity among children support the severity of this problem in underdeveloped countries, where in the 1- to 4-year-old age-group the death rate may be 20 to 50 times higher than in the United States.

Even in the United States, the PCM diseases of kwashiorkor and marasmus are reported in hospitals each year. They occur primarily (1) as a complication of an underlying disease process, (2) as a result of fad diets, such as vegetarianism, (3) from lack of parental education regarding infant nutrition, and (4) from inappropriate management of food allergy, for example, the use of high-fat, low-protein, nondairy creamer as a substitute for milk.

Vegetarianism. The importance of vegetarian diets and their relationship to potential nutritional deficiencies in children cannot be overemphasized. The stricter the vegetarian diet, the more difficult it is to ensure adequate nutrition for infants and children. The two major types of vegetarianism are:

lacto-ovovegetarians who exclude meat from their diet but eat milk and eggs and sometimes fish
pure vegetarians (vegans) who exclude any food of animal origin, including milk and eggs

RESULTS OF DEFICIENCY OR EXCESS	NURSING CONSIDERATIONS

Deficiency
Night blindness
Keratinization (hardening and scaling) of epithelium
  Xerophthalmia (hardening and scaling of cornea and conjunctiva)
  Phrynoderma (toadskin)
  Drying of respiratory, gastrointestinal, and genitourinary tracts
Defective tooth enamel
Retarded growth
Impaired bone formation
Decreased thyroxine formation
	Encourage foods rich in vitamin A, such as whole cow's milk
	As milk consumption decreases, encourage foods rich in vitamin A
	If cod liver oil is prescribed, suggest following method of preparation:
	  Prepare gelatin as directed on the package
	  Place a small amount (about ¼ cup) in a container
	  When the gelatin is soft set, mix in the cod liver oil; serve when completely jelled

Excess Early signs—irritability, anorexia, pruritus, fissures at corners of nose and lips Later signs—hepatomegaly, jaundice, retarded growth, poor weight gain, thickening of the cortex of long bones with pain and fragility, hard tender lumps in extremities and occiput of the skull NOTE: Overdose only results from ingestion of large quantities of the vitamin, not the provitamin; large amounts of carotene (carotenemia) cause yellow or orange discoloration of the skin (not the sclera as in jaundice), but none of the above symptoms	Emphasize correct use of vitamin supplements Investigate child's dietary habits to calculate approximate intake; if excessive, remove supplemental source

Continued.

TABLE 9-1. SUMMARY OF VITAMINS AND THEIR NUTRITIONAL SIGNIFICANCE—cont'd

VITAMINS	PHYSIOLOGIC FUNCTION	SOURCES
B_1 (thiamin)	Coenzyme (with phosphorus) in carbohydrate metabolism Needed for healthy nervous system	Pork, beef, liver, legumes, nuts, whole or enriched grains
B_2 (riboflavin)	Coenzyme (with phosphorus) in carbohydrate, protein, and fat metabolism Maintains healthy skin especially around mouth, nose, and eyes	Milk and its products, eggs, organ meats (liver, kidney, and heart), enriched cereals, some green leafy vegetables, legumes
Niacin (nicotinic acid, nicotinamide)	Coenzyme (with riboflavin) in protein and fat metabolism Needed for healthy nervous system, skin, and normal digestion	Meat, poultry, fish, peanuts, beans, peas, whole or enriched grains except corn and rice Milk and its products are sources of tryptophan (60 mg of tryptophan = 1 mg of niacin)
B_6 (pyridoxine)	Coenzyme in protein and fat metabolism Needed for formation of antibodies, hemoglobin Needed for utilization of copper and iron Aids in conversion of tryptophan to niacin	Meats, especially liver and kidney, cereal grains (wheat and corn), yeast, soybeans, peanuts
Folic acid (folacin; reduced form is called folinic acid or citrovorum factor)	Coenzyme for single-carbon transfer (purines, thymine, hemoglobin) Necessary for formation of red blood cells	Green leafy vegetables (spinach), asparagus, liver, kidney, nuts, eggs, whole grain cereals
B_{12} (cobalamin)	Coenzyme in protein synthesis; indirect effect on formation of red blood cells (particularly on formation of nucleic acids and folic acid metabolism) Needed for normal functioning of nervous tissue	Meat, liver, kidney, fish, milk, eggs, cheese (no vegetable source is known)
Biotin	Coenzyme in carbohydrate, protein, and fat metabolism Interrelated with functions of other B vitamins	Liver, kidney, egg yolk, tomatoes, legumes, nuts
Pantothenic acid	Coenzyme in carbohydrate, protein, and fat metabolism Synthesis of amino acids, fatty acids, and steroids	Liver, kidney, heart, salmon, eggs, vegetables, legumes, whole grains

RESULTS OF DEFICIENCY OR EXCESS	NURSING CONSIDERATIONS
Vitamin B complex deficiency	**Vitamin B complex**
Beriberi	Encourage foods rich in B vitamins
Gastrointestinal—anorexia, constipation, indigestion	Stress proper cooking and storage techniques to preserve potency, such as minimal cooking of vegetables in small amount of liquid; storage of milk in opaque container
Neurologic—apathy, fatigue, emotional instability, polyneuritis, convulsions and coma (in infants)	Advise against fad diets that severely restrict groups of food, such as vegetarianism
Circulatory—palpitations, cardiac failure, peripheral vasodilation, edema	Explore need for vitamin supplements when dieting or when using goat milk exclusively for infant feeding (deficient in folic acid)
Ariboflavinosis	
Lips—cheilosis (fissures at corners of lips), perlèche (inflammation at corners of lips)	
Tongue—glossitis	
Nose—irritation and cracks at nasal angle	
Eyes—burning, itching, tearing, photophobia, corneal vascularization, cataracts	
Skin—seborrheic dermatitis, delayed wound healing and tissue repair	
Pellagra	
Oral—stomatitis, glossitis	
Cutaneous—scaly dermatitis on exposed areas	
Gastrointestinal—anorexia, weight loss, diarrhea, fatigue	
Neurologic—apathy, anxiety, confusion, depression, dementia	
Death	
Scaly dermatitis, weight loss, anemia, retarded growth, irritability, convulsions, peripheral neuritis	
Macrocytic anemia, bone marrow depression, glossitis, intestinal malabsorption	
Pernicious anemia	
General signs of severe anemia	
Lemon yellow tinge to skin	
Spinal cord degeneration	
Deficiency	
Deficiency is uncommon because synthesized by bacterial flora	
Deficiency is uncommon because of its multiple food sources and synthesis by bacterial flora	

Continued.

TABLE 9-1. SUMMARY OF VITAMINS AND THEIR NUTRITIONAL SIGNIFICANCE—cont'd

VITAMINS	PHYSIOLOGIC FUNCTION	SOURCES
C (ascorbic acid)	Essential for collagen formation Increases absorption of iron for hemoglobin formation Enhances conversion of folic to folinic acid Affects cholesterol synthesis and conversion of proline to hydroxyproline Probably a coenzyme in metabolism of tyrosine and phenylalanine May play role in hydroxylation of adrenal steroids May have stimulating effect on phagocytic activity of leukocytes and formation of antibodies Antioxidant agent (spares other vitamins from oxidation)	Citrus fruits, berries, tomatoes, potatoes, melon, cabbage, green and yellow vegetables
D_2 (ergocalciferol) and D_3 (cholecalciferol)	Absorption of calcium and phosphorus and decreased renal excretion of phosphorus	Direct sunlight Cod liver oil, herring, mackerel, salmon, tuna, sardines Enriched food sources—milk, milk products, cereals, margarine, breads, many breakfast drinks

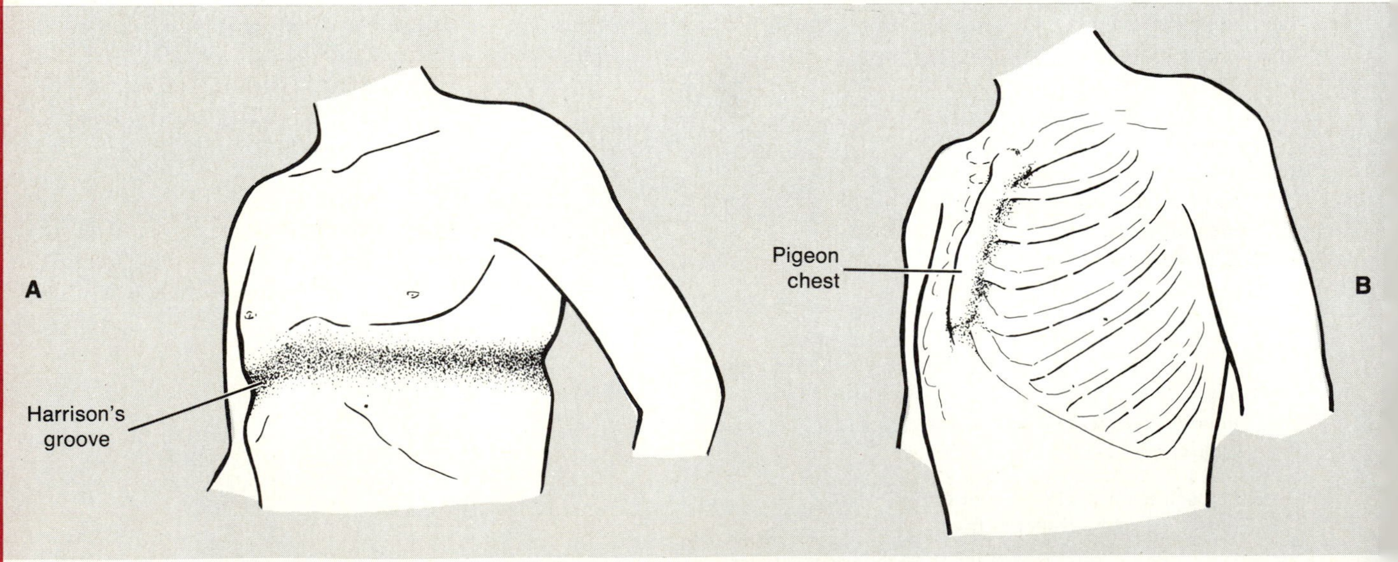

FIG. 9-1
Chest deformities in vitamin D deficiency. **A,** *Harrison's groove.* **B,** *Pigeon chest.*

RESULTS OF DEFICIENCY OR EXCESS	NURSING CONSIDERATIONS

Deficiency

Scurvy

Skin—dry, rough, petechiae, perifollicular hyperkeratotic papules (raised areas around hair follicles)

Musculoskeletal—bleeding into muscles and joints, pseudoparalysis from pain, swelling of joints, costochondral beading (scorbutic rosary)

Gums—spongy, friable, swollen, bleed easily, bluish red or black color, teeth loosen and fall out

General disposition—irritable, anorexic, apprehensive, in pain, refuses to move, assumes semi-froglike position when supine (scorbutic pose)

Signs of anemia

Decreased wound healing

Increased susceptibility to infection

Encourage foods rich in vitamin C

Investigate infant's diet for sources of vitamin, especially when cow's milk is principal source of nutrition

Stress proper cooking and storing techniques to preserve potency

Wash vegetables quickly; do not soak in water

Cook vegetables in covered pot with minimal water and for short time; avoid copper or cast iron cookware

Do not add baking soda to cooking water

Use fresh fruits and vegetables as soon as possible; store in refrigerator

Store juice in airtight opaque container

In caring for child with scurvy:

Position for comfort and rest

Handle very gently and minimally

Administer analgesics as needed

Prevent infection

Provide good oral care

Provide soft, bland diet

Emphasize rapid recovery when vitamin is replaced

Deficiency

Rickets

Head—craniotabes (softening of cranial bones, prominence of frontal bones) deformed shape (skull flat and depressed toward middle), delayed closure of fontanels

Chest—rachitic rosary (enlargement of costochondral junction of ribs), Harrison's groove (horizontal depression in lower portion of rib cage) (Fig. 9-1, *A*), pigeon chest (sharp protrusion of sternum) (Fig. 9-1, *B*)

Spine—kyphosis, scoliosis, lordosis

Abdomen—potbelly, constipation

Extremities—bowing of arms and legs, knock-knee, saber shins, instability of hip joints, pelvic deformity, enlargement of epiphysis at ends of long bones

Teeth—delayed calcification, especially of permanent teeth

Rachitic tetany—seizures

Encourage foods rich in vitamin D, especially fortified cow's milk

In breast-fed infants encourage use of vitamin D supplements if maternal diet inadequate or infant exposed to minimal sunlight

Emphasize importance of exposure to sun as source of vitamin

In caring for child with rickets:

Maintain good body alignment

Reposition frequently to prevent decubiti and respiratory infection

Handle very gently and minimally

Prevent infection

Institute seizure precautions

Have 10% calcium gluconate available in case of tetany

Observe for possibility of overdose from supplements

If prescribed, supervise proper use of orthopedic splints or braces

Excess

Acute—vomiting, dehydration, fever, abdominal cramps, bone pain, convulsions, and coma

Chronic—lassitude, mental slowness, anorexia, failure to thrive, thirst, urinary urgency, polyuria, vomiting, diarrhea, abdominal cramps, bone pain, pathologic fractures

Calcification of soft tissue—kidneys, lungs, adrenal glands, vessels (hypertension), heart, gastric lining, tympanic membrane (deafness)

Osteoporosis of long bones

Elevated serum levels of calcium and phosphorus

Same as vitamin A; may include low-calcium diet during initial therapy

Continued.

TABLE 9-1. SUMMARY OF VITAMINS AND THEIR NUTRITIONAL SIGNIFICANCE—cont'd

VITAMINS	PHYSIOLOGIC FUNCTION	SOURCES
E (tocopherol)	Production of red blood cells Muscle and liver integrity Coenzyme factor in tissue respiration Minimizes oxidation of polyunsaturated fatty acids and vitamins A and C in intestinal tract and tissues	Vegetable oils, wheat germ oil, milk, egg yolk, muscle meats, fish, whole grains, nuts, legumes, spinach, broccoli
K	Catalyst for production of prothrombin and blood clotting factors II, VII, IX, and X by the liver	Pork, liver, green leafy vegetables (spinach, kale, cabbage), tomatoes, egg yolk, cheese

The major deficiencies in the stricter vegetarian diets are (1) inadequate protein for growth, especially if complementary sources of nonanimal protein foods are not given, (2) inadequate calories for energy and growth, (3) poor digestibility of many of the natural, unprocessed foods, especially for infants, and (4) specific vitamin and mineral deficiencies of vitamin B$_{12}$, niacin, thiamine, riboflavin, vitamin D, iron, and zinc. In the United States, strict vegetarian diets are common among members of Black Muslim or Seventh Day Adventist faiths.

Kwashiorkor. Kwashiorkor is a deficiency of protein with an adequate supply of calories. The word comes from the Ghan language and means "the sickness the older child gets when the next baby is born." It is an appropriate name because it is a syndrome that develops in the first child, usually between 1 and 4 years of age, when he is weaned from the breast and fed a diet consisting mainly of starch grains or tubers once the second child is born. Such a diet provides adequate calories in the form of carbohydrates but an inadequate amount of high-quality proteins.

The child with kwashiorkor has thin, wasted extremities and a prominent abdomen from edema (ascites). The edema often masks the severe muscular atrophy, making the child appear less debilitated than he actually is. The skin is scaly and dry and has areas of depigmentation. Several dermatoses may be evident, partly resulting from the vitamin deficiencies. Permanent blindness often results from the severe lack of vitamin A. Mineral deficiencies are common, especially iron, calcium, and zinc. The hair is thin, dry, coarse, and dull. Depigmentation is common, and patchy alopecia may occur (Fig. 9-2).

Diarrhea frequently results from a lowered resistance to infection. Gastrointestinal disturbances occur, affecting the liver and spleen. Behavioral changes are evident as the child grows progressively more irritable, lethargic, withdrawn, and apathetic. Fatal deterioration may be caused by diarrhea and infection or as the result of circulatory failure.

Marasmus. Marasmus is the result of general malnutrition of both calories and protein. It is a common occurrence in underdeveloped countries during times of drought. Because children are fed last in these cultures, there is seldom enough food remaining for the younger ones.

Marasmus is usually a syndrome of physical and emotional deprivation and is not confined to geographic areas where food supplies are inadequate. It may be seen in failure-to-thrive children, where the cause is not solely nutritional but primarily emotional.

RESULTS OF DEFICIENCY OR EXCESS	NURSING CONSIDERATIONS

Deficiency
  Hemolytic anemia from hemolysis caused by shortened life of red blood cells, especially in premature infants, and focal necrosis of tissues
  Causes infertility in rats, but not in humans (does *not* increase human male virility or potency)
 	
Excess
  Little is known; less toxic than other fat-soluble vitamins but excess of water-soluble preparations has been fatal in premature infants
	Initiate early feeding in premature infants; may need supplementation

Deficiency
  Hemorrhage
 	
Excess
  Hyperbilirubinemia in infants
  Hemolytic anemia in individuals who are deficient in glucose-6-phosphate dehydrogenase
	Administer prophylactically to newborns
	Other indications include intestinal disease, lack of bile, prolonged antibiotic therapy, or use of anticoagulants such as heparin or dicumarol (bishydroxycoumarin), which are vitamin K antagonists

Marasmus is characterized by gradual wasting and atrophy of body tissues, especially of subcutaneous fat (Fig. 9-3). The child appears to be very old; his skin is flabby and wrinkled, unlike the child with kwashiorkor who appears more rounded from the edema. Fat metabolism is less impaired than in kwashiorkor, so that deficiency of fat-soluble vitamins is usually minimal or absent.

The child is fretful, apathetic, withdrawn, and so lethargic that prostration frequently occurs. Intercurrent infection with debilitating diseases such as tuberculosis, parasitosis, and dysentery is common.

Therapeutic management. Treatment of PCM includes providing a diet high in quality proteins and/or carbohydrates, vitamins, and minerals. Electrolyte imbalance requires immediate attention, and parenteral fluid replacement may be necessary initially to correct the dehydration and restore renal function. When oral fluids and food are not tolerated, hyperalimentation is life-saving. Coexisting problems, such as infection, diarrhea, parasitic infestation, and anemia, require prompt attention for optimum recovery.

Nursing considerations. Provision of essential physiologic needs, such as rest, individually tailored activity, and protection from infection, is paramount. Since the child is usually weak and withdrawn, he depends on others to feed him. Hygiene may be distressing because of the poor integrity of the skin, and decubiti are a constant threat. Appropriate developmental stimulation should be provided also.

The larger problem is the prevention of these conditions through education concerning the importance of high-quality proteins and adequate carbohydrates. Children can receive optimal nutrition from vegetarian diets with appropriate dietary counseling, such as prolonged breast-feeding, substitution of fortified soy milk if dairy products are excluded, and use of complementary incomplete proteins, such as grains and legumes.

ALLERGY

Allergy, or *atopy*, is an altered, adverse reaction to a foreign substance or antigen that usually produces no untoward effects in humans. An *antigen* is any substance capable of stimulating the production of antibodies and, subsequently, reacting with them to initiate the allergic response. Antigens enter the body through ingestion, inhalation, transepidermal penetration, or parenteral infusion. Development of the allergic state depends on the nature of

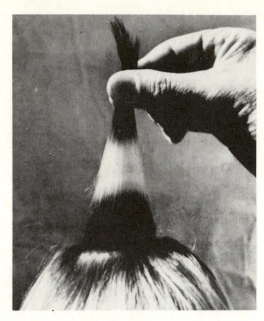

FIG. 9-2

Appearance of the hair in kwashiorkor. Pigmentation changes indicate periods of normal and abnormal growth of hair. (From Scrimshaw, N.S., and Béhar, M.: Malnutrition in underdeveloped countries, N. Engl. J. Med. 272:137, 1965. Reprinted by permission from The New England Journal of Medicine.)

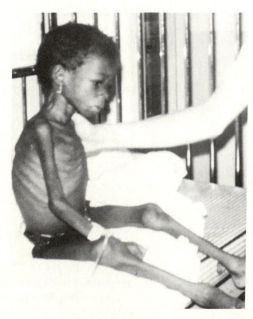

FIG. 9-3

Child with marasmus. (Courtesy Dr. Donald Anderson, Travis Air Force Base, Calif.; from Dodge, P.R., Prensky, A.L., and Feigin, R.D.: Nutrition and the developing nervous system, St. Louis, 1975, The C.V. Mosby Co.)

the antigen, the type of exposure, and the duration of contact.

One of the most important aspects of allergies is their genetic component. Although all individuals are potentially allergic, certain people have an inherited predisposition for the development of allergies. Studies have revealed that anywhere from 40% to 80% of allergic individuals have a positive family history for allergy.

Age is another important factor in the development of allergies. For example, foods are the most important allergens during the first 6 months of life. During infancy, eczema (atopic dermatitis) is frequent but asthma is rare. After the third year, eczema clears spontaneously and asthma and hay fever become dominant.

Nutritional allergies

Nutritional allergies can occur in anyone at any age, and frequently the allergic response is exhibited after the food has been ingested one or more times. Food allergies are most common during infancy, and the chief offenders are cow's milk, eggs, and wheat. Sensitivity to fish and nuts is also likely but is less often outgrown than allergy to the other substances.

Nutritional allergies during infancy are common because the infant is exposed to many new food antigens. Physiologically the intestinal tract is immature and is permeable to many more inadequately catabolized proteins, which, unlike the amino acids that compose them, are capable of producing an allergic response. This explains why the food allergy may disappear as the child grows older.

There is some evidence that nutritional allergies can be delayed and possibly prevented. Exclusive breast-feeding for 4 months or longer reduces the chances of developing antibodies to cow's milk protein, provided the mother avoids ingesting all milk products while breastfeeding. In a child with a strong family history for allergy, certain foods should be avoided during the first year.

Table 9-2 lists common foods that are potentially allergenic. Soy-based formula is recommended as a substitute for cow milk formulas in these infants. In addition, following careful schedules for introducing new foods can quickly identify the offending agent. If any local inflammation occurs, such as swelling of the lip or urticaria around the mouth, the food must be avoided and is usually not reintroduced for a period of 6 or more months.

Cow's milk sensitivity

Cow's milk sensitivity (milk allergy, milk intolerance) is a multifaceted disorder representing adverse systemic and local gastrointestinal reactions to cow's milk protein. It is

TABLE 9-2. HYPERALLERGENIC FOODS

FOOD	SOURCES	FOOD	SOURCES
Milk	Ice cream, butter, margarine, yogurt, cheese, pudding, baked goods, wieners, bologna, canned creamed soups, instant breakfast drinks, powdered milk drinks, milk chocolate	Fish or shellfish	Cod liver oil, pizza with anchovies, Caesar salad dressing, any food fried in same oil as fish
Eggs	Mayonnaise, creamy salad dressing, baked goods, egg noodles, some cake icing, meringue, custard, pancakes, french toast, root beer	Chocolate	Cola beverages, cocoa, chocolate-flavored drinks
		Buckwheat	Some cereals, pancakes
		Pork, chicken	Bacon, wieners, sausage, pork fat, chicken broth
Wheat	Almost all baked goods, wieners, bologna, pressed or chopped cold cuts, gravy, pasta, some canned soups	Strawberries, melon, pineapple	Gelatin, syrups
		Corn	Popcorn, cereal, muffins, cornstarch, corn meal
Legumes	Peanut butter, peanuts, beans, peas, lentils	Citrus fruits	Orange, lemon, lime, grapefruit; any of these in drinks, gelatin, juice, or medicines
Nuts	Chocolate, baked goods, cherry soda (may be flavored with a nut extract)	Tomatoes	Juice, some vegetable soups, spaghetti, pizza sauce, and catsup
		Spices	Chili, pepper, vinegar, cinnamon

the most common nutritional allergy during infancy, affecting 1% to 2% of all infants. It usually appears within the first 2 months of life following cow's milk feeding. Some newborns and exclusively breast-fed infants may be symptomatic following their first exposure to cow's milk, suggesting placental sensitization in utero or sensitization by cow's milk protein in breast milk from maternal ingestion of milk. Many children who are sensitive to cow's milk can tolerate it by 2 years of age.

Clinical manifestations of milk allergy are generally gastrointestinal disturbances, such as vomiting, diarrhea, and colic, but may include a wide variety of other symptoms, such as wheezing, rhinitis, or eczema. Diagnosis of milk allergy is based on disappearance of these symptoms following elimination of all milk products. Confirmation of the diagnosis should be determined by a trial period of reintroduction of milk to ascertain if the symptoms reappear. Only after careful investigation should appropriate dietary changes occur.

Milk allergy can be mistakenly diagnosed as galactosemia or as lactose intolerance, which is an inability to digest usual levels of milk lactose. Lactose intolerance is more common in those of Mediterranean, African, and Asian extraction and is less prevalent in young children than in adults.

Nursing considerations. The principal nursing objectives are identification of potential milk sensitivity and appropriate counseling of parents regarding substitute formulas. The initial alternative is soy milk, although approximately 1:5 children who are allergic to cow's milk are also sensitive to soy milk. Commercially available soy formulas include Prosobee and Isomil. Commercial formulas that are suitable cow's and soy milk substitutes include Meat Base Formula, Nutramigen, Pregestimil, and Vivonex. The latter three preparations contain hydrolyzed protein or amino acid mixtures. Goat's milk is not an acceptable substitute because it cross-reacts with cow's milk protein and is deficient in folic acid.

Infants are maintained on the diet until after 1 year of age, when very small quantities of milk are gradually reintroduced. Children with eczema or other allergic disorders may not be given milk for a considerably longer time.

If milk sensitivity is suspected, finding acceptable substitutions is frequently time-consuming, frustrating, and expensive. Parents are advised to purchase small quantities of the formula and to ask if unused portions can be returned. Frequently when parents are told to try a new formula, they purchase a case rather than a few cans. At the end of the trial period they have a large reserve of unused, costly formulas.

The protein hydrolysate formulas are less palatable than milk-based formulas. Consequently reluctance to accept the new formula may be a problem. This can be overcome by introducing the formula gradually over a few days using 1 ounce of new formula to 7 ounces of old formula, then 2 to 6 ounces, 3 to 4, and so on. Parents also need to be reassured that the infant will receive complete nutrition from the new formula and will suffer no ill effects from the absence of cow's milk.

The nurse also stresses that all associated milk products must be avoided (see Table 9-2). This requires carefully reading all food labels to avoid potential addition of milk products to the prepared food. If the infant is sensitive to soy, parents are advised that it is commonly found in baby junior foods and cereals. In addition, some medication, such as penicillin, vitamins, and diaper ointment, contain lactose as a filler or bulk agent. Parents should be advised to check with the pharmacist regarding this possibility when obtaining drugs. Since allergy to one protein may mean allergy to other proteins, particularly egg albumin and wheat, such foods should be restricted from the infant's diet for the first 9 to 12 months of life.

FEEDING PROBLEMS

A number of feeding difficulties can occur during the infant's first year. The most common cause of feeding problems is improper feeding technique and is corrected with guidance and demonstration. Others, such as spitting up, require little more than parental reassurance. Problems such as colic can disrupt a family tremendously, although the problem resolves spontaneously. Still other disorders, such as rumination, can be fatal even though there is no organic cause.

Regurgitation or "spitting up"

The return of small amounts of food after a feeding is a common occurrence during infancy. It should not be confused with actual vomiting, which can be associated with a number of disturbances, both insignificant and serious. For clarification the following terms are defined:

> **spitting up** dribbling of unswallowed formula from the infant's mouth immediately after a feeding
>
> **regurgitation** the return of undigested food from the stomach, usually accompanied by burping
>
> **vomiting** the forcible ejection of stomach contents, usually accompanied by nausea
>
> **projectile vomiting** vomitus ejected with such force that it projects as far as 2 to 4 feet from the child; the vomiting is not associated with nausea
>
> **rumination** regurgitation and rechewing of food

Persistent regurgitation necessitates medical evaluation to rule out gastroesophageal reflux.

Nursing considerations.   The insignificance of regurgitation or spitting up should be explained to parents,

especially to those who are unduly concerned about it. It can be reduced by some simple measures, such as frequent burping during and after feeding, minimal handling at feeding and after, and positioning the child on the right side with the head slightly elevated after feeding. The inconvenience of spitting up is managed with use of absorbent bibs on the infant and protective cloths on the parent.

Sometimes, frequent dribbling of formula causes excoriation of the corners of the mouth, chin, and neck. Keeping the area dry promotes healing but can be difficult to maintain. Helpful suggestions include applying a thin film of petrolatum jelly or A and D ointment to the affected areas after cleansing and using absorbent terrycloth bibs that are changed frequently.

Rumination

Rumination is the active, voluntary return of swallowed food into the mouth. The food is then rechewed, partially or completely reswallowed, or expelled. In some instances rumination may lead to progressive malnutrition and even death, since considerable food and fluid loss can occur.

Rumination differs from regurgitation, which is involuntary. The ruminating infant makes purposeful movements of the mouth, tongue, and stomach in an attempt to force food back into the oropharynx. On successful regurgitation the infant is obviously satisfied with the activity.

Organic causes for rumination are rarely found, although the possibility of gastroesophageal reflux should be investigated in the differential diagnosis. It may also be seen in profoundly retarded children. However, it most often is a result of a disturbance in the parent-child relationship. The factors culminating in the disorder are similar to those described in nonorganic failure to thrive.

Nursing considerations.   The primary objective is to terminate the ruminating behavior and restore normal feeding patterns. This is accomplished through a structured feeding plan. Generally the same guidelines apply to feeding the ruminating child as to feeding the failure-to-thrive child. In addition, emphasis should be placed on the following areas:

1. Assign the same nurse to feed the child as often as possible. This is even more critical than in failure to thrive.
2. Continue *positive* attention immediately after the feeding, since ruminating infants often vomit after a feeding once they are left unattended.
3. Introduce new foods slowly, with emphasis on texture, consistency, and flavor. These children are often "picky eaters," and new foods introduced too quickly can increase rumination.
4. If acceptance of solids is a problem, give the child a small quantity of milk (or juice), immediately followed by 1 teaspoon of solid food. Begin with pureed food, and

once accepted, advance to junior and adult foods. Gradually give fewer sips of milk and more spoonfuls of food until a regular diet for the child's age is achieved.

These children often require prolonged inpatient intervention to reduce their rumination. Positive stimulation programs must accompany the feeding plan. Parents need to be included in learning how to feed the child, and follow-up after discharge is essential to prevent a recurrence of the behavior.

Paroxysmal abdominal pain (colic)

Colic is generally described as paroxysmal abdominal pain or cramping that is manifested by loud, inconsolable crying and drawing the legs up to the abdomen. It is more common in young infants under the age of 3 months than in older infants. Despite the obvious behavioral indications of pain, the child tolerates the formula well, gains weight, and thrives.

Many theories have been investigated as potential causative factors, such as too rapid feeding, overeating, swallowing excessive air, improper feeding technique, especially in positioning and burping, and emotional stress or tension between parent and child. Generally colic is thought to be caused by excessive fermentation and gas production in the intestines. Excessive intake of carbohydrates causes flatus, but a change in diet rarely prevents the attacks of colic. Colic may be a sign of cow's milk sensitivity, and there is evidence that eliminating cow's milk products from the diet of lactating mothers can reduce the symptoms. Management of colic should begin with an investigation of such causes.

Although colic is considered a minor ailment, a colicky, crying, irritable infant can have an intense emotional impact on parent-child attachment and family relationships. Mothers often relate histories of the daily routine that are laden with feelings of frustration, anger, despair, guilt, fatigue, and helplessness. A vicious cycle ensues in which the parent's own anxiety may be transferred to the infant, which further increases his tension, irritability, and crying.

Nursing considerations. The initial step in managing colic is to take a thorough, detailed history of the usual daily events or to ask parents to keep a log for 48-72 hours. Areas that should be stressed include (1) diet of the breast-feeding mother, (2) time of day when attacks occur, (3) relationship of the attacks to feeding time, (4) presence of specific family members during attacks, (5) activity of the mother or usual caregiver before, during, and after the crying, and (6) measures used to relieve the crying. Of special emphasis is a careful assessment of the feeding process via *demonstration* by the mother.

In breast-feeding mothers a milk-free diet (see Table 9-2) should be followed for a minimum of 5 days in an attempt to reduce symptoms in the infant. If this is successful, the milk-free diet is continued, although mothers may need to take calcium supplements. Mothers need to be cautioned about some nondairy creamers that may contain calcium caseinate, a cow's milk protein.

Often no change is required in feeding practices. When no cause can be identified, it is preferable to determine the time of the onset of crying and attempt to manipulate the circumstances associated with it. For example, some infants have episodes of colic around the family's dinner time, when all household members are home and the mother is preoccupied with cooking. The overstimulating, more tense atmosphere may upset the infant. Encouraging the mother to prepare food items for dinner earlier in the day, such as salad, dessert, or vegetables, and feeding the infant in a more quiet area of the house may help reverse the environmental conditions that may have provoked the attack of colic. Other approaches for relieving colic are listed in the boxed material that follows. Parents are encouraged to try as many of them as possible because not all are effective for every infant. Mild sedation may be prescribed but should be delayed until other options are exhausted.

SUGGESTIONS FOR RELIEVING COLIC

Place the infant prone over a hot-water bottle, heated towel, or covered heating pad, taking precautions to avoid burning the skin

Massage the infant's abdomen or whole body; using lotion may be soothing

Provide smaller, frequent feedings; burp during and after feedings using the shoulder position, and place in an upright seat after feedings

Introduce a pacifier for added sucking

Try giving the infant warm, dilute herbal teas using one teaspoon fennel, chamomile, or anise

Change the infant's position frequently; walk him face down with his body across the parent's arm and hand under the abdomen applying gentle pressure ("colic carry")

Use a "snugli" or front carrier for transporting the infant

Swaddle the infant tightly with a soft, stretchy blanket

Place the infant in a wind-up swing

Play music; try different types of music

Take the infant for car rides or outside for a change in environment

Avoid overstimulating infant; for example, pick infant up but don't talk to him until he relaxes, then talk in soothing tones

Encourage parents to spend short periods of time away from infant whenever possible

One of the most important areas of nursing concern is the support of parents during the colic period. It is stressed that despite the crying and obvious pain, the infant is doing well. Colic disappears spontaneously, usually by 3 months of age, although guarantees should never be given because it may continue for much longer. The mother should be encouraged to leave the house and arrange for some free time. Most importantly, it should be emphasized that the colic is not an indicator of poor or inadequate mothering. The mother's negative feelings toward the infant and her insecurities regarding her mothering abilities are normal. She should be encouraged to talk about them, since active listening may do more to relieve the colic syndrome than offering stereotyped advice, remedies, and glib statements such as, "Don't worry-about it; your child will eventually outgrow the colicky spells."

FAILURE TO THRIVE (FTT)

The term *failure to thrive* is used to describe infants and children whose weight and sometimes height fall below the 5th percentile for their age. There are two distinct categories of failure to thrive:

> **organic failure to thrive** is the result of a physical cause, such as congenital heart defects, neurologic lesions, microcephaly, chronic urinary tract infection, gastroesophageal reflux, renal insufficiency, malabsorption syndrome, endocrine dysfunction, or cystic fibrosis.
>
> **nonorganic failure to thrive** is caused by psychosocial factors, the problem being a disturbed relationship between the child and primary caregiver, usually the mother. In this situation the lack of physical growth is secondary to the lack of emotional and sensory stimulation. It has been described under a variety of less acceptable names, including maternal deprivation, environmental deprivation, and deprivation dwarfism.

In the majority of children with FTT no organic cause is found for the condition, and the diagnosis of nonorganic FTT is usually made on the basis of exclusion of pathophysiologic findings. Unfortunately many of these children are unnecessarily subjected to exhausting, traumatic, and expensive diagnostic procedures. To prevent this, nonorganic FTT should be considered *early* in the differential diagnosis, when a careful history and physical examination rule out a gross medical cause.

Characteristics of FTT children and their families

Nonorganic FTT has traditionally been referred to as *maternal deprivation syndrome* because of the findings that mothers of FTT children have difficulty relating to and perceiving the needs of these children. However, the disturbance in the relationship involves at least two individuals: the child and the primary caregiver. Because complex physical, psychosocial, and emotional variables affect this relationship, it is probably more correct to refer to the problem as one of *parent-child attachment deprivation syndrome*. This broader term allows an understanding of the characteristics of the child, parent, and environment that are important in preventing, diagnosing, and treating nonorganic FTT syndrome.

The child. Besides the obvious signs of malnutrition and delayed development, the child seems to have a characteristic posture or "body language." In one extreme the child is unpliable, stiff, and rigid. He is uncomforted by and unyielding to cuddling or holding and is very slow in smiling or socially responding to others. The other extreme is the floppy infant, who is like a rag doll. Neither child molds to the holder's body, maintains sustained eye-to-eye contact, or shows signs of satisfaction or contentment during any care-giving procedures.

There is frequently a history of difficult feeding, vomiting, sleep disturbance, and excessive irritability. Difficulties in infant feeding may include poor appetite, poor suck, crying during feedings, vomiting, hoarding food in the mouth, ruminating after feeding, refusal to switch from liquids to solids, and aversion behavior, such as turning from food or spitting food. Ultimately these habit patterns become attention-seeking mechanisms to prolong the attention received at mealtime. In addition, chronic reduction in calories can lead to appetite depression, which compounds the problem.

An outstanding feature of FTT children is their irregularity (low rhythmicity) in activities of daily living. Some of these children typify the "difficult child pattern" (p. 238). However, another type is the passive, sleepy, lethargic child who does not wake up for feedings. Parents who have been advised of "demand feeding schedules" may be unsure of whether to wake the child or let him sleep. Because of their inexperience and lack of guidance, they may develop a pattern of infrequent feeding that is inadequate to meet the infant's nutritional needs. Likewise, the developmental stimulation may be considerably less than that given to a child who responds more actively to his environment.

One cannot assume that such characteristics in a child result in FTT. Rather, it is the degree of *fit* between the child's temperament and that of his parents that is critical. It is not unusual for a mother to have reared other offspring successfully and to bear a child who is more difficult to relate to. Since the personalities of infants can have definite effects on the mother-child attachment process, identifying such situations of incompatibility may be one approach toward prevention and anticipatory guidance.

The parents. Some parents are at increased risk for attachment problems because of (1) isolation and social crisis, (2) inadequate support systems, and (3) poor parenting as a child. Other factors that should be considered are lack of education; physical and mental health problems, such as retardation, depression, or drug dependence; immaturity, especially in adolescent parents; and lack of commitment to parenting, such as giving higher priority to career goals.

Frequently these parents and their families are under stress and in chronic emotional, social, and financial crises. Often there is marital discord; if fathers or husbands are present, they give little emotional support to their wives. Although the literature almost exclusively discusses characteristics of mothers of FTT children, it must be remembered that every child has a biologic father and that in some way he may have contributed to the parent-child disturbance either by his presence or absence. Frequently the father is not discussed because he is a covert partner, whereas the mother is usually the one visibly present and identifiable. Such mothers tend to lead lonely, solitary lives with few outside interests or friends who can relieve them of childrearing responsibilities in times of heightened stress.

Often the parents were maternally deprived as children and did not experience a warm, nurturing childhood. They have a need to be taken care of rather than to take care of another. They have a low self-esteem and feelings of inadequacy, which are strengthened by their inability to satisfy their infant.

Typically these parents have difficulty in perceiving and assessing their infants' needs. For example, they cannot distinguish "cries" of hunger, pain, or general dissatisfaction. They are unaware of what to expect developmentally from their child at a particular age and, consequently, do not know how to stimulate or play with the infant. The parent's reaction to the child's dissatisfied response to care-giving activities or social play is frustration and anger, resulting in a vicious, destructive cycle.

Many of these parents display negative maladaptive feelings toward the infant (see summary at end of this section). Ambivalence toward pregnancy can be an early clue when combined with other characteristics of high-risk parents. Being alert to such clues may avert a potential FTT situation by identifying these parents prenatally and planning interventions aimed at increasing satisfying parenting skills.

SUMMARY OF NURSING CARE OF THE CHILD WITH NONORGANIC FAILURE TO THRIVE

GOALS	RESPONSIBILITIES
Recognize characteristics of parents of failure-to-thrive children	Be alert to the following History of maternal deprivation as a child Low self-esteem; feelings of inadequacy Desire for dependency Loneliness, isolation Limited support system Multiple life crises and stress
Identify mothers (and fathers) at risk	Be alert to parental nonadaptive behaviors toward the infant Has persistent ambivalence or negative feelings about the fetus and the pregnancy during the prenatal period Makes no plans for obtaining basic infant supplies Appears indifferent to infant at time of delivery; may appear sad or angry; is expressionless Makes no effort to establish eye-to-eye contact with infant Handles infant only when necessary Makes few or no spontaneous movements with infant Asks few questions about care Sees infant as ugly or unattractive Displays disgust with infant's drooling and sucking sounds; is revolted by infant's body fluids Is annoyed with diaper changing Perceives infant's odor as revolting Holds infant with little support to head and body

Continued.

SUMMARY OF NURSING CARE OF THE CHILD WITH NONORGANIC FAILURE TO THRIVE—cont'd

GOALS	RESPONSIBILITIES
Identify mothers (and fathers) at risk—cont'd	Holds infant away from body during feeding or props bottle for feeding; seldom cuddles infant
	Does not coo or talk to infant
	Refers to infant in an impersonal manner
	Develops inappropriate responses to infant's needs, such as leaving infant in one place for long periods, leaving in room, overfeeding or underfeeding, overstimulating or understimulating infant, forcing or refusing eye contact, bouncing or tickling infant when he is fatigued
	Cannot discriminate between infant's signals for hunger, comfort, rest, body contact
	Is convinced the infant has a defect or disease even when reassured to the contrary
	Makes negative statements regarding mothering role
	Believes the infant is judging her and her efforts as an adult
	Believes the infant does not love her and exposes her as an unlovable and unloving parent
	Develops paradoxical attitudes and behavior toward the infant
	Determine whether pregnancy was planned or unplanned
	Determine whether there were any disturbing events associated with pregnancy or delivery of the child
Identify children who fail to thrive	Suspect parental deprivation in infants and young children who display characteristics such as
	Growth failure—below fifth percentile in height and weight
	Developmental retardation—social, motor, adaptive, language
	Apathy
	Poor hygiene
	Withdrawing behavior
	Feeding or eating disorders, such as vomiting, anorexia, voracious appetite, pica, rumination
	No fear of strangers (at age when stranger anxiety is normal)
	Avoidance of eye-to-eye contact
	Wide-eyed gaze and continual scan of the environment ("radar gaze")
	Stiff and unyielding or flaccid and unresponsive
	Minimal smiling
Provide optimum nutrients	Make feeding a priority goal
	Keep accurate record of intake to ensure ingestion of calculated daily calories
	Weigh daily and record to ascertain weight gain

Nursing considerations—families as patients

The priority nursing goals are (1) providing the infant with sufficient nutrients for growth and (2) structuring the environment for positive psychosocial interactions. Usually the physical and developmental retardation in FTT children is so great that hospitalization is required. Since these children are not ill with any physical disorder but debilitated from general malnutrition, they should be placed in a room with noninfectious children of a similar age.

Since part of the difficulty between parent and child was dissatisfaction and frustration, a consistent primary nurse for all three shifts with scheduled relief for days off is a priority. Only the same nurse caring for the child over a period of time can learn to perceive the child's cues and reverse the cycle of dissatisfaction, especially in the area of feeding.

Each child with FTT is responding to stimuli that have led to his negative feeding patterns. The first goal of care is to assess those patterns, tailor the feeding process to change negative habits, and replace them with positive

SUMMARY OF NURSING CARE OF THE CHILD WITH NONORGANIC FAILURE TO THRIVE—cont'd

GOALS	RESPONSIBILITIES
Introduce a positive feeding environment	Assign one nurse for feeding Maintain calm, even temperament; be persistent Provide a quiet, unstimulating environment Hold young child for feeding Maintain eye-to-eye contact with child Talk to child by giving appropriate directions and praise for eating Follow the child's rhythm of feeding Establish a structured routine and follow it consistently
Provide a nurturing environment for the hospitalized child	Assess child's developmental age Apply primary care concepts to assure continuity of care with a minimum number of caregivers Provide gentle, sure, and loving handling Perform physical care with as much holding, rocking, and cuddling as the child will respond to Encourage eye-to-eye contact Employ consistent schedule in meeting child's needs for food, hygiene, care, and rest Assign a foster grandparent or child life specialist to child Provide sensory stimulation and play appropriate to the child's developmental level
Reduce parental anxiety and provide education	Welcome parents and encourage, but do not push them to become involved in the child's care Teach parents about the child's physical care, developmental skills, and emotional needs through example, not lecture Afford parents the opportunity to discuss their lives and feelings toward the child Supply emotional nurturance without encouraging dependency Promote parents' self-esteem and confidence by praising their achievements with the child Prepare parents for adjustments with anticipatory guidance
Prepare for discharge	Assess home environment and relationships Continue interventions begun in the hospital Establish a consistent contact system through public health nurse Refer to appropriate agencies for assistance with financial, social, or other family needs

ones. Initially it is recommended that staff members feed these children. Parents are encouraged to visit often but not at mealtime until caloric intake and weight gain are adequate. Then they are taught by demonstration successful feeding techniques. Several general guidelines can be established for the feeding interaction:

1. **Provide a quiet, unstimulating atmosphere.** A number of these children are very distractible and their attention is diverted with minimal stimuli. Older children do well at a feeding table; younger children should always be

held. A single adult in the feeding situation is recommended.

2. **Maintain a calm, even temperament throughout the meal.** Negative outbursts may be commonplace in this child's habit formation. Limits on eating behavior definitely need to be provided, but they should be stated in a firm, calm tone. If the nurse is hurried or anxious, the feeding process will not be optimized.

3. **Talk to the child by giving directions about eating.** "Take a bite, Lisa" and "Don't spit the cereal out, Lisa" are appropriate and directive. The more distracti-

ble the child, the more directive the nurse should be to refocus attention on feeding. Positive comments about feeding are given actively.

4. **Follow the child's rhythm of feeding.** The child will set a rhythm when the previous conditions are met.

5. **Develop a structured routine.** FTT children are in particular need of routine feeding patterns. Disruption in their other activities of daily living have great impact on feeding responses, so these should also be structured. The same nurse should feed the child in the same way and place as often as possible. The length of the feeding should also be established (usually 30 minutes).

6. **Be persistent.** This is perhaps one of the most important guidelines. Parents often give up when the child begins negative feeding behavior. Calm perseverance through 10 to 15 minutes of food refusal will eventually diminish negative behavior. Although forced feeding is avoided, "strictly encouraged" feeding is essential.

7. **Maintain a face-to-face posture with the child when possible.** Encourage eye contact and remain with the child throughout the meal.

Foods appropriate to the child's age are selected. Supplements, such as Polycose, can be added to foods to increase caloric intake. FTT children who have been exclusively bottle fed often refuse all solids. They require the same feeding plan as children with rumination.

Besides attending to the physical needs of the child, the nurse must plan care for appropriate developmental stimulation. The word "appropriate" is emphasized because it refers to the child's developmental age, not to his chronologic age.

The Denver Developmental Screening Test (DDST) should be administered on admission to assess development. The DDST gives an approximate age for the child's present achievement in gross/fine motor, social-adaptive, and language skills. Only after objective measurements are available can a plan of care for stimulation be organized. Periodic testing is an excellent tool for evaluation of the child's developmental progress.

Nursing care involves a systems approach. In other words, for the entire family to become healthy, each member must be helped to change. To nurture the child back to physical, developmental, and emotional help during his hospitalization while neglecting the emotional needs of the parents does not solve the problem. Therefore, the nursing care plan must also include the parents. Fathers or significant other persons, who can be helped to be more emotionally, physically, and financially supportive to the family unit, can become the emotional reservoir needed by mothers to give nurturance to their child. Some hospitals have child life specialists or volunteer foster grandparents who spend scheduled, consistent periods of time with the infant as a surrogate mother.

Care of the mother is aimed at helping her increase her feelings of self-esteem through positive, successful mothering skills. Initially this necessitates providing an environment in which she feels welcomed and accepted. Because these women are often distrustful of authority figures, it may take some time before the mother develops any trust toward the nurse. One approach is to empathize with the parent about the difficulties of childrearing. For example, the nurse may state that many parents find adjusting to parenthood a trying time or that the demands of caring for an infant can become overwhelming.

Once the mother feels comfortable enough to visit with her infant, teaching infant care techniques are begun through *example* and *demonstration,* not by lecturing. As the nurse perceives the infant's cues, these are emphasized to the mother. For example, during a feeding the nurse might comment that the infant is still hungry because he sucks vigorously and looks at her. When he is satisfied, the nurse points out that the infant is signaling this by releasing the strong suck, closing his eyes, and breathing deeply and more slowly. By example, the child is gently placed in the crib for a nap.

At the same time the mother is offered an opportunity to care for the infant without making demands on her. For example, the nurse suggests that at the next feeding the mother offer her child the bottle. Whenever the mother participates, she is praised for her efforts and encouraged to continue caring for the child.

Before discharge, plans are made to continue these interventions at home. A public health referral is made, and if a foster grandparent was included, this person should also visit the family. Social agencies that can provide financial or housing assistance to lessen the stress of everyday life are also contacted.

SUDDEN INFANT DEATH SYNDROME (SIDS)

Sudden infant death syndrome, also referred to as cot or crib death, is defined as "the sudden death of any infant or young child, which is unexpected by history, and in which a thorough postmortem examination fails to demonstrate an adequate cause for death." It is the number one cause of death in children between the ages of 1 week and 1 year and claims the lives of 8000 to 10,000 infants annually. Table 9-3 summarizes the characteristics of SIDS.

Etiology

There are numerous theories regarding the etiology of SIDS. Presently the exact cause is unknown. However, evidence is accumulating that supports a relationship with prolonged periodic apnea and chronic hypoxia. The cause of the apneic spells is inconclusive, although they may be linked to a functional abnormality of the autonomic nervous system or delayed maturation of the cardiorespiratory system. Autopsies have revealed consistent pathologic findings that support the theory of chronic hypoxia. Thus the diagnosis SIDS can be definitively confirmed from an autopsy.

TABLE 9-3. CHARACTERISTICS OF SIDS

FACTORS	OCCURRENCE
Incidence	1.5 to 2:1000 live births
Peak age	2 to 4 months; 90% occur by 6 months
Sex	Higher percentage of males affected
Time of death	Usually during nighttime
Time of year	Increased incidence in winter
Racial	Greater incidence in nonwhites
Socioeconomic	Increased occurrence in lower socioeconomic class
Birth	Higher incidence in: Premature infants Multiple births Neonates with low Apgar scores Infants with central nervous system isturbances
Feeding habits	Not significant; breast-feeding does not prevent SIDS
Siblings	Ten times greater incidence

"Near-miss" infants and subsequent siblings

There are two groups who are at increased risk from SIDS. One is the "near-miss" infant—a child who has ceased breathing and seems to have died suddenly and unexpectedly but whose life is apparently saved by timely intervention, usually by a parent or baby-sitter. The more acceptable term for near-miss SIDS is *infantile apnea.* The other at-risk group includes the subsequent siblings of the SIDS infant, who have about a ten times greater risk of sudden death than infants in the general population.

Studies conducted on these two groups often demonstrate distinct differences in physiologic function from that of normal infants, especially cardiac and respiratory functions. Consequently there is much concern for the future survival of these at-risk groups. Many of these children undergo home apnea monitoring until they are past the age of vulnerability and demonstrate normal pneumocardiograms, which monitor and record breathing and heart rate patterns.

If home monitoring is required, the nurse can be a major source of support to the parents in terms of education about the equipment and cardiorespiratory resuscitation. To lessen the continuous responsibility of monitoring, other family members such as grandparents should be taught the procedures and encouraged to stay with the infant for regular periods to allow parents time away.

SUMMARY OF NURSING CARE OF THE FAMILY EXPERIENCING SUDDEN INFANT DEATH SYNDROME (SIDS)

GOALS	RESPONSIBILITIES
Support the parents on discovery of the dead infant	Recognize signs of SIDS and distinguish them from signs of deliberate abuse Inform parents that the child probably died from SIDS; explain the necessity of an autopsy in confirming the diagnosis Emphasize that SIDS cannot be predicted or prevented Ask as few questions as possible Avoid giving any indication of wrongdoing Make sensitive judgments concerning resuscitative efforts (if applicable) Arrange for parents and possibly siblings to accompany infant to hospital; arrange for support person to be with them
Allow parents the opportunity for a last visit with infant	Before parents see infant, remove any blood or emesis from child; tidy room Provide privacy Encourage expression of emotion Answer any questions honestly, emphasizing what is known about SIDS
Promote adjustment to the loss	Make home visit as soon as possible after the death Help parents gain an understanding of the disease Provide printed literature about SIDS Refer to local Foundation for SIDS, especially parent groups Encourage expression of emotion Explore issues such as subsequent child and reactions of siblings Schedule follow-up visits as needed

Nursing considerations—crisis intervention

Loss of a child from SIDS presents several crises with which the parents must cope. In addition to the grief and mourning for the death of their child, the parents must face a tragedy that was extremely sudden, unexpected, and unexplained. The psychologic intervention for the family must deal with these additional variables. It is the purpose in this discussion to stress primarily the objectives of care for families experiencing SIDS, rather than the process of grief and mourning, which is explored in Chapter 16.

One approach toward delineating the nursing care plan for these families is to base it on the usual sequence of events that occurs after the infant is found. This approach encompasses the different areas in which nurses may be involved with the family.

Finding the infant. It is usually the mother who finds the child dead in the crib. Typically the child is in a disheveled bed, with blankets over his head, and huddled into a corner. Frothy, blood-tinged fluid fills the mouth and nostrils, and the infant may be lying face down in the secretions, suggesting that he bled to death. The diaper is wet and full of stool, which is consistent with a cataclysmic type of death. The hands may be clutching the sheets, as if the child were in distress before he died. The initial appearance of the child combined with the shock of such an unexpected event adds to the horror and nightmare that the parents must face.

Frequently the mother is alone and must deal with her initial shock, panic, grief, questions of the other siblings, and the decision of where to find help. The first persons to arrive may be the police and ambulance attendants. Hopefully they will handle the situation by asking few questions, giving *no* indication of wrongdoing, abuse, or neglect, making sensitive judgments concerning the resuscitation efforts for the child, and comforting the members of the family as much as possible. The trend is toward public professional education of SIDS, particularly for those who arrive on the scene first. If properly informed, they should be able to recognize signs of SIDS and tell parents that their child probably died from a disease called sudden infant death syndrome, which cannot be predicted or prevented. A compassionate, sensitive approach to the family during the very first few minutes can help spare them some of the overwhelming guilt and anguish that frequently follow this type of death.

Arriving at the emergency room. The first contact that nurses have with these families is in the emergency room, when the infant is seen by a physician in order to be pronounced dead. Usually there is no attempt at resuscitation. During the time in the emergency room several aspects warrant special consideration. Parents are asked only factual questions, such as when they found the infant, how he looked, and who they called for help. Any remarks that may suggest responsibility, such as why didn't they go in earlier, didn't they hear him cry out, was his head buried in a blanket, or were the other siblings jealous of this child, are avoided.

The events that took place when help arrived are discussed. If resuscitation was attempted, the infant may have fractured ribs, internal bleeding, and traumatic bruising, which can simulate physical abuse. Also, if statements were made that were misguided, such as, ''This looks like suffocation,'' they can be corrected before parents harbor them in their minds as indications of their guilt. Since the diagnosis of SIDS can be definitively made on postmortem findings, autopsies of all suspected cases of SIDS should be performed. This subject should be approached positively by stating that SIDS is suspected but that it is a disease that must have an autopsy for a positive diagnosis to be made.

Another very important aspect of compassionate care toward these parents is allowing them to say good-bye to their child. A happy, beautiful, living part of themselves has suddenly been taken from them forever. Before they go into the examining room, any blood or emesis is removed from the child, he is covered partially with a sheet or blanket, and the room is put in order, especially if instruments and equipment were used. These are the parents' last moments with their child, and they should be as quiet, meaningful, peaceful, and undisturbed as possible. The child's belongings are packaged for the parents to take home if they wish. Nothing involved in the care of these grief-stricken people is complicated, difficult, or time-consuming; it only involves being human.

Returning home. When the parents return home, they should be visited by a competent, qualified professional as soon after the death as possible. A referral should also be made to the local Foundation of Sudden Infant Death. Printed material that contains excellent information about SIDS (available from the national* or local chapters) should be provided.

During the initial visit the parents are helped to gain an intellectual understanding of the disease. The nursing objectives are to assess what the parents have been told, what they think happened, and how they have explained this to the other siblings.

During the second visit the goal is to help the parents bring their feelings out into the open. This may require ''precipitating'' emotions by asking about crying and feeling sad, angry, or guilty. It is an attempt to provoke a display of emotion, not just an admission of a feeling. During this session the parents should be helped to explore their usual coping mechanisms and, if these are ineffectual, to investigate new approaches.

---

*National Foundation for Sudden Infant Death, Inc., 2 Metro Plaza, Suite 205, 8240 Professional Place, Landover, MD 20785.

The number of visits and plan for subsequent intervention needs to be flexible. For example, the siblings may initially appear accepting of the explanation and well adjusted but may later refuse to go to sleep or ask questions about graves or funerals, indicating their need for further help in dealing with the death. Parents facing the question of a subsequent child will need support.

Since the mourning process takes *at least* a year for completion of acceptance and social reorganization, nurses should call on the family periodically to evaluate their progress. Many families receive much solace and support from talking to other parents who have lost a child from SIDS. Parent groups have been formed throughout the United States and can be contacted through the national or local chapters of the Foundation of Sudden Infant Death.

INFANTILE AUTISM

Autism, the earliest form of psychosis in children, occurs in about five children per 10,000 and is approximately four times more common in males than in females. It is usually characterized by disturbances in the following areas: relationship with the social environment, use of speech for social expression and communication, developing a sense of personal identity, use of affect, and total integration and reorganization of personality. Autistic children exhibit bizarre, deviant behavior almost from birth.

Characteristics of autistic children

The most prominent characteristics of infantile autism are (1) the child's extreme interpersonal isolation and (2) an intense, abnormal concern for preservation of sameness. Their social development is retarded to the point that there is no advancement from the typical behavior of a 1-month-old child. They fail to develop a smiling response to others or the usual anticipatory movements, such as putting their arms out to be picked up, which signify their interest in their social environment. They are unyielding to cuddling and holding and fail to show any signs of satisfaction or pleasure in tactile contact. They have a blank, detached look in their eyes and do not respond to verbal stimulation, which may lead others to suspect deafness. Most notably, they fail to demonstrate the usual 6- to 8-month stranger anxiety and fear of separation from mother. In fact they have no difficulty in tolerating separation and seem unaware of the parent's absence. Autistic children are content to be left alone and provide no satisfaction or feedback to the parent or caregiver for any type of nurturing.

In sharp contrast to their detachment from social interaction is their intense preoccupation with the preservation of sameness and their attachment to mechanical objects. Typically during their second year they become engrossed in odd repetitive behaviors, such as flicking a light switch on and off, passing a toy back and forth from one hand to other, or walking around a room feeling the walls. If they are interrupted while engaged in these activities or if their environment is disturbed, such as if the crib is moved even a few inches, they will react with a violent temper tantrum. Other self-stimulatory behaviors include rocking, whirling, flapping of arms, or flicking of hands and fingers before their eyes while staring at bright lights.

Recognition of autism usually follows the appearance of the typical language and communication defects of this disorder, such as *echolalia* or *parrot speech*—the automatic repetition of words spoken to them; *pronominal reversal*—the tendency to use "you" for "I" and the striking absence of the first person to refer to oneself; and literal, concrete use of words, for example, "in" to mean "door." Although their phonation and articulation of sounds are clear, their highly individualized and specialized speech makes communication with others almost impossible.

Sensory deficits are common in autistic children, even though vision and hearing are usually intact. Autistic children often act as if they are deaf, yet a moment later may be overly sensitive to the same sound. They cover their ears and cringe from certain sounds but emit piercing sounds when annoyed. They are fascinated by music, light patterns, different textures, and sometimes offensive tastes and odors. They may be hyposensitive or hypersensitive to pain and have an aversion to touch.

Occasionally an autistic child may excel in one area, such as motor ability or unusual musical talent. However, despite such islets of normal to exceptional ability, the majority of autistic children are retarded. More than half have IQs of less than 50 and only 20% are in the mild to borderline range of retardation. Testing these children for their intellectual abilities is important because the prognosis for the borderline group is much better. Whatever the child's potential, his outcome will depend on appropriate training at home and special education programs geared to his needs. About 15% of autistic individuals can lead near-normal lives working at a trade and living independently.

Origins of infantile autism

The precise origin of autism is still an unanswered question. At one time several authorities believed that there was a psychogenetic basis for autism, which had its pathology in the mother-child relationship. Currently there is little evidence to support this view and increasing documentation for a biogenic theory that contends that autism results from damage to the central nervous system. Although the biogenic cause is unknown, supportive evidence shows that autistic children experience more prenatal and perinatal complications as compared with control children. These include breech delivery, the presence of amniotic meconium, low birth weight, low Apgar scores, elevated bilirubin levels, hemolytic disease, and respiratory distress syndrome.

One of the foremost hypotheses concerns abnormal left hemisphere functioning. This is supported by problems autistic children have in certain areas, such as in speech and perceptual skills, that are controlled by the left hemisphere of the brain. However, those functions thought to be mediated by the right hemisphere, such as visual-spatial skills and memory, are much less affected and may be well developed.

Nursing considerations

Therapeutic intervention for the autistic child is a specialized area of nursing. Several approaches, such as the use of the therapeutic one-to-one relationship, play therapy, and behavioral modification, have been attempted and advocated. In all instances the objective is to increase social awareness of others, teach verbal communication, and decrease unacceptable behavior.

Autism, like so many other chronic conditions, becomes a "family disease." Unfortunately the psychogenetic theory is well-known and although unsupported by current findings, greatly multiplies the parents' guilt. Stressing what is known about the disorder from a biologic standpoint as well as how little is known can help lessen guilt and shame. Carefully questioning parents about the infant's very early behavior usually yields evidence of autistic tendencies before significant parental or environmental factors could have negatively influenced the child.

Parents need expert counseling early in the course of the disorder and should be referred to the National Society for Autistic Children (NSAC).* NSAC is the most efficient clearinghouse for information about education, treatment programs and techniques, and specialized facilities such as camps and group homes.

When these children are hospitalized, they usually present many management problems for nurses. Decreasing stimulation by using a private or semiprivate room, avoiding extraneous auditory and visual distraction, and

*1234 Massachusetts Ave. NW, Washington, DC 20005.

encouraging parents to bring in possessions the child is attached to may lessen the disruptiveness of hospitalization. Since physical contact frequently upsets these children, minimal holding and physical care may be necessary to prevent temper tantrums. A thorough assessment of the child's usual routine and activities helps maintain an environment that is manageable and conducive to physical recovery.

A key principle in working with these children is to assume that the child is unable to name, define, or locate even ordinary experiences. For example, if another child is crying, it is necessary to point out to the autistic child that *he* is not crying. In the hospital setting it is necessary to define for the child what is happening in the environment, such as clarifying what sounds are being heard.

Because autistic children have difficulty organizing their behavior and redirecting their energy, they need to be told directly what to do. For example, if they are throwing toys, they are told to stop throwing them on the floor and instructed to drop them into a container. Moralizing about "breaking toys" or "hurting someone" is useless and only serves to confuse the child. Directions need to be precise and concrete. Through such approaches it may be possible for the child to develop some trust with people in his environment.

BIBLIOGRAPHY
Nutritional disturbances

American Academy of Pediatrics, Committee on Nutrition: Vitamin and mineral supplement needs in normal children in the United States, Pediatrics **66**(6):1015-1020, 1980.

Dietz, W.H., and Dwyer, J.T.: Nutritional implications of vegetarianism for children. In Suskind, R.M., editor: Textbook of pediatric nutrition, New York, 1981, Raven Press.

Goel, K.: Rickets: an old enemy returns, Nurs. Mirror **152**(13):16-18, 1981.

Johnston, P.K.: Getting enough to grow on, Am. J. Nurs. **84**(3):336-339, 1984.

Nurses' quick guide to nutritional disorders, Nursing 83 **13** (4):56-57, 1983.

Purvis, G.A.: Vegetarian nutrition in infancy, Pediatr. Basics **34**:1, 1982.

Solomons, N.W.: Zinc bioavailability: implications for pediatric nutrition, Pediatr. Basics **33**:4-11, 1982.

Thomas, K.: Folic acid deficiency related to the use of goat milk for infant feeding, Issues Compr. Pediatr. Nurs. **4**:37-43, 1980.

Viteri, F.E.: Primary protein-energy malnutrition: clinical, biochemical, and metabolic changes. In Suskind, R.M., editor: Textbook of pediatric nutrition, New York, 1981, Raven Press.

Allergies/cow's milk sensitivity

American Academy of Pediatrics, Committee on Nutrition: Soy-protein formulas: recommendations for use in infant feeding, Pediatrics **72**(3):359-363, 1983.

Bierman, C.W., and Furukawa, C.T.: Food allergy, Pediatr. Rev. **3**(7):213-220, 1982.

Brockwell, C.: Cow's milk allergy in babies—a review, Health Visitor **54**:236-237, June 1981.

Crook, W.G.: Tracking down hidden food allergy, Tennessee, 1980, Professional Books, Inc.

Kuzemko, J.A.: A review of pediatric allergies, Midwife Health Visit Commun. Nurse **15**(10):390-397, 1979.

White, J.E., and Owsley, V.B.: Helping families cope with milk, wheat, and soy allergies, Am. J. Maternal Child Nurs. **8**(6):423-428, 1983.

Feeding problems

Dixie, M.: Maternal food allergy as a cause of infantile colic in the breast fed baby, Health Visitor **54**(6):240- 241, 1981.

Fleisher, D.R.: Infant rumination syndrome, Am. J. Dis. Child. **133**:266-269, March 1979.

Imber, J.H.: Living and coping with colic, Am. Baby **42**:29, Dec. 1980.

Rowell, P.A.: Infantile colic: reviewing the situation, Pediatr. Nurs. **4**(3):20-21, 1978.

Waldman, W.H., and Sarsgard, D.: Helping parents to cope with colic, Pediatr. Basics **33**:12-14, 1982.

Failure to thrive (FTT)

Ayoub, C., Pfeifer, D., and Leichtman, L.: Treatment of infants with nonorganic failure to thrive, Child Abuse Neglect **3**:937-941, 1979.

Corcoran, M.: Nursing role and management of failure-to-thrive clients, Issues Compr. Pediatr. Nurs. **3**:29-40, Oct. 1978.

Gottsacker, J.: Maternal attachment in relation to failure to thrive. In Brandt, P.A., and others, editors: Current practice in pediatric nursing, vol. I, St. Louis, 1976, The C.V. Mosby Co.

Harrison, L.: The failure to thrive child. In Johnson, S.: High-risk parenting, Philadelphia, 1979, J.B. Lippincott Co.

Mira, M., and Cairns, G.: Intervention in the interaction of a mother and child with nonorganic failure to thrive, Pediatr. Nurs. **7**(2):41-46, 1981.

Norris, T.N., and Anderson, A.S.: Failure to thrive in infants and very young children, Pediatr. Basics **26**:4-7, March 1980.

Yoos, L.: Taking another look at failure to thrive, Am. J. Maternal Child Nurs. **9**(1):32-36, 1984.

Sudden infant death syndrome (SIDS)

Bakke, K., and Dougherty, J.: Sudden infant death syndrome and infant apnea: current questions, clinical management, and research directions, Issues Compr. Pediatr. Nurs., **5**: 77-88, 1981.

Clapp, L., and Price, J.H.: Sudden infant death syndrome, J. Nurs. Care **13**(3):13-17, 1980.

Cordell, A.S., and Apolito, R.: Family support in infant death, JOGN Nurs. **10**(4):281-285, 1981.

Deal, A., and Bordeaux, B.: The phenomenon of SIDS, Pediatr. Nurs. **6**(1):48-50, 1980.

DiMaggio, G.T., and Sheetz, A.H.: The concerns of mothers caring for an infant on an apnea monitor, Am. J. Maternal Child Nurs. **8**(4):294-297, 1983.

Duncan, J., and Webb, L.Z.: Teaching families home apnea monitoring, Pediatr. Nurs. **9**(3):171-175, 1983.

Kotsubo, C.Z.: Helping families survive S.I.D.S., Nursing 83 **13**(5):94-96, 1983.

Lundeen, K.W.: When baby makes three...challenges, Nursing 82 **12**(3):74-75, 1982.

Nikolaisen, S.: The impact of sudden infant death on the family: nursing intervention, Top. Clinical Nurs. **3**(3):45-53, 1981.

Rehm, R.: Teaching cardiopulmonary resuscitation to parents, Am. J. Maternal Child Nurs. **8**(6):411-414, 1983.

Webb, L.Z., and Duncan, J.A.: Selecting the right home apnea monitor, Pediatr. Nurs. **9**(3):179-182, 1983.

Williams, R.A., and Nikolaisen, S.M.: Sudden infant death syndrome: parents' perceptions and responses to the loss of their infant, Res. Nurs. Health **5**:55-61, 1982.

Infantile autism

Christian, W.P: Childhood autism. In Levine, M. and others, editors: Developmental-behaviora' pediatrics, Philadelphia, l983, W.B. Saunders Co.

Dudziak, D.: Parenting the autistic child, J. Psychosocial Nurs. Mental Health Services **20**(1):11-16, 1982.

Harris, M.: Understanding the autistic child, Am. J. Nurs. **78**(10):1682-1685, 1978.

Killion, S., and McCarthy, S.: Hospitalization of the autistic child. Part I—Assessment. Part II—Autistic children, intervention, Am. J. Maternal Child Nurs. **5**(6):412-423, 1980.

Moss, B.K.: When autism threatens family balance, Patient Care **15**:15-33, April 1981.

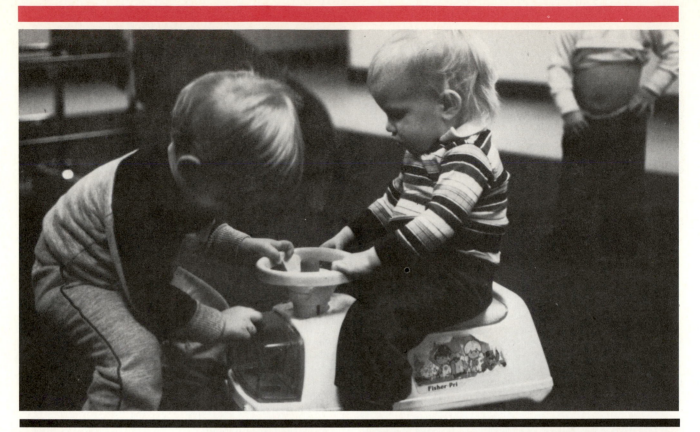

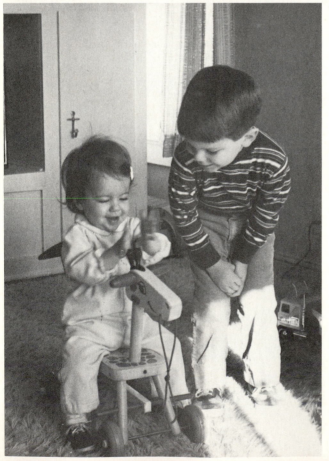

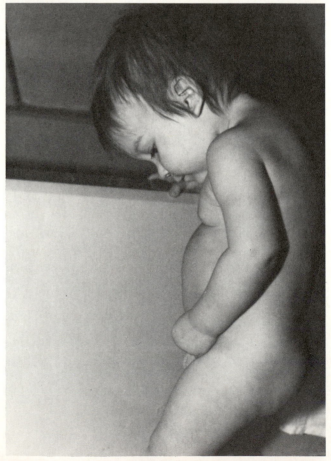

UNIT 5

EARLY CHILDHOOD

Early childhood comprises the years of toddlerhood and preschool. It is primarily a period of physical development and refinement, attainment of social skills, and achievement of independent behavior. Dramatic changes occur in the child as he leaves the dependent world of infancy and readies himself for the self-sufficient life of a school-age child. Chapters 10 and 11, *The Toddler Years* and *The Preschool Years,* are concerned with the biologic growth and psychologic development of the toddler and preschooler. Emphasis is placed on promoting optimum development during each phase of early childhood, especially through anticipatory guidance regarding nutrition, achievement of self-care activities, prevention of accidental injury, and specific parental concerns.

Chapter 12, *Health Problems of Early Childhood,* deals with health problems that commonly occur during early childhood. Although many of the disorders that occur during this period are caused by infectious processes, most of the child's care is implemented in the home, necessitating nursing guidance rather than direct intervention. The other conditions discussed are results of environmental and social factors to which toddlers and preschoolers are especially vulnerable or by which they are greatly influenced. In each of these health problems, emphasis is placed on prevention, recognition, and nursing interventions that return the child to an optimum physical and mental status following recovery.

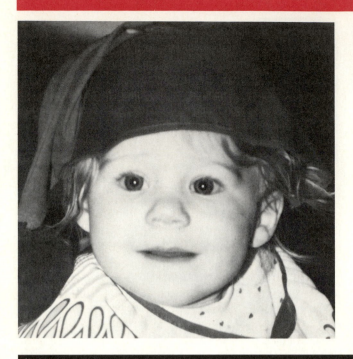

10

THE TODDLER YEARS

OBJECTIVES

On completion of this chapter the reader will be able to:

■ Identify the major biologic, psychosocial, cognitive, and adaptive developments during the toddler years

■ Relate separation anxiety and negativism to developmental tasks

■ Recognize signs of readiness for toilet training and offer parents guidelines for training

■ Prepare toddlers for birth of a sibling

■ Provide parents with guidelines for limit setting and discipline, including management of temper tantrums

■ Provide parents with feeding recommendations

■ Provide anticipatory guidance to parents regarding accident prevention based on the toddler's developmental achievements

■ Outline a preventive dental hygiene plan for toddlers

NURSING DIAGNOSES

Nursing diagnoses identified for the toddler include, but are not restricted to, the following:

Health perception–health management pattern

■ Infection, potential for, related to increased exposure outside the home

■ Injury, potential for (poisoning, suffocation, trauma), related to environmental hazards

Nutritional-metabolic pattern

■ Nutrition, alterations in: potential for more or less than body requirements, related to (1) knowledge deficit; (2) physiologic anorexia

The term *terrible twos* has often been used to describe the toddler years, a period from age 12 months to the completion of 2 years of age. It is a time of intense exploration of the environment as the child attempts to find out how things work, what the word "no" means, and how to control others with temper tantrums, negativism, and obstinacy. The phrase "he gets into everything" underestimates the toddler's voracity for adventure, but the very adventure of getting into things is his means of acquisition of learning and knowledge.

Although this can be a difficult time for parents and child as each learns to know the other better, it is also an extremely important period for developmental achievement and intellectual growth. Successful mastery of the tasks of this age requires a strong foundation of trust during infancy and frequently necessitates guidance from others when parent and toddler face the struggles of toilet training, limit setting and discipline, and sibling rivalry. Nurses who understand the dynamics of growth and development of the toddler can help parents deal effectively with the tasks of this age.

Activity-exercise pattern

■ Self-care deficit related to (1) developmental level; (2) toilet training; (3) self-feeding; (4) dental care

Sleep-rest pattern

■ Sleep-pattern disturbance related to (1) fear of separation from parents; (2) negativism

Self-perception—self-concept pattern

■ Anxiety related to (1) stranger fear; (2) separation; (3) regression

Role-relationship pattern

■ Family process, alteration in, related to sibling rivalry

■ Parenting, alteration in: potential, related to knowledge deficit (temper tantrums, negativism, regression)

Coping-stress tolerance pattern

■ Coping, family: potential for growth, related to successful parenting

GROWTH AND DEVELOPMENT

General concepts of growth and development, such as stages and patterns of development and individual differences, are discussed in Chapter 2. This chapter is primarily concerned with biologic, psychosocial, cognitive, and adaptive development of toddlers.

Biologic development

Biologic development and maturation of body systems are less dramatic during early childhood than during infancy. Growth slows considerably. The average weight gain is 1.8 to 2.7 kg (4 to 6 pounds) per year. The birth weight is quadrupled by 2½ years of age. The average weight at 2 years is 12 kg (27 pounds).

The rate of increase in height also slows. The usual increment is an addition of 7.5 cm (3 inches) per year and occurs mainly in elongation of the legs rather than the trunk. The average height of a 2-year-old is 86.6 cm (34 inches). In general, adult height is about twice the child's height at 2 years of age.

Accurate measurement of height and weight during the toddler years should reveal a steady growth curve that is steplike in nature rather than straight. This is characteristic of the growth spurts during the early childhood years.

Head circumference slows somewhat by the end of infancy and is usually equal to the chest circumference by 1 to 2 years of age. The usual increase in head circumference during the second year is 2.5 cm (1 inch). It continues to decrease until at age 5 years the increase is less than

1.25 cm (0.5 inch) per year. The anterior fontanel closes between 12 and 18 months of age.

Chest circumference continues to increase in size and exceeds head circumference during the toddler years. Its shape also changes as the transverse or lateral diameter exceeds the anteroposterior diameter. After the second year the chest circumference exceeds the abdominal measurement, which, in addition to the growth of the lower extremities, gives the child a taller, leaner appearance. However, the toddler retains a squat, "pot-bellied" appearance because of the less well-developed abdominal musculature and short legs (Fig. 10-1). The legs retain a slightly bowed or curved appearance during the second year from the weight of the relatively large trunk. This lateral curvature disappears by 3 years of age.

Most of the physiologic systems are relatively mature by the end of toddlerhood. The volume of the respiratory tract and growth of associated structures continue to increase during early childhood, lessening some of the factors that predisposed the child to frequent and serious infections during infancy. However, the internal structures of the ear and throat continue to be short and straight, and the lymphoid tissue of the tonsils and adenoids continues to be large. As a result, otitis media, tonsillitis, and upper respiratory infections are common.

The respiratory and heart rates slow and the blood pressure increases (see inside front cover). Respirations continue to be abdominal during the toddler years.

Under conditions of moderate variation in tempera-

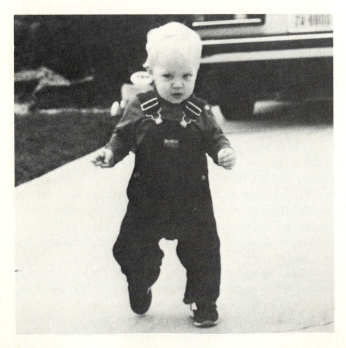

FIG. 10-1
Typical toddling gait.

ture, the toddler rarely has the difficulties of the young infant in maintaining body temperature. The mature functioning of the renal system serves to conserve fluid under times of stress, decreasing the risk of dehydration. The gastrointestinal tract can handle most foods consumed by adults, and the slower transit time also makes the toddler somewhat less vulnerable to dehydration from diarrhea.

The defense mechanisms of the skin and blood, particularly phagocytosis, are much more efficient in toddlers than in infants. The production of antibodies is well established. However, many young children demonstrate a sudden increase in colds and minor infections when entering nursery school or other group situations. Gradually their resistance increases, although their contact with heavily crowded areas, such as shopping centers or restaurants during holiday seasons, should be limited.

Psychosocial development

The toddler is faced with the mastery of several important tasks. If the need for basic trust has been satisfied, he is ready to give up dependence for control, independence, and autonomy. Some of the specific tasks to be dealt with include (1) differentiation of himself from others, particularly his mother, (2) toleration of separation from mother or parent, (3) ability to withstand delayed gratification, (4) control over bodily functions, (5) acquisition of socially acceptable behavior, (6) verbal means of communication, and (7) ability to interact with others in a less egocentric, autistic manner. Mastery of these goals is only begun during late infancy and toddler years, and such tasks as developing interpersonal relationships with others may not be completed until adolescence. However, crucial foundations for successful completion of such developmental tasks is laid during these early formative years.

Developing a sense of autonomy. According to Erikson, the developmental task of toddlerhood is to acquire a sense of *autonomy* while overcoming a sense of doubt and shame. As the infant gains trust in the predictability and reliability of his parents, his environment, and his interaction with others, he begins to discover that his behavior is his own and has a predictable, reliable effect on others. However, while he realizes his will and control over others, he is confronted with the conflict of exerting his autonomy and relinquishing his much-enjoyed dependence on others. In addition, exerting his will has definite negative consequences, such as verbal disapproval or punishment, whereas retaining dependent, submissive behavior is generally rewarded with affection and approval. However, continued dependency creates in the child a sense of doubt regarding his potential capacity to control his actions. This doubt is compounded by a sense of shame for feeling this urge to revolt against others' will and a fear that he will exceed his own capacity for manipulating his environment.

Just as the infant has the social modalities of grasping and biting, the toddler has the newly gained modality of holding on and letting go. To hold on and let go is evident with the use of the hands, mouth, eyes, and, eventually, the sphincters, when toilet training is begun. These social modalities are expressed constantly in the child's play activities, such as casting or throwing objects, taking objects out of boxes, drawers, or cabinets, holding on tighter when someone says, ''No, don't touch,'' and spitting out food as taste preferences become very strong.

Several characteristics are typical of toddlers in their quest for autonomy. Two of these, *negativism* and *ritualism,* are especially significant. As the toddler attempts to express his will, he is often contrary to everything around him. The words ''no'' or ''me do'' can be the sole vocabulary. Emotions become very strongly expressed, usually in rapid mood swings. One minute the toddler can be engrossed in an activity, and the next minute he might be violently angry because he was unable to manipulate a toy or open a door. If scolded for doing something wrong, he can have a temper tantrum and almost instantaneously pull at his mother's legs to be picked up and comforted. Often these swift changes are difficult for parents to understand and cope with. Many parents find the negativism exasperating and, instead of dealing with it, give into it, which further threatens the child in his search for learning acceptable methods of interacting with others (see also p. 296).

In contrast to negativism, which frequently disrupts the environment, ritualism becomes the needed buffer to maintain sameness and reliability. The toddler can venture out with security when he knows that familiar people, places, and routines still exist. One can easily understand why change, such as hospitalization, represents such a threat to these children. Without the comfortable rituals, there is little opportunity to exert autonomy. Consequently, dependency and regression occur (see also p. 292).

Erikson focuses on the development of the *ego* during this phase of psychosocial development. There is a struggle as the child deals with the impulses of the *id,* attempts to tolerate frustration, and learns socially acceptable ways of interacting with the environment. The ego, which may be thought of as reason or common sense, is evident as the child is able to tolerate delayed gratification.

There is also rudimentary beginning of the *superego* or conscience, which is the incorporation of the morals of society and the process of acculturation. With the development of the ego the child further differentiates himself from others and expands his sense of trust within himself. But as he begins to develop awareness of his own will and capacity to achieve, he also becomes aware of his ability

to fail. This ever-present awareness of potential failure creates fear of doubt and shame. Successful mastery of the task of autonomy necessitates opportunities for self-mastery while withstanding the frustration of necessary limit setting and delayed gratification. Opportunities for self-mastery are present in appropriate play activities, toilet training, the crisis of sibling rivalry, and successful interactions with significant others.

Cognitive development

By the beginning of the second year it is quite clear that the toddler ''thinks'' and ''reasons'' things out. There is deliberate trial and error experimentation to produce certain results. The mental abstracts of time, space, and causality begin to have meaning, but the child's conception of each is different from that of the adult's. The main cognitive achievement of early childhood is the acquisition of language, which represents mental symbolism.

Piaget classifies the period of 12 to 24 months as part of infancy, which completes the six stages of the sensorimotor phase. In the fifth stage, *tertiary circular reactions* (from 13 to 18 months), the child uses active experimentation to achieve previously unattainable goals. Newly acquired physical skills are increasingly more important for the function they serve rather than for the acts themselves. The child incorporates the old learning of secondary circular reactions and applies the combined knowledge to new situations, with emphasis on the results of the experimentation. In this way there is the beginning of rational judgment and intellectual reasoning. During this stage there is further differentiation of oneself from objects. This is evident in the child's increasing ability to venture away from his mother and to tolerate longer periods of separation.

Awareness of a causal relationship between two events is apparent. As the child flips a light switch, he is aware that a reciprocal response occurs. However, he is not able to transfer that knowledge to new situations. Therefore, every time he sees what appears to be a light switch, he must reinvestigate its function. Such behavior demonstrates the beginning of categorizing data into distinct classes, subclasses, and so on. There are innumerable examples of this type of behavior in toddlers as they continuously explore the same object each time it appears in a new place.

Since classification of objects is still rudimentary, the appearance of an object denotes its function. For example, if the child's toys are stored in a paper bag or large container, that toy receptacle is no different than the garbage pail or laundry basket. If the child is allowed to turn over the toy receptacle, he will just as quickly do the same to other similar containers because, for him, there is no difference. Expecting the child to judge which receptacles are permissible to explore and which are not is inappropriate for this age-group. Instead, the forbidden object such as the garbage pail should be placed out of reach.

The discovery of objects as objects leads to the awareness of their spatial relationships. The child is able to recognize different shapes and their relationship to each other. For example, he can fit slightly smaller boxes into each other (nesting) and can place a round object into a hole, even if the board is turned around, upside down, or reversed. He is also aware of space and the relationship of his body to dimensions such as height. He will stretch, stand on a low stair or stool, and pull a string to reach an object.

Object permanence has advanced. Although he still cannot find an object that has been invisibly displaced or moved from under one pillow to another pillow without his seeing the change, the toddler is increasingly aware of the existence of objects behind closed doors, in drawers, and under tables. Parents are usually acutely aware of this developmental achievement and find high places and locked cabinets the only places inaccessible to toddlers.

During ages 19 to 24 months the child is in the final sensorimotor stage, the *invention of new means through mental combinations*. This stage completes the more primitive, autistic thought processes of infancy and prepares the way for more complex mental operations during the phase of preoperational thought. One of the most dramatic achievements of this stage is in the area of object permanence. The child will now actively search for an object in several potential hiding places. Also, he can infer a cause when only experiencing the effect. He can infer that an object was hidden in any number of places even if he only saw the original hiding place.

Imitation displays deeper meaning and understanding. There is greater symbolization to imitation. The child is acutely aware of others' actions and attempts to copy them in gestures and in words. *Domestic mimicry* (imitating household activities) and sex-role behavior become increasingly common during this period and during the second year. Identification with the parent of the same sex becomes apparent by the second year and represents the child's intellectual ability to differentiate different models of behavior and to imitate them appropriately (Fig. 10-2).

The conception of time is still embryonic, but the child has some sense of timing in terms of anticipation, memory, and the limited ability to wait. He may listen to the command, "Just a minute," and behave appropriately. However, his sense of timing is exaggerated because for him 1 minute can last an hour. The toddler's limited attention span reflects his sense of immediacy and concern for the present. His whole world is for his satisfaction and benefit. However, there is advancement from the infantile form of narcissistic behavior in the child's ability to wait,

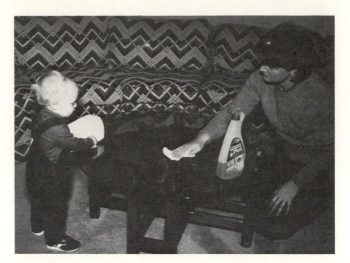

FIG. 10-2

Domestic mimicry and sex role behavior are common during the toddler years.

increased concern with pleasing mother, and awareness of outside controls on his actions.

At approximately 2 years of age the child enters the *preconceptual phase* of cognitive development, which spans the period of 2 to 4 years of age. In some of Piaget's writing, the preconceptual phase is part of a larger category, the *preoperational phase,* which includes the time span of ages 2 to 7 years. The period from ages 2 to 4 years is primarily one of transition, which bridges the purely self-satisfying behavior of infancy and the rudimentary socialized behavior of latency.

The 2-year-old child is in a state of continuous investigation. The primary focus of his attention is still egocentric. He sees, experiences, and lives every event in reference to himself. For example, if a person is positioned between him and another child, the toddler will explain that both children can see the middle person's face. He is unable to view the middle person from a different perspective.

Imaginary and symbolic play is rich in activities that involve total absorption with one's self. The child can be anyone, do anything, and experience everything just by thinking that it is so. *Magical thinking* is very prevalent during early childhood and explains the child's feelings of omnipotence and supreme authority. However, it also places him in the very vulnerable position of feeling guilty and responsible for bad thoughts, which may occur coincidently. A typical example is wishing a new sibling dead. If that sibling becomes ill or dies, the child thinks his wish caused the event. His inability to logically reason the cause and effect of illness or an accident makes it especially difficult for the child to understand such events.

The concept of causality is demonstrated in a phenomenon called *animism,* in which the child attributes to inanimate objects lifelike qualities. For example, if the child falls down the stairs, he blames the stairs for causing the accident and will frequently ''scold'' the stairs. Cause and effect is more related to the proximity of events than to anything else.

The child's reasoning is *transductive,* from the particular to the particular. For example, if he did not like one food on the table, he will not like any other food. This prelogic is often very difficult to understand and confusing for parents, who will respond to the previous example by stating, ''What does this food have to do with that food?'' As far as the child is concerned, his statement is logical because it is based on his own frame of reference. No amount of ''reasoning'' will reverse this logic.

Typical of toddlers' thinking is global organization of thought processes or, in other words, the idea that changing any part of the whole changes the entire whole. Behaviorally this is repeatedly demonstrated in the toddler's ritualistic and rigidly traditional world. Everything must remain the same for the entire event to remain constant. Changing the smallest detail disrupts the entire experience. For example, substituting a new dish for the usual one spoils the entire meal.

Within the second year the child increasingly uses language as symbols and is concerned with the ''why'' and ''how'' of things. For example, a pencil is ''something to write with,'' food is ''something to eat,'' and so on. Mental symbolization is closely associated with the prelogical reasoning. For instance, a needle is ''something that hurts.'' Through the rapid acquisition of language and the ability to associate causes, the child is able to speculate and anticipate future events. If he remembers the needle as something that hurts, he will anticipate any visit to the doctor as one that causes pain. Reminding young children about other visits that did not hurt or experiences that were pleasant will usually do little to change their frame of reference regarding such events.

Body image. As in infancy, the development of body image closely parallels cognitive development. With increasing motor ability toddlers recognize the usefulness of body parts and gradually learn their respective names. They also learn that certain parts of the body have various meanings. For example, the genitals become significant during toilet training. By 2 years of age there is recognition of sexual differences and reference to self by name and then by pronoun.

Once they begin preoperational thought, toddlers can use symbols to represent objects but their thinking may lead to inaccuracies. For example, if someone who is pregnant is called ''fat'' they will describe all ''fat'' ladies as having babies. There is probably some recognition of words used to describe physical appearance, such as ''pretty,'' ''handsome,'' ''big boy,'' and so on. Such expressions eventually influence how children view their own bodies.

Although there has been little research done on body image development in young children, it is evident that body integrity is poorly understood and that intrusive experiences are threatening. For example, during a physical assessment toddlers forcefully resist procedures such as examining the ear or mouth and taking a rectal temperature. While these same behaviors are evident during the preschool years, preparatory explanations can decrease these fears in preschoolers but not in toddlers.

Adaptive behaviors

Adaptive behaviors can be classified according to developmental achievement in the following areas—gross motor, fine motor, language, and personal-social behaviors. The key developmental ages for the toddler are 18 and 24 months, although the chronologic ages of 15 and 30 months are also significant. Fifteen months of age is a particularly integrative period of developmental achievement, since it represents the completion or fruition of many skills that were unperfected at 1 year of age. Table 10-1 presents a summary of the major features of growth and development for the age-groups of 15, 18, 24, and 30 months.

Gross and fine motor behavior. The major gross motor skill during the toddler years is the acquisition of locomotion. By age 15 months he walks alone, by age 18 months he tries to run but falls easily, and by age 2 years he walks well and runs fairly well, using a wide stance for extra balance.

Fine motor development is demonstrated in increasingly skillful manual dexterity. Once the pincer grasp is achieved, the toddler combines this skill with other developing sensory and cognitive abilities. Casting, or voluntarily throwing objects, and retrieving them become almost obsessive activities around 15 months of age.

Mastery of gross and fine motor skills is evident in all phases of the child's activity, such as play, dressing, language comprehension, response to discipline, social interaction, and proneness to accidents. Activities occur less in isolation and more in conjunction with other physical and mental abilities to produce a purposeful result. For example, the infant engages in many physical activities for the sheer joy of those activities, such as crawling for crawling's sake. Now the toddler employs a skill for a purpose. He walks to reach a new location, releases a toy to pick it up or to choose a new one, and scribbles to look at the image produced. The possibilities of the exploration, investigation, and manipulation of his environment seem endless.

TABLE 10-1. SUMMARY OF GROWTH AND DEVELOPMENT DURING THE TODDLER YEARS

AGE (months)	PHYSICAL	GROSS MOTOR	FINE MOTOR
15	Steady growth in height and weight Height 78.7 cm (31 inches) Weight 10.9 kg (24 pounds) Head circumference 48 cm (19 inches)	Walks without help (usually since age 13 months) Creeps up stairs Kneels without support Cannot walk around corners or stop suddenly without losing balance Assumes standing position without support Cannot throw ball without falling	Constantly casting objects to floor Builds tower of two cubes Holds two cubes in one hand Releases a pellet into a narrow-necked bottle Scribbles spontaneously Uses cup well but rotates spoon
18	Physiologic anorexia from decreased growth needs Anterior fontanel closed Able to control sphincters	Runs clumsily, falls often Walks up stairs with one hand held Pulls and pushes toys Jumps in place with both feet Seats self on chair Throws ball overhand without falling	Builds tower of three to four cubes Release, prehension, and reach well-developed Turns pages in a book two or three at a time In drawing, makes stroke imitatively Manages spoon without rotation
24	Head circumference 49 to 50 cm (19.6 to 20 inches) Chest circumference exceeds head circumference Lateral diameter of chest exceeds anteroposterior diameter Usual weight gain of 1.8 to 2.7 kg (4 to 6 pounds) Usual gain in height of 10 to 12.5 cm (4 to 5 inches) Adult height approximately double height at 2 years of age	Goes up and down stairs alone with two feet on each step Runs fairly well, with wide stance Picks up object without falling Kicks ball forward without overbalancing	Builds tower of six to seven cubes Aligns two or more cubes like a train Turns pages of book one at a time In drawing, imitates vertical and circular strokes Turns doorknob, unscrews lid

SENSORY	SPEECH/LANGUAGE	SOCIALIZATION/COGNITION
Able to identify geometric forms; places round object into appropriate hole Binocular vision well-developed Displays an intense and prolonged interest in pictures	Uses expressive jargon Says four to six words, including names "Asks" for objects by pointing Understands simple commands May use head-shaking gesture to denote "no" Says "no" even while agreeing to the request	Tolerates some separation from mother Less likely to fear strangers Beginning to imitate parents, such as cleaning house (sweeping, dusting, folding clothes) Feeds self using regular cup with little spilling May discard bottle Manages spoon but rotates it near mouth Kisses and hugs parents, may kiss pictures in a book Expressive of emotions, has temper tantrums Can find hidden objects, but only in first location Able to insert a round object into a hole Fits smaller objects into each other (nesting) Realizes that "out of sight" is not out of reach; opens doors and drawers to find objects
	Says ten or more words Points to a common object, such as shoe or ball, and to two or three body parts	Great imitator ("domestic mimicry") Manages spoon well Takes off gloves, socks, and shoes and unzips Temper tantrums may be more evident Beginning awareness of ownership ("my toy") May develop dependency on transitional objects, such as "security blanket" Searches for an object through several hiding places Will infer a cause by associating two or more experiences (such as candy missing, sister smiling) Follows directions and understands requests Uses words "up," "down," "come," and "go" with meaning Has some sense of time; waits in response to "just a minute"; may use word "now"
Accommodation well-developed Visual acuity, 20/40 In geometric discrimination, able to insert square block into oblong space	Has vocabulary of approximately 300 words Uses two- to three-word phrases Uses pronouns I, me, you Understands directional commands Gives first name; refers to self by name Verbalizes need for toileting, food, or drink Talks incessantly	Stage of parallel play Has sustained attention span Temper tantrums decreasing Pulls people to show them something Increased independence from mother Dresses self in simple clothing Thinking is characterized by global organization of thought, transductive reasoning, concept of animism, and magical thinking

Continued.

TABLE 10-1. SUMMARY OF GROWTH AND DEVELOPMENT DURING THE TODDLER YEARS—cont'd

AGE (months)	PHYSICAL	GROSS MOTOR	FINE MOTOR
	Respiratory rate 25 to 28 breaths/minute Heart rate approximately 110 beats/minute Blood pressure: systolic, 96 mm Hg; diastolic, 58 mm Hg Physiologic systems, except for endocrine and reproductive, stable and mature May have achieved readiness for beginning daytime control of bowel and bladder Primary dentition of 16 teeth		
30	Birth weight quadrupled Primary dentition (20 teeth) completed May have daytime bowel and bladder control	Jumps with both feet Jumps from chair or step Stands on one foot momentarily Takes a few steps on tiptoe	Builds tower of eight cubes Adds chimney to train of cubes Good hand-finger coordination; holds crayon with fingers rather than fist Can move fingers independently In drawing, imitates vertical and horizontal strokes, makes two or more strokes for cross

Language behavior. The most striking characteristic of language development during early childhood is the increasing level of comprehension. Although the number of words acquired—from about four at 1 year of age to approximately 300 at age 2 years—is notable, the ability to comprehend and understand speech is much greater than the number of words the child can say. This is particularly evident in bilingual families where the vocabulary may be delayed, but comprehension in either language is appropriate.

Regardless of cultural background, language development follows fairly well-delineated steps during early childhood. The infant progresses through the stages of undifferentiated crying, differentiated crying, cooing, babbling, lallation or imperfect imitation, and echolalia (imitation of the sounds of others). During the second year he may use expressive jargon, a term that refers to a string of utterances that sound like sentences. During most of these stages the child is acquiring a repertoire of sounds that eventually become words, phrases, and sentences. At age 1 year the child uses one-word sentences or holophrases. The word "up" can mean "pick me up" or "look up there." For the child the one word conveys the meaning of a sentence, but to others it may mean many things or nothing. During this age about 25% of the vocalizations are intelligible. By the age of 2 years the child uses multiword sentences by stringing together two or three words, such as the phrase, "mama go bye-bye" or "all gone," and approximately 66% of the speech is understandable.

Personal-social behavior. One of the most dramatic aspects of development in the toddler is his personal-social interaction. Parents frequently wonder why their manageable, docile, lovable infant has turned into a determined, strong-willed, volatile-tempered little tyrant. In addition the tyrant of the terrible twos can swiftly and unpredictably revert back to the adorable infant. All of this is part of his "growing up" and is evident in such areas as dressing, feeding, tolerating brief periods of separation, developing fears, playing, especially with older children, and establishing self-control.

The toddler still fears strangers and depends on his mother for security, but he ventures away from her voluntarily to explore the environment. Verbal and visual reassurance from the parent gradually replace some of the previous need to be physically close to the parent for comfort. The toddler is more willing to meet strangers and will tolerate longer periods of separation. There is less of the extreme fear of separation that was prominent during the latter half of infancy.

The toddler is also developing skills of independence, which are evident in all areas of behavior. The 15-month-old child feeds himself, drinks well from a regular household cup, and manages a spoon, with considerable spilling. By age 18 months he uses a spoon well and may be using a fork, but "finger feeding" is usually preferred (Fig. 10-3). Between ages 2 and 3 years he eats with the family, likes to help with chores such as setting the table or removing dishes from the dishwasher, but lacks table

SENSORY	SPEECH/LANGUAGE	SOCIALIZATION/COGNITION
	Gives first and last name	Separates more easily from mother
	Refers to self by appropriate pronoun	In play, helps put things away, can carry breakable objects, pushes with good steering
	Uses plurals	Begins to notice sex differences; knows own sex
	Names one color	May attend to toilet needs without help except for wiping

manners and may find it difficult to sit through the family's entire meal.

Dressing also demonstrates strides in independence. The 15-month-old child helps his mother by putting his arm or foot out for dressing and pulls his shoes and socks off. The 18-month-old child removes his own gloves, helps with pullover shirts, and may be able to unzip. By age 2 he removes most of his clothing and puts on his socks, shoes, and pants without regard for right or left and back or front. Skills in undressing facilitate the learning of toileting, since independence helps prevent accidents.

Play

Play magnifies the toddler's physical and psychosocial development. Interaction with people becomes increasingly important. The solitary play of infancy (see Chapter 8) progresses to *parallel* play. The toddler plays alongside, not with, other children. Although sensorimotor play is still prominent, there is much less emphasis on the exclusive use of one sensory modality. The toddler inspects the toy, talks to the toy, tests its strength and durability, and invents several uses for it. Imitation is one of the most distinguishing characteristics of play and dictates the most appropriate toys for children in this age-group. With less emphasis on sex-stereotyped toys, play objects such as dolls, dollhouses, dishes, cooking utensils, child-sized furniture, trucks, and dress-up clothes are suitable for both sexes.

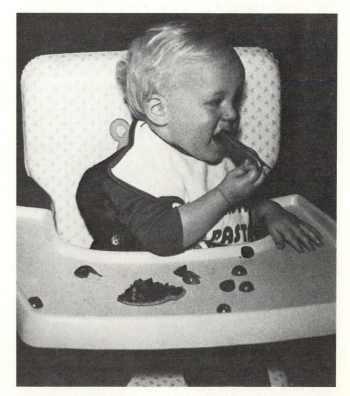

FIG. 10-3
Toddlers enjoy "finger feeding."

Increased locomotive skills make push-pull toys, stick horses, straddle trucks or cycles, a small, low gym and slide, varied size balls, and rocking horses appropriate for the energetic toddler. Finger paints, thick crayons, chalk, blackboard, paper, and puzzles with large simple pieces use the developing fine motor skills. Blocks in varied sizes and shapes provide hours of fun and, during later years, are useful objects for creative and imaginative play.

Because the toddler is experimenting with self-control and independence, feelings of anger and frustration are common and frequently have no suitable outlet other than screaming and temper tantrums. Toys such as drums, play nails and hammer, clay, and Play-Doh provide alternative methods of dissipating psychic energy. They also begin to teach socially acceptable ways of dealing with feelings of aggression.

Talking is a form of play for the toddler, who enjoys musical toys such as play phonographs, "talking" dolls and animals, and play telephones. Appropriate children's television programs are excellent for children in this age-group, who learn to associate words with visual images. Toddlers also enjoy "reading" stories from a picture book and imitating the sounds of animals.

Tactile play is also important for the exploring toddler. Water toys, a sandbox with pail and shovel, finger-paints, soap bubbles, and clay provide excellent opportunities for free creative and manipulative recreation. Parents sometimes forget the fascination of feeling slippery cream, catching airy bubbles, squeezing and reshaping clay, or smearing paints. But these kinds of unstructured activities are equally as important as educational play in order to allow children freedom of expression.

Selection of appropriate toys must involve safety factors, especially in relation to size and sturdiness. The oral activity of toddlers makes them at risk for aspirating small objects. Parents need to be especially vigilant of toys played with in other children's homes or those of older siblings. Toys are a potential source of serious bodily damage to toddlers, who may have the physical strength to manipulate them but not the knowledge to appreciate their danger.

PROMOTING OPTIMUM DEVELOPMENT

The toddler years can be one of the most trying and confusing periods for parents. Behaviorally the toddler can be described as untiringly energetic, insatiably inquisitive, annoyingly negative, and obstinately ritualistic. Understanding these behaviors helps parents realize the necessity of the behaviors and allows the parents to effectively deal with the developmental tasks of children in this age-group.

Separation anxiety

A major task of the toddler period is differentiation of the self from the environment. There is increased understanding and awareness of permanence and some ability to withstand delayed gratification and to tolerate moderate frustration. As a result, toddlers react differently to strangers than do infants. The appearance of unfamiliar persons does not represent such a significant threat to their attachment to mother. They have learned from experience that parents exist when physically absent. Repetition of events such as going to bed without mother but waking to find her there again reinforces the reliability of such brief separations. Consequently toddlers are able to venture away from their parents for brief periods of time because of the security of knowing that the parent will be there when they return.

This is also the age for transitional objects, such as a special blanket or stuffed toy. These objects provide extra security for the child, especially when he is alone or tired (Fig. 10-4).

Learning to tolerate and master brief periods of separation is an important developmental task of children in this age-group. In addition it is a necessary component of parenting, because brief periods of separation from toddlers allow parents to recoup their energy and patience. Without such outlets for physical and emotional relief, their irritations and frustrations may be directed toward the children.

Although the specific reaction of young children to the separation that results from hospitalization is discussed in Chapter 18, it is worthwhile to explore how they behave in response to separation for any reason. Toddlers show less fear of strangers than do infants when their parents are present but are very fearful and angry when their parents leave. When alone, they are acutely anxious with strangers, manifest depressive behavior, such as crying and withdrawal, may become restless, hyperactive, or passive, and may revert to regressive behaviors. Such reactions may be evident the first time a child is left with a baby-sitter or during the first day of nursery school. These behaviors are not harmful if parents realize how desperately their children need them. Sensitive, perceptive parents will be aware of the child's need for increased love, affection, and attention when they are together.

Regression

Regression is the retreat from one's present pattern of functioning to past levels of behavior. It usually occurs in instances of discomfort or stress, when one attempts to conserve his psychic energy by reverting to patterns of behavior that were successful in earlier stages of development. Regression is common in toddlers, because almost

behavior. Children are saying, ''We can't cope with this present stress and perfect this skill as well, but we will if given patience and understanding.'' For this reason it is not advisable to attempt new areas of learning when an additional crisis is present or expected. An excellent example is beginning toilet training shortly before a sibling is born or attempting new areas of learning during a brief period of hospitalization.

Toilet training

One of the major tasks of toddlerhood is toilet training. Voluntary control of the anal and urethral sphincters is achieved sometime after the child is walking, probably between ages 18 and 24 months. However, complex psychophysiologic factors are required for readiness. The child must be able to recognize the urge to let go and hold on and be able to communicate this sensation to the mother. In addition, there is probably some necessary motivation in the desire to please mother by holding on, rather than pleasing oneself by letting go.

Usually physical and psychologic readiness is not complete until the later half of the second year. By this time the child has mastered the majority of essential gross motor skills, can communicate intelligibly, is less in conflict with self-assertion and negativism, and is aware of his ability to control his body and please his mother. One of the most important responsibilities of nurses is to help parents identify readiness in their child (Table 10-2).

Bowel training is usually accomplished before bladder training because of its greater regularity and predictability. There is a stronger sensation for defecation than urination, which can be brought to the child's attention. Nighttime bladder training may not be completed until 4 or 5 years of age. Daytime accidents are also not uncommon, particularly during periods of intense activity. Preschoolers become so engrossed in play activity that if they are not reminded they will wait until it is too late to make it to the bathroom. Boys master the stand-up position after they have been toilet trained for some time. Imitating father during the preschool years is a powerful motivating force.

Child-rearing theories are also filled with various helpful techniques to encourage the child's cooperation. Some advocate the use of a free-standing potty-chair, which allows the child a feeling of security. Others suggest a portable seat attached to the regular toilet to facilitate the transition from potty-chair to regular toilet (Fig. 10-5). If a potty-seat is not available, having the child sit *facing* the toilet tank provides added support. Using positive reinforcement through the use of training pants or fancy panties and encouraging imitation by watching others also works for some children. Forcing the child to sit on the potty for long periods of time, spanking him for having

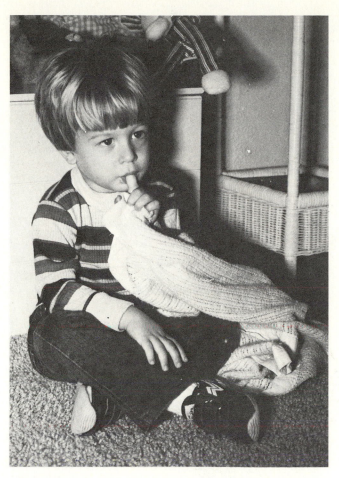

FIG. 10-4

Transitional objects, such as a warm and fuzzy blanket and a finger, are sources of security to a toddler.

any additional stress lessens their ability to master present developmental tasks. Any threat to their autonomy, such as illness, hospitalization, separation, or adjustment to a sibling, represents a need to revert to earlier forms of behavior, such as increased dependency, refusal to use the potty-chair, temper tantrums, demand for the bottle, stroller, or crib, and loss of newly learned motor, language, social, and cognitive skills.

At first such regression appears acceptable and comfortable for children, but on closer inspection one realizes that the loss of newly acquired achievements is frightening and threatening, because children are aware of their total helplessness in the recent past. Parents, too, become frightened about regressive behavior and frequently in their efforts to deal with it force the child to cope with an additional source of stress, the pressure to live up to expected standards.

When regression does occur, the best approach is to ignore it, while praising existing patterns of appropriate

TABLE 10-2. INDICATIONS OF READINESS FOR TOILET TRAINING

PHYSICAL READINESS	MENTAL READINESS	PSYCHOLOGICAL READINESS	PARENTAL READINESS
Voluntary control of anal and urethral sphincters, usually by 18 to 24 months Ability to stay dry for 2 hours Gross motor skills of sitting, walking, and squatting Fine motor skills to remove clothing	Recognizes urge to defecate or urinate Verbal or nonverbal communicative skills to indicate when wet or has urge to defecate or urinate Cognitive skills to imitate appropriate behavior and follow directions	Expresses willingness to please parent Able to sit on toilet for 5 to 10 minutes without fussing or getting off	Recognizes child's level of readiness Willing to invest the time required for toilet training Absence of family stress or change, such as a divorce, moving, new sibling, or imminent vacation

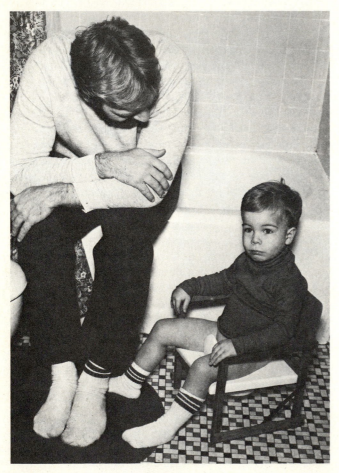

FIG. 10-5
Toddler on a free-standing potty chair.

accidents, or other methods of negative control are avoided.

Sibling rivalry

The arrival of a new infant into the family represents a crisis for even the best prepared toddler, especially the firstborn, who has experienced the wonderful position of being number one. The toddler does not hate or resent the infant but the change that this additional sibling produces. Mother and father now share their love and attention with someone else, the usual routine is disrupted, and the toddler may lose his crib—all at a time when he thought he was in control of his world.

Preparation of a child for the birth of a sibling is quite individual, but age dictates some important considerations. Time for toddlers is a vague concept. Preparing children too soon for the birth may lessen their interest by the time the event occurs. Toddlers are aware of something when mother's belly gets large and changes have taken place within the house. A month or two in advance is ample time for preparing the child.

Toddlers also need to have a realistic idea of what newborns are like. Telling him that a new playmate will come home soon is foolish, since it is untrue and sets up unrealistic expectations. Rather, parents should stress the activities that will take place when the baby arrives home, such as diapering, bottle- or breast-feeding, bathing, and dressing. At the same time they should emphasize which routines will stay the same, such as reading stories or going to the park. If the toddler has had no contact with an infant, it is a good idea to introduce him to one, if that is feasible.

Frequently other preparations, such as introducing the toddler to a regular bed or moving him to a different room, should be made earlier. If these changes are done well in advance, they will not be associated with the infant's arrival.

Pregnancy is an abstraction for toddlers. They need concrete illustrations of how the baby is growing inside the mother. It is an excellent opportunity for introducing aspects of reproduction and sexuality. Showing simple pictures of the uterus and fetus, allowing the child to feel the fetus move, and involving the child in care-giving activities after the infant is born help him feel part of the experience (Fig. 10-6).

How children exhibit jealousy is complex. Some will overtly hit the infant, push him off mother's lap, or pull the bottle or breast from his mouth. More often the expressions of hostility and resentment are much more subtle and covert. Toddlers may verbally express a wish that the infant "go back inside mommy," or they will revert to more infantile forms of behavior, such as demanding a bottle, soiling their diaper, clinging for attention, using baby talk, or aggressively acting out toward others. For this reason infants must be protected by supervising the interaction between the siblings.

Limit setting and discipline

While these two terms are often used interchangeably, they can also refer to different concepts. *Limit setting* refers to establishing the rules or guidelines for behavior, whereas *discipline* is the action taken to enforce the rules when the child does not comply. Generally the clearer the limits are set and consistently enforced, the less need there is for discipline. Therefore, the initial nursing goal is to help parents establish realistic and concrete "rules."

Limit setting and discipline are positive, necessary components of childrearing. They serve several useful functions as they help children to (1) test their limits of control, (2) achieve in areas appropriate for mastery at their level, (3) channel undesirable feelings into constructive activity, (4) protect them from danger, and (5) teach socially acceptable behavior.

Children want and need limits. Unrestricted freedom is a tremendous threat to their security and safety. Through testing the limits imposed on them, they learn how far they can manipulate their environment as well as gain reassurance from knowing that others will be there to protect them from potential harm.

Limit setting also circumscribes areas of success and mastery for children. When allowed to play with toys that are suitable to their developmental age, children have the opportunity to master a task and feel satisfaction. When they are aware of what pleases their parents, they are certain of love and approval. Limit setting is part of establishing a routine scheduled environment for toddlers.

General guidelines. Certain principles govern the

effectiveness of any type of discipline. The first is *consistency* and *firmness*. Once a limit is set, parents must consistently practice the rule. A pattern of intermittent or "sometime" enforcement of limits actually prolongs the undesired behavior because the toddler knows that if he got his way once, he can do it again.

Another principle is *timing*. For punishment to have meaning, it must occur immediately after the wrongdoing. A common example of delayed punishment is telling the child, "Wait until your father comes home." Not only is this ineffectual, but it also conveys negative connotations about the other parent.

Limit setting and discipline should be *positive* and *teach appropriate behavior*. Requests for appropriate behavior are made in a positive statement such as, "Put the book down," rather than, "Don't touch the book."

Finally, discipline should be combined with *praise* for something the child did right. Sometimes, especially with toddlers who seem to be in the wrong places and doing the wrong things, parents can be disciplining almost constantly. To avoid attending to the child only at these times, parents should find something positive to praise.

Types of discipline. Once the limits are set, parents need guidelines for appropriate disciplinary action when the rules are broken. There are numerous theories regarding types of discipline. Among the most common ones are (1) corporal punishment, (2) reasoning and scolding, (3) ignoring or extinction, and (4) time-out. The following is a brief overview of the use and limitations of each.

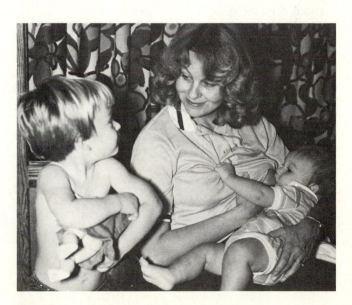

FIG. 10-6

Toddlers enjoy participating in care-giving activities for the new sibling, such as this toddler who is "breast-feeding" his doll.

Corporal punishment. Corporal punishment most often takes the form of spanking. Although there is much controversy regarding the use and abuse of corporal punishment, there are some instances when it is effective, especially in young children who refuse to listen to the verbal command. For example, slapping the child's hand while saying, ''No, don't touch,'' reinforces the meaning of the statement. A good rule when using mild physical punishment is that only one slap is given because the first slap is for the child; additional slaps are for the punisher.

Reasoning and scolding. Reasoning involves explaining why an act is wrong. Although it is always a good practice to explain why limits are based on the moral issue behind a wrong act, it is foolish to expect young children to understand the explanation.

Reasoning is almost always combined with scolding, which sometimes takes the form of shame. For example, the parent may state, ''You are a bad boy; I am very disappointed in you.'' Unfortunately children take such remarks seriously and personally, believing that *they* are bad. It is important to always disapprove of the *behavior,* not the child, with such statements as, ''That was a wrong thing to do. I am disappointed when you act that way.''

Ignoring or extinction. Ignoring is based on the behavioral theory that if an act is consistently ignored, the lack of attention will eventually extinguish the behavior. Although this approach sounds very simple, it is extremely difficult to adhere to it. Parents frequently ''give in'' and resort to old patterns of discipline, since they lack the perseverance to do nothing. Consequently the behavior is actually reinforced because the child learns that his persistence gained their attention.

Time-out. Time-out is actually a refinement of the common practice of ''sending the child to his room.'' It is also based on the premise of removing the reinforcer, that is, the satisfaction or attention the child is receiving from the activity. By placing the child in an unstimulating and isolated place, he becomes bored and consequently agrees to behave in order to reenter the family group. A rule for the length of time-out is *1 minute per year of age; a* kitchen timer should be used to record the time rather than a watch. Time-out avoids many of the problems of the other disciplinary approaches because no physical punishment is involved, no reasoning or scolding is given, and the parent is usually not present for all of the time-out, facilitating his ability to consistently apply the punishment.

All of these approaches teach the child what not to do. Therefore, it is the parents' responsibility to discuss with children what they did wrong that deserved punishment and how they should behave next time to avoid punishment.

Temper tantrums

Toddlers may assert their independence by violently objecting to discipline. They may lie down on the floor, kick their feet, and scream at the top of their lungs. Some have learned the effectiveness of holding their breath until the parent relents. Although holding one's breath may cause fainting from the lack of oxygen, the accumulation of carbon dioxide will stimulate the respiratory control center, resulting in no physical harm.

The best approach toward extinguishing such attention-seeking behavior is to ignore it, provided the behavior is not injuring the child, such as violently banging his head on the floor. The parent should remain close by, however. When the tantrum has subsided, the child needs to feel some control and security. At this time a different toy or a favorite activity can be substituted for the ungranted request.

Frequently temper tantrums can be avoided by giving the child advance warning of a request. For example, a popular time for tantrums is before bed. Active toddlers often have trouble slowing down and when placed in bed, resist staying there. One approach is to establish limited rituals that signal readiness for bed, such as a bath or story. Parents can reinforce the pattern by stating, ''After this story it is bedtime,'' and consistently carrying through the routine.

Negativism

One of the more difficult aspects of rearing children in this age-group is their persistent negative ''no'' response to every request. The negativism is not an expression of being fresh or insolent, but a necessary assertion of self-control. One method of dealing with the negativism is reducing the opportunities for a ''no'' answer. Asking the child, ''Do you want to go to sleep now?'' is an almost certain example of a question that will be answered with an emphatic ''no.'' Instead, tell the child that it is time to go to sleep and proceed accordingly.

In their attempt to exert control, children like to make choices. When confronted with appropriate choices, such as, ''You can have a peanut butter and jelly sandwich or chicken noodle soup for lunch,'' they are more likely to choose one than automatically say no. However, if their response is negative, parents should make the choice for the child.

HEALTH PROMOTION DURING THE TODDLER YEARS

Physical and psychosocial changes in toddlers affect two major areas of health maintenance and promotion, namely, nutrition and accident prevention. As the growth rate slows, young children require fewer calories and demonstrate this through increased fussiness and decreased appetite. Their negativism and awareness of food as a control mechanism pose potential problems for parents.

Gross and fine motor skills are so well developed that toddlers seem vulnerable to almost every kind of accident. It is not difficult to appreciate the facts that accidents are the number one cause of death and that nearly half of all poisonings occur in children less than 5 years of age. Parents' ability to safeproof the environment and to set reasonable limits is the major component in preventing accidents.

Another area of health maintenance is dental hygiene. Care of the teeth becomes important during late infancy and toddlerhood, when primary dentition is completed. The principal objective is teaching parents aspects of diet and dental hygiene to prevent loss of teeth.

Nutritional requirements and counseling

During the period from 12 to 18 months of age, the growth rate slows, decreasing the child's need for calories, protein, and fluid. However, the protein and calorie requirements are still relatively high to meet the demands for muscle tissue growth and high activity level. Need for minerals such as iron, calcium, and phosphorus is still high, particularly when one considers the poor food habits of children in this age-group and the increased mineralization within bones. The number of servings in each food group and suggested portions are given in Table 10-3.

At approximately 18 months of age, most toddlers manifest this decreased nutritional need in a phenomenon known as *physiologic anorexia*. They become picky, fussy eaters with strong taste preferences. They may eat voraciously one day and almost nothing the next. They are increasingly aware of the nonnutritive function of food: the pleasure of eating, the social aspect of mealtime, and the control of refusing food. They are influenced by factors other than taste when choosing food. If a family member refuses to eat something, the child is likely to imitate that response. If the plate is overfilled, he is likely to push it away, overwhelmed by its size. If food does not appear or smell appetizing, he will probably not agree to try it. In essence mealtime is more closely associated with psychologic components than nutritional ones.

Consequently, the method of serving food is important. Toddlers need to feel control and achievement in their abilities. Giving them large, adult-size portions contributes to their feeling overwhelmed. In general what is eaten is much more significant than how much is consumed. Small amounts of meat and vegetables supply greater food value than a large consumption of bread or potato. Young chil-

TABLE 10-3. SERVINGS PER DAY FOR TODDLERS BASED ON BASIC FOUR FOOD GROUPS*

FOOD GROUP	SERVINGS PER DAY

Milk or equivalent
½ cup whole milk equals:
  1 ounce cheese
  ½ cup cottage cheese,
    yogurt, milk pudding
	3
	Usual serving, ¾ cup

Meat, fish, poultry, or
  equivalent
1 ounce meat equals:
  1 egg
  1 ounce cheese
  2 tablespoons peanut
    butter
  ¼ cup tuna fish
  ½ cup legumes
	2
	Usual serving, 1 egg or
	  1 to 2 ounces meat

Vegetables and fruits
  Citrus equivalents:
  1 orange or tomato
  ½ cup orange or grape-
    fruit juice
  ¾ cup strawberries
	4 (one citrus daily; one
	  yellow or dark green
	  vegetable every other
	  day)
	Usual serving, 4 ounces

Breads and cereals
1 slice enriched bread
  equals:
  ¾ cup dry cereal
  ½ cup cooked pasta,
    rice, or cereal
	4 or more
	Usual serving, ½ slice
	  bread

*Fats and carbohydrates should be served sparingly to meet caloric needs.

dren tend to like less spicy, bland food, although this is culturally determined in many instances. Substitutions should be provided for foods that they do not enjoy. The ritualism of this age also dictates certain principles in feeding practices. Toddlers like the same dish, cup, or spoon every time. They may reject a favorite food simply because it is served in a different utensil. Since toddlers are unpredictable in their table manners, it is best to use plastic dishes and cups, both for economic and safety reasons. A regular mealtime schedule also contributes to their desire and need for predictability and ritualism.

Eating habits established in the first 2 or 3 years of life tend to have lasting effects on subsequent years. If food is used as a reward or sign of approval, it is possible that the person may overeat for this reason. If food is forced and mealtime is consistently unpleasant, one may never develop the usual pleasure associated with eating. Mealtimes should be enjoyable rather than times for discipline or family arguments. The social aspect of mealtime may be distracting for young children; therefore, an earlier feeding hour may be appropriate. Young children are unable to sit through a long meal and become fidgety and disruptive. This is particularly common when children are brought to the table just after active play. Calling them in from play 15 minutes before mealtime allows them ample opportunity to get ready for eating while settling down their active minds and bodies.

Most children by 12 months of age are eating the same food prepared for the rest of the family. However, appetite and food preferences are sporadic. Often the interest in food parallels a growth spurt so that periods of good eating are interspersed with phases of poor eating. ''Food jags'' are common.

Such food fads do not ensure a well-balanced diet, but attempts to alter them are usually unsuccessful. It is preferable to accept such extremes and offer other foods in small portions. Introducing at least three items from the basic four food groups at each meal helps develop a variety of taste preferences and well-balanced habits.

Accident prevention

The statistics concerning accidents in children 1 to 4 years old attest to the seriousness of this problem. More children in this age-group die from accidents than from the combined deaths in the next seven leading causes of mortality. In addition, the accident rate has remained relatively unchanged during the past decade, whereas the corresponding rates from all other causes combined have declined.

Mortality from accidental causes tells only part of the story. Disability is another dominant factor. Approximately one third of the entire population under 6 years of age suffers some injury requiring medical attention or involving 1 day's restricted activity. About two thirds of all these accidents occur in the home, and almost all accidents are preventable. Their prominence as the leading cause of death among toddlers and preschoolers underscores the need to emphasize safety awareness among parents. Child protection and parent education are key determinants in every health professional's battle against accidents.

Table 10-4 summarizes specific categories of accidents according to the major developmental achievements of toddlers and preschoolers and presents appropriate prevention for each.

Motor vehicle accidents. Motor vehicle fatalities dominate the accident mortality of all pediatric age-groups after 1 year of age. Such deaths cause almost one half of all accidental deaths among children ages 1 to 4 years. Many of the deaths are caused by accidents within the car in which restraints have not been used or have been used improperly.

Nurses have a responsibility for educating parents regarding the importance of car restraints and their proper use. Four types of restraints are available: (1) infant rearward-facing device, (2) older child car seat, (3) shield, and (4) harness with or without a booster seat. Since the infant-type restraints are discussed in Chapter 8, only the remaining types are included here.

The older child car seat is designed for children who can sit by themselves and who are over 7.7 to 9 kg (17 to 20 pounds). It consists of a molded hard plastic or metal frame with energy-absorbing padding and a five-point harness system (Fig. 10-7). Some models require the use of a top anchor (tether) strap to prevent the child from pitching forward in a crash. If the tether strap is not used, up to 90% of the restraint's protection is lost. Instructions for proper installation of the tether strap and permanent bracket are included with the car restraint. If parents object to drilling holes in the car to install the bracket, it is advisable that they select a model without this feature.

The shield-type car restraint is composed of high-impact plastic and a padded interior (Fig. 10-8). Some of the models sit directly on top of the car seat; others incorporate a raised seat into their design. The shield is anchored to the car seat by the lap belt. The shield has the major advantage of convenience because the child can climb in unassisted and no harness is needed. However, children can also climb out easily, which may reduce its effectiveness. The shield may not be suitable for children who wear eyeglasses.

The third type of car restraint is the safety harness and booster seat designed for older children who have outgrown the conventional restraints (Fig. 10-9). The harness requires permanent installation similar to the top anchor strap. The booster seat is not safe if used with a lap belt alone and should not be used once the midpoint of the child's head exceeds the height of the back of the vehicle seat.

Children should use their restraints until they have outgrown them. The ''rule of fours'' is a guide to when this occurs: the child weighs about 40 pounds (18 kg), is 40 inches (100 cm) tall, or is 4 years old. From then until the child is 55 inches (123 cm) tall, a standard lap belt is used. Once the child is over 55 inches, the seat belt/shoulder harness system is used. The safest area of the car for children in child or auto restraint systems is the middle of the backseat.

When purchasing a restraint, parents should consider cost and convenience. The convertible-type seats, which can by used for infants and older children, are more expensive initially but cost less than two separate systems. Convenience is a major factor because a cumbersome restraint may be used less and improperly. Before buying a restraint, it it best to test out different models. For exam-

TABLE 10-4. ACCIDENT PREVENTION DURING EARLY CHILDHOOD

MAJOR DEVELOPMENTAL TASK	ACCIDENT PREVENTION
Walks, runs, and climbs Able to open doors and gates Can ride tricycle Can throw ball and other objects	**Motor vehicles** Use federally approved car restraint; if restraint is not available use lap belt Supervise children while playing outside Do not allow to play on curb or behind a parked car Do not permit to play in pile of leaves, snow, or large cardboard container in trafficked area Supervise tricycle riding Lock fences and doors if not directly supervising children Teach children to look for a car before crossing, recognize color of traffic lights, and obey traffic officers
Able to explore if left unsupervised Has great curiosity Helpless in water; unaware of its danger; depth of water has no significance	**Drowning** Supervise closely when near any source of water Have fence around swimming pool and lock gate Teach swimming and water safety
Able to reach heights by climbing, stretching, and standing on toes Pulls objects Explores any holes or opening Can open drawers and closets Unaware of potential sources of heat or fire Plays with mechanical objects	**Burns** Turn pot handles toward back of stove Place guard rails in front of radiators, fireplaces, or other heating elements Store matches and cigarette lighters in locked or inaccessible area Place burning candles, incense, hot foods, and cigarettes out of reach Do not let tablecloth hang within child's reach Do not let electric cord from iron or other appliance hang within child's reach Cover electrical outlets with protective plastic caps Keep electrical wires hidden or out of reach Do not allow child to play with electrical appliance Stress danger of open flames; teach what ''hot'' means Always check bathwater; adjust hot-water temperature to 52° C (125° F) or lower; do not allow to play with faucets
Explores by putting objects in mouth Can open drawers, closets, and most containers Climbs Cannot read labels	**Poisoning** Place all potentially toxic agents out of reach or in a locked cabinet Replace medications and poisons immediately; replace child-protector caps properly Administer medications as a drug, not as a candy Do not store large surplus of toxic agents Promptly discard empty poison containers; never reuse to store a food item or other poison Never remove labels from containers of toxic substances Know when and how to use ipecac syrup Know number and location of nearest poison control center
Able to open doors and some windows Goes up and down stairs Depth perception unrefined	**Falls** Keep screen in window, nail securely, and use guard rail Place gates at top and bottom of stairs Keep doors locked when there is danger of falls (stairwells, porches) Keep crib rails fully raised and mattress at lowest level Place carpeting under crib and in bathroom Keep child restrained in vehicles; never leave unattended in shopping cart Supervise at playgrounds; select safe play areas with soft ground cover Check child's shoes and trousers

Continued.

TABLE 10-4. ACCIDENT PREVENTION DURING EARLY CHILDHOOD—cont'd

MAJOR DEVELOPMENTAL TASK	ACCIDENT PREVENTION
Puts things in mouth May swallow hard or nonedible pieces of food	**Aspiration and asphyxiation** Avoid large chunks of meat, such as whole hot dogs Avoid fruit with pits, fish with bones, dried beans, hard candy, chewing gum, and nuts Choose large sturdy toys without sharp edges or small removable parts Discard old refrigerators, ovens, and so on If storing an old appliance, remove the doors Keep automatic garage door transmitter in inaccessible place Select safe toy boxes or chests without heavy, hinged lids
Still clumsy in many skills	**Bodily damage** Avoid giving toddler sharp or pointed objects, especially when walking or running Do not let toddler have lollipops or similar objects in mouth when walking or running Teach safety precautions, for example, to carry knife or scissors with pointed end away from face Store all dangerous tools, garden equipment, and firearms in locked cabinet Alert parents to danger of unsupervised animals and household pets

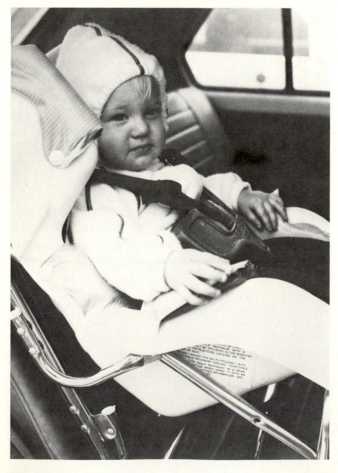

FIG. 10-7
Child car-seat restraint.

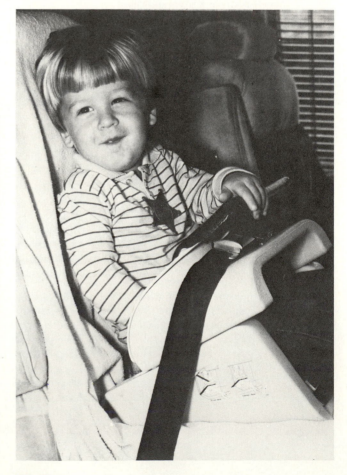

FIG. 10-8
Shield car-seat restraint.

ple, some types are too large for subcompact cars. Asking neighbors about the advantages and disadvantages of their restraints is helpful. Some service clubs and hospitals have loan programs for restraints. Information about approved models is available from Physicians for Automotive Safety* and the U.S. Department of Transportation.†

The most important component of any restraint is that

---

*50 Union Ave., Irvington, NJ 07111.
†National Highway Traffic Safety Administration, Washington DC 20590.

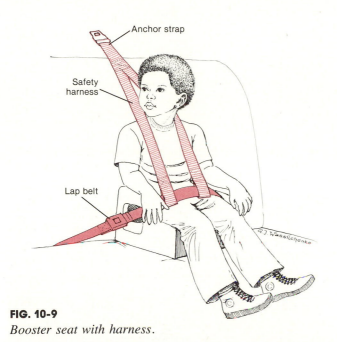

FIG. 10-9
Booster seat with harness.

it be used. Children who are introduced to them during infancy usually have little difficulty tolerating the seat. To ensure compliance, certain ''rules of riding'' should be practiced:

1. Do not start the car until *everyone* is properly restrained.
2. *Always* use the restraint, even for short trips.
3. If the child begins to climb out or undo the harness, firmly say, ''No.'' It may be necessary to stop the car and/or slap his hand to reinforce the expected behavior.
4. Decrease boredom on long trips. Keep special toys in the car for quiet play; talk to the child; point out objects and teach the child about them. Stop periodically. If the child wishes to sleep, make sure he stays in the restraint.

Children riding in car seats are generally much better behaved than children left unrestrained. This can be a major benefit to parents and should be stressed as an additional advantage of safety restraints.

Children over age 3 years are most often involved in pedestrian traffic accidents. Because of their gross motor skills of walking, running, and climbing and their fine motor skills of opening doors and fence gates, they are able to leave most restricted areas when unsupervised. Unaware of danger and unable to approximate the speed of a car, they are hit by moving vehicles (Fig. 10-10, *A*). Running after a ball, playing in a pile of leaves or snow, playing inside a cardboard box, riding a tricycle, and playing behind a parked car or near the curb are common activities that may result in a vehicular tragedy (Fig. 10-10, *B*).

Preventing vehicular accidents involves protecting and educating the child about the danger from moving or parked vehicles. Although preschool children are too young to be trusted to always obey, emphasis on looking

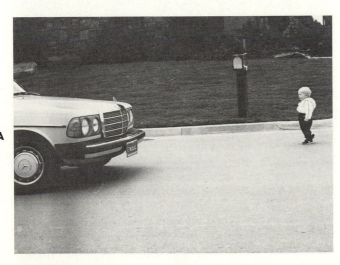

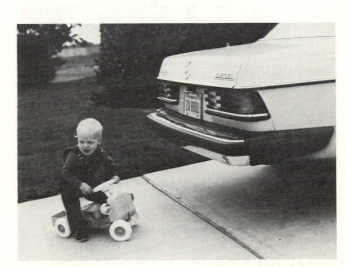

FIG. 10-10
*Young children are frequent victims of pedestrian vehicular accidents when they **A,** run in front of a moving car or **B,** play behind a parked car.*

for moving vehicles before crossing the street, recognizing the color of traffic lights for stop and go, and following traffic officers' signals is important. Most of all, practice what is preached. Children learn through imitation, and consistency reinforces learning.

Drowning. Drowning, not including drowning from water transportation, ranks second among preschool boys and third among preschool girls as a cause of accidental death. With well-developed skills of locomotion they are able to reach potentially dangerous areas, such as bathtubs, swimming pools, and lakes. Their intense drive for exploration and investigation, combined with an unawareness of the danger of water and helplessness in water, makes drowning always a threat. It is also one category of accidents that results in death within minutes, diminishing the chance for rescue and survival. Supervising children when near any source of water and teaching swimming and water safety help eliminate this potential fatality.

Burns. Burns rank second among preschool girls and third among preschool boys as cause of accidental death. A major contributing factor to the sex difference is that girls tend to play indoors and imitate sex-related functions, such as cooking at the stove. Their ability to climb, stretch, and reach objects above their head makes any hot surface a potential source of danger. Scalds from pulling pots on top of themselves are a major source of accidents. Pot handles should be turned toward the back of the stove. Ideally the knobs for controlling the range burners should be out of reach, not on the front panel where nimble fingers can turn them on and accidently touch the hot burner. Oven doors should be closed whenever the oven is turned on or when it is cooling. The outside of doors of some automatic self-cleaning ovens may become hot and, if touched, could cause a burn. Other sources of heat, such as radiators, fireplaces, accessible furnaces, kerosene heaters, or wood-burning stoves, should have guards placed in front of them. The tops of some of these heaters are designed to become hot enough to boil water to provide humidity. They are hazardous if touched or if the pan of water is spilled. Portable electric heaters must be placed in a high area, well out of reach of climbing young children.

Hot objects, such as candles, incense, cigarettes, pots of tea or coffee, or irons must be placed away from children. The flame of the candle and the smoke of a cigarette invite investigation from young children. Ashtrays with a center well should be used to prevent the cigarette from falling off the rim. Tablecloths should not be used; if they are used, the edges should be placed out of reach to prevent accidents from both burns and falling objects.

Electrical burns also represent an immediate danger to children. With preschoolers' ability to manipulate small, thin objects, they are able to insert hairpins or other conductive articles into electrical sockets. Young toddlers may explore outlets and wires by mouthing them. Since water is an excellent conductor, the chance for a severe circumoral electrical burn is great. Electrical outlets should have protective guards plugged into them when not in use or be made inaccessible by placing furniture in front of them when feasible (Fig. 10-11). Children should not be allowed to play with electrical cords or appliances, which should be kept out of reach as much as possible.

Scald burns are the most common type of thermal injury in children. Among toddlers and preschoolers a significant type of scalding burn is caused by high-temperature tap water, either as a result of turning on the hot-water faucet, falling into a bathtub of hot water, or deliberate abuse. Besides the obvious prevention of always supervising youngsters when they are near tap water and checking bathwater temperatures, a recommended passive prevention is to limit household water temperatures to less than 52° C (125° F). At this temperature it takes 2 minutes for exposure to the water to cause a full-thickness burn. Setting the temperature only 3° C lower raises the time necessary for a third-degree burn to 10 minutes. Conversely, water temperatures of 54° C (130° F), the usual setting of most water heaters, exposes household members to the risk of full-thickness burns within 30 seconds. Nurses can help prevent such burns by advising parents of this common household danger and recommending that they readjust the water heater to a safe temperature of 49° to 52° C (120° to 125° F). A meat or candy thermometer is a convenient way to measure water temperature. A special "Frog Prince" thermometer, which changes color to show water temperature, is also available at nominal cost.*

Poisoning. Ingestion of toxic agents is extremely common during early childhood. The highest incidence occurs in children in the 2-year-old age-group. Although in many instances poisoning does not result in mortality, it may cause significant morbidity, such as esophageal stricture from lye ingestion. Mouthing activity continues to be prevalent after 1 year of age and exploring objects by tasting them is part of children's curious investigation. Almost every nonfood substance is potentially harmful, including many house plants, and toddlers by 2 years of age are able to climb most heights, open most drawers or closets, and unscrew most lids. By trial and error younger children also manage to undo tops of bottles, plastic containers, aerosol cans, and jars. Legislature has mandated the use of child-guard tops on articles such as prescription drugs, but many young children have outwitted such "safe" caps. In addition, pharmacists often transfer drugs to regular containers for the elderly who may have difficulty with child-guard closures. Therefore, such drugs can be hazardous if accessible to young children.

The major cause of poisoning is improper storage (Fig. 10-12). The guidelines suggested in Chapter 8 apply

---

*Clinitemp, Inc., PO Box 40273, Indianapolis, IN 46240.

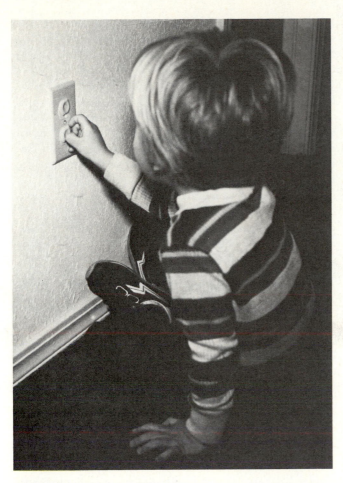

FIG. 10-11
Special plastic caps in electrical sockets prevent young fingers from exploring dangerous areas.

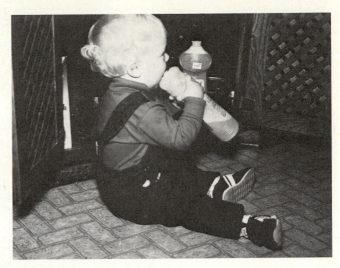

FIG. 10-12
No unlocked cabinet is safe for young children.

to children in this age-group as well. However, unlike the infant who was confined to certain heights and unable to unlatch inventive locks, preschoolers manage to find access to many high-level, tight-security places. Sometimes it is necessary to test a lock or high shelf by challenging the child to undo or reach it. Uncovering potential loopholes in one's security system now prevents tragedies later. Emergency measures for accidental poisoning are discussed in Chapter 12.

Falls. Falls are still a hazard to children in this age-group, although by the later part of early childhood, gross and fine motor skills are well developed, decreasing the incidence of falls down stairs, from chairs, or out of windows.

However, playground accidents become common. Children need to be taught safety at play areas, such as no horseplay on high slides or jungle gyms, *sitting* on swings, and staying away from moving swings. Passive prevention includes placement of grass, sand, or wood chips under play equipment. If loose organic material is used, it will require replacement as it pulverizes. Swing seats should be

made of plastic, canvas, or rubber rather than wood and have smooth or rounded edges. Slides should not exceed an incline of 30 degress, have evenly spaced rungs for climbing, and have protective "tunnels."

The climbing and running of the typical toddler are complicated by his total neglect for and lack of appreciation of danger. Gates must be placed at both ends of stairs. Accessible windows that are left open during warm weather must be screened or guarded with a rail. Falling from open windows is a major cause of accidental death in urban lower socioeconomic groups. Doors leading to stairwells or porches must be locked, since preschool children can easily open them. A convenient type of lock is a sliding bar or hook that can be attached to the door and frame at a level higher than the child can reach. One must be careful that inventive youngsters do not pull a chair over to unlatch the hook or bar.

Another source of falls is from cribs and vehicles. Besides crib rails being fully raised, the mattress is kept at the lowest position and toys or bumper pads that may be used as steps to climb out are removed. Ideally the floor should be carpeted. Once the child reaches a height of 89 cm (35 inches) he should sleep in a bed rather than a crib. To prevent falls from vehicles, children should always be properly restrained. They should never ride in the open back of a truck; the danger of falls can be compounded by another vehicle striking the child. An unrecognized hazard is grocery shopping carts. Children left unattended can easily fall out.

Clothing can also increase the chance of falling. Slippery shoes or socks, rubber-soled shoes that "catch" on the floor and rug, and loose or cuffed pants can easily make a child fall. Simple safety measures, such as checking clothing and shoes and keeping shoelaces tied with double knots, can prevent such needless accidents.

Aspiration and asphyxiation. Usually by 1 year of age children chew well, but they may have difficulty with large pieces of food, such as meat and whole hot dogs, and with hard foods, such as nuts or dried beans. Young children cannot discard pits from fruit or bones from fish as older children can. It takes practice to learn how to chew gum without swallowing it. Play objects for toddlers must still be chosen with an awareness of danger from small parts. Large, sturdy toys without sharp edges or removable parts are safest. Coins, paper clips, pull-tabs on cans, thumbtacks, nails, screws, jewelry, and all type of pins are household objects that can cause significant harm if swallowed. Because of the danger of aspiration, parents should be taught emergency procedures for choking (p. 631).

Another cause of death by traumatic asphyxiation is from electrically operated garage doors. Young children playing in the garage may become trapped under the door. Although the automatic doors should reverse when striking an object, they may not do so when hitting a flexible object or one that is very close to the ground. Precautions to lessen the chances of this accident occurring include placing controls where they are inaccessible to children, such as high on a wall and in a locked car, and instructing children that the transmitter is not a toy.

Suffocation is less frequent from causes seen during infancy but is an ever-present threat from old refrigerators, ovens, and other large appliances. Toddlers can climb inside these appliances and if they close the door behind them can be trapped inside. Discarding old appliances and removing all doors during storage prevent such tragic accidents. Toddlers may also suffocate when unsafe toy box lids accidently close on their head or neck. Parents should be advised of this danger and encouraged to buy storage chests with lightweight, removable covers.

Bodily damage. Toddlers are still clumsy in many of their skills and can seriously harm themselves when walking while holding a sharp or pointed object or having food or objects, such as spoons, in their mouth. Foreseeing such potential accidents is the best approach. For the older child, teaching safety is most important. The child should be taught that when walking with a pointed object, such as a knife or scissors, the pointed end is held away from the face. Dangerous garden or workshop equipment and all firearms should be stored in a locked cabinet. Safety education should include respect for firearms and their proper appropriate use. In addition, the child should be warned of and protected against potential danger from animals, including household pets, such as dogs and cats.

Dental care

The importance of oral hygiene in preserving the teeth and maintaining healthy gums cannot be overemphasized or begun too early. Dental care begins as soon as the first tooth erupts by wiping its surfaces with a cloth. Regular brushing, flossing, and dental examinations should begin by the time the primary dentition is completed, usually by 2½ years of age. Use of fluoride should begin shortly after birth.

The objective of oral hygiene is removal of *plaque,* soft bacterial deposits that adhere to the teeth and cause dental caries (cavities) and periodontal (gum) disease. The most effective methods for plaque removal are brushing and flossing. Several brushing techniques exist. One that is suitable for cleaning the primary teeth is the *scrub* method. The tips of the bristles are placed firmly at a 45-degree angle against the teeth and gums and moved back and forth in a vibratory motion. The ends of the bristles should be wiggling but not moving forcefully back and forth, which can damage the gums and enamel. All the surfaces of the teeth are cleaned in this manner except the lingual (inner) surfaces of the anterior teeth. To clean these surfaces, the toothbrush is placed vertical to the teeth and moved up and down. Only a few teeth are brushed at one time, using six to eight strokes for each section. A systematic approach is used so that all surfaces are thoroughly cleaned.

For young children the most effective cleaning is done by parents. Several positions can be used that facilitate access to the mouth and help stabilize the head for comfort, such as sitting on a couch or bed with the child's head in the parent's lap or sitting on a floor or stool with the child's head straddled between the parent's thighs (Fig. 10-13). The latter position is advantageous because the child can be kept amused watching television during the brushing.

For effective cleaning, a small toothbrush with soft, rounded, multitufted nylon bristles that are short and uniform in length is recommended. Nylon bristles dry more rapidly after use and retain their shape better than natural bristles. Children should have at least two toothbrushes, which are used alternately to allow them to dry thoroughly. Wet bristles are less resilient and consequently less effective in removing plaque. Toothbrushes are replaced as soon as the bristles are frayed or bent.

After the teeth have been cleaned, flossing with unwaxed dental floss is done to remove plaque and debris from between the teeth and below the gum margin where brushing is ineffective. Since young children do not have the dexterity to manipulate the floss, parents are taught the procedure. A disclosing agent is helpful to identify areas where plaque remains. It also helps motivate children to clean their teeth because plaque is difficult to see.

Ideally, the teeth should be cleaned after each meal and especially before bedtime and the child given nothing to eat or drink after the night brushing except water. At those times when brushing is impractical, the ''swish and

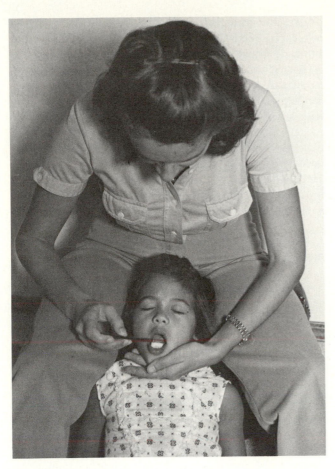

FIG. 10-13
Position that facilitates parent's brushing of child's teeth.

TABLE 10-5. SUPPLEMENTAL FLUORIDE DOSAGE SCHEDULE (mg/day*)		
	CONCENTRATION OF FLUORIDE IN DRINKING WATER (ppm)		
AGE	**<0.3**	**0.3-0.7**	**0.7**
2 weeks-2 years	0.25	0	0
2-3 years	0.50	0.25	0
3-16 years	1.00	0.50	0

From Committee on Nutrition American Academy of Pediatrics; Fluoride supplementation: Revised dosage schedule, Pediatrics **63**:150, 1979.
*2.2 mg sodium fluoride contains 1 mg fluoride

swallow'' method of cleaning the mouth is taught; the child rinses his mouth with water and swallows, repeating the procedure three to four times.

The kind of toothpaste is important mainly in terms of fluoride. A fluoride dentifrice reduces caries even if the water supply is fluoridated. However, a concern with fluoride toothpaste is ingestion by the young child and the possibility of fluorosis or mottled enamel. As a safeguard the child's use of toothpaste should be supervised to prevent swallowing of excessive amounts. Fluoride rinses are not recommended for toddlers and preschoolers because they are unable to safely rinse the mouth with the liquid.

In communities where the water supply is not fluoridated, oral fluoride supplements are recommended (Table 10-5). Because fluoride has both topical and systemic beneficial effects, the supplement should remain in contact with the teeth for a short time before it is swallowed. For young children the tablets are chewable, and they are instructed to chew them and then forcefully swish the solution around the teeth. A helpful suggestion is to persuade the child to ''color'' the teeth by moving the tongue to deposit the solution on all tooth surfaces.

Nurses have a responsibility to ensure that fluoride is a regular part of the oral health program. This necessitates a knowledge of the fluoride content of the community water supply, especially in rural areas, and appropriate supplementation as needed.

One advantage of supplements is that the child receives a known quantity of fluoride daily. This is in contrast to fluoridated water, where the supply depends on the amount of water consumed. Consequently parents need to be encouraged to use water to prepare drinks and foods such as soup. For example, instead of using prepared orange juice, it is better to purchase the concentrate and dilute it with tap water. Such measures ensure that the child is receiving sufficient fluoride.

Diet is critical to good teeth. Foods rich in sugar promote caries and ideally should be eliminated. This includes natural foods, such as honey, molasses, and corn syrup, and dried fruits such as raisins, which are highly cariogenic. Since this is often impractical, some suggestions can be helpful. Parents should be advised that *the frequency with which sugar is consumed is more important than the total amount eaten.* For example, the more cariogenic foods are sticky or hard candies, which remain in the mouth longer periods of time. If sweets are eaten, they are less damaging when consumed immediately after a meal, rather than as a snack between meals. When sweets are served as the dessert, the teeth can be cleaned afterward, decreasing the amount of time the sugar is in the mouth.

Another cause of dental caries that is less common but rarely considered is the cariogenicity of several liquid medications, such as Lanoxin, Dilantin, Actifed, Pen-Vee-K, and several vitamin preparations. Obviously children taking these medications for prolonged periods are most at risk. However, educating parents regarding the need to clean the teeth after each dose could decrease the caries potential. A minimal step is rinsing the mouth with water after giving the drug. Ideally the teeth should be brushed

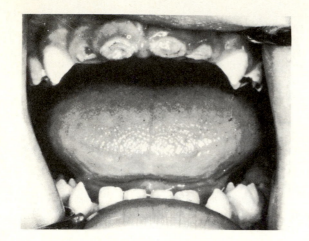

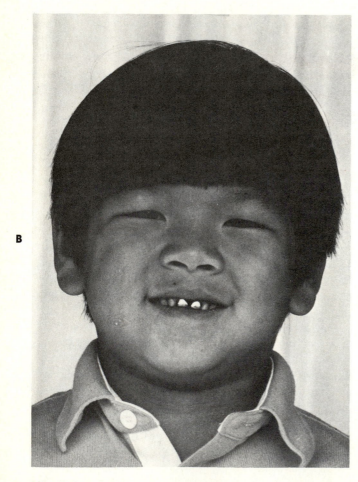

FIG. 10-14

A, *Nursing bottle caries. Note the extensive carious involvement of maxillary primary incisors.* **B,** *Stainless steel bands may be used to restore teeth affected by nursing bottle caries.* (**A** *from McDonald, R., and Avery D.: Dentistry for the child and adolescent, ed. 4, St. Louis, 1983, The C.V. Mosby Co.).*

as well. Administering medication with meals, if this is not contraindicated, also lessens the number of times the teeth are exposed to the sugar.

A special form of tooth decay in children between 18 months and 3 years is "nursing bottle caries" (also called "bottle-mouth caries"). It occurs when the child is routinely given a bottle of milk or juice at nap or bedtime. Frequent nocturnal breast-feeding for prolonged periods also leads to extensive destruction of the teeth. The liquid pools in the mouth, bathing the teeth for several hours. The maxillary (upper) incisors and molars are affected most, since the mandibular (lower) incisors are protected by saliva, which dilutes the sugar-containing beverage (Fig. 10-14, *A*). Severely damaged teeth may require stainless steel bands until the permanent teeth erupt (Fig. 10-14, *B*).

Prevention of nursing bottle caries involves eliminating the bedtime bottle completely, feeding the last bottle before bedtime, substituting a bottle of water for milk or juice, or limiting the frequency and duration of nocturnal breast-feeding. Juice in bottles, especially commercially available ready-to-use bottles, should be discouraged. Juice should always be offered in a cup in order to avoid prolonging the bottle-feeding habit.

Another aspect of oral hygiene is regular dental examinations. Ideally the child should see a dentist (or pedodontist) soon after the first teeth erupt and no later than by 2½ years when primary dentition is completed. Initial visits to the dentist (or pedodontist) should be nontraumatizing. Since toddlers react negatively to new and potentially frightening experiences, the initial visit can center around meeting the dentist, seeing the equipment, and sitting in the chair. If the child is cooperative, the dentist may just look at the teeth but reserve a more thorough examination for another visit. This type of conditioning is very important in preparing the child for future experiences.

ANTICIPATORY GUIDANCE—CARE OF PARENTS

Understanding toddlers is fundamental to successful child-rearing, regardless of the approach used. Nurses, particularly those in ambulatory or child health centers, are in a most favorable position to assist parents in meeting the tasks and needs of children in this age-group. It seems to be an almost universal phenomenon that prevention yields better results than treatment. Anticipatory guidance in each of the areas presented in the box on the facing page is paramount if one wishes to prevent future problems.

Advice is sometimes not the only answer. Actual assistance, such as being available for home visiting or telephone consulting, should be part of nurses' flexible reper-

PARENTAL GUIDANCE DURING TODDLER YEARS

Age (months)	Guidance
12-18	Prepare parents for expected behavioral changes of toddler, especially negativism and ritualism
	Assess present feeding habits and encourage gradual weaning from bottle and increased intake of solid foods
	Stress expected feeding changes of physiologic anorexia, presence of food fads and strong taste preferences, need for scheduled routine at mealtimes, inability to sit through an entire meal, and lack of table manners
	Assess sleep patterns at night, particularly habit of a bedtime bottle, which is a major cause of dental caries, and procrastination behaviors that delay hour of sleep
	Prepare parents for potential dangers of the home, particularly motor vehicular, poisoning, and falling accidents; give appropriate suggestions for safeproofing the home (Table 10-4)
	Discuss need for firm but gentle discipline and ways in which to deal with negativism and temper tantrums; stress positive benefits of appropriate discipline
	Emphasize importance for both child and parents of brief, periodic separations
	Discuss new toys that use developing gross and fine motor, language, cognitive, and social skills
18-24	Stress importance of peer companionship in play
	Explore need for preparation for additional sibling; stress importance of preparing child for new, and potentially frightening, experiences
	Emphasize need for dental supervision, types of basic dental hygiene at home, and food habits that predispose to caries; stress importance of supplemental fluoride
	Discuss present discipline methods, their effectiveness, and parents' feelings about child's negativism; stress that negativism is important aspect of developing self-assertion and independence and is not a sign of spoiling

Age (months)	Guidance
18-24—cont'd	Discuss signs of readiness for toilet training; emphasize importance of waiting for physical and psychologic readiness
	Discuss development of fears, such as darkness or loud noises, and of habits, such as security blanket or thumb-sucking; stress normalcy of these transient behaviors
	Prepare parents for signs of regression in times of stress
	Assess child's ability to separate easily from parents for brief periods of separation under familiar circumstances
	Allow parents opportunity to express their feelings of weariness, frustration, and exasperation; be aware that it is often difficult to love toddlers at times when they are not asleep!
	Point out some of the expected changes of the next year, such as longer attention span, somewhat less negativism, and increased concern for pleasing others
24-36	Discuss importance of imitation and domestic mimicry and need to include child in activities
	Discuss approaches toward toilet training, particularly realistic expectations and attitude toward accidents
	Stress uniqueness of toddlers' thought processes, especially through their use of language, poor understanding of time, casual relationships in terms of proximity of events, and inability to see events from another's perspective
	Stress that discipline still must be quite structured and concrete and that relying solely on verbal reasoning and explanation leads to accidents, confusion, and misunderstanding
	Discuss investigation of nursery school or day-care center toward completion of second year

toire of interventions. Whether parents are experiencing the rearing dilemmas of a first or subsequent child, they benefit from sharing their feelings, frustrations, and satisfactions. They need adult companionship, freedom from childrearing responsibilities, and periodic separations from their children. Sometimes they lose perspective of the needs of each other in the marital relationship and fail to communicate effectively. Part of nurses' responsibility is to provide opportunities for ventilation of parents' feelings and guidance in personal areas such as marital needs, career fulfillment, and peer companionship.

BIBLIOGRAPHY
Growth and development

Ames, L.B., and Ilg, F.L.: Your two-year-old: terrible or tender, New York, 1979, Delacorte Press.

Brown, M., and Murphy, A.: A child grows. Part II. How the child grows and develops psychologically, socially and culturally, Pediatr. Nurs. 1(2):22-30, 1975.

Brown, M., and Murphy, A.: A child grows. Part III. The child's cognitive development, Pediatr. Nurs. 1(3):7-12, 1975.

Brown, M., and Murphy, A.: A child grows. Part IV. The child's perceptual and linguistic development, Pediatr. Nurs. 1(4):9-15, 1975.

Illingworth, R.S.: Development of the infant and young child, ed. 7, New York, 1980, Churchill Livingstone, Inc.

Knoblich, H., and Pasamanick, B.: Gesell and Amatruda's developmental diagnosis, New York, 1974, Harper & Row, Publishers, Inc.

Maier, H.: Three theories of child development, ed. 3, New York, 1978, Harper & Row, Publishers, Inc.

Selekman, J.: The development of body image in the child: a learned response, Topic Clin. Nurs. 5(1):12-21, l983.

Toilet training

Euler, M.M., and McClellan, M.A.: Toilet training: ready or not? Pediatr. Nurs. 7(1):15-20, 1981.

Euler-Horner, M.M.: The challenge of toilet training — bowel management for the child with psychogenic encopresis or neurogenic deficit, Pediatr. Basics 32:4-10, 1982.

Sibling rivalry

Bahr, J.E.: Canine and feline rivalry: another form of sibling rivalry, Pediatr. Nurs. 7(4):14-15, 1981.

Gates, S.: Children's literature: it can help children cope with sibling rivalry, Am. J. Maternal Child Nurs. 5:351-352, Sept./Oct. 1979

Malinowski, J.S.: Answering a child's questions about sex and a new baby, Am. J. Nurs. 79:1965-1968, Nov. 1979.

Sweet, P.T.: Helping children to accept and welcome a new baby, Am. J. Maternal Child Nurs. 4(2):82-83, 1979.

Vestal, K.W.: Siblings: adapting to accommodate the neonate, Issues Health Care Women 1:13-25, 1979.

Limit setting and discipline

American Academy of Pediatrics, Committee on Psychosocial Aspects of Child and Family Health: The pediatrician's role in discipline, Pediatrics 72(3):373-374, 1983.

Hammer, D., and Drabman, R.S.: Child discipline: what we know and what we can recommend, Pediatr. Nurs. 7(3):31-35, 1981.

Melichar, M.M.: Using crisis theory to help parents cope with a child's temper tantrums, Am. J. Maternal Child Nurs. 5(3):181-185, 1980.

Murphy, M.: When parents ask about discipline, Pediatr. Nurs. 2(6):28-32, 1976.

Nutritional requirements/nutritional counseling

Dwyer, J.: Diets for children and adolescents that meet the dietary goals, Am. J. Dis. Child. **134:**1073-1080, Nov. 1980.

Henneman, A., and Koziol, J.: Preschool feeding problems: it's not nutritious unless they eat it, Issues Compr. Pediatr. Nurs. **4:**7-12, Dec. 1980.

Pipes, P.: Nutrition in infancy and childhood, ed. 2, St. Louis, 1981, The C.V. Mosby Co.

Williams, S.R.: Nutrition and diet therapy, ed. 4, St. Louis, 1981, The C.V. Mosby Co.

Wurtman, J.J.: What do children eat? Eating styles of the preschool, elementary school, and adolescent child. In Suskind, R.M., editor: Textbook of pediatric nutrition, New York, 1981, Raven Press.

Accident prevention

Elfert, H.: Helping preschool children learn to be safe, Can. Nurse **75:**26-29, Dec. 1979.

Hot water frogs, Am. J. Maternal Child Nurs. **6:**213, May/June 1981.

Macknin, M.L.: Dog and cat bites, Pediatr. Basics **35:**7-11, l983.

Maddocks, G.: Accidents in childhood, Nurs. Mirror **152**(21):2-15, 1980.

Marcus, D.F.: Child car seats: a must for safety, Pediatr. Nurs. **7**(3):13-17, 1981.

McAtee, J.M.: How to help your kids play it safe, Family Safety **41**(2):12-13, 1982.

Meyer, R.J.: Save that child: children and automobile restraints, Public Health **71**(2):122-123, 1981.

Righi, F.C., and Krozy, R.E.: The child in the car: what every nurse should know about safety, Am. J. Nurs. **83**(10):1421-1424, 1983.

Surveyer, J.A., and Halpern, J.: Age-related burn injuries and their prevention, Pediatr. Nurs. **7**(5):29-34, 1981.

Dental care

Coutts, L.: Dental health education for mothers of pre-school children, Midwife Health Visit Commun. Nurse **16**(8):328-331, 1980.

Hennon, D.K.: Nutrition and dental health. In McDonald, R.E., and Avery, D.R., editors: Dentistry for the child and adolescent, ed. 4, St. Louis, 1983, The C.V. Mosby Co.

Horowitz, A.M.: Oral health education for pediatric patients. In Forrester, D.J., Wagner, M.L., and Fleming, J., editors: Pediatric dental medicine, Philadelphia, 1981, Lea & Febiger.

Kilmon, C., and Helpin, M.L.: Update on dentistry for children, Pediatr. Nurs. **7**(5):41-44, 1981.

Kilmon, C., and Helpin, M.L.: Recognizing dental malocclusion in children, Pediatr. Nurs. **9**(3):204-208, 1983.

Starkey, P.E.: Toothbrushing, flossing, and oral hygiene instruction. In McDonald, R.E., and Avery, D.R., editors: Dentistry for the child and adolescent, ed. 4, St. Louis, 1983, The C.V. Mosby Co.

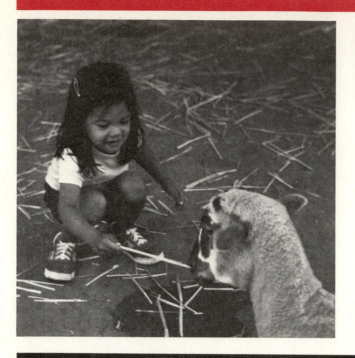

THE PRESCHOOL YEARS

OBJECTIVES

On completion of this chapter the reader will be able to:

- Identify the major biologic, psychosocial, cognitive, spiritual, and adaptive developments during the preschool years
- List the benefits of imaginary playmates
- Prepare preschoolers for nursery or daycare experience
- Provide parents with guidelines for sex education
- Provide parents with guidelines for dealing with fears and sleep problems
- Recognize cause of stuttering during the preschool years
- Offer parents suggestions for preventing speech problems
- Recognize feeding patterns of preschoolers
- Provide anticipatory guidance to parents regarding accident prevention based on the preschooler's developmental achievements

NURSING DIAGNOSES

Nursing diagnoses identified for the preschooler include, but are not restricted to, the following:

Health perception–health management pattern

- Infection, potential for, related to increased exposure outside the home
- Injury, potential for (poisoning, suffocation, trauma), related to environmental hazards

Nutritional-metabolic pattern

- Nutrition, alterations in: potential for more or less than body requirements, related to (1) knowledge deficit; (2) food habits

Activity-exercise pattern

- Self-care deficit, related to developmental level

The preschool years, a period from 3 years of age to the completion of 5 years of age, comprise the end of early childhood. It is an age of discovery, inventiveness, curiosity, and developing sociocultural patterns of behavior. In some ways it is a period of ease and comfort for parents, particularly when many of the child-rearing tasks, such as toileting, independence, and self-caring abilities, have been mastered. Preschoolers usually have less difficulty in tolerating separation, adjusting to change, behaving appropriately, and accepting compromise than toddlers. Their world is no longer confined to the home environment and the immediate family. They need and enjoy the companionship of other children.

Many authorities believe that the most critical period of emotional and psychologic development extends from birth to before entering school. Successful mastery of trust, autonomy, and initiative are foundational for further personality maturation, and failure to complete these stages may result in deep-seated, long-range problems in later life. During this period parental influence on the formation of the child is greatest. Helping parents realize and understand the pliability and malleability of young children as early as possible is one method of preventing problems in subsequent years.

GROWTH AND DEVELOPMENT

The combined biologic, psychosocial, cognitive, spiritual and adaptive achievements of children in this age-group prepare preschoolers for their most significant change in life-style—entrance into school. Their control of bodily systems, experience of brief and prolonged periods of separation, ability to interact cooperatively with other children and adults, use of language for mental symbolization, and increased attention span and memory ready them for the next major period—the school years. Successful mastery of previous levels of growth and development is essential for preschoolers to refine many of the tasks that were begun during the toddler years.

Physical development

Physical growth continues to slow and stabilize during the preschool years. Average weight gain remains about 2.3 kg (5 pounds) per year. The average weight at 3 years is 14.5 kg (32 pounds), at 4 years 16.4 kg (36 pounds), and at 5 years 18.6 kg (41 pounds).

Height also remains steady at a yearly increase of 6.75 to 7.5 cm (2.5 to 3 inches) and generally occurs in elongation of the legs rather than of the trunk. The average height at 3 years is 95.7 cm (37.7 inches), at 4 years 103 cm (40.5 inches), and at 5 years 109 cm (43 inches).

Bodily proportions no longer resemble those of the

Sleep-rest pattern

■ Sleep-pattern disturbance related to (1) fears; (2) high activity level

Self-perception—self-concept pattern

■ Anxiety related to (1) fears; (2) separation, especially preschool experience; (3) sexual curiosity

Role-relationship pattern

■ Communication, impaired verbal, potential, related to parental anxiety with speech hesitancy

■ Parenting, alteration in: potential, related to knowledge deficit

Coping-stress tolerance pattern

■ Coping, family: potential for growth, related to successful parenting

squat, potbellied toddler. The preschooler is slender but sturdy, graceful and agile, with erect posture. There is little difference in physical characteristics according to sex, except as dictated by dress, hair style, and so on.

Most bodily systems are mature and stable and can adjust to moderate stress and change. Motor development consists mostly of increases in strength and refinement of previously learned skills, such as walking, running, and jumping. However, muscle development and bone growth are still far from mature. Excessive activity and overexertion can injure delicate tissues. Properly fitting shoes, good posture, appropriate exercise, and adequate rest are essential for optimal development of the musculoskeletal system.

Psychosocial development

By the time children reach 3 years of age their gross and fine motor abilities are sufficiently developed to enable them to pursue almost limitless activities. If they have been allowed to express their independence and negativism constructively, they are ready to direct their energy toward new learning. They learn how to interact and relate to other children and adults; they learn appropriate sex role functions and socially acceptable behavior; they learn right and wrong and the types of rewards or punishment associated with each. However, learning does not necessarily imply success. Without appropriate guidance and reinforcement, children can learn unacceptable behavior and, instead of feeling accomplishment, feel inadequacy, guilt, and inferiority.

Developing a sense of initiative. If preschoolers have mastered the tasks of the toddler period, they are ready to face the developmental endeavors of this stage. Erikson maintains that the chief psychosocial task of the preschool period is acquiring a sense of *initiative*. The child is in a stage of energetic learning. He plays, works, and lives to the fullest and feels a real sense of accomplishment and satisfaction in his activities. Conflict arises when the child oversteps the limits of his ability and inquiry and experiences a sense of *guilt* for not having behaved or acted appropriately. Feelings of guilt, anxiety, and fear may also result from thoughts that differ from expected behavior.

A particularly stressful thought is wishing one's parent dead (a phenomenon sometimes referred to as the Oedipus complex). As a sense of rivalry or competition develops between the child and same sex parent, the child may think of ways to rid himself of the interfering parent. In most situations this is resolved by strongly identifying with the same sex parent and peers during the school years. However, if that parent dies before the identification process is completed, the preschooler can be overwhelmed with feelings of guilt for having wished and, therefore, caused the death. Clarifying for children that wishes cannot and do not make events occur is essential in helping them overcome their guilt and anxiety.

Developing a conscience. Development of the *superego,* or *conscience,* has its beginnings toward the end of the toddler years and is a major task for preschoolers. Learning right from wrong and good from bad is the beginning of morality. Children in this age-group are generally unable to understand the reasons for why something is acceptable or nonacceptable. They are aware of appropriate behavior mainly through punishment or reward and rely almost religiously on parental principles for developing their own moral judgment. However, verbal enforcement of limits is much more effective. For example, the toddler needed to be supervised, fenced in, and told not to run into the street to prevent accidents. The preschooler is much more aware of danger and can be relied on to listen and obey in most instances. If allowed to disagree and question, he will develop socially acceptable behavior as well as independence in thought and action.

Developing a conscience implies *learning the sociocultural mores* of the family's heritage. Depending on the type of attitudes conveyed, the child will learn not only appropriate behaviors but also tolerant, biased, or prejudiced values concerning his ethnic, religious, and social background and that of other groups. Much of this influence may remain dormant until he associates with children or adults of a different heritage. Then, depending on the particular group, he may be accepted or isolated for his attitudes.

Cognitive development

One of the tasks related to the preschool period is *readiness for school and scholastic learning*. Many of the thought processes of this period are crucial for achieving such readiness. Piaget's cognitive theory actually does not include a period specifically of 3 to 5 years. The *preoperational* phase comprises the age span from 2 to 7 years and is divided into two stages, the *preconceptual* phase, ages 2 to 4 years, and the phase of *intuitive thought,* ages 4 to 7 years. One of the main transitions during each of these two phases is the shift from totally egocentric thought to social awareness and regard for others.

Piaget's concept of *conservation,* or the idea that a mass can be changed in size, shape, volume, or length without losing or adding to the original mass, is not understood by prelogical children. Rather, they judge what they see by the immediate perceptual clues given them. For example, if two lines of equal length are presented in such a way that one appears longer than the other, the child will state that one line is longer, even if he measures both lines with a ruler or yardstick and finds that each has the same length.

Understanding this prelogical thinking in young children helps other persons, such as nurses, interact with them in the most efficacious manner. One example of how manipulating matter according to the child's understanding can facilitate performing an activity concerns administration of drugs. If the child is to receive 5 ml of liquid medication, it is advisable to give it in a small medicine cup, rather than a large cup, since the child will imagine that the large vessel contains more liquid. Since he is unable to perceive the two dimensions of height and width simultaneously, the child will choose one dimension and measure the amount according to that standard. If the child refuses the medicine in the small cup, he may accept it once it is poured into a large cup because the liquid will appear less in a tall, wide container.

There are many everyday examples of how the young child's inability to conserve matter influences his behavior. Probably one of the most common situations involves eating and the amount of food placed on a dish. If the same amount of food is placed on a small and a large plate, the child may state that the large plate contains more food and may feel overwhelmed by the apparently large quantity. Parents are usually "taught" this by their children and "learn" ways to use this thinking. Meat that is cut thin and flat appears to be more in quantity than the same amount of meat that is cut thick, and the child will generally consume more of the thicker portion. The opposite also has its advantages. Giving a child a large, flat cookie will please and satisfy him more than giving him a small, thick one.

Language continues to develop during the preschool period. Speech remains primarily a vehicle of egocentric communication. The child assumes that everyone thinks as he does and that a brief explanation of his thinking makes his entire thought understood by others. Because of this self-referenced, egocentric verbal communication, it is frequently necessary to explore and understand the young child's thinking through other nonverbal approaches. For children in this age-group, the most enlightening and effective method is play.

Preschoolers increasingly use language without comprehending the meaning of words, particularly concepts of right or left, time, and causality. The child may use the concepts correctly but only in the circumstances he has learned them. For example, he may know how to put on his shoes by remembering that the buckle is always on the outside of the foot. However, if different shoes have no buckles, he cannot reason which shoe fits which foot. In other words he does not understand the concept of right and left.

Preschoolers believe in the power of words and accept their meaning literally. A significant example of this type of thinking is calling the child "bad" because he did something wrong. In his mind, telling him that he is bad means that he is bad. For this reason it is better to relate such words to the act, by saying, for example, "That was a bad thing to do."

Superficially, *causality* resembles logical thought. The child explains a concept as he heard it described by others, but his understanding is limited. An example is the concept of time. Since *time* is still incompletely understood, the child interprets it according to his own frame of reference, such as "A long time means until Christmas." Consequently, time is best explained in relationship to an event, such as "Your mother will visit you after you finish your lunch." Avoiding terms such as yesterday, tomorrow, next week, Tuesday, and so on to express when an event is expected to occur and associating time with usual expected daily occurrences help children learn about temporal relationships, while increasing their trust in others' predictions.

The preschooler's thinking is often described as *magical*. Because of his egocentrism and his transductive reasoning (association of one event with a simultaneous event), the child believes that his thoughts are all-powerful. A classic example is the development of fears during this period (see p. 322). Because the child need not base his thinking on logical facts, any explanation that he contrives to explain an event is acceptable to him. If two events occur at the same time, his thoughts are even more strengthened. For example, if he has an injury that necessitates emergency medical attention, he may assume that the treatment is punishment for wrongdoing rather than a necessary intervention.

Body image. The preschool years play a significant role in the development of body image. With increasing comprehension of language preschoolers recognize that individuals have more or less desirable appearances. They recognize differences in skin color and racial identity and are vulnerable to learning prejudices and biases. They are aware of the meaning of words, such as "pretty" or "ugly," and reflect the opinion of others regarding their appearance. For example, by 5 years of age children compare their size to their peers and can become conscious of being large or short, especially if others refer to them as "so big or so little for your age."

Despite the advances in body image development, preschoolers have poorly defined body boundaries and little knowledge of their internal anatomy. Intrusive experiences are frightening, especially those that disrupt the integrity of the skin, such as injections and surgery. There is a fear that if the skin is "broken" all their blood and "insides" can leak out. Therefore, bandages are critical to "keeping everything from coming out."

Sexual identity is developing beyond gender recognition and modesty may become a concern, as well as fears of mutilation. There is sex role imitation, and "dressing up" like mommy or daddy are important activities. Attitudes and responses of others to the child's role-playing can condition him to views of himself or others. For example, comments such as ''boys shouldn't play with dolls'' can influence his self-concept of masculinity. Perhaps this is a time when children begin forming ideal images of how they would want to look as adults.

Spiritual development

Children's knowledge of faith and religion are learned from significant others in their environment, usually from the religious practices of the parents. However, the young child's understanding of spirituality is influenced by his cognitive level. Preschoolers have a concrete conception of a God with physical characteristics who is often like an imaginary friend. They understand simple Bible stories and memorize short prayers but their understanding of the meaning of these rituals is limited. They benefit from concrete representations of religious practices, such as picture Bible books and small statues, such as the Nativity scene.

Development of the conscience is strongly linked to spiritual development. At this age children are learning right from wrong and behave correctly to avoid punishment. Wrongdoing provokes feelings of guilt, and preschoolers often misinterpret illness as a punishment for real or imagined misdeeds. It is important that God be viewed as bestowing unconditional love, rather than as a judge of good or bad behavior. Praying to God and observing religious traditions, such as prayers before meals or bedtime, can help a child through stressful periods, such as hospitalization.

Adaptive development

By 3 years of age the child has made tremendous strides from the dependency of infancy and the negativism of toddlerhood. The preschooler has excellent gross and fine motor control. Few physical barriers are obstacles. He is a very social and domesticated being. He cares for himself almost completely and enjoys doing simple household chores. He deliberately attempts to please others and is aware of manners and social amenities. Language use is a

TABLE 11-1. THE MAJOR DEVELOPMENTAL ACHIEVEMENTS OF CHILDREN 3, 4, AND 5 YEARS OF AGE

AGE (years)	PHYSICAL	GROSS MOTOR	FINE MOTOR	SENSORY	LANGUAGE
3	Heart rate approximately 105 beats/minute Respiratory rate approximately 24 breaths/minute Blood pressure: systolic 96 mg Hg; diastolic 58 mm Hg Usual weight gain of 1.8 to 2.7 kg (4 to 6 pounds) Usual gain in height of 5 to 6.25 cm (2 to 2.5 inches) May have achieved nighttime control of bowel and bladder	Rides tricycle Jumps off bottom step Stands on one foot for a few seconds Goes up stairs using alternate feet, may still come down using both feet on the step Broad jumps May try to dance, but balance may not be adequate	Builds tower of nine to ten cubes Builds bridge with three cubes Adeptly places small pellets in narrow-necked bottle In drawing, copies a circle, imitates a cross, names what he has drawn, cannot draw stick man but may make circle with facial features	Able to copy geometric figures Can place geometric forms into respective opening if form board is reversed Reading readiness may be present	Has vocabulary of about 900 words Uses primarily ''telegraphic'' speech Uses complete sentences of three to four words Talks incessantly regardless of whether anyone is paying attention Repeats sentence of six syllables Constantly asks questions

vehicle of communication, learning, and self-expression. The vocabulary is relatively extensive, almost completely intelligible, and fairly grammatically correct. The major developmental achievements for 3-, 4-, and 5-year-old children are summarized in Table 11-1.

Gross and fine motor behavior. Walking, running, climbing, and jumping are well established by age 36 months. Refinement in eye-hand and muscle coordination is evident in several areas. At age 3 years the preschooler rides a tricycle, walks on tiptoe, balances on one foot for a few seconds, and broad jumps. By 4 years of age he skips and hops proficiently on one foot and catches a ball reliably. By age 5 years he skips on alternate feet, jumps rope, and begins to skate.

Fine motor development is evident in the child's increasingly skillful manipulation, such as in drawing and dressing. These skills provide readiness for learning and independence for entry to school.

Language behavior. Language during the preschool years is quite sophisticated and complex. It also becomes a major mode of communication and social interaction. Vocabulary increases dramatically, from 900 words at age 3 years to over 2100 words at the end of 5 years of age. Sentence structure, grammatical usage, and intelligibility also advance to a nearly adult level.

Between 3 and 4 years of age children form sentences of about three to four words and include only the most essential words to convey a meaning. Such speech is often termed ''telegraphic'' for its brevity in length. Three-year-old children ask many questions and use plurals, correct pronouns, and the past tense of verbs. They name familiar objects, such as animals, parts of the body, and relatives or friends. They can give and follow simple commands. They talk incessantly, regardless of whether anyone is listening or answering them. They enjoy musical or talking toys or dolls and imitate new words proficiently.

From 4 to 5 years of age preschoolers use longer sentences of four to five words and more words than are used to convey a message, such as prepositions, adjectives, and a variety of verbs. They follow simple directional commands, such as ''Put the ball on the chair,'' and can carry out three requests at a time. They answer questions, such

SOCIALIZATION	COGNITION	FAMILY RELATIONSHIPS
Dresses self almost completely if helped with back buttons and told which shoe is right or left	Is in preconceptual phase	Attempts to please parents and conform to their expectations
Buttons and unbuttons accessible buttons	Is egocentric in thought and behavior	Is less jealous of younger sibling; may be opportune time for birth of additional sibling
Pulls on shoes	Has beginning understanding of time; uses many time-oriented expressions, talks about past and future as much as about present, pretends to tell time	Is aware of family relationships and sex role functions
Has increased attention span		
Feeds self completely		Boys tend to identify more with father or other male figure
Pours from a bottle or pitcher	Has improved concept of space as demonstrated in understanding of prepositions and ability to follow directional command	Has increased ability to separate easily and comfortably from parents for short periods
Can prepare simple meals, such as cold cereal and milk		
Can help to set table, dry dishes without breaking any	Has beginning ability to view concepts from another perspective	
Likes to ''help'' entertain by passing around food		
May have fears, especially of dark and going to bed		
Knows own sex and appropriate sex of others		
In play, parallel and associative phase; begins to learn simple games and meaning of rules, but follows them according to self-interpretation; speaks to doll, animal, truck, and so on; begins to work out social interaction through play; able to share toys, although expresses idea of ''mine'' frequently		

Continued.

TABLE 11-1. THE MAJOR DEVELOPMENTAL ACHIEVEMENTS OF CHILDREN 3, 4, AND 5 YEARS OF AGE—cont'd

AGE (years)	PHYSICAL	GROSS MOTOR	FINE MOTOR	SENSORY	LANGUAGE
4	Pulse and respiration decrease slightly Blood pressure remains same Height and weight gain remain constant Length at birth is doubled	Skips and hops on one foot Catches ball reliably Throws ball overhand Walks down stairs using alternate footing	Imitates a gate with cubes Uses scissors successfully to cut out picture following outline Can lace shoes, but may not be able •to tie bow In drawing, copies a square, traces a cross and diamond, adds three parts to stick figure	Maximum potential for development of amblyopia	Has vocabulary of 1500 words or more Uses sentences of four to five words Questioning is at peak Tells exaggerated stories Knows simple songs May be mildly profane if he associates with older children Obeys four prepositional phrases, such as "under," "on top of," "beside," "in back of" or "in front of" Names one or more colors Comprehends analogies, such as "If ice is cold, fire is _____" Repeats four digits Uses words liberally but frequently does not comprehend meaning
5	Pulse and respiration decrease slightly Blood pressure remains same Growth rate is similar to that of previous year Eruption of permanent dentition may begin, especially if deciduous tooth eruption was early (before age 6 months)	Skips and hops on alternate feet Throws and catches ball well Jumps rope Skates with good balance Walks backward with heel to toe Jumps from height of 12 inches, lands on toes Balances on alternate feet with eyes closed	Ties shoelaces Uses scissors, simple tools, or pencil very well In drawing, copies a diamond and triangle; adds seven to nine parts to stick man; prints a few letters, numbers, or words, such as his first name	Minimum potential for development of amblyopia Visual acuity approaches 20/20 (may not be completely achieved until 8 years of age)	Has vocabulary of about 2100 words Uses sentences of six to eight words, with all parts of speech Names coins (nickel, dime, and so on) Names four or more colors Describes drawing or pictures with much comment and enumeration

SOCIALIZATION	COGNITION	FAMILY RELATIONSHIPS
Very independent	Is in phase of intuitive thought	Rebels if parents expect too much from him, such as impeccable table manners
Tends to be selfish and impatient	Causality still related to proximity of events	
Aggressive physically as well as verbally	Understands time better, especially in terms of sequence of daily events	Takes aggression and frustration out on parents or siblings
Takes pride in accomplishments	Unable to conserve matter	Do's and don'ts become important
Has mood swings	Judges everything according to one dimension, such as height, width, or first	May have rivalry with older or younger siblings, may resent older's privileges and younger's invasion of privacy and possessions
Boasts and tattles		
Shows off dramatically, enjoys entertaining others		
Tells family tales to others with no restraint	Immediate perceptual clues dominate judgment	May run away from home
Still has many fears	Can choose longer of two lines or heavier of two objects	Identifies strongly with parent of opposite sex
In play, is cooperative and associative; imaginary playmates common; uses dramatic, imaginative, and imitative devices; works through unresolved conflicts, such as jealousy toward sibling, anger toward parent, or unconquered fear in himself; sexual exploration and curiosity demonstrated through play, such as being ''doctor'' or ''nurse''	Is beginning to develop less egocentrism and more social awareness	Is able to run errands outside the home
	May count correctly but has poor mathematic concept of numbers	
	Still believes that thoughts cause events	
	Obeys because parents have set limits, not because of understanding of reason behind right or wrong	
Less rebellious and quarrelsome than at age 4 years	Begins to question what parents think by comparing them to age-mates and other adults	Gets along well with parents
More settled and eager to get down to business		Doesn't run away from home
Not as open and accessible in thoughts and behavior as in earlier years	May notice prejudice and bias in outside world	May seek out mother more often than at age 4 years for reassurance and security, especially when entering school
Independent but trustworthy, not foolhardy	Is more able to view other's perspective, but tolerates differences rather than understands them	
Has fewer fears, relies on outer authority to control the world		Is upset not to find parent, for example, when he comes home from school
Eager to do things right and to please, tries to ''live by the rules''	Tends to be matter-of-fact about differences in others	
Acts ''manly'' or ''womanly''	May begin to show understanding of conservation of numbers through counting objects regardless of arrangement	Tolerates siblings, but finds 3-year-old children a special nuisance
Takes increased responsibility for his actions		Begins to question parents' thinking and principles
Has fairly consistent and polished manners		
Cares for himself totally, occasionally needing supervision in dress or hygiene	Uses time-oriented words with increased understanding	Strongly identifies with parent of same sex, especially boys with their fathers

Continued.

TABLE 11-1. THE MAJOR DEVELOPMENTAL ACHIEVEMENTS OF CHILDREN 3, 4, AND 5 YEARS OF AGE—cont'd

AGE (years)	PHYSICAL	GROSS MOTOR	FINE MOTOR	SENSORY	LANGUAGE
	First permanent teeth to erupt are four molars, which come in behind the last temporary teeth (often mistaken for temporary molars) Handedness is established (about 90% are right-handed)				Asks meaning of words Asks inquisitive questions Can repeat sentence of ten syllables or more Knows names of days of week, months, and other time-associated words Defines words using action as well as description Knows composition of articles, such as, ''A shoe is made of _____'' Can follow three commands in succession

as ''What do you do when you are hungry?'' by describing the appropriate action. Asking questions is at its peak, and children usually repeat the question until they receive an answer.

By the end of age 5 years children use all parts of speech correctly, except for deviations from the rule. They can define simple words by describing their use, shape, or general category of classification, not only by stating their outward appearance. For example, they define a ball as ''round, something you bounce, or a toy,'' rather than by its color.

Personal-social behavior. The pervasive ritualism and negativism of toddlerhood gradually diminish during the preschool years. Although self-assertion is still a major theme, preschoolers demonstrate their sense of autonomy differently. They are able to verbalize their request for independence, as well as perform independently, because of their much refined physical and cognitive development. They fully care for themselves by 4 or 5 years of age, needing little, if any, assistance with dressing, eating, or toileting. They can also be trusted to obey warnings of danger, although the 3- or 4-year-old child may exceed his boundaries at times. They are also much more sociable and willing to please. They have internalized many of the standards and values of the family, and their conscience dictates many of their actions. By the end of early childhood they begin to question parental values and compare them to those of the peer group and other authority figures; as a result they may be less willing to abide by the family's code of conduct.

Preschoolers have relinquished much of the stranger anxiety and fear of separation of earlier years. They relate to unfamiliar people easily and tolerate brief separations from parents with little or no protest. However, they still need parental security, reassurance, guidance, and approval, especially when entering nursery or regular school. Prolonged separation, such as that imposed by illness and hospitalization, is difficult, but preschoolers respond very well to anticipatory preparation and concrete explanation. They can cope with changes in daily routine much better than toddlers, but they may develop more imaginary fears. They gain security and comfort from familiar objects, such as toys, dolls, or photographs of family members. They are able to work through many of their unresolved fears, fantasies, and anxieties through play, especially if guided with appropriate play objects such as dolls or puppets that represent family members, medical and nursing staff, and other children.

SOCIALIZATION	COGNITION	FAMILY RELATIONSHIPS
May complain over minor injuries but tries to be brave for major pain In play, cooperative; likes rules and tries to follow them but may cheat to avoid losing; begins to notice group conformity and sense of belonging; very industrious, tries to accomplish a goal and feels pride and satisfaction, as well as unhappiness and discontent; may demand to watch television more now that he understands programs better; not ready for concentrated close work or small print because of slight farsightedness and still unrefined eye-hand coordination; imitative play mimics the portrayed adult like a mirror image; wants to use real objects during play, such as actual ingredients to make cookies rather than sand or mud	Very curious about factual information regarding his world	Enjoys doing activities, such as sports, cooking, shopping, and so on, with parent of same sex

Play

Play is the young child's work and life. Play has an autotherapeutic value as the child grows and learns. Various types of play, particularly cooperative and associative, are typical of preschoolers (see Chapter 2) (Fig. 11-1).

Imaginary playmates.   Play is so much a part of the young child's life that reality and fantasy become blurred. The make-believe is reality during play and only becomes fantasy when the toys are put away or the dress-up clothes are removed. It is no wonder that imaginary playmates are so much a part of this age period.

The appearance of imaginary companions usually occurs between the ages of 2½ to 3 years, and for the most part such playmates are relinquished when the child enters school. There seems to be a relationship between the level of intelligence and the presence of the imaginary companion. The more intelligent children tend to have the more vivid and complex pretend playmates.

Imaginary companions serve many purposes—they become friends in times of loneliness, they accomplish what the child is still attempting, and they experience what the child wants to forget or remember. It is not unusual for the "friend" to have a myriad of vices and to be blamed for wrongdoing. Sometimes the child hopes to es-

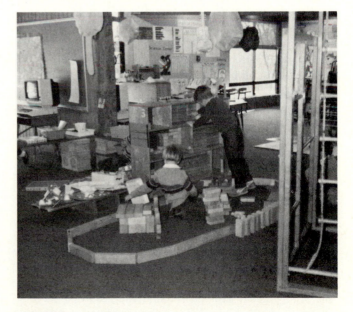

FIG. 11-1
Associative play is typical of preschoolers who enjoy lending and borrowing without the rigid rules of more structured play.

cape punishment by saying, "My friend George broke the glass." At other times he may fantasize that the companion misbehaved and the child plays the role of parent. This becomes a way of assuming control and authority in a safe situation.

Parents often worry about the imaginary playmates, not realizing how normal and useful they are. They need to be reassured that children's fantasy is a sign of health that helps them differentiate between pretend and reality. Parents can acknowledge the presence of the imaginary companion by calling him by name and even agreeing to simple requests such as setting an extra place at the table, but they should not allow the child to use the playmate to avoid punishment or responsibility. For example, if the child blames the companion for messing his room, the parent needs to state clearly that the child is the only one he sees and therefore he is responsible for cleaning up.

Selection of play materials. Play activities for children in this age-group should provide for *physical growth and refinement of motor skills,* such as jumping, running, and climbing. Tricycles, trucks, wagons, gym and sports equipment, sandbox, wading pool, and winter sleds help develop muscles and coordination. Activities such as swimming, skating, and skiing teach safety as well as muscle development and coordination.

Manipulative, constructive, creative, and *educational toys* provide for quiet activities, fine-motor development, and self-expression. Easy construction sets, large blocks of various sizes and shapes, a counting frame, paints, crayons, simple carpentry tools, musical toys, illustrated books, simple sewing or handicraft sets, large puzzles, and clay are suitable toys. Electronic games such as Speak & Spell* and educational computer programs for television are especially valuable in helping children learn basic skills such as letters and simple words.

Probably the most characteristic and pervasive preschooler activity is *imitative, imaginative,* and *dramatic play.* Dress-up clothes, dolls, housekeeping toys, dollhouses, play store toys, telephones, farm animals and equipment, village sets, trains, trucks, cars, planes, hand puppets, and doctor and nurse kits provide hours of self-expression (Fig. 11-2). Even in households where there is a blurring of the traditional sex roles, children identify with certain feminine or masculine behaviors, which are demonstrated in almost all heterosexual relationships. Probably at no other time is the reproduction of the behavior of significant adults so faithful and absorbing as in 4- and 5-year-old children. Toward the end of the preschool period, children are less satisfied with make-believe or pretend objects and enjoy actually doing the activity, such as cooking and carpentry.

Television and the television computer games also

have a place in children's play. Unfortunately, more often than not, these forms of play foster social isolation. Supervised selection of programs and scheduled hours of the day for quiet activity should guide how television is used. Children in this age-group enjoy and learn from educational children's programs, which are purposely shown before dinner or after meals to provide a quiet activity. The exact influence of television on children's development and attitudes toward sex, violence, crime, and so on is a much disputed subject. However, few authorities disagree on the fact that television should only be one part of children's total repertoire of social and recreational activities.

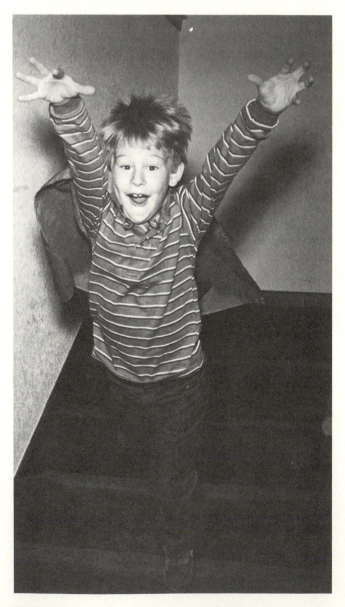

FIG. 11-2

Dress-up clothes such as this cape are all that are necessary for a preschooler to become a "super hero."

---

*Texas Instruments, Dallas, TX

PROMOTING OPTIMUM DEVELOPMENT

In many respects the preschool years present few child-rearing problems. The preschooler is quite independent, listens and obeys most of the time, clings less to adults, and enjoys peers for playmates. However, he also faces new challenges, such as entry into nursery school. He is increasingly inquisitive into new areas of learning, such as sex education, which may cause parents embarrassment. While trying to act grown up, he is vulnerable to fears and sleep problems. Nursing goals are aimed at helping parents understand and cope with these issues as they arise during the preschool period.

Preschool or daycare experience

The effects of early education and stimulation on children have increasingly gained recognition and importance. These first few years are foundational for personality development, social awareness, concept formation, and language. Since social development widens to include age-mates and other significant adults, preschool provides an excellent vehicle for expanding children's experiences with others.

In nursery school or day-care centers, children are exposed to opportunities for learning group cooperation, adjusting to various sociocultural differences, and coping with frustration, dissatisfaction, and anger. If activities are tailored to provide mastery and achievement, children increasingly feel success, self-confidence, and personal competence.

Nursery school is particularly beneficial for children who lack a peer group experience, such as an only child, and for children from culturally deprived homes. Nursery school provides extensive stimulation for language, physical, and social development. It also is an excellent preparation for entrance into regular school.

The disadvantages of out-of-home care for young children have not been clearly defined. However, evidence is accumulating that daycare centers pose an increased risk of infection among children, especially in centers that care for children under 2 years of age. Outbreaks of hepatitis A are not uncommon and are related to hygienic measures. Nurses who are associated with daycare centers can assist in minimizing this risk by stressing the importance of handwashing by children and staff and proper cleaning of diaper changing areas, including the diaper changing surface and accessory items that may become contaminated during a diaper change.

Children need preparation for the preschool experience, whether it is a formal nursery school, organized day-care center, or casual gathering in a neighbor's home. For young children it represents a change from their usual home environment and prolonged separation from parents.

Before the child begins the school experience, the parents should present the idea as exciting and pleasurable. Talking to the child about activities such as painting, building with blocks, or enjoying swings and other outdoor equipment allows the child to fantasize about the forthcoming event in a positive manner (Fig. 11-3). When the day arrives to begin school, the parents should behave confidently with no hesitancy or self-doubt about the decision, lest such feelings be transmitted to the child and influence his adjustment. Such behavior necessitates that the parents work through their own feelings regarding the nursery school or day-care center experience.

Parents should introduce their child to the teacher and familiarize him with the school. In some instances it is helpful to remain for at least some part of the first day until the child is comfortable and at ease. Other specific actions that can help lessen separation anxiety include providing the school with detailed information about the child's home environment, such as familiar routines, favorite activities, food preferences, names of siblings or pets, and personal habits. Such information helps the child feel familiar in the strange surroundings. When schools automatically request this information, the parent has a valuable clue to evaluating the quality of the program since the request represents the staff's awareness of each child's needs. Transitional objects such as a favorite toy or blanket may also help the child bridge the gap from home to school.

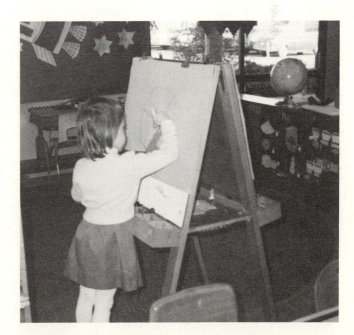

FIG. 11-3

Emphasizing the positive aspects of preschool can help the child feel comfortable in a new environment.

Sex education and sexual curiosity

Preschoolers have absorbed and experienced a tremendous amount of information during their short lifetimes. Although their thinking may not be adultlike, they search constantly for explanations and reasons that are logical and reasonable to them. The word "why" seems to supplant the word "no," which was common in toddlerhood. It is only natural that as they learn about "me" they will also want to know "why me," "how me," and so on. Questions such as "Where do babies come from?" are sexual in content but informational in intent. Such inquiries are as casual as "Why is the sky blue?" "What makes it rain?" or "Who is that?" It is the *way* in which questions about procreation are answered that conditions children, even the youngest, to separate these questions from others about their world.

Probably two rules govern answering questions about sex. The first is to *find out what the child thinks*. By investigating the theories he has conjured in his mind as a reasonable explanation, parents can not only give correct information but also help the child understand why his explanation is inaccurate. Another reason for ascertaining what the child thinks before offering any information is that the "unasked for" answer may be given. For example, 4-year-old Sally asked her father, "Where did I come from?" Both parents quickly took this inquiry as a clue for offering sex education. After a lengthy miniobstetric course, Sally exclaimed, "I don't know about all that! All I know is Mary came from New York and I want to know where I was born."

The second rule for giving information is *honesty*. It is true that much of the correct information will be forgotten or misunderstood by the preschooler, but what is more important is that the correct information can be restated until the child absorbs and comprehends the facts. Even though the correct anatomic words may be hard to pronounce or even more difficult to remember, they become foundational content for explaining other concepts later on.

Honesty does not imply bombarding children with every fact of life or allowing excessive permissiveness in sexual curiosity. When children ask one question, they are looking for one answer, not the entire procreation cycle. When they are ready, they will ask about the other "unfinished" parts of the story. Sooner or later they will wonder how the "sperm meets the egg" and "how the baby gets out," but it is best to wait until they ask.

Regardless of whether children are given sex education, they will engage in games of sexual curiosity and exploration. At about 3 years of age children are aware of the anatomic differences between the sexes and are very concerned with how the other "works." This is not really "sexual" curiosity, because many children are still unaware of the reproductive function of the genitals. Their curiosity is for the eliminative function of the anatomy.

Little boys wonder how girls can urinate without a penis, so they watch girls go to the bathroom. Since they cannot see anything but the stream of water coming out, they want to observe further for what makes it come out. "Doctor play" is often a game invented for just such investigation. Little girls are no less curious about boys' anatomy. It is very intriguing to have a closer inspection of this "thing" that girls do not have.

One question that parents often have is how to handle such sexual curiosity. A positive approach is neither to condone nor condemn the sexual curiosity but to express that if the child has questions he should ask his parents, and then encourage the child to engage in some other activity. In this way children can be helped to understand that there are ways other than through playing investigative games that their sexual curiosity can be satisfied. This in no way condemns the act but stresses alternate methods to seek solutions. Allowing children unrestricted permissiveness only intensifies their anxiety and concern since exploring and searching usually yield little evidence to satisfy their questions.

Another concern for some parents is masturbation, or self-stimulation of the genitals. This occurs at any age for a variety of reasons and, if not excessive, is normal and healthy. For preschoolers it is a part of sexual curiosity and exploration. If parents are concerned with masturbation in their children, it is essential for nurses to investigate the circumstances associated with the activity, because it may be an expression of anxiety, boredom, or unresolved conflicts. For example, a boy who repeatedly touches his penis is not masturbating for pleasure but may be reassuring himself that it is intact. Also, children who openly and publicly masturbate are inviting a reaction, such as discipline, punishment, or criticism. They may be overwhelmed by their sexual feelings and asking others to help them channel them into more constructive outlets. Since masturbation, like other forms of sex play, is a private act, parents should emphasize this to children as part of teaching them socially acceptable behavior.

Fears

As a result of magical thinking, all kinds of fears become real and logical in the minds of young children. Parents often become perplexed about handling the fears because no amount of logical persuasion, coercion, or ridicule will send away the ghosts, boogeymen, monsters, and devils.

The best way to help children overcome their fears is by actively involving them in finding practical methods to deal with the frightening experience. This may be as simple as keeping a dim night-light on in the child's bedroom to assure him that no monsters lurk in the dark. Exposing children to the feared object in a safe situation also provides a type of conditioning or desensitization. For instance, children who are afraid of dogs should never be forced to approach or touch one, but they may be gradually introduced to the experience by watching other children play with the animal. This type of *modeling*, demonstrating fearlessness in others, can be very effective if the child is allowed to progress at his own rate.

Usually by 5 or 6 years of age children relinquish these old fears. If told about a previous fear, such as believing in ghosts, they will typically remark that they do not believe in or fear them because they have never seen one. This is quite logical and very concrete and helps explain away many of the fears of younger years. Explaining the developmental sequence of fears and their gradual disappearance may help parents feel more secure in handling preschoolers' fears.

Sleep problems

Young children sometimes have trouble going to sleep. After so much activity and stimulation during the day, some are unable to abruptly "shut off their motors." Others may have bedtime fears, wake during the night, or have nightmares. Still others may prolong the inevitable through elaborate rituals.

After a careful assessment of the events surrounding the problem, a recommended approach involves counseling the parent about the importance of a consistent bedtime ritual and emphasizing the normalcy of this type of behavior in young children. Attention-seeking behavior is ignored, and the child is not taken into the parents' bed or allowed to stay up past a reasonable hour. If nightmares occur, the child is comforted but left in his own bed. Sometimes the child's door must be locked in order to enforce the limits, although the safety of this procedure in case of a fire must always be considered. Other measures that may be helpful include keeping a light on in the room, providing transitional objects, such as a favorite toy, or leaving a drink of water by the bed.

Helping the child slow down before bedtime also contributes to less resistance to going to bed. Reading the child a story, playing with him in the bath, and letting him sit in the caregiver's lap while listening to television or music are quieting activities. If extra stimulation such as having visitors arrive at bedtime is disruptive to the child's routine, it is advisable to settle the child in bed beforehand.

Speech problems

The most critical period for speech development occurs between 2 and 4 years of age. During this period the child is using his rapidly growing vocabulary to interact with the environment. However, the rate of vocabulary acquisition does not keep pace with the advancing mental ability or the degree of comprehension. Consequently, it can result in the child's stuttering or stammering as he tries to say the word he is already thinking about. This hesitancy or nonfluency in speech pattern is a *normal* characteristic of language development.

However, when parents or other significant persons place undue emphasis or stress on this pattern of dysfluency, an abnormal speech pattern may result. Chances for reversal of stuttering are good until about 7 years of age. Therefore, prevention must begin early. The nurse discusses with parents the normal dysfluencies in children's speech. When stuttering does occur, parents are advised to use the suggestions listed in the boxed material that follows to prevent inadvertently reinforcing this pattern. If excessive concern on the part of the parent or frustration and struggling behavior from the child are noted, they are referred for language and speech evaluation. The critical point to remember is that the dysfluency must be

---

SUGGESTIONS FOR PARENTS REGARDING STUTTERING IN CHILDREN

To be encouraged

Viewing the hesitancy and dysfluency as a normal part of speech development

Giving the child plenty of time and the impression that you are not rushed or in a hurry

Looking directly at the child while he is talking; being patient and never ridiculing or criticizing

Speaking clearly and articulating well but not stressing that all sounds must be perfected too early

Identifying situations when stuttering increases and avoiding them or ignoring the hesitancy

Capitalizing on periods of fluent speech with positive reinforcement

To be avoided

The natural tendency to "help" the child by supplying the word when he is having a block

Telling him to stop and start over, to think before he speaks, or to take it easy and go slowly

Showing great concern, embarrassment, or disapproval for the hesitancy

Anything that emphasizes the stuttering and calls the child's attention to his speech skills

arrested before the child develops an awareness or anticipation of the difficulty and begins to mistrust his speech skills.

Children who are pressured into producing sounds ahead of their developmental level may develop dyslalia (articulation problems) or revert to using infantile speech. Prevention involves discussing with parents the usual achievement of speech production during childhood. The Denver Articulation Screening Examination (DASE) is an excellent tool to assess articulation skills in the child and to explain to parents the expected progression of sounds (Appendix C).

The DASE employs the word-imitative procedure. The child repeats 22 words but pronounces 30 different sound elements. The raw score, or the number of correctly pronounced sounds, is then compared to the percentile rank for children in that age-group. The examiner must be careful to evaluate the specific sound, rather than the quality of the entire word. For beginning examiners it is helpful to validate the final score by comparing the results with a different examiner, ideally a speech therapist. The child is also scored on intelligibility, by selection of one of four possible categories: (1) easy to understand, (2) understandable half of the time, (3) not understandable, or (4) cannot evaluate. The DASE is a reliable, effective screening tool for nurses because it requires only 10 minutes to perform and it is designed to discriminate between significant delay and normal variations in the acquisition of speech sounds.

The best therapy for speech problems is prevention. One of the most essential factors involves anticipatory preparation of parents for the expected hesitation in speech during the preschool period and discussion of developmental achievements characteristic of young children.

HEALTH PROMOTION DURING PRESCHOOL YEARS

Health promotion mainly involves nutritional guidance and accident prevention. A brief discussion of each is presented to emphasize the particular needs or differences of preschoolers and toddlers. (For a more comprehensive understanding the reader is urged to also review the material presented in Chapter 10 under ''Health promotion during the toddler years.'')

Nutritional guidance

Nutritional requirements for preschoolers are fairly similar to those for toddlers. The requirement for calories per unit of body weight continues to decrease slightly. Fluid requirements may also decrease slightly but depend on activity level, climatic conditions, and state of health. Protein consumption is more than adequate if it comprises 15% of the total caloric intake. Although the optimum protein requirement is not known, a daily consumption of approximately 30 g is recommended.

Parents sometimes worry about the quantity of food preschoolers consume. In general the quality is much more important than the quantity, a fact that should be stressed during nutritional counseling. Young children often consume more food than parents realize. One approach toward lessening this parental concern is advising parents to keep a weekly record of everything the child eats. In particular the need for measuring the amount of food, such as setting aside ½ cup of vegetables, and serving the child from this premeasured amount should be stressed. In this way, there is a more accurate estimate of food intake at each meal. Usually, by the end of the week's food chart, parents are amazed at how much the child has consumed, even though at each meal the amount seemed minimal. In general preschoolers consume only slightly more than toddlers, or about half of an adult's portion.

Some preschoolers still have food habits that are typical of toddlers, such as food fads and strong taste preferences. Four years of age seems to be another period for resurgence of finicky eating, which is generally characteristic of the more rebellious and rowdy behavior of children in this age-group. By age 5 years children are greatly influenced by the food habits of others and are more agreeable to trying new foods, especially if encouraged by an adult who also experiments with a new taste or different dish.

Mealtimes can become battlegrounds if parents expect impeccable table manners. Usually the 5-year-old child is ready for the ''social'' side of eating, but the 3- or 4-year-old child still has difficulty in sitting quietly through a long family meal.

Accident prevention

Because of improved gross and fine motor skill, coordination, and balance, preschoolers are less prone to falls than toddlers. They tend to be less reckless, listen more to parental rules, and are aware of potential danger, such as hot objects, sharp instruments, dangerous heights, and so on. Putting objects in the mouth as part of exploration has all but ceased, although poisoning is still a danger. Pedestrian motor vehicle accidents increase from activities such as playing in the street, riding tricycles, running after balls, or forgetting safety regulations when crossing streets.

In general the guidelines suggested for accident prevention in Table 10-4 are applicable to children in this age-group as well. However, emphasis is now on *education* for safety and potential hazards, in addition to appropriate protection. Since preschoolers are great imitators, it is especially essential that parents set a good example by ''practicing what they preach.'' Children are very quick to observe discrepancies in what they are told to do and what they see others do. Since they faithfully and unquestioningly believe in their parents' values and rules, this is an excellent opportunity for parents to practice and teach safe, cautious habits in daily living.

ANTICIPATORY GUIDANCE—CARE OF PARENTS

Although the preschool years present fewer childrearing difficulties than earlier years, this stage of development is facilitated by appropriate anticipatory guidance in the areas already discussed. (See also the boxed material shown below.) There is a shift in childrearing practices from protection to education. An occasional spanking during the toddler years may have been effective, but it now ceases to teach any lesson for why certain behavior is wrong or not acceptable. Likewise, accident prevention previously focused on safeguarding the immediate environment with less emphasis on reasoning. Now the protective guardrails or electrical outlet caps are substituted with verbal explanations of why danger exists and how to avoid it with appropriate judgment and understanding.

During this period an emotional transition between parent and child is also occurring. Although children are still attached to their parents and accepting of all their values and beliefs, they are nearing the period of life when they will question previous teachings and prefer the companionship of peers. Entry into school marks a separation from home for parents as well as for children. Parents need help in adjusting to this change, particularly if the mother has focused her daily activity primarily on home responsibilities. As preschoolers begin nursery or regular school, mothers may need to seek activities beyond the family, such as community involvement or pursuing a career. In this way all family members are adjusting to change, which is part of the process of growth and development.

PARENTAL GUIDANCE DURING THE PRESCHOOL YEARS	
AGE	**GUIDANCE**
3 years	Prepare parents for child's increasing interest in widening relationships
	Encourage enrollment in nursery school
	Emphasize importance of setting limits
	Prepare parents to expect exaggerated tension-reduction behaviors, such as need for ''security blanket''
	Encourage parents to offer the child choices when the child vacillates
	Expect marked changes at 3½ years when the child becomes less coordinated (motor and emotional), becomes insecure, exhibits emotional extremes, and develops behaviors such as stuttering
	Prepare parents to expect extra demands on their attention as a reflection of the child's emotional insecurity and fear of loss of love
	Warn parents that the equilibrium of the 3-year-old will change to the aggressive out-of-bounds behavior of the 4-year-old
	Anticipate a more stable appetite with more expansive food selection
4 years	Prepare for more aggressive behavior including motor activity and shocking language
	Expect resistance to parental authority
	Explore parental feelings regarding child's behavior
	Suggest some kind of respite for the primary caregiver such as placing the child in nursery school for part of the day
	Prepare for increasing sexual curiosity
	Emphasize importance of realistic limit setting on behavior
	Discuss discipline
	Prepare parents for the highly imaginary 4-year-old who indulges in ''tall tales'' (to be differentiated from lies) and for the child's acquisition of imaginary playmates
	Suggest swimming lessons if not begun earlier
	Explain Oedipus feelings and reactions
	Expect nightmares or an increase in them and suggest they make certain the child is fully awakened from a frightening dream
	Provide reassurance that a period of calm begins at 5 years of age
5 years	Expect a tranquil period at 5 years
	Prepare and assist child through initial entrance into school environment
	Make certain immunizations are up to date before entering school

BIBLIOGRAPHY

(References specific to preschoolers are included here; additional references can be found in Chapter 10.)

Growth and development

Ames, L.B., and Ilg, F.I.: Your three-year-old: friend or enemy, New York, 1980, Delacorte Press.

Ames, L.B., and Ilg, F.I.: Your four-year-old: wild and wonderful, New York, 1981, Delacorte Press.

Ames, L.B., and Ilg, F.I.: Your five-year-old: sunny and serene, New York, 1981, Delacorte Press.

Betz, C.: Faith development in children, Pediatr. Nurs. **7**(2):22-25, 1981.

Kay, P.: The imaginary companion: review of the literature, Maternal Child Nurs. J. **9**:8-11, 1980.

Mitchell, S.: Imaginary companions: friend or foe? Pediatr. Nurs. **6**(6):29-30, 1980.

Sahler, O.J., and McAnarney, E.R.: The child from three to eighteen, St. Louis, 1981, The C.V. Mosby Co.

Shelly, J.: The spiritual needs of children, Illinois, 1982, Inter-Varsity Press.

Selekman, J.: The development of body image in the child: a learned response, Topic Clin. Nurs. **5**(1):12-21, 1983.

Preschool or daycare experience

Baker, J., and Proett, P.: One hospital's response: a child care referral service, Am. J. Nurs. **83**(4):550-551, 1983.

Ballard, P.: Selecting child care, Issues Compr. Pediatr. Nurs. **5**:219-231, 1981.

Chabin, M.: Hospital-supported child care, Am. J. Nurs. **83**(4):548-551, 1983.

Mayer, G.: Choosing daycare, Am. J. Nurs. **81**(2):346-348, 1981.

Payne, P.A.: Day care and its impact on parenting, Nurs. Clin. North Am. **12**(3):525-533, 1977.

Richardson, J.: Nursery schools, Midwife Health Visit Community Nurse **16**(6):256, 1980.

Watkins, S.: The day care decision, Pediatr. Nurs. **4**(3):9-11, 1978.

Sex education

Calderone, M.S.: Sexual health and the child, Compr. Ther. **6**(12):3-7, 1980.

Children's books on sex and siblings, Am. J. Nurs. **79**:1968, Nov. 1979.

Gallo, A.: Early childhood masturbation, Pediatr. Nurs. **5**(5):47-49, 1979.

Malinowski, J.S.: Answering a child's questions about sex and a new baby, Am. J. Nurs. **79**(11):1965-1968, 1979.

Fears/sleep problems

Hewitt, K.E.: Sleeping problems in pre-school children: what to ask and what to do, Health Visitor **54:**100-101, March 1980.

Inglis, S.: The nocturnal frustration of sleep disturbance, Am. J. Maternal Child Nurs. **1**(5):280-287, 1976.

Miller, S.R.: Children's fears: a review of the literature with implications for nursing research and practice, Nurs. Res. **28**(4):217-223, 1979.

Prescott-Day, S.: Sleep variations of the pre-school child, Health Visitor **52:**465-468, Nov. 1979.

Schowalter, J.E.: Emotional disorders in children: children are different. Behavioral Development Monograph Series number 4, Columbus, Ohio, 1983, Ross Laboratories.

Schumann, M.J.: A method for inducing sleep in young children, Pediatr. Nurs. **7**(5):9-13, 1981.

Speech problems

Brown, M.S.: Testing of a young child for articulation skills, Clin. Pediatr. **15**(7):639-644, 1976.

Rommel, J.: Referral of children with speech problems, Pediatr. Nurs. **2**(2):28-32, 1976.

Schwartz, A.H., and Murphy, M.W.: Cues for screening language disorders in preschool children, Pediatrics **55**(5):717-722, 1975.

Van Hattum, R.J.: Communication disorders in children: a guide for detection and referral, Nursing 75 **5**(3):12-15, 1975.

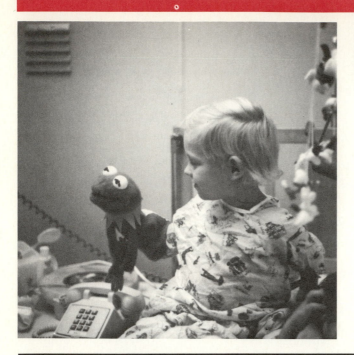

HEALTH PROBLEMS OF EARLY CHILDHOOD

OBJECTIVES

On completion of this chapter the reader will be able to:

■ Describe the major characteristics of communicable diseases of childhood

■ List three principles of nursing care of children with communicable disease

■ Describe the postoperative nursing care of the child with a tonsillectomy

■ Describe the nursing care of the child with otitis media

■ Describe the nursing care of the child with conjunctivitis

■ Identify the principles in the emergency treatment of poisoning

■ Describe the nursing care of the child with lead poisoning

■ State three factors known to be associated with child abuse

■ State four areas of the history that should arouse suspicion of abuse

■ Describe the nursing care of the abused child

NURSING DIAGNOSES

Nursing diagnoses identified for health problems during early childhood include, but are not restricted to, the following:

Health perception-health management pattern

■ Health maintenance, alteration in, related to poisoning

■ Infection, potential for, related to exposure of contacts to communicable disease

■ Injury, actual (poisoning), related to inadequate prevention; potential (trauma), related to continued abuse

■ Noncompliance related to knowledge deficit

Nutritional-metabolic pattern

■ Oral mucous membranes, alteration in, related to poor hygiene after tonsillectomy

Elimination pattern

■ Urinary elimination, alteration in patterns, related to lead poisoning

Activity-exercise pattern

■ Activity intolerance, related to anemia (lead poisoning)

■ Breathing patterns, ineffective, related to salicylate poisoning

■ Home maintenance management, impaired, related to knowledge deficit

■ Self-care deficit related to (1) developmental level; (2) illness

Cognitive-perceptual pattern

■ Comfort, alterations in: pain, related to (1) tonsillectomy; (2) otitis media

■ Knowledge deficit (parenting), related to child abuse

Self-perception—self-concept pattern

■ Anxiety, related to hospitalization (tonsillectomy)

■ Fear, related to (1) injections (lead poisoning); (2) continued abuse

■ Powerlessness, related to child abuse

■ Self-concept, disturbance in, related to parenting abilities

Role-relationship pattern

■ Family process, alterations in, related to temporary illness in child

■ Parenting, alterations in: actual, related to (1) lead poisoning; (2) child abuse

Coping-stress tolerance pattern

■ Coping, family: potential for growth, related to (1) prevention of further poisoning; (2) successful resolution of abuse

■ Coping, ineffective family: compromised, related to child abuse

■ Coping, ineffective individual, related to (1) illness; (2) abuse

This chapter is concerned with health problems that occur most frequently during the early childhood years, such as poisoning and child abuse, and with diseases or illnesses that necessitate intervention, such as tonsillitis or communicable disease. The influence of growth and development on each health problem is of special concern, since the cause or the treatment may be directly affected by the child's age. Optimum care includes knowledge of the pathologic, psychologic, developmental, and familial variables of the health problem in order to plan and provide individualized care to meet each child's particular needs.

COMMUNICABLE DISEASES

The incidence of common communicable diseases of childhood has declined tremendously since the advent of immunizations. Serious complications resulting from such infections have been further reduced with the use of antibiotics and antitoxins. However, infectious diseases do occur and in most cases are prevalent during early childhood when resistance to infectious agents may still be low but when exposure is beginning to increase as a result of social involvement outside the home. Therefore, the nurse must be familiar with the infectious agent in order to recognize

TABLE 12-1. INFECTIOUS DISEASES THAT OCCUR DURING EARLY CHILDHOOD*

DISEASE

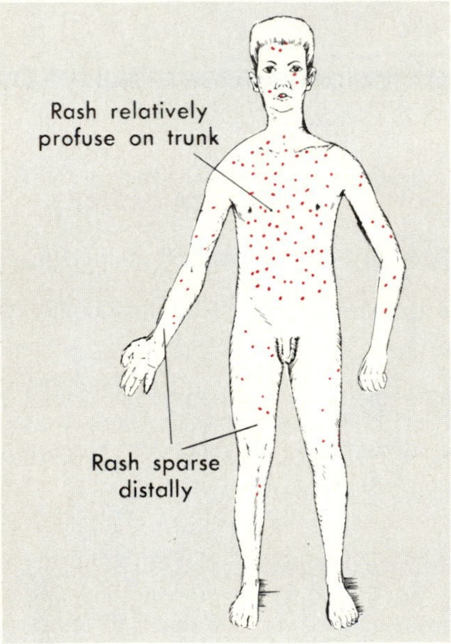

Rash relatively profuse on trunk

Rash sparse distally

FIG. 12-1

Chickenpox (Fig. 12-1)
Agent: varicella zoster
Source: primary secretions of respiratory tract of infected persons; to a lesser degree skin lesions (scabs not infectious)
Transmission: direct contact, droplet spread, and contaminated objects
Incubation period: 2 to 3 weeks, commonly 13 to 17 days
Period of communicability: probably 1 day before eruption of lesions (prodromal period to 6 days after first crop of vesicles when crusts have formed)

Diphtheria
Agent: Corynebacterium diphtheriae
Source: discharges from mucous membranes of nose and nasopharynx, skin, and other lesions of infected person
Transmission: direct contact with infected person, a carrier, or contaminated articles
Incubation period: usually 2 to 5 days, possibly longer
Period of communicability: variable; until virulent bacilli are no longer present (identified by three negative cultures); usually 2 weeks but as long as 4 weeks

*Figs 12-1 to 12-4 from Krugman, S., and Katz, S.: Infectious diseases of children, ed. 7, St. Louis, 1981, The C.V. Mosby Co.

the disease and institute appropriate preventative and nursing interventions (Table 12-1).

Nursing considerations

The principal nursing goals are (1) identification of the communicable disease, (2) prevention of complications, and (3) prevention of spread to others. For most of the diseases care is chiefly symptomatic, and the nursing intervention is to help parents cope with the symptoms to provide comfort for the child.

Identification. Identification of the infectious agent is of primary importance in order to prevent exposure to susceptible individuals. Nurses in ambulatory care settings, such as emergency rooms, health maintenance centers, nursery or regular schools, and physicians' offices, are often the first persons to see signs of a communicable disease, such as a rash or sore throat. The nurse must operate under a high index of suspicion for common childhood diseases in order to identify potentially infectious cases and to recognize diseases that require medical intervention. An illustrative example is the common complaint

CLINICAL MANIFESTATIONS	THERAPEUTIC MANAGEMENT/COMPLICATIONS	NURSING CONSIDERATIONS

Prodromal stage: slight fever, malaise, and anorexia for first 24 hours; rash highly pruritic; begins as macule, rapidly progresses to papule and then vesicle (surrounded by erythematous base, becomes umbilicated and cloudy, breaks easily and forms crusts); all three stages (papule, vesicle, crust) present in varying degrees at one time
Distribution: centripetal, spreading to face and proximal extremities but sparse on distal limbs
Constitutional signs and symptoms: elevated temperature from lymphadenopathy, irritability from pruritus
	Specific: none
	Supportive: Diphenhydramine hydrochloride or antihistamines to relieve itching; skin care to prevent secondary bacterial infection
	Complications:
	  Secondary bacterial infections (abscesses, cellulitis, pneumonia, sepsis)
	  Encephalitis
	  Varicella pneumonia
	  Hemorrhagic varicella (tiny hemorrhages in the vesicles and numerous petechiae in the skin)
	  Reye's syndrome
		Isolation of child in home until vesicles have dried (usually 1 week after onset of disease) and isolation of high-risk children
		Administer skin care: give daily bath, change clothes and linens daily; administer topical application of calamine lotion or paste of baking soda and water; keep child's fingernails short and clean; apply mittens if child must scratch
		Lessen pruritus; keep child occupied
		Remove loose crusts that rub and irritate skin
		Teach child to apply pressure to pruritic area rather than scratch it
		If older child, reason with him regarding danger of scar formation from scratching

Varies according to anatomic location of pseudomembrane
Nasal: resembles common cold, serosanguineous mucopurulent nasal discharge without constitutional symptoms; may be frank epistaxis
Tonsillar/pharyngeal: malaise; anorexia; sore throat; low-grade fever; pulse increased above expected for temperature within 24 hours; smooth, adherent, white or gray membrane; lymphadenitis possibly pronounced (bull's neck); in severe cases, toxemia, septic shock, and death within 6 to 10 days
Laryngeal: fever, hoarseness, cough, with or without previous signs listed; potential airway obstruction, apprehensive, dyspneic retractions, cyanosis
	Antitoxin (usually intravenously); preceded by skin or conjunctival test to rule out sensitivity to horse serum
	Antibiotics (penicillin or erythromycin)
	Complete bed rest (prevention of myocarditis)
	Tracheostomy for airway obstruction
	Treatment of infected contacts and carriers
	Complications:
	  Myocarditis (second week)
	  Neuritis
		Maintain *strict* isolation
		Participate in sensitivity testing; have epinephrine available
		Administer antibiotics; observe for signs of sensitivity to penicillin
		Administer *complete* care to maintain bed rest
		Use suctioning as needed
		Regulate humidity for optimum liquefaction of secretions
		Observe respirations for signs of obstruction

Continued.

TABLE 12-1. INFECTIOUS DISEASES THAT OCCUR DURING EARLY CHILDHOOD—cont'd

DISEASE

Erythema infectiosum (fifth disease)
Agent: probably virus
Source: infected persons
Transmission: presumably direct contact by droplet infection
Incubation period: 6 to 14 days
Period of communicability: uncertain; most outbreaks subside in 1 to 2 months

Exanthema subitum (roseola)
Agent: probably virus
Source: unknown
Transmission: unknown (virtually limited to children between 6 months and 2 years of age)
Incubation period: unknown
Period of communicability: unknown

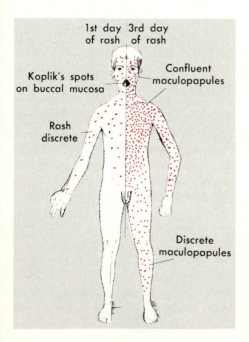

Measles (rubeola) (Fig. 12-2)
Agent: virus
Source: respiratory tract secretions, blood, and urine of infected person
Transmission: usually by direct contact with droplets of infected person
Incubation period: 10 to 20 days
Period of communicability: from 4 days before to 5 days after rash appears but mainly during prodromal (catarrhal) stage

FIG. 12-2

CLINICAL MANIFESTATIONS	THERAPEUTIC MANAGEMENT/COMPLICATIONS	NURSING CONSIDERATIONS
Rash appears in three stages: *I*—erythema on face, chiefly on cheeks, "slapped face" appearance; disappears by 1 to 4 days *II*—about 1 day after rash appears on face, maculopapular red spots appear, symmetrically distributed on upper and lower extremities; rash progresses from proximal to distal surfaces and may last a week or more *III*—rash subsides but reappears if skin is irritated or traumatized (sun, heat, cold, friction)	None necessary *Complications:* Self-limited arthritis and arthralgia	Reassure parents regarding benign nature of condition
Persistent high fever for 3 to 4 days in child who appears well Precipitious drop in fever to normal with appearance of rash *Rash:* discrete rose-pink macules or maculopapules appearing first on trunk, then spreading to neck, face, and extremities; nonpruritic, fades on pressure, lasts 1 to 2 days *Associated signs and symptoms:* cervical/postauricular lymphadenopathy, injected pharynx, occasionally catarrhal otitis media	None specific Antipyretics to control fever Anticonvulsives for child with history of febrile seizures *Complications:* Febrile seizures	Teach parents measures for lowering temperature (antipyretic drugs and tepid sponge baths) If child is prone to seizures, discuss appropriate precautions Reassure parents regarding benign nature of illness

Prodromal (catarrhal) stage: fever and malaise, followed in 24 hours by coryza, cough, conjunctivitis, Koplik's spots (small, irregular red spots with a minute, bluish white center first seen on the buccal mucosa opposite the molars) 2 days before rash; symptoms gradually increase in severity until second day after rash appears, when they begin to subside
Rash: appears 3 to 4 days after onset of prodromal stage, begins as erythematous maculopapular eruption on face and gradually spreads downward; more severe in earlier sites (appears confluent) and less intense in later sites (appears discrete); after 3 to 4 days assumes brownish appearance, and fine desquamation occurs over areas of extensive involvement
Constitutional signs and symptoms: anorexia, malaise, generalized lymphadenopathy
	Supportive: bed rest during febrile period; antipyretics
	Antibiotics to prevent secondary bacterial infection in high-risk children
	Complications:
	  Otitis media
	  Pneumonia
	  Bronchiolitis
	  Obstructive laryngitis and laryngotracheitis
	  Encephalitis
		Isolation until fifth day of rash; if hospitalized, institute respiratory precautions
		Maintain bed rest during prodromal stage; provide quiet activity
		Fever: instruct parents to administer antipyretics and cool sponge bath; avoid chilling; if child is prone to seizures, institute appropriate precautions (fever spikes to 40°C [104°F] between fourth and fifth days)
		Eye care: dim lights if photophobia present; clean eyelids with warm saline solution to remove secretions or crusts; keep child from rubbing his eyes; examine cornea for signs of ulceration
		Coryza/cough: use cool mist vaporizer; protect skin around nares with layer of petrolatum; encourage fluids and soft bland foods
		Skin care: keep skin clean; use tepid baths as necessary

Continued.

TABLE 12-1. INFECTIOUS DISEASES THAT OCCUR DURING EARLY CHILDHOOD—cont'd

DISEASE

Mumps
Agent: virus
Source: saliva of infected persons
Transmission: direct contact with or droplet spread from an infected person
Incubation period: 14 to 21 days
Period of communicability: most communicable immediately before and after swelling begins

Pertussis (whooping cough)
Agent: Bordetella pertussis
Source: discharge from respiratory tract of infected persons
Transmission: direct contact or droplet spread from infected person; indirect contact with freshly contaminated articles
Incubation period: 5 to 21 days, usually 10
Period of communicability: greatest during catarrhal stage before onset of paroxysms and may extend to fourth week after onset of paroxysms

CLINICAL MANIFESTATIONS	THERAPEUTIC MANAGEMENT/COMPLICATIONS	NURSING CONSIDERATIONS
Prodromal stage: fever, headache, malaise, and anorexia for 24 hours, followed by "earache" that is aggravated by chewing *Parotitis:* by third day, parotid gland(s) (either unilateral or bilateral) enlarges and reaches maximal size in 1 to 3 days; accompanied by pain and tenderness *Other manifestations:* submaxillary and sublingual infection, orchitis, and meningoencephalitis	*Symptomatic and supportive:* analgesics for pain and antipyretics for fever Intravenous fluid may be necessary for child who refuses to drink or vomits because of meningoencephalitis *Complications:* Sensorineural deafness Postinfectious encephalitis Myocarditis Arthritis Hepatitis Sterility (in adult males)	Isolation during period of communicability; institute respiratory isolation during hospitalization Maintain bed rest during prodromal phase until swelling subsides Give analgesics for pain; if child is unwilling to chew medication, use elixir form Encourage fluids and soft, bland foods; avoid foods requiring chewing Apply hot or cold compresses to neck, whichever is more comforting To relieve orchitis, provide warmth and local support by means of tight-fitting underpants (stretch bathing suit works well)
Catarrhal stage: begins with symptoms of upper respiratory infection, such as coryza, sneezing, lacrimation, cough, and low-grade fever; symptoms continue for 1 to 2 weeks, when dry, hacking cough becomes more severe *Paroxysmal stage:* cough that most commonly occurs at night consists of a series of short, rapid coughs followed by a sudden inspiration that is associated with a high-pitched crowing sound or "whoop"; during paroxysms cheeks become flushed or cyanotic, eyes bulge, and tongue protrudes; paroxysm may continue until a thick mucous plug is dislodged; vomiting frequently follows an attack; stage generally lasts 4 to 6 weeks, followed by convalescent stage	Antimicrobial therapy (such as erythromycin) Administration of pertussis-immune globulin *Supportive treatment:* hospitalization required for infants, children who are dehydrated, or those who have complications Bed rest Increased oxygen intake and humidity Adequate fluids Intubation possibly necessary *Complications:* Pneumonia (usual cause of death) Atelectasis Otitis media Convulsions Hemorrhage (subarachnoid, subconjunctival, epistaxis) Weight loss and dehydration Hernia Prolapsed rectum	Isolation during catarrhal stage; if hospitalized, institute respiratory isolation Maintain bed rest as long as fever is present Keep child occupied during the day (interest in play is associated with fewer paroxysms) Reassure parents during frightening episodes of whooping cough Provide restful environment and reduce factors that promote paroxysms (dust, smoke, sudden change in temperature, chilling, activity, excitement); keep room well ventilated Encourage fluids; offer small amount of fluids frequently; refeed child after vomiting Keep child in Croupette with high humidity; suction gently but often to prevent choking on secretions Observe for signs of airway obstruction (increased restlessness, apprehension, retractions, cyanosis) Involve public health nurse if child is cared for at home

Continued.

TABLE 12-1. INFECTIOUS DISEASES THAT OCCUR DURING EARLY CHILDHOOD—cont'd

DISEASE

Poliomyelitis

Agent: enteroviruses, 3 types; type 1—most frequent cause of paralysis, both epidemic and endemic, type 2—least frequently associated with paralysis, type 3—second most frequent in association with paralysis

Source: feces and oropharyngeal secretions of infected persons, especially young children

Transmission: direct contact with persons with apparent or inapparent active infection; spread is via fecal-oral and pharyngeal-oropharyngeal routes

Incubation period: usually 7 to 14 days, with range of 5 to 35 days

Period of communicability: not exactly known; virus is present in throat and feces shortly after infection and persists for about 1 week in throat and 4 to 6 weeks in feces

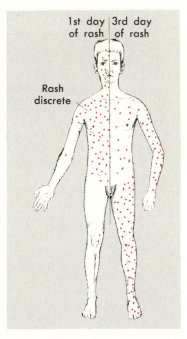

FIG. 12-3

Rubella (German measles) (Fig. 12-3)

Agent: virus

Source: primarily nasopharyngeal secretions of persons with apparent or inapparent infection; virus also present in blood, stool, and urine

Transmission: direct contact and spread via infected person; indirectly via articles freshly contaminated with nasopharyngeal secretions, feces, or urine

Incubation period: 14 to 21 days

Period of communicability: 7 days before to about 5 days after appearance of rash

CLINICAL MANIFESTATIONS	THERAPEUTIC MANAGEMENT/COMPLICATIONS	NURSING CONSIDERATIONS
May be manifest in three different forms: ***Abortive or inapparent***—fever, uneasiness, sore throat, headache, anorexia, vomiting, abdominal pain; lasts a few hours to a few days ***Nonparalytic***—same manifestations as abortive but more severe, with pain and stiffness in neck, back, and legs ***Paralytic***—initital course similar to nonparalytic type, followed by recovery and then signs of central nervous system paralysis	No specific treatment, including antimicrobials or gamma globulin Complete bed rest during acute phase Assisted respiratory ventilation in case of respiratory paralysis Physical therapy for muscles following acute stage ***Complications:*** Permanent paralysis Respiratory arrest Hypertension Kidney stones from demineralization of bone during prolonged immobility	Maintain complete bed rest Administer mild sedatives as necessary to relieve anxiety and promote rest Participate in physiotherapy procedures (use of moist hot packs and range of motion exercises) Position child to maintain body alignment and prevent contractures or decubiti; use footboard Encourage child to move; administer analgesics for maximum comfort during physical activity Observe for respiratory paralysis (difficulty in talking, ineffective cough, inability to hold breath, shallow and rapid respirations); report such signs and symptoms to physician; have tracheostomy tray at bedside
Prodromal stage: absent in children, present in adults and adolescents; consists of low-grade fever, headache, malaise, anorexia, mild conjunctivitis, coryza, sore throat, cough, and lymphadenopathy; lasts for 1 to 5 days, subsides 1 day after appearance of rash ***Rash:*** first appears on face and rapidly spreads downward to neck, arms, trunk, and legs; by end of first day body is covered with a discrete, pinkish red maculopapular exanthema; disappears in same order as it began and is usually gone by third day ***Constitutional signs and symptoms:*** occasionally low-grade fever, headache, malaise, and lymphadenopathy	No treatment necessary other than antipyretics for low-grade fever and analgesics for discomfort ***Complications:*** Rare (arthritis, encephalitis, or purpura); most benign of all childhood communicable diseases; greatest danger is teratogenic effect on fetus	Reassure parents of benign nature of illness Employ comfort measures as necessary Isolate child from pregnant women

Continued.

TABLE 12-1. INFECTIOUS DISEASES THAT OCCUR DURING EARLY CHILDHOOD—cont'd

DISEASE

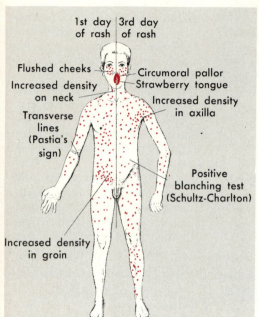

1st day | 3rd day
of rash | of rash

Flushed cheeks
Increased density on neck
Transverse lines (Pastia's sign)

Circumoral pallor
Strawberry tongue
Increased density in axilla

Positive blanching test (Schultz-Charlton)

Increased density in groin

FIG. 12-4

Scarlet fever (Fig. 12-4)
Agent: group A β-hemolytic streptococci
Source: usually from nasopharyngeal secretions of infected persons and carriers
Transmission: direct contact with infected person or droplet spread; indirectly by contact with contaminated articles, ingestion of contaminated milk or other food
Incubation period: 2 to 4 days, with range of 1 to 7 days
Period of communicability: during incubation period and clinical illness approximately 10 days; during first 2 weeks of carrier phase, although may persist for months

Tuberculosis
Agent: Mycobacterium tuberculosis
Source: respiratory secretions of actively infected persons
Transmission: direct contact with infected persons
Incubation period: from infection to primary lesion, about 4 to 6 weeks
Period of communicability: as long as bacilli are discharged

of sore throat. Although most often a symptom of a minor viral infection, it can signal diphtheria or a streptococcal infection, such as scarlet fever. Each of these conditions requires appropriate medical treatment to prevent serious sequelae.

Several important factors are helpful in identifying potentially communicable diseases: (1) recent exposure to a known case, (2) a history of prodromal symptoms or evidence of constitutional symptoms, such as a fever or rash (see Table 12-1), (3) a history of previous immunizations, and (4) a previous history of having the disease. Since immunizations are available for several of the diseases and in almost each case an attack confers lifelong immunity, one can rule out the possibility of many infectious agents based on these two criteria.

Prevention of complications. Many of the diseases require only supportive measures until the illness

runs its course. Children are usually cared for at home until they are no longer communicable and until they feel well enough to resume normal activity. However, there are groups of children who are at risk for serious, even fatal, complications from communicable diseases, especially those of viral etiology. Such children include those who are undergoing steroid or other immunosuppressive therapy, those who have a generalized malignancy, such as leukemia or lymphoma, or those who have an immunologic disorder. The nurse immediately refers children who have signs of a communicable disease to a physician. School nurses who are aware of such susceptible children have the responsibility of warning their parents of recent outbreaks of a communicable disease in order to prevent their exposure to known cases. In most instances the child is kept out of school until the outbreak is over. At the present time chickenpox is the most frequent disease re-

CLINICAL MANIFESTATIONS	THERAPEUTIC MANAGEMENT/COMPLICATIONS	NURSING CONSIDERATIONS

Prodromal stage: abrupt high fever, pulse increased out of proportion to fever, vomiting, headache, chills, malaise, abdominal pain
 	
Enanthema: tonsils enlarged, edematous, reddened, and covered with patches of exudate; in severe cases appearance resembles membrane seen in diphtheria; pharynx is edematous and beefy red; during first 1 or 2 days tongue is coated and papillae become red and swollen (white strawberry tongue); by the fourth or fifth day white coat sloughs off, leaving prominent papillae (red strawberry tongue); palate is covered with erythematous punctate lesions
 	
Exanthema: rash appears within 12 hours after prodromal signs; red pinhead-sized punctate lesions rapidly become generalized but are absent on the face, which becomes flushed; rash is more intense in folds of joints; by end of the first week desquamation begins, which may be complete by 3 weeks or longer
	Treatment of choice is a full course of penicillin (or erythromycin in penicillin-sensitive children); fever should subside 24 hours after beginning therapy
	
	Antibiotic therapy for newly diagnosed carriers (nose or throat cultures positive for streptococci)
	
	Supportive measures: bed rest during febrile phase, analgesics for sore throat
	
	Complications:
	  Otitis media
	  Peritonsillar abscess
	  Sinusitis
	  Rheumatic fever
	  Glomerulonephritis
		Institute respiratory isolation until 24 hours after initiation of treatment
		
		Ensure compliance with oral antibiotic therapy (intramuscular benzathine penicillin G [Bicillin] may be given if parents' reliability in giving oral drugs is questionable)
		
		Maintain bed rest during febrile phase; provide quiet activity during convalescent period
		
		Relieve discomfort of sore throat with analgesics, gargles, lozenges, antiseptic throat sprays (Chloraseptic), and inhalation of cool mist
		
		Encourage fluids during febrile phase; avoid irritating liquids (citrus juices) or rough foods; when child is able to eat, begin with soft diet
		
		Advise parents to consult physician if fever persists after beginning therapy
		
		Discuss procedures for preventing spread of infection

Usually asymptomatic Diagnosis confirmed by demonstration of bacilli in sputum or gastric washings. In infants and children with advanced disease, may see fever, pallor, weakness, weight loss, cough, hoarseness, and tachypnea	Chemotherapy with combined drugs, usually isoniazid (INH) and rifampin Avoid further contact with infected persons *Complications:* Dissemination of bacilli in various sites, for example, meninges, skeleton, lymph nodes	Participate in TB screening programs Teach parents and child about disease and treatment Encourage compliance with long-term drug therapy Promote optimum general health, especially maintaining nutrition and preventing infection

quiring isolation of high-risk children because no immunization is available.

Prevention of spread. Prevention consists of the following two components: prevention of the disease and control of spread of the disease to others. Primary prevention rests almost exclusively on immunization. (The nurse's role in immunization of children is discussed in Chapter 8.)

Control measures to prevent spread of the disease include appropriate isolation and early definitive treatment when necessary. The nurse is responsible for instructing parents regarding isolation techniques. The most important procedure to stress is handwashing. Persons directly caring for the child or handling contaminated articles must wash their hands before and after leaving the room. The child should be instructed to practice good handwashing technique after toileting and before eating. He should be con-

fined to his room (preferably alone, but not necessarily so) until the period of communicability is over.

With the exception of those diseases requiring strict isolation, no special precautions need to be observed in cleaning the child's room, intimate articles, or clothing. However, the child should use disposable tissues that are discarded in a sealed plastic bag. His eating and drinking utensils should not be shared by others, unless washed thoroughly beforehand. His room should be aired and cleaned without spraying dust in the air. Vacuuming is preferable to using a dust mop, and sheets should be collected and placed in a receptacle, not shaken in the room.

For those diseases spread by droplets, the nurse instructs parents in measures aimed at reducing airborne transmission. If the child is old enough, he should cover his face during coughing or sneezing; otherwise the parent should cover the child's mouth with a tissue and then dis-

SUMMARY OF NURSING CARE OF THE CHILD WITH A COMMUNICABLE DISEASE

GOALS	RESPONSIBILITIES
Assist in identifying etiologic agent	Recognize exanthema associated with communicable diseases (Table 12-1) Operate under a high index of suspicion for children who are susceptible to infectious diseases Identify high-risk children to whom communicable disease may be fatal; in case of an outbreak, advise parents to confine child to the home Assist in performing tests used to identify the organism, such as collection of specimens for culture Be aware of significance of test results in terms of the etiologic agent and child's level of immunity
Prevent occurrence of the disease	Participate in public education regarding prophylactic immunizations, method of spread of communicable diseases, and proper preparation and handling of food and water supplies Participate in immunization programs or screening program to identify streptococcal infections
Prevent spread of the disease	Institute appropriate isolation procedures Post isolation procedures on door to child's room Make referral to public health nurse when necessary to ensure appropriate isolation procedures in the home Work with families to ensure compliance with therapeutic regimens Identify close contacts who may require prophylactic treatment (specific immune globulin or antibiotics) Report disease to local health department
Prepare child for isolation	Explain reason for confinement and use of any special precautions Allow child to play with gloves, mask, and gown Always introduce yourself to child and allow him to see your face before donning protective clothing Provide diversionary activity Encourage parents to remain with child during hospitalization Help child view isolation experience as challenging rather than solely negative Discontinue isolation as soon as period of communicability is over; discuss this with parents if child is at home
Provide comfort measures	Schedule analgesics and antipyretics for maximum relief of discomfort Maintain bed rest; administer complete care as needed Keep mucous membranes moist with use of cool-mist vaporizer, gargles, and lozenges Apply petrolatum to chapped lips or nares Clean eyes with physiologic saline solution Keep skin clean (change bedclothes and linens at least daily) Administer oral hygiene
Prevent complications	Ensure compliance with therapeutic regime (bed rest, antibiotics, adequate hydration) Institute seizure precautions if febrile convulsions are a possibility Monitor temperature; unexpected elevations may signal a secondary infection Attend to good body hygiene Prevent child from scratching the skin; keep nails short and clean; apply mittens or elbow restraints Ensure adequate hydration with small frequent sips of water or favorite drinks and soft, bland foods (gelatin, pudding, ice cream, soups); refeed after vomiting; observe for signs of dehydration
Provide emotional support	Recognize loneliness imposed by isolation; encourage contact with friends via telephone (in hospital can use intercom between room and nurse's station) Reinforce parents' effort to carry out plan of care Provide assistance when necessary, such as visiting nurse to help with home care Keep parents aware of child's progress; stress rapidity of recovery in most cases

card it. Persons who are susceptible to the disease should not come close to the child unless special precautions are taken.

Whenever the child is hospitalized, rigid adherence to appropriate isolation procedures is required. It is the nurse's responsibility to ensure that the correct isolation procedures are instituted and properly implemented. In the case of a child who is admitted with an undiagnosed exanthema, strict isolation is instituted until a diagnosis is established. To facilitate nursing care and minimize the possibility of spread of infection, nursing activities are organized to allow for the least number of trips in and out of the room. Suggestions for preparing the child for isolation are discussed in Chapter 18.

In suggesting isolation procedures for the home, the nurse considers the family's cultural and socioeconomic background. For example, it is useless to recommend confining the child to his own room if the entire family sleeps together. A more appropriate suggestion would be to select a sleeping area, such as a couch or one end of the bed, that is not in direct contact with the other members. Ideally the best approach is to make a home visit and suggest practical measures based on the family's living situation. During a visit the nurse also questions other family members about symptoms suggestive of the disease.

Nursing care of the child with a communicable disease is summarized in the boxed material (opposite); since most of the diseases are associated with skin manifestations, the reader is also referred to Chapter 27 for a discussion of nursing care in dermatologic conditions.

TONSILLITIS

The *tonsils* are masses of lymphoid tissue located in the pharyngeal cavity. Their function is to filter and protect the respiratory and alimentary tracts from invasion by pathogenic organisms. They also may have a role in antibody formation. Although the size of tonsils varies, children generally have much larger tonsils than adolescents or adults. This difference is thought to be a protective mechanism at a time when young children are especially susceptible to upper respiratory infection.

Several pairs of tonsils encircle the pharynx (Fig. 12-5). The *palatine* or *faucial* tonsils are located on either side of the oropharynx, behind and below the pillars of the fauces (opening from the mouth). A free surface of the palatine tonsils is usually visible during oral examination. The palatine tonsils are the pair of tonsils usually removed surgically during tonsillectomy. Above these are the *pharyngeal* tonsils, also known as the *adenoids*. They are located in the posterior wall of the nasopharynx, opposite the posterior nares. Their proximity to the nares and eus-

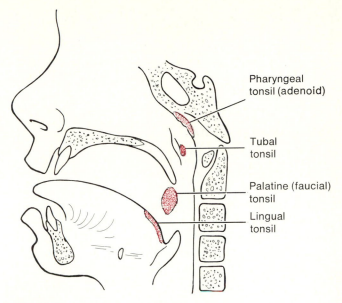

FIG. 12-5
Location of the various tonsillar masses.

tachian tubes causes difficulties in instances of inflammation. The *lingual* tonsils are located at the base of the tongue and only rarely are removed. The *tubal* tonsils are found near the posterior nasopharyngeal opening of the eustachian tubes.

Etiology

Tonsillitis usually occurs as a result of pharyngitis—inflammation of the structures of the pharynx. Because of the normally abundant amount of lymphoid tissue and the frequency of upper respiratory infection in young children, tonsillitis is a very common cause of morbidity. The causative agent may be viral or bacterial. About 15% of the cases of pharyngitis are caused by group A β-hemolytic streptococci.

Pathophysiology and clinical manifestations

The pathology and clinical manifestations of tonsillitis are chiefly caused by inflammation. As the palatine or faucial tonsils enlarge as a result of edema, they may meet in the midline (sometimes called kissing tonsils), obstructing the passage of air or food. The child has difficulty in swallowing and breathing. Enlargement of the adenoids blocks the space behind the posterior nares, making it difficult or impossible for air to pass from the nose to the throat. As a result the child breathes through the mouth.

If mouth breathing is continuous, the mucous membranes of the oropharynx become dry and irritated. There may be an offensive mouth odor, and the senses of taste and smell are impaired. Because air cannot be trapped for proper speech sounds, the voice has a nasal and muffled quality. A persistent, harassing cough is also common. Because of the proximity of the adenoids to the eustachian tubes, this passageway is frequently blocked in adenoiditis. As a result normal drainage is impaired and otitis media frequently occurs.

Diagnostic evaluation

Diagnosis of tonsillitis is easily confirmed on visualization of the oropharynx. However, it is often difficult to diagnose which cases are viral and which are bacterial from clinical manifestations alone. Table 12-2 contrasts some of the more typical findings characteristic of viral or bacterial pharyngitis. The only reliable method for differentiating the specific cause is a throat culture, which is read within 24 hours.

Therapeutic management

Treatment of viral pharyngitis is symptomatic, because the illness is self-limiting. Throat cultures that are positive for group A β-hemolytic streptococci warrant antibiotic treatment. A 10-day schedule of oral drug therapy, such as penicillin, is necessary to totally eradicate the bacilli. However, noncompliance is a major problem in the efficacy of this treatment. For this reason many physicians advocate administering an intramuscular dose of parenteral benzathine penicillin G, which maintains substantial blood levels for at least 10 days.

Surgical treatment of chronic tonsillitis is a controversial subject. Tonsillectomy is the most frequently performed pediatric surgical procedure. Many authorities believe they are unnecessary, except in selected cases. These include persons who have persistent chronic sore throats that result in significant morbidity, those who have respiratory distress from retropharyngeal obstruction, or those who are carriers of diphtheria.

Generally, removal of the tonsils should occur after 3 or 4 years of age because of the problem of excessive blood loss in small children and the possibility of regrowth or hypertrophy of lymphoid tissue. The tubal and lingual tonsils often enlarge to compensate for the lost lymphoid tissue, resulting in continued pharyngeal and eustachian tube obstruction.

Adenoidectomy (removal of the adenoids) is recommended for children with recurrent otitis media to prevent hearing loss and for those children in which hypertrophied adenoids obstruct nasal breathing. Their removal may be warranted in the child under 3 years of age and should be performed without a tonsillectomy. Follow-up after adenoidectomy should include assessment of hearing, smell, and taste for expected improvement.

Nursing considerations

Nursing care of the child with tonsillitis and/or pharyngitis mainly involves providing comfort. A soft to liquid diet is generally preferred. A cool-mist vaporizer helps keep the mucous membranes moist during periods of mouth breathing. Warm, saltwater gargles, throat lozenges, and analgesic/antipyretic drugs such as acetaminophen (Tylenol) are useful to promote comfort.

If antibiotics are prescribed, parents need counseling regarding their correct administration (see p. 567) and the necessity of completing the treatment period. If injections are given, they must be administered deeply into a large muscle mass, such as the vastus lateralis or the gluteus muscle in older children. Parents need to be aware of the residual tenderness, which may cause the child to limp for a day or two. Local applications of heat are helpful in relieving some of the discomfort.

If surgery is indicated, the child requires the same psychologic preparation and physical care needed for any other operation (see Chapter 19). The following discussion focuses on the nursing care that is specific for tonsillectomy and adenoidectomy.

Preoperative care. A complete history is taken, and since the operative site is highly vascular, special notation is made of any bleeding tendencies. Bleeding and clotting times are included in the usual blood work. The

TABLE 12-2. COMPARISON OF SIGNS AND SYMPTOMS OF VIRAL vs BACTERIAL PHARYNGITIS (TONSILLITIS)

VIRAL PHARYNGITIS	BACTERIAL (STREPTOCOCCAL) PHARYNGITIS
Gradual onset	More abrupt onset
Low-grade fever	Fever increased to 40° C (104° F)
Headache, rhinitis, cough, and hoarseness occur after 1 or 2 days of fever	Conjunctivitis, rhinitis, cough, or hoarseness uncommon
	Headache, severe sore throat, and abdominal pain more common
Slight erythema of pharynx and slight or moderate enlargement of tonsils	White exudate on posterior pharynx and tonsils; erythema and enlargement of tonsils
Firm, tender cervical lymph nodes may be present	Localized firm, tender cervical lymph nodes common
Child is moderately ill for 1-5 days	Child is acutely ill for as long as 2 weeks

presence of any loose teeth is noted during physical assessment.

Postoperative care. Postoperative nursing objectives include measures to relieve the pain, positioning to avoid aspiration, and observation of signs of hemorrhage. The throat is very sore after surgery. An ice collar may provide relief, but many children find it bothersome and prefer not to have it. Analgesics are usually ordered but may need to be given rectally or intramuscularly to avoid the oral route. If children are very irritable, mild sedation is helpful to lessen crying, which irritates the operative site, increasing the chance of bleeding.

Before the child is fully awake he is placed on his abdomen or side to facilitate drainage of secretions. If suctioning is needed, it is performed carefully to avoid any trauma to the oropharynx. When alert the child may prefer sitting up, although he should remain in bed for the rest of the day. Some secretions are common, particularly dried blood from surgery. Dark brown blood is usually present in the emesis, as well as in the nose and between the teeth. If parents do not expect this, they may be frightened at a time when they need to be calm and reassuring for the child.

Food and fluid are restricted until the child is fully alert and there are no signs of hemorrhage. Cool water or fruit juice is given first, although fluids with a red or brown color are avoided in order to distinguish fresh or old blood in emesis from the ingested liquid. The use of straws has been advised against because sucking may precipitate bleeding, however, this is not universally accepted. Citrus juice is usually poorly tolerated because of the discomfort it causes. Milk, ice cream, and pudding are not offered until after clear fluids are retained, because milk products coat the mouth and throat, causing the child to try and clear the throat more often, which may initiate bleeding. Soft foods, particularly gelatin, cooked fruits, sherbet, soup, and mashed potatoes, are started on the first or second postoperative day or as the child tolerates them. Eating promotes healing because it increases the blood supply to the tissues.

Postoperative hemorrhage is not usual, but it can occur. The most obvious early sign is the child's continuous swallowing of the trickling blood. The nurse directly observes the throat for bleeding, using a good source of light and if necessary, carefully inserting a tongue depressor. If the child is asleep, the frequency of swallowing is noted. Other signs of hemorrhage include increased pulse (above 120 beats/minute), pallor, frequent clearing of the throat, and vomiting of bright red blood. Restlessness, an indication of hemorrhage, may be difficult to differentiate from general discomfort after surgery. Decreasing blood pressure is a later sign and signals impending shock.

SUMMARY OF NURSING CARE OF THE CHILD WITH A TONSILLECTOMY

GOALS	RESPONSIBILITIES
Preoperative Prepare for hospitalization and surgery	(See preparations for hospitalization and surgery in Chapter 18 and 19) Order bleeding and clotting time Explain to the child that he will have a sore throat when he awakens but will be able to talk Explain what he can expect when he returns to his room, especially his positioning in bed and expectoration of blood and mucus Emphasize adventurous aspect of the experience, such as riding a gurney, seeing new places
Postoperative Assess general status	(See general postoperative care, Chapter 19)

Detect extent of bleeding	Take pulse and respiration frequently
	Assess skin color
	Be alert for
	   Restlessness
	   More than usual frequency of swallowing
	   Frequent clearing of throat
	   Nausea and vomiting
	Inspect throat for signs of oozing
	   Insert tongue depressor carefully
	   Use good light source
	Inspect any vomitus for evidence of fresh bleeding (blood-tinged mucus expected; may be small amounts of old blood)

Continued.

SUMMARY OF NURSING CARE OF THE CHILD WITH A TONSILLECTOMY—cont'd

GOALS	RESPONSIBILITIES
Prevent bleeding	Discourage child from coughing frequently or clearing his throat Avoid use of gargles or hard objects in mouth such as toothbrush
Provide adequate hydration	Monitor intravenous infusion (if any) Offer fluids as tolerated after child has fully recovered from anesthetic and shows no evidence of bleeding Avoid fluids with red or brown color that may be confused with bleeding Assess state of hydration

Provide nourishment	Offer diet as tolerated
	   Cool liquid diet for 12 to 24 hours
	   Soft diet thereafter
	   Advance to regular diet as recommended
	Avoid substances that irritate denuded areas

Facilitate drainage	Position child on his side or stomach while sleeping

Promote comfort	Offer cool, soothing liquids as appropriate
	Avoid irritation to tonsillar area
	Administer analgesics as prescribed
	Apply cool compresses or ice collar to throat if desired or tolerated
	Keep perioral area clean and free of mucus and blood
	Change child's clothing and linen as soon as soiled or damp from perspiration
	   Place plastic-lined pads or other easily removed protected covering under head
	   Provide meticulous mouth care, avoiding insertion of hard objects into mouth (except tongue depressor to inspect pharynx)

Reduce anxiety	Explain source of discomfort Remain with child or allow significant persons to be with child Anticipate needs Keep child and bed free from any blood-tinged excretions Reassure the child regarding any blood-tinged drainage Keep emesis basin within easy reach Make certain the child has call light or other signal device within reach

If continuous bleeding is suspected, the physician is notified immediately since surgery may be required to ligate the bleeding vessel. Airway obstruction may occur as a result of edema or accumulated secretions and is indicated by progressive cyanosis. Suction equipment should always be set up at the bedside after tonsillectomy.

Discharge instructions include (1) avoiding foods that are irritating or highly seasoned, (2) avoiding the use of gargles or vigorous toothbrushing, (3) discouraging the child from coughing or clearing the throat, and (4) using mild analgesics or an ice collar for pain. Hemorrhage may occur 5 to 10 days after surgery, as a result of tissue sloughing from the healing process. Any sign of bleeding warrants immediate medical attention. Objectionable mouth odor and slight ear pain with a low-grade fever are common occurrences for a few days postoperatively. How-

ever, persistent severe earache, fever, or cough necessitates medical evaluation. The child's voice may be altered for some time after surgery. Most children are ready to resume normal activity within 1 to 2 weeks after the operation.

Emotional care. A tonsillectomy and/or adenoidectomy often represent the first hospitalization experience for the child. Since the surgery is usually an elective procedure, there is ample opportunity to prepare both the child and parents for this event. Both need reassurance regarding what to expect at the time of admission, before and after surgery, and at discharge. Parents are encouraged to visit often or room in if possible and participate in the child's care if they wish. The child is honestly appraised of postoperative discomfort and reassured that he will be able to talk. Sometimes children believe that the operation will

SUMMARY OF NURSING CARE OF THE CHILD WITH A TONSILLECTOMY—cont'd

GOALS	RESPONSIBILITIES

Reassure parents	Explain what to expect
	    Appearance of child following surgery
	    Expectoration of blood-tinged mucus
	    Temporary alteration in voice
	    General morbidity
	Answer questions
	Explore fears and anxieties regarding child's status and expectations
	Explain what child is permitted to do

Instruct parents regarding home care	
Expected signs and symptoms	Appearance of wound area—white membrane covering denuded area Sore throat for 7 to 10 days Child may complain of ear discomfort, especially on swallowing These minor complaints may awaken child at night
Unexpected signs and symptoms	Bleeding—if occurs, will be either day of surgery or 5th to 10th day postoperatively when membrane sloughs from operative site Infection
Diet	Provide liquids and soft foods as tolerated for 1 week; general diet thereafter Avoid acid foods (citrus fruit, fruit juices) and foods that may irritate wound area (toast crusts, raw vegetables, potato chips)
Activity	Encourage quiet activities Keep quiet and indoors for first 3 days Child may be outside if weather permits for next week Child may return to school at approximately 10 to 14 days postoperatively Avoid exposure to persons with infections
Discomfort	Administer analgesics Provide cool liquids
Assistance	Make certain parents know where to call for help if needed Remind regarding checkup appointment, usually 2 weeks following surgery

immediately "make the throat all better" and are dismayed to find that it still hurts after the surgery. Ideally, the child should have an opportunity to discuss his experiences to gain a feeling of mastery and to overcome any fears or misconceptions.

OTITIS MEDIA (OM)

Otitis media, middle ear infection, is one of the most common early childhood diseases, particularly as a complication of upper respiratory infection, respiratory allergy, adenoiditis, or unrepaired cleft palate. The classifications of otitis media are:

1. *Acute or chronic suppurative otitis media,* in which bacterial or viral agents cause a purulent exudate to accumulate behind the eardrum in the space of the middle ear.

2. *Serous (secretory) or nonsuppurative otitis media,* in which a nonpurulent sterile mucoid effusion collects as a result of blocked eustachian tubes. When the effusion is thick, serous otitis media is sometimes referred to as *glue ear.*

Etiology

Acute suppurative otitis media is frequently caused by *Hemophilus influenzae,* pneumococci, or streptococci. Chronic suppurative otitis media is most often a result of inadequately treated acute otitis media, recurrent adenoiditis, or unrepaired cleft palate. The etiology of the serous type is unknown, although it frequently results from blocked eustachian tubes from the edema of allergic rhinitis or hypertrophic adenoids.

Pathophysiology

Otitis media is primarily the result of dysfunctioning eustachian tubes. The eustachian tube connects the middle ear to the nasopharynx. Normally it is closed and flat, preventing organisms from the pharyngeal cavity from entering the middle ear. It opens to allow drainage of secretions produced by the middle ear mucosa and to equalize air pressure between the middle ear and outside environment.

If the tubes are blocked these protective functions cannot occur. With drainage impaired, the normal secretions are retained (serous type). The air that cannot escape or equalize through the blocked tube is absorbed through the vascular circulation, causing a negative pressure within the middle ear. If the tube opens, bacteria are swept up through the tube into the middle chamber as a result of this difference in pressure. Once inside the middle ear, the organisms quickly proliferate and invade the mucosa (suppurative type).

Clinical manifestations

As purulent fluid accumulates in the small space of the middle ear chamber, pain results from the pressure on surrounding structures. Infants become irritable and indicate their discomfort by holding or pulling at their ears and rolling their head from side to side. Young children will usually verbally complain of the pain. A temperature as high as 40° C (104° F) is common. Postauricular and cervical lymph glands may be enlarged. Rhinorrhea, vomiting, and diarrhea as well as signs of concurrent respiratory or pharyngeal infection may also be present. Anorexia is common, and sucking or chewing tends to aggravate the pain. As the exudate accumulates and as pressure increases, the tympanic membrane may rupture spontaneously. As a result there is an immediate relief of pain, a gradual decrease in temperature, and the presence of purulent discharge in the external auditory canal.

Severe pain or fever is usually absent in serous otitis media, and the child may not appear ill. Instead there is a feeling of "fullness" in the ear, a popping sensation during swallowing, and a feeling of "motion" in the ear if air is present above the level of fluid. Since chronic serous otitis media is the most frequent cause of conductive hearing loss in young children, audiometry may reveal deficient hearing.

Diagnostic evaluation

In acute otitis media, otoscopy reveals an intact membrane that appears bright red and bulging, with no visible bony landmarks or light reflex. In the serous type, otoscopic findings may include a slightly injected, dull gray membrane, obscured landmarks, and a visible fluid level or meniscus behind the eardrum, if air is present above the fluid.

Tympanometry may be used to measure the change in air pressure in the external auditory canal from movement of the eardrum. In otitis media, membrane mobility is decreased.

If purulent discharge is present, it should be cultured and a specific antibiotic chosen for that organism. Tympanocentesis (aspiration of middle ear fluid) is indicated for children with persistent infection.

Therapeutic management

Treatment of suppurative otitis media is administration of antibiotics, especially ampicillin. In some cases of otitis media aspiration of the fluid, surgical incision of the eardrum (myringotomy), or drainage of the middle ear with insertion of myringotomy tubes (also called tympanostomy tubes, pressure-equilizer [PE] tubes, grommets, or dottles) may be indicated. These tubes are usually inserted while the child is under general anesthesia in an outpatient surgical department. Mechanical drainage promotes better healing of the membrane and prevents scar formation and loss of elasticity. In cases of chronic otitis media, the tubes are left in place indefinitely.

Other measures include the use of analgesic/antipyretic drugs such as aspirin or acetaminophen to reduce the pain and fever. Although ear drops may promote comfort, they may not be used because they obscure a clear view of the tympanic membrane.

The medical management of serous otitis media is uncertain and controversial. The widespread use of decongestants and antihistamines to shrink the mucous membranes and increase eustachian tube function is of unproven benefit. In selected instances of chronic serous otitis media the insertion of myringotomy tubes may be necessary to continually drain and ventilate the middle ear. In any case the underlying cause should be investigated and properly treated.

Nursing considerations

Nursing objectives include relief of pain, facilitation of drainage when possible, and prevention of complications or recurrence. Analgesics are often very helpful to reduce the severe earache. Although acetaminophen is usually recommended for children, aspirin may be more effective in alleviating the pain. High fever, particularly in infants, should be reduced with antipyretic drugs and/or cool sponges to avoid febrile convulsions. The application of heat with a heating pad or hot water bottle wrapped in a towel may reduce the discomfort. Local heat should be placed over the ear with the child lying on the affected side. This position also facilitates drainage of the exudate

SUMMARY OF NURSING CARE OF THE CHILD WITH ACUTE OTITIS MEDIA (OM)

	RESPONSIBILITIES
Recognize overt and covert signs and symptoms	Assess for evidence of discomfort Be alert to sudden relief of pain from rupture of drum Inspect external auditory canal and observe for drainage Inspect tympanic membrane for redness, bulging, and/or puncture Assess for hearing impairment
Eliminate infective agent	Administer antibiotics as prescribed Promote compliance to medication regimen Emphasize to parents the importance of regular administration and completion of the course of therapy
Promote comfort	Position for comfort according to needs of individual child (usually lying on unaffected side or supine) Administer analgesics as needed and as prescribed at regular intervals for maximum comfort Apply external heat (with heating pad on low setting) or cool compresses Avoid chewing by offering liquid or soft foods
Reduce fever	Administer antipyretic drugs as needed Provide external cooling via tepid baths or sponges

Facilitate drainage when appropriate	Position with affected ear in dependent position, with child lying on affected side
	Maintain wick
	   Insert loosely
	   Change as needed

Prevent skin breakdown	Keep skin around ear and pinna clean and dry Protect skin with protective coat of zinc oxide or petrolatum (if permitted) Change ear wicks when soiled or wet (if used)
Prevent recurrence	Impress on caregiver the importance of following directions for administering medications Feed in upright position Encourage gentle nose blowing Teach Valsalva's maneuver Eliminate tobacco smoke and known allergens from environment
Educate parents	Teach correct administration of medications Refer to community agencies as appropriate Stress importance of regular hearing tests to assess early signs of impairment Teach to recognize signs of hearing impairment in the infant or child (see Chapter 17) Avoid excessive water in ear if myringotomy tubes were part of the therapy

if the eardrum has ruptured or if myringotomy was performed. An ice bag placed over the affected ear may also be beneficial since it reduces edema and pressure. If the child is cooperative either procedure can be tried to determine which offers maximum relief.

If the ear is draining, the external canal may be cleaned with sterile cotton swabs or pledgets soaked in hydrogen peroxide. If ear wicks or lightly rolled sterile gauze packs are placed in the ear after surgical treatment, they should be loose enough to allow accumulated drainage to flow out of the ear; otherwise the infection may be transferred to the mastoid process. Parents should be told to keep these wicks dry during shampoos or baths. Occasionally drainage is so perfuse that the auricle and the skin surrounding the ear become excoriated from the exudate. This is prevented by frequent cleansing and application of petrolatum or zinc oxide to the area.

A concern presented with the use of myringotomy tubes is the possibility of water entering the middle ear. Small amounts of water pose little hazard. However, a factor affecting the danger of water entering the ear is potential for introducing bacteria. Water from baths, showers, swimming pools, and fresh waters lakes is contaminated. In these situations, most ear plugs, while not water tight, prevent total flooding of the external canal and provide sufficient protection (Strome, 1983). Parents should be aware of the appearance of a grommet (usually tiny, white plastic spool-shaped tube) so that they can observe if it falls out. They are reassured that this is normal and requires no immediate intervention, although they should notify the physician.

Prevention of recurrence necessitates adequate parent education regarding antibiotic therapy. Antibiotics are frequently regarded as "miracle" drugs or as the "one-dose" cure for everything. Since the symptoms of pain and fever usually subside within 24 to 48 hours, the rapid outward signs of recovery support such thinking. Nurses must emphasize that, although the child looks well, the infection is not completely eradicated until all the prescribed medication is taken. Although one does not want to alarm parents, it is important to stress the potential complications of otitis media that can be prevented with adequate treatment and follow-up care. Such complications include (1) conductive hearing loss, (2) a perforated and scarred eardrum, (3) mastoiditis, an inflammation of the mastoid air cell system, (4) cholesteatoma, a cystlike lesion that can invade and destroy surrounding auditory structures, and (5) intracranial infections, such as meningitis.

The chances of otitis media may be reduced by sitting or holding the child upright for feedings, encouraging gentle nose blowing, especially during a cold, and promoting aeration of the middle ear through the modified Valsalva's maneuver, which involves pinching the nose, closing the lips, and forcing air up the eustachian tube. Young children can blow balloons or chew sugarless gum to accom-

plish the same goal. Eliminating tobacco smoke and known allergens is also recommended.

CONJUNCTIVITIS

Acute conjunctivitis in children is a common condition. It occurs from a variety of causes that are typically age related. For example, in the newborn period, chemical conjunctivitis is a frequent sequela of silver nitrate administration. In infants, recurrent conjunctivitis may be a sign of nasolacrimal duct obstruction. In children past infancy the usual causes are viral, bacterial, allergic, or related to a foreign body.

Clinical manifestations

The most common cause of conjunctivitis is a virus, usually in association with an upper respiratory infection. The eye appears swollen and reddened, and there is a serous (watery) drainage.

Bacterial conjunctivitis is often called "pink eye" and can be caused by a number of bacteria, including staphylococci. The distinguishing symptom is purulent drainage, causing crusting of the eyelids on awakening. The conjunctiva is inflamed and the lids are swollen. Frequently both eyes are infected.

A moderate conjunctivitis is associated with allergic causes. There is a watery to viscous stringy discharge, lid redness, swelling, and periorbital itching. Usually other signs of allergy such as sneezing are also present.

The chief sign of conjunctivitis caused by a foreign body is the limitation of symptoms to only one eye. In this case, the eye should be carefully examined.

Therapeutic management

Treatment of conjunctivitis depends on the cause. Viral conjunctivitis is self-limiting and treatment should be limited to removal of the accumulated secretions and avoidance of topical antibiotics or steroids.

Bacterial conjunctivitis is usually treated with topical antibacterial agents, such as sulfacetamide. Administration of ophthalmic drops every 1 to 2 hours is required since tears wash out the antibiotic solution. At bedtime an ointment preparation is preferred because it remains in the eye longer. Ointments are usually not used in the daytime because they blur vision.

Nursing considerations

Nursing goals primarily include keeping the eye clean and properly administering the ophthalmic medication. Accumulated secretions are always removed by wiping from the inner canthus downward and outward, away from the opposite eye. Warm moist compresses, such as a clean wash-cloth wrung out with hot tap water, are helpful in removing the crusts. Compresses are *not* kept on the eye because an occlusive covering promotes bacterial growth. Medication should be instilled immediately after the eyes have been cleaned and according to correct procedure (see Chapter 19).

Prevention of infection in other family members is an important consideration with bacterial conjunctivitis. The child's washcloth and towel are kept separate from those used by others. Tissues used to clean the eye are disposed of properly. The child should refrain from rubbing his eye and is instructed in good handwashing.

INGESTION OF INJURIOUS AGENTS

The high incidence of poisoning in children attests to the importance of its prevention and immediate treatment. The developmental factors predisposing the vulnerable high-risk group of toddlers and preschoolers to this accident and appropriate suggestions for prevention are discussed in Chapter 10.

Children are poisoned by a variety of ingested substances, including plants, soaps, detergents, household cleaners, vitamins, minerals, and drugs. This section is primarily concerned with the immediate emergency treatment of ingestion of injurious agents and the management of plant, salicylate, acetaminophen, and lead poisoning.

PRINCIPLES OF EMERGENCY MANAGEMENT

The first and most important principle in dealing with a child who has been poisoned is to treat the child first, not the poison. This necessitates an immediate concern for life support, including respiratory assistance, circulatory support, or control of seizures.

Termination of exposure

The initial step in emergency treatment is to terminate the exposure to the toxic substance. This includes (1) emptying the mouth of pills, plant parts, or other material, (2) thoroughly flushing the eyes and/or skin with tap water if they were involved, (3) removing contaminated clothing (for example, if gasoline had spilled), and (4) bringing the victim of an inhalation poisoning into fresh air. If a poison was swallowed, the child can be given water to dilute it. However, large amounts are contraindicated, since this may enhance the drug's escape through the py-

lorus. Once in the small intestine, absorption of the poison is rapid.

Identification

The next step is identifying the poison so that appropriate treatment can be instituted. This may involve searching for an empty bottle, an opened container, or other visible evidence of the ingested substance. Any substance from the child's body such as vomitus, stool, or urine is brought to the hospital. Likewise, the partial or completely empty container is also kept for possible clues to the exact composition of the toxic substance.

Since parents or baby-sitters are the most likely people to learn of the accident, they should be advised of these measures when they call the emergency squad, hospital, or poison control center (usually listed in the front of the telephone directory). When taking a call, the nurse should obtain the name and telephone number of the caller so contact can be reestablished if the connection is interrupted.

Removal

In general, the immediate treatment is to remove the ingested poison by inducing vomiting. The preferred method is to administer ipecac syrup, an emetic that exerts its action by direct stimulation of the vomiting center and an irritant effect on the gastric mucosa. Proper administration of this nonprescription drug is essential. The usual dose for children over 1 year of age is 15 ml (3 teaspoons) with one or two large glasses of water, which enhances the local irritant effect. A reduced dose can be given to infants, but only as prescribed by the physician. If emesis fails to occur within 20 minutes, a second dose is given *once*.

Gastric lavage may also be done to empty the stomach of the toxic agent. For example, it may be used in young infants when ipecac is contraindicated or when certain antiemetics have been ingested, which can inactivate the ipecac. Some authorities also advocate lavage in selected cases of petroleum distillate poisoning, but this is controversial. When lavage is performed, the largest diameter tube that can be inserted is used to facilitate passage of gastric contents.

The use of an emetic is generally contraindicated in the following instances:

1. If the person is comatose, in severe shock, or convulsing, or if he has lost the gag reflex, since any of these conditions increases the risk of aspiration
2. If the poison is a low-viscosity hydrocarbon, because if aspirated it can cause a severe chemical pneumonitis
3. If the poison is a strong corrosive (acid or alkali), because emesis of the corrosive redamages the mucosa of the esophagus and pharynx

Another method of decontaminating the stomach is the use of activated charcoal, an odorless, tasteless, fine black powder that adsorbs many compounds, creating a stable complex. It is used within 1 hour of the poisoning but *after* giving an emetic, since it will also adsorb the emetic, preventing its pharmacologic effect. It is mixed with water or saline cathartic to form a slurry, but it is often accepted more readily if disguised with flavoring agents, such as cherry syrup, and served through a straw.

When toxic substances cannot be removed, treatment is aimed at preventing further damage. With caustic or corrosive substances, the immediate action is to dilute the agent with water. Neutralization with vinegar or lemon juice is not recommended because the neutralizing reaction may produce heat, thus causing a thermal burn in addition to the chemical burn. Other aspects of care include providing a patent airway if necessary, administering analgesics for pain, and giving the child nothing by mouth or a liquid diet if tolerated. Long-term care may involve surgery to correct an esophageal stricture.

The immediate danger from hydrocarbons is aspiration, because even small amounts aspirated into the lungs can cause a severe, sometimes fatal, chemical pneumonitis. However, adverse systemic effects from gastrointes-

SUMMARY OF NURSING CARE OF THE CHILD WITH ACUTE POISONING

GOALS	RESPONSIBILITIES
General Identify that a poisoning has occurred	Call local poison control center, emergency facility, or physician for immediate advice regarding treatment Save all evidence of poison (container, vomitus, urine, and so on)
Remove poison	Dilute with water Induce vomiting except as contraindicated Administer ipecac syrup, 15 ml with 1 to 2 glasses of water; if vomiting has not occurred, repeat *once* in 20 minutes Administer activated charcoal only *after* inducing vomiting Prepare appropriate equipment for potential medical use, such as gastric lavage
Prevent aspiration of vomitus	Keep child's head lower than chest, place head between his legs, or position him on his side
Observe for latent symptoms and complications of poisoning	Treat as appropriate, for example, institute seizure precautions, keep warm and position correctly in case of shock, reduce temperature if hyperpyrexic, and so on
Support child and parent	Keep calm and quiet Do not admonish or accuse child or parent of wrongdoing
Prevent occurence and/or recurrence	Assess possible contributing factors in occurrence of accident, such as discipline, parent-child relationship, developmental ability, environmental factors, and behavior problems Institute anticipatory guidance for possible future accidents based on child's age and maturation level Refer to visiting nurse agency to evaluate home environment and need for safe-proofing measures Provide assistance with environmental manipulation when necessary
Petroleum distillates (hydrocarbons) Prevent ingestion	Teach parents proper storage of petroleum distillate products (kerosene, turpentine, gasoline, lighter fluid, furniture polish, metal polish, benzene, naphtha, some insecticides, cleaning fluid)

tinal absorption are usually mild. If small amounts have been ingested, treatment is symptomatic. In particular, the child is kept calm and relaxed to avoid the possibility of vomiting. Removal is indicated only when large amounts have been ingested or if the petroleum distillate is a vehicle for a more toxic substance (for example, a pesticide.

Treatment of symptoms

Treating the symptoms is another important aspect in the supportive management of poisoning. The increased re-

covery from acute poisonings is largely attributable to vigorous use of supportive measures after symptoms have begun. Since shock is a complication of several types of household poisons, particularly the petroleum distillates and corrosives, measures to reduce the effects of shock, such as elevation of legs and head to level of heart to promote venous drainage and provision of warmth and rest, are important. Maintenance of respiratory function may require mouth-to-mouth resuscitation or insertion of an airway and/or mechanical ventilation.

SUMMARY OF NURSING CARE OF THE CHILD WITH ACUTE POISONING—cont'd

GOALS	RESPONSIBILITIES
Identify ingestion of distillates	Recognize signs of toxicity Gagging, choking, and coughing; nausea; vomiting; alterations in sensorium, such as lethargy; weakness; respiratory symptoms of pulmonary involvement, such as tachypnea, cyanosis, retractions, grunting
Prevent further irritation	Avoid causing emesis Implement gastric lavage or emesis *only* as indicated
Treat pulmonary complications	(See nursing care of the child with pneumonia in Chapter 20)
Corrosives Prevent ingestion	Teach parents proper storage of corrosive products (oven and drain cleaners, electric dishwasher granules, strong detergents)
Identify ingestion	Recognize signs of toxicity Severe burning pain in mouth, throat, and stomach White, swollen mucous membranes, edema of lips, tongue, and pharynx (respiratory obstruction) Violent vomiting (hemoptysis) Signs of shock Anxiety and agitation
Maintain patent airway	Examine pharynx for burns Observe for respiratory difficulty Provide airway if necessary; have emergency equipment available Administer steroids if prescribed
Prevent further irritation	Avoid causing emesis Dilute with water if advised Give nothing by mouth except as ordered and tolerated
Provide comfort	Administer analgesics as needed

Nursing considerations

The emergency room nurse's responsibility is to be prepared for immediate intervention with any of the necessary equipment. Since time and speed are critical factors in recovery from several poisonings, anticipation of potential problems and complications may mean the difference between life and death.

Emotional support. A poisoning is more than a physical emergency for the child. It usually represents an emotional crisis for the parent, particularly in terms of guilt, self-reproach, and insecurity in the parenting role. The emergency room is no time to admonish the parent for negligence, lack of appropriate supervision, or failure to safe-proof the home. Rather it is a time to calm and support the child and parent while unaccusingly exploring the circumstances of the accident. If the nurse prematurely attempts to discuss ways of preventing such an accident from recurring, the parent's anxiety will block out any suggestions or offered guidance. Instead, it is preferable to delay the discussion until the child's condition is stabilized or, if the child is discharged immediately after emergency treatment, to make a public health referral.

Prevention of recurrence. The ultimate objective is to prevent poisonings from occurring or recurring. This involves counseling the parent regarding those events that increased the risk of poisoning and appropriate education to reduce future risk. One method of identifying risk areas is to ask specific questions about the events of the actual poisoning, such as where the poison was stored. In this way the nurse can provide constructive advice based on identification of an area that needs improvement. The subject of accident prevention is introduced in a nonjudgmental, nonaccusing manner for the parent to accept the information and incorporate the suggestions in the home. One method of accomplishing effective counseling for accident prevention is first to discuss the difficulties of constantly watching and safeguarding young children. In this way the monumental task of raising children is shared as a common problem, with accident prevention as one part of the parental role, not as the central issue.

PLANTS

Ingestion of plant parts is a very common cause of childhood poisoning. Fortunately, most of these children are not seriously affected and do not require hospitalization. However, some are severely, even fatally, poisoned. Given the abundance of plants both in and outside the home, it is essential that parents be advised of this danger. Table 12-3 lists some of the more common poisonous plants as well as non-toxic varieties that can be safely grown. Other preventive measures include (1) placing houseplants out of young children's reach, such as on high

TABLE 12-3. POISONOUS AND NONPOISONOUS PLANTS

POISONOUS PLANTS	TOXIC PARTS	NONPOISONOUS PLANTS
Apricot	Leaves, stem, seed pits	African violet
Azalea	Foliage and flowers	Aluminum plant
		Boston fern
Buttercup	All parts	Coleus
Cherry (wild or cultivated)	Twigs and foliage	Gardenia
		Grape ivy
		Jade plant
		Piggyback begonia
Daffodil	Bulbs	Piggyback plant
Dumb cane, Dieffenbachia	All parts	Prayer plant
		Rubber tree
		Snake plant
Elephant ear	All parts	Spider plant
Foxglove	Leaves, seeds, flowers	Wax plant
		Zebra plant
Holly, mistletoe	Berries	
Hyacinth	Bulbs	
Ivy	Leaves	
Oak tree	Acorn, foliage	
Philodendron	All parts	
Poinsettia	Leaves	
Poison ivy, poison oak	Leaves, fruit, stems, smoke from burning plants	
Rhubarb	Leaves	
Tulip	Bulbs	
Water hemlock	All parts	
Wisteria	Seeds, pods	

shelves or in hanging baskets, (2) teaching children *never* to eat anything without parental permission, and (3) avoid making teas or homemade medicines from plants. In the event of a poisoning, the same measures as outlined for emergency treatment are followed.

SALICYLATE POISONING

Aspirin ranks as one of the most frequently ingested drugs among children. One of the reasons for this is the readily available source of aspirin in most homes and the stimulus of observing parents readily take aspirin themselves. It may also result from children's inability to differentiate between candy and medicine. Children's aspirin has a delicious, orange flavor, and parents sometimes induce children to take tablets by emphasizing the appealing taste.

Under present law, children's aspirin is packaged in small quantities in a safety-cap bottle as a preventive measure to reduce the chance of overdose. However, no such regulation pertains to adult strength aspirin, and, even with child guard caps, some children are able to open the container and ingest the contents. Since the adult 5-grain tablets are four times stronger than the children's preparation, it takes fewer adult strength aspirin to cause toxicity.

Time-released aspirin is a particularly lethal preparation for children since symptoms are delayed for several hours. In addition this type of aspirin is frequently used by people with arthritis who find the safety caps very difficult to open. As a result they may transfer the drug to an ordinary container or incorrectly replace the safety cap. Either of these possibilities increases the chance of young children gaining access to the drug and accidentally ingesting it.

Etiology

Salicylate poisoning usually results from acute overdose. The *toxic* dose is approximately 2 grains/pound (4.4 grains/kg) of body weight, and the *lethal* dose is from 3 to 4 grains/pound (6.6 to 8.8 grains/kg). For a child who weighs 20 pounds (9 kg), toxicity occurs with eight adult aspirin or 32 baby aspirin (1.25 grains).

Another cause is therapeutic overdose, which results in chronic poisoning. It can occur when parents give the child frequent doses of aspirin for several days or combine it with other aspirin-containing drugs, such as cold preparations. The symptoms of chronic poisoning are similar to acute overdose but are more subtle in onset and may be confused with the illness being treated. Therefore, this is more difficult to diagnose.

Pathophysiology and clinical manifestations

Toxic amounts of salicylates directly affect the respiratory system. Hyperventilation, the most impressive clinical manifestation of salicylate overdose, causes loss of carbon dioxide and respiratory alkalosis. Signs of respiratory alkalosis include confusion, loss of consciousness, and, if not treated, coma and death from respiratory failure.

Salicylates also increase metabolism, resulting in greater oxygen consumption, carbon dioxide production, and heat production, which is manifest as hyperpyrexia. Metabolic acidosis occurs from the accumulation of ketones and other organic acids and results in symptoms of anorexia, vomiting, and diaphoresis.

In chronic overdose, salicylates can cause bleeding tendencies since aspirin inhibits platelet aggregation and prothrombin production.

Diagnostic evaluation

Aspirin exerts its peak effect in 2 to 4 hours, and its effects may last for as long as 18 hours. There is usually a delay of up to 6 hours before evidence of toxicity is noted. This delay represents a serious diagnostic problem, since by the time symptoms are evident, pathophysiologic disturbances are fairly advanced.

Because of the delay in symptoms, laboratory tests to determine serum salicylate levels are essential. These levels are compared to a special chart (nomogram) that determines the degree of toxicity from the time of ingestion.

Therapeutic management

The immediate treatment of salicylism is to remove the drug from the stomach either by forced emesis or gastric lavage. Since an appreciable amount may have been absorbed before the stomach was emptied and because side effects are slow to develop, the child should be observed for 12 to 24 hours.

Further therapy depends on the clinical manifestations. The acid-base disturbances are treated with appropriate electrolyte transfusions. Intravenous administration of sodium bicarbonate facilitates salicylate excretion. Calories and fluids are supplied to meet the increased metabolic rate. The hyperpyrexia is controlled with cool sponges or hypothermia blankets to reduce the possibility of convulsions. Vitamin K may be administered to decrease the bleeding tendencies. In extreme cases of salicylate poisoning, external removal of the drug may be attempted through peritoneal dialysis or hemodialysis, but such intervention is usually reserved for cases of life-threatening salicylism.

A major problem exists after accidental ingestion of time-released aspirin, since symptoms may not arise until 6 to 16 hours have elapsed. Cathartics and colonic irrigations are helpful in removing the unabsorbed drug, and in severe cases dialysis may be necessary.

Nursing considerations

The major nursing objectives are removal of the poison, observation of latent effects of overdose, assistance with any medical treatments of the complications, prevention of recurrence of the poisoning, and emotional support of the child and parents.

Parents of children suffering from chronic overdose need an understanding of the potential danger in giving too much aspirin and instruction regarding correct dosage (see Table 19-2). They should be advised to call a physician if symptoms such as fever or pain persist, rather than continuing to treat them with multiple doses of aspirin.

SUMMARY OF NURSING CARE OF THE CHILD WITH SALICYLATE POISONING (SALICYLISM)

GOALS	RESPONSIBILITIES
Prevent salicylate poisoning	Educate parents regarding safe storage of aspirin Teach parents to take aspirin or other drugs out of the sight of children Teach children the hazards of ingesting nonfood items without supervision Caution family against leaving aspirin within reach of children Caution against keeping large amounts of the drug on hand, especially children's varieties Discourage transferring aspirin to containers without safety caps Discuss problems of discipline and children's noncompliance Instruct parents regarding correct administration of aspirin for therapeutic purposes and to discontinue drug if evidence of mild toxicity

Identify salicylate overdose	Recognize signs of mild salicylate toxicity: ringing in the ears, dizziness, disturbances of hearing and vision, sweating, nausea, vomiting, diarrhea, delirium
	Recognize signs of salicylate poisoning
	    Evidence of ingestion of the drug, such as empty bottle
	    Hyperventilation, hyperpyrexia, and vomiting
	Order or obtain blood for analysis of salicylate levels
	Obtain urine specimen

Empty stomach	Induce vomiting Administer ipecac syrup Assist with gastric lavage, if appropriate
Adsorb drug remaining in stomach	Administer activated charcoal after ipecac syrup
Increase excretion of salicylates	Administer saline cathartic Assist with peritoneal dialysis, hemodialysis, or exchange transfusion, if necessary Administer intravenous fluids as prescribed
Correct electrolyte imbalance	Assess blood gases and serum electrolyte concentration frequently Administer sodium bicarbonate and administer electrolytes as indicated
Prevent and/or detect bleeding	Administer vitamin K Insert nasogastric tube to detect any gastric bleeding Assess stools for occult blood (guaiac test)
Maintain hydration	Monitor intravenous infusion Measure intake and output Check urine specific gravity
Reduce temperature	Administer tepid sponges Place on cooling blanket
Monitor status	Take vital signs frequently Obtain serial blood and urine specimens Assess level of consciousness and other neurologic signs
Control seizure activity	Administer anticonvulsants Implement seizure precautions
Support child	Explain procedures and tests according to developmental level of the child Allow for expression of feelings Provide comfort measures Encourage parents to visit (For care of the unconscious child, see Chapter 25)
Support parents	Allow expression of feelings regarding circumstances related to poisoning Provide reassurance as appropriate Explain therapies and tests Keep informed of child's progress Avoid placing blame

ACETAMINOPHEN POISONING

Acetaminophen is used increasingly as a mild analgesic/antipyretic drug, especially as a substitute drug for aspirin. The extensive availability of this nonprescription medication increases the probability of accidental ingestion of toxic quantities by infants and children. Like aspirin, acetaminophen is available in many palatable forms that are well accepted by youngsters.

Etiology

Acetaminophen poisoning occurs from acute overdose. Unlike aspirin, which can result in overdose from chronic therapeutic use, acetaminophen does not cause toxicity from continued use of recommended dosages. Recommended dosages for children are listed in Table 19-3. The precise toxic dose is uncertain, though dosages significantly greater than recommended levels can produce toxicity.

Pathophysiology

Acute overdose of acetaminophen results in hepatic damage. The damage is not from the drug itself but from one of its metabolites, which in large quantities binds to the liver cells. Over a period of days there may be liver dysfunction and possible hepatic failure.

Clinical manifestations

During the first 12 to 24 hours there are signs of nausea, vomiting, anorexia, sweating, and pallor. Some patients recover completely at this point, but others experience a latent phase of up to 4 days, when signs of liver involvement begin. The first sign is pain in the right upper quadrant followed by signs of hepatic damage. If the toxicity is not treated, hepatic failure, coma, and death can occur.

Diagnostic evaluation

Because of the initially mild symptoms, diagnosis is confirmed by serum acetaminophen levels (similar to aspirin). Liver and renal function tests are performed to assess the pathologic effect of toxicity on these organs.

Therapeutic management

Initial management is removal of the drug with emesis or lavage. Activated charcoal is not given because it interferes with the definitive treatment—the use of the antidote *N*-acetylcysteine (Mucomyst). *N*-acetylcysteine binds with the metabolite so that the liver is protected. It is given orally (mixed with cola or fruit juice) or via nasogastric tube. Because of its offensive odor (similar to rotten eggs) it may be accepted more readily if given by the nasogastric route. If vomiting occurs within 1 hour of administration of *N*-acetylcysteine, the dose is repeated.

Nursing considerations

Nursing goals are essentially the same as those discussed under salicylate poisoning. The nurse needs to be familiar with acetaminophen preparations in order to identify pos-

---

SUMMARY OF NURSING CARE FOR THE CHILD WITH ACETAMINOPHEN POISONING

GOALS	RESPONSIBILITIES
Prevent overdose	See salicylism, (p. 354)
Identify acetaminophen overdose	Recognize signs of overdose: profuse sweating, nausea and vomiting, skin eruptions, weakness, cyanosis, slow, weak pulse, depressed respirations, decreased urine output, hypothermia, circulatory collapse, coma Order or obtain serum acetaminophen level
Decrease absorption of drug	Induce vomiting with ipecac Assist with lavage Employ caution in fluid administration Administer antidote (*N*-acetylcysteine) if ordered
Monitor status	Attach to electrocardiograph monitor Measure intake and output Take vital signs frequently Obtain blood for hepatic and renal function tests
Support child and family	See salicylism, p. 354

sible ingestion. For example, cold remedies may contain acetaminophen in excessive amounts. However, if the nurse is unaware of this, the potential source of an acute overdose may be missed.

As with any poisoning, the primary goal is prevention. With the present emphasis on acetaminophen as a "safe" substitute for aspirin, it is important to stress that in excess this drug, like any other, is capable of toxic and lethal side effects.

HEAVY METAL POISONING

Heavy metal poisoning can occur from a variety of substances. The most common is lead. Other sources are iron from medicinal supplement preparations and mercury, found mostly in excessive quantities of seafood harvested from polluted waters. Another source of mercury poisoning is from the elemental form found in thermometers. Elemental mercury is nontoxic when ingested but poisonous when inhaled.

Heavy metals have an affinity for certain essential tissue chemicals, which must remain free for adequate cell functioning. When metals are bound to these substances, cellular enzyme systems are inactivated. Consequently the pathologic effects and treatment are similar to those for lead poisoning.

Lead poisoning (plumbism)

Lead poisoning is a prevalent pediatric problem. In 1980 more than 25,000 children were identified as having lead toxicity, and the Centers for Disease Control (1981) conclude that this in an underestimate of the magnitude of the problem. Black children have a six times greater incidence than white children. The peak age is from 2 to 3 years, and most poisoning occurs in warm weather months.

Etiology. The exact reason why children ingest lead is unknown; however, several factors usually influence the ingestion of lead-containing substances.

Environmental characteristics. The first necessary factor is the availability of lead in the environment. Lead enters the system either by ingestion or inhalation; the boxed material lists the more common sources. Lead-based paint from dilapidated housing remains the most frequent high-dose source of lead. Although the child's immediate environment is usually the source of lead, other living conditions should be investigated, such as nursery or daycare centers. A few chips of paint may contain several hundred times the usual safe daily ingestion of lead.

Characteristics of child. Developmentally young children are at risk for lead poisoning because of their high level of oral activity. Particularly during late infancy and toddlerhood children explore their environment by putting

POTENTIAL SOURCES OF LEAD	
INGESTED	**INHALED**
Lead-based paint	Burning of leaded objects
Interior: walls, windowsills, floors, furniture	Automobile batteries
	Newspaper logs of colored paper
Exterior: door frames, fences, porches, siding	Sanding and scraping of lead-based painted surfaces
Plaster, caulking	Automobile exhaust
Unglazed pottery	Cigarette smoke
Colored newsprint	Sniffing leaded gasoline
Painted food wrappers	Dust
Cigarette butts and ashes	Poorly cleaned urban housing
Water from leaded pipes	Contaminated clothing and skin of household members working in smelting factories
Foods or liquids from cans soldered with lead	
Household dust	
Soil, especially along heavily trafficked roadways	
Food grown in contaminated soil	

objects in their mouth. This normal hand-to-mouth activity contributes to the amount of lead they ingest in dust and dirt. In addition, the child who ingests lead often practices *pica*, the habitual, purposeful, and compulsive ingestion of nonfood substances. By virtue of their size, young children inhale air that is closer to the ground, which is more heavily contaminated with lead.

Lead poisoning is not confined to the young child who ingests the substance. It can also occur in older children who habitually sniff leaded gasoline. The nurse must be aware of children experimenting with drugs or other psychotropic substances and the possibility of gasoline sniffing, which is especially prevalent among American Indian children on reservations.

Parental characteristics. Parent-child interaction is another significant variable in the ingestion of lead. Many mothers whose children have the pica habit also demonstrate the behavior. It is postulated that a child's high level of oral activity may be reinforced by a mother with similar oral interests and that it is probably associated with relief of anxiety.

The most common maternal pattern seen in these families is dependency. Such mothers have a history of despair and passivity to everyday life. As a result they are usually unable to stimulate or discipline the child to more constructive forms of activity. Another frequent pattern is the parent who is unaware of the child's pica, either from ignorance that ingestion of such substances is harmful or

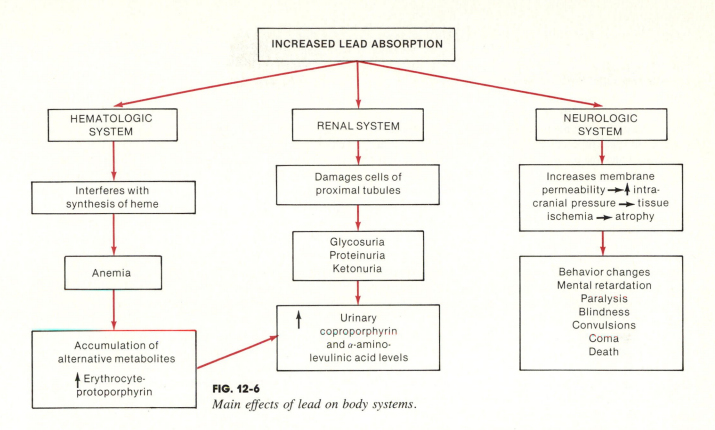

FIG. 12-6
Main effects of lead on body systems.

from lack of supervision and knowledge of the child's usual behavior.

Pathophysiology and clinical manifestations. Normally lead is poorly absorbed by the body and is very slowly excreted. Retained lead is largely stored in bone. However, under conditions of chronic ingestion, the excess lead is deposited in the tissues, affecting several body systems (Fig. 12-6).

Hematologic system. Lead is extremely toxic to the biosynthesis of heme, preventing the formation of hemoglobin and causing its precursors, especially protoporphyrin, coproporphyrin, and δ-aminolevulinic acid (ALA), to increase in the body. Free-erythrocyte protoporphyrin (FEP) is elevated in the blood when the blood-lead concentration is only minimally increased. The latter two intermediary metabolites are excreted in the urine in excessive amounts.

Reduction of the heme molecule in the red blood cell results in anemia, one of the initial signs of the disease. The pathologic changes in the bone marrow are reversed when lead leaves the soft tissue and is excreted in urine or stored in bone.

Renal system. Lead damages the cells of the proximal tubules, resulting in abnormal excretion of glucose, protein, amino acids, and phosphate. With adequate treatment kidney damage is usually reversible.

Central nervous system. The most serious and irreversible side effects of lead intoxication are on the nervous system. Initially, behavioral changes indicate lead toxicity. These include hyperactivity, aggression, impulsiveness, decreased interest in play, lethargy, irritability, delay or reversal in verbal maturation, loss of newly acquired motor skills, clumsiness, deficits in sensory perception, learning difficulties, short attention span, and distractibility. As toxic damage to the brain progresses, more serious complications develop, including convulsions, mental retardation, paralysis, blindness, and, ultimately, coma and death.

Nonspecific signs. Other, vague symptoms are acute crampy abdominal pain, vomiting, constipation, anorexia, headache, and fever.

Diagnostic evaluation. Several tests are available to detect the presence of toxic amounts of lead in the body. The most frequently used procedures for routine screening are the blood-lead concentration and the erythrocyte-protoporphyrin level. Various protocols based on the results of these two tests are available for suggesting when children should be treated. Most agree that when the blood-lead level exceeds 50 μg/100 ml, chelation therapy should be initiated.

Other tests that are helpful in determining the presence of lead in the body are (1) radiographs of the long bones for "lead lines," caused by deposition of lead and of the abdomen for presence of recently ingested lead, (2) urinalysis for increased lead and the metabolites coproporphyrin and δ-aminolevulinic acid, and (3) blood studies for evidence of anemia and basophilic stippling, which indicates the number of immature circulating erythrocytes. Another diagnostic characteristic is black lines along the gums.

Therapeutic management. The objective of treatment is to remove the lead from the blood and soft tissues by enhancing its deposition in bones and its excretion in the urine. The main vehicle for accomplishing these goals is the use of chelation therapy, which involves the removal of the metal by combining it with another substance.

Calcium disodium edetate (CaNaEDTA) is the principal chelating agent used. It forms a fairly stable, highly soluble compound that causes free lead to be readily excreted in the urine. It may be used singly or in combination with the chelating drug dimercaprol, also called BAL (British antilewisite). A combination of these drugs is thought to result in fewer side effects and better removal of lead from the brain. Success of treatment is measured by urinary excretion of lead.

The exact course of therapy differs according to the severity of the child's condition and the preferred method of the physician. However, a commonly accepted regimen involves the intramuscular administration of one or both drugs six times a day for a period of 5 days. For this treatment children are hospitalized and any supportive measures related to the child's symptoms are instituted. Children with less severe lead poisoning may be treated with oral penicillamine (Cuprimine, Depen) on an outpatient basis.

Symptomatic treatment largely involves controlling seizures and anemia. If shock is present, immediate intravenous replacement of blood is begun. If the child's clinical condition is stable, oral or intramuscular iron is used. Supplemental oxygen is helpful in situations of low hemoglobin levels. Kidney function is carefully monitored because nephrotoxicity is a side effect of plumbism and CaNaEDTA. Decreased kidney function severely limits the effectiveness of chelation therapy. Blood calcium and phosphorus levels are measured frequently since chelation agents also remove calcium from the body, predisposing to the risk of hypocalcemia.

Various other treatments may be part of the total therapy. Sometimes exchange transfusions are used to remove lead rapidly from the body. Vitamin D, calcium, and phosphorus may be given to enhance deposition of lead in bones. Cleansing enemas are ordered for episodes of acute lead ingestion or when lead is visible on radiologic examination in the gastrointestinal tract. Every effort is made to prevent infection and maintain adequate hydration.

Nursing considerations. The goals of nursing care are many in plumbism. The first is primary prevention of lead poisoning. However, this involves a multidisciplinary approach of pediatrician, nurse, social worker, and social services to intervene in all three factors involved in lead poisoning—the child, the parent, and the environment.

For the child who must undergo chelation therapy, the nurse has several priority objectives. Certainly one of the most significant objectives is preparation of the child for the tremendous number of injections that he will receive. For example, if CaNaEDTA and BAL are to be administered as separate injections every 4 hours for 5 days, the child will receive a total of 60 injections. The nurse prepares the child through needle play on a doll or stuffed toy before the therapy begins and after receiving each injection (see Chapter 19). It is important to allow the child an outlet for the pain and anger he feels and to emphasize the reason for the drugs, particularly that it is not a punishment for eating lead or paint. The parents are also prepared for the drug treatment and forewarned of the child's possible psychologic and physical reactions to it.

CaNaEDTA and BAL are both viscous solutions. For adequate absorption, each must be administered deeply into a different large muscle mass. Planning a rotation schedule for each series of injections is essential to prevent tissue damage and to ensure maximum tissue absorption.

A complication of multiple injections in one site is the development of hard, painful areas of fibrotic tissue. The nodules feel firm and almost circular when palpated. It is advisable practice to routinely feel the muscle mass before preparing the injection site to avoid administering additional medication into the same area.

Sometimes, a local anesthetic such as procaine is injected simultaneously with the CaNaEDTA or BAL to help lessen the pain during administration. If this is done, the chelating agent is drawn into the syringe, followed by the anesthetic. In this way the anesthetic is the first medication to be injected into the tissue. It is introduced slowly in order to allow some time for it to exert its deadening effect. An air bubble at the top of the syringe flushes the needle of any remaining medication, thereby decreasing the chance of tracking the drug through the layers of the skin on withdrawal of the syringe.

Since the injections are painful, the child's activity is tailored to allow adequate rest and physical stimulation that does not aggravate the painful sites. Local application of warm soaks or insulated hot packs helps relieve the discomfort, although the pain may persist and be severe enough to limit movement.

CaNaEDTA is also a calcium-chelating agent; therefore, calcium is removed with the lead from the body. Although calcium is replaced in the calcium disodium edetate preparation, the nurse observes for signs of hypocalcemia, especially tetany and convulsions. Calcium gluconate should be readily available as the emergency antidote to calcium deficiency. Seizure precautions, such as those discussed in Chapter 25, are instituted for all children hospitalized with plumbism.

Since chelating agents, particularly CaNaEDTA, are

SUMMARY OF NURSING CARE OF THE CHILD WITH LEAD POISONING (PLUMBISM)

GOALS	RESPONSIBILITIES
Identify lead poisoning	Assist in screening and diagnostic procedures Recognize behavioral indications of asymptomatic or borderline lead poisoning Identify high-risk groups, especially "pica" child, "dependent" mother, and "lead" environment
Eliminate lead from body	Administer chelating agent Assist with exchange transfusion if appropriate
Prepare child for multiple injections	Give reason for injection, while emphasizing that it is not a punishment for eating lead (paint) Use dramatic needle play with preschooler Involve parents in comforting child after injection
Prevent complications from multiple injections into same site	Schedule rotation of site, using recommended muscle areas for each individual child Palpate muscle area before preparing site to locate and avoid fibrosed tissue from previous injections
Provide relief from pain at site of injection	Apply warm soaks or heating pad to injection site Avoid activity that places undue strain or exertion on painful muscle area, for example, use wheelchair for transportation Inject local anesthetic slowly as first drug (draw up last in syringe and do not mix)
Observe for signs of encephalopathy or toxicity of chelating agents	Have seizure precautions and emergency respiratory arrest equipment at bedside Evaluate urinary functioning (intake and output record and periodic urinalysis)
Maintain hydration	Encourage child to drink fluids Measure intake and output Monitor intravenous infusion if appropriate
Assess success of therapy	Collect urine specimens and blood work as needed
Provide rest (depending on physical status)	Tailor activity to suit child's energy level Encourage quiet recreational activity that is stimulating and educational yet geared to present developmental level Provide supplemental oxygen as needed if anemia is severe
Educate parents	Discuss with parents dangers of lead ingestion, particularly for prevention of recurrence Inform parents of type of treatment and possible physical and psychologic reactions from child
Support parents	Suggest ways to help parents relate to their child in a more constructive manner in order to decrease pica behavior Help parents deal with additional crises in order to devote more energy to childrearing responsibilities Locate potential child-care services to relieve some parental responsibilities, while increasing supervision of child outside the home
Acquire needed services	Refer to public health nurse, social worker, and other agencies who can assist in overall management of complex problem
Prevent occurrence and/or recurrence	Educate public about dangers of lead ingestion, signs and symptoms indicating intoxicity, and need for treatment Assist in renovation of home to remove sources of lead, as well as measures to improve parenting Participate actively in social/political movement to provide suitable housing for everyone

toxic to the kidneys, records are kept of intake and output and frequent urinalysis is performed to evaluate gross renal functioning. If renal damage is suspected, a urine sample is sent for laboratory analysis.

Comprehensive management of the child with lead poisoning involves ''treating'' the environment to prevent recurrence after hospital discharge. However, this is not part of discharge planning but rather a priority objective as soon as diagnosis of lead poisoning is made. When it is not possible for the family to move to better housing or expensively refurbish the present home, some simple, inexpensive measures can be used. As much of the old flaking paint as possible is scraped from the walls, ceilings, and floors. Since a new coating of lead-free paint does not prevent additional chips from falling away from the plaster, the walls are covered with wallpaper, contact paper, fabric, or burlap.

In addition, the children must be supervised and guided toward activity other than pica. Helping parents learn methods of stimulating their children, locating preschool or day-care centers, or helping parents organize a play group are methods of improving parenting and, consequently, lessening those factors that contribute to plumbism.

NONACCIDENTAL INJURIES

Unfortunately, children may succumb to injuries deliberately inflicted by adults. Such injuries are generally considered under the broad term, child abuse. Another form of child abuse is sexual molestation, which is discussed separately in Chapter 15.

CHILD ABUSE

In the broadest sense, child abuse is a term that includes physical abuse and/or emotional abuse or neglect, or sexual molestation. When defined in this manner, the statistics for abused and neglected children in the United States become staggering: a total of more than *1 million cases* a year and approximately *4,000 children* killed by neglect and abuse.

Abuse or battered child syndrome is defined as a clinical condition in young children who have received serious physical abuse, generally from a parent or foster parent.

Emotional neglect is generally considered failure on the part of the parents to provide the child with the emotional support necessary for the development of a sound personality. This may result when the home lacks warmth and security and when a child is met with overt or subtle rejection and is made to feel unwanted and inferior to others.

Another form of abuse is *sexual molestation,* which frequently results from incestuous relationships.

Etiology

The exact cause of child abuse is not known, but three major criteria—parental characteristics, characteristics of the child, and environmental characteristics—are necessary in order for a child to be physically injured or neglected by his parents or guardian.

Parental characteristics. Although no two abusing individuals are exactly alike, there are several common factors that help identify potential abusers. One of the most significant is the type of parenting they received as a child. Most abusing parents were themselves abused. As children they learned that no matter how hard they tried to be good or provide for their parents' needs, it was never enough. They eventually believed that they were no good and deserved to be maltreated. As a result they developed a poor self-image and low self-esteem. As parents they transfer this belief to their children, who they believe must also be punished in order to perform according to parental expectations.

Since their parents had a distorted concept of what children were like or realistically could accomplish, abusing parents also have little knowledge of normal developmental achievements. For example, they may be unaware that an infant needs to be fed every 3 or 4 hours, be unable to cook a meal, or not know what constitutes a nutritious meal. The most serious lack of knowledge is failure to recognize emotional nurturing as an essential need of children. Instead, they expect the children to nurture and parent them. When the child fails to meet their needs, the parents literally strike out at the child as a method of releasing their increasing frustration and anxiety.

Another consequence of inadequate knowledge of children's development is the expectation that children have the maturity and responsibility of an adult. For example, very young children may be left alone with a 4- or 5-year-old child because the parent assumes that the preschooler is capable of looking after them. Another instance is the parent who fails to safeguard the house because of the belief that ''warning the child about the danger'' is sufficient. This lack of parental judgment often leads to serious or fatal accidents.

When abusing parents were children they never mastered the task of forming trust. Consequently they live in social isolation and find little pleasure and satisfaction from interpersonal relationships. With such needs unmet, they seek gratification in a marriage partner, who may be the abuser or who condones the abuse by not interfering with it.

Characteristics of the child. The child also contributes to the abusing situation. In families of two or more children, it is usual to find only one child as the victim of abuse. This child's temperament, position in the family, additional physical needs if ill, activity level, or sensitivity to parental needs all in some way contribute to why he escapes or fosters physical abuse.

Not infrequently the abused child is illegitimate, unwanted, brain damaged (especially in situations where the parents cannot accept the retardation), hyperkinetic, physically disabled, or from a broken home. Sometimes the child is abused because he reminds the parent of someone the parent dislikes, for example, a younger brother or sister who received all the attention from their own parents. Premature infants are at risk for maltreatment because of the possible failure of parent-child bonding during early infancy.

Often the precipitating factor for the abuse is not an identifiable stress but an ordinary task of childrearing, such as toilet training, speech development, or self-help skills. With no realistic knowledge of children's age-appropriate capabilities, the parent expects learning to take place automatically. For example, the parent may decide that the 1-year-old child is ready for toilet training and expect that once the child is put on the potty-chair he will immediately learn to control elimination. When the child fails, the parent punishes him for not complying with the expected behavior.

Although one child is usually the victim in an abusing family, if that child is removed for his own protection, the parents quickly replace him with another victim. Child abuse is not confined to one child because of a disturbed parent-child relationship but is the result of dysfunctioning parenting, which can involve any child. Therefore, no child is safe if left in the abusing environment unless the parents can be helped in some way to learn new parenting skills and to meet their needs and release their frustration through alternatives other than attacking their children.

Environmental characteristics. The environment is an integral part of the potential abusing situation. Typically it is one of chronic stress, including financial, emotional, physical, and marital crises. The social milieu of the abusive family is one devoid of adequate support systems. The environment becomes a trap from where there is no emotional exit except to direct the anger and frustration toward a helpless victim, the child.

Although most reporting of abuse has been from lower socioeconomic populations, child abuse is by no means a problem of any one societal group. Concealed crises can be present in upper class families. For example, a wealthy family experiencing major life changes, such as relocating, birth of an additional child, or marital discord, may have sufficient environmental stressors imposed on them to produce a potentially abusing situation. Nurses need to be aware of such factors in order to identify the hidden sources of child abuse and neglect.

Identification of abuse or neglect

A thorough physical examination and a careful, detailed history are the diagnostic tools. Nurses have a very special role because they may be the first person to see the child and parent and because they may be the consistent caregiver if the child is hospitalized.

Evidence of maltreatment. Physical abuse may be evident from obvious marks on the body. Some of the more common forms of physical injury include small, round burns or scars from cigarettes; localized burns on the buttocks or soles of the feet from being placed against a radiator or immersion in hot water; slap marks resembling the shape of a hand; welts from beatings with a belt, belt buckle, chains, or hangers; and circular abrasions around the ankles or wrists from tying the child down.

A form of abuse that leaves no visible marks but causes severe pain from damage to the muscles and subcutaneous tissue is flogging the child with a wet towel. Another abusive act is vigorously shaking the child, which may result in a whiplash type of injury to the neck and can cause brain damage. Other evidence of abuse includes radiologic findings of healed or new fractures or dislocation of the extremities, especially the shoulder, from pulling the child or throwing him against a hard surface.

Neglect or emotional abuse is much more difficult to recognize and document. Neglect is suspected when the child is unbathed, poorly nourished, inadequately dressed for the weather, or wearing old or torn clothing. Emotional abuse may be evident when signs of failure to thrive are seen (see Chapter 9). Another clue is also the type of parent-child relationship, especially when the parent verbally abuses the child or continually belittles him in front of others.

In order to identify sexual molestation, health professionals must be willing to investigate the possibility of its existence. Besides the routine physical examination for signs of abuse or neglect, the child is carefully inspected for evidence of oral and/or anal penetration, as well as genital contact. Laboratory tests are done to detect the presence of semen and venereal disease. With the exception of congenital syphilis or gonoccocal conjunctivitis in newborns, the presence of venereal infection in children should be considered an indication of possible sexual abuse.

History pertaining to the incident. Besides observable evidence of abuse, the type of history revealed by the parents or other caregiver, such as the baby-sitter or mother's boyfriend, is a significant diagnostic factor. Those areas of the history that should arouse suspicion of abuse include (1) conflicting stories about the ''accident'' from the parents or child, (2) an injury inconsistent with the history, such as a concussion and broken arm from falling off a bed, (3) a complaint other than the one associated with signs of abuse, for example, a chief complaint of a cold when the child has evidence of first- and second-degree burns on his body, (4) inappropriate parental concern for the degree of the injury, such as an exaggerated or absent emotional response, (5) refusal of the parents to sign for additional tests or to agree to necessary treatment, and (6) absence of the parents for questioning.

Parental behaviors. Certain behavioral responses of the parents to their child and to the interviewer should alert the nurse to the possibility of maltreatment. Typically the parents have difficulty in showing concern toward their child. They maintain that the child injured himself and, if asked any question regarding their responsibility of protecting or supervising the child, become hostile and aggressive. Their entire perception of the incident is in terms of how it affects them, not the child, which is an indication of their preoccupation with their own needs and their inability to give any support to others.

Child behaviors. Battered children also exhibit behaviors that are not typical of those of well-nurtured children. They show no expectation of being comforted by their parents. When admitted to the hospital unit they are less afraid of strangers than are their age-mates, and they tend to settle in quickly. They may form ''friends'' almost immediately, but there is little selectivity or preference in their attachments.

Maltreated children rarely betray their parents by confessing to the abuse they received. Whether they respond this way out of fear is uncertain. However, the child knows what he has in his parents. Even if the parent-child relationship is distorted, the child has a home, a family, and, in a sense, security. Between abusing events the child may receive attention and love from his parents, even if it is a result of his attending to their needs. If he betrays his parents, he loses all of this and is uncertain of what may be in its place. So he protects his parents because, in his thinking, a little love is better than none.

Nursing considerations

The principal goal in care of the abused child is protection from further injury. However, prevention of abuse and education of the family after abuse are equally important functions.

Prevention. Prevention involves identifying potential abusers and instituting supportive intervention before the occurrence of an abusive act. This involves helping the parents identify with the child, teaching them effective child-rearing practices, and promoting their self-esteem.

Identification and protection from further abuse. Initially, identification of cases of suspected abuse or neglect is essential. Signs that indicate abuse, such as the physical findings, specific parent or child behaviors, inconsistencies in the history, and contributing familial and environmental factors, must be recognized by the nurse. *The priority is to remove the child from the abusive situation to prevent further injury.*

All states have laws for mandatory reporting of child maltreatment. Referrals usually come to the Bureau of Child Welfare and are assigned to a caseworker in an agency such as the Child Protective Services. In most states, once a referral has been made, there is an automatic court order, which gives the agency the right to keep the child in protective custody for 72 hours to investigate the report.

In some states a court proceeding is necessary before the child can be placed in an institution. When the courts are involved, they usually require first-hand testimony by the referring parties. This may mean that nurses are subpoenaed or that their records are introduced as evidence. In either case the nurse has a great responsibility in reporting facts, not hearsay or subjective opinion, particularly when writing nurses' notes.

Care of the child. Frequently children suspected of abuse are hospitalized for medical management of their injuries. Their needs are the same as those of any hospitalized child but are multiplied by their situation. Even though they tend to adjust easily to their new environment and make friends quickly, they need a consistent caregiver. The goal of the consistent nurse-child relationship is to (1) foster a therapeutic environment for the child in which he learns to trust in one individual and (2) provide a role model for the parents in helping them to relate positively and constructively to their child.

Hospitalization is often extended as eventual placement is arranged. Frequently this is much longer than that necessary for recovery from the injury or neglect. The child is guided toward physical and mental wellness during this period. He is treated as a child with the usual physical needs, developmental tasks, and play interests—not as a dramatic victim of abuse.

Discharge planning should begin as soon as the legal disposition for placement has been decided, which may be temporary foster home placement, return to the parents, or permanent termination of parental rights. The last is the most drastic resolution, but it is necessary in situations of repeated abuse. Whenever children are remanded to a foster home or juvenile institution, they must be allowed the opportunity to ventilate their feelings. No matter how severe the abuse, they usually mourn the loss of their parents. They need help to understand why they must not return home and that this new home is in no way a punishment. Whenever possible, foster parents should be encouraged to visit, and the nurse should take an active role in helping these parents understand the child.

Care of parents. One of the most difficult, yet essential, components of success with abusing parents is the quality of the therapeutic relationship. It must be one of genuine concern and treatment, not one of accusation and punishment. Nurses must examine their personal feelings toward these parents. Unless the nurse's attitude is positive, abusing parents will not be motivated to change, since they will not be working with a trusting person who demonstrates the kind of behavior that is being asked of them.

Since these parents have unrealistic expectations of children's capabilities, the nurse fosters knowledge and understanding of normal growth and development. The nurse demonstrates how to handle children, how to teach them at their age level, and what realistically to expect from them. Since these parents are very sensitive to criticism or domination and already possess a very low self-esteem, teaching is done through demonstration and example, rather than through lecturing. Any competent parenting abilities they demonstrate are praised in an attempt to promote their sense of parental adequacy. Abusing parents desperately need ''mothering'' in order to be able to mother or father their own children. The nurse attends to their needs for security, trust, release from responsibility, and so on.

The solution to child abuse is not an easy one. Success is never certain, and failure may well be a child's life. However, there are services available, such as Parents Anonymous,* psychiatric or mental health intervention, and group therapy sessions, that help parents achieve major changes within themselves. Nurses have a responsibility to work with those families they care for in the hospital or community in terms of establishing a supportive and trusting relationship and to refer parents for additional help whenever possible.

---

*2030 West Imperial Highway, Inglewood, CA 90303.

SUMMARY OF NURSING CARE OF THE ABUSED CHILD

GOALS	RESPONSIBILITIES
Prevent abuse	Identify families at risk for potential abuse Promote parental attachment to child Emphasize child-rearing practices, especially effective methods of discipline Increase parents' feeling of adequacy and self-esteem Encourage support systems that lessen stress and total responsibility of child care on one or both parents Be available for assistance
Identify suspected cases of child abuse or neglect	Be alert to signs that may indicate abuse or neglect Report suspicions to appropriate authorities Keep factual, objective records of the child's physical condition; behavioral response to parents, others, and environment; and interviews with family members
Determine extent of injuries	Perform physical assessment Assess emotional state and evaluate behaviors Assist with diagnostic procedures
Protect from further abuse	Assist in removing child from unsafe environment and establishing a safe environment Establish protective measures for the hospitalized child as indicated
Promote therapeutic environment during hospitalization	Provide consistent caregiver Demonstrate acceptance of child while not expecting same in return Show attention while not reinforcing inappropriate behavior Plan appropriate activities with nurse, other adults, and other children; use play to work through relationships Avoid displacing anger on child, such as shouting or yelling, as method of dealing with own frustration toward child's negative behavior Praise child's abilities in order to promote his self-esteem

Continued.

SUMMARY OF NURSING CARE OF THE ABUSED CHILD—cont'd

GOALS	RESPONSIBILITIES
Relieve anxiety in child	Treat child as one who has a specific physical problem for hospitalization, not as "abused" victim Avoid asking too many questions; use play, especially family or dollhouse activity, to investigate kind of relationships perceived by child; child should relate to one consistent person regarding events of abuse Foster healthy aspects of parent-child relationship, encourage child to talk about parents in positive sense; avoid criticizing parents' actions to child
Promote wellness in child	Besides physical needs related to injury or neglect, focus on developmental needs such as sensory stimulation and education Accept temporary regression as necessary mechanism to cope with present crisis
Promote a sense of parental adequacy during child's hospitalization	Orient parents to hospital unit and help them feel welcomed and an important part of child's care and recovery Reinforce competent child-care activities Focus on the abuse as a problem that requires therapeutic intervention, not as a behavior characteristic or deficiency of the parent Empathize with difficulties of rearing children, especially with additional life crises, while not condoning the act of abuse or neglect
Plan for discharge	Prepare for discharge as soon as disposition is finalized If child is being placed in foster home, encourage family members to visit child before discharge; stress to them child's need to regress in order to complete missed stages of development If child is returning to his own home, encourage parents to visit as much as possible; plan for close supervision and counseling of family If parents' rights are being terminated permanently, help child grieve this loss, especially if it entails separation from siblings (long-term counseling is optimum goal)
Prevent recurrence	Collaborate efforts of multidisciplinary team to continually evaluate progress of child in foster home or in return to own family As public health or school nurse, actively look for signs of continued abuse or neglect Help parents identify those circumstances that precipitate an abusive act and ways in which to deal with the release of anger in ways other than attacking child
Support parents	Provide "mothering" by directing attention to parent, taking over child-care responsibilities until parents feel ready to participate, and focusing on parent's needs Refer parents to Parents Anonymous (initially may need to attend with parents as their advocate) or special "hot line" services Help identify a support group for parents, such as extended family or nearby neighbors; help these significant others understand their important role in also preventing further abuse
Teach parents	Teach realistic expectations of child's behavior and capabilities Emphasize alternate methods of discipline, such as reward and verbal disapproval Suggest methods of handling developmental problems or goals, such as toddler negativism, toilet training, and independence Teach through demonstration and role modeling rather than lecture; avoid authoritarian approach
Lessen environmental crises	Refer to social agencies who can provide assistance in financial support, adequate housing, employment, and so on

REFERENCES

Centers for Disease Control: Lead poisoning, Morbid. Mortal. Weekly Report, Annual Summary, 1980, **29**(54):110, 1981.

Strome, M.: Must children with tympanotomy tubes avoid swimming? Pediatr. Alert **8**(7):28, 1983.

BIBLIOGRAPHY

Communicable diseases

American Academy of Pediatrics: Report of the Committee on Infectious Diseases, Evanston, Ill., 1982, The Academy.

Fleming, J.W.: How to differentiate dermatologic conditions—often confusing and difficult—in infants and school-age children, Am. J. Maternal Child Nurs. **6**(5):346-354, 1981.

Hayman, L.L.: Varicella, Nursing 83 **13**(4):41, 1983.

Krugman, S., and Katz, S.L.: Infectious diseases of children, ed. 7, St. Louis, 1981, The C.V. Mosby Co.

Shahan, M.R.: Mumps, Nursing 83 **13**(2):43, 1983.

Wiswall, J.: Update on common exanthematous communicable diseases, Pediatr. Nurs. **4**(5):50-51, 1978.

Tonsillitis, otitis media, and conjunctivitis

Adams, J., Evans, G., and Roberts, J.: Diagnosing and treating otitis media with effusion, Am. J. Maternal Child Nurs. **9**(1):22-28, 1984.

Castiglia, P., Aquilina, S., and Kemsley, M.: Nonsuppurative otitis media, Pediatr. Nurs. **9**(6):427-431, 1983.

Corkery, C.M.: Removal of a child's tonsils and adenoids, Nurs. Times **75**:742-743, May 1979.

Dupont, J.: EENT emergencies, Nursing 79 **9**(11):65-70, 1979.

Gladwin, B.: Adenotonsillectomy: bearing up with Paddington, Nurs. Mirror **150**(6):42-44, 1980.

Havener, W.: Synopsis of ophthalmology, St. Louis, ed. 5, 1979, The C.V. Mosby Co.

Kass, J.R., and Beebe, M.E.: Serous otitis media, Nurse Pract. **4**(2):25-28, 1979.

Moore, R., and Schmitt, B.: Conjunctivitis in children, Clin. Pediatr. **18**(1):26-32, 1979.

Sataloff, R.T., and Colton, C.M.: Otitis media: a common childhood infection, Am. J. Nurs. **81**(8):1480-1483, 1981.

Study identifies children at risk for otitis media, AORN J. **31**(6):1014-1015, 1980.

Ingestion of injurious agents

Arena, J.M.: Prevention of poisoning in children, Public Health Currents **23**(1):1-4, 1983.

Centers for Disease Control: Preventing lead poisoning in young children, J. Pediatr. **93**(4):709-720, 1978.

Driggers, D.A., and Johnson, R.: Initial management of pediatric poisoning, Pediatr. Basics **35**:4-6, 1983.

Drummond, A.H., Jr.: Lead poisoning in children, J. School Health **51**(1):43-47, 1981.

Foster, S.D.: In case of an emergency: ipecac syrup, Am. J. Maternal Child Nurs. **7**(4):227, 1982.

Gever, L.N.: A new treatment for a new problem: acetaminophen overdose, Nursing 80 **10**(6):57, 1980.

Gillies, C.: Management of pediatric poisoning, role of the nurse practitioner, Pediatr. Nurs. **6**(5):33-35, 1980.

Keim, K.A.: Preventing and treating plant poisonings in young children, Am. J. Maternal Child Nurs. **8**(4):287-289, 1983.

Langner, B., and Modrcin-McCarthy, M.A.: Lead poisoning: an ongoing pediatric nursing concern, Issues Compr. Pediatr. Nurs. **4**(3):23-36, 1980.

Lovejoy, F.: Management of pediatric poisoning. Part I, Pediatr. Nurs. **6**(5):37-39, 1980.

Miller, S.J.: Nursing care of the lead-burdened child: a problem oriented approach, Pediatr. Nurs. **7**(5):47-52, 1981.

Schiffhauer Erler, M.: Iron poisoning, J. Emerg. Nurs. **6**(2):40-42, 1980.

Temple, A.: Management of pediatric poisoning. Part II, Pediatr. Nurs. **6**(5):40-43, 1980.

Child abuse

Bittner, S., and Newberger, E.H.: Pediatric understanding of child abuse and neglect, Pediatr. Rev. **2**(7):197-207, 1981.

Deitch, E.A., and Staats, M.: Child abuse through burning, J. Burn Care Rehab. **3**(2):89-94, 1982.

Fontana, V.J.: The maltreated child, ed. 4, Springfield, Ill., 1979, Charles C Thomas, Publisher.

Gray, J.D., and others: Prediction and prevention of child abuse, Semin. Perinatol. **3**:85-88, 1979.

Heindl, M.C., editor: Child abuse and neglect, Nurs. Clin. North Am. **16**(1):101-188, 1981.

Helberg, J.L.: Documentation in child abuse, Am. J. Nurs. **83**(2):238-239, 1983.

Helfer, R.E.: Preventing the abuse and neglect of children, Pediatr. Basics **23**:4-7, April 1979.

Holter, J.C.: Child abuse, Nurs. Clin. North Am. **14**(3):417-427, 1979.

Josten, L.: Prenatal assessment guide for illuminating possible problems with parenting, Am. J. Maternal Child Nurs. **6**(2):113-117, 1981.

Kauffman, C.K., and Neill, M.K.: The abusive parent. In Johnson, S.J.: High-risk parenting, Philadelphia, 1979, J.B. Lippincott Co.

Kempe, C.H., and Helfer, R.E., editors: The battered child, ed. 3, Illinois, 1982, University of Chicago Press.

McKittrick, C.A.: Child abuse: recognition and reporting by health professionals, Nurs. Clin. North Am. **16**(1):103-115, 1981.

Newberger, E.H.: Understanding child abuse, Child Care Newsletter **1**:3-6, Fall 1981.

Ortman, E.: Attachment behaviors in abused children, Pediatr. Nurs. **5**(4):25-29, 1979.

Scharer, K.M.: Rescue fantasies: professional impediments in working with abused families, Am. J. Nurs. **78**:1483-1484, 1978.

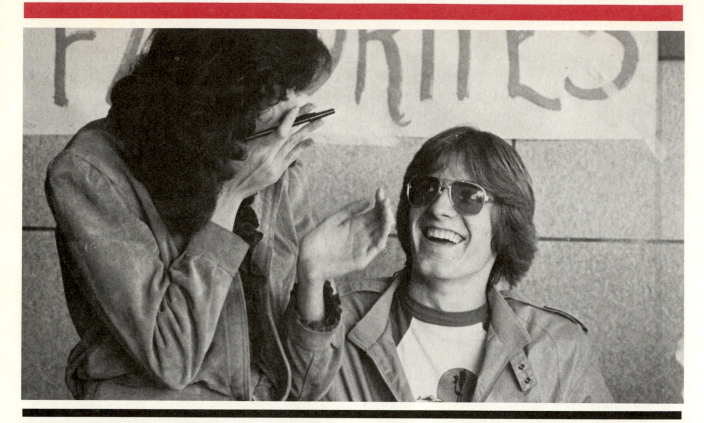

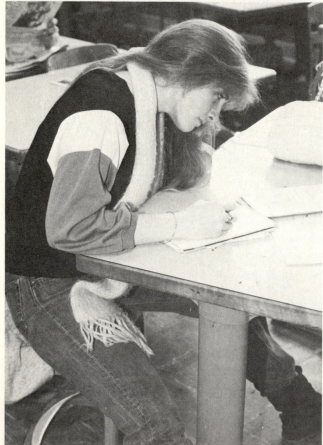

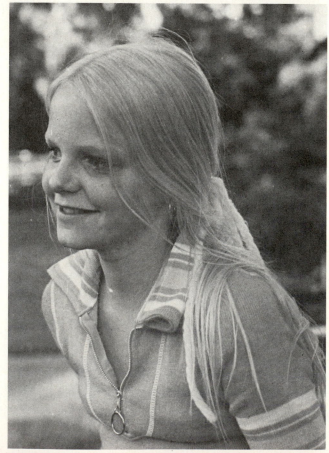

unit 6

MIDDLE CHILDHOOD AND ADOLESCENCE

Children in the middle childhood years enjoy a relatively stable period of slow but steady growth and maturation with few physical or emotional stresses. It is a comfortable period of adjustment with a developmental pace sufficiently slow to meet the physical and psychologic demands placed on them. It is a period of broadening horizons when children encounter a wider sphere of influence—school, peers, and multiple opportunities for social interaction. During this period children learn the fundamental skills of their culture and develop inner resources for coping with larger social units. The emphasis during this period is on competence in physical and mental tasks and on the equally important changes in social relationships.

Adolescence is a period of transition that is based on childhood experiences and accomplishments and that has a goal of mature, independent, and responsible functioning. This transition is a biologic, emotional, and social process, a preparatory period requiring the accomplishment of defined developmental tasks in order to attain satisfactory adjustment to adulthood. The early years of adolescence are concerned with individuation from previous dependency roles and a gradual movement toward peer-group identity. The peer group is the focus of the adolescent's world—the persons in his life who are going through the same transition and who understand the problems and frustrations he is experiencing. Later years of adolescence are centered around acquiring a personal identity, completing the separation process from family, and career-directed activity.

Chapter 13, *The School-Age Years,* provides a brief overview of the developmental changes that take place in middle childhood, including a lengthy summary of the major characteristics of each age within the period of middle childhood. Chapter 14, *The Adolescent Years,* provides an overview of the transitional adolescent period during which youth must adjust to rapid body changes, establish a personal identity, gain emotional and (for some) economic freedom from their parents, and evolve a set of values uniquely their own. Chapter 15, *Health Problems of Middle Childhood and Adolescence,* outlines the more common health problems encountered during these years. Few major illnesses are associated with middle childhood, although children during this time are still subject to many of the problems that characterize the earlier childhood years, and, with the wider social relationships, communicable diseases continue to be prevalent. Health problems associated with adolescence result from either the changes related to biologic maturation or the psychologic adjustments imposed by these changes and the expectations of society.

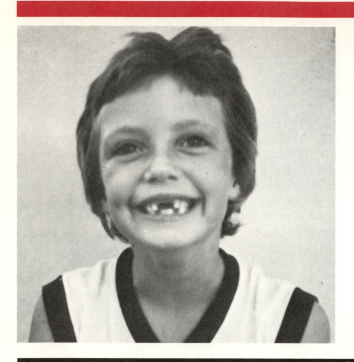

13

THE SCHOOL–AGE YEARS

OBJECTIVES

On completion of this chapter the reader will be able to:

- Describe the physical, cognitive, and moral changes that take place during the middle childhood years

- Describe ways to assist a child in developing a sense of accomplishment

- Demonstrate an understanding of the changing interpersonal relationships of the school-age child

- Discuss the role of the peer group in the socialization of the school-age child

- Outline an appropriate health teaching plan for the school-age child

- Identify the causes and discuss the preventive aspects of accidents in middle childhood

- Plan a sex education session for a group of school-age children

NURSING DIAGNOSES

Nursing diagnoses identified for the school-age child include, but are not restricted to, the following:

Health perception-health management pattern

- Infection, potential for, related to increased contact with persons outside the home

- Injury, potential for, related to (1) environmental hazards; (2) immature musculature and coordination; (3) immature reasoning and judgment; (4) natural propensity for vigorous activity

Nutritional-metabolic pattern

- Nutrition, alteration in: potential for more than body requirements related to inactivity (some children)

Activity-exercise pattern

■ Self-care deficit, partial, related to (1) developmental level; (2) knowledge deficit; (3) disinclination to engage in hygienic activities

Sleep-rest pattern

■ Sleep pattern disturbance related to nightmares

Self-perception—self-concept pattern

■ Anxiety related to (1) strange environment; (2) previous experience(s); (3) perception of impending events; (4) separation; (5) knowledge deficit; (6) intrafamily stresses; (7) stressful interpersonal relationships

■ Powerlessness related to dependence-independence conflict

■ Self-concept, disturbance in, related to (1) perception of others' evaluations; (2) inability to meet expectations of others; (3) inability to compete with age-mates satisfactorily; (4) perceived imperfections; (5) injury (specify)

Role-relationship pattern

■ Family process, alteration in, related to situational crises

■ Parenting, alterations in: potential, related to (1) skill deficit; (2) family stress

■ Social isolation related to (1) peer rejection; (2) physical illness; (3) absence from school; (4) personality characteristics

Coping-stress tolerance pattern

■ Coping, ineffective individual, related to (1) knowledge deficit; (2) inexperience

Value-belief pattern

■ Spiritual distress related to (specific situation)

The segment of the life span that extends from age 6 years to approximately age 12 years has been tagged with a variety of labels, each of which describes an important characteristic of the period. These middle years are most often referred to as *school-age* or the *school years*. This period begins with entrance into the wider sphere of influence represented by the school environment, which has a significant impact on development and relationships. The term *gang age* describes the child's affiliation with agemates and learning the culture of childhood. With peer groups children establish the first close relationships outside the family group. From a psychoanalytic point of view, this is the period of *latency,* which has been considered to be a time of sexual tranquility between the Oedipal phase of early childhood and the eroticism of adolescence. It is during this time that children experience the intimacy of relationships with same-sex peers, following the indifference of earlier years and preceding the heterosexual fascination that accompanies the changes of puberty.

Physiologically the middle years begin with the shedding of the first deciduous tooth and end at puberty with the acquisition of the final permanent teeth (with the exception of the wisdom teeth). During the preceding 5 to 6 years, the child has progressed from a helpless infant to a sturdy, complicated individual with the capacity to communicate, conceptualize in a limited way, and become involved in complex social and motor behavior. Physical growth has been equally rapid. In contrast, the period of middle childhood, between the rapid growth of early childhood and the turmoil of the prepubescent growth spurt, is a time of gradual growth and development with steadier and more even progress in both its physical and emotional aspects. Physical health is generally good, and it is a comfortable period of physical adjustment. Physiologic processes in general have attained a stage of development that permits their maintenance at stable levels under ordinary conditions and their ready adjustment to changing needs and stresses. Under normal circumstances these children are usually well able to meet the physical and psychologic demands that are placed on them.

There is a special quality about the middle childhood years. This is the period of childhood that the adult remembers with fond recollections. The school-age child likes this age period, and it is the one to which the preschooler eagerly looks ahead and for which the adolescent yearns. In the Western world the school-age child has a good deal of freedom and few responsibilities.

With a firm foundation of trust, autonomy, and initiative, the child is ready and eager for the wider world of learning and competition associated with developing a sense of industry. The child moves from the egocentricity of early childhood to the subperiod of cognitive domain described as concrete operations. Until recently middle childhood has generated the least interest and preoccupation among psychologists and others concerned with the effects of childhood experiences on later adjustments. However, it has been found that this period makes an important contribution to the child's learning the fundamental skills of his culture and the development of competence and self-esteem. It is a time of intellectual growth, investment in work, and the first real commitment to a social unit outside of and larger than the family.

BIOLOGIC DEVELOPMENT

During middle childhood growth in height and weight assumes a slower but steady pace as compared with the earlier years and the years immediately ahead. Between ages 6 and 12 years, children will grow an average of 2½ to 5 cm (1 to 2 inches) per year to gain 30 to 60 cm (1 to 2 feet) in height and will almost double in weight, increasing 1½ to 3 kg (3 to 6 pounds) per year. The average 6-year-old child is about 117 cm (46 inches) tall and weighs about 22 kg (48 pounds); the average 12-year-old child stands about 150 cm (59 inches) tall and weighs approximately 38 kg (84 pounds). During this age period girls and boys differ very little in size, although boys tend to be slightly taller and somewhat heavier than girls. Toward the end of the school-age years both boys and girls begin to increase in size, although most girls begin to surpass boys in both height and weight (to the acute discomfort of both).

Proportional changes

School-age children are more graceful than they were as preschoolers, and they are steadier on their feet. Their body proportions take on a slimmer look, with longer legs, varying body proportion, and a lower center of gravity. Posture improves over that of the preschool period to facilitate locomotion and efficiency in using the arms and trunk. These proportions make climbing, bicycle riding, and other activities much easier. Fat gradually diminishes and its distribution patterns change, contributing to the thinner appearance of the child during the middle years. Accompanying the skeletal lengthening and fat diminution is an increase in the percentage of body weight represented by muscle tissue. By the end of this age period, both boys and girls will double their strength and physical capabilities and their steady and relatively consistent acquisition of refined coordination will increase their poise and skill. However, this increased strength can be misleading. Although strength increases, muscles are still functionally immature when compared with those of the adolescent, and they are more readily damaged by muscular injury caused by overuse.

The most pronounced changes, and those that seem best to indicate increasing maturity in children, are a decrease in head circumference in relation to standing height, a decrease in waist circumference in relation to height, and an increase in leg length related to height. These observations often provide a clue to a child's degree of maturity that has proved useful in predicting his readiness for meeting the demands of school. There appears to be a correlation between physical indications of maturity and success in school.

Facial changes. Certain physiologic and anatomic characteristics are typical of children in the years of middle childhood. Facial proportions change as the face grows faster in relation to the remainder of the cranium. The skull and brain grow very slowly during this period and increase little in size thereafter. Since all of the primary (deciduous) teeth are lost during this age span, middle childhood is sometimes known as the *age of the loose tooth* and the early years of middle childhood as the *ugly duckling stage,* when the new secondary (permanent) teeth appear to be much too large for the face.

Maturation of systems

Development of all body systems continues during middle childhood to become more efficient and adult-like in function.

Gastrointestinal tract. Maturity of the gastrointestinal system is reflected in fewer stomach upsets, better maintenance of blood sugar levels, and an increased stomach capacity, which permits retention of food for longer periods of time. The school-age child does not need to be fed as carefully, as promptly, or as frequently as before. Caloric needs in relation to stomach size are less than they were in the preschool years and less than they will be during the coming adolescent growth spurt.

Renal system. Physical maturation is evidenced in other body tissues and organs. Bladder capacity, although differing widely among individual children, is generally greater in girls than in boys. There are individual variations in frequency of urination and differences in one child according to circumstances such as temperature, humidity, time of day, amount of fluids ingested, and emotional state.

Heart. The heart grows more slowly during the middle years and is smaller in relation to the rest of the body than at any other period of life. Consequently, many believe that strongly competitive sports with prolonged, intense physical exertion may be damaging to the school-age child. The heart and respiratory rates steadily decrease and the blood pressure increases during the ages from 6 to 12 years (inside front cover).

Eyes. The shape of the eye changes during growth; the normal farsightedness of the preschool child is gradually converted to 20/20 vision during middle childhood. There is still controversy regarding the age at which 20/20 vision is achieved, although it appears to be well established by 9 to 11 years of age. To aid vision throughout the school years, large print is recommended for reading matter and regular vision testing should be a part of the school health program.

Bones. Bones continue to ossify throughout childhood, but, since mineralization is not completed until maturity, bones resist pressure and muscle pull less than mature bones. Consequently, care must be taken to prevent alterations in bone structure, such as providing well-fitted shoes and seeing that chairs and desks allow correct sitting posture, with the feet able to reach the floor and the hips able to fit well back in the seat. Children should have ample opportunity to move around, and they should observe appropriate caution in carrying heavy loads. For example, they should shift books from one arm to the other, and newscarriers who carry heavy loads of newspapers slung from the shoulders should alternate the load from one shoulder to the other to avoid developing a low shoulder or spine curvature.

Sex differences. There are wider differences between children at the end of middle childhood than at the beginning; such differences are sometimes striking. These differences become increasingly apparent and, if extreme or unique, may create emotional problems unless the associated characteristics of height and weight relationships, rapid or slow growth, and other important features of development are recognized and explained to children and their families. Also, physical maturity is not necessarily correlated with emotional and social maturity. The 7-year-old child who looks like a 10-year-old child will, in fact, think and act like a 7-year-old child. To expect behavior appropriate for a 10-year-old child from him is unrealistic and can be detrimental to his development of competence and self-esteem. Conversely, to treat a 10-year-old as though he were 7 years old is an equal disservice to the child.

Toward the end of middle childhood the discrepancies in growth and maturation between boys and girls begin to be apparent. On the average there is a difference of approximately 2 years between girls and boys in the age of onset of pubescence. The average age of onset for girls is about 10 years; for boys it is about 12 years. There are wide differences between individuals, and some girls may display characteristics of puberty or experience developmental changes as early as 8 years of age. Because of this discrepancy, some authors define the middle childhood or school-age years as 6 to 10 years for girls and 6 to 12 years for boys.

Physical activity

The improved capabilities and adaptability of the school-age child permit greater speed and effort in motor activities, and larger, stronger muscles with greater efficiency and skill permit longer and increasingly strenuous play without exhaustion. During this age period children acquire the necessary coordination, timing, and concentration that are required to participate in adult-type activities, even though they may be deficient in the strength, stamina, and control of the adolescent and adult. Consequently a larger amount of physical activity should be expected and encouraged during the school years. However, it must be kept in mind that, although school-age children are large and appear to be strong, they may not be prepared yet for strenuous competitive athletics. A great deal of controversy has surrounded the trend toward earlier participation in competitive athletics and the questions of the amount and type of competitive sports that are appropriate for children in the elementary grades. At present most authorities do not discourage participation in Little League baseball, soccer, swimming, and other sports for school-age children. However, it is important for those involved with children in this age-group to understand the child's physical limitations and to teach the proper techniques and safety in order to avoid injury to developing bones and muscles. Equipment should be maintained in safe condition, and protective apparatus should be worn to prevent serious accidents.

All growing children need some regular exercise and should be afforded opportunities of various kinds that provide satisfying experiences to meet individual likes and dislikes. Appropriate activities that promote coordination and development during the school-age years include running, skipping rope, swimming, roller skating, ice skating, and bicycle riding. Positive reinforcement achieved by experiencing increasingly smooth, rhythmic, and efficient use of the body conditions the child toward regular physical activity.

Acquisition of skills

School-age children also demonstrate increasing capacities in fine muscle facility and complex artistic skills. Handedness is well established by the beginning of the school years, and the child makes great strides in writing and drawing during this age period. It is a period of energetic and vibrant creative productivity. With the tools of language and reading, children can create poems, stories, and plays. With more advanced fine motor skills, they are able to master an unlimited variety of handicrafts, such as ceramics, needlework, wood carving, and beadwork. They avidly pursue these skills in solitude (Fig. 13-1), with a friend, or in programs offered through organizations such as boys' or girls' clubs, scouting, or the YWCA and YMCA, which use crafts as a means to occupy, entertain, and educate children (Fig. 13-2).

The school-age child is capable of assuming respon-

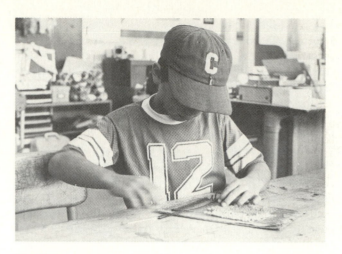

FIG. 13-1
School-age children are motivated to complete tasks working alone.

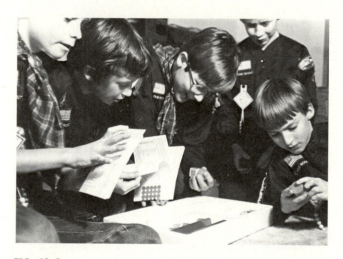

FIG. 13-2
School-age children cooperate to complete tasks working with others.

sibility for his own needs, although his distaste for soap and water and "dress" clothes is legendary. School-age children can and want to assume their share of household tasks, which usually are related to the male and female roles that have been defined by their culture, and many assume responsibility for tasks outside the home, such as baby-sitting or paper routes.

PSYCHOLOGIC DEVELOPMENT

There is no concept more difficult to assess or more elusive than that of the personality or the "self." Most persons draw inferences regarding children's personalities

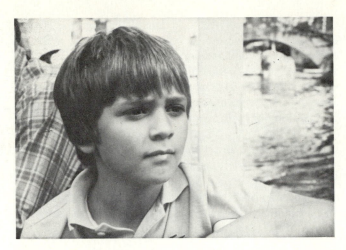

FIG. 13-3

In middle childhood the child broadens his understanding of the world and begins to see things from the point of view of another.

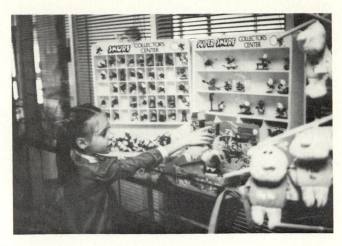

FIG 13-4

School-age children are avid collectors

from observation of their behaviors. These behaviors are based on many different innate and acquired characteristics, the way in which these characteristics are organized, and the manner in which each characteristic modifies or alters the other to contribute to the unique quality of each child. Personality is reflected in the way in which the child reacts to himself and others, the way in which others react to him, and the way in which he adjusts to his environment. Development of the personality involves a number of different types of development—physical, intellectual, social, emotional—all of which are profoundly influenced by the environment in which the child grows and develops.

Cognitive development

Somewhere around the beginning of the school years, children begin to acquire the ability to relate a series of events and actions to mental representations that can be expressed both verbally and symbolically. This is the stage in development that Piaget describes as *concrete operations,* wherein the child is able to use his thought processes to experience events and actions. His rigid, egocentric outlook is replaced by thought processes that allow him to see things from the point of view of another (Fig. 13-3).

During this stage the child develops an understanding and use for relationships between things and ideas. He progresses from making judgments based on what he sees (perceptual) to making judgments based on what he reasons (conceptual). He is increasingly able to master symbols and to use his memory store of past experiences in evaluating and interpreting the present.

One of the major cognitive tasks of the school-age child is mastering the concept of *conservation.* Early (about 5 to 6 years) he grasps the concept of reversibility

of numbers as a basis for simple mathematic problems (for example, $2 + 4 = 6$ and $6 - 4 = 2$). He learns that certain properties of the environment are not changed simply by altering their disposition in space, and he becomes able to resist perceptual cues that suggest such alterations in the physical state of an object. For example, he recognizes that changing the shape of a substance such as a lump of clay does not alter its total mass. He no longer perceives a tall, thin glass of water as containing a greater volume than a short, wide glass; he can distinguish between the weight of items regardless of their size. He recognizes that the size is not necessarily related to weight or volume. There appears to be a developmental sequence in the child's capacity to conserve matter. Conservation of mass usually is accomplished earliest (7 to 8 years), weight some time later (9 to 10 years), and volume last (11 to 12 years).

The school-age child now has the ability to classify, to place things in a sensible and logical order, to group and sort, and, in doing so, to hold a concept in his mind while he makes decisions based on that concept. It is characteristic of middle childhood that children derive a great deal of enjoyment from classifying and ordering their environment. They become occupied with numerous and varied collections of objects, such as wrappers, stamps, shells, dolls, cars, stones, and anything that is classifiable (Fig. 13-4). They even begin to order friends and relationships, such as first best friend, second best friend, and so on.

They develop the ability to understand relational terms and concepts, such as bigger and smaller; darker and paler; heavier and lighter; to the right of and to the left of; first, last, and intermediate relationships (fourth, second, and so on); and more than and less than. They can see family relationships in terms of reciprocal roles—for example, in order to be a brother, one must have a sibling.

They learn the alphabet and the ever-widening world of symbols called words that can be arranged in terms of structure and their relationship to the alphabet. They learn to tell time, to see the relationship of events in time (history) and places in space (geography), and to combine time and space relationships (geology and astronomy).

The most significant skill, the ability to read, is acquired during the school years and becomes the most valuable tool for independent inquiry. The child's capacity for exploration, imagination, and expansion of knowledge is enhanced with the ability to read, as he progresses from the repetition and confusion of early efforts to increasing facility and comprehension.

Developing a sense of accomplishment

Successful mastery of Erikson's first three stages of psychosocial development is probably the most important accomplishment in terms of development of a healthy personality (see p. 35). Successful completion of these stages implies that a child has attained a confidence in an environment of loving relationships within a stable family unit that has prepared him to engage in experiences and relationships beyond this intimate group. It has been suggested that the individual's fundamental attitude toward work is established during middle childhood.

A sense of industry, for which a more descriptive term is the *stage of accomplishment,* is achieved somewhere between age 6 years and adolescence. It involves an eagerness for building skills and participating in meaningful and socially useful work. It is acquired through the process of education—formal and self-directed. Interests expand in the middle years and, with a growing sense of independence, the child wants to engage in tasks that can be carried through to completion. Children gain a great deal of satisfaction from independent behavior in exploring and manipulating their environment and from interaction and peers. Extrinsic sources of reinforcement in the form of grades, material rewards, additional privileges, and recognition provide encouragement and stimulation. Peer approval is a strong motivating power.

A sense of accomplishment also involves the ability to cooperate and to compete with others—to cope more effectively with people. Middle childhood is the time when children learn the value of doing things alongside and with others and the benefits derived from division of labor in the accomplishment of goals.

The danger inherent in this period of personality development is the imposition of situations that might result in a sense of inadequacy or inferiority. This may happen if the previous stages have not been successfully achieved or if the child is incapable of or unprepared for assuming the responsibilities associated with developing a sense of accomplishment. Feelings of inferiority or lack of worth

can be derived from the child himself or from the social environment. However, no child is able to do well in everything, and children must learn that they will not be able to master each skill that they attempt. All children, even children who in most instances have positive attitudes toward work and their own capabilities, will feel some degree of inferiority in regard to a specific skill that they cannot master.

Children need and want real achievement. When they have access to tasks that need to be done, that they are able to do well despite individual differences in their innate capacities and emotional development, and for which they are suitably rewarded, children will be able to achieve a sense of industry and accomplishment.

Moral development

As children move from egocentrism to the more logical patterns of thought, they also move through stages in development of conscience and moral standards. Young children do not believe that standards of behavior come from within themselves but that rules are established and set down by others. They learn the standards for acceptable behavior, act according to these standards, and feel guilty when they violate the standards. Although children of 6 or 7 years of age know the rules and behaviors expected of them, they do not understand the reasons behind them. Rewards and punishment guide their judgment; a "bad act" is one that breaks a rule or does harm. Young children may believe that what other people tell them to do is right and that what they think of themselves is wrong. Consequently, children 6 or 7 years old are more likely to interpret accidents and misfortunes as punishment for misdeeds.

Older school-age children are able to judge an act by the intentions that prompted it rather than just by the consequences. Rules and judgments become less absolute and authoritarian and begin to be founded more on the needs and desires of others. For older children a rule violation is apt to be viewed in relation to the total context in which it appears; reactions are influenced by the situation as well as by the morality of the rule itself. While a younger child can judge an act only according to whether it is right or wrong, older children will take into account a different point of view to make a judgment. They are able to understand and accept the concept of doing as one would be done by.

Spiritual development

Children at this age think in very concrete terms but are avid learners and have a great desire to learn about their God. They picture God as human and tend to describe him in terms of character traits such as loving and helping. He is a very important person in the lives of many children. They are fascinated by hell and heaven and, with a developing conscience and concern about rules, they fear going to hell for misbehavior. School-age children want and expect to be punished for misbehavior but, if given the option, tend to choose a punishment that ''fits the crime.'' Often they view illness or injury as a punishment for a real or imagined misdeed. The beliefs and ideals of family and religious personages are more influential than their peers in matters of faith.

School-age children begin to learn the difference between the natural and the supernatural but have difficulty understanding symbols. Consequently religious concepts must be presented to them in concrete terms. They are comforted by prayer or other religious rituals and, if this is a part of their daily lives, these activities can help them cope with threatening situations. Their petitions to their God in prayers tend to be for very tangible rewards and, although younger children expect their prayers to be answered, as they get older they begin to recognize that this does not always occur and become less concerned when prayers are not answered. They are able to discuss their feelings about their faith and how it relates to their lives.

Self-evaluation (self-esteem)

Closely associated with developing a sense of industry is developing a concept of one's value and worth. At first a child's self-concept is formed exclusively from what he perceives to be his parents' evaluation of him. During middle childhood the opinions of peers and teachers provide further input. The difficulty that children encounter in the attempt to assess their own abilities is their inclination to rely on their own expectations or on the expectations expressed by others regarding their performance. A child's self-concept is composed of his own critical self-assessment plus what he interprets as the opinions of members of his family and outside social contacts.

The significant adults in a child's life can often manage, unseen, to manipulate the child's environment so that he meets with success. Each small success increases the child's self-image a little. The more positive he feels about himself, the more confident he feels in trying again for success. Every child profits from a feeling that he is in some way special to a significant adult. A positive self-concept makes him feel likable, worthwhile, and someone with a valuable contribution to make in his world. Such feelings lead to self-respect, self-confidence, and a general feeling of happiness.

Body image. An important part of the development of self-esteem is development of a body image. As the child's social environment expands, he continually compares his attributes and abilities with those of his peers. He is acutely conscious of the way he looks to others and is highly aware of deviations from the normal in himself and others. At this time, physical impairments such as hearing or visual defects, ears that ''stick out,'' or birthmarks assume greater importance. Increasing awareness of these differences, especially when accompanied by unkind comments and taunts from other children, may cause him to feel inferior and less desirable. This is especially true if the defect interferes with his ability to participate in childhood games and activities.

PREADOLESCENCE

The preadolescent years, roughly ages 10 to 13, are years of transition. This is a period of rapid growth, especially for girls; for boys (and some girls, too) it is generally a period of steady growth in height and weight.

There is no universal age at which children assume the characteristics of preadolescence. The first physiologic signs begin to appear at about 9 years of age (particularly in girls) and are usually clearly evident in 11- to 12-year-old children. Although the preadolescent child does not want to be different, at this age the variability in physical growth and physiologic changes between children of the same sex, between the two sexes, and even within each individual child is often striking. This variability, especially in relation to the onset of secondary sexual characteristics, is of utmost concern to the preadolescent. Either early or late appearance of these characteristics is a source of embarrassment and uneasiness to both sexes.

Preadolescence is a time when there is a good deal of overlapping of developmental characteristics with elements of both middle childhood and early adolescence. However, there is a sufficient number of unique characteristics to set this period apart as an age category, even with the wide range of variability in the ages 11 and 12 years (or even 9 to 13 years in some children). Generally, the earliest age at which puberty begins is 10 years in girls and 12 years in boys, although there has been an increase in the number of girls reaching puberty at 9 years of age. The average age of puberty in girls is 12 years, and for boys it is 14 years. Boys experience little sexual maturation during preadolescence.

SOCIETY OF CHILDREN

One of the most important socializing agents in the life of the child is the peer group with whose members he explores ideas and the physical environment around him. Although it has neither the traditional authority of the parents nor the legal authority of the schools for imparting information, the peer group manages to convey a substantial amount of material to its members. Children have a culture all their own, with secrets, mores, and codes of ethics with which they promote feelings of group solidarity and detachment from adults. Through peer relationships children learn ways in which to deal with dominance and hostility and to relate to persons in positions of leadership and authority.

Identification with peers appears to be a strong influence in the child's gaining independence from parents. The aid and support of the group provides the child with enough security to risk the moderate parental rejection brought about by each small victory in his development of independence.

Much of the child's concept of the appropriate sex role is acquired through relationships with peers. During the early school years there is little difference relative to sex in play experiences of children. Games and many other activities are shared by both girls and boys. However, in the later school years the differences become marked. Boys and girls grow more intolerant of each other, especially on the surface.

Social relationships and cooperation

Daily relationships with age-mates provide the most important social interactions in the life of school-age children. For the first time children are able to join in group activities with unrestrained enthusiasm and steady participation when, formerly, interactions had been limited to short periods under considerable adult supervision. With increased skills and wider opportunities, children are able to become involved with one or several peer groups in which they can gain status as respected members.

There are valuable lessons to be learned from daily interaction with age-mates. First, children learn to appreciate the numerous and varied points of view that are represented in the peer group. As the child interacts with peers who see the world in ways that are somewhat different from the way he sees it, he becomes aware of the limits of his own point of view. Because age-mates are peers and are not forced to accept each other's ideas as they are expected to accept those of adults, other children have a significant influence on decreasing the egocentric outlook of the child. Consequently he learns to argue, persuade, bargain, cooperate, and compromise in order to maintain friendships.

Second, the child becomes increasingly sensitive to the social norms and pressures of the peer group. The peer group establishes standards for acceptance and rejection, and the child may be willing to modify his behavior in order to be accepted by the group. The need for peer approval becomes a powerful influence toward conformity. The child learns to dress, talk, and otherwise behave in a manner acceptable to the group. A variety of roles, such

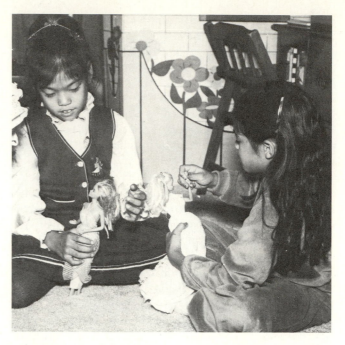

FIG. 13-5
Age-mates involved in quiet play.

as class joker or class hero, may be assumed by individual children in order to gain approval from the group.

Third, the interaction among peers leads to the formation of intimate friendship between same-sex peers. School-age is the time when children have "best friends" with whom they share secrets, private jokes, and adventures; they come to one another's aid in times of trouble. In the course of these friendships children also fight, threaten, break up, and reunite. These dyadic relationships, in which the child experiences love and closeness for a peer, seem to be important as a foundation for heterosexual relationships in adulthood (Fig. 13-5).

Gangs. One of the outstanding characteristics of middle childhood is the formation of formalized groups, or gangs, a prominent feature of which is the rigid rules imposed on the members. There is an exclusiveness in the selection of persons who have the privilege of joining. Acceptance in the group is often determined on a pass-fail basis according to social or behavioral criteria. Conformity is the core of the gang structure. There are often secret codes, shared interests, and special modes of dress, and each child must abide by a standard of behavior established by the group. Understanding of and conformity to the rules provide the child with a feeling of security and relieve him of the responsibility of making decisions. By merging his identity with that of his peers, the child is able to move from the family group to an outside group as a step toward seeking further independence. He substitutes conformity to a peer-group pattern for conformity to a family pattern while he is still too shaky and insecure to function independently.

During the early school years gangs are rather small, loosely organized groups with changing membership and little formal structure and without the more prolonged cohesiveness characteristic of gangs in later school years. As a rule, girls' gangs are less formalized than boys' gangs, and, although there may be a mixture of both sexes in the earlier school years, the gangs of later school years are composed predominantly of children of the same sex. Common interests are a frequent basis around which a gang is structured.

Ethical misconduct

During the middle childhood it is not uncommon for children to engage in what is considered to be antisocial behavior. Lying, stealing, and cheating may manifest in previously well-behaved children. It is especially disturbing to parents who may have difficulty coping with this behavior.

Lying. Preschool children often have difficulty distinguishing between fact and fiction. By the time they reach school age they still tell stories but can distinguish between what is real and what is make-believe. Often children will exaggerate a story or situation as a means to impress their family or friends. Younger children will lie to escape punishment or get out of some difficulty even when the evidence of their misbehavior is before their eyes. Older ones may lie in order to meet expectations set by others to which they have been unable to measure up. They are much concerned with the wrongness of lying and cheating—especially in their friends.

Cheating. Cheating is most common in young children aged 5 to 6. They find it difficult to lose at a game or contest and cheat in order to win. They have not yet acquired the full realization of the wrongness of this behavior and do it almost automatically. It usually disappears as they mature.

Stealing. Like other ethical behavior stealing is not an unexpected event in the younger child. Between 5 and 8 years children's sense of property rights is limited and they tend to take something simply because they are attracted to it or to take money for what it will buy. They are equally likely to give away something valuable that belongs to them. When young children are caught and punished they are penitent, "didn't mean to," and promise "never to do it again," but it is quite likely that they will repeat the performance the following day. Often they not only steal but will lie about it as well or attempt to justify the act with excuses. It is seldom helpful to trap children into admission by asking directly if they did the offensive

thing. Children do not take a responsibility such as that until nearer the end of middle childhood.

There are several reasons why children steal: lack of a sense of property rights, to acquire the means with which to bribe favors from other children, a strong desire to own the coveted item, or as a means for revenge in order to "get back at someone" (usually a parent) for what they consider to be unfair treatment. Older children may steal to supplement an inadequate income from other sources. Sometimes stealing is an indication that something is seriously wrong or lacking in the child's life. For example, a child may steal to make up for love or other satisfaction which he feels is lacking.

It is difficult for many parents to cope with these behaviors in their children. However, in most situations it is best not to attempt to find a hidden or deep meaning to the stealing. An admonition together with an appropriate and reasonable punishment, such as having the older child pay back the money or return stolen items, will ordinarily take care of the majority of cases. Most children can be taught to respect the property rights of others with little difficulty despite the temptations and opportunities presented to them. Some children simply need more time to learn the importance of the culture's rules regarding private property.

Relationships with parents

Although the peer group is highly influential and necessary to normal child development, the parents are still the primary influence in shaping the child's personality, setting standards for behavior, and establishing a value system. It is the family values that usually predominate when parental and peer value systems come into conflict.

Peer associations seem to remain within the social class systems, and, not infrequently, there may be discrimination in membership on the basis of ethnic or racial origin.

The child will want to spend more time in the company of his peers and may seem anxious to leave the house; he will often prefer activities of the gang to family activities. This can be very disturbing to parents. The child becomes intolerant and critical of the parents and their ways when they deviate from those of the gang.

Although increased independence is the goal of middle childhood, children are not yet prepared to abandon parental control. They feel more secure knowing that there is an authority greater than themselves to implement controls and restrictions. Children may complain loudly about the restrictions and try their best to break down parental barriers, but they are uneasy if they can succeed in doing so. They respect the adults on whom they can rely to prevent them from acting on each and every urge. Children sense in this behavior an expression of love and concern for their welfare.

Children also need their parents as adults, not as pals. Sometimes parents, hurt at their children's rejection, attempt to maintain their love and gratitude by assuming the role of "pals." Children need the stable, secure strength provided by mature adults to whom they can turn during troubled relationships with peers or stressful changes in their world. During a disruption in their lives, such as times of failure, periods of illness, or a move that separates them from the security of friends, children need the firm, secure anchor of parental interest and concern. With a secure base in a loving family, children are able to develop the confidence in themselves and the maturity needed to break loose from the gang and stand independently.

School experience

The schools serve as agents for transmitting the values of the society to each succeeding generation of children and as the setting for much of their relationships with peers. As a socializing agent second only to the family, schools exert a profound influence on the social development of children. Until school entrance at approximately 5 or 6 years, the primary sphere of influence of the child is the family, in which his interactions are with parents and siblings. Neighborhood children provide broader relationships, but parents serve as the only continuous adult contact, those with whom he is most intimately involved and who set the pattern of his daily life. School entrance marks a sharp change in the child's experiences with others. His world at once becomes more complex, requiring adjustments to a new set of interpersonal contacts and authority figures. In addition, he is separated from the parents and siblings for a substantial portion of the day.

School entrance constitutes a sharp break in the structure of the child's world (Fig. 13-6). For many children it is their first experience in conforming to a group pattern imposed by an adult who is not a parent and who has responsibility for too many children to be constantly aware of each child as an individual. Children want to go to school and usually adapt to the new conditions with little difficulty. Successful adjustment is directly related to the physical and emotional maturity of the child and the mother's readiness to accept the separation associated with school entrance. Unfortunately some mothers express their unconscious attempts to delay the child's maturity by clinging behavior, particularly with their youngest child.

By the time they enter school, the majority of children have a fairly realistic concept of what school involves. The child receives information regarding the role of pupil from parents, playmates, and the communication media. In ad-

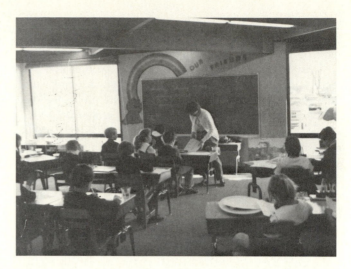

FIG. 13-6
School provides a wider range of social relationships and a new authority figure.

dition, most children have had some experience with kindergarten, and some with nursery school as well.

Although most children have had some experience with schooling before they enter first grade, the extent to which they are prepared differs. Middle-class children have fewer adjustments to make and less to learn about expected behavior, since the school tends to reflect dominant middle-class customs and values. If the child has attended a preschool program the emphasis of the program significantly affects the child's adjustment. Some provide custodial care only, while others emphasize emotional, social, and intellectual development as well.

To facilitate the transition from home to school, educators select teachers, usually women, with personality characteristics that allow them to deal with potential problems of young children. As a mother surrogate the teacher in the early grades performs many of the activities formerly assumed by the mother, such as recognizing the children's personal needs (such as a need to go to the bathroom or help with clothing) and helping to develop their social behavior (for example, manners).

Teachers, like parents, are concerned about the psychologic and emotional welfare of the child. Although the functions of teachers and parents differ, both place constraints on behavior and both are in a position to enforce standards of conduct. The teacher shares the parental influence in determining the child's attitudes and values. Teachers serve as models with whom children identify and whom they try to emulate. Teacher approval is sought; teacher disapproval is avoided. The teacher is a very significant person in the life of the early school child, and hero worship of a teacher may extend into late childhood and preadolescence (Fig. 13-7).

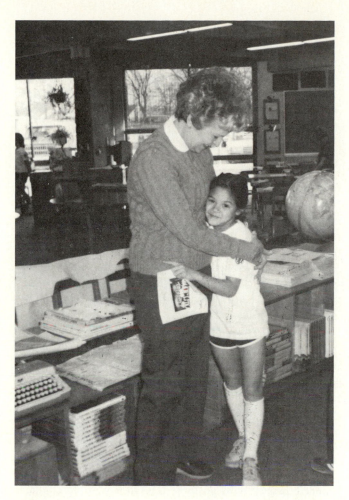

FIG. 13-7
Children develop a close relationship to their teachers.

Play

As children enter the school years, their play takes on new dimensions that reflect this new stage of development. Not only does play involve increased physical skill, intellectual skill, and fantasy, but, as they form gangs and cliques, children begin to evolve a sense of team or club. To belong to a group is of vital importance.

Rules and ritual. The need for conformity in middle childhood is strongly manifested in the activities and games that are so important in the life of school-age children. Up to this point, they have played games they have invented themselves, or they have played in the company of a friend or an adult, when rules more or less evolved with the game. Now they begin to see the need for rules, and the games they begin to play have fixed and unvarying rules that may be bizarre and extraordinarily rigid (especially those made up by the group). Clubs and secret societies become part of the culture of childhood.

Conformity and ritual permeate the play of school-age children. Not only are they present in games, but they are also evident in much of the children's behavior and language. Childhood is full of chants and taunts, such as "Eeeny, meeny, miney, mo," "Johnny's mad and I'm glad," "Last one is a rotten egg," and "Step on a crack, break your mother's back." Children derive a great deal of pleasure from such sayings, which have been handed down with few changes through generations.

Team play. A more complex form of play that evolves from group consciousness is the team games and sports that are part of the life of the early school years. The rules of a team game may even require the presence of a referee, umpire, or person of authority, in order that the rules can be followed more accurately. Through team play children learn to subordinate personal goals to goals of the group and the concept that division of labor is an effective strategy for attaining a goal. They learn about the nature of competition and the importance of winning—an attribute highly valued in the United States.

Team play can also contribute to children's social, intellectual, and skill growth. A child will work hard to develop the skills needed to become a member of a team, to improve his contribution to the group effort, and to anticipate the consequences of his behavior for the group. Team play helps stimulate cognitive growth, as children are called on to learn many complex rules, make judgments about those rules, plan strategies, and assess the strengths and weaknesses of members of their own team and the opposing team.

Quiet games and activities. Although the play of school-age children is highly active, they also enjoy many quiet and solitary activities. The middle years are the time for collections, which constitute another ritual. The early school-age child's collections are an odd assortment of unrelated objects in messy, disorganized piles. Collections of later years are more orderly and selective, and they are organized neatly in scrapbooks, on shelves, or in boxes.

School-age children become fascinated with increasingly complex board or card games, such as monopoly and rummy, that they can play with a best friend or a group. As in all games, their adherence to rules is fanatic. There is usually much discussion and argument, but the disagreement is easily resolved through reading the appropriate rule of the game.

The newly acquired skill of reading becomes increasingly satisfying as school-age children become able to expand their knowledge of the world through books (Fig. 13-8). School-age children never tire of stories and, just as preschool children, they love to have stories read aloud. Sewing, cooking, carpentry, gardening, and creative activities such as painting are other activities that these children enjoy. Many of the creative skills, as well as athletic skills such as swimming, riding, hiking, dancing, and skating, that are learned and delighted in during childhood are continued to be enjoyed into adolescence and adulthood.

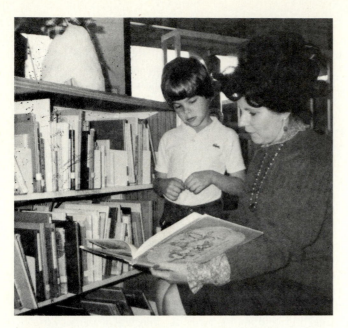

FIG. 13-8
Selecting a book with the assistance of an adult.

Ego mastery. Play also affords children the means to acquire representational mastery over themselves, their environment, and others. Through play they can feel as big, as powerful, and as skillful as their imaginations will allow, and they can attain vicarious mastery and power over whomever and whatever they choose. They need to feel in control in their play. School children still need the opportunity to use large muscles in exuberant outdoor play and the freedom to exert their newfound autonomy and initiative. They need space in which to exercise large muscles and to work off tensions, frustrations, and hostility. Physical skills practiced and mastered in play help them develop a feeling of personal competence, which contributes to a sense of accomplishment and helps provide a place of status in the peer group.

HEALTH PROMOTION DURING MIDDLE CHILDHOOD

Health supervision of children, begun in early childhood, is continued in middle childhood; it includes the periodic ongoing health assessment and guidance advised for children 6 to 12 years of age. Since regular health checkups and prophylactic measures such as immunizations are a routine function of health supervision, this need not be reiterated.

When school-age children enter school, they leave the relatively protected environment of home and neighborhood and experience interpersonal contacts with a larger number of children. Many childhood illnesses can be prevented by careful health supervision. For example, most of the communicable diseases, formerly a cause of high morbidity in school children, can be prevented by immunization. The body's natural defenses against illness can be supported through careful attention to diet, rest, and exercise and protection from extreme mental and physical stress.

Sleep and rest

The amount of sleep and rest that is required during middle childhood is a highly individual matter. There is no specific amount needed by a child at any given age. The amount depends, rather, on the child's age, the activity level, and other factors, such as his state of health. The growth rate has slowed; therefore, less energy is expended in growth than was expended during the preceding periods and than will be required during the adolescent growth spurt.

During the school years children usually do not require a nap, but they sleep an average of 11 to 12 hours nightly at age 6 years and 9 to 10 hours a night at 11 or 12 years. Although there are fewer bedtime problems with advancing years, there are still occasional difficulties associated with the necessary bedtime ritual. Usually there is little problem for children 6 and 7 years old, and the task of going to bed can be facilitated by encouraging quiet activity before bedtime, such as coloring and reading. However, most children in middle childhood must be reminded frequently to go to bed; 8- to 9-year-old children and 11-year-old children are particularly resistant. Often the child is unaware that he is tired; if he is allowed to remain up later than usual, he is fatigued the following day. Sometimes the bedtime resistance can be resolved by allowing a later bedtime in deference to his advancing age. Twelve-year-old children usually offer no difficulty in relation to bedtime. Some even retire early in order to enjoy slow preparations for bed, to read, or to listen to the radio.

Nutrition

Although caloric needs are diminished in relation to body size during middle childhood, resources are being laid down for the increased growth needs of the adolescent period. It is important to impress on children and their parents the value of a diet that is balanced to promote growth. Since the child usually eats as the family does, the quality of his diet depends to a large extent on the family's pattern of eating.

Likes and dislikes established at an early age continue in middle childhood, although the propensity for single food preferences begins to end and children acquire a taste for an increasing variety of foods. However, with the influence of the mass media and the temptation of an immense variety of "junk food," it is all too easy for children to fill up on empty calories—foods that do not promote growth, such as sugars, starches, and excess fats. The easy availability of high-calorie foods, combined with the tendency toward more sedentary activities, is contributing to an increasing prevalence of childhood obesity. This problem is discussed further in Chapter 15.

Nutrition education can and should be integrated throughout the child's school years as part of classroom learning. In school the basic food groups and the elements of a wholesome diet are learned, as well as how food products are grown, processed, and prepared. The school nurse can take an active role in nutrition education by working with teachers to plan and implement units of nutrition instruction and with parents and children to give nutritional guidance.

Exercise and activity

Exercise is essential for developmental progress in a number of areas, including muscle development and tone, refinement of balance and coordination, gaining strength and endurance, and stimulating body functions and metabolic processes. Children need ample space in which to run, jump, skip, and climb and safe facilities and equipment to use both inside and outside. Most children need little encouragement to engage in physical activity. They have so much energy that they seldom know when to stop.

Children with handicapping conditions or those who hesitate to become involved in active play, such as obese children, require special assessment and help so that activities that will appeal to them, that are compatible with their limitations, and that, at the same time, meet their developmental needs can be determined.

Television. For some time child development specialists and parents have been concerned about the effects that television has on child development and behavior. There is no doubt that children learn from television, but the values and attitudes are not always realistically displayed and often conflict with those they have been taught. The inability to distinguish fantasy from reality is a problem with the preschool child but does not disturb the school-age child, who has had sufficient life experience to be able to view much of television fare with skepticism. However, television rarely depicts the reality of day-to-day situations that confront the child.

The greatest criticism of television, however, centers around violence. Children imitate the behavior of role models and may eventually incorporate the observed aggressive behavior into their own behavior unless it is tempered by the presence of a calm adult to point out the inappropriateness and consequences of undesirable behaviors. Otherwise the child may become more aggressive in his play.

Sports. A great deal of controversy has surrounded the trend toward earlier participation in competitive athletics and regarding the amount and type of competitive sports that are appropriate for children in the elementary grades. The current view is that virtually every child is suited for some type of sport, and authorities do not discourage participation if the child is matched to the type of sport appropriate to his abilities and to his physical and emotional constitution. School-age children enjoy competition and, when those involved with children in this age-group understand the child's physical limitations and teach him the proper techniques and safety to avoid injury to developing bones and muscles, a safe and appropriate sport can be found for even the most unskilled and nonaggressive child (Fig. 13-9).

During the school-age years girls have the same basic structure as boys and thus have a similar response to systematic exercise training. At puberty, when boys become larger and have more muscle mass, it is usually recommended that girls compete only against other girls. Before puberty there is no essential difference in strength and size between girls and boys, making these precautions unnecessary (Shaffer, 1980).

The same principles apply to children with chronic illnesses such as diabetes, epilepsy, asthma, or allergies if the disorder is mild and can be controlled with medication. Mentally retarded children need not be excluded from sports competition if they are matched evenly against other children of equal abilities and provided with skilled supervision and coaching. Sometimes the activities need to be modified to accommodate the limitations of these children.

Accidents

As in all age-groups, accidental injury is closely related to the developmental characteristics associated with normal growth and maturation. With new capabilities children are often tempted to test these abilities in activities that may not be appropriate. Because school-age children have developed more refined muscular coordination and control and can apply their cognitive capacities to a more judicious course of action, the incidence of accidents is diminished in children in this age-group when compared with the incidence in early childhood.

The most common cause of severe accidental injury and death in school-age children is motor vehicle accidents—either as pedestrian or passenger. It is imperative that nurses continue to emphasize the importance of the three safety measures that have been found to reduce the severity of injuries: effective restraint systems, door lock mechanisms, and appropriate passenger seating locations in the motor vehicle.

The school-age child's penchant for riding bicycles increases the risk of injury on streets and byways, and other

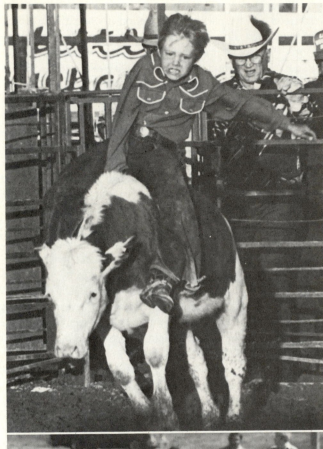

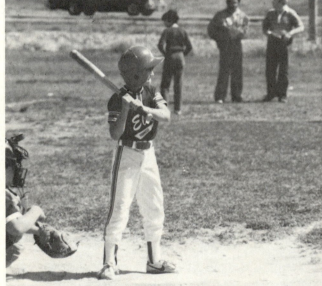

FIG. 13-9

The activities engaged in by school-age children vary according to interest and opportunity. **A,** *Little Britches Rodeo competitor.* **B,** *Little League competitors.*

serious injuries associated with moving conveyances include accidents on skateboards, roller skates, skis, and other sports equipment. The most effective means of prevention is education of the child and family regarding the hazards of risk taking and improper use of the equipment. Safety helmets are strongly recommended for children engaged in active sports in which they are not required equipment. For example, falls from bicycles and skating devices are the cause of an impressive number of head injuries in school-age children.

Physically active, school-age children are highly susceptible to cuts and abrasions, and the incidence of childhood fractures, strains, and sprains is impressive. The incidence is significantly higher in school-age boys than in school-age girls, and most occur in or near the home or school. Accidental injuries of serious nature are discussed as appropriate elsewhere in the book—burns (p. 921), eye trauma (p. 484), near drowning (p. 613), and head injuries (p. 820)—and need not be elaborated here. The prevalence of accidents depends on the dangers present in the environment, the protection offered by adults, and the behavior patterns of the children.

The accident-prone child. Although causative factors are controversial, there is a group of children who appear to be *accident-prone,* that is, they suffer significantly more accidents than the overall childhood population. There appear to be personality characteristics that are more prominent in these children. One type of accident-prone child is overreactive, restless, and impulsive. These children become increasingly impulsive and disorganized during periods of stress, often to the point that they are unable to recognize or heed danger signals. Resentful, hostile children and immature children who attempt to compete with others beyond their capacities in a hazardous environment represent other types of children who have many accidents. The quality of parent-child relationships appears to be a significant factor in these children. Parents of these children provide less supervision, appear more distant with their children, and are casual in their attitudes toward the injuries.

It has been shown that children undergoing stressful changes in their lives are more susceptible to accidents. In addition, there is concern regarding some accidental injuries in school children, such as poisoning, that are considered to be nonaccidental unless specifically reported otherwise. The "accident" may be a manifestation of a significant mental health problem.

Dental health

Since it is during the school-age years that the permanent teeth erupt, good dental hygiene and regular attention to dental caries are vital parts of health supervision during

SUMMARY OF ACCIDENT PREVENTION DURING SCHOOL-AGE YEARS

MAJOR DEVELOPMENTAL CHARACTERISTICS	ACCIDENT PREVENTION

Is developing increasing independence
Has increased motor skills
Needs strenuous physical activity
Is interested in acquiring new skills and perfecting attained skills
Is daring and adventurous
    Frequently plays in hazardous places
Confidence often exceeds physical capacity
Desires group loyalty and has strong need for peer approval
    Attempts hazardous feats
    Accompanies peers to potentially hazardous facilities
Motor ability variable, especially fine motor
Delights in physical activity
Is likely to overdo
Linear growth exceeds muscular growth and coordination
	Motor vehicles
	Educate regarding proper use of seat belts while a passenger in a vehicle
	Maintain discipline regarding deportment while a passenger in a closed vehicle, for example, keep arms inside, do not lean against doors, jump about, or interfere with driver
	Emphasize safe pedestrian behavior
	Teach safety and maintenance of two-wheeled vehicles
	Insist on wearing of safety apparel (e.g., helmet) where applicable
	
	Drowning
	Teach to swim
	Teach basic water safety
	
	Burns
	Instruct in behavior in the areas involving contact with potential burn hazards, for example, gasoline, matches, bonfires or barbecues, firecrackers, lighters, cooking utensils, chemistry sets; avoid climbing around high-tension wires
	Instruct in proper behavior in the event of fire (e.g., fire drills at home, school, and so on)
	Teach proper behavior if clothing becomes ignited
	Advise regarding excessive exposure to sunlight (ultraviolet burn)
	
	Poisoning
	Educate regarding hazards of taking nonprescription drugs, including aspirin and alcohol
	Keep potentially dangerous products in properly labeled receptacles—preferably out of reach
	
	Falls
	Instruct in proper use of playground equipment
	Instruct in proper use and care of sports equipment, especially the more hazardous devices (skateboards, trampolines, skis, and so on)
	Emphasize use of protective equipment when engaged in individual activities such as skateboarding and cycling and team sports such as soccer, hockey, and so on
	
	Bodily damage
	Help provide facilities for supervised activities
	Encourage playing in safe places
	Keep firearms safely locked up except during adult supervision
	Teach proper care of, use of, and respect for devices with potential danger (power tools, firecrackers, and so on)
	Stress eye protection when using potentially hazardous objects or devices
	Teach safety regarding use of corrective devices (glasses); if child wears contact lenses, monitor duration of wear to prevent corneal damage

this period. Correct brushing techniques should be taught or reinforced, and the role that fermentable carbohydrates play in production of dental caries should be emphasized. It is also important to be alert to possible malocclusion problems that may result from irregular eruption of permanent teeth and that may impair function. Regular dental supervision and continued fluoride supplementation are as essential as regular medical supervision and should be an integral part of the overall health maintenance program.

Brushing. One of the most effective means of preventing dental caries is a regimen of proper oral hygiene tailored to the individual child by his dentist. The child should be taught to carry out his own dental care with the supervision and guidance of the parents. Parents should learn the brushing technique along with the child, and they should inspect his efforts until he can assume full responsibility for his own care.

One regimen advocated by authorities includes staining the teeth with a plaque-disclosing agent, followed by thorough brushing with plain water and flossing. After the teeth have been inspected with the aid of a mirror under adequate light, they are again cleansed, this time with a fluoridated dentifrice to freshen the mouth and provide further protection. This procedure may be carried out regularly or occasionally, according to instructions from the child's dentist.

For the school-age child with mixed and permanent dentition the best toothbrush is one of soft nylon bristles with an overall length of about 6 inches. The design of the brush is of little importance; it is usually left to the child's preference. The horizontal brushing method, well suited to the preschool child, is not appropriate for the older child. The brushing method for the school-age child is selected according to the needs of the individual child, as evaluated by the dentist.

A relatively simple and effective technique acceptable to most dentists is the roll method of toothbrushing. The bristles of the brush are placed as high as possible between the gums and the buccal surface, with the sides of the bristles touching the gingiva. Lateral pressure is exerted against the gingival tissues with the sides of the bristles; then the brush is moved in the direction of the occlusive surfaces of the teeth. The brush is turned slowly so that the ends of the bristles come into contact with the enamel as the brush nears the plane of occlusion. This rolling motion is repeated eight times in the same place; then the brush is moved to a new area. The same procedure is followed until all areas have been brushed.

Dental caries. Dental caries is one of the most common chronic diseases that afflict humans at all ages; it is the principal oral problem in children and adolescents. Reducing the incidence and consequences of the disorder is of great importance in childhood because dental caries, if untreated, results in total destruction of involved teeth.

The ages of greatest vulnerability are 4 to 8 years for the primary dentition and 12 to 18 years for the secondary or permanent dentition (see p. 33 for sequence of tooth eruption).

Dental caries is a multifactorial disease; it involves susceptible teeth, cariogenic microflora, and an appropriate oral environment. The incidence of lesions and the likelihood of progressive invasion vary considerably and depend on a number of factors being present in the right combination. Oral inspection is an integral part of the nursing assessment of the child. If there is any evidence of dental caries or other unhealthy state, the child is referred for dental services. The family may have a family dentist or a pedodontist who can provide needed care. An alarming number of children do not receive regular dental supervision, and a significant number reach adulthood without having been examined or treated by a dentist.

Malocclusion. When teeth of the upper and lower dental arches approximate in the proper relationships, the physiologic function of mastication is more effective and the cosmetic effect is more pleasing. Teeth that are uneven, crowded, or overlapping, or that otherwise interfere with their ability to meet their opponents in the opposite jaw in the appropriate relationships, may be predisposed to disease in later years.

Orthodontic treatment is usually most successful when it is started in the later school-age years or the early teenage years, after the last primary teeth have been shed and before growth ceases. However, referral should be made as soon as malocclusion is evident, since some deformities can be corrected at an earlier age.

Sex education

Evidence indicates that many children experience some form of sex play during or prior to preadolescence as a response to normal curiosity, not as a result of love or sexual urge. Children are experimentalists by nature, and this play is incidental and transitory. Any adverse emotional consequences or guilt feelings depend on how the behavior is managed by the parents, if it is discovered, or whether the child views his actions as wrong in the eyes of significant persons, particularly the parents.

Much of the child's attitude toward sex that is acquired indirectly at a very early age affects the way in which he responds to sexual information presented at a later time. Middle childhood appears to be an ideal time for formal sex education, and many authorities believe that the topic is best presented from a life-span approach. Initial curiosity about differences in body structure between boys and girls and between children and adults has arisen in the preschool years, and the next stage, adolescence, will arouse both anxiety and excitement about sexual encounters. Information about sexual maturation and the process of reproduction presented during middle childhood helps to minimize the child's uncertainty, embarrassment, and feelings of isolation that often accompany the events of puberty.

Nurse's role in sex education. No matter where nurses practice, they can provide information on human sexuality to both parents and children. Nurses can help parents by first becoming knowledgeable about human sexuality themselves, including the common myths and misconceptions associated with sex and the reproductive process. Because parents often either repress or avoid the child's sexual curiosity, the sexual information that he receives is acquired almost entirely from his peers. When peers are the primary source of sexual information, it is transmitted and exchanged in secret, clandestine conversation and contains a large amount of misinformation. Children's questions about sex should be answered to the same extent as their questions about any other topic—honestly and at their level of understanding.

During encounters with parents, nurses can be open and available for questions and discussion. They can set an example by the language they use in discussing body parts and their function and by the way in which they deal with problems that have emotional overtones, such as exploratory sex play and masturbation. Parents need to be helped to understand normal behaviors and to view sexual curiosity in their children as a part of the developmental process. Assessing the parents' level of knowledge and understanding of sexuality provides cues to their need for supplemental information that will better prepare them for the increasingly complex explanations that will be needed as their children grow older.

School health problems

Child health maintenance is ultimately the responsibility of the parents; however, the public schools and health departments in the United States have contributed to the im-

---

SUMMARY OF GROWTH AND DEVELOPMENT DURING SCHOOL-AGE YEARS

AGE (years)	PHYSICAL AND MOTOR	MENTAL AND SOCIAL	ADAPTIVE	PERSONAL-SOCIAL
6	Growth and weight gain slower Central mandibular incisors erupt Weight: 16-23.6 kg (35½-58 pounds); height: 106.6-123.5 cm (42-48 inches) Gradual increase in dexterity Active age; constant activity Often returns to finger feeding More aware of hand as a tool Likes to draw, print, and color	Counts 13 pennies Knows whether it is morning or afternoon Defines common objects such as fork and chair in terms of their use Obeys triple commands in succession Shows right hand and left ear Says which is pretty and which is ugly of a series of drawings of faces Describes the objects in a picture rather than simply enumerating them Period of more tension but is intellectually more stimulating Giggles a lot Attends first grade More independent, probably influence of school Has own way of doing things Increased socialization Tries out own abilities	At table, uses knife to spread butter or jam on bread At play, cuts, folds, pastes paper toys, sews crudely if needle is threaded Enjoys making simple figures in clay Takes bath without supervision; performs bedtime activities alone Reads from memory; enjoys oral spelling game Likes table games, checkers, simple card games	Can share and cooperate better Great need for children of own age Will cheat to win Often engages in rough play Often jealous of younger brother or sister Does what he sees adults doing Often has temper tantrums Is a boaster Has difficulty owning up to misdeeds Sometimes steals money or attractive items

Continued.

SUMMARY OF GROWTH AND DEVELOPMENT DURING SCHOOL-AGE YEARS—cont'd

AGE (years)	PHYSICAL AND MOTOR	MENTAL AND SOCIAL	ADAPTIVE	PERSONAL-SOCIAL
7	Begins to grow at least 2 inches a year Maxillary central incisors and lateral mandibular incisors erupt Weight: 17.7-30 kg (39-66½ pounds); height: 111.8-129.7 cm (44-51 inches) Gross motor actions are cautious but not fearful More cautious in approaches to new performances Repeats performances to master them Posture more tense and unstable; maintains one position longer	Notices that certain parts are missing from pictures Can copy a diamond Repeats three numbers backward Reads ordinary clock or watch correctly to nearest quarter hour; uses clock for practical purposes Attends the second grade Takes part in group play Boys prefer playing with boys; girls prefer playing with girls More mechanical in reading; often does not stop at the end of a sentence, skips words such as it, the, he, and so on	Uses table knife for cutting meat; may need help with tough or difficult pieces Brushes and combs hair acceptably without help or "going over"	Is becoming a real member of the family group Likes to help and have a choice Less resistant and stubborn Spends a lot of time alone; doesn't require a lot of companionship Stealing may still be a problem
8-9	Continues to grow at 5 cm (2 inches) a year Lateral incisors (maxillary) and mandibular cuspids erupt Weight: 19.6-39.6 kg (43-87 pounds); height: 117-141.8 cm (46-56 inches) Movement fluid; often graceful and poised Always on the go; jumps, chases, skips Increased smoothness and speed in fine motor control Dresses self completely Likely to overdo; hard to quiet down after recess	Gives similarities and differences between two things from memory Counts backward from 20 to 1 Repeats days of the week and months in order; knows the date Describes common objects in detail, not merely their use Makes change out of a quarter Attends third and fourth grades Goes about home and community freely, alone or with friends Likes to compete and play games	Makes use of common tools such as hammer, saw, or screwdriver Uses household and sewing utensils Helps with routine household tasks such as dusting, sweeping Assumes responsibility for share of household chores Looks after all of own needs at table Buys useful articles; exercises some choice in making purchases Runs useful errands Likes pictorial magazines Likes school; wants to answer all the questions	Easy to get along with at home Likes the reward system Dramatizes Is more sociable Is better behaved Interested in boy-girl relationships but will not admit it

provement of child health by providing a healthful school environment, health services, and health education that emphasizes sound health practices. Most of these functions constitute major components of community health services and involve large amounts of public funds and large numbers of health professionals, including nurses, on either a full-time or a part-time basis. School health programs contribute to the goals of the community for the education and development of the children.

A school health program is also involved in ongoing health maintenance through assessment, screening, and referral activities. Routine health services provided by most

SUMMARY OF GROWTH AND DEVELOPMENT DURING SCHOOL-AGE YEARS—cont'd

AGE (years)	PHYSICAL AND MOTOR	MENTAL AND SOCIAL	ADAPTIVE	PERSONAL-SOCIAL
		Shows preference in friends and groups Plays mostly with groups of own sex but is beginning to mix Reads classic books, but also enjoys comics	Greater reader; may plan to wake up early just to read More aware of time; can be relied on to get to school on time Afraid of failing a grade; ashamed of bad grades More critical of self	
10-12	Slow growth in height and rapid weight gain; may become obese in this period Posture is more similar to an adult's; will overcome lordosis Pubescent changes may begin to appear Rest of teeth will erupt and tend toward full development Weight: 24.3-58 kg (54-128 pounds); height: 127.5-162.3 cm (50-64 inches) Body lines soften and round out in girls	Does occasional or brief work on own initiative around home and neighborhood Is sometimes left alone at home or at work for an hour or so Is successful in looking after own needs or those of other children left in his care Attends fifth to seventh grades Writes occasional short letters to friends or relatives on own initiative Uses telephone for practical purposes Responds to magazine, radio, or other advertising by mailing coupons Reads for practical information or own enjoyment—stories or library books of adventure or romance, or animal stories	Makes useful articles or does easy repair work Cooks or sews in small way Raises pets Writes brief stories Produces simple paintings or drawings Washes and dries own hair Is responsible for a thorough job of cleaning hair, but may need reminding to do so Likes his family; family really has meaning Likes mother and wants to please her in many ways Demonstrative of affection Likes dad too; he is adored and idolized Respects parents Loves friends; talks about them constantly Boys like large playgrounds	Fond of friends Chooses friends more selectively Loves conversation Beginning interest in opposite sex More diplomatic

schools include health appraisal, emergency care and safety, communicable disease control, and counseling and follow-up care. Health education of school children is primarily directed toward providing knowledge of health and influencing habits, attitudes, and conduct in relation to health and accident prevention. The variety of topics for health instruction is endless, and eager minds are ready and willing to learn.

Traditionally, school nurses have been viewed from a limited perspective that placed them in the role of disease detector, applier of Band-Aids, and official caregiver in cases of illness and injury. Although these are still impor-

PARENTAL GUIDANCE DURING THE SCHOOL-AGE YEARS

AGE (years)	GUIDANCE
6	Expect strong food preferences and frequent refusals of specific food items
	Expect increasingly ravenous appetite
	Prepare parents for emotionality as child experiences erratic mood changes
	Anticipate increase in susceptibility to illness and more sickness than at previous ages
	Teach accident prevention and safety, especially bicycle safety
	Respect the child's need for privacy; provide a room of his own if possible
	Prepare for increasing interests outside the home
	Encourage interaction with peers
7-10	Expect improvement in health with fewer illnesses; however, allergies may increase or become apparent
	Prepare for increase in minor accidents
	Emphasize caution in selection and maintenance of sports equipment and re-emphasize teaching safety
	Expect increased involvement with peers and interest in activities outside the home
	Encourage independence but maintain limit-setting and discipline
	Expect more demands upon mother at 8 years
	Expect increasing admiration for father at 10 years; encourage father-child activities
	Prepare for prepubescent changes in girls
11-12	Prepare child for body changes of pubescence
	Expect a growth spurt in girls
	Make certain the child's sex education is adequate with accurate information
	Expect energetic but stormy behavior at 11 to become more even-tempered at 12
	Encourage child's desire to "grow up" but allow regressive behavior when needed
	Expect an increase in masturbation
	May need increased amount of rest
	Educate child regarding experimentation with potentially harmful activities or substances

tant functions and their importance is not to be minimized, this traditional role is acquiring much broader dimensions. School nurses are being prepared to provide primary health care on a broader scale that includes assessment of physical, psychomedical, psychoeducational, behavioral, and learning disorder problems and to provide comprehensive well-child care. The school nurse practitioner is also concerned with development, implementation, and evaluation of health care plans and programs.

REFERENCES

Erikson, E.H.: Childhood and society, ed. 2, New York, 1963, W.W. Norton & Co., Inc.

Shaffer, T.E.: The young athlete: new guidelines in sports medicine, Pediatr. Consult. 1(5):1-12, 1980.

BIBLIOGRAPHY
General

Allen, M.T.: An overview of the type A behavior pattern in children and adolescents, Pediatr. Nurs. 9:407-412, 1983.

Belkengren, R.P., and Sapala, S.: Physical fitness from infancy through adolescence, Pediatr. Nurs. 8(4):A-I, 1982.

Cameron, C.O., Juszczak, L., and Wallace, N.: Using creative arts to help children cope with altered body image, Children's Health Care 12:108-112, 1984.

Dansky, K.H.: Assessing children's nutrition, Am. J. Nurs. 77:1610-1611, 1977.

Havighurst, R.J.: Developmental tasks and education, ed. 3, New York, 1972, David McKay Co., Inc.

Kaluger, G., and Kaluger, M.F.: Human development: the span of life, ed. 3, St. Louis, 1984, The C.V. Mosby Co.

LaMontagne, L.L.: Three coping strategies used by school-age children, Pediatr. Nurs. 10(1):25-28, 1984.

McCown, D.: TV: its problems for children, Pediatr. Nurs. 5(2):17-19, 1979.

Mussen, P.H., Conger, J.J., and Kagan, J.: Child development and personality, ed. 5, New York, 1979, Harper & Row, Publishers, Inc.

Newman, B.M., and Newman, P.R.: Development through life: a psychosocial approach, Homewood, Ill., 1979, The Dorsey Press.

Pipes, P.L.: Nutrition in infancy and childhood, ed. 2, St. Louis, 1981, The C.V. Mosby Co.

Stone, L.J., and Church, J.: Childhood and adolescence, ed. 5, New York, 1983, Random House, Inc.

Sutterly, D.C., and Donnelly, G.F.: Perspectives in human development, ed. 2, Philadelphia, 1980, J.B. Lippincott Co.

Williams, S.R.: Nutrition and diet therapy, ed. 4, St. Louis, 1981, The C.V. Mosby Co.

Accidents

Betz, C.L.: Bicycle safety: opportunities for family education, Pediatr. Nurs. **9:**111, 1983.

Narins, D.M., Belkengren, R.P., and Sapala, S.: Nutrition and the growing athlete, Pediatr. Nurs. **9**(3):163-168, 1983.

Thomas, K.A.: Screening the child for sports participation, Issues Compr. Pediatr. Nurs. **5:**179-194, 1983.

Dental health

Babington, M.A., and Spadaro, D.C.: Cariogenic medications, Pediatr. Nurs. **8**(3):165-169, 1982.

Boraz, R.A.: Preventive dentistry for the pediatric patient, Issues Compr. Pediatr. Nurs. **5:**89-97, 1981.

Cormier, J.F., and Trammel, H.: Fighting tooth decay: the fluoride plan, Pediatr. Nurs. **5**(3):18-22, 1979.

Kilmon, C., and Helpin, M.L.: Recognizing dental malocclusion in children, Pediatr. Nurs. **9**(3):204-208, 1983.

Slattery, J.: Dental health in children, Am. J. Nurs. **76:**1159-1161, 1976.

Smith, J.T.: Promoting childhood dental health, Pediatr. Nurs. **2**(3):16-19, 1976.

Sex education

Czarniecki, L.: The integration of sex education in pediatric nursing practice, Pediatr. Nurs. **2**(2):12-16, 1976.

Edelman, S.K.: Sex and life education in rural school, Am. J. Nurs. **77:**233-239, 1977.

Ehrman, M.: Sex education for the young, Nurs. Outlook **23:**538-585, 1975.

Rybicki, L.L.: Preparing parents to teach their children about human sexuality, Am. J. Maternal Child Nurs. **1:**182-185, 1976.

Southall, C.: Family life and sex education, Am. J. Nurs. **77:**1473-1476, 1977.

School health

Fine, L.L., and Bellaire, J.M.: The school nurse: an obsolete professional revisited, Pediatr. Nurs. **1:**25, 1975

Garner, G.: Modifying pupil self-concept and behavior, Today's Educ. **63:**24-28, 1974.

Hordin, D.: The school-age child and the school nurse, Am. J. Nurs. **74:**1476-1478, 1974.

Oda, D.: A viewpoint on school nursing, Am. J. Nurs. **81:**1677-1678, 1981.

Robinson, T.: School nurse practitioners on the job, Am. J. Nurs. **81:**1674-1676, 1981.

Switzer, K.H., and Kelly, J.T.: The nurse: a member of the school team, Am. J. Maternal Child Nurs. **6:**289-293, 1981.

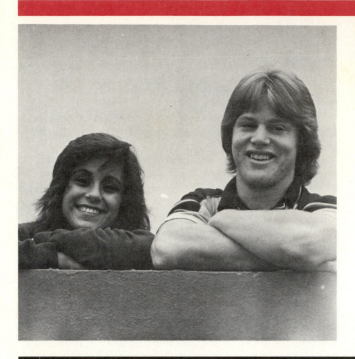

14

THE ADOLESCENT YEARS

OBJECTIVES

On completion of this chapter the reader will be able to:

- Describe the physical changes that occur at puberty in the male and the female

- Discuss the reactions of the adolescent to physical changes that take place at puberty

- Demonstrate an understanding of the processes by which the adolescent develops a sense of identity

- Discuss the significance of the changing interpersonal relationships and the role of the peer group during adolescence

- Outline a health teaching plan for adolescents

- Identify the causes and discuss the preventive aspects of accidents in adolescence

- Plan a sex education session for a group of adolescents

NURSING DIAGNOSES

Nursing diagnoses identified for the adolescent include, but are not restricted to, the following:

Health perception-health management pattern

- Health maintenance, alteration in, related to knowledge deficit

- Infection, potential for, related to deficient health and hygienic practices

- Injury, potential for, related to knowledge deficit

Nutritional-metabolic pattern

- Nutrition, alterations in: less than body requirements related to (1) increased need for nutrients (e.g., protein, iron); (2) eating practices

- Nutrition, alterations in: more than body requirements related to (1) inactivity; (2) eating practices

- Skin integrity, impairment of: potential related to (1) peer practices (e.g., ear piercing, use of make-up); (2) hormonal changes

Activity-exercise pattern

- Activity intolerance related to (1) nutritional deficits; (2) over-exertion; (3) insufficient rest; (4) lack of motivation

- Self-care deficit related to lack of motivation

Sleep-rest pattern

- Sleep pattern disturbance related to involvement in activities

Cognitive-perceptual pattern

- Knowledge deficit related to (1) inexperience; (2) unfamiliarity with information resources

Self-perception—self-concept pattern

- Anxiety related to (1) perception of changing body structure and function; (2) perception of impending events; (3) relationships with members of opposite sex; (4) role confusion; (5) relationship with parents; (6) career selection

- Powerlessness related to feelings of dependency

- Self-concept, disturbance in, related to (1) perception of developmental changes; (2) inability to meet expectations of self and/or others

Role-relationship pattern

- Family process, alterations in, related to (1) independence-dependence conflicts; (2) situational crisis

- Parenting, alterations in: potential related to (1) skill deficit; (2) family stress; (3) knowledge deficit

- Social isolation related to (1) inability to conform; (2) personality characteristics; (3) peer rejection

Sexuality-reproductive pattern

- Sexual dysfunction related to (1) immaturity; (2) knowledge deficit

Coping-stress tolerance pattern

- Coping, ineffective individual, related to (1) situational crises; (2) knowledge deficit; (3) deficient problem-solving skills

Value-belief pattern

- Spiritual distress related to inner conflicts

Adolescence is a period of transition between childhood and adulthood; a time of physical, social, and emotional maturing as the boy prepares for manhood and the girl for womanhood. The precise bounderies of adolescence are difficult to define, but this period is customarily viewed as beginning with the gradual appearance of secondary sex characteristics at about 11 or 12 years of age and ending with cessation of body growth at 18 to 20 years.

Several terms are commonly used in reference to this particular stage of growth and development. *Puberty* primarily refers to the maturational, hormonal, and growth process that occurs when the reproductive organs begin to function and the secondary sex characteristics develop. This process is sometimes delineated as *pubescence,* the period of about 2 years immediately prior to puberty when the child is developing preliminary physical changes that herald sexual maturity and when he is experiencing the prepubertal growth spurt; *puberty,* the point at which sexual maturity is achieved, marked by the first menstrual flow in girls but by less obvious indications in boys; and *postpubescence,* a 1- to 2-year period following puberty during which skeletal growth is completed and reproductive functions become fairly well established. *Adolescence,* which literally means ''to grow into maturity,'' is generally regarded as the psychologic, social, and maturational process initiated by the pubertal changes. The term *teenage years* is used synonymously with adolescence to describe ages 13 through 19.

Adolescence is a period of life that presents special problems of adjustment. With the impetus of their internal changes and the pressures of society, children must progress to emotional independence from their parents, consider prospects of economic independence, and learn the meaning of a more intimate heterosexual companionship. They learn to work with age-mates on common interests, to subordinate personal differences as they pursue a common goal, and to become responsible persons who are in control of their lives and who possess a knowledge of who they are in relation to the world.

PHYSICAL DEVELOPMENT

The physical changes of puberty are primarily the result of hormonal activity under the influence of the central nervous system, although all aspects of physiologic functioning are mutually interacting. The very obvious physical changes are noted in increased physical growth and the appearance and development of secondary sex characteristics; less obvious are physiologic alterations and neurogonadal maturity, accompanied by the ability to procreate. Physical distinction between the sexes is determined on the basis of distinguishing characteristics: *primary sex characteristics* are the external and internal organs that carry on the reproductive functions; *secondary sex characteristics* are the characteristics that distinguish the sexes from each other but play no direct part in reproduction.

Physical growth

A constant phenomenon associated with sexual maturation is a dramatic increase in growth. The final 20% to 25% of linear growth is achieved during puberty, and most of this growth occurs during a 24- to 36-month period—the adolescent growth spurt. This accelerated growth occurs in all children but, as in other areas of development, is highly variable in age of onset, duration, and extent. The growth spurt begins earlier in girls, usually between ages 10 and 14 years; on the average it begins between ages 12 and 16 years in boys. During this period the average boy will gain 10 to 30 cm (4 to 12 inches) in height and 7 to 30 kg (15 to 65 pounds) in weight; the average girl, in whom the growth spurt is slower and less extensive, will gain 5 to 20 cm (2 to 8 inches) in height and 7 to 25 kg (15 to 55 pounds) in weight. Growth in height commonly ceases at 16 or 17 years in girls and 18 to 20 years in boys (Figs. 14-1 and 14-2).

This increase in size is acquired in a characteristic sequence of changes. Growth in length of extremities and neck precedes growth in other areas, and, since these parts are first to reach adult length, the hands and feet appear larger than normal during adolescence. Increases in hip and chest breadth take place in a few months, followed several months later by an increase in shoulder width. These changes are followed by increases in length of the trunk and depth of the chest. It is this sequence of changes that is responsible for the characteristic long-legged, gawky appearance of the early adolescent child.

Sex differences in general growth patterns. Sex differences in general growth and distribution patterns are apparent in skeletal growth, muscle mass, adipose tissue, and skin. Skeletal growth differences between boys and girls are apparently a function of hormonal effects at puberty and are evident primarily in limb length. The earlier cessation of growth in girls is caused by epiphyseal unity under the potent effect of estrogen secretion, and the hormonal effect on female bone growth is much stronger than the similar effect of testosterone in males. In boys, the prolonged growth period prior to puberty and the less rapid epiphyseal closure are reflected in their greater overall height and longer arms and legs. Other skeletal differences are increased shoulder width in boys and broader hip development in girls.

Hypertrophy of the laryngeal mucosa and enlargement of the larynx and vocal cords occur in both boys and girls to produce voice changes. Girls' voices become slightly deeper and considerably fuller, but the effect in boys is striking. The ''change of voice'' in adolescent boys is one

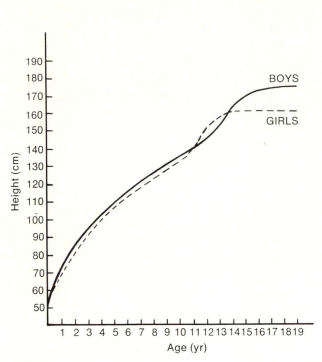

FIG. 14-1

Linear growth throughout childhood. (From Tanner, J.M., Whitehouse, R.H., and Takaishi, M.: Arch. Dis. Child. **41**:454-471, 1966.)

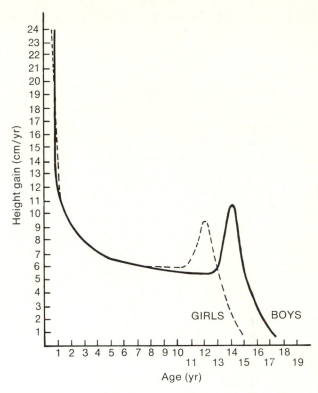

FIG. 14-2

Linear growth in centimeters per year. (From Tanner, J.M., Whitehouse, R.H., and Takaishi, M.: Arch. Dis. Child. **41**:454-471, 1966.)

of the most noticeable traits of puberty, with the voice often shifting uncontrollably from deep to high tones in the middle of a sentence.

Growth of lean body mass, principally muscle, which tends to occur after the bone growth spurt, takes place steadily during adolescence. Lean body mass is both quantitatively and qualitatively greater in males than in females at comparable stages of pubertal development. Muscle development, under the influence of androgenic hormones, increases steadily. Muscles become remarkably well developed in boys, whereas in girls muscle mass increase is proportionate to general tissue growth.

Nonlean mass, primarily fat, is also increased but follows a less orderly pattern. There may be a transient increase in subcutaneous fat just prior to the skeletal growth spurt, especially in boys, which is followed 1 to 2 years later by a modest to marked decrease, again more marked in boys. Later, variable amounts of fat are deposited to fill out and contour the mature physique in patterns characteristic of the adolescent's sex.

Hormonal influences during puberty cause an acceleration in growth and maturation of the skin and its structural appendages. Sebaceous glands become extremely active at this time, especially those on the genitals and in the "flush areas" of the body—that is, the face, neck, shoul-

ders, and upper back and chest. This increased activity and the structural nature of the glands are extremely important in the pathogenesis of a common problem of puberty, acne. The eccrine sweat glands, present almost everywhere on the human skin, become fully functional and respond to emotional as well as thermal stimulation. Heavy sweating appears to be more pronounced in boys than in girls. The apocrine sweat glands, nonfunctional in childhood, reach secretory capacity during puberty. Unlike the eccrine sweat glands, the apocrine glands are limited in distribution and grow in conjunction with hair follicles in the axillae, around the areola of the breast, around the umbilicus, on the external auditory canal, and in the genital and anal regions. Apocrine glands secrete a thick secretion as a result of emotional stimulation that, when acted on by surface bacteria, becomes highly odoriferous.

Body hair assumes very characteristic distribution patterns and texture changes during puberty. Under the influence of gonadal and adrenal androgens, hair coarsens, darkens, and lengthens at sites related to secondary sex characteristics. Pubic and axillary hair appears in both sexes, although pubic hair is more extensive in males than in females. Beard, mustache, and body hair on the chest, upward along the linea alba, and sometimes on other areas (such as the back and shoulder) appear in males. Extremity hair appears in varying amounts in both males and females but is also more prolific in the male.

Physiologic changes

A number of physiologic functions are altered in response to some of the pubertal changes. The size and strength of the heart, blood volume, and systolic blood pressure increase, whereas the pulse rate and basal heat production decrease (see inside front cover). Blood volume, which has increased steadily during childhood, reaches a higher value in boys than in girls, a fact that may be related to the increased muscle mass in pubertal boys. Adult values are reached for all formed elements of the blood. Respiratory rate and basal metabolic rate, decreasing steadily throughout childhood, reach the adult rate in adolescence.

Through progressive maturation of the body as it reaches adult size, the adolescent develops the ability to respond to physical stresses and strains equal to or in excess of adult competence. During this period physiologic responses to exercise change drastically—performance improves, especially in boys, and the body is able to make the physiologic adjustments needed for normal function after exercise is completed. These capabilities are a result of the increased size and strength of muscles and the increased level of cardiac, respiratory, and metabolic functioning. Adolescents enjoy physical activity, and there appears to be a positive relationship between regular exercise and physical conditioning activities and good general health, endurance, and appearance.

Reproductive endocrine system

It is generally accepted that the events of puberty are caused by hormonal influences and controlled by the anterior pituitary (adenohypophysis) in response to a stimulus from the hypothalamus. Stimulation of the gonads has a dual function: (1) production and release of gametes—production of sperm in the male and maturation and release of ova in the female—and (2) secretion of sex-appropriate hormones—estrogen and progesterone from the female ovaries and testosterone from the male testes.

Sex hormones. Sex hormones are secreted by the ovaries, testes, and adrenals, and are produced in varying amounts by both sexes throughout the life span. The adrenal cortex is responsible for the small amounts secreted during the prepubescent years, but the sex hormone production that accompanies maturation of the gonads is responsible for the variety of biologic changes observed during pubescence and puberty.

Estrogen, the feminizing hormone, is found in low quantities during childhood; it is secreted in slowly increasing amounts until about age 11 years. In males this gradual increase continues through maturation. In females the onset of estrogen production in the ovary causes a pronounced increase that continues until about 3 years after the onset of menstruation, at which time it reaches a maximum level that continues throughout the reproductive life of the female.

Androgens, the masculinizing hormones, are also secreted in small and gradually increasing amounts up to about 7 or 9 years of age, at which time there is a more rapid increase in both sexes, especially boys, until about age 15 years. These hormones appear to be responsible for most of the rapid growth changes of early adolescence. With the onset of testicular function, the level of androgens (principally testosterone) in males increases over that in females and continues to increase until a maximum is attained at maturity.

Development of reproductive function in females. Approximately 1 to 2 years before the onset of menstruation in the female, the secretion of estrogen assumes a cyclic pattern. The initial appearance of menstruation *(menarche)* occurs about 2 years after the first appearance of pubescent changes. The normal age range of menarche is usually considered to be 10 to 15 years, with the average age being 12.5 years for North American girls. Menarche has been related to a critical point in body weight (48 kg or 106 pounds) but may vary with race. During the establishment of the ovarian cycle, the menstrual periods are usually scanty and irregular and may not be accompanied by ovulation. Ovulation usually occurs 12 to 24 months after menarche.

Development of reproductive function in males. Unlike the cyclic germ cell production in the female, spermatogenesis is a continuous process that is usually well established by 17 years of age. There is no sudden physical change to indicate puberty such as the menarche in girls. The overt signal in boys is the beginning of nocturnal emissions of seminal fluid, which occur spontaneously during sleep at intervals of approximately 2 weeks. Nocturnal emissions will persist into adulthood and will occur whenever there is a buildup of semen in the genital ducts. As with girls, mature germ cells may not be produced for several months. The average age range at which boys attain puberty is 12.5 to 16.5 years, with a mean of 14.5 years.

Determination of sexual maturity

The visible evidence of sexual maturation is achieved in orderly sequence, and the state of maturity can be estimated on the basis of the appearance of these external manifestations. The age at which these changes are observed and the time required to progress from one stage to another may vary considerably between individual children. From the appearance of breast buds to full maturity may range from 1½ to 6 years for adolescent girls; male genitalia may take from 2 to 5 years to reach adult size. The stages of the development of secondary sex characteristics and genital development have been defined as a guide for estimating sexual maturity.

The usual sequence of appearance of maturational changes in girls is as follows: rapid increase in height and weight, breast changes, increase in pelvic girth, growth of pubic hair, appearance of axillary hair, menstruation (which usually begins 2 years after first signs), and an abrupt deceleration of linear growth.

The usual sequence of appearance of maturational changes in boys is as follows: increase in weight; enlargement of testicles; rapid increase in height; growth of pubic hair, axillary hair, hair on upper lip, hair on face and elsewhere on body (facial hair usually appears about 2 years after appearance of pubic hair); changes in the larynx and, consequently, the voice, which usually take place concurrently with growth of the penis; nocturnal emissions; and an abrupt deceleration of linear growth.

ADOLESCENT'S REACTION TO BODY IMAGE CHANGES AT PUBERTY

Physical growth and maturation during adolescence occur so rapidly that these young people have difficulty in adjusting to a changing body image. Adolescence is the time when young persons' self-awareness reaches a peak and, as a result of sexual awareness, when much of their thought and concern is turned inward. The sudden growth that takes place in early adolescence creates feelings of confusion about their bodies. Teenagers are acutely aware of their appearance as they begin to acquire images of themselves as adults, but they see discrepancies between their ideal and actual skills and abilities.

Strange and unfamiliar feelings press on them as inner urges announce a sexual awakening. Sexuality is not the same for boys as it is for girls, and it has different psychic overtones that influence behavior and adaptation. Although it appears that the intensity of the sexual drive is different in adolescent boys and girls, this has not been conclusively demonstrated. Current findings indicate that the difference may be related to the physiologic nature of the sex drive rather than to its intensity. Sexual arousal in males is very direct and centered in the genitals, whereas in females it is more vague, diffuse, and closely linked to their total personality.

Boys' responses to puberty

The early adolescent increases in height and muscle mass are welcomed by the adolescent boy, whose growth, for several months, has lagged significantly behind that of his female age-mates. Although his more mature physique brings a highly valued increase in strength and more mature athletic skills, this rapid growth is uneven and he therefore has some trouble adjusting. When bones grow faster than muscles, muscles are taut and respond with quick, jerky movements; when muscles grow faster than bones, they become somewhat loose and sluggish. For a period of time he is awkward and uncoordinated.

The development of secondary sex characteristics, especially the growth of facial and body hair, has psychologic and social meaning to the adolescent boy. This, more than any other secondary characteristic, is associated with the masculine sex role, and the ritual act of shaving at the slightest evidence of growth is a way for the young boy to validate his identification with this role. Shaving also provides a legitimate excuse to gaze at and admire the broadening shoulders and altered features of his changing body image.

The growth of the penis and testes creates some important problems for the adolescent male. Unlike the reproductive organs in the female, the male reproductive organs are readily visible and provide the boy with concrete evidence of his masculine character. He knows by the sensations localized within these organs that he is now a man. His reproductive organs become very sensitive to sexual stimulation. Sexual feelings are directly related to the genitals, desire is urgent, and he seeks rapid relief from pressure and tension through ejaculation. Spontaneous ejaculations are frequently puzzling, troublesome, and embarrassing events. Unless he has been prepared in advance for this eventuality, the boy often finds it difficult to seek an explanation from his parents; therefore, he turns to friends or reading material to gain information, or he may puzzle about the meaning in his own mind.

The opportunity for gratification of these genital urges through heterosexual expression is often limited by Western cultural standards, early premarital sexual involvement is fraught with many problems and conflicts, and homosexual activities are generally condemned by society. As a consequence, the teenage boy resorts to masturbation, the manipulation of the genitals for the purpose of ejaculation, to relieve him of the accumulated pressures in his genital organs. It is essentially a normal activity, and almost every boy masturbates alone or in relation to sexual experimentation with others of the same sex. However, this too is often associated with guilt and anxiety. Misconceptions still dominate the feelings of many people who believe masturbation to be evil, unmanly, or "not nice" and who attribute a wide assortment of ills to the practice. Current enlightenment accepts that to engage in the practice from time to time is normal and temporarily helps provide the young man with important information about how his body works and how adult physical sexuality and reproduction are accomplished.

Girls' responses to puberty

As girls begin the pubertal changes, they, too, become very body conscious. Because in girls the onset of puberty is almost 2 years in advance of that in boys, their initial reaction to increased height may be embarrassment, as they find themselves towering above their male classmates. They worry about becoming too tall. Adolescent girls often slouch or adopt a hunched posture in an attempt to minimize this increased height—especially early-maturing girls, who are normally of above-average height. The increase in weight and the normal plumping of features with fat deposition are predominant concerns of the pubescent girl. They perceive these changes to be evidence of a tendency toward obesity; many attempt to avoid them by strict and rather faddish dieting. This ill-timed strategy can deprive their bodies of essential nutrients during a period of rapid body development.

The young girl is interested in her changing form and feminine curves. The average girl looks on her budding breasts with pleasure as a sign of approaching maturity and evidence of her femininity. She observes and may even measure the progress of her developing breasts and continually compares her own progress with that of her friends and classmates. She begins to wear a brassiere. Some girls are sensitive about their breast development and attempt to hide it, whereas others are delighted with their new figures and wear tight sweaters and clothes that accentuate their curves.

Development of some of the secondary sex characteristics may be less pleasing to girls than they are to boys, particularly the growth of body hair. A culture in which smooth-skinned females are preferred makes it necessary for the girl to shave her underarms and legs regularly to meet the standards for feminine appearance. The girl becomes increasingly conscious of the feminine ideal and, in an effort to approach this standard, experiments with a variety of cosmetics and hairstyles. Alone and together, she and her friends spend endless hours before the mirror posing, applying cosmetics, and combing their hair.

The advent of menstruation, that exclusive feature of female puberty, provides the greatest impetus toward full realization and acceptance of female sexuality. Menstruation is positive evidence of womanhood and the potential for pregnancy and childbearing. Most girls are adequately prepared for the event and take this new function in stride, looking forward to menstruation, feeling satisfaction at its onset, and seeing it as the symbol of their passage from childhood to womanhood. Others find it distressing, frightening, and difficult to accept.

Unlike the adolescent boy, strong sexual feelings in the adolescent girl are not usually centered in the genital region but are more generalized and ill defined. Her reproductive apparatus, less obvious than that of the boy, contributes in only a vague way to sexual awareness. The girl in early adolescence may experience pleasant sensations and even tingling in the genital area, but these feelings are diffuse and difficult to separate from other body sensations. Her sexual feelings are centered less on the genitals and erotic gratification with release of tension than on manipulating a pleasant state with romantic feelings about love. Sexual impulses tend to be secondary rather than primary as they are in the boy. However, with the more open, liberal views regarding female sexual responses, it is being revealed that much of the nature of the adolescent girl's sexual arousal may have a cultural rather than a biologic basis.

In the adolescent girl, the urge for self-stimulation is not as strong as it is in the male. Although many girls handle the genitals for the pleasant sensation that is evoked, not all carry the activity to a climax. Masturbation is frequently combined with fantasy.

PSYCHOLOGIC AND EMOTIONAL DEVELOPMENT

While adolescents are adjusting to physical changes that may contribute to or detract from their feelings of self-worth, they are learning how to use their developing mental capacities. Their ability to reason, to assess and evaluate, and to use divergent thinking to come up with new ideas increases during this period of life. The adolescent begins to think beyond the present and into the future. However, these capacities and the ability to make good judgments are still limited by inexperience and as yet insufficient knowledge from which to gain an adequate perspective for problem solving.

Cognitive development

Progression in the realm of cognitive thinking culminates with the capacity for abstract thinking. This stage, the period of formal operations, is Piaget's fourth and last stage. Living in the nonpresent as well as the present, they are no longer concerned with and restricted to the real and actual, which was typical of the period of concrete thought, but they are also concerned with the possible. They now think beyond the present. At this time their thoughts can be influenced by more logical principles than by their own perceptions and experiences. They now become capable of scientific reasoning and formal logic. Without having to center attention on the immediate situation, they can imagine the possible—a sequence of events that might occur, such as college and occupational possibilities; how things might change in the future, such as relationships with parents; and the consequences of their actions, such as dropping out of school.

Young people are now able to think about their own thinking and the thinking of others. They wonder what opinion others have of them, and they are increasingly able to imagine the thoughts of others. With this capacity comes the ability to differentiate between others' thoughts and their own and to interpret thoughts of others more accurately. Thus they are able to see themselves and the world in a more relativistic way. As they come to know that other cultures and communities have different norms and standards from their own, it becomes easier to accept members of these other cultures and the decision to behave in their own culture in an accepted manner becomes a more conscious commitment to that culture.

Search for identity

Traditional psychosocial theory holds that the developmental crisis of adolescence leads to the formation of a sense of identity (Erikson, 1963). Throughout childhood individuals have been going through the process of identification as they concentrate on various parts of the body at specific times. During infancy the child identifies himself as separate from the mother, during early childhood he establishes a gender role identification with the appropriate-sex parent, and in later childhood he establishes who he is in relation to others. In adolescence he comes to see himself as a distinct individual, somehow unique and separate from every other individual. In the light of their observations, some authorities see the central conflict of identity vs role diffusion of adolescence as being resolved in two stages (Newman & Newman, 1979). The early period of adolescence begins with the onset of puberty and extends to relative physical and emotional stability at or near graduation from high school. During this time the adolescent is faced with the crisis of *group identity* vs alienation. In the period that follows, the individual hopes to attain autonomy from the family and develop a sense of *personal identity* as opposed to role diffusion. A sense of group identity appears to be essential as a prelude to a sense of personal identity. Young adolescents must resolve questions concerning relationships with a peer group before they are able to resolve questions about who they are in relation to family and society.

Group identity. During the early stage of adolescence the pressure to belong to a group is intensified. Teenagers find it essential to have a group to which they feel they can belong and which provides them with status. Belonging to a crowd helps adolescents to define the differences between themselves and their parents. They dress as the group dresses and wear makeup and hairstyles according to group criteria—all of which are different from those of the parental generation. Language, music, and dancing reflect a culture that is exclusive to the adolescent. When adults begin to emulate these fashions and interests, the style changes immediately. The evidence of adolescent conformity to the peer group and nonconformity to the adult group provides teenagers with a frame of reference in which they can display their own self-assertion while they reject the identity with their parents' generation.

Individual identity. The quest for personal identity is part of the ongoing identification process. As the child establishes identity within a group, he is also attempting to incorporate multiple body changes into a concept of the self. Body awareness is part of self-awareness, and for some time the adolescent will engage in assimilating the self represented by this dimension. It has been determined that the body image established during adolescence is the one that the individual retains throughout life. Much of the adolescent's search for identity takes place before a mirror as he tries to read from the reflected features just who he is and what he looks like to other people (Fig. 14-3). The adolescent practices facial expressions and postures, tries out hair arrangements, worries about a pimple, and in other ways attempts to assess the best means to achieve a maximum effect—to reveal the "true self."

In this search for identity, adolescents take into consideration the relationships that have developed between themselves and others in the past as well as the directions they hope to be able to take in the future. Significant others hold certain expectations for the behavior of the adolescent. Often these expectations or demands are persistent enough to induce certain decisions that might be made differently or not at all if the individual could be solely re-

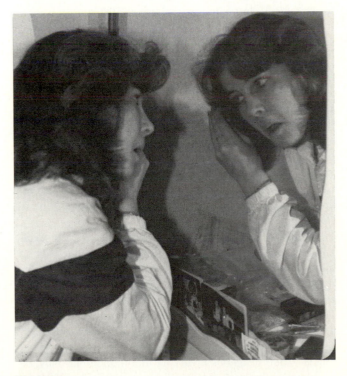

FIG. 14-3
Time spent before a mirror helps a teenager acquire a personal identity.

sponsible for identity formation. It is all too easy to slip into the roles that are expected by these external influences without incorporating personal goals or questioning these decisions in relation to the developing personality. Thus the individual becomes what parents or others wish him to be based on these premature decisions. Also, a young person might form a negative identity when society or his culture provides him with a self-image that is contrary to the values of the community. Labels such as "juvenile delinquent," "hood," or "failure" are applied to certain adolescents, who then accept and live up to these labels with behaviors that validate and strengthen them.

The process of evolving a personal identity is time-consuming and fraught with periods of confusion, depression, and discouragement. To determine an identity and a place in the world is a critical and perilous feature of adolescence. However, as the pieces are gradually shifted and settled into place, a positive identity eventually emerges from the confusion. Role diffusion results when the individual is unable to formulate a satisfactory identity from the multiplicity of aspirations, roles, and identifications.

Sex-role identity. Adolescence is the time for consolidation of a sex-role identity. During early adolescence the peer group begins to communicate some expectations regarding heterosexual relationships, and, as development progresses, adolescents encounter expectations for mature sex-role behavior from both peers and adults. Expectations such as these vary from culture to culture, between geographic areas, and between socioeconomic groups.

Moral development

Late adolescence is characterized by a serious questioning of existing moral values and their relevance to society and the individual. Adolescents can easily take the role of another. They understand duty and obligation based on reciprocal rights of others, as well as the concept of justice that is founded on making amends for misdeeds and repairing or replacing what has been spoiled by wrongdoing. However, they seriously question established moral codes, often as a result of observing that adults verbally ascribe to a code but do not adhere to it.

Whereas the younger child merely accepts the decisions or point of view of adults, the adolescent, to gain autonomy from adults, must substitute his own set of morals and values. When old principles are challenged but new and independent values have not yet emerged to take their place, young people search for a moral code that preserves their personal integrity and guides their behavior, especially in the face of strong pressure to violate the old beliefs. Their decisions involving moral dilemmas must be based on an internalized set of moral principles that provides them with the resources to evaluate the demands of

the situation and to plan a course of action that is consistent with their ideals.

Spiritual development

As youngsters move toward independence from parents and other authorities, some begin to question the values and ideals of their families. Others cling to these values as a stable element in their lives as they struggle with the conflicts of this turbulent period. Adolescents need to work out these conflicts for themselves, but they also need support from authority figures and/or peers for their resolution. Often the peer group is more influential than parents, although values acquired during the formative years are usually maintained.

Adolescents are capable of understanding abstract concepts and of interpreting analogies and symbols. They are able to empathize, philosophize, and think logically. Most are searching for ideals and speculate about illogical statements and conflicting ideologies. Their tendency toward introspection and emotional intensity at this age often makes it difficult for others to know what they are thinking. They tend to keep their thoughts private fearing that no one will understand these feelings that they perceive to be unique and special. It is not uncommon for them to reveal deep spiritual concerns and then become silly and deny these feelings (Shelly, 1982). They need support and encouragement in their struggle for understanding and the freedom to question without censure.

Emotionality and adolescent behavior

The pubertal changes in physical appearance are accompanied by changes in emotional control and response. The stability of the prepubescent period is replaced by the turmoil precipitated by the physical and psychologic alterations that teenagers experience. They are deluged with new sensations and feelings that they cannot understand. The behavior of adolescents is bewildering to others and often to the adolescents themselves. They vacillate between emotional states and between considerable maturity and childlike behavior. One minute they are exuberant and enthusiastic; the next minute they are depressed and withdrawn. Unpredictable, but essentially normal, outbursts of primitive behavior appear as the teenager loses control over instinctual drives. As the tension is relieved, emotion is brought under control and the individual retreats in order to review what has happened, to attempt to master his anger, and in the overall process to grow in his ability to control his emotions and gain from the new experience.

Teenagers begin to take hold of themselves in later adolescence. Their emotions are better controlled, they can approach problems more calmly and rationally, and, although they are still subject to periods of depression, their feelings are less vulnerable and they are beginning to demonstrate the more mature emotions of later adolescence. Whereas early adolescents react immediately and emotionally, older adolescents can control their emotions until socially acceptable times and places for expression present themselves. They are still subject to heightened emotion, and, when it is expressed, their behavior reflects feelings of insecurity, tension, and indecision.

Interests and activities

During early adolescence the interests and activities of girls and boys are in rather sharp contrast. Boys spend a great deal of time in active outdoor sports or ''just going out with the guys.'' They enjoy hobbies and clubs, and television takes up a good part of their time. Girls and mixed-sex activities are of interest to boys but do not become prominent concerns until their development more nearly approaches that of the more rapidly maturing girls. As their bodies gain strength and size, ''making the team'' is a major concern for many youths, and a boy may spend an excessive amount of time in attempting to perfect athletic skills. The essential bicycle of middle childhood is replaced by the automobile, the symbol of status to the adolescent. If a car cannot be acquired, a motorcycle or motorbike is preferable to walking, riding the bus, or the humiliation of being chauffeured by a parent or sibling. Most boys avidly seek part-time employment, many because of economic necessity.

Although girls' leisure interests involve many outdoor activities, an increased interest in parties and social activities is evident. They are interested in hobbies and volunteer activities, and many seek part-time jobs through necessity or in order to purchase more clothes and other teenage ''necessities.'' They are avid conversationalists and spend much of their time in the company of other girls, talking, listening to records, and experimenting with makeup, hairstyles, and clothes. They enjoy shopping for clothes, but there is seldom agreement between mother and daughter regarding types and styles of clothing. Many of their thoughts and feelings are confessed in a diary. Daydreaming is a prominent characteristic of the adolescent girl.

Members of both sexes enjoy movies, rock concerts, dancing, and other communal activities and entertainment (Fig. 14-4). Girls seem to prefer sentimental, romantic films when they are available, whereas boys would rather see sports, mystery, or action films. The X-rated movie theaters are crowded with adolescents.

Reading is still a favorite occupation of teenagers and may serve to satisfy some of their needs for vicarious experiences. Reading is more purposeful at this stage than at

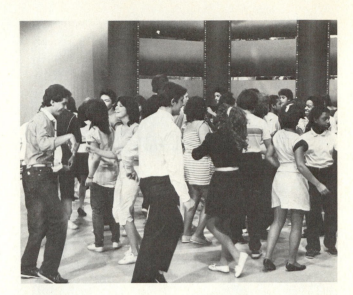

FIG. 14-4
Adolescents enjoy the activity and social aspects of dancing.

earlier ages, and most adolescents prefer to read magazines rather than books.

Television viewing declines in adolescence, and many teenagers have a decided preference for the radio (Fig. 14-5). Teenagers often are avidly addicted to the transistor radios that accompany many of their other activities—studying, walking, and so on. Closely associated with the radio is the stereo, which assumes an important role in teenagers' lives. Much of their money is spent on records and tapes, which are collected in much the same way as books.

When they are not engaged in other activities, they are probably participating in ''rap sessions'' or in endless telephone conversations. The telephone provides that essential link between peers when they are physically removed from one another. It is a means for fulfilling the need for flight from parents to peers without leaving the home. For boygirl conversations, the telephone provides a way to experience closeness without the fear of complications that physical proximity may engender.

Teenage interests and activities are subject to rapid change. Each succeeding ''generation'' of teenagers has its own peculiar characteristics, which are evidenced in behavior, vocabulary, dress, and other external manifestations that reflect and establish a clear line of separateness, although superficial, between the peer and the adult cultures. The rapidity with which these external trappings change is often astonishing.

Sports. The importance of sports activities during the teens cannot be underestimated. Both girls and boys participate in recreational sports and many are actively involved in competitive athletics either in conjunction with

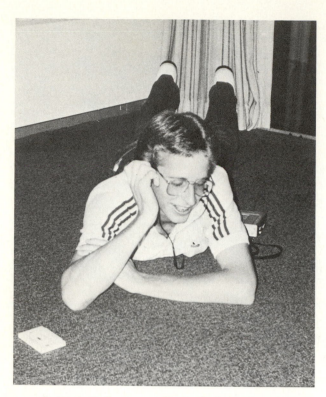

FIG. 14-5
Teenagers spend endless hours listening to music.

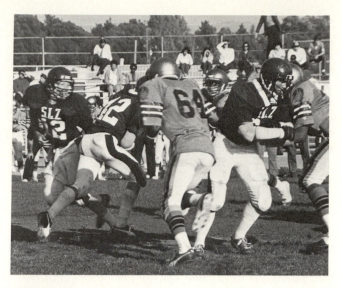

FIG. 14-6
Participation in school athletics is a primary goal of most adolescents.

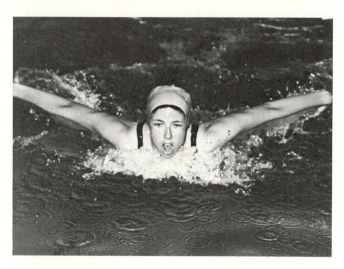

FIG. 14-7
Many sports activities can be both competitive and recreational.

school (Fig. 14-6) or as members of amateur athletic associations. As with younger children, the sport should be one suited to the youngster and they should have proper training, supervision, and equipment. The chance of injury is significantly reduced if the youngster is physically prepared for the activity. Nurses can encourage their participation as an excellent means for health promotion and building of self-esteem (Fig. 14-7). However, no youngster should be encouraged to engage in physical activity that is beyond his physical or emotional capacity.

INTERPERSONAL RELATIONSHIPS

To achieve full maturity, adolescents must free themselves from family domination and define an identity independent of parental authority. However, this process is fraught with ambivalence on the part of both teenagers and their parents. Adolescents want to grow up and to be free of parental restraints, yet they are fearful as they try to comprehend the responsibilities that are linked with independence. Part of this emancipation involves developing social relationships outside the family that help teenagers identify their role in society.

Adolescents and their parents

During adolescence the parent-child relationship changes from one of protection-dependency to one of mutual affection and equality. The process of achieving independence often involves turmoil and ambiguity as both parent and adolescent learn to play new roles and work toward this end while, at the same time, resolving the often painful series of rifts essential to establishing the ultimate relationships.

Most of the behavior observed in the adolescent is related to the struggle for independence and the external restrictions and checks that are placed on this spontaneous maturation process. On the one hand, adolescents are accepted as maturing preadults. They are allowed privileges heretofore denied, and they are provided with increasing responsibilities. On the other hand, because of their unpredictability and insecurity in evaluating situations and making sound judgments, they must conform to regulations and restrictions set by adults. This state of affairs is particularly exemplified by the struggle between parents and adolescents concerning the nightly curfew.

The teenager's earliest attempts to achieve emancipation from parental controls are manifested in a period of rejection of the parents. Adolescents are critical, argumentative, and generally remote with both parents. They absent themselves from home and family activities and spend an increasing amount of time with the peer group. They are less close and confiding in relationships with parents. This rejection is not consistent, however, and varies with mood changes.

With advancing adolescence, teenagers become more competent, and with this competence comes a need for more autonomy. However, although they are psychologically better prepared for independence, they are often thwarted in their efforts by lack of money or by other parental barriers. Much conflict arises from the teenager's outside activities and the elements of privacy and trust. To gain the respect and trust of their adolescent, parents must respect his privacy and show an honest and sincere interest in what he believes and feels.

The recent trends in society in terms of equality and relaxation of previous moral standards have made the adjustments of teenagers and parents increasingly difficult. The so-called generation gap is widening in relation to a number of attitudes, values, and beliefs. Parents can no longer find guidance from their own experiences in understanding the needs of today's teenagers.

Peer relationships and influence

Although parents remain the primary influence in their lives, for the majority of adolescents peers assume a more significant role in adolescence than they did during childhood. The peer group serves as a strong support to teenagers, individually and collectively, providing them with a sense of belonging and a feeling of strength and power. It forms that transitional world between dependence and autonomy.

Peer group. Adolescents have always been social, gregarious, and group minded. Except in a few small, homogeneous high schools, teenagers distribute themselves into a relatively predictable social hierarchy. The largest

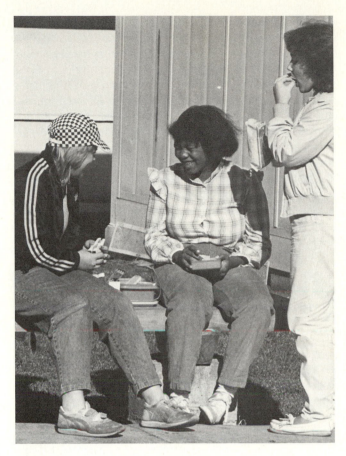

FIG. 14-8
Teenagers like to gather in small groups.

social division is the set. Both boys and girls are members of the crowd, but for some occasions and activities they separate into like-sex crowds. The adolescents know to which set they and others belong, although in large schools they may not all know each other.

Within the set are smaller, distinct, and rather exclusive crowds or cliques of selected close friends, based on common tastes, interests, and background, who are emotionally attached to each other. Although cliques may become formalized, most remain informal and small. But each has an identifying feature that proclaims its difference from others and its solidarity within itself, in much the same manner as the adolescent generation as a whole sets itself apart from the adult generation. Cliques are usually made up of one sex, and girls tend to be more cliquish than boys and to have a greater need for close friendships (Fig. 14-8). Within the intimacy of the group adolescents gain support in learning about themselves, consideration for the feelings of others, and increased ego development and self-reliance.

Best friends. Personal friendships of the one-to-one variety usually develop between like-sex adolescents. This relationship is closer and more stable than it is in middle childhood, and it is important in the quest for identity. A best friend is the best audience on whom to try out possible roles and identities that an adolescent wants to test. Best friends may try a role together, each providing support for the other. Each cares about what the other thinks and feels. Since a sense of intimacy grows within a permanent relationship, the stability of this like-sex friendship is an important link in the progress toward an intimate heterosexual relationship in young adulthood.

Heterosexual relationships. During adolescence relationships with members of the opposite sex take on new importance. Although there seems to be a trend toward earlier dating, on the *average,* dating activities begin in the seventh and eighth grades and are usually "crowd" dates at organized school functions. For example, a group of girls just happens to be around a certain group of boys at most activities. By the ninth grade crowd dates are still popular, but now there is more pairing off of couples. In the tenth grade paired crowd dates, in which some boys and girls come as couples and join the crowd consisting of several couples and perhaps a few unattached friends, are the rule. Double-dating follows group dating and is the more common practice in the eleventh grade; both double-dating and single-pair dating are common by the twelfth grade. Most adolescents are dating to some degree by the time they leave high school.

The type and degree of seriousness of heterosexual relationships vary. The initial stage is usually noncommittal, extremely mobile, and seldom characterized by any deep romantic attachments. Crushes, those strong feelings of at-

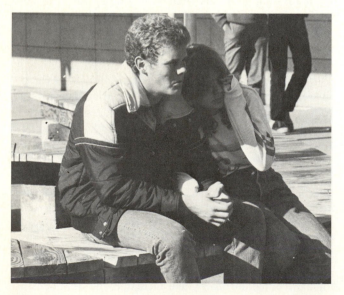

FIG. 14-9
Heterosexual friendships are characteristic of adolescence.

tachment to an important or well-liked adult in the youngster's life, are common in early adolescence; one of the earliest "love" attachments. With advancing adolescence and a more firm sexual identity, steady dating and boy-girl love relationships with deeper commitment become more numerous among teenage youngsters. Steady dating is evidence of adolescent insecurity and uncertainty—an escape from loneliness and from being left out—and provides a sense of belonging. The relationship continues until misunderstanding or boredom ends the association, and the process is often repeated with another partner.

Authorities disagree regarding the value of early opposite-sex relationships in the development of a sexual identity. Some believe that longer like-sex relationships are necessary to fully develop the characteristics of their own sex, whereas others believe that dating provides adolescents with experience in human relationships, promotes social skills, and enhances their ability to choose a mate wisely (Fig. 14-9).

Sexual codes. Heterosexual codes among teenage youngsters have undergone a notable change in recent years. The extent to which adolescents engage in intimate sexual relationships is not known precisely.

Some degree of permanent commitment is needed before sexual intimacy is considered appropriate. Most adolescents have indulged in petting, including transient, exploratory homosexual petting, and petting is generally more acceptable than intercourse as a form of sexual expression. However, available information indicates that at least 40% of girls and 80% to 95% of boys experience coitus by the end of adolescence. The prevalence increases with advancing age so that the largest numbers of sexually active youngsters are college students.

Adolescents engage in sexual relationships for pleasurable sensations, to satisfy sexual drives, to satisfy curiosity, as a conquest, as an expression of some degree of affection, or from inability to withstand pressures to conform. Often the urge to belong and gain reassurance and the wish to really belong to someone provoke a series of increasingly intimate physical contacts with a favored boyfriend or girlfriend, with each contact being more sexually provocative than the last. Eventually sexual intercourse becomes established as a behavior pattern and a method for ensuring social participation—or even as an end in itself.

The current trend toward greater permissiveness regarding adolescent sexual behavior will undoubtedly have an effect on the adolescent developmental experience. It is quite likely that young people will be accorded progressively more decision-making authority concerning control over their bodies. These alterations in the attitudes and value systems toward sex will have important implications for health professionals.

HEALTH PROMOTION DURING ADOLESCENCE

Adolescents are, on the whole, healthy individuals. The disease level is low during this age period, but there is heightened concern about the body. Most of the health problems and the more common illnesses are in some way related to the body changes of puberty.

Health promotion in persons in this age-group is primarily one of health teaching and guidance. Adolescents as a group are eager to learn about themselves, and nurses who are truly interested in them, who respect them as persons, and who are willing to listen to them will be able to gain their confidence and trust. Individual counseling provides adolescents with a knowledgeable adult in whom they can confide without the threat of an intimate relationship.

Personal care

The body-conscious teenager is highly amenable to discussion and counseling about personal care and hygiene. Body changes associated with puberty bring with them special needs for cleanliness. The hyperactive sebaceous glands and newly functioning apocrine glands make the daily bath imperative, and underarm deodorants assume an important place in personal care. The adolescent will find that hair requires more frequent shampooing, and girls will have questions about hair removal, use of cosmetics, and menstrual hygiene. Many group discussions center around the virtues of particular products or methods. Adolescents are continually bombarded with messages from the media regarding the best means to enhance their popularity and appeal to the opposite sex. Nurses are in a position to help them evaluate the relative merits of commercial products.

Teenagers vary in their need for sleep and rest. The rapid physical growth, tendency toward overexertion, and the overall increased activity of this age contribute to fatigue in adolescents. They find it very difficult to get out of bed in the mornings, and they sleep late at every opportunity. Adequate sleep and rest at this time are important to a total health regimen.

Ear piercing. The currently popular trend of ear piercing may sometimes create a health problem in the uninformed teenager. It is a nursing responsibility to caution girls or boys against the practice of having their ears pierced by friends, mothers, or themselves. Although in most cases there are few if any serious side effects, there is always a danger of complications such as infection, cyst or keloid formation, bleeding, dermatitis, or metal allergy. Therefore, the procedure should be performed by a physician or qualified nurse using proper sterile technique. This is especially important if a youngster has a history of diabetes, allergies, or skin disorders. Teenagers are prone to develop keloids, particularly if there is a history of keloid formation.

Vision. Regular vision testing is an important part of health care and supervision during adolescence. At this time the incidence of visual refractive difficulties reaches a peak that is not exceeded until the fifth decade. Adolescents may not have poorer vision than children or adults, but the increased demands of schoolwork make good vision important for academic success.

Smoking. The problem of smoking among teenagers is becoming an increasingly serious one. The habit appears to be spreading among teenagers even as the evidence of the relationship between smoking and health problems and other harmful effects increases. The latest statistics indicate not only that the incidence of smoking among teenagers 12 to 18 years of age has increased but also that the proportion of girls who smoke regularly equals or surpasses the proportion of boys who smoke regularly. Consequently the ways of dealing with the problem become more important.

A variety of methods has been employed to deal with the problem. Communication through posters, charts, displays, and statistics and the use of examples of actual damaged lungs all have their supporters and doubters. Anything that will make the habit distasteful to young people offers hope. If a significant number of influential peers can "sell" their classmates on the idea that the habit is not popular, the followers will imitate their behavior. Another ploy that seems to be meeting with some success is emphasizing the effect of smoking on personal appearance, such as the unattractive stains on teeth and hands and the unpleasant odor that smoking gives to the breath. The appeal to the youngster's capacity to participate in sports is sometimes effective. Reduced lung capacity and function are deterrents to optimum athletic prowess. Nurses in schools and other agencies of the community are in a position to implement and reinforce teaching, to serve as consultants and counselors to student, teacher, and parent groups, and to be advocates in all areas in which antismoking campaigns might be effective.

Nutrition

The rapid and extensive increase in height, weight, muscle mass, and sexual maturity of adolescence is accompanied by new and greater nutritional requirements. Since nutritional needs are closely related to the increase in body mass, the peak requirements occur in the year of maximum growth, during which time the body mass almost doubles. This period occurs between the tenth and twelfth years in girls and about 2 years later in boys. The calorie and protein requirements during this year are higher than at almost any other time of life. As a result of this increased ana-

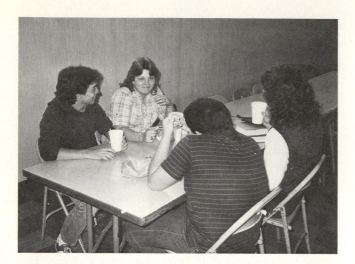

FIG. 14-10
A small group gathers for lunch.

bolic need, the adolescent is highly sensitive to caloric restrictions.

Adolescents want food, their appetites soar, and their capacity to consume food is often awe-inspiring, as any parent of a teenage boy can attest. A fast-growing boy may never get filled up. His stomach may be too small to accommodate the amount of food he requires to meet his growth needs unless he eats at very frequent intervals. Not only do teenagers eat at every pause in the day's activities, but they enjoy food and the pleasures related to its consumption. Food is part of the attraction of the ''hangouts'' and gathering places that teenagers frequent (Fig. 14-10).

The nutritional needs of adolescents are difficult to determine, because of meager nutritional information on members of this age-group. This difficulty is further complicated by the influence of emotional and other stress factors affecting nutrient utilization and the psychologic factors that influence eating habits. In addition, the wide variations in growth rates during adolescence and the equally wide variations in ages at which these changes take place complicate any attempt to set minimum dietary standards for this age-group. Consequently the Recommended Dietary Allowances for teenagers include a safety factor that attempts to allow for these differences under average circumstances.

Protein intake remains a constant need throughout childhood and adolescence to meet continual growth needs. There is usually sufficient intake to meet these needs except in those young people who limit their food intake because of economic problems or in an attempt to lose weight.

There is a substantial increase in the need for the minerals calcium, iron, and zinc during periods of rapid growth. Calcium for skeletal growth, iron for expansion of

muscle mass and blood volume, and zinc for the generation of both skeletal and bone tissue. Girls may be especially susceptible to iron deficiency at menarche.

Eating habits and behavior. Eating and behavior toward food are primarily family centered during early and middle childhood, and food habits are largely related to cultural and individual family preferences and patterns. With adolescence and the move toward independence, family influences on the child change. Children's interests, attitudes, and routines are altered as an increasing number of meals is eaten away from home. These changes are largely a result of the high value that teenagers place on peer acceptability and sociability; therefore, their eating habits are easily influenced by their associates.

Omitting breakfast or eating a breakfast that is nutritionally poor in quality is frequently a problem, and pressure for time and their commitments to activities adversely affect the teenager's eating habits. Snacks, usually selected on the basis of accessibility rather than nutritional merit, become more and more a part of the habitual eating pattern during adolescence. Adolescents characteristically reject or only infrequently eat a sufficient amount of fresh fruits and vegetables, especially those that are rich in ascorbic acid. Milk is usually passed over in favor of soft drinks, the appropriate social drink of the peer culture.

Overeating or undereating during adolescence presents special problems. As they experience the normal increase in weight and fat deposition of the growth spurt, teenage girls often resort to dieting. The desire for the admired slim figure and a fear of becoming ''fat'' prompt teenage girls to embark on nutritionally inadequate reducing regimens that sap their energy and deprive their growing bodies of essential nutrients. They resort to diets on their own or with peers in an effort to conform. Many adopt the current fad diets and are victims of food misinformation. Boys are less inclined to undereat. They are more concerned about gaining in size and strength. However, they tend to eat foods high in calories but low in other essential nutrients.

Nursing considerations. Nothing can make adolescents eat wisely. Since their food habits reflect many influences and conditions, these must be considered when planning nutritional education and guidance.

In helping teenagers select a nutritious diet, it is best to begin where they are and actively involve them in the process. Teenagers dislike being talked down to or preached to, but they do respond when their independence is respected and they are given the opportunity to make their own decisions regarding food choices.

In general, adolescents are body-conscious and concerned about their appearance. When diet is associated with clear skin, firm flesh, and glossy hair, the teenager is more likely to be receptive to nutritional education. However, helping young persons arrive at a decision for change is more difficult than providing information. They respond best when the counselor provides straightforward information, talks with them and not at them, and listens to what they have to say.

Posture

The process of normal development during adolescence does little to promote good posture in the teenage girl or boy. The rapid skeletal growth that is usually associated with a significant lag in muscular growth leads to weakness, easy fatigability, and awkwardness. This situation predisposes youngsters to slumping and makes them less inclined to stand or sit erectly. A relative reduction in physical activity, which often accompanies the rapid skeletal growth, aggravates the situation, especially in teenage girls. The adolescent who is routinely engaged in vigorous physical activity appears to have fewer problems with posture.

The best approach to counseling teenagers about posture is to show, not tell, them and to serve as a proper model. Good posture can be demonstrated best when the adolescent is standing before a full-length mirror. Postural defects and desired alterations can be pointed out in full view of both the young person and the nurse. A sunken chest, winged scapulas, swayback, protruberant abdomen, and drooping head and shoulders are clearly visible, and the nurse is able to demonstrate the simple corrections that can transform the youngster into a more attractive and, ultimately, healthier person. Adolescents will need reassurance that the fatigue they feel when attempting to maintain correct posture is a transient effect caused by weak muscles, especially those of the back, and that they will soon acquire the strength and endurance to maintain the desired posture. If they concentrate on assuming correct positioning several times each day, with regular practice it will eventually become a permanent aspect of their person.

Serious postural defects, detected in the process of a physical assessment, will require early medical intervention. Scoliosis is usually intensified during adolescence, and tight muscles often produce postural problems that need special attention. Nurses can refer a youngster to the appropriate source, such as the family physician, pediatrician, or health clinic, for evaluation and implementation of corrective therapy.

Accidents

Accidents are the greatest single cause of death in the adolescent age-group and claim more lives than all other causes combined. The most vulnerable ages are the years 15 to 24, when accidents account for 61% of deaths in boys and 39% of deaths in girls. The tragedy of this is that the figures remain fairly constant from year to year and almost all fatal accidents are preventable.

During adolescence, peak physical, sensory, and psychomotor function gives teenagers a feeling of strength and confidence that they have never experienced before and the physiologic changes of puberty give impetus to many basic instinctual forces. One manifestation of this is an increase in energy that simply must be discharged through action, often at the expense of logical thinking and other control mechanisms. Their propensity for risk-taking behavior plus feelings of indestructibility make adolescents especially prone to accidents.

Motor vehicle accidents. Almost half the accidents in the adolescent age-group are motor vehicle accidents. The adolescent's newly acquired ability to drive and the normal developmental need for independence and freedom make the automobile an attractive, if not necessary, part of adolescents' lives. Most fatal accidents involving adolescent drivers occur because of improper driving or poor judgment on the part of the driver. These young people, delighted with the freedom that a driver's license affords them, are less concerned about the new responsibilities associated with this freedom.

The recent upsurge in the use of drugs, including alcohol, by adolescents has further compounded the problem of motor vehicle accidents involving youth. Overindulgence in alcohol is known to impair the ability of the best driver. The combination of inexperience, lack of defensive driving skills, and inexperience with drinking is a lethal one, and the unfortunate consequences are predictable.

Firearms. Improper use of firearms continues to be one of the leading causes of accidental death in the adolescent age-group. Most of these deaths occur in or on home premises. The natural interest in gun-related activities is accelerated at this time, when almost half the victims of firearm fatalities are between the ages of 15 and 24 years. Most accidental injuries can be prevented when proper safety precautions are taken in the use and storage of firearms. For example, loaded guns should never be permitted in or around the home, and guns and ammunition must be stored where only appropriate adults have access to them.

Sports injuries. Adolescents probably spend more time and energy practicing and participating in sports activities than members of any other age-group. Because the degree of physical maturation, size, coordination, and endurance varies greatly among adolescents of the same age, sports competition between young people who differ markedly in strength and agility is unfair and hazardous. Matching candidates for sports should be done relative to physical maturity, height, weight, and physical fitness and skills, particularly in a sport involving rigorous body contact. Age is a less important consideration.

Every sport has some potential for injury—whether one participates in serious competition or is actively en-

SUMMARY OF ACCIDENT PREVENTION DURING ADOLESCENCE

MAJOR DEVELOPMENTAL CHARACTERISTICS	ACCIDENT PREVENTION

Need for independence and freedom
Testing independence
Propensity for risk-taking
Feeling of indestructibility
Age permitted to drive a motor vehicle (varies)
Need for discharging energy, often at expense of logical thinking and other control mechanisms
Peak incidence for practice and participation in sports
Strong need for peer approval; may attempt hazardous feats
Access to more complex tools, objects, and locations
Can assume responsibility for own actions
	Motor vehicles
	Pedestrian—emphasize and encourage safe pedestrian behavior
	Passenger—promote appropriate behavior while riding in a motor vehicle
	Driver—provide competent driver education; encourage judicious use of vehicle, discourage drag racing, "chicken," and so on; maintain vehicle in proper condition (e.g., brakes, tires)
	Teach and promote safety and maintenance of two-wheeled vehicles
	Promote and encourage wearing of safety apparel such as helmet, long trousers
	Reinforce the dangers of drugs (including alcohol) when operating a motor vehicle)
	
	Drowning
	Teach to swim (if unable to do so)
	Teach basic rules of water safety
	    Judicious selection of places to swim
	    Sufficient water depth for diving
	    Swimming with companion
	
	Burns
	Reinforce proper behavior in areas involving contact with burn hazards (e.g., gasoline, electric wires, fires)
	Advise regarding excessive exposure to sunlight (ultraviolet burn)
	Discourage smoking
	
	Poisoning
	Educate in hazards of drug use, including alcohol
	
	Falls
	Teach and encourage general safety measures in all activities
	
	Bodily damage
	Promote acquisition of proper instruction in sports and use of sports equipment
	Promote use of appropriate arena for sports activities
	Instruct in safe use of and respect for firearms and other devices with potential danger (power tools, firecrackers, and so on)
	Provide and encourage use of protective equipment when using potentially hazardous devices
	Promote access to and/or provision of safe sports and recreational facilities
	Be alert for signs of depression (potential suicide)
	Discourage use of and/or availability of hazardous sports equipment (e.g., trampoline, surfboards)
	Instruct regarding proper use of corrective devices such as glasses, contact lenses, hearing aids
	Encourage and foster judicious application of safety principles and prevention

gaged in the activity for pure enjoyment. Serious injury is not limited to the athlete who competes in rough contact sports; a large number of severe or fatal injuries occur to persons who are not physically prepared for the activity. The increase in strength and vigor in adolescence may tempt youngsters to overextend themselves, especially boys who are egged on by teammates or are stimulated by the admiration of female observers.

Not only does the activity itself pose a hazard, but the environment and the sports or recreational equipment provide additional risks. Some of the sports that contribute to adolescent accidental injuries by their activity and equipment are bicycling, football, basketball, baseball, snow skiing, hockey, trampoline jumping, and water activities such as swimming, diving, and fishing. The range of injuries sustained in sports or recreational activities can involve any part of the body and extend from relatively minor cuts, bruises, and abrasions to totally incapacitating central nervous system injuries or death.

Nursing considerations. Accident prevention is an ongoing part of nursing responsibility throughout the childhood years. Anticipatory guidance to parents regarding the expected problems and hazards related to growth and development does not end as the child nears maturity. They need the same education in basic safety precautions, encouragement to acquire proper instruction in skills required in performance of activities, handling motor vehicles and firearms, and proper maintenance of equipment. However, at adolescence health and safety education and guidance are more effective when the young people are involved directly, but parents and health professionals can emphasize the importance of safety in the execution of activities and skills and the proper conditioning and preparation for sports.

Dental health

Dental health should not be neglected during adolescence, although the rate of caries formation is not as great as it was in childhood. Early adolescence is usually the time when corrective orthodontic appliances are worn, and these are frequently a source of embarrassment and concern to the youngster. Reassurance regarding the temporary nature of the annoyance and anticipation of an improved appearance help to make the inconvenience tolerable. It is also important to reinforce the orthodontist's directions regarding use and care of the appliances and to emphasize careful attention to brushing during this time.

Sex education and guidance

Contemporary adolescents are constantly exposed to sexual symbolism and erotic stimulation from the mass media. At the same time the development of primary and secondary sex characteristics and the increased sensitivity of the genitals produce thoughts and fantasies about heterosexual relationships. Although many adolescents have received sex education from parents and school throughout childhood, they are not always adequately prepared for the impact of puberty. A large portion of their knowledge is acquired from peers, provocative illustrations, and inscriptions on the walls of public restrooms. Consequently much of the sex information they accumulate is incomplete, inaccurate, riddled with cultural and moral values, and not very helpful.

Sex education should consist of instruction concerning a normal body function, and it should be presented in a straightforward manner using correct terminology. However, the questions of who is responsible for teaching and how the teaching can be best accomplished must be con-

---

SUMMARY OF GROWTH AND DEVELOPMENT DURING ADOLESCENCE (ages 13 to 18)

PHYSICAL AND MOTOR	MENTAL AND SOCIAL	ADAPTIVE
Maximum growth increase, especially in height: gain in height is abrupt at the onset and continues at a rapid rate the first 2 years, followed by a deceleration	Tends toward intellectual maturity	Performs responsible routine chores without prodding
	May be passionate and idealistic	Does share of household work
	Able to generally use money with common sense	May have conflicts with parents
Girls have more subcutaneous tissue so may be more obese	Writes business and social letters that are more than matter of routine	Plans for future; saves money
Boys develop larger muscles		May receive advice, but makes own decisions
Appears long-legged and gangling	Discusses general news, sports, events and follows these	Authority comes from parents mostly
Girls become relatively broad-hipped about the age of 12	Transition from dependent childhood to independent adult life	Accepts one's physique; uses the body effectively
Boys grow rapidly in shoulder breadth from about 13 years	Is achieving appropriate peer relations	Is achieving emotional independence and assurance of future economic independence
Complete secondary sex characteristics	Takes part in games requiring skills such as card games, tennis, swimming	Is setting up own values

Continued.

SUMMARY OF GROWTH AND DEVELOPMENT DURING ADOLESCENCE (ages 13 to 18)—cont'd

PHYSICAL AND MOTOR	MENTAL AND SOCIAL	ADAPTIVE
Girls are generally 2 years ahead of boys in development at first Beginning of menses Bones increase in size; ossification speeds up Coordination improves until approximately 14, when it reaches a plateau, and child may then appear awkward Boys experience nocturnal emissions Muscles develop faster than bones grow in boys Skeletal frame mature and ossification completed Coordination improves steadily with age in boys	Is an active member of athletic team or other organization Attends parties, dances, and other activities with persons of own age without adult direction Goes outside limits of hometown and makes own arrangements Shows personal interest in the opposite sex; starts dating Experiences feelings of ambivalence Great dependence on peer groups Conforms to peer group norms Identifies with small select group Crushes are prevalent in this period Anxiety is often produced by strong sex drives Conscience develops more fully	Understands scoring and abides by the rules Strives for independence while still desiring dependence Experiences conflicts with parents over independence-dependence Develops standards for life and images of marriage partners

PARENTAL GUIDANCE DURING ADOLESCENCE

AGE (years)	GUIDANCE
12-15	Support and reassure the adolescent Be available to the adolescent when needed but avoid pressing him too far Expect turbulent, unpredictable behavior Explain that rejecting behavior is a manifestation of the struggle for independence Provide undemanding love Allow increasing independence but maintain suitable limit-setting for the adolescent's safety and well-being Suggest parents acquire outside interests for themselves Allow parents to express feelings regarding the sometimes frustrating experience of coping with an adolescent
15-18	Help the adolescent prepare for the adult role Assist in selection of career goals Help parents have realistic expectations of the adolescent and avoid "pushing" him in a direction unsuited to his capabilities Help parents recognize that present times are different from those of their youth Help parents cope with the multiple and diversified problems of relationships with adolescents Provide support and reassurance

sidered. Sex education is, and has been, assumed by parents, schools, churches, community agencies such as Planned Parenthood–World Population, and health professionals.

The most comprehensive approach to sex education is offered by the Sex Information and Education Council of the United States (SIECUS), an interdisciplinary organization founded to establish sexuality as a health entity and to dignify it by openness of approach, study, and scientific research. SIECUS maintains that every sex education program should present the topic from six aspects: biologic, social, health, personal adjustments and attitudes, interpersonal associations, and the establishment of values.

Whether nurses counsel young people on an individual basis, in mixed groups, or in groups segregated by sex makes little difference. Some nurses and teenagers are uneasy in mixed groups for discussions of sexuality, and no hard-and-fast rule prevails. Ideally boys and girls should be able to discuss sex objectively with one another and in groups, but this is not always possible. The difference in the rate of maturation between boys and girls and between different members of the same sex often makes it desirable to discuss certain aspects of sexuality in segregated groups. As a general rule, the need for separate discussion groups diminishes as young people progress toward maturity.

When discussing sex and sexual activities, nurses should use simple but correct language—not street language, highly scientific terminology, or evasive jargon. Once the meanings of biologic terms such as uterus, testicles, vagina, and so on are understood, teenagers prefer to use them in their discussions.

Both boys and girls need to know more about what is going on in their bodies than they are able to see. Although most girls are adequately prepared for menstruation, they do not always understand its relationship to the total process of reproduction. Many are under the impression that the ''safe'' time for sexual intercourse is midway between menstrual periods. Whether they are sexually active or not, adolescents should receive accurate information about pregnancy, including when and how it occurs and ways by which it can be avoided. They need to know about venereal diseases, the manner in which they are transmitted, symptoms, and how to get treatment if one becomes infected.

REFERENCES

Erikson, E.H.: Childhood and society, ed. 2, New York, 1963, W.W. Norton & Co., Inc.

Newman, B.M., and Newman, P.R.: Development through life, a psychosocial approach, rev. ed., Homewood, Ill., 1979, Dorsey Press.

Shelly, J.A.: The spiritual needs of children, Downers Grove, Ill., 1982, Inter-Varsity Press.

BIBLIOGRAPHY

Adams, G.: The sexual history as an integral part of the patient history, Am. J. Maternal Child Nurs. 1(3):170-175, 1976.

Amenta, M.M.: Free clinics change the scene, Am. J. Nurs. 74:284, 1974.

American Academy of Pediatrics, Committee on Accident and Poison Prevention and Committee on Pediatric Aspects of Physical Fitness, Recreation and Sports: Trampolines II, Pediatrics 67(3):438, 1980.

Anderson, F.J.: The developmental experience of adolescence, Issues Compr. Pediatr. Nurs. 1:1-16, 1976.

Belkengren, R.B., and Sapala, S.: Physical fitness from infancy through adolescence, Pediatr. Nurs. 8(4):A-I, 1982.

Brown, B.S.: A nonsmoking generation is not a pipe dream, Pediatr. Nurs. 8(5):295, 1982.

Bullough, V., and Bullough, B.: PNPs, patients, parents, and sexuality, Pediatr. Nurs. 8(3):A-I, 1982.

Caghan, S.B.: The adolescent process and the problem of nutrition, Am. J. Nurs. 75:1728-1731, 1975.

Cohen, M.T.: The process of adolescence: its psychologic and physiologic basis, Pediatr. Nurs. 4(6):27-29, 1978.

Davis, R.C.: The family with an adolescent. In Hymovich, D.P., and Barnard, M.U., editors: Family health care, vol. II, New York, 1979, McGraw-Hill Book Co.

Dylag, H.: How difficult the ''I'': the adolescent maturation of critical identity. In Hall, J.E., and Weaver, B.R.: Nursing of families in crisis, Philadelphia, 1974, J.B. Lippincott Co.

Frankle, R.T., and Heussanstamm, F.K.: Food zealotry and youth, Am. J. Public Health 64:11-17, 1974.

Garrick, J.G.: The sports medicine patient, Nurs. Clin. North Am. 16:759-766, 1981.

Giuffra, M.J.: Demystifying adolescent behavior, Am. J. Nurs. 75:1724-1727, 1975.

Graf, C.M.: Sex and the adolescent, Issues Compr. Pediatr. Nurs. 1:31-41, 1976.

Kaluger, G., and Kaluger, M.F.: Human development: the span of life, ed. 3, St. Louis, 1984, The C.V. Mosby Co.

Kuhnen, K.K., and others: Barny: a computer for teaching sex education, Am. J. Maternal Child Nurs. 8:350-353, 1983.

Latinis, B.: Frequent sports injuries of children: etiology, treatment, and prevention, Issues Comp. Pediatr. Nurs. 6:167-178, 1983.

Mahon, N.E.: Developmental changes and loneliness during adolescence, Topics Clin. Nurs. 5(1):66-76, 1983.

Marks, A.: Health screening of the adolescent, Pediatr. Nurs. 4(4):37-41, 1978.

Mercer, R.T.: Perspectives in health care, Philadelphia, 1979, J.B. Lippincott Co.

Narins, D.M., Belkengren, R.P., and Sapala, S.: Nutrition and the growing athlete, Pediatr. Nurs. 9(3):163-168, 1983.

Nelms, B.C.: What is a normal adolescent? Am. J. Maternal Child Nurs. 6:402-406, 1981.

O'Boyle, C.M.: Sports injuries in adolescents: emergency care, Am. J. Nurs. 75:732-739, 1975.

Osguthorpe, N.C., and Osguthorpe, J.D.: Scuba diving hazards: emergency management, Am. J. Nurs. 81:1456-1458, 1981.

Ostaszewski, T.M., and Marshall, J.L.: Prevention and treatment of sports injuries, Am. J. Nurs. 75:1737, 1975.

Reres, M.E.: Stressors in adolescence, Fam. Comm. Health 2(4):31-41, 1980.

Sapala, S., and Strokosch, G.: Adolescent sexuality: use of a questionnaire for health teaching and counseling, Pediatr. Nurs. 7(6):33-35, 1981.

Throne, B.P: A nurse helps prevent sports injuries, Am. J. Maternal Child Nurs. 7:236-239, 1982.

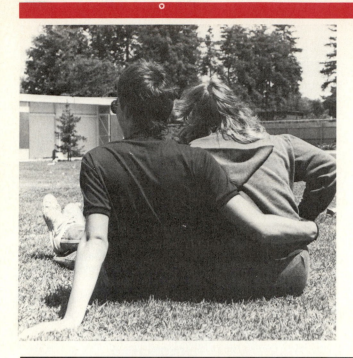

HEALTH PROBLEMS OF MIDDLE CHILDHOOD AND ADOLESCENCE

OBJECTIVES

On completion of this chapter the reader will be able to:

- Describe the most common causes of growth and/or maturation failure in later childhood

- Demonstrate an understanding of common disorders of the male and female reproductive systems

- Demonstrate an understanding of health problems related to sexuality

- Outline a plan of care for the child or adolescent with a health problem

- Outline a plan of care for the child or adolescent with an eating disorder

- Discuss the manifestations and nursing management of selected emotional and/or behavioral problem

NURSING DIAGNOSES

Nursing diagnoses identified for the school-age child or adolescent with health problems include, but are not restricted to, the following:

Health perception-health management pattern

- Health maintenance deficit related to (1) knowledge deficit; (2) depression

- Injury, potential for, related to (1) impaired judgment (drugs); (2) suicidal intent

- Noncompliance related to (1) knowledge deficit; (2) denial of illness; (3) altered thought processes (substance abuse); (4) established eating habits

Nutritional-metabolic pattern

- Nutrition, alterations in: less than body requirements related to (1) decreased calorie intake; (2) distorted body image (anorexia nervosa); (3) knowledge deficit

- Nutrition, alterations in: more than body requirements related to (1) diminished activity; (2) excess calorie intake

- Skin integrity, impairment of: potential, related to (1) altered nutritional state; (2) injection of substances

Elimination pattern

■ Bowel elimination, alterations in: constipation related to (1) drug ingestion; (2) nutritional inadequacies

■ Bowel elimination, alterations in: diarrhea related to (1) drug ingestion; (2) nutritional peculiarities

■ Urinary elimination, alteration in patterns, related to nocturia

Activity-exercise pattern

■ Activity in tolerance, related to (1) inadequate nutrition; (2) obesity

■ Breathing pattern, ineffective, related to (1) overweight; (2) substance abuse

■ Diversional activity deficit related to prolonged illness

■ Home maintenance management, impaired, related to deficient cognitive functioning (drugs)

■ Self-care deficit, related to (1) impaired cognitive functioning; (2) depression

Sleep-rest pattern

■ Sleep-pattern disturbance related to (1) personal stress; (2) nocturia

Cognitive-perceptual pattern

■ Knowledge deficit related to (1) cognitive limitations; (2) ingestion of injurious chemical agents; (3) unfamiliarity with information sources

■ Powerlessness related to (1) sexual assault; (2) depression

■ Sensory-perceptual alterations related to (1) ingestion of injurious chemicals; (2) depression

■ Thought processes, alterations in, related to (1) disease process (e.g., anorexia nervosa); (2) ingestion of injurious chemical substances

Self-perception—self-concept pattern

■ Anxiety related to (1) self-image alterations; (2) perceived powerlessness; (3) perception of impending events

■ Fear related to (1) rape trauma; (2) knowledge deficit

■ Self-concept, disturbance in, related to (1) perceived body image; (2) health problem (specify, e.g., enuresis, obesity, rape trauma, pregnancy, growth disturbances)

Role-relationship pattern

■ Communication, impaired verbal, related to cognitive impairment

■ Family process, alterations in, related to (1) situational crisis; (2) temporary family disorganization

■ Parenting, alterations in: potential, related to (1) skill deficit; (2) knowledge deficit

■ Social isolation related to (1) body image disturbance; (2) pregnancy; (3) restricted mobility; (4) cognitive impairment

■ Violence, potential for, related to impaired perception (substance abuse)

Sexuality-reproductive pattern

■ Rape trauma syndrome related to sexual abuse

■ Sexual dysfunction related to misinformation

Coping-stress tolerance pattern

■ Coping, ineffective individual, related to (1) knowledge deficit; (2) problem-solving deficit; (3) inadequate support systems; (4) inadequate coping mechanisms

As a group, both school-age children and adolescents are relatively healthy individuals, especially when compared to children in infancy and early childhood. The ages 9 to 12 are the healthiest years and this state of health continues into pubescence. Most youngsters in these age-groups have either contracted the communicable diseases of childhood or have been immunized against them. Their excellent appetites, adequate rest, and sufficient physical exercise further contribute to their general good health. During the school years respiratory illnesses and gastrointestinal upsets are the most common illnesses. Most health problems of adolescents are related to the physical changes taking place in their bodies and the crucial psychosocial crisis of identity formation. Other conditions that are not uncommon are accidental injuries (see Chapters 13 and 14) and emotional or behavior disorders.

ALTERATIONS IN GROWTH AND/OR MATURATION

The absence of physical and/or sexual maturation at a time when other children are experiencing positive evidence of sexual development and its associated spurt in growth and physical strength is a matter of concern to both the parents and their affected child. Fortunately in most instances the delay in development is a simple physiologic or constitutional delay that merely represents one end of the normal genetically influenced variation of pubertal growth. These children will go through a delayed but normal puberty to finally catch up, in their late teens, with their more rapidly developing age-mates. Less benign causes of delayed development may be of endocrine origin or caused by chromosomal aberrations. In other situations delayed development may be a result of chronic diseases such as malabsorption, chronic asthma, and poorly controlled diabetes mellitus that are serious enough to retard the developmental process.

The rate of maturation is important during the school years, but at puberty it assumes gigantic proportions to the youngster and often to his parents as well. Girls or boys who lag behind their peers in physical maturation are painfully aware of their shortcomings. The adolescent girl feels out of place among her companions whose hips and bosoms are developing, feels cheated because she has not yet menstruated, and feels that she is not a part of the giggling and boy-talk of her friends. The adolescent boy feels weak and small compared with his muscular companions with whom he can no longer compete, and his high voice sounds childish in contrast to the deep tones around him. Slow-maturing youngsters need much support and reassurance that they are not abnormal and need only to be patient

until the time comes when they, too, will develop the characteristics for which they yearn.

ENDOCRINE DYSFUNCTION

The child with endocrine or genetic disorders that interfere with the maturation process needs special help. The major hormones that promote physical growth are thyroid hormone, growth hormone, and sex hormones. Insulin can be said to promote growth by its effect on carbohydrate metabolism, whereas cortisol inhibits growth. Therefore, deficiencies of growth-promoting hormones or an excess of cortisol can cause growth retardation in children. Endocrine deficiencies can be the result of abnormal secretory function in the glands responsible for their production, the pituitary hormones that stimulate their secretion, or the releasing factors from the hypothalamus. (See Chapter 26 for disorders associated with endocrine dysfunction.)

Cortisol excess as a result of organic causes or of prolonged cortisone therapy also has an adverse effect on growth in children. Because of the growth-suppressing effect of cortisone in excess of minimal requirements, therapy is limited to short-term administration whenever possible.

TALL OR SHORT STATURE

Variations in height are expression of genetic diversity among all populations. Most often the diversity is simply a manifestation of the person's genetic constitution, but it may be caused by a physiologic or emotional disorder. To the person on the extremes of height it can be a source of intense discomfort and anxiety. Boys are more distressed over short stature; girls are more likely to be disturbed by tall stature.

Tall stature

Despite the fact that the average height of both boys and girls is steadily increasing, there is still a small group of children who, because of some organic disorder or a familial tendency, are excessively tall when compared with their contemporaries. To some it can be a source of pride or a source of intense anxiety and a severe social handicap.

When the rate of height change before puberty suggests the probability of excessive adult height, treatment with hormones may be considered, although there is a great deal of controversy regarding its use for this purpose. The selection of children for hormonal therapy is made on the basis of a careful evaluation of physical, psychologic, and social factors.

Short stature

A small group of children suffer delay of growth or onset of adolescence because of disorders that may or may not be amenable to treatment. From a worldwide point of view, the most common cause of short stature and/or delayed development is probably inadequate nutrition; however, the major disorders that produce delayed development are chronic diseases, endocrine dysfunction, and syndromes of primary gonadal failure.

Chronic diseases can interfere with growth, but, unless the illness is unduly prolonged, catch-up growth will occur. Diseases and disorders that usually cause some degree of growth delay include asthma, cystic fibrosis, gastrointestinal diseases (such as parasitic infestations), malabsorption syndromes, cardiac anomalies, and chronic renal disturbances. It appears that the duration of the illness is more significant than the intensity in its effect on growth, although the precise length of time necessary to affect growth permanently has not been determined.

Skeletal disorders that affect growth in stature are principally those described as dwarfism. Most are caused by a variety of congenital defects and disorders, such as achondroplasia, and some of the inborn errors of metabolism, such as Hurler or Hunter syndromes.

Psychosocial dwarfism Psychosocial, or deprivation, dwarfism is a term applied to children who are significantly retarded in growth because of environmental circumstances. When these children are removed from the deprived environment, their growth proceeds at a normal or increased rate. (See also nonorganic failure to thrive p. 270.)

Nursing considerations

Deviation from the normal course of puberty is always of concern to the affected adolescent, and to some it assumes monumental proportions. Most of the problems of delayed development are those caused by simple constitutional delay of puberty, and in this situation the child can be assured that the normal course of events will eventually take place.

One of the difficulties related to a size that is incongruent with chronologic and mental age is the manner in which others, especially adults, relate to the child. People quite naturally respond to children with short stature as though they are younger than their age. Consequently these children often react with babyish or juvenile behavior, thus setting in motion a circular pattern of behavior and response. Conversely children who are tall or physically advanced for their age are treated as though they are more advanced than their years. They are often considered to be retarded or behaviorally immature when they actually perform according to the normal behavioral expectations for their age.

Listening to distressed adolescents and conveying to them genuine interest and concern are prerequisite to any successful intervention. Counseling and therapy are individualized to meet the needs of each youngster and his problems. Encouraging these children to accentuate the positive aspects of their body and personality with sound health practices and good grooming helps foster a more positive self-image.

SYNDROMES OF PRIMARY GONADAL FAILURE

The most frequently seen disorders associated with primary gonadal failure are the sex chromosomal defects categorized collectively as gonadal dysgenesis, principally Turner syndrome. Impairment of male sexual function caused by a chromosome defect is most commonly caused by Klinefelter syndrome. (See p. 53 for discussion of the genetic aspects of these disorders.)

Turner syndrome

Turner syndrome is caused by absence of one of the X chromosomes. The incidence of the condition in the population has been variously estimated at 1 in 1500, 1 in 3000, to 1 in 10,000 live female births. Although this disorder is often recognized at birth, it is diagnosed most frequently at puberty because of three outstanding features: short stature, sexual infantilism, and amenorrhea (see also p. 414). Definitive diagnosis is confirmed on the basis of a negative sex chromatin test; chromosomal analysis is rarely necessary.

Therapy is always individualized for these girls and consists primarily of hormone treatment and psychologic counseling for both child and parents. Linear growth often can be increased by the administration of anabolic steroids followed by estrogen therapy to promote the development of secondary sex characteristics. Responses to estrogen therapy vary from girl to girl, but gradual feminization is accomplished to some degree in most individuals.

Klinefelter syndrome

The most common of all chromosomal abnormalities, Klinefelter syndrome, is caused by the presence of one or more additional X chromosomes. Young boys with this disorder are seldom seen before puberty, at which time varying degrees of failure of adolescent virilization occur. Some males are not detected until they appear for evaluation for infertility. All have absence of sperm in the semen (azoospermia), small testes, and defective development of secondary sex characteristics. The incidence of Klinefelter syndrome is estimated to be approximately 1 in 500 live male births. In 80% of these boys there is a chromatin-positive buccal smear and the extra chromosome is apparent on chromosomal analysis.

The major effort in medical treatment is directed toward enhancing the masculine characteristics through the administration of male hormones, principally testosterone. Cosmetic surgery will eliminate embarrassment for the boy with gynecomastia.

Nursing considerations

The nursing care of children with Turner or Klinefelter syndromes is primarily supportive. Nurses assist in diagnosis, explain tests and therapies to children and families, and provide support and encouragement. Since both disorders render the individual unable to reproduce, psychologic counseling will be an important aspect of care as well as modification of sex education.

GYNECOMASTIA

Some degree of bilateral or unilateral breast enlargement frequently occurs in young boys during puberty. In most instances it is a transient phenomenon that subsides spontaneously with achievement of male development. Occasionally, however, it is associated with abnormalities such as Klinefelter syndrome or endocrine dysfunction; therefore, these possibilities are ruled out by appropriate diagnostic examination.

Treatment usually consists of assurance to the boy and his parents that this is a benign and temporary situation. If the condition persists or is extensive enough to cause acute embarrassment or to produce doubts about gender identity in the young boy, plastic surgery is indicated for cosmetic and psychologic considerations. Administration of testosterone has no effect on breast development or regression and may even aggravate the condition. Since the boy is distressed about his physical integrity and masculinity, he will need reassurance regarding this apparently incongruous development.

DISORDERS OF THE MALE REPRODUCTIVE SYSTEM

It is fortunate for the male that most of the parts of the reproductive system are external and therefore visible and palpable. Therefore, most obvious anomalies such as hypospadias, hydrocele, phimosis, and cryptorchidism have been identified and corrective measures instituted during early childhood. The most frequent problems related to the reproductive organs in later childhood are (1) infections, such as urethritis; (2) hematuria; (3) penile problems, such as nonretractable foreskin in uncircumcised males, carci-

noma, and trauma; (4) scrotal conditions, such as varicocele (elongation, dilation, and tortuosity of the veins superior to the testicle); and (5) testicular torsion (a condition in which the testicle hangs free from its vascular structures which can result in partial or complete venous occlusion with rotation). Tumors of the testes are not a common condition, but when manifested in adolescence, they are generally malignant and demand immediate evaluation.

Nursing considerations

The adolescent male is extremely self-conscious about his changing body and often refuses a genital examination. The most successful approach is to assume a matter-of-fact attitude to the examination, explain precisely what will take place, and maintain a continuous commentary about what is being done and the findings at each phase of the examination. The adolescent male is approached as someone important as a person, with the nurse interested in his concerns. To supplement routine health assessment, every adolescent male should be taught frequent testicular self-examination (TSE) to familiarize him with his own anatomy and to ensure early detection of any abnormality.

DISORDERS OF THE FEMALE REPRODUCTIVE SYSTEM

Unlike the male, the reproductive organs of the female are located internally; therefore, abnormalities are less apparent and more difficult to detect. Infections are a major source of morbidity, especially those described as sexually transmitted diseases. However, the problems most often brought to the attention of health professionals are those related to menstruation—menstrual delay, irregularities, or discomfort. A menstrual history and gynecologic examination should be a routine part of the assessment of the adolescent girl and any of her concerns is worthy of consideration and understanding from health professionals.

Amenorrhea

It is not unusual for an adolescent to skip a menstrual period or two when establishing normal menstrual and ovulatory cycles. Delay in initiation of menstruation is ordinarily a temporary problem resulting from late onset of puberty and requires no intervention. This is of little concern unless it creates undo anxiety on the part of the girl and her parents, which can ordinarily be allayed by explanation and reassurance. Careful examination will reveal any congenital defects of the genital tract (a rare cause).

Primary amenorrhea (when menarche is delayed beyond age 17 years) may be the result of absence or malformation of the female genital structures or the inability of normal structures to respond to hormonal stimulation.

The most common cause of secondary amenorrhea (prolonged absence of menstruation for 12 months or more between periods in the first 2 years following menarche or when more than three periods have been missed after menses have become established) are emotional disturbances and pregnancy, which is accompanied by the signs and symptoms associated with this state.

Dysfunctional uterine bleeding

Irregularities in the timing, length, or amount of menstrual flow are common conditions in adolescent girls and are caused primarily by either imbalance in the secretion of hormones that control menstrual function or variability in responsiveness of the target organs in adolescence. Anovulatory menstruation is characteristic of the early menstrual periods following menarche and is self-limited for the majority of teenage girls. Ordinarily only reassurance and attention to general health status are needed, with emphasis on a well-balanced diet, adequate rest, and moderate exercise.

Dysmenorrhea

A certain amount of discomfort during the first day or two of the menstrual flow is extremely common. Most girls experience cramping, abdominal pain, backache, and leg ache, but in a few the pain is intolerable and incapacitating. The term *primary dysmenorrhea* is applied to these symptoms when there is no pelvic disease to account for the cramping discomfort. When the discomfort can be attributed to endometriosis, infection, adhesions from peritonitis, or other pelvic disease, the complaint is described as *secondary dysmenorrhea*.

No specific etiology of primary dysmenorrhea is known; however, some contributory factors are recognized. In all instances of primary dysmenorrhea is the occurrence of prior ovulation. There is also a relationship between uterine contractility and the secretion of prostaglandins. However, in some girls the discomfort may be a result of low pain tolerance.

A thorough gynecologic examination is carried out to exclude any pelvic abnormalities, and a careful history is taken regarding the type and duration of pain, its relationship to menstrual flow, and any associated symptoms. These questions not only provide information to the examiner but also serve to provide the girl with evidence that her problem is being taken seriously. An explanation of the physiology of menstruation helps to give reassurance.

Treatment consists of administration of prostaglandin inhibitors. Aspirin has proved effective when begun a few days before the onset of the menses—approximately 11 days after ovulation. The relief appears to be the result of prostaglandin inhibitory (rather than analgesic) effect.

Some relatively new prostaglandin inhibitors, such as mefenamic acid and naproxen, provide relief and can be taken at the start of menses. Simple exercises similar to those recommended for relief of prenatal discomfort, such as pelvic rocking, assuming the knee-chest position, and breathing exercises, may also be beneficial. The girl is encouraged to practice good hygiene and participate in regular activities. Sometimes cyclic estrogen therapy to prevent ovulation provides dramatic and predictable relief from pain.

Vaginitis and vulvitis (vulvovaginitis)

A small quantity of vaginal mucus is normal and in adolescent girls usually increases at the time of ovulation and before the onset of menstruation. It is characteristically clear and, except in rare instances when it appears in large amounts, causes no discomfort. However, some teenagers mistakenly believe it to be a sign of vaginal infection. Following an examination, the girl can generally be reassured.

Exposure to diethylstilbestrol

Intrauterine exposure to diethylstilbestrol (DES) has been associated with the development of clear-cell adenocarcinoma of the genital tract in girls during adolescence. The disease is rare in girls under 14 years of age, but the incidence increases, reaches a peak at age 19, and drops rapidly thereafter. Therefore, all daughters exposed to DES during their mother's pregnancy should have annual screening examinations beginning no later than menarche or age 14.

Nursing considerations

The nurse is most frequently the person to whom a young girl turns for advice regarding menstrual problems or problems related to vaginal discharge. Usually all the youngster needs is reassurance about this normal function, but this also provides an opportunity for the nurse to listen to what the adolescent is saying and to engage in health teaching concerning menstrual physiology and hygiene and the importance of a well-balanced diet, exercise, and general health maintenance. It is a time to dispel any myths the girl may have in relation to menstruation and her femininity. When assessment indicates a potential problem and need for her evaluation, the girl is referred to a physician, health service, or clinic.

One of the most difficult experiences facing the adolescent girl is the gynecologic examination. Whether it is her first experience or not, she is most likely filled with apprehension. Almost all adolescents are extremely self-conscious about their bodies and the changes taking place. She will need continuing support in the form of anticipatory guidance regarding what she can expect and suggestions of what she can do to help herself relax during the procedure. Usually the stressful experience of being placed in stirrups for the pelvic examination can be avoided. The youngster who is relaxed may be examined in the supine position. If a female nurse is not the examiner, it is essential for her to remain with the patient during the examination to offer support and guidance.

HEALTH PROBLEMS RELATED TO SEXUALITY

The child entering and progressing through the multiple physical and emotional changes of puberty is subject to some medical problems associated with these changes. The increasing incidence of adolescent pregnancy, sexually transmitted disease, and sexual trauma make it imperative that health professionals have an understanding of these disorders.

ADOLESCENT PREGNANCY

One of the consequences of adolescent experimentation, acting-out, the need to conform, impulsivity, and the search for a sexual identity is pregnancy. Although the incidence of adolescent pregnancy is influenced by the availability of contraception and abortion, pregnant teenagers present a population at risk—medically, socially, economically, and educationally.

With better facilities available for care, the mortality rates for teenage pregnancies are decreasing, but the morbidity still remains high. Teenage girls and their unborn infants are at greater risk for complications of both pregnancy and delivery. The most frequent complications are premature labor and infants of low birth weight, high neonatal mortality, toxemia of pregnancy, iron-deficiency anemia, fetopelvic disproportion, and prolonged labor. There may be a greater incidence of weight gain in young mothers and, in younger girls, a competition in the nutritional needs for growth between the fetus and the teenage girl.

Nursing considerations

The most important goal in nursing care of the pregnant teenager is to obtain medical care for her if she has not already done so. The importance of early prenatal care is well known for the welfare of both mother and infant when the girl chooses to continue the pregnancy and to facilitate a safe abortion when she elects this option. For guidelines, teaching, and general support measures during pregnancy,

SEXUALLY TRANSMITTED DISEASES	
Traditional	**New inclusions**
Syphilis	Scabies
Gonorrhea	Pediculosis
Chancroid	Herpes progenitalis
Lymphogranuloma venereum	Condyloma acuminatum (genital warts)
Granuloma inguinale	*Hemophilus vaginalis*
	Trichomonas infection
	Chlamydia trachomatis
	Cytomegalovirus
	Monilial vaginitis
	Molluscum contagiosum of the genitalia
	Nongonococcal urethritis

the reader is directed to the excellent textbooks available on nursing care throughout the maternity cycle.*

CONTRACEPTION

Family planning services in general have developed and expanded during recent years, and, with the increase in sexual activity among the teenage population, there is also an increased awareness of the need for contraceptive services as a part of the health care of adolescents.

The choice of a contraceptive method, to be safe and effective, must be suited to the individual. The choice is based on the youngster's preference and the physician's judgment. Although a girl may prefer to use the pill, if her menstrual pattern suggests that she is not ovulating normally, she will be guided to another method. Also, the girl must be motivated to use whatever method is recommended or prescribed. No matter what method is selected, the provision of a birth control device is only part of a comprehensive sex education program.

SEXUALLY TRANSMITTED DISEASES

Traditionally known as venereal diseases, newer terminology designates them as sexually transmitted diseases (STD). They are among the most prevalent and dangerous of the communicable diseases and are now epidemic in the United States, with a disproportionate number occurring in adolescents and young adults. Sexually active adolescents are particularly at risk because they are often late in seeking medical attention. Traditional sexually transmitted diseases and those that are now also designated as such in the

*Bobak, I.M., and Jensen, M.D.: Essentials of maternity nursing, St. Louis, 1984, The C.V. Mosby Co.

TABLE 15-1. SEXUALLY TRANSMITTED DISEASES

DISEASE	MANIFESTATIONS		THERAPY	NURSING CONSIDERATIONS
Gonorrhea (*Neisseria gonorrhoeae*)	Male:	urethritis—dysuria with profuse yellow discharge, frequency, urgency, nocturia	Penicillin with probenecid	Find and treat sexual contacts Educate young people regarding facts of the disease and its spread Encourage use of barrier in sexually active young people High rate of mixed disease; therefore, treat also for chlamydia (recommended)
	Female:	cervicitis (postpubertal)—may be associated with discharge, dysuria, dyspareunia; vulvovaginitis (prepubertal)		
Chlamydia (*Chlamydia trachomatis*)	Male:	meatal erythema, tenderness, itching, dysuria, urethral discharge	Oral tetracycline	Same as above
	Female:	mucopurulent cervical exudate with erythema, edema, congestion		
Syphilis (*Treponema pallidum*)	Primary stage: chancre—a hard, painless, red, sharply defined lesion with indurated base, raised border, eroded surface, and scanty yellow discharge; usually located on penis, vulva, or cervix Secondary stage: systemic influenza-like symptoms and lymphadenopathy, rash; usually appears 1 to 3 weeks after healing of chancre		Penicillin	Viability of organism outside body is short Rapidly killed by oxygen, soap, common bacterial agents, and drying About 95% transmitted sexually; affected person most infectious during first year of disease
Herpes progenitalis (Herpesvirus hominis—type II)	Small (usually painful) vesicles on genital area, buttocks, and thighs; itching usually initial symptom; when vesicles break, shallow, circular, extremely painful lesions remain		No known cure Acyclovir (Zovirax) ointment decreases healing time and pain	Pregnancy should be avoided in sexually active girls Infection can be transmitted to infant during birth
Trichomoniasis (*Trichomonas vaginalis*)	Pruritus and edema of external genitalia; foul-smelling, greenish vaginal discharge; sometimes postcoital bleeding May be asymptomatic, especially in males		Oral metronidazole	May be contracted by self-infection from toilet bowls, bathtubs, or swimming pools (not total agreement on this) Patient should not consume alcohol while taking medication and for at least 48 hours following last dose
Candidiasis, or moniliasis (*Candida albicans*)	Edema and erythema of vulva and thick white, cheesy vaginal discharge May be satellite lesions on groin, thighs, and buttocks Cutaneous lesions on penis May be asymptomatic		Nystatin vaginal suppositories Miconazole vaginal cream	Possibility of predisposing factors such as oral contraceptives (which alter vaginal environment) or antibiotics Increased risk of neonatal thrush

adolescent age-group are listed in the box on p. 416. It is important that when a patient has one of these conditions, the history and examination should encompass the others.

The most prevalent STDs in the adolescent and adult populations are gonorrhea and chlamydial infections; therefore, they will be described briefly. These and other diseases that are seen less frequently are outlined in Table 15-1. Disorders such as scabies and pediculosis are discussed elsewhere in relation to infestations (see p. 912).

Gonorrhea

Gonorrhea (also known as the whites, clap, the drips, and the dose) is a disease that occurs primarily in larger metropolitan areas and is more prevalent in nonwhite than in white populations. There are three times as many males affected as females. An attack of gonorrhea confers no immunity to reinfections by the same untreated partner or any infected sexual partner. It is almost always genitally contracted, although pharyngeal and rectal infections in some persons reflect variant modes of sexual contact.

A genuine prophylaxis against gonorrheal infection is not yet available; therefore, preventive efforts must be directed toward finding and treating affected persons, locating and examining contacts of affected persons, educating young people regarding the facts of the disease and its spread, and encouraging the use of barriers in sexually active young people.

Chlamydial infection

Recent evidence indicates that chlamydial infection is a major type of sexually transmitted disease in adolescents and young adults and is as important as gonorrhea in its incidence, transmission, range of infection sites, and carrier state. It is suggested that all patients with gonorrhea receive a course of tetracycline therapy because of the high rate of mixed gonococcal and chlamydial infections. Treatment of sexual partners is also an essential part of therapy.

Nursing considerations

Nursing responsibilities encompass all aspects of sexually transmissible disease education, prevention, and treatment. Part of the sex education of young people should include information about these diseases, such as their symptoms and treatment, and dispelling the myths associated with their mode of transmission. It is true that most persons in the vulnerable teenage population are uninformed or misinformed about these diseases. Helping to promote the inclusion of venereal disease information in schools is an important function of the nurse.

SEXUAL TRAUMA

Sexual trauma, sexual abuse, and sexual assault involve situations in which children or adolescents "are pressured into sexual activity by a person who stands in a power position over them as through age, authority, or some other way" (Burgess & Holmstrom, 1975). Sexual assault can consist of manual, genital, or oral contact with the genitalia of the victim without consent, usually perpetrated by force, drugs, fraud, or threats of retaliation. Definitions of several types of sexual assault follow:

rape sexual assault in which the penis is forced into the genitalia of the victim. Fitting the penis between the labia without disruption of the hymen or evidence of ejaculation is also considered sufficient penetration to constitute rape.

statutory rape this may be charged when the victim is unable to give consent legally by virtue of age (age varies from state to state, but is usually less than 16 years of age), mental deficiency, psychosis, or an altered state of consciousness caused by sleep, drugs (including alcohol), or illness.

molestation sexual assault without intercourse.

incest sexual intercourse between persons too closely related to contract a marriage legally and/or culturally.

Assault

Adolescent females are the victims in approximately half of the reported rapes. They are frequently selected at random because they are apparently helpless and are usually in a vulnerable situation. The assailant may be someone who knows the victim and has waited for an opportunity when the victim is defenseless, such as the teenager at home alone with an uncle or cousin or the baby-sitter being driven home.

In the case of younger adolescents and children, the offender is known to the victims or their families in the majority of instances and is often a friend, relative, neighbor, or someone in a position of authority. In a significant number of cases concerning young victims, the sexual abuse has taken place repeatedly over a period of weeks or months. Families are often ambivalent about reporting abuse to avoid disgrace, or they may not believe the victim.

Physical force, including roughness, nonbrutal beating (slapping), brutal beating (slugging, kicking, beating repeatedly with fists), and choking or gagging, is present in a large number of cases. The predominant reaction of the victim is fear—of the rape and of injury. Thus the victim is faced with the dilemma of submission or resistance.

Young victims. In contrast to adult victims, young children and many adolescents are largely "accessories to sex." Most offenders are family members or friends who stand in a relationship of dominance over the victim and who pressure the victim into being an accessory to the sexual activity through various means. The methods of pressure are such that the child may be totally unaware that sexual activity is part of the offer.

The successful sex offender also employs means to pressure the victim into secrecy regarding the activity. It is not uncommon for the child to reveal the fear that their parents would not believe them if they told, especially if the offender is a trusted member of the family. Some fear they will be blamed for the situation, and many young children with limited vocabulary have difficulty in describing the activity when they do have the courage or opportunity to complain.

Therapeutic management

Adolescents who have been raped arrive at the emergency room or physician's office under a variety of circumstances. They are usually brought in by parents, friends, or police, but some girls may seek medical help on their own. It is advisable to obtain parental consent for examination, but the examination may be performed without consent if the adolescent is mature and the parents are unavailable. A nurse should be present during the history and examination. Since rape is a legal matter to be determined by the courts, medical examination merely provides evidence of penetration, ejaculation, and, when possible, use of force. The last is difficult to determine since many young women are left physically unmarked when forced to comply at the point of a gun or other weapon.

History. The history should be as complete as possible and must be taken and presented in the patient's own words. Information includes date, time, location, and an accurate description of all types of sexual contact. All related activities are included. For example, evidence can be altered if the victim has bathed, urinated, defecated, douched, or changed clothing; therefore, these activities should be recorded. Use of a condom by the alleged assailant can alter evidence. For adequate care, other important data include data of last menstrual period, date of last intercourse (where applicable), use of contraception, and any possibility of a preexisting pregnancy or venereal disease. Behavior and emotional state should be recorded also, since reponses range from outward calm and controlled behavior and affect to excessive agitation or hysteria.

Examination. The physical examination is carried out as soon as possible, since physical evidence deteriorates rapidly. The victim is examined thoroughly, including nongenital areas for evidence of injury that might substantiate the use of force. Sometimes the stress of the incident makes the girl unaware of physical trauma or even

serious injury. Physical injury varies greatly in victims of rape.

Specimens are obtained from the vaginal cul-de-sac, and a hang-drop preparation is examined immediately to assess sperm mobility. A Papanicolaou (Pap) smear is prepared and sent to the laboratory. Vaginal secretions are also tested for acid phosphatase, since this enzyme is not normally present in the female genital tract but is found in high concentrations in semen.

A baseline serology is drawn, and a gonococcal culture is obtained to prove that the victim did not have any preexisting infection. The child is reexamined at appropriate intervals (4 to 6 weeks for syphilis; 2 to 3 days for gonorrhea) to determine if the child acquired disease from the assailant.

Treatment. Any injuries sustained by the victim that require surgical treatment are repaired. Lacerations of the vagina are not uncommon. Most physicians prescribe, and many of the victims and/or their parents prefer the girl to receive, prophylactic administration of penicillin at the time of initial examination. Pregnancy prophylaxis, usually diethylstilbestrol, is offered to the victim who is not using oral contraceptives, pregnant, or menstruating.

Nursing considerations

In no other area of nursing practice is there greater need for understanding and compassion toward patients and their families. When a child is seen initially it is extremely important for the health personnel to take time with the child and attempt to help her through this crisis. Many girls feel uncomfortable with a male physician or nurse and are unwilling to have them examine them after a sexual assault. A female nurse should remain with the child during the examination, and she is frequently the person able to elicit the necessary information from the child.

Although many children are able to talk spontaneously about the incident, others find if difficult. The child is encouraged to talk not only to provide needed information but also because talking makes people feel better, and children are no exception. It is often easiest to begin the interview with neutral questions dealing with such things as the child's reaction to the hospital and then to proceed to a discussion of the incident in general terms. Sometimes the parents are able to help the child to describe the incident, and questions can become directed to the circumstances of the assault. It is usually difficult for young people to express feelings verbally. Talking in physical rather than sexual terms helps to facilitate discussion.

It is extremely important in this instance that the nurse and the physician take time to explain exactly what is to be done to the child clearly, thoroughly, and in language the child can understand. The physical examination is quite upsetting to the child, and she will be frightened of physical contact, especially in the genital area and other painful areas. Often young girls will cry before, during, and after the examination. The roles of the nurse and the physician should be explained to the child as well as the procedures to be performed.

After the questioning, physical examination, and any medical or surgical treatment required, it is important to discuss the situation with the parents and elicit their feelings and reaction to the assault. The family's need to discuss the incident and their feelings are essential in order that they can provide the support needed by the child. They are the strongest support system available to the child, and their ability to cope with the situation determines the degree to which they can be supportive.

Prevention. One aspect of sexual assault that is rarely given the significance that it deserves is prevention. Ideally, educating children regarding "anyone touching them in private parts of the body" should be just as commonplace as the admonition, "Don't go with strangers," and should be included in sex education. It must be remembered that children, especially preschoolers and school-age children, have little concept of sexual activities and easily succumb to statements such as, "I just want to be nice to you. This is our little secret." Bewildered, the child agrees to the act, often with familiar "nice" people, and remains secretive, sometimes for years, especially in incestuous relationships.

Children need reassurance that no matter what the other person says or does, the parents want to know and will not punish them for reporting questionable behavior. In addition, parents need to be made aware that "nice" people, including friends and relatives, can be molesters; parents should carefully observe how others act toward their children. Health professionals can alert parents to the dangers inherent in some adult behaviors and guide them toward an appreciation of the problem and providing concrete guidelines for child education and protection.

DISORDERS OF LATER CHILDHOOD

There are some disorders that seem to be more prevalent in the school years or that are first recognized during this period. The closer contact of many adolescent youngsters make infectious disorders more easily transmitted. Sexually transmitted diseases and the usual communicable diseases have already been discussed and will not be mentioned further. Infectious mononucleosis appears to be disease that affects children in later childhood, and hypertension is diagnosed with increasing frequency in the later childhood years (see Chapter 22).

INFECTIOUS MONONUCLEOSIS

Infectious mononucleosis is an acute, self-limiting infectious disease presumed to be of viral etiology that is common among young persons up to 25 years of age. The disease is characterized by an increase in the mononuclear elements of the blood and general symptoms of an infectious process. The course is usually mild but occasionally can be severe or, rarely, accompanied by serious complications.

Etiology and pathophysiology

Recent evidence implicates the herpes-like EB (Epstein-Barr) virus as the cause of infectious mononucleosis. It appears in both sporadic and epidemic forms, the sporadic cases being most common. The mechanism of spread has not been proved, although it is believed to be transmitted by direct intimate contact with oral secretions. It also appears to be only mildly contagious, and the period of communicability is unknown. The incubation period following exposure is 2 to 6 weeks.

Clinical manifestations

The onset of symptoms appears anywhere from 10 days to as much as 6 weeks following exposure and may be acute or insidious. The common presenting symptoms of infectious mononucleosis vary greatly in type, severity, and duration. The characteristics of the disease are malaise, sore throat, and fever with generalized lymphadenopathy and splenomegaly that may persist for several months. Most often the symptoms appear insidiously with fatigue, lack of energy, and sore throat that may not become prominent. The youngster's chief complaint is often difficulty in maintaining his usual level of activity. This is frequently attributed to lack of sleep, an upper respiratory infection, or both.

A skin rash is present in a few cases, most often a discrete macular eruption most prominent over the trunk. Other symptoms may include headache, epistaxis, and abdominal pain. The tonsils may be enlarged, reddened, and sometimes covered with a diphtheria-like membrane. Hepatic involvement to some degree is almost always present, often associated with jaundice, which may cause the disease to be confused with infectious hepatitis.

Diagnostic tests

The leukocyte count may be normal or low, but usually lymphocyte leukocytosis develops; of these, approximately 10% are atypical lymphocytes.

The heterophil antibody test determines the extent to which the patient's serum will agglutinate sheep red blood cells. In infectious mononucleosis, a titer of 1:160 is considered diagnostic, although a rising titer during the earlier stages is the best indicator.

The more recent "spot test" (Monospot), a slide test of high specificity, has been developed for the diagnosis of infectious mononucleosis. It is rapid, sensitive, inexpensive, easy to perform, and has the advantage that it can detect significant agglutinins at lower levels, thus enabling earlier diagnosis.

Therapeutic management

There is no specific treatment for infectious mononucleosis. Common symptoms are ordinarily relieved by simple remedies. Aspirin is usually sufficient to relieve the bothersome symptoms of headache, fever, and malaise. Bed rest is encouraged for fatigue but is not imposed for any specified period of time. Affected youngsters are instructed to regulate activities according to their own tolerance, unless complicating factors are present. If the spleen is enlarged, for example, activities in which they might receive a blow to the abdomen or chest should be avoided.

A short course of oral penicillin is sometimes prescribed for sore throat, especially if β-hemolytic streptococci are present. Sore throat can be relieved by gargles, hot drinks, analgesic troches, or aspirin. Some physicians favor the use of corticosteroids for suppression of high fever and/or severe sore throat but usually limit its use to the period of more intense symptoms or if the youngster is severely ill.

The course of infectious mononucleosis is self-limiting and usually uncomplicated. Contrary to popular belief, mononucleosis is not necessarily a difficult, prolonged, disabling disease, and the prognosis is generally good. Acute symptoms usually disappear within 7 to 10 days, and the persistent fatigue subsides within 2 to 4 weeks. A number of affected youngsters may need to restrict activities for 2 or 3 months; the disease rarely extends for longer periods.

Nursing considerations

Nursing responsibilities are directed toward comfort measures to relieve the symptoms and helping the affected youngster and his family determine appropriate activities according to the stage of the disease and his interests. They may need diet counseling to select foods that contain sufficient calories to meet growth and energy needs and yet are easy to swallow. Every effort should be made to prevent a secondary infection; therefore, the adolescent is counseled to limit exposure to persons outside the family, especially during the acute phase of illness.

The protracted nature of the illness and its associated weakness and fatigue frequently cause depression and resentment on the part of the usually vigorous, active teenager. It is important to spend time with the youngster to listen to his concerns and to allow him to express his feelings and vent his anger. The adolescent needs to be reassured that the limitations are only temporary and that social activities, so essential at this stage of development, can be resumed after the acute phase and that he will have sufficient autonomy to determine the extent of his capabilities and the rate of resumption of activities.

EATING DISORDERS

Eating disorders are among the most frequently encountered health problems in childhood and adolescence. Overeating often begins in infancy and continues throughout childhood; undereating usually does not become apparent until later childhood or adolescence. Either overeating or undereating can have a detrimental effect on health and well-being and, especially in the case of undereating, can be a decided threat to life.

OBESITY

There is probably no problem related to childhood and adolescence that is so obvious to others, is so difficult to treat, and has such long-term effects on psychologic and physical health status as obesity. It is the most common nutritional disturbance of children and one of the most challenging contemporary health problems at all ages.

Obesity is an increase in body weight resulting from an excessive accumulation of fat or simply the state of being too fat. *Overweight* refers to the state of weighing more than average for one's height and body build, which may or may not include an increased amount of fat. It is possible for two children to have the same height and weight and for one to be obese whereas the other is not.

Pathophysiology

Obesity results from a caloric intake that consistently exceeds calorie requirements and expenditure. The causes that produce this disequilibrium are complex and may involve a variety of influences including metabolic, hypothalamic, hereditary, social, cultural, and psychologic factors (Fig. 15-1).

It is known that the metabolism of glucose plays an important role in the regulation of fat deposition, since excess calories from carbohydrates are stored as fat and a lack of glucose prompts the release of fat as a source of energy. It appears that the obese are able to store fat easily

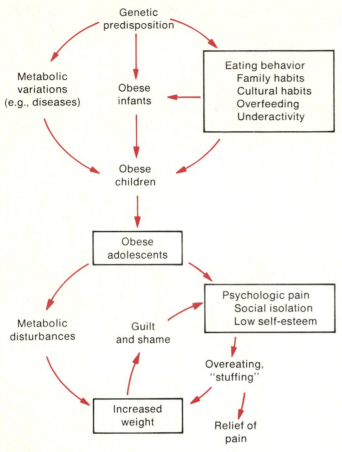

FIG. 15-1

Complex relationships in adolescent obesity.

but are unable to release this fat or burn it for energy.

Heredity has been demonstrated to be a factor in the development of obesity in some cases and eating patterns are culturally and socially based in most instances.

Psychologic factors may provide a basis for eating patterns in childhood. In infancy the child first experiences relief from discomfort through feeding and learns to associate eating with feelings of well-being, security, and the comforting presence of the mothering person. Soon eating is deeply associated with the feeling of being loved. Many parents use food, such as candy and other ''treats,'' as a positive reinforcer for desired behavior or as a way to compensate for their own feelings of guilt, especially if the child was unwanted or overvalued because of loss of a previous child. This practice soon acquires symbolic significance to the extent that the child continues to use food as a reward, a comfort, and a means by which to deal with feelings of depression or hostility.

Diagnostic evaluation

The presence of obesity is obvious from appearance alone, and a gross determination can be made by a rough com-

parison of height and weight with standard growth charts. Children who are 20% over the normal for their height and weight should be further evaluated. Evaluation includes height and weight history of the child, parents, and siblings as well as eating habits, appetite and hunger patterns, and physical activities engaged in. Appropriate diagnostic tests rule out suspected metabolic and endocrine disorders.

It is useful to have an estimation of the degree of fatness in order to have some idea of the component of body weight that can be modified. Several tests, both scientific and unscientific, can be employed to assess obesity. Simple screening tests for use in older children and adolescents include weight tables, observation, anthropometric measurements, and the pinch test, in which a fold of skin and subcutaneous fat can be lifted free, between thumb and forefinger, from underlying tissues. A fold significantly greater that 18 to 22 mm, or approximately 1 inch, indicates an excess of subcutaneous fat.

Nursing considerations in therapeutic management

Medical and nursing management are considered together since nearly all successful weight-reduction programs involve professional nurses. Few physicians are able or inclined to devote the time to the long-term supportive care needed to maintain the motivation of obese youngsters.

Motivation to lose weight is the key to success. The reasons behind the teenager's desire to lose weight need to be explored with him, but success is rarely achieved unless the youngster is motivated to lose weight and takes personal responsibility for his dietary habits and exercise program. Teenagers who are forced by parents to seek help are seldom sufficiently motivated, become rebellious of parental nagging, and are unwilling to control dietary intake. A rigid approach and one that is based on parental enforcement of the regimen is usually doomed from the start.

Diet. Planning caloric restriction for the adolescent during the rapid growth period requires a careful design. Since obesity is usually a lifelong problem, it is best to provide the individual with a diet that can be maintained throughout life with the emphasis on restricting calories. The most successful diets are those that use ordinary foods in controlled portions rather than diets that require the avoidance of any specific food. The youngster is taught how to incorporate favorite foods into the diet and how to select substitutes that are also satisfying. The dieting youngster should eat what the rest of the family eats, but less of it, and should not be deprived of favorite foods. These can be allowed—in small amounts. There are a multitude of restricted calorie diets available from a number of sources, such as the American Dietetic Association, and the caloric values for a wide variety of commercial foods are available to facilitate meal planning.

For children, especially the teenager, snacking is an integral part of the daily routine, which makes dieting particularly difficult for the obese child. They have little concept of the caloric content of even the most commonplace snack foods. Vending machines are usually stocked with high-calorie, low nutrient temptations, they are readily accessible, and the children have ample pocket money with which to purchase these items. Following pressures from concerned parents and nutritionists, many school cafeterias are providing more wholesome "treats" such as fruit, juices, and raw vegetables in vending machines in school cafeterias. However, the favorite gathering places for children and teens are the fast-food establishments, which are often located curiously near to large schools. See Table 15-2 for the caloric values for some of the fast food items and snack foods.

TABLE 15-2. CALORIC VALUES FOR SELECTED FAST FOODS

FOOD	CALORIC VALUE	FOOD	CALORIC VALUE
Burger King		**Taco Bell**—cont'd	
Cheeseburger	350	Beefy Tostada	291
Hamburger	290	Brazier Chili Dog	330
Whopper, regular	630	Super Brazier Dog	518
w/cheese	740	w/cheese	593
Double beef, plain	850	Super Brazier Chili Dog	555
w/cheese	950	Brazier Fries, small	200
French fries, regular	210	**Pizza Hut**	
Onion rings, regular	70	Thin 'n Crispy:	
Chocolate shake	365	Standard cheese, ¼ med.	340
McDonald's		Superstyle cheese, ¼ med.	410
Big Mac	563	Standard pepperoni, ¼ med.	370
Hamburger	255	Superstyle pepperoni, ¼ med.	430
Cheeseburger	307	Thick 'n Chewy:	
Chicken McNuggets, 1 serv.	332	Standard cheese, ¼ med.	390
Quarter pounder	424	Superstyle cheese, ¼ med.	450
w/cheese	524	Standard pepperoni, ¼ med.	450
Egg McMuffin	327	Superstyle pepperoni, ¼ med.	490
French fries, regular	220	Supreme, ¼ med.	480
Filet-O-Fish	432	Super Supreme, ¼ med.	590
Milk shake, vanilla	352	**Fruit**	
chocolate	383	Apple w/skin 2½ in. diam.	66
Wendy's		Banana, medium	100
Hamburger, single	470	Peach w/skin, 2 in. diam.	38
w/cheese	580	**Cookies and cakes**	
Hamburger, double	670	Hostess, 1 cup cake	
w/cheese	800	orange	151
Hamburger, triple	850	chocolate	166
w/cheese	1040	Hostess twinkie, 1	147
French fries	330	Oreo, each	50
Frostie	390	Chocolate chip	50-80
Long John Silver's		Brownie	200
Fish w/batter, 2 pieces	366	Fig Newton, 1	60
3 pieces	549	Doughnut, regular, 1 oz. pc.	113
Fish sandwich	337	Old fashioned, 1 oz. pc.	151
French Fryes	288	Powdered, 1 oz. pc.	117
Cole slaw	138	**Crackers**	
Hushpuppies (3)	153	Cheese balls & curls, 1 oz.	160
Taco Bell		Corn chips, 1 oz.	150-160
Beef Burrito	466	Graham crackers, 1 piece	30
Burrito Supreme	457	Pretzels, 1 oz.	110-116

Continued.

TABLE 15-2. CALORIC VALUES FOR SELECTED FAST FOODS—cont'd

FOOD	CALORIC VALUE	FOOD	CALORIC VALUE
Rye Krisp, 1 triple	110-116	Nuts	
Saltine, 1 piece	25	Almonds, 1 oz.	170-178
Tortilla Chips, 1 oz.	12-18	Peanuts, dry roasted, 1 oz.	160-173
Trisket, 1 piece	130-140	oil roasted, 1 oz.	179
Wheat Thins, 1 piece	20	Pecans, 1 oz.	190-220
	9	Pistachio, 1 oz.	174
Candy		Pumpkin seeds, unshelled, 1 oz.	116
Heath, 2¼ oz.	334	Sunflower, shelled, 1 oz.	164
Hershey's, 1.2 oz bar	187	unshelled, 1 oz.	86
Nestle's, 1.1 oz. bar	159	Dessert snacks	
Hershey's Kisses, 1 piece	27	Popsicle, 1 twin pop	70
Krackle bar, .35 oz.	52	Turnover	310-340
Life Savers, 1 piece	10	Pop Tart	200-220
Milk Duds, ¾ oz. box	89	Baskin-Robbins	
1¼ oz. box	148	Ice cream, 1 scoop	
M & Ms		Vanilla	147
Peanut, 1½ oz.	219	French vanilla	181
Plain, 1½ oz.	202	Chocolate	165
Mr. Goodbar, 1½ oz.	233	Chocolate fudge	178
Snickers, 1.8 oz.	247	Sherbet, 1 scoop	99-139
Crackerjack, ¾ oz.	90	Beverages	
Chewing Gum		Chocolate milk, 8 oz.	213
Any brand, 1 stick	10	Skim milk, 8 oz.	88
Dentyne, 1 stick	4	Whole milk, 8 oz.	159
Chicklets, Beechies, 1 piece	6	Coca Cola, 8 oz.	96
Miscellaneous snacks		Sprite, 8 oz.	95
Potato chips, 1 oz.	150-160		
Pringles, 1 oz.	172		
Yogurt, plain, 8 oz.	150-160		
Fruit, 8 oz.	230-262		
Popcorn, plain, 1c.	54		

No child or adolescent should be encouraged to initiate a reduction diet without a health assessment, evaluation, and counseling. It is also important to emphasize the undesirable nature of the fad diets and crash programs that continually appear in various publications. Although some success has been achieved with low-carbohydrate, high-fat diets, their unpalatability and dietary boredom contribute to a high failure rate. Exotic diets have not been successful, and their unbalanced nature makes them potentially dangerous for growing children or adolescents. To be successful from all aspects, a dietary program should be nutritionally sound with sufficient satiety value, produce the desired weight loss, and be accompanied by nutrition education and continued support.

Exercise. Since weight loss will occur only when caloric expenditure is greater than caloric intake, physical activity in the form of regularly scheduled exercise, progressively increased over the child's usual activity, is an integral part of a weight-reduction program. Activities should be those that stress self-improvement rather than competition, and teenagers need continued psycholgic support and encouragement to prevent the beginning of the destructive cycle of passivity, withdrawal, and rejection.

Drugs. A variety of preparations have been introduced as a means for achieving weight loss, ostensibly to decrease appetite to help the individual follow a reduction diet or to utilize energy more effectively and to a greater degree. Most authorities agree that drugs have limited value in achieving permanent weight loss and are transient in action, useless, or actually harmful. They are used occasionally as a matter of convenience or as a supportive measure for a short period during the initial phase of therapy.

Surgical techniques. Surgical techniques are available that bypass substantial portion of the intestine or occlude a large segment of the stomach to produce a marked diet restriction and, hence, weight loss. These shunting techniques are hazardous surgical procedures with

SUMMARY OF NURSING CARE IN ASSESSMENT AND MODIFICATION OF EATING HABITS

GOALS	RESPONSIBILITIES
Identify eating patterns and behaviors	Keep a record of everything eaten, including 　Time eaten 　Amount eaten 　Where food was consumed, for example, table, chair, in front of television, and so on 　Activity engaged in while eating 　With whom the food was eaten or if it was eaten alone 　Feelings at the time food was eaten, for example, angry, depressed, lonely, elated, and so on Analyze preceding data for patterns of eating and relationships of other factors as a basis for making adjustments
Control eating patterns	Eat only at specific times Eat only in a specific place (selected according to the family's eating pattern) Do nothing else while eating, such as watching television, reading, talking, talking on the telephone (it is easy to consume more than intended when distracted from eating) Prepare low-calorie foods in an attractive, inviting way Get rid of junk foods Put snacks out of sight and put away remaining food after meal or snack preparation (such as sandwich makings) before beginning to eat Avoid purchase of problem foods
Change the act of eating	Slow pace of eating Use smaller plates to make amount of food seem larger Leave a small amount of food on the plate Serve food from stove or other place out of reach of the established eating place to make seconds more difficult
Use methods other than eating to deal with emotional stress, boredom, and fatigue	Substitute other activities for eating in response to these feelings: activities help divert attention from food, for example, sewing, working at a hobby, taking a short walk, straightening up the room, and so on Become involved in activities out of the house and away from food
Give positive reinforcement for accomplishments	Provide a system of rewards for changes in eating behavior, exercise, and weight loss 　Point system 　Tangible rewards such as a trip, a new record, a concert Think positively (overweight individuals are negative thinkers) Have a family member serve as a monitor at home to help in progress toward goals and to encourage youngster with positive statements daily

many metabolic complications. Most authorities believe that the complex metabolic effects need clarification and that certainly this procedure should be restricted to those massively obese youngsters in whom other therapies have failed and whose obesity is life-threatening in disease states that demand weight loss for effective management.

Behavioral therapy. Probably the most successful method for treating obesity is diet combined with behavior modification, which emphasizes identification and elimination of inappropriate eating habits. Although the long-term effects of this method are still in need of evaluation,

it appears to hold promise for the treatment of obesity in adolescents. Some of the techniques used in this approach are listed in the boxed material on above.

Group involvement. Some persons on weight-reduction programs find that support and mutual reinforcement provided by a group of persons with a similar problem help them to adjust to the changes needed for successful accomplishment of their goals, including weight loss. Commercial groups such as Weight Watchers, TOPS, or diet workshops composed primarily of adults may be helpful to a few, but, for teenagers, a group composed of persons their own age is more acceptable. Some types of teenage groups include summer camps designed for obese youngsters and conducted by health professionals, school groups organized and led by the school nurse, and groups associated with special clinics.

The group is concerned not only with weight loss but also emphasizes the development of a positive self-image. Nutrition education and diet planning are essential elements of the group function, but equally important are discussions centered around better grooming and improvement of social skills. Improvement is measured by positive changes in all aspects of endeavor. Group support and reinforcement are basic to success.

ANOREXIA NERVOSA

Anorexia nervosa (AN) is the term applied to a long-recognized disorder characterized by severe weight loss in the absence of obvious physical cause. The term "anorexia nervosa" inaccurately describes the disorder in which emaciation occurs as a result of self-inflicted starvation. Anorexia nervosa occurs predominantly in adolescent and young adult females, and the incidence appears to be increasing significantly.

The onset of anorexia nervosa generally takes place at or near menarche, but it may begin in preadolescence or in adulthood. The peak ages are 12 and 13 years, with another peak occurring around ages 19 to 20 years or in the mid-twenties.

Clinical manifestations

Young women who have this disorder are most frequently from the upper or middle socioeconomic groups, are often described as "good children," are academically high achievers, are conforming, are conscientious, and have a high energy level, even with marked emaciation. These girls are usually strongly dependent on their parents, and frequently an ambivalent mother-daughter relationship is present. The etiology of the disorder remains unclear. There is a distinct psychologic component, and the diagnosis is based primarily on psychologic and behavioral criteria. Nevertheless, the physical manifestations of anorexia lend support to possible organic factors in the etiology.

In the wake of the severe weight loss, these young girls exhibit signs of altered metabolic activity. They develop secondary amenorrhea if they have attained menarche or primary amenorrhea if not, bradycardia, lowered body temperature, decreased blood pressure, and cold intolerance. They have dry skin and brittle nails and develop lanugo hair. The changes are usually reversible with adequate weight gain and improved nutritional status.

Psychologic aspects

Dominating the psychologic aspects of anorexia nervosa are a relentless pursuit of thinness and a fear of fatness, usually preceded by a period of a year or two of mood disturbances and behavior changes. The weight loss is usually triggered by a typical adolescent crisis such as the onset of menstruation or traumatic interpersonal incidents that precipitate serious dieting that continues out of control. Frequently there is an exaggerated misinterpretation of the normal fat deposition characteristic of the early adolescent period, or someone may comment that the adolescent girl is putting on weight. The weight loss may be a response to teasing, some change in her life (such as changing schools or going off to college), or an incident that requires an independent decision that she is unprepared to make (such as a career choice).

Nursing considerations related to therapeutic management

The treatment and management of anorexia nervosa are directed toward correction of the severe state of malnutrition and resolution of the psychologic disorganization. Because of the psychogenic nature of the disorder, treatment is difficult and requires long-term management. All of those involved in therapy must keep in mind the adolescent's distorted sense of body image and self-awareness and her feelings of self-doubt, ineffectiveness, and helplessness that prompt such bizarre behavior in order to feel in control of her own body functions.

The initial goal is to treat the life-threatening malnutrition with strict adherence to dietary requirements, which sometimes necessitates intravenous and tube feedings. The most successful approach uses simple operant conditioning that emphasizes positive reinforcement for weight gain. A clearly defined behavior modification plan is communicated to the child and maintained through a unified team approach by all persons involved in her care. Children whose disorder can be clearly related to a dysfunctional family situation respond to therapy best when separated from the family. Many of those whose therapy plan is implemented in the hospital need a continued behavior modification program after discharge in order to maintain the desired weight.

Psychotherapy is aimed at helping the child resolve the adolescent identity crisis, particularly as it relates to a distorted body image. Nurses need to adopt and maintain a kind, supporting, yet firm manner in managing the care of an anorectic child. The child requires the sustained support and reassurance as she copes with ambivalent feelings related to her own body concept and the desire to see herself as cooperative, reliable, and worthy of the kindness she receives. Encouraging the child with education and ac-

SUMMARY OF NURSING CARE OF THE ADOLESCENT WITH ANOREXIA NERVOSA

GOALS	RESPONSIBILITIES

Recognize anorexia nervosa	Observe for signs of
	    Malnutrition
	    Behaviors associated with the disorder
	    Evidence of hormonal changes, especially those associated with pubertal changes
	Obtain complete history
	Explore patient's body image perception

Restore nutritional status	Implement high-calorie diet as prescribed Explain nutritional plan to patient and family With dietitian and patient select balanced diet with the prescribed incremental increase in calories Help patient prepare a dietary diary Maintain and monitor nasogastric feedings or hyperalimentation schedule, if prescribed
Enforce behavior modification plan (if implemented)	Make certain all members of the health team understand the therapeutic plan Make certain that the patient and family understand the conditions of the plan Involve patient in plans Ensure consistent application of plan by involved health professionals Consult with patient regarding progress Avoid coercive techniques Avoid extensive discussion of food
Reduce energy expenditure	Monitor physical activity Supervise selection and performance of activity Be alert to evidence of secretive exercising
Prevent relapse	Maintain consistency in therapeutic approach selected Maintain vigilance to detect signs of sabotaging the therapeutic plan, such as self-induced vomiting, hoarding food, disposing of food, placing weighted material in clothing for weigh-in Provide positive reinforcement for progress Be alert for signs of depression Support psychotherapeutic measures Help arrange for follow-up care
Monitor progress	Obtain baseline information Observe and record emotional status Observe and record interactions with family and peers
Provide patient with appropriate feeling of control	Channel need for control and feeling of effectiveness in appropriate directions (rather than control of weight) Obtain psychiatric referral as indicated Encourage patient to monitor own care as appropriate
Support patient	Maintain open communications with patient Convey an attitude of caring and protection to patient Avoid conveying an attitude of intrusion Encourage participation in own care
Resolve disturbed pattern of family interaction	Observe family interaction Explore feelings and attitudes of family members Support psychotherapeutic measures for redirecting malfunctioning family processes Help arrange for referral to individuals and groups that further therapeutic goals
Prepare for home care	Make certain both patient and family understand therapeutic plan Arrange for follow-up care

tivities that strengthen her self-esteem facilitates her resocialization process and social acceptance among her peers. Additional information and support for parents can be obtained from any of the national organizations*.

BULIMIA

Bulimia, bulimarexia, or bulimia nervosa is a newly recognized clinical syndrome of self-induced vomiting as a means of weight control. The affected persons characteristically display a powerful and intractable urge to overeat, attempt to avoid the fattening effects of this overindulgence by induced vomiting and/or use of laxatives, and have a morbid fear of becoming fat. The bulimic patients are usually young women (mean age 24 years) but approximately 20% are older adolescents, and it is believed that the disorder frequently begins in adolescence.

Most patients are in the normal weight range but are afraid of gaining weight and most report that they persistently feel fat. The self-induced vomiting takes place at least once daily. It is highly secretive and associated with extreme guilt, which makes it difficult to detect. Many persons who practice bulimia have the characteristics of depression and express a sense of hopelessness. A number of anorexia nervosa sufferers indulge in the practice and some believe it may be a phase of that disorder.

Therapy is indefinite. Some have benefitted from psychotherapy, some from weight reduction or other support groups, and others from antidepressants. All need support and understanding.

BEHAVIOR DISORDERS IN SCHOOL-AGE CHILDREN

A number of classification systems have been employed to outline the various problems of middle childhood that interfere with development, learning, and social relationships. Although there is no universal categorization, most authorities seem to broadly classify behavioral disorders in some manner that identifies mental subnormality, learning disabilities, neuroses, psychoses, and antisocial behavior. Many disorders have a major organic or developmental component, whereas others are seen almost exclusively in

*American Anorexia-Bulimarexia Association, 133 Cedar Lane, Teaneck, NJ 07666

Anorexia Nervosa and Associated Disorders, Suite 2020, 550 Frontage Rd., Northfields IL 60093

National Anorexic Aid Society, Box 29461, Columbus, OH 43229

National Association of Anorexia Nervosa and Associated Disorders, Box 271, Highland Park, IL 60035

children of school-age. Still others are primarily problems of adolescence and many extend throughout the course of childhood. Very often a change in behavior is one of the manifestations of an organic disease; at other times emotional problems produce somatic symptoms of greater or lesser seriousness.

ATTENTION DEFICIT DISORDER (ADD)

A good deal of confusion surrounds the definitions and relationships of various behavior problems that in some way impair the child's capacity to profit from new experiences. Most of the confusion is related to the category of behaviors for which many overlapping terms have emerged—"hyperkinetic reaction of childhood," "hyperactive child syndrome," "minimal brain dysfunction," "specific learning disabilities," "neurologic handicap," "hyperkinetic syndrome," and "developmental dyslexia," for example. Other points of confusion are in relation to manifestations that overlap in the way in which the behaviors vary according to the activity being observed, the setting in which it is observed, and the criteria or measurement tools being employed.

Because the behavior most consistently observed in these children is attention difficulties, the term "attention deficit disorder" (ADD) is now accepted as the correct terminology. ADD is further delineated into two subtypes: (1) attention deficit disorder with hyperactivity and (2) attention deficit disorder without hyperactivity. The term "specific learning disabilities," which refers to the behavioral outcomes of impaired functioning in central processing such as dyslexia, dysphasia, and inability to calculate or draw, is primarily an educational concern.

Early identification of affected children is needed since the characteristics of the disorder significantly interfere with the normal course of emotional and psychologic development. Many of these children, in the attempt to cope with cerebral dysfunction, develop maladaptive behavior patterns that are a deterrent to psychosocial adjustment. Their behavior evokes negative responses from others, and repeated exposure to negative feedback adversely affects the child's self-concept.

Clinical manifestations

The behaviors exhibited by the child with ADD are not unusual aspects of child behavior. The difference lies in the quality of motor activity and developmentally inappropriate inattention, impulsivity, and hyperactivity the child displays. The manifestations may be numerous or few, mild or severe, and will vary with the developmental level of the child. Any given child will not have every manifestation that is characteristic of a syndrome, and the degree

DIAGNOSTIC CRITERIA IN IDENTIFYING THE CHILD WITH ATTENTION DEFICIT DISORDER

A. **Inattention.** At least three of the following:
   1. Often fails to finish things he starts
   2. Often does not seem to listen
   3. Easily distracted
   4. Has difficulty concentrating on schoolwork or other tasks requiring sustained attention
   5. Has difficulty sticking to a play activity
B. **Impulsivity.** At least three of the following:
   1. Often acts before thinking
   2. Shifts excessively from one activity to another
   3. Has difficulty organizing work (not a result of cognitive impairment)
   4. Needs a lot of supervision
   5. Frequently calls out in class
   6. Has difficulty awaiting turn in games or group situations
C. **Hyperactivity.** At least two of the following:
   1. Runs about or climbs on things excessively
   2. Has difficulty sitting still or fidgets excessively
   3. Has difficulty staying seated
   4. Moves about excessively during sleep
   5. Is always ''on the go'' or acts as if ''driven by a motor''
D. Onset before age 7
E. Duration of at least 6 months
F. Not caused by schizophrenia, affective disorder, or severe or profound mental retardation

Modified from American Psychiatric Association: Diagnostic and statistical manual of mental disorders, ed. 3 (DSM III), Washington, D.C., 1980, American Psychiatric Association.

of severity is highly variable. The diagnostic criteria for identifying the child with ADD is outlined in the box above.

Therapeutic management

Management of the child with ADD usually involves a multiple approach that includes family education and counseling, medication, remedial education, environmental manipulation, and sometimes psychotherapy for the child.

Medication. Extensive experience with central nervous stimulants has demonstrated them to be highly effective in reducing many of the symptoms in children with attention deficit disorder. The most prominent of these are amphetamines, such as amphetamine sulfate (Benzedrine) and dextroamphetamine sulfate (Dexedrine), and methylphenidate hydrochloride (Ritalin). However, not all children benefit from medications. Those who do may respond to only one medication or to a combination of two medications, and the effective dosage varies from child to child.

In recent years there has been interest in diet and hyperkinesis. There are those who believe that the observed behavioral patterns are related to an innate sensitivity to certain food items and/or food additives. Although this theory does not have wholehearted support, a few children do show improvement when certain foods are eliminated from their diet, particularly those containing salicylates and those with specific additives such as artificial coloring, sweetening, and preservatives.

Environmental manipulation. The child's environment is simplified by decreasing external stimuli, reducing alternatives, encouraging desired patterns of behavior, and, sometimes, controlling his diet. The child needs an environment in which distractions and external stimuli are reduced to a minimum. Also, the more the environment is controlled, the less medication is required.

Remedial education. Special training activities in the schools are designed to offer a direct attack on such areas of deficit as visual perception, auditory perception, and other areas involving integration and coordination. The purpose of programs for children with special learning disabilities is to assist them toward more successful achievement, personal adjustment, and eventual retention in the regular classroom.

Nursing considerations

Nurses are active participants in all aspects of management of the child with ADD. Nurses in the community setting work with families in the home on a long-term basis to help plan and implement therapeutic regimens and to evaluate the effectiveness of therapy.

ENURESIS

Enuresis is a common and troublesome disorder that is difficult to define because of the variable ages at which children achieve bladder control. In a broad sense enuresis can be defined as repeated involuntary urination (usually nocturnal) in children who are beyond the age when voluntary bladder control should normally have been acquired. Some authorities place 4 years as an arbitrary age by which diurnal and nocturnal bladder control is normally accomplished, although 5 years of age is probably more accurate. The incidence is approximately 5% to 17% in otherwise normal children between 3 and 15 years of age. Enuresis is more common in boys than in girls.

Organic causes that may be related to enuresis should be ruled out before psychogenic factors are considered. These include structural disorders of the urinary tract, urinary tract infection, major neurologic deficits, nocturnal epilepsy, disorders such as diabetes mellitus and diabetes insipidus that increase the normal output of urine, and disorders such as chronic renal failure or sickle cell disease that impair the concentrating ability of the kidneys. In other cases the enuresis is influenced by emotional factors, although it is doubtful that they are causative factors.

In most enuretic children nocturnal bed-wetting is a primary maturational problem and usually ceases between 6 and 8 years of age, although it sometimes continues into adolescence. The predominant symptom is urgency that is immediate and accompanied by acute discomfort, restlessness, and sometimes urinary frequency. Nocturnal enuresis is most common and is occasionally accompanied by diurnal wetting; diurnal wetting without nocturnal bed-wetting is unusual.

Various therapeutic techniques are employed in the management of enuresis. These include anticholinergic drugs, bladder training, restriction or elimination of fluids after the evening meal, interruption of sleep to void, and some type of electrical device designed to establish a conditioned reflex response to waken the child at the initiation of micturition.

Nursing considerations

No matter what techniques are employed, the nurse can help both child and parents to understand the problem of enuresis, the treatment plan, and the probable difficulties they may encounter in the process. More important, the nurse can provide consistent support and encouragement to help sustain them through the inconsistent and unpredictable treatment process. The child needs to believe that he is helping himself and to sustain feelings of confidence and hope.

ENCOPRESIS

Encopresis is the repeated voluntary or involuntary passage of feces of normal or near-normal consistency into places not appropriate for that purpose in the individual's own sociocultural setting and not the result of any physical disorder. The disorder is less common than enuresis, but the two may coexist. It is seldom an isolated symptom and is commonly clustered with other somatic symptoms—social withdrawal, antisocial-aggressive behaviors, affective-dependent behaviors, and somatic manifestations.

Primary encopresis is identified by age 4 when the child has not achieved fecal continence for at least a year. Secondary encopresis is fecal incontinence occurring between ages 4 and 8 that has been preceded by a period of fecal continence. Predisposing factors seem to be inadequate, inconsistent toilet training and psychosocial stress, such as entering school or the birth of a sibling. The dis-

order is more common in males than in females. When incontinence is involuntary, it frequently occurs secondary to constipation, impaction, or retention of feces with subsequent overflow. It is not unusual for soiling to take place after bathing because of reflex stimulation.

School performance and attendance is affected as the child's offensive odor becomes a target for scorn and derision from classmates. This causes further withdrawal and other behavioral manifestations. Therapeutic management is similar to that employed in the psychologic treatment of enuresis. Frequently psychotherapeutic intervention with the child and the family becomes necessary.

RECURRENT ABDOMINAL PAIN

Recurrent abdominal pain is one of the somatic complaints of childhood that is almost always attributed to a psychogenic etiology, although it can be a symptom of either psychosomatic or organic disease.

The characteristic feature of the disorder is abdominal pain that the child usually locates in the periumbilical area. However, on palpation the pain is more likely to be experienced in the epigastric area or in the lower right or left quadrant and is accompanied by vague tenderness without muscle guarding. The pain is irregular in time, duration, and intensity and is associated with either loose or pellet-formed stools. Other symptoms that may accompany the abdominal pain are headache, pallor, dizziness, and dysuria.

Support for the psychologic aspects of this disorder is based on observations of aggravation of symptoms during times of tension or stress. Children with recurrent abdominal pain tend to be highly sensitive, have a poor self-image, and are uncomfortable with expressions of anger or argument, especially in those persons who are significant in their life. School attendance is adversely affected, and these children generally exhibit poor learning performance. It is not uncommon for symptoms to be aggravated during school days.

Treatment is difficult. Hospitalization may be necessary, and the child frequently shows improvement in the hospital environment. Initial efforts are directed toward ruling out organic causes of the pain, relieving discomfort, and attempting to determine the situations that precipitate attacks. When simple measures are ineffective, an antispasmodic drug such as propantheline bromide may be prescribed to relieve the muscle spasm.

Nursing considerations

Once the diagnosis has been established, the parents and the child need an explanation of the pain, which can be compared to a skeletal muscle cramp or ''charley horse'' for easier comprehension. Reassurance that the symptoms are not unique to their child and that the pain can be expected to subside is helpful in relieving parental fears and anxieties. When parents are reassured that there is no organic cause of the pain, they will need some guidance regarding what they can do during a pain episode. All too often they feel helpless and anxious, which tends to compound the child's distress.

The simple expedient of putting the child at rest by having him lie down in a peaceful, quiet environment and providing comfort will often relieve the symptoms in a short time. A heating pad may also help ease the discomfort. If pain is not relieved by these simple measures, the parents are taught how to administer antispasmodics, if prescribed. For example, if pain is precipitated by meals, having the child take the medication 20 to 30 minutes before mealtime may prevent an episode.

The most valuable measures that the nurse can provide are support and reassurance to the family. When open communication is established and families are able to see a relationship between stress-provoking situations and the child's symptoms, the chance for remedial action is enhanced. Follow-up care and continued support are essential because the symptoms tend to remit and exacerbate; therefore, the availability of a supportive health professional can be a source of comfort to the child and family.

CONVERSION REACTION

Conversion reaction, also known as hysteria, hysterical conversion reaction, and childhood hysteria, is a psychophysiologic disorder with a sudden onset that can usually be traced to a precipitating environmental event. The manifestations involve primarily the voluntary musculature and special senses and include abdominal pain, fainting, pseudoseizures, paralysis, headaches, and visual field restriction. The most commonly observed symptom is seizure activity, which can be differentiated from those of neurogenic origin by formal tests, the most useful of which is the finding of a normal electroencephalogram.

It has been observed that nearly all children with conversion reaction have experienced a major family crisis before the onset of symptoms, such as loss of a parent or other significant person through death, divorce, or moving. Nursing care is similar to that for the child with recurrent abdominal pain.

SCHOOL PHOBIA

School phobia is a term used to describe children, other than beginning students, who resist going to school because of dread of the school situation, concerns with leaving home, or both. Anxiety—especially anxiety over separation from the mother— that frequently verges on panic is a constant manifestation. Some children are afraid the mother will not be home when they get there. Simple reassurance is often sufficient for these children.

Children can develop symptoms as a protective mechanism to keep them from facing the situation that distresses them. Physical symptoms are prominent and may affect any part of the body—anorexia, nausea, vomiting, diarrhea, dizziness, headache, leg pains, or abdominal pains, to name a few. There may even be a low-grade fever. A striking feature of school phobia is the prompt subsiding of symptoms when it is evident that the child can remain at home. Another significant observation is absence of symptoms on weekends and holidays unless they are related to other places such as Sunday school or parties. Occasional mild reluctance is not uncommon among school children, but if the fear continues for longer than a few days it must be considered as a serious problem—a warning of an important personality problem. The goal is to keep the child in school even if this requires an alternative schedule such as half-day classes. If the problem persists, professional help is recommended.

CHILDHOOD DEPRESSION

Depression in childhood is often difficult to detect. They may be unable to express their feelings and tend to act out their problems and concerns. *Acute depression* is almost always precipitated by a traumatic event such as a period of hospitalization, loss of a parent through death or separation, loss of a significant relationship with something (a pet), someone (a friend or family member), or a place (move from a familiar home, neighborhood, or city).

The easily identified manifestations include a sad, downcast face, tearfulness, irritability, and withdrawal from previously enjoyed activities and relationships. The child tends to spend more time in solitary activities, especially television viewing, and schoolwork is impaired. Some children become more dependent and clinging; others become more aggressive and disruptive. Sleeplessness and/or anorexia are not uncommon reactions. The manifestations may last a few days or weeks, usually resolving spontaneously.

Less common than acute depression, *chronic depression* has no apparent precipitating event but there is often a history of frequent disruptions in important relationships. Commonly there is also a history of depressive illness in one or both parents during the child's lifetime. Manifestations are as varied as those observed in acute depression but occur more frequently and extend over a longer period of time.

Masked depression is the term applied to a disorder

whereby children display acting-out behavior to hide or cover up their feelings of depression. The behavior can take the form of behavior such as aggression, hostility, poor school performance, psychosomatic or hypochondriacal complaints, or delinquent behavior that may be uncovered occasionally to reveal their depressed feelings. Authorities do not agree on the concept of masked depression, however.

The management of childhood depression is usually psychotheraputic and highly individualized. Nurses should be aware that depression is a problem that can easily be overlooked in the school-age child and one that can interrupt normal growth and development. Recognizing depression and making appropriate referrals is an important nursing function. Identification of the depressed child requires a careful history (health, growth and development, social, and family health), interviews with the child, and observations by the nurse, parents, and teachers.

CHILDHOOD SCHIZOPHRENIA

Childhood schizophrenia is a term used to describe severe deviations in ego functioning and is generally reserved for psychotic disorders that appear after the first 4 or 5 years of life. Schizophrenia in adults occurs with relative frequency, and, although childhood psychosis is not as common, it is by no means rare.

Childhood schizophrenia is characterized by a gradual onset of neurotic symptoms that show wide variation according to each affected child's developmental level, the age of onset, the nature of early childhood experiences, and the type of defense mechanisms used. However, the basic core disturbance is a lack of contact with reality and the subsequent development of a world of the child's own. Secondary characteristics represent impairment in a wide number of areas of development including cognition, perception, emotion, language, and physical motor control. The most common manifestations involve language disturbances, impaired interpersonal relationships, and inappropriate affect (outward expression of emotion).

Nursing of psychotic children is a highly specialized area, but since these problems are being recognized with increasing frequency, nurses should be alert to the possibility. A child who consistently demonstrates abnormal behavior should be referred for evaluation.

SERIOUS HEALTH PROBLEMS OF LATER CHILDHOOD AND ADOLESCENCE

The transition to adulthood with its prescribed developmental tasks produces a sense of diffuse discomfort within some adolescents, who respond with faulty problem solving in their search for relief from the discomfort and stress of this transitional period of life. Some of the more serious health problems may arise during this time of developmental stress although there is an increased incidence of suicide and substance abuse among school-age children.

SUBSTANCE ABUSE

The use of drugs and other substances by children and adolescents to produce an altered state of consciousness is widespread and is believed to reflect the variety of changes taking place in their lives and the stresses engendered by these changes. Drug abuse is the regular use of drugs for other than the accepted medical purposes and to the extent that it results in physical or psychologic harm to the user and/or is used in a way that is detrimental to society.

Most drugs to which young people turn induce changes in perception, a feeling of well-being, and a sense of closeness. To most, they provide a feeling of happiness. With the exception of some stimulant drugs used for practical purposes, such as working better, studying, or increasing cognitive effectiveness, the drugs used are simply pleasure-promoting chemicals used in the hope for altered consciousness or the attainment of a different level of functioning. In the majority of cases drug use begins with experimentation. The individual may try a drug only once, it may be used occasionally, or it may become an integral part of a drug-centered life-style.

Motivation

There are several common motives for drug use. Children and adolescents try drugs out of curiosity, for kicks. Drugs produce for some persons a dreamy state of altered consciousness and a feeling of power, excitement, heightened acuity, or confidence. Others seek visual hallucinatory experiences and sexual sensation. Many youngsters use drugs not only for the perceptual and sensory experiences but also for the social aspects. They use drugs because others use them and because they want to "turn on" or "tune in" to the drug culture. Teenagers are highly influenced by fads and fashions within their society, and they are, developmentally, sensation-hungry risk takers. It is characteristic that they are eager to test their mental and physical capabilities to the utmost.

Types of drugs abused

Any drug can be abused, and most are potentially harmful to youngsters still going through formative life experiences. Although rarely conceived as drugs by society, the chemically active substances most frequently abused are the xanthines and theobromines contained in chocolate and in common beverages such as tea, coffee, and colas. Common analgesics such as aspirin, propoxyphene hydrochloride (Darvon compound), and butalbital (Fiorinal); ethyl alcohol; and nicotine are others that, although recognized as drugs, are sanctioned by society. Any of these can produce mild to moderate euphoric and/or stimulant effects and can lead to physical and psychic dependence.

Drugs with mind-altering capacity that are available on the black market and that are of medical and legal concern are the hallucinogenic, narcotic, hypnotic, and stimulant drugs. In addition, those of concern to the health professionals are alcohol and various volatile substances, such as antifreeze, plastic model airplane cement, typewriter correction fluid, and organic solvents, that are inhaled to achieve altered sensation in the user. Drugs available on the street are often mixed with other compounds and fillers so that the purity of the drug, its strength, and the nature of additives are highly variable.

Narcotics. Narcotic drugs include opiates such as heroin, morphine, meperidine hydrochloride (Demerol), and codeine. They produce a state of euphoria by removing painful feelings and creating a pleasurable experience of specific quality and a sense of success accompanied by clouding of consciousness and a dreamlike state. Physical signs of narcotic abuse include constricted pupils, respiratory depression and, often, cyanosis. Needle marks may be visible on arms or legs in chronic users. Withdrawal from opiates is extremely unpleasant unless controlled with supervised substitution of methadone.

Central nervous system depressants. A variety of hypnotic drugs that produce physical dependence and withdrawal symptoms on abrupt discontinuance may be used by adolescents. They create a feeling of relaxation and sleepiness but impair general functioning. Drugs in this category include barbiturates, nonbarbiturates (such as methaqualone [Quaalude]), and alcohol.

Alcohol consumption by youthful drinkers is not a new phenomenon, but because of its easy accessibility, alcohol appears to have become the drug of choice among youth. It is the most widely accepted drug, can be purchased legally by adults, is relatively inexpensive, is often used as part of a meal (wine, beer), and is approved of by adults throughout the world when used in moderation.

The most noticeable effects of alcohol are on the central nervous system—incoordination, emotional lability, and impaired judgment, memory, and perception. Youthful alcoholics enjoy the effect of the alcohol and look forward to becoming intoxicated. They drink rapidly to obtain a "high" emotional state, often drink alone, cannot predictably control their use of alcohol, and protect their supply, afraid that they will be caught without anything to drink. Not all of these characteristics are observed in the alcoholic but if several of the signs are evident, the youngsters should be considered at risk and detoxification therapy initiated to assure safe and complete withdrawal from the drug.

Central nervous system stimulants. Amphetamines and cocaine do not produce strong physical dependence and can be withdrawn without much danger. However, psychologic dependence is strong and acute intoxication can lead to violent aggressive behavior or psychotic episodes manifest by paranoia, uncontrollable agitation, and restlessness. When combined with barbiturates, the euphoric effects are particularly addictive.

Mind-altering drugs. Hallucinogens (psychedelic, psychotomimetic, psychotropic, or illusionogenic) are drugs that produce vivid hallucinations and euphoria. These drugs do not produce physical dependence, since they can be abruptly withdrawn without ill effect. However, acute and long-term effects are variable, and in some individuals the dissociative behavior may be unduly protracted. This category includes cannabis (marijuana, hashish) and lysergic acid diethylamide (LSD).

Hydrocarbons and fluorocarbons. Glue "sniffing," the inhalation of plastic cement, and inhalation of other volatile substances that youngsters breathe and rebreathe in paper or plastic bags produce euphoria and altered consciousness. They are extremely hazardous to the individual, causing rapid loss of consciousness and respiratory arrest. Many persons taking these drugs do not have time to remove the bag from their heads and quickly become asphyxiated.

Nursing considerations related to therapeutic management

Nurses in almost every setting are increasingly likely to have contact with youthful drug abusers or to be in a position to serve as educator and patient advocate. The nurse most often encounters youthful drug abusers when they are (1) experiencing overdose symptoms, (2) experiencing withdrawal symptoms, (3) manifesting bizarre behavior or confusion secondary to drug ingestion, or (4) worried that they are becoming or will become addicted.

Nurses may encounter drug use in relation to other health problems. Nurses caring for adolescents in the hospital or under treatment for other illnesses need to know if the youngsters use drugs compulsively, since withdrawal phenomena can seriously complicate the illness. They should be able to recognize physical or behavioral clues that indicate the onset of withdrawal or the effects of drugs that might have been brought to the youngster secretly by well-meaning relatives or friends.

Acute care. Adolescents experiencing toxic drug effects or withdrawal symptoms are frequently seen as emergencies. Experienced emergency room personnel are familiar with the management of acute drug toxicosis; the signs, symptoms, and behavioral characteristics of a variety of substances; and differences and similarities among them. When the drug is questionable or unknown, knowledge of these factors facilitates handling of the youngster and implementation of a treatment regimen. Often observation of or description of the behavior is of more value than a report by patients or their friends as to the chemical agent taken.

The treatment for drug toxicity or withdrawal varies according to the drug and the method used. Every effort should be made to determine the type and amount of drug taken, the time it was taken, the mode of administration, and factors related to the onset of presenting symptoms. It is helpful to know that patient's pattern of use. For example, if two types of drugs are involved they may require different treatments. Gastric lavage may be employed when the drug has been ingested recently and the cough reflex is intact but would be of little value when the drug has been administered by the intravenous (''mainlined'') or intranasal (''sniffed'') route. Since the actual content of most street drugs is highly questionable, other pharmaceutical agents are administered with caution, except perhaps the narcotic antagonists in cases of suspected opiate overdose. It is necessary to assess for possible trauma that might have been sustained while under the influence of the drug.

Long-term management. A major factor in the treatment and rehabilitation of the young drug user is careful assessment, in the nonacute stage, to determine the function that the drug plays in the youngster's life. The adolescent needs help to identify the problem that motivated him to resort to drugs and to recognize his own role in self-destructive, inappropriate drug-abuse behavior before he can embark on a rehabilitation program.

Rehabilitation begins when a youngster has decided that, with the help of concerned and supportive adults, he can and is willing to change. Rehabilitation implies not only environmental manipulation and involvement therapy but also commitment on the part of the patient to substitute dependency on people for his dependency on drugs and to explore alternative mechanisms for problem solving and coping with stress. Persons working with troubled youth must be prepared for recidivism, or the tendency to relapse, and maintain a plan for reentry into the treatment process.

Prevention. Drug abuse in adolescence is both an individual and a community problem, and nurses play an important role in education and legislation as well as in individual observation, assessment, and therapy. In this drug-oriented society, patterns of drug use may be established through parental models and the influence of the media as an effective means to make the user ''feel better.'' Impressionable youth need to be educated regarding appropriate use of chemicals. More important, those associated with adolescents should listen to what they are saying, determine what is bothering them, and try to help

them meet these needs through alternative methods before they resort to drugs.

SUICIDE

Suicide is defined as the deliberate act of self-injury with the intent that the injury should kill. Of successful suicides in children of both sexes, aged 10 to 14 years, firearms and hanging account for the largest number of deaths. The predominant method at ages 15 to 19 years is the use of firearms by males and poisons by females.

In the pediatric population there is a direct relationship between the rate of suicide and advancing age. Suicide is nonexistent in children less than 5 years of age and most unusual, or not reported, in children aged 5 to 9 years, although a large number (about 10%) of those who do attempt to kill themselves are successful. The rate of suicide increases in ages 9 to 14 years, and the rate and number have been rising steadily each year. At age 14 years there is a sharp rise, and in ages 15 to 19 years the rate increases eightfold to tenfold and doubles again at ages 20 to 24 years. The greatest increase in suicides is among young men 15 to 24 years of age, where it ranks as one of the leading causes of death.

In all age-groups three times as many males commit suicide as females and the males are generally successful in the first try. The rate is reversed for attempted suicides, where females outnumber males three to one. The reason for this is not entirely clear; however, males tend to use more violent means and those that are more likely to succeed, such as firearms, hanging, and explosives. Females, on the other hand, use less violent methods that allow time for rescue, such as ingesting pills or poisons.

Sometimes an adolescent will threaten suicide in order to manipulate the environment. Unfortunately, with no self-destructive intent, a youngester may make a halfhearted attempt that leads to death. The high incidence of accidental death in the adolescent age-group has led some to speculate that many of these young people intentionally or unintentionally invite injury or become victims of homicide.

Motivation

Suicidal behavior is generally divided into (1) primarily ''acting-out'' behavior, representing a cry for help, and (2) a true death wish. Most suicidal gestures are impulsive acts committed to force parents or other significant persons in their lives to pay attention to the need for help. The attempt usually is the culmination of a behavioral pattern. These youngsters often have a history of attention-getting behaviors that range from minor acts to increasingly dramatic ones. With the ultimate act of attempted suicide, the child finally makes himself heard. He seldom actually plans a suicidal act because he really wants to die; successful suicides are committed either impulsively or accidentally.

Occasionally there are adolescents who are so severely depressed that suicide appears to them to be the only means of release from their despair. These youngsters rarely give evidence of their intent, concealing their suicidal thoughts for fear of outside intervention. Sometimes this self-destructive behavior on the part of adolescents is a desire to punish themselves for guilt-filled actions, such as masturbation or, more often, thoughts. Peer pressure, too, has convinced many young persons that there is something wrong with them if they feel lonely or depressed; therefore, they direct these feelings inward to avoid the risk of rejection. Social isolation is seen in many suicidal adolescents, but it appears to be the most significant factor in distinguishing those who will kill themselves from those who will not. It is more characteristic of those who complete suicide than of those who make attempts or threats.

Suicidal threats should be taken very seriously. It has often been a general tendency to dismiss a suicide attempt as an impulsive act resulting from a temporary crisis or depression. If this drastic move to gain attention fails to draw attention to their problems or makes them worse, adolescents may conclude that taking their lives is their only means to solve these escalating, unsolvable, and unbearable problems.

Nursing considerations

Care of the suicidal adolescent includes early recognition, management, and prevention. Probably the most important aspect of management is the recognition of prodromal signs that indicate that a youngster is troubled and might attempt to take his life. Health professionals need to be alert to the signs of adolescent depression, and any youngster who exhibits such behavior, subtle or overt, should be referred for thorough psychologic assessment. Depression can be manifest in two ways: youngsters who feel depressed may talk about suicide and feelings of worthlessness or they may build themselves a solid defense against such intolerable feelings of depression with behavioral or psychosomatic disturbances. A sudden change in behavior from depression to cheerfulness can be mistaken for apparent adjustment but should be investigated. It frequently indicates that the child has reached the decision to take his life.

Too often suicidal threats or minor attempts are confused with bids for attention. No threat of suicide should be ignored or challenged in any way. It is a symptom that must be taken seriously. The child needs to know that someone cares and must be provided with swift and efficient crisis intervention. Most larger communities have

24-hour service in the form of "hot lines"—telephone communication that is within reach of troubled youngsters or their families where they can make ready contact with someone to listen to them. The function of the hot line is to help them through the immediate crisis. Through skillful questioning, but without imposing a solution on the caller, the listener helps the caller arrive at a course of action that will contribute to a solution for his problem.

REFERENCE

Burgess, A.W., and Holmstrom, L.L.: Sexual trauma of children and adolescents, Nurs. Clin. North Am. **10**:551-563, 1975.

BIBLIOGRAPHY
General

Jelneck, L.J.: The special needs of the adolescent with chronic illness, Am. J. Maternal Child Nurs. **2**(1):57-61, 1977.
Kalafatich, A.J.: Approaches to the care of adolescents, New York, 1975, Appleton-Century-Crofts.
Lore, A.: Adolescents: people, not problems, Am. J. Nurs. **73**:1232, 1973.
Mercer, R.T.: Perspectives on adolescent health care, Philadelphia, 1979, J.B. Lippincott Co.
Stein, R.F.: The hospitalized adolescent's dilemma. In Reinhardt, A.M., and Quinn, M.D., editors: Current practice in family-centered community nursing, vol. 1, St. Louis, 1977, The C.V. Mosby Co.
Torre, C.T.: Nutritional needs of adolescents, Am. J. Maternal Child Nurs. **2**:118-127, March/April 1977.

Alterations in growth and/or maturation

Ballard, P.: Menstrual disorders in adolescence, Issues Compr. Pediatr. Nurs. **2**(6):21-33, 1978.
Chard, M.: An approach to examining the adolescent male, Am. J. Maternal Child Nurs. **1**:41-43, 1976.
Gault-Catarrinho, P.L.: Testicular cancer, Crit. Care Update **10**(2):32-35, 1983.
Gever, L.N.: From arthritis pain to dysmenorrhea: a new indication for prostaglandin inhibitors, Nursing **10**(4):81, 1980.
Lauver, D.: Irregular bleeding in women: causes and nursing intervention, Am. J. Nurs. **83**:396-401, 1983.
Meyer, M.R.: Adolescent gynecology: problems and ponderings, Pediatr. Nurs. **4**(4):43-47, 1978.
Petres, R.E., Coogan, E.M., and Mendez-Picon, J.: Practical approach to adolescent gynecologic office problems, Pediatr. Nurs. **3**(6):7-9, 1977.
Wells, G.M.: Reducing the threat of a first pelvic exam, Am. J. Maternal Child Nurs. **2**:304-306, 1977.

Adolescent pregnancy

Abbott, M.I.: Parenting group for teen-agers fails, Pediatr. Nurs. **6**(5):54-65, 1980.
Abbott, M.I: Teens having babies, Pediatr. Nurs. **4**(3):23-26, 1978.
Abrams, B.: Helping pregnant teenagers eat right, Nursing 81 **11**(3):46-47, 1981.
Admire, G., and Byers, L.: Counseling the pregnant teenager, Nursing 81 **11**(4):62-63, 1981.

Brown, C.A.: Teen-age mother's well-child clinic, Pediatr. Nurs. **4**(3):27-31, 1978.

Brown, J.T., and Clancy, B.J.: Meeting the needs of teens regarding their sexuality, Issues Compr. Pediatr. Nurs. **1**:29-44, 1976.

Burke, P.J.: A community health model for pregnant teens, Am. J. Maternal Child Nurs. **8**:340-344, 1983.

Clarke, B.A.: Improving adolescent parenting through participant modeling and self-evaluation, Nurs. Clin. North Am. **18**:303-311, 1983.

Daniels, M.B., and Manning, D.: A clinic for pregnant teens, Am. J. Nurs. **83**:68-71, 1983.

Dibble, J.C.: ABC for teens: parent education after the baby comes, Pediatr. Nurs. **7**(4):21-23, 1981.

Dickerson, P.S., and Ouellette, M.D.: Prenatal education for adolescents in a delinquent youth facility. J. Obstet. Gynecol. Neonatal Nurs. **11**:39-44, 1982.

Donlen, J., and Lynch, P.L.: Teenage mother: high-risk baby, Nursing 81 **11**(5):51-56, 1981.

Frye, B.A., and Barham, B.: Reaching out to pregnant adolescents, Am. J. Nurs. **75**:1502-1504, 1975.

Harvey, K.: Caring perceptively for the relinquishing mother, Am. J. Maternal Child Nurs. **2**:24-28, 1977.

Kendell, N.: The unwed adolescent pregnancy: an accident? Am. J. Nurs. **79**:2112-2114, 1979.

Mercer, R.: Becoming a mother at sixteen, Am. J. Maternal Child Nurs. **1**:44-52, Jan./Feb. 1976.

Poole, C.J.: Adolescent mothers: can they be helped? Pediatr. Nurs. **2**:7-11, March/April 1976.

Poole, C.J., and Hoffmann, M.: Mothers of adolescent mothers: how do they cope? Pediatr. Nurs. **7**(1):28-31, 1981.

Sewall, K.S.: Peer-group reality therapy for the pregnant adolescent, Am. J. Maternal Child Nurs. **8**:67-69, 1983.

Smith, P.B., Mumfort, D.M., and Hamner, L.E.: Child-rearing attitudes of single teenage mothers, Am. J. Nurs. **79**:2115-2116, 1979.

Tauer, K.M.: Promoting effective decision-making in sexually active adolescents, Nurs. Clin. North Am. **18**:275-292, 1983.

Contraception

Babington, M.A.: Adolescent use of oral contraceptives, Pediatr. Nurs. **10**:111-114, 1984.

Cowart, M., and Newton, D.W.: Oral contraceptives: how best to explain their effects to patients, Nursing 76 **6**:44-45, 1976.

Gara, E.: Nursing protocol to improve the effectiveness of the contraceptive diaphragm, Am. J. Maternal Child Nurs. **6**:41-45, 1981.

Huxall, L.K.: Update on IUDs, Am. J. Maternal Child Nurs. **5**:186-190, 1980.

Peach, E.H.: Counseling sexually active very young adolescents, Am. J. Maternal Child Nurs. **5**:191-195, 1980.

Taylor, D.: A new way to teach teens about contraceptives, Am. J.Nurs. **1**:378-383, 1976.

Sexually transmitted diseases

Bettoli, E.J.: Herpes: facts and fallacies, Am. J. Nurs. **82**:924-929, 1982.

Brown, M.S.: Syphilis and gonorrhea: an update for nurses in ambulatory settings, Nursing 76 **6**:71-74, 1976.

Campbell, C.E., and Herten, R.J.: VD to STD: redefining venereal disease, Am. J. Nurs. **81**:1629, 1981.

Hamm, P., and Jemison-Smith, P.: Chlamydia, Crit. Care Update **8**(3):34-36, 1981.

Hamm, P., and Jemison-Smith, P.: Herpesvirus hominus, Crit. Care Update **8**(8):34-37, 1981.

Larson, E.: Intransigent genital infection? Suspect chlamydiae, RN **46**(1):42-43, 1984.

Perley, N.Z., and Bills, B.J.: Herpes genitalis and the childbearing cycle, Am. J. Maternal Child Nurs. **8**:213-217, 1983.

Sexual trauma

Burgess, A.W., and Holmstrom, L.L.: Sexual trauma of children and adolescents: pressure, sex, and secrecy, Nurs. Clin. North Am. **10**:551-564, 1975.

Burgess, A.W., Holmstrom, L.L., and McCausland, M.P.: Counseling the child rape victim, Issues Compr. Pediatr. Nurs. **1**:45-57, 1976.

Cline, F.: Dealing with sexual abuse of children, Nurs. Pract., pp. 52-54, May/June 1980.

Geiser, R.L., and Norberta, M.: Sexual disturbance in young children, Am. J. Maternal Child Nurs. **1**:186-194, 1976.

Gorline, L.L.: The nurse and the sexually assaulted child. In Chinn, P.L., and Leonard, K.B., editors: Current practice in pediatric nursing, vol. III, St. Louis, 1980, The C.V. Mosby Co.

Hall, N.M.: Group treatment for sexually abused children, Nurs. Clin. North Am. **13**:701-705, 1978.

Laughlin, J.A., and Meacham, M.C.: Rape: victim counseling. In Kniesl, C.R., and Wilson, H.S., editors: Current perspectives in psychiatric nursing, vol. 1, St. Louis, 1976, The C.V. Mosby Co.

Leaman, K.: The sexually abused child, Nursing 77 **7**(5):68, 1977.

Sgroi, S.M.: Sexual molestation of children, Child. Today **4**:18, 1975.

Sisney, K.F.: Breaking the link: nursing intervention in the incestuous family, Issues Comp. Pediatr. Nurs. **4**(4):51-59, 1980.

Infectious mononucleosis

Belkengren, R.P., Sheldon, S.H., and Sapala, S.: Infectious mononucleosis, Pediatr. Nurs. **4**(6):16-19, 1978.

Obesity

Carman, D.D.: Infant and childhood obesity: guidelines for prevention and treatment, Pediatr. Nurs. **2**(6):33-38, 1976.

Cecere, M.C.: PIP (Positive image program): a group approach for obese adolescents, Nurs. Clin. North Am. **18**:249-256, 1983.

Hagenbuch, V.E.G.: Obesity and the school-age child, Nurs. Clin. North Am. **17**:207-216, 1982.

Jonides, L.: Childhood obesity: a treatment approach for private practices, Pediatr. Nurs. **8**:320-322, 1982.

Kaufmann, N.A., and others: Eating habits and opinions of teenagers on nutrition and obesity, J. Am. Diet. Assoc. **66**:264-268, March 1975.

Lasky, P.A.: Implications, considerations, and nursing interventions of obesity in neonatal and preschool patients, Nurs. Clin. North Am. **17**:199-205, 1982.

Mowery, B.D.: Family oriented approach to childhood obesity, Pediatr. Nurs. **6**(2):40-44, 1980.

Peckos, P.: The treatment of adolescent obesity, Issues Compr. Pediatr. Nurs. **1**:17-30, 1976.

Pipes, P.L.: Nutrition in infancy and childhood, ed. 2, St. Louis, 1981, The C.V. Mosby Co.

Rowe, N.R.: Childhood obesity: growth charts vs. calipers, Pediatr. Nurs. **6**(2):24-27, 1980.

White, J.H.: An overview of obesity: its significance to nursing, Nurs. Clin. North Am. **17**:191-198, 1982.

Winick, M.: Childhood obesity, Nutr. Today **9**(3):6-12, 1974.

Other eating disorders

Bhanji, S.: Anorexia nervosa: two schools of thought, Nurs. Times **76**(1):324-325, 1980.

Carino, C.M.: Disorders of eating in adolescence: anorexia nervosa and bulimia, Nurs. Clin. North Am. **18**:343-352, 1983.

Ciseaux, A.: Anorexia nervosa: a view from the mirror, Am. J. Nurs. **80**:1468-1472, 1980.

Claggett, M.S.: Anorexia nervosa: a behavioral approach, Am. J. Nurs. **80**:1471-1472, 1980.

Dexter, J.M.: Anorexia nervosa, Nurs. Times, **76**(1):325-327, 1980.

Marks, R.G.: Anorexia and bulimia: eating habits that can kill, RN **46**(1):44-47, 1984.

McNab, W.L.: Anorexia and the adolescent, J. School Health **53**:427-430, 1983.

Melton, J.H.: A boy with anorexia nervosa, Am. J. Nurs. **74**:1649-1651, 1974.

Misik, I.M.: When the anorectic patient challenges you, Nursing 81 **11**(12):46-49, 1981.

Potts, N.L.: Eating disorders. The secret pattern of binge/purge, Am. J. Nurs. **84**:32-35, 1984.

Richardson, T.F.: Anorexia nervosa: an overview, Am. J. Nurs. **80**:1470-1471, 1980.

Sanger, E., and Cassino, T.: Eating disorders: avoiding the power struggle, Am. J. Nurs. **84**:31-33, 1984.

Schmidt, M.P.W., and Duncan, B.A.B.: Modifying eating behavior in anorexia nervosa, Am. J. Nurs. **74**:1646-1648, 1974.

Behavior disorders in school-age children

Fond, K., and Brosnan, J.: School phobia: the school anxiety symptom, Pediatr. Nurs. **6**(5):9-13, 1980.

Nelms, B.C., and Brady, M.A.: Assessment and intervention: the depressed school-age child, Pediatr. Nurs. **6**(4):15-19, 1980.

Attention deficit disorder

Bassett, L.B., Gudas, L.J., and McAnulty, E.H.: The learning disabled child: recognition, evaluation, and management, Pediatr. Nurs. **8**(5):323-330, 1982.

Bowers, J.E.: Can you recognize childhood learning disorders? Nursing 77 **7**(11):26-29, 1977.

Brown, R.T., and Wynne, M.E.: Sustained attention in boys with attention deficit disorder and the effect of methylphenidate, Pediatr. Nurs. **10**:35-39, 1984.

Cantwell, D.P.: Recognition, evaluation, and management of the hyperactive child, Pediatr. Nurs. **5**(5):11-22, 1979.

Feingold, B.F.: Hyperkinesis and learning disabilities linked to artificial food flavors and colors, Am. J. Nurs. **75**:797-803, 1975.

Holmberg, N.J.: Serving the child with MBD and his family in a health maintenance organization, Nurs. Clin. North Am. **10**:381-392, June 1975.

Huber, C.J., and Dalldorf, J.S.: Minimal brain dysfunction syndrome, Nurs. Clin. North Am. **15**:551-569, 1980.

Robinson, L.A.: Food allergies, food additives, and Feingold diet, Pediatr. Nurs. **6**(6):38-39, 1980.

Rogers, M.: Early identification and intervention of children with learning problems, Pediatr. Nurs. **2**:21-26, Jan./Feb. 1976.

White, J.E.: Special nursing needs of hospitalized children with learning disabilities, Am. J. Maternal Child Nurs. **8**:209-212, 1983.

Woodward, P.B., and Brodie, B.: The hyperactive child: who is he? Nurs. Clin. North Am. **9**:727-746, 1974.

Enuresis and encopresis

Christophersen, E.R., and Berman, R.: Encopresis treatment, Issues Compr. Pediatr. Nurs. **3**(4):51-66, 1978.

Christophersen, E.R., and Rapoff, M.A.: Enuresis treatment, Issues Compr. Pediatr. Nurs. **2**(6):35-52, 1978.

Ruble, J.: Childhood nocturnal enuresis, Am. J. Maternal Child Nurs. **6**(1):26-31, 1981.

Younger, J.B., and Hughes, L.S.: No-fault management of encopresis, Pediatr. Nurs. **9**:185-187, 1983.

Substance abuse

Blades, S: Clinical notes on adolescent drug abuse, Issues Compr. Pediatr. Nurs. **1**:59-64, 1976.

Burton, J.: Intoxication by centrally acting substances. Part I, Crit. Care Update **10**(9):34-35, 45, 1983.

Notaro, C.: Adolescents and alcohol, Issues Compr. Pediatr. Nurs. **1**:50-58, 1976.

Palmer-Erbs, V.K., and DeForge, V.M.: Interventions with the adolescent drug user and the family, Issues Compr. Pediatr. Nurs. **3**(5):15-24, 1979.

Rehrig, M.: Cocaine look-alikes, Crit. Care Update **10**(2):47-49, 1983.

Rice, M.A., and Kibbee, P.E.: Review: identifying the adolescent substance abuser, Am. J. Maternal Child Nurs. **8**:139-142, 1983.

Tennant, F.S., and La Cour, J.: Children at high risk for addiction and alcoholism: identification and intervention, Pediatr. Nurs. **6**(1):26-27, 1980.

Thompson, W.L.: Drug overdose victims, Crit. Care Update **6**(6):24-28, 1979.

Woolf, D.S., Vourakis, C., and Bennett, G.: Guidelines for management of acute phencyclidine intoxication, Crit. Care Update **7**(6):17-24, 1980.

Yankelovich, D.: Drug users vs. drug abusers: how students control their drug crisis, Psychol. Today **9**:39-42, Oct. 1975.

Suicide

Blomquist, K.B.: Nurse, I need help: the school nurse's role in suicide prevention, J. Psychiatr. Nurs. Ment. Health Serv. **12**:22-26, 1974.

Carmack, B.J.: Suspect a suicide? Don't be afraid to act, RN **46**(4):43-45, 90, 1983.

Hafen, B.Q.:, and Peterson, B: Preventing adolescent suicide, Nursing 83 **13**(9):47-48, 1983.

Hart, N.A., and Keidel, G.C.: The suicidal adolescent, Am. J. Nurs. **79**:80-84, 1979.

Hart, N.A.C., and Prophit, P., Sr.: Adolescent suicide, Pediatr. Nurs. **5**(6):22-28, 1979.

Hoff, L.A., and Resing, M.: Was this suicide preventable? Am. J. Nurs. **82**:1107-1111, 1982.

Keidel, G.C.: Adolescent suicide, Nurs. Clin. North Am. **18**:323-332, 1983.

Marthas-Sampson, M.: Adolescents who commit suicidal acts: suicidogenic factors, Issues Compr. Pediatr. Nurs. pp. 49-64, 1976.

Nursing Grand Rounds: Nursing care of a suicidal adolescent, Nursing 80 **8**(4):56-59, 1980.

Reubin, R.: Spotting and stopping the suicide patient, Nursing 79 **9**(4):83-85, 1979.

Valente, S.: Suicide in school aged children: theory and assessment, Pediatr. Nurs. **9**:25-29, 1983.

Westercamp, T.M.: Suicide, Am. J. Nurs. **75**:260-262, 1975.

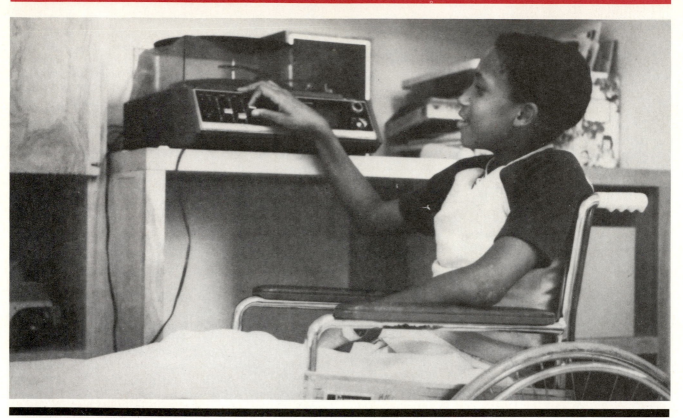

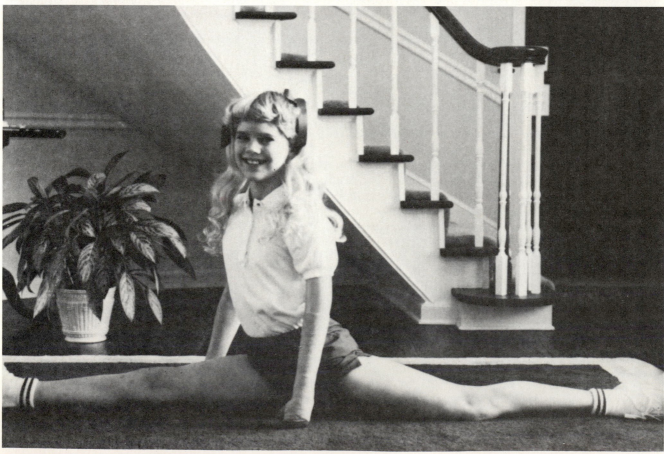

UNIT 7

THE CHILD WITH LONG-TERM PHYSICAL OR DEVELOPMENTAL PROBLEMS

Units 3 through 6 have focused on the growth and development of the well child. Most of the health problems discussed for each age-group have been ones that temporarily incapacitate a child. Unit 7 is concerned with the child who has a permanent or chronic physical and/or developmental problem. Such children need to master the same developmental tasks that well children master in accordance with their potential abilities and despite the handicapping or disabling conditions. Families of these children, likewise, are faced with exceptional challenges for which there is little guidance or few role models to emulate. As a result the entire family is highly vulnerable to psychologic and sometimes physical problems that arise from unsuccessful attempts to deal with the primary condition.

Chapter 16, *The Child Who is Handicapped, Chronically Ill, or Potentially Terminally Ill,* is an overview of the reactions of the child and family to such conditions and nursing interventions that assist each family member in adjusting and developing to his fullest despite the disability. This chapter serves as a basis for understanding the stresses and needs of the family when a child is chronically or terminally ill, physically disabled, or mentally retarded or when he has a sensory impairment. Chapter 17, *The Child with Mental or Sensory Dysfunction,* is primarily concerned with the retarded, deaf, or blind child; it discusses the classification of mental retardation, causes of each disability, and the nursing interventions required to help the child become independent. Emphasis is placed on the effect of the impairment on development, detection of the disorder, and nursing interventions that promote rehabilitation.

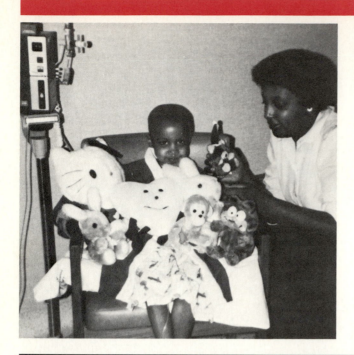

16

THE CHILD WHO IS HANDICAPPED, CHRONICALLY ILL, OR POTENTIALLY TERMINALLY ILL

OBJECTIVES

On completion of this chapter the reader will be able to:

■ Identify the scope of and changing trends in care for chronically or terminally ill and handicapped children

■ Define the stages of adjustment to the diagnosis of an exceptional problem

■ Recognize the impact of the illness or disability on the developmental stages of childhood

■ Identify the major reactions of and effects on the family with a child with an exceptional problem

■ Outline nursing interventions that promote the family's optimal adjustment to the child's chronic disorder

■ Define the stages of grief for the anticipated loss of a child

■ Outline nursing interventions that support the family during each stage of dying

NURSING DIAGNOSES

Nursing diagnoses identified for the child who is handicapped, chronically ill, or potentially terminally ill include, but are not restricted to, the following:

Health perception-health management pattern

■ Noncompliance related to knowledge deficit

Nutritional-metabolic pattern

■ Nutrition, alterations in: potential for more or less than body requirements related to (1) loss of appetite; (2) physical handicap; (3) excessive intake versus energy output

Activity-exercise pattern

■ Diversional activity deficit related to (1) lack of motivation; (2) depression; (3) lack of knowledge

■ Home maintenance management, impaired, related to knowledge deficit

■ Mobility, impaired physical, related to handicap

■ Self-care deficit (specify level: feeding, bathing/hygiene, dressing/grooming, toileting) related to (1) developmental level; (2) illness or handicap

This chapter focuses on the child who has one or more of the following conditions:

1. *Handicap*—permanent loss of a physical or sensory ability or a developmental disability, such as mental retardation, behavioral disorder, or learning disability
2. *Chronic illness*—any illness with an extended course; it can either be progressive and fatal or nonprogressive and associated with a relatively normal life span
3. *Terminal illness*—any illness, of long or short duration, with a life-threatening outcome

Throughout the chapter these three conditions are collectively referred to as *exceptional problems*.

Such conditions may occur at birth, or they may be acquired at any time during childhood. Because nurses are involved in every type of health deviation, it is inevitable that they will be responsible for some part of the care of children with these conditions. One must be familiar with family members' reactions to the loss of a "perfect" child and with the process of adjusting to a disability.

Self-perception—self-concept pattern

■ Anxiety, related to (1) loss of function; (2) death of child

■ Powerlessness, related to lack of knowledge

■ Self-concept, disturbance in, related to loss of function

Role-relationship pattern

■ Family process, alterations in, related to (1) illness or handicap; (2) death of child

■ Grieving, anticipatory, related to death of child

■ Parenting, alterations in: potential, related to (1) knowledge deficit; (2) lack of role models; (3) complexity of diagnosis

Coping-stress tolerance pattern

■ Coping, family: potential for growth, related to successful parenting of handicapped or ill child

Value-belief pattern

■ Spiritual distress, related to (1) guilt; (2) anger; (3) grief

SCOPE OF THE PROBLEM

Statistics regarding exceptional problems are formidable. It is estimated that as many as 10% to 15% of all children under 18 years of age have some type of chronic illness, including sensory impairments. The most frequent chronic childhood conditions are diseases of the respiratory system, chiefly asthma and bronchitis, neurologic diseases, and a variety of musculoskeletal disorders. Broadly expanding the definition of chronic conditions to include speech, learning, and behavioral disorders yields an estimated 30% to 40% of children who are suffering from a significant long-term disorder.

In addition to this group, 3% of the population has some form of mental retardation, and a larger percentage has sensory problems. Each year approximately 200,000 infants are born who survive with significant birth defects, thus increasing the population of children with long-term problems.

Terminal illness also significantly adds to the number of children with exceptional problems. Cancer is the leading cause of death from disease in children ages 3 through 14 years. It claims the lives of approximately 2500 children each year. However, because of advances in the treatment of several types of cancer, many children survive for long periods and experience problems commonly associated with chronic illness.

CHANGING TRENDS IN CARE

Several changes have occurred in the provision of services to children with handicaps. One is the focus on the child's *developmental* age, rather than his chronologic age. Using the developmental approach emphasizes the child's abilities and strengths rather than his disability.

Another principle that is increasingly employed is that of *normalization*, which refers to the establishment of a normal pattern of living. For example, traditionally the mentally retarded person performed all his activities in one room—unlike normal individuals, who conduct activities in various places. However, as a result of the principle of normalization, the environment for the retarded child is being "normalized" and "humanized."

Paralleling normalization has been a trend toward *mainstreaming*, or integrating children with exceptional problems into regular classrooms. These children then have the advantages of learning and socializing with a wide group of peers. In addition, there has been an increased focus on individualization, as the academic needs of these children are planned along with those of the regular students. A variety of supplemental programs has been designed in school systems to accommodate their special needs, thus providing them with an equal educational opportunity. This change has largely been a result of the passage of Public Law 94-142, the Education for All Handicapped Children Act of 1975.

FAMILIES OF CHILDREN WITH EXCEPTIONAL PROBLEMS

Families of children with exceptional problems are faced with the crisis of losing a perfect child and the task of adjusting to and accepting the child and his handicap or disorder. Many of the responses of parents to the birth of a child with a congenital anomaly are similar to those observed when the diagnosis of an exceptional problem is made later in a child's life. Nurses who understand the responses to the diagnosis and the usual effects the diagnosis has upon each family member are able to emotionally support the family, anticipate and prevent potential problems, and foster growth despite the handicap or disorder.

Response to diagnosis

When a diagnosis of an exceptional problem is made, the family progresses through a fairly predictable sequence of stages, regardless of the nature of the condition. These include (1) shock, (2) adjustment, (3) reintegration and acceptance, and in some instances (4) freezing out (Fig. 16-1). Not all families experience the last two stages, and family members vary widely in the time they need to progress through this process.

Shock. The initial stage is a period of shock and intense emotion. It may be accompanied by denial, especially if the condition is not obvious, as in a chronic illness. If the defect is highly obvious and overwhelming, such as the loss of eyesight or a limb, this period may be characterized by disintegration, because the emotional demands for dealing with the diagnosis leave no reserve for dealing with realistic problems.

Denial as a defense mechanism is a necessary cushion to prevent disintegration. Probably all parents experience various degrees of adaptive denial as they learn of the impact that the diagnosis has on their lives. Denial becomes maladaptive when it prevents recognition of treatment or rehabilitative goals necessary for the child's optimum survival. For example, denial of diabetes mellitus that results in failure to administer insulin has life-threatening consequences. However, such a failure is not infrequently seen in diabetic children, who may forget to give themselves the drug or eat excessive quantities of carbohydrates. Other common examples of parental denial are discussed on p. 460.

The response of a family to mental retardation may differ from the responses discussed in the preceding paragraphs, because as long as the family can maintain a fiction of normality and handle the deviance within the present familial roles and values, there may exist no recognition of the diagnosis. Instead the problem may be explained as slow maturation or as an easily remedied disorder. The denial may be enforced by the child's social development, which belies the degree of motor and speech

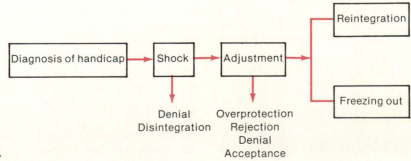

FIG. 16-1
Reactions to diagnosis.

retardation. Not infrequently this ability to rationalize delayed development is successful until the child enters school, when he is compared to other children and his differences become blatantly evident. At this point the family may begin to recognize the diagnosis as a crisis and react with shock and disbelief.

Adjustment. Adjustment follows shock and is usually characterized by an open admission that the condition exists. This stage is one of "chronic sorrow" and only partial acceptance. This period is manifest by several responses, probably the most universal of which are *guilt* and *self-accusation.* Guilt is often greatest when the cause of the condition is directly traceable to the parent, as in genetic diseases or accidental injuries. However, it occurs even without any scientific or realistic basis for parental responsibility. Frequently the guilt stems from a false assumption that the problem is a result of personal failing or wrongdoing. The ability to master resentful and self-accusatory feelings of having "caused" the child's disorder is a crucial factor in the parents' acceptance of their handicapped child.

Other common reactions are *bitterness* or *anger* because the child is an obstacle interfering with parental goals, and *envy* toward those who are not burdened with a handicapped child. Because the real reason for such feelings is usually unacceptable to parents, the emotions may be directed toward others, such as health professionals, for not "curing" their child.

A number of other reactions are typical, especially in parents who have a retarded child. These include:

1. *Loss of self esteem,* in which parents perceive a defect in their child as a defect in themselves; their life goals may be abruptly and dramatically altered, and they lose the fantasy of immortality through their child
2. *Shame,* in which parents anticipate social rejection, pity, or ridicule and related loss of social prestige and may experience social withdrawal
3. *Ambivalence,* in which the simultaneous experience of love and hatred normally experienced by parents toward their children is likely to be greatly intensified
4. *Depression,* in which parents experience chronic feelings of sorrow as a reaction to having an affected child
5. *Self-sacrifice,* in which parents adopt a "martyr" attitude and focus their total interest on the child, often to the detriment of other family members
6. *Defensiveness,* in which parents become acutely sensitive to implied criticism of their child and may react with resentment and belligerence, or they may deny the existence of the problem and seek professional opinions to substantiate their own belief that "there is really nothing wrong with him"

During the period of adjustment, there are four types of parental reactions to the child:

1. *Overprotection,* in which the parents fear letting the child achieve any new skill, avoid all discipline, and cater to every desire to prevent frustration
2. *Rejection,* in which the parents detach themselves emotionally from the child but usually provide adequate physical care or constantly nag and scold the child
3. *Denial,* in which parents act as if the handicap does not exist or attempt to have the child overcompensate for it
4. *Gradual acceptance,* in which parents place necessary and realistic restrictions on the child, encourage self-care activities, and promote reasonable physical and social abilities

The most common initial response, especially among mothers, is *benevolent overreaction*. It is usually a consequence of unresolved guilt or fear, such as ambivalent feelings about wanting the child during pregnancy, feeling responsible for the disorder, believing that the child would die at the time of birth or diagnosis, or reactivated feelings about a previous death of a loved one. Benevolent overreaction results in a vicious cycle of overprotective, permissive parent and dependent, demanding child (Fig. 16-2). It prevents the child from developing self-control, independence, initiative, and self-esteem. Fortunately it is a reaction that responds to early intervention and prevention.

Reintegration and acceptance. This stage is characterized by realistic expectations for the child and reintegration of family life, with the child's condition in proper perspective. Since a large portion of the adjustment phase is one of grief for a loss, total resolution is not possible until the child dies. Therefore, one can regard adjustment to chronic sorrow as "increased comfortableness" with everyday living.

This stage is also one of social reintegration, in which the family broadens its activities to include relationships outside of the home, with the child being an acceptable and participating member of the group. This last criterion often differentiates the reaction of gradual acceptance during the adjustment period from total acceptance.

One of the most important aspects of acceptance for health professionals to understand is that it is not an "all-or-none" phenomenon. Rather, it is interspersed with periods of intensified sorrow for the loss. Grieving is most likely seen at each period of the child's development, such as entry into school and onset of puberty. Consequently even families who have achieved a high level of adjustment and acceptance are at predictable times in need of professional support.

Freezing-out phase. If strategies of coping cannot be employed to minimize the stress and disorganization of maintaining the child within the home and to hold them to tolerable levels, the child may be placed outside the home in some type of residential setting, usually an institution. The evolvement of this phase is directly related to the degree of physical and mental handicap.

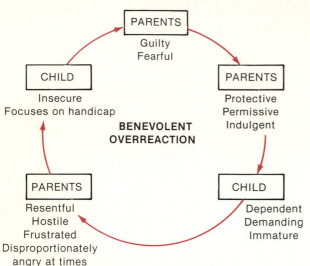

FIG. 16-2
*Common cyclical response between parents and handicapped child. (Redrawn from Boone, D.R., and Hartman, B.H.: The benevolent over-reaction, Clin. Pediatr. **11**(5):268-271, May 1972.)*

This phase is not necessarily one of maladjustment. Placement may be the only strategy that will preserve the integrity of the family. Aging parents may be forced to accept this alternative as a result of progressive inability to meet the demands of a severely retarded or multihandicapped offspring. Relinquishing the role of primary caregiver is followed by an initial sense of loss, relief, guilt, and ambivalence. The pattern of reactions is not unlike that seen in bereavement following the death of a terminally ill child (see p. 462).

Impact of chronic illness or disability on the child: developmental aspects

The impact of a chronic illness or disability is influenced by the age of onset. Chronic illness affects children of all ages, but the developmental aspects of each age group dictate particular stresses and risks for the child. An understanding of these factors facilitates planning care to support the child and minimize the risks.

Infancy. During infancy the child is engaged in the task of developing trust, which necessitates a reciprocal satisfying relationship between child and parent. When illness or disability strike, this relationship is potentially affected. For example, a visible defect can retard parent-child bonding as the parent mourns the loss of the perfect child. In addition, prolonged illness may impose separations that prevent the child and parent from attaching and deprives the infant from the nurturing relationship.

The illness itself affects the infant, especially since sensorimotor experiences are critical at this age. Illness and/or disability often impair the child's motor abilities, confining him to a crib and lessening his contact with the environment. Certainly the messages transmitted to the infant about his body are influenced by the amount of pain and discomfort he experiences. This lack of pleasurable sensations can lead to an irritable and unhappy child. Consequently, parents may interpret the behaviors as evidence that they are inadequate in meeting his physical and emotional needs, which further affects the parent-child relationship and the acquisition of trust.

To compensate for some of these feelings, parents, especially the mother, may become overly involved with the infant and promote increased dependency. This is significant during infancy when one of the tasks is separation and individuation from the parent. Such a response hinders the child's future development of self and often leads to the pattern of marked dependency, fearfulness, and passivity. One of the critical aspects of this pattern is that it is amenable to change if intervention is begun *early*.

Toddler. The toddler is in the stage of autonomy; the need for mastery of locomotor and language skills is paramount. As the child learns to walk and talk he progresses toward becoming a separate person, both physically and psychologically. However, illness or disability can hinder mobility and deprive the child of mastery. In addition the parents' overprotection can magnify the problem by setting limits on the child's exploration and experimentation for fear of his hurting or exerting himself. Even the most basic self-help skills, such as feeding and dressing, may be performed for the child. Age-appropriate tasks such as toilet training may be delayed. With such limited opportunities for testing his ability the child soon fears to venture on his own and develops little confidence in his ability. Over time these feelings are incorporated into a sense of low self-esteem.

Illness can impose separations that are detrimental to the toddler. Like the infant, separation is the most anxiety-producing event for toddlers. A chronic illness or disability can necessitate repeated hospitalizations and painful procedures. If the need to preserve the parent-child relationship is not appreciated, the child may become depressed and eventually detach from the parent. Such a response to separation has been associated with long-term consequences, such as the inability to form other close relationships (see also Chapter 18). Children seem to have a tremendous capacity to withstand stress provided their attachment to the parent is preserved.

Preschooler.   The preschooler is in the stage of initiative; numerous tasks are achieved during this age that can be severely hampered by chronic illness and disability. Impairment can limit the preschooler's learning about his environment, especially in terms of social development. Rather than being encouraged to play with peers and participate in nursery school activities, the chronically ill preschooler may be confined to the home with socialization limited to the secure and tolerant family. He may be allowed immature behavior because age-appropriate standards and discipline are not enforced. Consequently, when paired with children his own age or placed in school, he is deficient in knowing how to act and can easily be criticized by peers who view him as a "baby." In fact, his illness or disability may provoke much less criticism than his inappropriate behavior. Faced with such reactions from others in contrast to the security of the home the child may gradually choose a life of social isolation and loneliness, especially during the school-age years.

One of the major tasks of this period is establishing sexual identity and one of the principle methods is through imitation of sex-related activities. However, the sick child may have fewer opportunities to engage in such activity and may view the parent predominantly in the care-giving role, since this may be the focus of their relationship.

In addition to sexual identity, the child's image of his body is forming. The child's knowledge of his body is limited to what he sees, feels, and uses. If the child is chronically ill, his awareness of his body is focused on causing him pain and anxiety. For example, the young child may lose control over certain bodily functions, such as newly acquired bowel and bladder function, and feel embarrassed and inferior. The disabled child may have difficulty forming a mental image of impaired body parts, such as paralyzed extremities. Their poorly developed sense of body integrity makes them especially fearful of intrusive or mutilating experiences, which can be frequent during prolonged illness.

One of the more critical influences of chronic illness or disability on the preschooler is the feeling of guilt that he "caused" the condition by a real or imagined misdeed. This is probably less of a factor if the child is born with the disorder than if it occurs during the preschool years.

Unlike the child with a temporary physical impairment who has additional opportunities for achieving mastery and thus overcoming feelings of guilt and inferiority, the chronically ill or disabled child experiences continual insults. Unless situations are structured for him to succeed, life can become a series of failures—of never being strong enough or good enough to compete with peers.

School-age child.   The child of school age is striving to achieve a sense of accomplishment while overcoming a sense of inferiority. Successful mastery of this task depends on the child's ability to cooperate and to compete with others. Consequently, physical impairments can greatly affect their ability to achieve and compete (Fig. 16-3). For example, physical handicaps may hinder participation in sports and repeated absences from school due to illness can place the child at an academic disadvantage. To repeat a grade can saddle the child with feelings of shame, inadequacy, and inferiority. However, the decision to remain in the same grade can also enhance feelings of success because the work requirements may be easier and new classmates provide a second chance for forming friendships.

During this age there is a transition from relationships with family members to strong identification with peers. Peers increasingly influence school-age children's view of themselves and their self-esteem. Anything that labels the child as "different" can affect his sense of belonging to the group. Many handicapped children cope with their "differentness" by retreating from socialization. As they draw farther from the group their sense of belonging diminishes and intense loneliness and isolation dominates. However, if they are helped to deal with their feelings of not being "normal and perfect" and to recognize their unique abilities, these children can cope very well. It is to be expected that all children are unable to master every task and they will feel some degree of inferiority. If this is stressed to children with physical impairment, the burden to achieve is lessened.

As school-age children identify more with the peer group and authority figures outside the home, there is a concurrent striving for independence from the family. However, the ill child may be forced into an extended period of dependency either from the disorder or parental overprotectiveness. Attempts to demonstrate independence may be manifest as resentment toward the parents, refusal to comply with treatment, or risk-taking behavior, such as cheating on the special diet. If parents can understand that these behaviors are representative of a normal phase of development, they may be more tolerant and able to find appropriate outlets for independence, such as increasing the child's responsibility for home care.

Adolescence.   The major task of the adolescent is to establish an identity of his own. Pubertal changes must

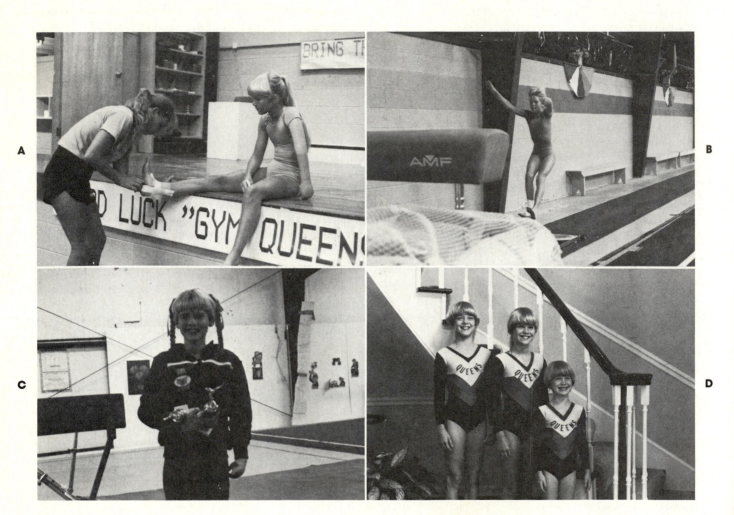

FIG. 16-3

Children with any type of handicap should have the opportunity to develop their skills in a wide range of intellectual, creative, and athletic pursuits. Frequently the handicap is only a ''minor inconvenience.'' Despite her prosthetic left arm, this youngster excels in competitive sports. However, children need **A,** *guidance in achieving a goal,* **B,** *an opportunity to demonstrate their skills,* **C,** *rewards for achieving, and* **D,** *a feeling of belonging.*

be integrated into the self-image while the teenager is gaining control and mastery over his increased physical capabilities and sexuality. During early adolescence this takes place primarily within the peer group. Illness or injury at this time interferes with the teenager's sense of mastery and control over his changing body. He is different at a stage of development when being different is unacceptable to the peer group, who may view a disability in one member as a threat to the established uniformity by which all are measured. At no time of life is an individual so vulnerable to the emotional stress of biologic impairment. Appearance, skills, and abilities are highly valued by peers; a teenager who is limited in any of these qualities is subject to rejection by this important group. This is especially marked when a physical disability interferes with sexual attractiveness.

Chronically ill teenagers are faced with the task of incorporating their disability into the changing self-concept. The youngster who develops the illness or acquires the disability during the crucial adolescent years has more difficulty accomplishing this task than does the teenager who has been affected since childhood. It appears that the earlier the onset of a limiting condition, the better the individual is able to adapt to it. The youngster with a newly acquired disorder will have the additional task of grieving for his lost "perfection" while adjusting to the changes taking place as a natural course of events. He often feels rejected because of his appearance or his inability to engage in activities expected of a healthy adolescent. The threat is greatest during middle adolescence when the teenager has less available energy to cope with illness, since his emotional resources are being used to meet the normal demands of this developmental phase.

The severity, type, and visibility of the illness also influence the adjustment process. Limitations are imposed by long-standing debilitating disorders, such as severe cardiac disease, inflammatory bowel disease, and uncontrolled epilepsy, which render the teenager unable to achieve in the same manner as age-mates. Dramatic alterations in body integrity that accompany acquired disfigurement, such as severe burns, the advent of a colostomy, or the dramatic and sudden dependency of paralysis from a spinal cord injury, can have devastating effects on the teenager's self-image and identity formation. However, there is often less distortion of reality in a highly visible disorder, even though there is a greater risk of devaluation by peers and others. Nonvisible conditions, such as diabetes or cardiac disease, create few problems of peer acceptance but pose limitations on activities or cause problems of compliance with therapeutic regimens because of the teenager's frequently distorted perception of the seriousness of the condition. Denial of the implications of an illness is a frequent response to a nonvisible defect.

Adolescence is also a time for achieving independence from the family and planning for future goals and responsibilities. Enforced dependency from physical impairment can exacerbate the parent-child conflicts surrounding independence. Lack of understanding from both parties can result in bitter feelings and intrafamilial turmoil. The tendency toward rebellion may be directed at the disorder with decreased compliance with treatment and risk-taking behavior that can place the teenager in jeopardy, such as driving a car despite a handicap that increases the chance of an accident. Fostering independence and autonomy is particularly important at this time. This can be accomplished by encouraging the teenager to assume responsibility for making and keeping appointments (ideally alone), by encouraging self-management of his disease, and by helping him make decisions regarding his life whenever possible. Planning for the future is a prominent concern, and future plans should be explored and modified to accommodate the handicap.

Reactions of and effects on family members

Each family that has a child with an exceptional problem is intimately involved. No member remains unaffected by the experience. The child's reactions and the siblings' reactions are usually direct consequences of the parents' responses.

Parents' responses at the time of birth. When a child is born with a congenital anomaly, parents must mourn the loss of the anticipated "perfect" child and accept a child who has an imperfection. To understand their reactions, it is helpful to review the parents' attachment to the unborn child.

Preparation for childbirth involves fantasies and images of the expected infant. Normally every parent wishes for a perfect child but, at the same time, fears that the infant will be abnormal. This fear is often expressed by parents who state that their concern is not whether the child is to be a girl or a boy, just that it is healthy. One of the first things parents want confirmed at the time of birth is, "Is our baby all right?"

In most instances there is some discrepancy between the parent's idealized child and the newborn—for example, the birth of a boy when a girl was hoped for. Resolution of this discrepancy is a developmental task of parenthood, and it is essential to the establishment of a healthy parent-child relationship. If the discrepancy is too great, as in the birth of an infant with a gross defect or when the wishes of the parent are unrealistic, the resulting emotional stress may be overwhelming.

The birth of a defective child abruptly ends the psychologic attachment the parents have formed for the child they idealized during pregnancy. They must now deal with loss of this wished-for, healthy child. Their fears have been realized, and they are faced with meeting the demands of this child for care and affection. The parents' grief for the loss of the expected child while adapting to the care of the handicapped child places overwhelming demands on them, especially for the mother whose own psychologic and physiologic resources have been depleted by the birth experience.

When parents are unable to face the reality of the infant's condition, they withdraw from the situation either physically or emotionally. Parents often extend this avoidance behavior to include the infant. They are unable to face the infant and do not visit the child in the nursery or the pediatric unit. Sometimes it takes time for the parents to master their own feelings before they are able to deal constructively with the situation. A more subtle form of isolation is seen in parents who are very objective in their behavior toward the infant and his defect. They are intellectually concerned with their infant's medical care, but they display no emotional involvement. Their attention is focused on the abnormality, not on the infant.

Parental reactions depend to a large extent on the type and severity of the defect. A gross, visible anomaly, especially one involving the face, elicits a more intense emotional response than one that is less apparent, such as a heart defect. The extent of the impairment cannot be used as a criterion to determine the degree of parental depressive reactions. Also, because of their limited contact with congenital defects, the parents' perception of the situation may be distorted; much depends on feelings they may have experienced with a similar abnormality. Therefore, their reactions may seem out of proportion to the actual extent and severity of the impairment as viewed by health professionals.

Parents' responses following birth or discovery of the diagnosis. Besides grieving for the loss of a perfect child, parents of a child with severe handicaps may be less likely than other parents to receive positive feedback from transactions with their child. Parenting such children may be a series of unrewarding experiences, which continually reinforce the parents' feelings of inadequacy and failure. These responses may be most evident in mothers who are responsible for the child's care. For example, they may become preoccupied with the ability to carry out certain procedures, overlooking the child's personal comfort and satisfaction or failing to praise him for anything less than perfect cooperation or performance. For these mothers it may be beneficial to reduce the quantity of time spent with the child, in order to increase the quality of the relationship.

Although a great deal of emphasis has been placed on the mother's reaction, little research has focused on the father's response. The available findings indicate that the main concerns of fathers of chronically ill children are for the child's future and the unpredictable nature of the illness (McKeever, 1981). Some also feel they are less competent than other parents. They have been found to lack gratifying relationships with their children and to experience significant stress even though they may have other, healthy children. Fathers, compared to mothers, generally have fewer opportunities to do something directly helpful for their children, such as taking them to the physician, the drugstore, the physical therapist, the special school, or other special health services. Organizations for parents may offer fewer services to fathers. As a result fathers have fewer opportunities available to mourn the loss of the perfect child and to deal with lowered self-esteem. Their need to adjust to the loss of a perfect male child may be particularly great, since the expectations of immortality through a son can no longer be realized.

Excessive demands may be placed on parents' time, energy, and financial resources. The wife often receives the brunt of the time and energy demands and the husband the financial responsibilities. However, with changing sex roles these responsibilities may be shared, or they may be shifted more heavily to one parent. For example, the working mother may feel the need to continue employment to help defray expenses, but she also incurs the burden of additional child and home responsibilities. The result can eventually be marital conflicts as one partner views his or her share as unequal. In addition, the partner who is not included in the care-giving activities may feel neglected, since all the attention is being directed toward the child. Without active participation in the care of the child, the parent has little appreciation of the time and energy involved in such activities. Whereas one parent feels neglected, the other feels resentful because of the increased responsibility and the other parent's noninvolvement.

Each partner may direct feelings of resentment, anger, and bitterness toward the other for having their life-style disrupted by the child's condition, while being unaware of the true reason for such feelings. For example, a mother who is forced to terminate a career in order to assume full-time child care responsibilities may express her feelings of resentment and bitterness as anger toward her husband for not sharing more in the household chores. Even if he participates more, she may continue to be angry with him because of her need to express the other unresolved feelings. He, in turn, may refuse to participate, since nothing he does can satisfy her. As a result communication breaks down and neither is able to support the other.

Reports differ concerning divorce rates among families with handicapped, chronically ill, or terminally ill children. While some studies report a divorce rate similar to that of the general population, they also stress the high level of marital discord between the partners. Feelings of low self-esteem and helplessness, as well as unmet dependency needs, are prevalent (Lansky and others, 1978). For those marriages that are dissolved, some of the contributing factors include avoidance of sex for fear of conceiving another affected child, financial stress, and disagreement regarding expectations from the affected offspring.

The child's responses.   The child's reaction to his condition depends to a great extent on the reactions of significant others to him and to his disability, the child's developmental level, his available coping mechanisms, and, to a lesser extent, on the condition itself. Four patterns of behavior that directly relate to parental responses to child-rearing are evident: (1) marked dependency, especially on the mother, fearfulness, inactivity, and lack of outside interests; (2) overactivity, defiance, and risk-taking behavior; (3) resentment and hostility, especially to normal individuals; and (4) dependence or independence appropriate for age and responsibility and achievement commensurate with limitation, pride, confidence, and self-esteem.

Because it is often easier to recognize the child who adjusts poorly to his condition, it is worthwhile to delineate the behaviors that characterize the well-adjusted child. The well-adjusted child slowly learns to accept his physical limitations and finds achievement in a variety of compensatory motor and intellectual pursuits. He functions well at home, at school, and with peers. He has an understanding of his disorder that allows him to accept his limitations, assume responsibility for care, and assist in treatment and rehabilitation regimens.

He expresses appropriate emotions, such as sadness, anxiety, and anger, at times of exacerbations but confidence and guarded optimism during periods of clinical stability. He is able to identify with other, similarly affected individuals, promoting positive self-images. The well-adjusted person displays pride and self-confidence in his ability to lead a productive, life despite the disability.

When a child experiences a serious disability, he proceeds through three predictable stages. The first stage, which occurs immediately, is *withdrawal,* in which the child becomes depressed and nonresponsive. The second is *preoccupation with self,* in which he focuses on his disability and loss of previous abilities. The third is a *gradual return to reality,* which is closely linked to the parents' ability to adjust to the problem.

The type of disability influences the emotional response. Because of the level of cognitive ability in children, and the fact that abstract thinking is not achieved until adolescence, it is likely that an obvious handicap is easier to accept than one that is not obvious, because its limitations are concrete. For example, the blind or crippled child is constantly reminded of his inability to run. However, the hemophiliac child not only must live by rules he does not understand, but also senses his illness only vaguely and occasionally—for example, when he runs and accidently initiates a bleeding episode.

The onset of a crippling condition generates a state of confusion for a young child, who may have trouble differentiating between his actual body functions and his image

of his body. He may also experience problems in distinguishing between himself and extensions of himself in the form of wheelchairs, braces, crutches, or other mechanical or prosthetic devices. In addition, he may have tremendous difficulty in accepting such functional aids.

Chronically ill children experience the emotional stress associated with long-term illness. Pain in young children is often perceived as punishment for some real or imagined transgression. Children may believe that they became ill because their parents failed to protect them. Diseases transmitted by hereditary factors may cause strain in the parent-child relationship once children discover the etiology of the disorder. During frequent and lengthy hospitalizations that result in separations from family, school, and friends, which can temporarily cut off needed sources of support, children may resent the need to be helped with bathing, feeding, or toileting. Painful procedures such as injections and surgery often reactivate fears of bodily mutilation and fantasies of punishment.

Repeated relapses in children with life-threatening disorders increase their anxiety regarding recovery and heighten their fear of death. Even very young children and children who have not been explicitly told their prognoses react to parental anxieties during relapses. Younger children tend to express their anxiety symbolically and physiologically, whereas older boys tend to act out their anxieties and older girls become depressed and withdrawn.

Although children with exceptional problems frequently learn to use aspects of their illness or disability to control members of the family, they also may feel responsible for much of the stress created by their condition, such as marital discord, financial problems, additional responsibilities for other family members, interruption of previous life-style, and interference with future goals. They may also feel insecure in terms of their true worth to the family. For example, it is not unusual for the child to wonder if the concern and attention focused on him result from his disorder. He may question his real worth as a person, especially if his disability has received more emphasis than his abilities.

Siblings' responses.   Siblings are deeply affected by the child's membership in the family. They often feel anger and resentment toward him and the parents for the loss of routine and parental attention. Although siblings are forced to cope with a disrupted family life, they are sometimes given no rewards and, often, inadequate explanations. It is difficult for older children and almost impossible for younger children to comprehend the plight of the affected child. Their perception is of a brother or sister who has the undivided attention of their parents, who is showered with special privileges and gifts, and who is the focus of everyone's concern.

Younger siblings in particular may be affected, because they are uprooted and displaced more than older children. For example, even though a retarded child may be the firstborn, he becomes the "youngest" by virtue of his developmental age. Conversely, the secondborn becomes the oldest, often assuming adultlike responsibilities and achieving parental expectations that would have been reserved for the eldest. Therefore, it is not uncommon for siblings to express the same feelings of depression, envy, bitterness, and so on that were described earlier for parents.

Siblings are likely to show symptoms of irritability, social withdrawal, and fear for their own health. In fact, healthy siblings may have a wide variety of physical complaints, such as headache, abdominal pain, or symptoms mimicking those of the sick or handicapped child, as a reflection of their anxiety and fear.

Siblings' reactions to a child with exceptional problems often do not parallel the severity of the condition. For example, siblings of children with obvious but less serious physical problems may have greater adjustment difficulties than siblings of children with less visible but more life-threatening illnesses.

For siblings of a child who has a potentially fatal disease that is inherited, such as muscular dystrophy or cystic fibrosis, there is the fear of being affected by the illness. As they observe their brother or sister's condition deteriorate, they are faced with the emotional task of coping with feelings about their own welfare and about that of the brother or sister.

Most parents can identify specific behaviors in the well children that have a negative effect on the family, such as jealousy, increased competition and fighting among siblings, anger, hostility, social withdrawal, attention-seeking behavior, and a decline in school performance. However, positive behaviors are also cited, such as increased nurturing, cooperation, sensitivity, compassion, and mastery of new skills. A common pattern among the siblings is periods of good adjustment alternating with times of poorer adjustment.

Siblings reveal feelings of isolation, deprivation, inferiority, and inadequate knowledge about the child's condition. Their lives are most affected in terms of the parent-child relationship, the medical care and treatment, and play and socialization. For example, the greatest effect of the ill child on the well siblings is a feeling of isolation and of being outside the parents/sick child dyad. This is often increased by social restriction in peer relationships because of additional responsibilities in the home. Siblings feel left out and uninvolved in the child's care, especially when the child is cared for away from home. In particular they report feeling ignored by health care members. One study found that only one sibling out of 25 had received information directly from a health care professional (Taylor, 1980).

Such findings emphasize that although positive, maturing attitudes can form in siblings of handicapped children, the responsibility of health professionals is to involve the entire family unit in the adjustment process.

Responses of extended family and society. Although extended family relationships and relationships with friends are often helpful to parents in rearing a child with an exceptional problem, they may also be sources of stress. Grandparents may have far more difficulty in accepting the diagnosis than do the parents themselves, and parents may have concerns about the best way in which to respond to the grandparents' anger over the diagnosis or criticism regarding parental care. For example, grandparents or other well-meaning relatives may attempt to reassure the parents that the child "will grow out of" his slowness at a time when the parents are struggling to accept reality.

Although society's views are changing toward a more accepting, nonjudgmental, and open attitude, parents, siblings, and the child himself frequently are victims of prejudice, ostracism, or criticism. A great deal of this stems from public ignorance and fear, which constitute a crucial area for intervention by health professionals.

NURSING CONSIDERATIONS

The major goal of the nurse is to help the family remain intact and functioning at maximum levels throughout the child's life. This involves more than supporting the child and his parents during the critical period of the newborn phase, when the infant's condition is being diagnosed, or when the parents encounter problems in the child of preschool or school age. It also involves facilitating better communication and alleviating feelings of inadequacy in the parents and inferiority in the child. This approach invites the parents' early input and encourages them to be more accountable and responsible for the child's care. It reinforces the fact that it is not so much the disorder itself that affects the child's progress and developmental outcomes as the family's ability to cope successfully with the child's problems. Thus long-term, comprehensive, systematic, family-centered approaches must be applied to meet these goals.

Assess the family's strengths

Since the nurse may meet a family during any phase of the rehabilitation process, it is essential that the family members' individual strengths and reactions to the child be assessed. The following are some of the important areas to assess in determining the family's strengths and possible weaknesses or risks:

1. Available support systems, particularly the relationship between the spouses, but also the existence of secondary supportive people, such as relatives and neighbors
2. Perception of the event, or in other words, its meaning and significance, which can be influenced by:
   a. Knowledge of the exceptional problem
   b. Past experiences with a similar event
   c. Religious beliefs
   d. Imagined cause of the condition
   e. Perceived effects of the event on the family
3. Coping mechanisms that family members are using to respond to the current situation and that they have used in previous crises; presence of concurrent stresses, such as marital or financial difficulties

The nurse also assesses the parents' reaction to the child. Questions that may be helpful include the following: "How is this child different from his siblings?" "Do you find yourself being a little more cautious with this child than your other children?" "How has your life-style changed since you learned of the diagnosis?" "When you think of your child's future, what thoughts do you have?" and "Describe your child's personality."

The degrees to which the parents and the child understand the condition are other significant assessment areas. Although they may be apparent in discussions with the family, often they are not, necessitating direct inquiry. One way of eliciting information is to ask a parent how he would explain the child's condition to a stranger. This approach frequently eliminates the use of medical jargon that family members have learned to conveniently cover up their true feelings.

While inquiring about the parents' level of understanding, the nurse also focuses on the knowledge of the child and the siblings. It is not unusual for parents who appear well adjusted and knowledgeable to state that they have never told the children the truth. Although this is less of a problem when the handicap is visible, it may occur when the disability can be cloaked in terms such as "a little behind" or "slow learner." Conflict arises when the child or the siblings learn of the diagnosis from nonparental sources.

Provide support at time of diagnosis

The impact of the crisis is usually greatest at the time of the diagnosis, which may be revealed at the time of birth, after a long period of physical and/or psychologic testing, or immediately after a tragic accident. It is a critical time for parents. Although they may not hear or remember all that is said to them, they frequently sense a certain attitude of acceptance, rejection, hope, or despair on the part of the informant.

Parents are encouraged to be together when they are informed of their child's condition, thus avoiding the problem of one parent having to interpret complex findings and deal with the initial emotional reaction of the other. This also gives the nurse an opportunity to observe the interaction between the parents as they are confronted with the tragedy of discovering an exceptional problem in their child. The parents' emotional needs are acknowledged by expressing acceptance of crying, sadness, anger, disappointment, and so on. Emotional support is offered by having tissues ready when one of the parents cries, and demonstrating understanding through facial and body language that indeed this is a difficult and painful period. The atmosphere of the informing session should be one in which parents feel free to express their own emotion. If their feelings can be expressed and acknowledged, the parents can be helped to deal openly with them and their need for further counseling can be determined.

Finally, the informing conference should not end with presentation of devastating news. Instead the child's strengths, his appealing behaviors, his potential for development, and available rehabilitation efforts or treatment are stressed. Although it may not be the time to discuss orthopedic appliances, special schools, or corrective surgical procedures in depth, it is appropriate to emphasize the positive future expectations for the child. The nurse also communicates to parents that life with their child is very similar to life with other children. Their experiences should be thought of as a series of problem-solving processes that they are capable of handling, particularly with available professional feedback. The parents are assured that the nurse or another health professional will be available to answer questions and to provide further assistance as it is needed in the future.

The preceding paragraphs have presented guidelines for discussing exceptional problems in general. However, some situations involve special problems. The following are brief discussions of special considerations based on the diagnosis.

Congenital anomaly. The first indication that all is not well occurs at the time of delivery. The atmosphere of happy anticipation suddenly changes to one laden with anxiety. Even when parents are unable to see the infant, they sense with terrified awareness the heightened and prolonged tension in the room, which conveys that something is seriously wrong. Personnel unprepared for this disturbing experience find it difficult to cope with their own feelings and react with feelings of frustration and resentment toward a situation that they are powerless to change. As a result they may forget about or retreat from the parents, who, at this moment, are suffering the most.

Most physicians believe that it is their responsibility to inform the parents of a congenital anomaly. Nurses and physicians need to clarify their roles in regard to revealing information, so that parents will be supported immediately after the birth of their child. For example, at the time of delivery, unless a pediatrician is in attendance, communication with the mother is delayed while the physician is involved with the mother's care. During this period the mother, unable to see her child and feeling the tense atmosphere, will believe either that the child is normal but that others do not share her enthusiasm or that the condition of the child is so terrible that the professional people in the room are unable to talk about it. A nurse, the person who is most likely to be free to support the mother and who is familiar with most common congenital anomalies, can make truthful statements about the defect.

The manner in which the infant is presented to the parents may well set the tone for the early parent-child relationship. It is best to explain briefly to them in simple language what the defect is and something concerning the immediate prognosis before the infant is shown to them, when they are more apt to "hear" what is said. Parents attach a great deal of meaning to the behavior of others during this critical period and watch the facial expressions of others closely for signs of revulsion or rejection. Presenting the infant as something precious, although incomplete, and emphasizing the well-formed aspects of the infant's body provide some reassurance to parents in this crisis period. It is important to allow time and opportunity for the parents to express their initial response to the situation. They are encouraged to ask questions and should receive honest, straightforward answers without undue optimism or pessimism.

Mental retardation. Unless mental retardation is associated with other physical handicaps, it is often easy for parents to miss clues to its presence or to make defensive excuses regarding diagnosis. Since the impact of a diagnosis is associated with the reactions of shock and denial, it is important to help parents develop awareness of the handicap. The best approach is planning situations that help them become aware of the problem. This may deliberately involve a prolonged period of evaluation to help the parents gain an appreciation of the child's strengths and weaknesses.

Without offering diagnostic opinions, the nurse encourages parents to discuss their observations of the child. For example, the parents are asked how this child's development compares with that of other siblings or peers, how he is doing in school, if the parents have any concerns about his progress, or what they have been told by others. By focusing on what the child can do and appropriate interventions to help him progress, such as infant-stimulation programs, the nurse involves parents in their child's care while helping them gain an awareness of his disability.

Physical disability. Loss of a motor or sensory ability is usually readily apparent. The challenge lies in helping the child and parents through the period of shock and grief and toward the phase of acceptance and reintegration. One of the most helpful interventions is to institute early rehabilitation, such as using a prosthetic limb, learning to read braille, or learning to read lips. However, physical rehabilitation usually precedes psychologic adjustment. Therefore, persons working with crippled or sensory-impaired children must bear in mind that even though a child is proficient in compensatory skills, he may still be grieving for his loss and in great need of emotional support.

When the cause of the disability is an accident, parental and child guilt can be overwhelming. It is imperative at the time of diagnosis to avoid implying that the parents or the child was responsible for the injury.

Multiple handicaps. The multihandicapped child may present special challenges because the child or the parents may require additional time for the shock phase. The child or the parents may only be able to attend to one diagnosis before hearing significant information regarding another handicap. The informing conference is structured to prevent overwhelming the family.

When an obvious handicap and a more hidden handicap coexist, such as cerebral palsy and mental retardation, the nurse must be sure that the parents understand and accept both diagnoses. Not infrequently the parents rationalize that any retarded development is the result of the physical impairment and resist accepting the intellectual deficit.

The nurse must also appreciate the devastating consequences of two or more handicaps to a child, especially if they interfere with expressive-receptive abilities. The overwhelming example is the blind and deaf child. Although both these defects may be present at birth, they may have different onsets—for example, partial deafness at birth, with progressive loss of vision. In this situation the child's experiences with the outside world are severely limited. The nurse must rely heavily on the ability to observe facial and bodily expressions as cues to the child's feelings and on the ability to use touch as a method of communication.

Chronic illness. Realization of the true impact of a diagnosis of chronic illness may take months or years. Conflict between the parents' concerns and the child's concerns may result in serious problems. For example, while parents worry about preventing bleeding episodes and joint deformity, the hemophiliac child may only focus on the activity restriction. Unless each member is able to gain an appreciation of the other's concerns, it is likely that no one's needs will be met.

When the illness is inherited, parents may blame themselves, and the child may blame the parents. This problem should be discussed with parents at the time of diagnosis, to lessen guilt and accusatory feelings on any person's part.

Terminal illness. A particular dilemma arises when the diagnosis indicates a potentially life-threatening disorder. Sometimes parents wish to conceal the diagnosis from the child. They may reason that the child is too young to know, that he will not be able to cope with the information, or that he will become despondent and lose his will to live. A decision not to tell the child has several disadvantages. It deprives the child of the opportunity to openly discuss his feelings and ask questions, it incurs the risk of the child's learning the truth from outside and sometimes less tactful sources, and it may lessen the child's trust and confidence in his parents once he learns the truth.

While the decision to "tell or not to tell" ultimately belongs to the parents, they can be guided to see the potential problems involved in fostering a conspiracy. One way of approaching the subject is by asking, "*How* will you tell your child about the diagnosis?" rather than "*What* will you tell him?" The former question implies truthfulness. One can also stress the difference between "cruel" truth and "gentle" truth. To tell someone that he has a potentially fatal disease and that he may die is cruel. However, telling a child the name of the illness and the reason for treatment instills hope, provides support from others, and serves as a foundation for explaining and understanding subsequent events.

Parents also need an explanation of how children of various ages view death. Children's understanding of death parallel their cognitive and psychosocial development. Death has the least significance to infants younger than 6 months of age. However, once parent-child attachment and the development of trust have been well established, the loss, even temporarily, of that significant person elicits profound resistance from the child. Therefore, separation is the major fear associated with death.

Children between 3 and 5 years of age have usually heard the word "death," and they have some idea of its meaning. They see death as a departure, possibly as a kind of sleep. They may recognize the fact of physical death, but they do not see that it involves the loss of the abilities a person has in life. The dead person in the coffin still breathes, eats, sleeps, and so on. Death is temporary and gradual; life and death can change places with one another. Because of their immature concept of time, there is no real understanding of the universality and inevitability of death. Words such as "forever" and "everyone" have meaning only in the child's egocentric thinking.

Much of what pertains to the preschool period regarding the understanding of death also relates to school-age children, particularly those near 6 or 7 years of age. However, these children have a deeper understanding of death in the concrete sense. They attempt to ascribe a more comprehensible meaning to the event by personifying death as a devil, God, a ghost, a bogeyman, and so on. As some of these names imply, there is a destructive connotation to death. These children particularly fear the mutilation and punishment they associate with death.

By 9 or 10 years of age most children have an adult concept of death. They realize that it is inevitable, universal, and irreversible. Their attitudes toward death are greatly influenced by the reactions and attitudes of others, particularly their parents.

Table 16-1 summarizes childrens' concepts of and reactions to death and outlines supportive interventions for each developmental stage.

Help the family cope

In order for the family to meet the stresses involved in optimum adjustment to the child's condition, each member must be individually supported so that each part of the family system is strong. Although the family unit can indefinitely support a member who is in need of assistance, its greatest strength lies in every member supporting the others. The nurse should bear in mind that the "member in need" is not necessarily the child but may be a parent or sibling who is dealing with stresses that require intervention.

Parents. Nurses who understand the grief response will be prepared to support the parents through this necessary process. This process is particularly important in the case of the birth of a defective child, because the parents cannot begin to invest any feeling for the child until they are able to talk about and work through their feelings of disappointment, resentment, guilt, and helplessness. Parents need to talk, and the supportive nurse is one who creates and maintains an atmosphere that encourages expression of feelings. Open expression is difficult for many people, and the parent(s) may hesitate to display intense feelings. Containing those feelings utilizes a great deal of energy that would be better used later to develop a relationship with the infant. Nurses, therefore, need to listen closely for cues that indicate areas of discomfort or readiness to talk. They can initiate discussion about matters that have been of concern to others in similar situations and help the parents to know that their feelings are natural. Parents are allowed silence and solitude if that is their wish. Most of all, nurses need to promote communication within the family and help strengthen family interpersonal relationships.

Mothers are very uneasy about handling infants with exceptional problems and require support and encouragement in their mothering tasks. A longer period of dependency is needed by these mothers to regroup their resources for coping. Although the mother should not feel forced to care for the infant until she is ready for the responsibility, she can be given opportunities to assume care of the infant as soon as possible, to help her deal with the reality of the infant's condition. Mothers' responses are highly individual and must be evaluated on this premise. However, all mothers need sympathetic, patient, and un-

TABLE 16-1. CHILDREN'S UNDERSTANDING OF AND REACTIONS TO DEATH

CONCEPTS OF DEATH	REACTIONS TO DEATH	INTERVENTIONS
Infants and toddlers Death has least significance to children under 6 months. After parent-child attachment and the development of trust is established, the loss, even temporary, of the significant person is profound. Prolonged separation during the first several years is thought to be more significant in terms of future physical, social, and emotional growth than at any subsequent age. Toddlers are egocentric and can only think about events in terms of their own frame of reference—living. Their egocentricity and vague separation of fact and fantasy make it impossible for them to comprehend absence of life. Instead of understanding death, this age-group is affected more by any change in life-style.	In the death of someone else, they may continue to act as though the person is alive. As the child grows older, he will be increasingly able and willing to let go of the dead person. Ritualism is important; a change in life-style could be anxiety producing. This age-group reacts more to the pain and discomfort of a serious illness than to the probable fatal prognosis.	Help parents deal with their feelings, allowing them more emotional reserve to meet the needs of their children. Encourage the parents to remain as near to the child as possible, yet be sensitive to the parents' needs. Maintain as normal an environment as possible to retain ritualism. If a parent has died, encourage a consistent caregiver for the child. If parents are unable to visit frequently, assign a primary nurse.
Preschool children Believe their thoughts are sufficient to cause death; the consequence is the burden of guilt, shame, and punishment. Their egocentricity implies a tremendous sense of self-power and omnipotence. Usually have some connotation of its meaning. Seen as a departure, a kind of sleep. May recognize the fact of physical death but do not separate it from living abilities. Seen as temporary and gradual; life and death can change places with one another. No understanding of the universality and inevitability of death.	If they become seriously ill, they conceive of the illness as a punishment for their thoughts or actions. May feel guilty and responsible for a death of a sibling. Greatest fear concerning death is separation from parents. May engage in activities that seem strange or abnormal to adults. Because of their fewer defense mechanisms to deal with loss, young children may react to a less significant loss with more outward grief than to the loss of a very significant person. The loss is so deep, painful, and threatening that the child must deny it for the present in order to survive its overwhelming impact. Behavior reactions such as giggling, joking, attracting attention, or regressing to earlier developmental skills indicate the child's need to distance himself from tremendous loss.	Help parents deal with their feelings, allowing them more emotional reserve to meet the needs of their children. Help parents to understand behavioral reactions of their children. Encourage the parents to remain near the child as much as possible, to minimize their great fear of separation from parents. If a parent has died, encourage a consistent caregiver for the child. If parents are unable to visit frequently, assign a primary nurse.

TABLE 16-1. CHILDREN'S UNDERSTANDING OF AND REACTIONS TO DEATH—cont'd

CONCEPTS OF DEATH	REACTIONS TO DEATH	INTERVENTIONS
School-age children Still associate misdeeds or bad thoughts with causing death and feel intense guilt and responsibility for the event. Because of their higher cognitive abilities, they respond well to logical explanations and comprehend the figurative meaning of words. Have a deeper understanding of death in a concrete sense. Particularly fear the mutilation and punishment they associate with death. By 9 or 10, children have an adult concept of death, realizing that it is inevitable, universal, and irreversible. Personify death as devil, monster, or bogeyman.	Because of their increased ability to comprehend, they may have more fears, for example: —the reason for the illness —communicability of the disease to themselves or others —consequences of the disease —the process of dying and death itself Their fear of the unknown is greater than the known. The realization of impending death is a tremendous threat to their sense of security and ego strength. Likely to exhibit fear through verbal uncooperativeness rather than actual physical aggression. Very interested in postdeath services. May be inquisitive about what happens to the body.	Help parents deal with their feelings, allowing them more emotional reserve to meet the needs of their children. Encourage the parents to remain near the child as much as possible, yet be sensitive to the parents' needs. Because of their fear of the unknown, anticipatory preparation is very important. Since the developmental task of this age is industry, helping children maintain control over their bodies and increasing their understanding allows them to achieve independence, self-worth, and self-esteem and avoids a sense of inferiority. Encourage children to talk about their feelings and provide aggressive outlets. Encourage parents to honestly answer questions about dying rather than avoiding or fabricating euphemisms. Encourage parents to share their moments of sorrow with their children. Provide preparation for postdeath services.
Adolescents Have a mature understanding of death. Still very much influenced by "remnants" of magical thinking and are subject to guilt and shame. Likely to see deviations from accepted behavior as reasons for their illness.	Straddle transition from childhood to adulthood. Have the most difficulty in coping with death. Least likely to accept cessation of life, particularly if it is their own. Concern is for the present much more than for the past or the future. May consider themselves alienated from their peers and unable to communicate with their parents for emotional support—feeling alone in their struggle. Adolescents' orientation to the present compels them to worry about physical changes even more than the prognosis. Because of their idealistic view of the world, they may criticize funeral rites as barbaric, money-making, and unnecessary.	Help parents deal with their feelings, allowing them more emotional reserve to meet the needs of their children. Avoid alliances with either parent or child. Structure the hospital admission to allow for maximum self-control and independence. Let the patient get to know you. Answer adolescents' questions honestly, treating them as mature individuals, and respecting their needs for privacy, solitude, and personal expressions of emotions. Help parents understand their child's reactions to death/dying, especially that concern present crises, such as loss of hair, may be much greater than for future ones, including possible death.

derstanding help to gain feelings of adequacy in the care of their children and to facilitate development of a positive relationship with the infant later on. Nurses must be prepared to accept parental reactions and defenses—anger, hostility, rejection, dependency—without anger and without withdrawing from the situation. If nurses make themselves available to the parents, they can often find nonthreatening ways to help, comfort, and support them.

Most families can be helped to feel adequate about their roles and responsibilities. Family members should understand from the beginning that they can shape their child's outcome. At the same time, the lack of stable cultural practices on which they can rely may make parents feel insecure in their roles, inadequate, burdened, and anxious. The nurse's role is to help alleviate these feelings by pointing out the parents' and the child's strengths. For example, a handicapped infant may be more demanding if he has difficulty in eating and needs more feedings. The child might be less responsive than the parents thought he would be. Therefore, the parent-infant relationship is vulnerable from the beginning. The nurse can support the parents in these concerns and supply information about what to expect from the infant in various phases of development.

Since mothers and fathers of handicapped children have few role models to imitate, they need support to help them adjust. Above all, the nurse ensures that the parents and siblings learn to perceive the handicapped child as a child first with unique and individual needs. How one interacts with, approaches, touches, or holds the child makes this obvious. Any signs of rejection of the child, though subtle in nature, are readily interpreted by parents. This attitude of liking, concern for, and acceptance of the child should begin in early infancy and continue throughout the handicapped child's life.

Parents are asked for suggestions on care planning, implementation, and evaluation. The nurse plays a valuable role in ensuring that the child learns about his handicap and fostering communication between the child and his parents so that he shares his concerns with them. The parents are helped to realize the child's level of maturity and understanding. The parents must stress to the child the hopeful aspects of his condition, as well as the problems. Careful consideration is given to avoid overwhelming him and to supporting him as he reacts to information about himself.

Parents are encouraged to discuss their feelings toward the handicapped child, the impact of this event on their marriage, and associated stresses, such as financial burdens. It is important to listen nonjudgmentally, avoiding any urge to align with one parent's feelings. Rather both parents are provided an equal opportunity to discuss their perceptions of events and relationships in the family.

Every effort is made to include the father in visits, such as to the nursery, clinic, special school, stimulation programs, and so on. His relationship with the child is observed, noting verbal interactions, tendency to assist the child, ability to give praise or set limits, and sensitivity to the child's needs. He is included in the assessment process with specific emphasis on having him describe the child's strengths and difficulties. It is not unusual to find two parents who have found opposing views of the child's abilities, especially in the area of developmental disabilities.

The father is encouraged to express his expectation for the child now and in the future. Because fathers tend to repress their feelings and feel less competent, the nurse acknowledges their difficulties and strengths, such as parenting skills and problem-solving abilities.

The child. Through ongoing contacts with the child, the nurse (1) observes the child's responses to his handicap, ability to function, and adaptive behaviors within the environment and with significant others, (2) explores the child's own understanding of the nature of his illness or condition, and (3) supports him while he learns to cope with his feelings. He is encouraged to express his concerns rather than allowing others to express them for him, since open discussions may reduce anxiety.

Parents sometimes convey the concern that the child cannot express the anxieties *he feels*. If the child cannot or will not talk, the nurse may have the child play out his feelings. He can be provided with toys to allow him to express threatening or stressful emotions. The nurse may find that the child responds best to drawing pictures or telling stories. Puppets can also be used to help him express himself. (See Chapter 4 for a discussion of communication techniques.)

Since school and peer relationships are so meaningful to a child, a child who must be hospitalized or stay at home should have some means of maintaining contact with his peers. The nurse and the school teacher can plan care to create and maintain an environment that meets this need. Besides periodic visits, peer contact can be fostered through telephone calls, letter writing, special cards, or the use of tape recordings.

One of the most important interventions is alleviating the child's feeling of being different and normalizing his life as much as possible. The following principles underlie this normalizing process (Krulik, 1980):

1. **Preparation.** Prepare the child in advance for changes that may occur from the illness or disability; for example, the child is told in advance of the possible side effects of drug therapy.
2. **Participation.** Include the child in as many decisions as possible, especially those relating to his care regimen; for example, the child is responsible for taking his medications or scheduling his home treatments.
3. **Sharing.** Allow both family members and the child's peers to be a part of the care regimen whenever possible; for example, the child is given his medication when the

other siblings receive their vitamins; mother cooks the same menu for the whole family; and if the child is invited to another's home, the mother advises the family of the child's dietary restrictions.

4. **Control.** Identify areas where the child can be in control so that feelings of uncertainty, passivity, and helplessness are decreased; for example, the child identifies activities that are appropriate to his energy level and chooses to rest when he is fatigued.

Siblings.   As pointed out previously, the presence of a child with an exceptional problem in a family may result in parents paying less attention to the other children or expecting older siblings to take on greater responsibility for the care of the child. The siblings may respond by developing negative attitudes toward the child or by expressing anger in various forms. The nurse can help by using ''anticipatory guidance''—questioning the parents about what they believe is the best way to have siblings respond to the child and about whether they have any concerns about the way in which they are assigning responsibility to older siblings. This questioning should take place before serious negative effects occur.

Siblings may also experience embarrassment associated with the stigma of a handicap such as mental retardation. Parents are then faced with the difficulty of responding to this embarrassment in an understanding and appropriate manner without punishing the siblings for feeling the way they do. Parents should talk with the siblings about how they view their affected brother or sister. For example, siblings of a retarded child may express fears about their ability to bear normal children. Adolescents in particular may not be able to discuss these vital issues with their parents and may prefer to consult with the nurse. The nurse emphasizes to parents that such questioning is natural for adolescents and that it should not be misconstrued as rebelliousness or rejection.

Many parents express concern about when and how to inform the other children in the family about the birth or the presence of a child who has an exceptional problem. The answer depends on each child's level of sophistication and understanding. However, it is usually best to inform the siblings before a neighbor or other non–family member does so. Nurses can show by their behavior that they see the parents as being capable, in their own unique way, of imparting information about the condition. However, they should make it clear that if the parents postpone informing the siblings they run the risk of hindering the siblings' ability to develop a realistic understanding of the problem. Uninformed siblings may fantasize or develop apprehensions that are out of proportion to the child's actual condition. Furthermore, if parents choose to be silent or deceptive about the issue, they are setting a negative precedent for the siblings to follow, rather than encourag-

ing them to cope with the experience in a healthy and nurturing way.

The nurse must be sensitive to the reactions of siblings and whenever possible intervene to promote more positive adjustments. For example, siblings often mention that they are expected to take on additional responsibilities to help the parents care for the child. It is not unusual for siblings to express a positive reaction to assuming the extra duties but to feel unappreciated for assuming them. Such feelings can often be remedied by encouraging the siblings to discuss the situation with the parents and by suggesting to parents ways of showing gratitude, such as an increase in allowance, special privileges, and, most significantly, verbal praise.

Extended family and people outside the family.   The nurse must also be sensitive to the family's cues regarding sources of stress from extended family members, such as grandparents. For example, the nurse may encourage the parents to invite the grandparents to be present during one of the child's visits to a clinic, during the diagnostic workup, or at a parent conference. Including grandparents in a discussion in which they can convey their concerns may help them deal with their feelings, thus reducing stress on the entire family. The nurse can help the grandparents understand the effects of their behavior on the family with an appropriate statement, such as, ''Your daughter is currently experiencing a great deal of pain and anguish. We realize that this is difficult for you as well as your daughter; however, you can be of tremendous help by being supportive toward her.''

Considerable stress can also arise from nonfamilial sources, such as friends, neighbors, or strangers. Inability to cope with comments about the disorder or curious stares by others may foster the tendency to isolate and protect the child within the home. The family needs guidance in preparing for these inevitable experiences. One approach is encouraging parents to dress the child as much as possible like other children. Good grooming is very important in minimizing differences in appearance. Through role playing, parents can practice responses to comments such as ''Is your child retarded?'' or ''Has he always been crippled?'' Through parent groups, family members can share experiences and learn from each other how they successfully deal with probing questions or unkind remarks. Such interventions must include the siblings and the child, who also must face and deal with these events.

Foster reality adjustment

Fostering a reality adjustment primarily involves (1) education of the parents regarding the condition and the developmental needs of the child and (2) realistic goal setting. Ideally, education should be aimed at preventing problems, rather than at relearning to change existing dilemmas. Like the interventions previously discussed, this goal requires an ongoing process that is part of assessment and emotional support of the family.

Supply information. Parents need accurate, up-to-date information in language they can understand. Since they do not hear all that is said the first time it is told to them, they want careful explanations about the child's defect, the treatments outlined, and what will be expected of them. Parents often misinterpret information and, therefore, require repeated explanations. Often the nurse's responsibility is to explain, interpret, and clarify information that has been given by the physician and to answer questions. Following basic concepts of interviewing, the nurse determines what the parents know and proceeds from that point. One cannot assume that the parents' failure to ask questions means they understand. Most parents have little or no knowledge of basic anatomy or physiology; therefore, pictures and other visual aids can be used effectively to explain both normal and deviant structures.

Parents also need guidance in how the condition may interfere with or alter activities of daily living, such as eating, dressing, sleeping, and toileting. One area frequently affected by chronic or terminal illness or developmental disability is nutrition. The most common problems are (1) undernutrition, as a result of loss of appetite or motor deficits that interfere with feeding, and (2) overnutrition, which is usually caused by a caloric intake in excess of energy expenditure or by boredom and lack of stimulation in other areas.

Teaching the parents to provide the special care that is frequently required is an important nursing responsibility. Special feeding, holding, and positioning techniques need to be explained and demonstrated. Anticipatory guidance regarding problems that are peculiar to each abnormality reduces apprehension and stimulates the parents to institute preventive measures and to make alert observations.

Another critical component for normal child development is discipline. Unfortunately, this is one of the earliest child rearing practices eliminated when parents react with "over benevolence." Not only does lack of discipline destroy the child's security, because he has no boundaries on which to test out his behavior, but also it fails to teach the child socially acceptable behavior and creates resentment and hostility among the siblings if different standards are applied to each child. One of the most effective approaches to discipline, especially with developmentally disabled children, is the use of behavior modification.

The nurse's responsibility is to help parents learn successful methods of controlling behavior before it becomes a problem. Simple limit-setting measures that should be applied to the child include a regular bedtime or nap hour, routine feeding schedule, preferably with the family, dressing in the morning, and scheduled playtime, including, for example, outdoor activity or limited television viewing. Such measures not only enforce certain expectations from the child but also encourage "normalization."

Referral to agencies and organizations that offer services for the specific defect can provide parents with help to deal with ongoing problems and to plan for those they will encounter in raising a child with an exceptional problem, including financial burdens. Public health agencies, social services, mental health clinics, and parent groups all have unique and specialized services that are designed to help support the family and to aid parents in their problem solving.

Several official and volunteer agencies offer special services. Many of these are discussed elsewhere in this book, under specific diagnoses.* Parents' organizations are especially helpful because they provide information and mutual support to their members.† The nurse who is aware of families whose situations are similar can be instrumental in organizing a self-help parent group. Sometimes the only effort necessary is identifying one or two parents as leaders, sharing with them the names, telephone numbers, and addresses of other families, and guiding them in how to initiate a first meeting.

Parents also need to be aware of the importance of communicating the child's condition in the event of a medical emergency. Young children are unable to give information about their disorder and although older children may be reliable sources, in an accident they may be physically unable to speak. Therefore, all children with any type of chronic condition that may affect medical care should wear some type of identification, such as a Medic Alert bracelet,‡ which lists the medical condition and a collect phone number for emergency medical records and other personal information, or a MediScope,§ a cylinder-shaped pendant which contains a microfilm medical record and a magnifying lens.

Set realistic goals. One of the most difficult adjustments is setting realistic future goals for the handicapped child and for those who must assume his continued care. Sometimes the impact of such decisions does not surface until the child finishes school or the parents near retirement. At such a time another crisis can arise because the family roles and relationships that maintained stability are being disrupted.

---

*A comprehensive list of books and pamphlets for parents and teachers of handicapped children is available from The National Easter Seal Society, 2023 W. Ogden Ave, Chicago, IL 60612. A bibliography of references for parents and children on life-threatening illness, especially cancer, is included at the end of this chapter.

†A parents' group for children with cancer is The Candlelighters, 2025 I Street, N.W., Washington, DC 20006; a group for bereaved parents is The Compassionate Friends, P.O. Box 1347, Oak Brook, IL 60521.

‡P.O. Box 1009, Turlock, CA 95381.

§MicroDesign Systems, P.O. Box 188, Arverne, NY 11692.

Planning for the future should be a gradual process. The parents should cultivate realistic vocations for the child. For example, if the child has a physical handicap, he should be directed to intellectual, artistic, or musical pursuits. If the child is developmentally disabled, he should be taught a manual skill that can be used in a special workshop. In this way the child's development proceeds in the direction of self-support through gainful employment.

Unfortunately, vocational pursuits are not realistic for every handicapped person. Multihandicapped or severely handicapped persons may require lifelong care and assistance. In these situations parents must look to the future, when they will no longer be able to care for their child. Residential placement may be very difficult unless the family mutually participates in the decision-making and planning process. Institutionalization should not be viewed as abandonment. Not infrequently it is the only way to preserve the family unit. The nurse should help the family members investigate suitable placements, discuss their feelings regarding this topic, and explore measures to maintain meaningful communication with the handicapped person. Alternatives to home care are described in Chapter 17.

GRIEF PROCESS IN EXPECTED DEATH AND UNEXPECTED DEATH

Grief is the normal response to a significant loss. For parents, it may be the loss of a child or of the "perfect" child; for the child, it may be loss of an ability, a body part, or a state of health. Unfortunately, not all children with exceptional problems survive. Some face the possibility of death from the time of diagnosis; others may suddenly develop complications that are fatal.

In *expected* death one must involve the patient and his family in the plan for intervention both before and after the death. In *unexpected* death the survivors face the tremendous task of integrating the loss into their lives, with no opportunity for anticipatory grief. However, in either situation nurses can facilitate the grief process by being aware of expected psychologic and somatic reactions and supporting the grievers through each stage.

Expected death

When death is expected, there is time for *anticipatory grieving*. This does not mean that the actual loss hurts less, but that the period of acute grief and mourning following the loss may be shortened. Many parents reflect that the physical absence of the child is the most difficult aspect of the death to bear.

In long-term, potentially fatal illnesses, the grief for anticipated loss becomes chronic. The parents mourn the loss of their child long before he dies. Unlike parents who experience a sudden loss, these family members are unable to resolve their grief until the child is considered cured or until he is dead. Each time they see the pain the child must endure or experience the sudden loss of hope that results from a relapse, they are reminded of their child's uncertain future.

However, the prolonged period of grief provides families with the precious opportunity to complete all "unfinished business," such as helping the child and siblings understand and cope with a fatal prognosis. Many families reflect on their changed perspective of time after learning of the diagnosis, particularly their heightened awareness of the value and worth of each day. As one father said, "I used to plan ahead for a better job, more money, and more prestige. But now I find myself wanting to stay home to be with my family. I never before realized how important time really is. Now I only wish we had more of it."

Unexpected death

In sudden, unexpected death the family does not have the advantages of anticipatory grief. There is no opportunity to prepare oneself or others for the death. Because of this lack of time to prepare, many families feel great guilt and remorse for not having done something differently or for not having done something at all. For example, they may berate themselves for not having prevented the accident or for depriving the child of some desired material object or privilege. It is important to assess how parents feel about the events just prior to the tragedy, to help them work through their feelings so that they may progress to the resolution of grief. Specific reactions to unexpected death are presented in the discussion of sudden infant death syndrome in Chapter 9.

SYMPTOMATOLOGY OF GRIEF

Several symptoms, both somatic and psychologic, characterize the reactions of each individual's response to the loss of significant others. The box on p. 460 summarizes the five characteristics of the normal grief syndrome.

Distortions of normal grief, or *morbid grief reactions*, such as delay or postponement of grief, may occur. However, through appropriate intervention it is possible to transform these potentially pathologic responses into normal reactions that result in successful resolution of acute grief.

Intervention. Health professionals can use this theoretic framework to support individuals who are grieving. One approach toward providing emotional support to a be-

CHARACTERISTICS OF NORMAL REACTION TO GRIEF

Sensations of somatic distress
Feeling of tightness in the throat
Choking, with shortness of breath
Marked tendency toward sighing
Empty feeling in abdomen
Lack of muscular power
Intense subjective distress described as tension or mental pain

Preoccupation with image of the deceased
Hears, sees, or imagines that the dead person is present
Slight sense of unreality
Feeling of emotional distance from others
May believe that he is approaching insanity

Feelings of guilt
Searches for evidence of failure in preventing the death
Accuses himself of negligence or exaggerates minor
  omissions

Feelings of hostility
Loss of warmth toward others
Tendency toward irritability and anger
Wish not to be bothered by friends or relatives

Loss of usual pattern of conduct
Restlessness, inability to sit still, aimless moving
  about
Continual searching for something to do or what he
  thinks he ought to do
Lack of capacity to initiate and maintain organized patterns of activity

Adapted from Lindemann, E.: Symptomatology and management of acute grief, Am. J. Psychiatry **101:**141-143, 1944. Copyright 1944 American Psychiatric Association.

reaved person is to emphasize that reactions such as hearing the dead person's voice, feeling distant from others who want to help, or seeking reassurance that he did everything possible for the lost person are *normal*, *necessary*, and *expected* responses. They in no way signify insanity or approaching mental breakdown. On the contrary, such behaviors following the loss signify that the survivor is working through the acute grief and that he will probably satisfactorily resolve the loss and resume a meaningful role in his social environment.

STAGES OF DYING

Elisabeth Kübler-Ross (1969) has identified five stages that people experience in terms of expected death. These stages represent a set of *ever-changing* behaviors that surface as the need for them arises within individuals' attempts to cope with expected loss. Each stage pertains to the dying person and to those experiencing this person's expected death. In the case of a child, the "patient" is the ill child, the parents, and the siblings.

Denial

In the first stage, denial, the person responds with shock and disbelief. The "no, not me" reaction occurs regardless of whether the person is explicitly told his diagnosis. The duration of the denial depends on the coping mechanisms used by the person in previous crises, the support systems available to the person to help him give up the use of denial, and the reactions of others, especially physicians and nurses, to the resistance that is demonstrated. Unfortunately, the need of others to deny the reality of the situation may be so great that it supports and fosters the patient's own denial and retards his progression to other stages.

Examples of denial may include the following: physician shopping, attributing the symptoms of the illness to a minor condition, refusal to believe the diagnostic tests, delay in agreeing to treatment, acting very happy and optimistic despite the revealed diagnosis, refusing to tell or talk to anyone about the condition, insisting that no one is telling the truth regardless of others' attempts to do so, denying the reason for admission to the hospital, and not asking questions about the diagnosis, treatment, or prognosis. Each of these mechanisms allows individuals to distance themselves from the onslaught of a tremendous emotional blow and to collect and mobilize their energies toward goal-directed, problem-solving behaviors.

Partial denial, such as seeking additional professional consultations or occasionally acting as if nothing were wrong, is used by most people throughout the dying process to cope with the constant emotional drain of anticipating their own deaths or the death of a family member. To a parent, anticipating the death of his child is the same as anticipating the loss of part of his personal hope for achievement, prestige, and accomplishment.

Denial is probably the least understood and most poorly dealt with reaction. Nurses and physicians typically label denial as "maladaptive" and actively attempt to strip it away by repeated and sometimes blunt explanations of prognosis. In children, the importance of denial has repeatedly been demonstrated as a factor in their positive coping with the diagnosis. Researchers have found that children who use denial to cope with illness are able to deal with anxiety and have a productive attitude about life (O'Malley and others, 1979).

Denial allows an individual to maintain hope in the face of overwhelming odds. Like hope, denial may be an adaptive mechanism for dealing with loss that persists until a family or patient is ready or needs other responses.

Intervention.   The nurse's response to denial is a critical component of the individual's need for sustaining this defense mechanism. The helping person's role in all stages of dying is to support the individual in his current stage, not to maneuver him from one stage to another. If support is truly therapeutic, the strength gained from this active intervention will help the person proceed on his own to another stage.

The most effective method of support is active listening. Silence neither reinforces nor rejects denial (or any other stage of dying) but implies a willingness and acceptance of the person's need for this behavior. However, silence alone can be misinterpreted. For example, if the person demonstrates denial, perhaps by saying, "I am sure the doctors made a mistake," and the nurse responds with silence and leaves, the person may infer disapproval, agreement, avoidance, or rejection. To be effective, silence and listening must be accompanied by physical and mental concentration and use of body language to communicate interest and concern. Direct eye contact, touching, physical closeness, and body posture, such as sitting and leaning slightly forward, demonstrate silent but effective communication. Sometimes this type of support is sufficient to give the patient or family members enough strength to relinquish the denial and deal with the impact of reality.

If hope and denial are important elements in adjusting to a potential loss, then communication must allow for them. This does not imply keeping facts from families or patients but revealing them in such a way that if there is a margin for reversal, remission, or even partial recovery, this is emphasized. Information about prognosis should be conveyed in such a way that the "uncertainty" of the future is stressed rather than the omnipotence of having all the answers.

Anger

The second stage in the dying process is anger, which usually follows denial, but may occur or recur at any time during the dying process. When denial fails and the reality of the situation penetrates consciousness, the person's reaction is, "Why me?" Anger, rage, and hostility may be directed at oneself or at others, notably members of the medical and nursing staff, and envy or resentment may be displayed toward people who are not in his situation. However, unlike denial, anger is not socially approved or condoned. Frequently the person is harshly judged for his angry refusal to accept the diagnosis and is further isolated.

When one thinks about why the dying person or the parent of a dying child becomes enraged and resentful, one only begins to imagine the tremendous consequences of loss. Dreams, hopes, and expectations are now only painful memories. He is angry with those who are physically strong, who can make the dreams reality, and who live without pain or suffering. He is not angry at such people themselves but at the things they represent, which for the dying person are no longer possible.

Intervention.   The angry person needs to express these feelings but without feeling guilty or being judged by others. Sometimes the freedom to express angry thoughts is in itself therapeutic. The following steps encourage expression of emotions:

1. Describe the behavior: "You seem angry at everyone."
2. Give evidence of understanding: "Being angry is only natural."
3. Give evidence of caring: "It must be difficult to endure so many painful procedures."
4. Help focus on feelings: "Sometimes people wonder why things like this happened to them."

One essential element to the successful implementation of this process is to wait for the person to respond to a statement before proceeding to the next step. Since the objective of each statement is for the person to speak freely, the statements should not encourage the "yes" or "no" type of answer.

Bargaining

The next stage, and one that is often difficult to identify, is bargaining. It is the dying person's attempt to postpone the inevitable. The bargaining for additional time may be with God, with oneself, or with the most significant other person. One way of exploring a person's silent bargaining is to ask, "If you could do one more thing, what would that be?" Frequently the answer will reveal a hidden desire.

Intervention.   Because bargaining may be associated with guilt, it is always important to explore the reasons behind the expressed wish. One mother who prayed that God would make her daughter live a little longer later revealed that the child was illegitimate. Unfortunately the child died shortly after the diagnosis was made. The mother was convinced that her death was a sign of God's revenge for the out-of-wedlock pregnancy. She refused to accept the child's death and acted as if she were still alive. Although members of the nursing staff had been aware of the implications of this child's failure to recover, they were powerless in their attempts to help the mother, who isolated herself from everyone.

Bargaining also occurs in children. The dying child may wish for additional time for himself. One must listen very carefully to children in order to understand their symbolic language. One child who had recently been told that he had had a relapse of leukemia casually said to his mother, "Do you know what I wished for on my last birthday? Another birthday.'' The mother was certain that this was the child's way of bargaining for more time against the odds that he knew existed.

Depression

Without the protection of denial, the anger to displace the emotional anxiety, and the bargaining to postpone the inevitable, the person eventually experiences depression. Generally, there are two types of depression: that experienced because of past losses and that experienced because of anticipated or impending losses.

In a chronic terminal illness there are many reasons for the first kind of depression, such as loss of hair from therapy, loss of a body part or function, restricted physical ability, and change in life-style. The second kind of depression signals preparation for the impending loss of all love objects as the dying person realizes the enormity of his loss. Unlike the survivors, who are saying good-bye to one person, the dying person is saying good-bye to everyone and everything he ever loved.

Intervention. Dealing with each loss in a constructive, positive manner can greatly relieve the first type of depression. For example, purchasing an attractive wig, emphasizing one's ability rather than one's disability, and manipulating one's life-style to accommodate physical changes help the person deal with the depression of each crisis.

During the period characterized by the second type of depression, which could be considered preparatory grief, there is little need for verbal reassurances. Attempts to ''lighten the mood'' or ''cheer up the person'' not only are ineffective but also may burden him with the additional task of trying to appear happy in order to meet the needs of those around him. It is a time of listening and of being physically present with the dying person. Toward the terminal stage the person may request the company of only one or two significant people. Children usually desire the presence of their parents more than anyone else.

Acceptance

The final stage of dying is acceptance. The person is no longer angry or depressed. If bargaining occurs, it is usually for a peaceful, painless death rather than for prolongation of life. It is a time of inner peace and resolution that death is a certainty. The person may signal his acceptance by displaying a lack of interest in present or future events and being preoccupied with past events, preferring few visitors, and wanting quiet and solitude.

Intervention. Such behavior may be very upsetting to others close to him, including health personnel who have not reached the same level of acceptance. One critical objective is to recognize the behaviors of acceptance in the

patient and help others understand their relevance. Often the medical plan calls for continued treatment and does not allow the patient the opportunity to accept the inevitable end. Nurses can be instrumental in planning care with all members of the health team, with the patient and family's wishes receiving priority. For some families the alternative of hospice-type home care is a very significant and fulfilling means of sharing their child's final days.*

BEREAVEMENT: ACCEPTING THE FINAL LOSS

Families can prepare themselves for the expected loss, but when it occurs there is a period of acute grief, followed by an extended phase of mourning.

Brief shock

When death occurs, there is a brief period of shock. As one parent explained, ''We were as prepared for our son's death as anyone could be, but it was a shock when in a moment his life was finished. I just can't get over the rapidity with which life ends.'' Following the death, the family members need a period of time to say good-bye to the child. The body should be left in the room. If there is any reason to clean the body or remove medical equipment, the nurse should do so as quickly and calmly as possible. It is important for family members to remember the child in quiet, peaceful, pleasant surroundings.

Review of relationship

During the period immediately after the death, there is a tendency to review the events of the child's life and to evaluate the effectiveness of the parents' efforts to care for him. Parents will frequently look for validation of their efforts from the nurses who were with the child during his final hospitalization. It is important to support all parental actions and to listen for any feelings of guilt, which may delay the resolution of grief.

Indecision

Intervention is necessary after the child's death, because new conflicts, such as whether to have additional children, may arise. Many parents fear the recurrence of the condition in subsequent children. Although nurses cannot make such a decision for parents, they can assess their readiness for another pregnancy. The successful resolution of mourning is characterized by decreased preoccupation with the deceased, development of a realistic memory of him,

---

*Information on hospice care for children is available from Children's Hospice International, 501 Slater's Lane, #207, Alexandria, VA 22314.

establishment of new interests, and resumption of self-enjoyment and pleasure.

Social reintegration

The final resolution of grief is not only reintegration within the immediate family but also resumption of social attachments. This is particularly relevant for the mother, who suffers a double loss—loss of her child and loss of the mothering role. Part of her resolving the grief is finding a substitute role that is fulfilling and rewarding. Nurses can be instrumental in this process by (1) preparing the mother for anticipating the *normal* feelings of emptiness, loneliness, and sometimes even failure, (2) helping her reevaluate her role as parent and spouse, stressing that giving up the lost child must occur before she can reestablish emotional relations, (3) encouraging her to explore fulfilling activities that utilize her special interests, talents, and qualifications, and (4) supporting her as her role changes, particularly assisting with communication between family members who are affected (Wong, 1980).

REFERENCES

Krulik, T.: Successful "normalizing" tactics of parents of chronically ill children, J. Adv. Nurs. **5**(6):573-578, 1980.

Kübler-Ross, E.: On death and dying, New York, 1969, Macmillan, Inc.

Lansky, S., and others: Childhood cancer: parental discord and divorce, Pediatrics **62**(2):184-188, 1978.

McKeever, P.T.: Fathering the chronically ill child, Am. J. Maternal Child Nurs. **6**(2):124-128, 1981.

O'Malley, J.E. and others: Psychiatric sequelae of surviving childhood cancer, Am. J. Orthopsychiatry **49**(4):608-616, 1979.

Taylor, S.C.: The effects of chronic childhood illnesses upon well siblings, Am. J. Maternal Child Nurs. **9**(2):109-116, 1980.

Wong, D.: Bereavement: the empty-mother syndrome, Am. J. Maternal Child Nurs. **5**(6):385-389, 1980.

BIBLIOGRAPHY
Congenital anomalies

Brown, M.S.: The Gordons needed all the help they could get, Nursing 77 **7**(10):40-43, 1977.

Clay, C.: There is something wrong with your baby. In McNall, L.K., and Galeener, J.T., editors: Current practice in obstetric and gynecologic nursing, vol. 1, St. Louis, 1976, The C.V. Mosby Co.

Darling, R.B., and Darling, J.: Children who are different: meeting the challenges of birth defects in society, St. Louis, 1982, The C.V. Mosby Co.

Gracely, K.A.: Parental attachment to a child with a congenital defect, Pediatr. Nurs. **3**(5):15-17, 1977.

Horan, M.L.: Parental reaction to the birth of an infant with a defect: an attributional approach, Adv. Nurs. Sci. **5**(1):57-68, 1982.

Irvin, N.A., Kennell, J.H., and Klaus, M.H.: Caring for parents of an infant with a congenital malformation. In Klaus, M.H., and Kennell, J.H.: Parent-infant bonding, ed. 2, St. Louis, 1982, The C.V. Mosby Co.

Mercer, R.T.: Crisis: a baby born with a defect, Nursing 77 **7**(11):45-47, 1977.

Mills, G.C.: Supporting parental needs after birth of a defective infant. In Brandt, P.A., Chinn, P.L., and Smith, M.E., editors: Current practice in pediatric nursing, vol. 1, St. Louis, 1976, The C.V. Mosby Co.

Pi, E.H.: Congenitally handicapped children and their families: short- and long-term intervention, Pediatr. Basics **31**:10-14, 1981.

Waechter, E.H.: Bonding problems of infants with congenital anomalies, Nurs. Forum **16**(3,4):298-318, 1977.

Young, R.K.: Chronic sorrow: parent's response to the birth of a child with a defect, Am. J. Maternal Child Nurs. **2**(1):38-42, 1977.

Handicap/chronic illness

Bernard, B., and others: Exercise for children with physical disabilities, Issues Compr. Pediatr. Nurs. **5**:99-107, 1981.

Burton, L.: The family life of sick children, Boston, 1975, Routledge and Kegan Paul of America, Ltd.

Coupey, S., and Cohen, M.: A developmental approach to the chronically ill adolescent, Feelings Med. Signif. **22**(2): 7-10, 1980.

Craft, M.: Help for the family's neglected "other" child, Am. J. Maternal Child Nurs. **4**(5):297-300, 1979.

Crummette, B.: Assessing the impact of illness upon an adolescent and family, Matern. Child Nurs. J. **12**(3):155-167, 1983.

Fostel, C.: Chronic illness and handicapping conditions: coping patterns of the child and the family. In Brandt, P., and others, editors: Current practice in pediatric nursing, vol. 2, St. Louis, 1978, The C.V. Mosby Co.

Frauman, A.C., and Sypert, N.S.: Sexuality in adolescents with chronic illness, Am. J. Maternal Child Nurs. **4**(6):371-375, 1979.

Holaday, B.: Parenting the chronically ill child. In Brandt, P., and others, editors: Current practice in pediatric nursing, vol. 2, St. Louis, 1978, The C.V. Mosby Co.

Hymovich, D.P.: The chronicity impact and coping instrument: parent questionnaire, Nurs. Res. **32**(5):275-281, 1983.

Isaacs, J., and McElroy, M.R.: Psychosocial aspects of chronic illness in children, J. Sch. Health **50**(6):318-321, 1980.

Jelneck, L.J.: The special needs of the adolescent with chronic illness, Am. J. Maternal Child Nurs. **2**(1):57-61, 1977.

Kawasaki, M.A.: Summer camp and the disabled child, Pediatr. Nurs. **7**(4):9-12, 1981.

Lloyd, J.K.: Dietary problems associated with the care of the chronically sick children, J. Hum. Nutr. **33**(2):135-139, 1979.

Pattullo, A.W.: The socio-sexual development of the handicapped child, Nurs. Clin. North Am. **10**:361-369, 1975.

Pierce, P.M., and Giovinco, G.: Reach: self-care for the chronically ill child, Pediatr. Nurs. **9**(1):37-40, 1983.

Sahin, S.: The physically disabled child. In Johnson, S., editor: High-risk parenting, Philadelphia, 1979, J.B. Lippincott Co.

Seidle, A.H., and Altshuler, A.: Interventions for adolescents who are chronically ill, Child. Today **8**(6):16-19, 1979.

Shelly, J.A.: Spiritual care...planting seeds of hope, Crit. Care Update **9**(12):7-15, 1982.

Slonim, M.B.: Depression in the chronically ill or handicapped, Am. J. Maternal Child Nurs. **6**(4):266-273, 1981.

Stearns, S.E.: Understanding the psychological adjustment of physically handicapped children in the classroom, Child. Today **10**:12-15, Jan./Feb. 1981.

Zamerowski, S.T.: Helping families to cope with handicapped children, Top. Clin. Nurs. **4**:41-56, July 1982.

Zelle, R.S.: The developmentally disabled child and the family. In Hymovitch, D.P., and Barnard, M.U., editors: Family health care, New York, 1979, McGraw-Hill Book Co.

Terminal illness

Arnold, J.H., and Gemma, P.B.: A child dies: a portrait of family grief, Maryland, 1983, Aspen Systems Corp.

Dolan, M.B.: If your patient wants to die at home, Nursing 83 **13**(4):50-55, 1983.

Edstrom, S., and Miller, M.W.: Preparing the family to care for the cancer patient at home: a home care course, Cancer Nurs. **4**(1):49-52, 1981.

Everson, S.: Sibling counseling, Am. J. Nurs. **77**(4):644-646, 1977.

Fochtman, D., and Foley, G., editors: Nursing care of the child with cancer, Boston, 1982, Little, Brown & Co.

Garfield, C., editor: Stress and survival: the emotional realities of life-threatening illness, St. Louis, 1979, The C.V. Mosby Co.

Geltman, R.L., and Paige, R.L.: Symptom management in hospice care, Am. J. Nurs. **83**(1):78-85, 1983.

Greene, P.E.: The child with leukemia in the classroom, Am. J. Nurs. **75**(1):86-87, 1975.

Gyulay, J.E.: The forgotten grievers, Am. J. Nurs. **75**(9):1476-1479, 1975.

Iles, J.P.: Children with cancer: healthy siblings' perceptions during the illness experience, Cancer Nurs. **2**(5): 371-377, 1979.

Johnson-Soderberg, S.: The development of a child's concept of death, Oncol. Nurs. Forum **8**(1):23-26, 1981.

Klopovich, P., Suenram, D., and Cairns, N.: A common sense approach to caring for children with cancer: the community health nurse, Cancer Nurs. **3**(3):201-208, 1980.

Krulik, T.: Helping parents of children with cancer during the midstage of illness, Cancer Nurs. **5**(6):441-445, 1982.

Lindamood, M.M., and others: Groups for bereaved parents—how they can help, J. Fam. Pract. **9**(6):1027-1033, 1979.

Martinson, I.M.: Symposium on child psychiatric nursing. Caring for the dying child, Nurs. Clin. North Am. **14**:467-474, Sept. 1979.

Mills, G.: Books to help children understand death, Am. J. Nurs. **79**(2):291-295, 1979.

Moldow, D.G., and Martinson, I.M.: From research to reality—home care for the dying child, Am. J. Maternal Child Nurs. **5**(3):159-166, 1980.

Moore, I.M., and Triplett, J.L.: Students with cancer: a school nursing perspective, Cancer Nurs. **3**(4):265-270, 1980.

Sahler, O. J., editor: The child and death, St. Louis, 1978, The C.V. Mosby Co.

Shelton, R.L.: The patient's need of faith at death, Top. Clin. Nurs. **3**(3):55-59, 1981.

Shuler, S.: Death during childhood: reactions in parents and children. In Brandt, P., and others: Current practice in pediatric nursing, vol. 2, St. Louis, 1978, The C.V. Mosby Co.

Spinetta, J.J., and Deasy-Spinetta, P., editors: Living with childhood cancer, St. Louis, 1981, The C.V. Mosby Co.

Williams, H.A., Frederick, P.R., and Rothenberg, M.B.: The child is dying: who helps the family?, Am. J. Maternal Child Nurs. **6**(4):261, 1981.

Wong, D.: The terminally ill child. In Johnson, S., editor: High-risk parenting, Philadelphia, 1979, J.B. Lippincott Co.

Books for children and parents on life-threatening disorders

Baker, L.: You and leukemia: a day at a time, Philadelphia, 1978, W.B. Saunders Co.

Candlelighters Foundation Quarterly Newsletter, Candlelighters Foundation, Suite 1011, 2025 Eye Street, N.W., Washington, D.C. 20006.

Candlelighters Foundation Youth Newsletter, Candlelighters Foundation, Suite 10100, 2025 Eye Street, N.W., Washington, D.C. 20006.

Coping with cancer: an annotated bibliography of public, patient, and professional information and education materials, Bethesda, Maryland, 1980, Cancer Information Clearinghouse, Office of Cancer Communications, NIH Pub. No. 80-2129.

Coping with cancer: a resource for the health professional, Bethesda, Maryland, 1980, Cancer Information Clearinghouse, Office of Cancer Communications, NIH Pub. No. 80-2080.

Davis, A.J.: Please see my need, Charles City, Iowa, 1981, Satellite Books.

Diet and nutrition: a resource for parents of children with cancer, U.S. Department of Health, Education, and Welfare, Public Health Service, NIH Pub. No. 80-2038.

"Easing the way"....a resource guide for parents of children with cancer, New Jersey, 1982, American Cancer Society, N.J. Division.

*Fassler, J.: My grandpa died today, New York, 1971, Human Sciences Press, Inc.

Frantz, T: When your child has a life-threatening illness, Washington, D.C., 1983, Association for the Care of Children's Health.

Grollman, E.: Talking about death: dialogue between parent and child, Boston, 1976, Beacon Press.

Help yourself: tips for teenagers with cancer, National Cancer Institute, Office of Cancer Communications, 9000 Rockville Pike, Bldg. 31, Rm. 10A18, Bethesda, Maryland 20205.

Hospital days-treatment ways: hematology-oncology coloring book, Ohio, 1978, The Ohio State University Comprehensive Cancer Center.

Manning, D.: Don't take my grief from me, Hereford, Texas, 1979, Insight Books, Inc.

Our child died: an attempt to help you endure by some who have, 1981, Virginia Baptist Hospital, 3300 Rivermont Avenue, Lynchburg, Virginia 24503.

Pochedly, C.: Cancer in children: reasons for hope, Port Washington, New York, 1979, Ashley Books, Inc.

Roach, N.: The last day of April, New York, 1974, The American Cancer Society.

Schiff, H.: The bereaved parent, New York, 1977, Crown Publishers, Inc.

Schweers, E., and others: Parents' handbook on leukemia, New York, 1977, The American Cancer Society.

Sherman, M.: The leukemic child, U.S. Department of Health, Education and Welfare, NIH Pub. No. 78-863.

*Stein, S.: About dying: an open family book for parents and children together, New York, 1974, Walker and Co.

Students with cancer: a resource for the educator, U.S. Department of Health, Education, and Welfare, NIH Pub. No. 80-2086.

Temes, R.: Living with an empty chair, New York, 1980, Irvington Publishers, Inc.

Wolf, A.: Helping your child to understand death, New York, 1973, Child Study Press.

Young people with cancer: a handbook for parents, U.S. Department of Health and Human Services, NIH Pub. No. 82-2378. (Included is an excellent annotated list of additional reading materials.)

*Zolotow, C.: My grandson Lew, New York, 1974, Harper & Row, Publishers, Inc.

Additional reading materials

Selected pamphlets and books from The Compassionate Friends, Inc., P.O. Box 1347, Oak Brook, Ill. 60521:
Caring for surviving children
Church, M.J., Chazin, H. and Ewald, F.: When a baby dies
Grieving, healing, growing
Levy, E.: Children are not paper dolls: a visit with bereaved siblings
Miles, M.: The grief of parents
Stillbirth, miscarriage and infant death: understanding grief
Suggestions for doctors and nurses
LaTour, K: For those who live
Understanding grief
When a child dies...

---

*Story books for children about death.

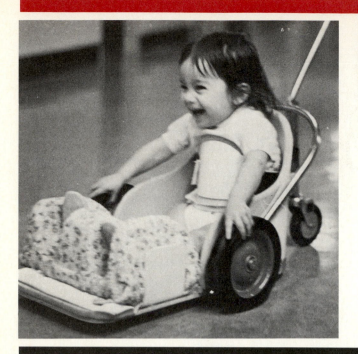

17

THE CHILD WITH MENTAL OR SENSORY DYSFUNCTION

OBJECTIVES

On completion of this chapter the reader will be able to:

- Define the classifications of mental retardation

- Outline nursing interventions for the retarded child that promote optimum development, including during hospitalization

- Identify the major biologic and cognitive characteristics of the child with Down syndrome

- Outline nursing interventions for the child with Down syndrome

- List the general classifications of hearing impairment and the effect on speech

- Outline nursing interventions for the child with hearing impairment, including during hospitalization

- List the common types of visual disorders in children

- Outline nursing interventions for the child with visual impairment, including during hospitalization

- Outline nursing interventions for the child with retinoblastoma

NURSING DIAGNOSES

Nursing diagnoses identified for the child with mental retardation or sensory impairments include, but are not restricted to, the following:

Health perception-health management pattern

- Health maintenance, alteration in, related to cognitive or sensory impairments

- Infection, potential for, related to (1) immobility; (2) dermatologic changes; (3) retention of respiratory secretions in Down syndrome

- Noncompliance, potential for, related to (1) knowledge or skill deficit; (2) denial of condition; (3) lack of support systems

Nutritional-metabolic pattern

- Nutrition, alteration in: potential for more than body requirements related to immobility

- Nutrition, alteration in: potential for less than body requirements related to feeding difficulties

- Skin integrity, impairment of: potential, related to (1) immobility; (2) dermatologic changes in Down syndrome

Elimination pattern

- Bowel elimination, alterations in: constipation related to (1) impaired abdominal musculature; (2) decreased activity in Down syndrome

Activity-exercise pattern

- Airway clearance, ineffective, related to (1) nasal obstruction; (2) impaired musculature in Down syndrome

- Diversional activity deficit related to cognitive or sensory impairment

- Home maintenance management, impairment of: potential related to (1) child's specific disability; (2) knowledge deficit; (3) lack of role modeling; (4) inadequate support systems

- Self-care deficit related to (1) cognitive or sensory impairment; (2) developmental level

Cognitive-perceptual pattern

- Knowledge deficit related to cognitive or sensory impairments

- Sensory-perceptual alteration, related to hearing or vision impairment

Self-perception—self-concept pattern

- Anxiety, related to (1) loss of hearing or vision; (2) hospitalization

- Powerlessness, related to perceived inability to control event

- Self-concept, disturbance in, related to unrealistic self-expectations

Role-relationship pattern

- Communication, impaired verbal: related to cognitive or hearing impairment

- Family process, alteration in, related to handicapped child

- Grieving, anticipatory, related to potential loss of child with retinoblastoma

- Parenting, alterations in: potential, related to (1) lack of support system; (2) unrealistic expectations of child; (3) knowledge deficit

- Social isolation, related to lack of peer group

Sexuality-reproductive pattern

- Sexual dysfunction, potential for, related to (1) misinformation or lack of knowledge; (2) values conflict

This chapter is concerned with two types of handicaps: mental retardation and sensory impairments, in particular, impairments of hearing and vision. Each poses special threats to a child's developmental potential. Without assistance in dealing with the impairments, these children are vulnerable to lifelong disadvantages.

Parents are the major rehabilitators of the child. However, they need guidance and support from specially trained professionals to help the child learn. The nurse is often in a strategic position to prevent and identify mental or sensory disorders, support the family in adjusting to the handicap, and assist them in learning methods of overcoming or compensating for the disability. The major goal is for the child to be valued and reared as a child with unique abilities and as much as possible for the disability to be viewed as a surmountable inconvenience.

MENTAL RETARDATION

Mental retardation is one of the most prevalent handicapping conditions in the United States. An estimated 6.5 million persons, or 3% of the entire population, are mentally retarded. Since mentally retarded children are no longer automatically admitted into institutional settings but often remain at home, parents need role models and adequate preparation to effectively teach the child to function optimally within his environment. Nurses are in a strategic position to assume a vital role in assisting these parents with observation, problem solving, and decision making.

GENERAL CONCEPTS

The most commonly accepted definition of mental retardation by the American Association on Mental Deficiency (AAMD) states that "mental retardation refers to significantly sub-average general intellectual functioning existing concurrently with deficits in adaptive behavior and manifested during the developmental period" (Grossman, 1977). An important aspect of this definition is that it emphasizes both intelligence and behavior as criteria for mental retardation.

According to the AAMD definition, subaverage intelligence is defined as an intelligence quotient (IQ) below a score of 83 or 84, depending on the scale used. According to this one criterion, nearly 16% of the population can be classified as mentally retarded, which provides educational opportunities for a group of children who are usually neglected, such as those defined as "slow learners" or "borderline intelligent."

Classification

Mentally retarded children can be classified according to several criteria. The most useful is classification based on educational potential or symptom severity. The approximate range of IQ for each category is given to familiarize the nurse with scoring standards usually used to diagnose subaverage intelligence. However, the nurse should refrain from using numbers as the criterion for assessing or evaluating the child's abilities, since they provide little value in counseling parents or training retarded children.

Borderline* (IQ 68-83)†. Borderline mentally retarded children are usually called *slow learners*. Although they often exhibit no abnormal delays in development, they tend to achieve marginal success in the regular classroom. Many are found in classes for the educationally handicapped or learning disabled. They usually require special educational assistance within the regular classroom to achieve academic success. They are capable of graduating from high school, learning gainful skilled or semi-skilled labor, and adjusting to social relationships, including marriage and childrearing. However, they may need additional support during major stressful periods during their life.

Mildly retarded (IQ 52-67). Mildly mentally retarded children are also referred to as *educable,* because they are able to benefit from educational programs. They can achieve a mental age of 8 to 12 years. Although they may develop slowly, they have the potential to be assimilated into their community economically and socially. They require educational programs directed toward their adjustment to accepted social interaction patterns and realistic occupational goals, as well as supportive guidance in selecting and holding suitable jobs. On occasion they may require special assistance and guidance to cope with major life crises, but generally they are capable of working in competitive situations and living independent lives. They function well in compatible marital relationships but are usually unable to cope with the responsibilities of childrearing.

Moderately retarded (IQ 36-51). Moderately retarded individuals are referred to as *trainable,* because they can be taught to independently care for their own needs. They can achieve a mental age of 3 to 7 years. Although they may require supervision and support throughout life, they can learn to do meaningful tasks at home and work at appropriate simple jobs such as those in sheltered workshops maintained by community agencies for special work training. Some of these persons may live in special residential care centers, which are available to

---

*Based on classification from American Association on Mental Deficiency.
†According to Stanford-Binet scale.

them when no responsible relative or significant others can be responsible for them.

Severely retarded (IQ 20-35). Children with severe retardation are limited in their language, social skills, motor capabilities, and communication abilities and may have associated physical handicaps. They may have impaired judgment and require help in making important life decisions for themselves. They are certainly capable of learning selected self-care skills and learning to protect themselves within their environment. Although they may need to be placed in residential facilities for various reasons, many of them can live at home under the supervision of their parents.

Profoundly retarded (IQ 0-19). Children who are profoundly retarded generally need complete custodial care or supervision. They exhibit major impairments in physical coordination and in sensorimotor development. They generally require supervised living, whether they live at home or in a specially designed residential facility. They may acquire minimal speech development, but their chances for achieving self-sufficiency are extremely limited.

No matter which set of criteria characterize a retarded child, it is crucial that both nurses and parents capitalize on the child's unique capabilities, strengths, and abilities and carefully evaluate those areas in which he requires help. An individual approach is essential to the child's optimum development.

Causes

In the majority of instances the exact cause of mental retardation is unknown. However, there are general categories of events that may lead to retardation:

1. Infection and intoxication, such as congenital rubella, syphilis, maternal drug consumption (such as excessive alcohol), or chronic lead ingestion
2. Trauma or physical agent, namely injury to the brain suffered during the prenatal, perinatal, or postnatal period
3. Inadequate nutrition and metabolic disorders, such as phenylketonuria
4. Gross postnatal brain disease, such as neurofibromatosis and tuberous sclerosis
5. Unknown prenatal influence, including cerebral and cranial malformations, such as microcephaly and hydrocephalus
6. Gestational disorders, including prematurity, low birth weight, and postmaturity
7. Psychiatric disorders that have their onset during the child's developmental period up to age 18 years
8. Environmental influences, including evidence of a deprived environment associated with a history of mental retardation among parents and siblings
9. Chromosomal abnormalities, such as Down syndrome

NURSING CONSIDERATIONS WITH MENTALLY RETARDED CHILDREN

The goal of caring for retarded children is to promote their optimum development as individuals within a family and community. The nurse is in a vital position to teach parents how to foster learning in their child. The following discussion focuses on principles involved in (1) educating these children, (2) teaching self-care skills, (3) promoting optimum development, (4) helping families adjust to future care, and (5) caring for hospitalized retarded children.

Educate mentally retarded children

In order to teach mentally retarded children, it is necessary to investigate their learning abilities and deficits. This is important for the nurse who may be involved in a home care type of program or who may be caring for the retarded child in a health care setting. The nurse who understands how these children learn can effectively teach them basic skills or prepare them for various health-related procedures.

Retarded children have a marked deficit in their ability to discriminate between two or more stimuli because of difficulty in paying attention to relevant cues. However, these children can learn to discriminate if the cues are presented in an exaggerated concrete form and all extraneous stimuli are eliminated. For example, the use of colors to emphasize visual cues can help them learn. Their deficit in discrimination also implies that concrete ideas are learned much more effectively than abstraction. Therefore, demonstration is preferable to verbal explanation, and learning should be directed toward mastering a skill rather than understanding scientific principles underlying the procedure.

Another deficit of retarded children is in short-term memory. Whereas normal children can remember several words, numbers, or directions at one time, these children are unable to do so. Therefore, they need simple one-step directions. Learning through a step-by-step process requires a *task analysis*, in which each task is separated into its necessary components and each step is taught completely before proceeding to the next activity.

Motivation is also lacking in these children, and reinforcers are often necessary to stimulate their interest in pursuing an activity. Advances in technology have greatly aided in providing reinforcement. With the use of specially designed switches the child is given control of some event in his environment, such as turning on the television (Fig. 17-1). The television becomes reinforcement for activating the switch. Repetitive use of these switches provides an early, simplistic association with a technical device that may progress to increasingly more complex aids. Numerous types of switches are available that enable children

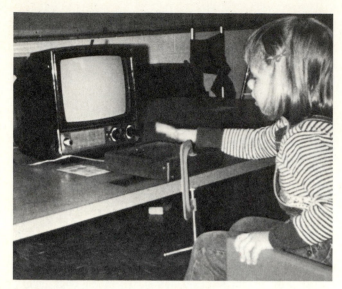

FIG. 17-1

A single push panel allows a retarded child to turn a television on and off.

with physical disabilities to manipulate equipment (Fig. 17-2.)

Promote independent self-help skills

The principal self-help skills are feeding, toileting, dressing, and grooming. Teaching these skills to retarded children requires a basic knowledge of the developmental sequence in learning the skills by normal children. For example, one would not expect a retarded child to be independent in toileting at the usual age for a normal child.

It also necessitates a working knowledge of the individual steps needed to master a skill. For example, before beginning a self-feeding program a task analysis is done. Following a task analysis, the child is observed in a particular situation, such as eating, to determine what skills he possesses and his developmental readiness to learn the task. Parents are included in this process because their ''readiness'' is as important as the child's.

Numerous self-help aids are available to facilitate independence (Fig. 17-3).* While they are not strictly for retarded children, they can be most helpful in eliminating some of the difficulties of learning, such as using a plate with suction cups to prevent accidental spills. They should always be considered when physical impairments also exist.

Specific stimulation programs for learning self-help skills and gross motor development are described in *Nurs-*

---

*One resource is the Professional Self-Help Aids Catalog from Fred Sammons, Inc., Box 32, Brookfield, IL 60513-0032.

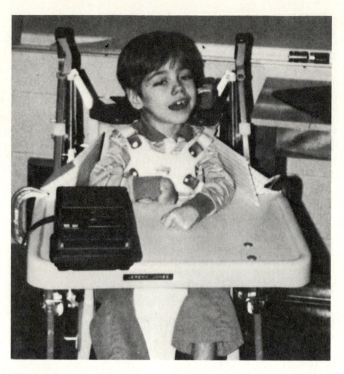

FIG. 17-2

A blade switch allows a retarded child with physical impairments to control a tape recorder.

ing Care of Infants and Children, Chapter 23 (Whaley and Wong, 1983), and other texts devoted to the care of developmentally disabled children. The reader is encouraged to review these sources for a more in-depth discussion of the subject.

Promote optimum development

Optimum development involves more than achieving independence. It requires appropriate guidance for establishing acceptable social behavior and personal feeling of self-esteem, worth, and security. These attributes are not simply learned through a stimulation program; rather they must arise from the genuine love and caring that exists among family members. However, parents need guidance in providing an environment that fosters optimum development. Often it is the nurse who can provide assistance in these areas of childrearing.

Another important area for promoting optimum development and self-esteem is ensuring the child's physical well-being. Any congenital defects should be repaired, such as cardiac, gastrointestinal, or orthopedic anomalies. Plastic surgery should be considered in situations where the child's appearance may be substantially improved. Dental health is very significant, and orthodontic and restorative procedures can immensely improve facial appearance.

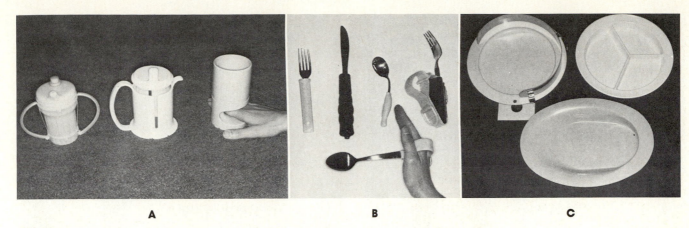

A   B   C

FIG. 17-3

Self-help aids for feeding: **A,** *(from left to right) modified drinking cup, glass with holder and lid, pedestal cup;* **B,** *(from left to right) soft built-up handle utensil, weighted knife, child's bent spoon, Quad-Quip utensil holder (holds most household utensils), (at bottom) vertical palm self-handle utensil;* **C,** *(from left to right, top) plastic plate with suction feet and optional metal food guard, partitioned scoop dish, (at bottom) scoop dish.*

Play. The retarded child has the same needs for play as any other child. However, because of his slower development, parents may be less aware of the need to continue appropriate stimulation. Therefore, the nurse guides parents toward selection of suitable toys and interactive activities. Since play has been discussed for children in each age-group in earlier chapters only the exceptions for the retarded child are presented.

Play is based on the child's developmental age. For the retarded child, the need for sensorimotor play may be prolonged for several years. Parents should use every opportunity to expose the child to as many different sounds, sights, and sensations as possible.

Toys should be selected for their educational value. For example, a large inflatable beach ball is a good water toy, encourages interactive play, and can be used to learn motor skills, such as balance, rocking, kicking, and throwing. Toys should be simple in design so that the child can learn to manipulate them without help. Toys that are too complicated are frustrating to the child. Adapted toys with simple on-off switches provide opportunities for these children to play with a much wider variety of toys (Fig. 17-4).

Safety is a major consideration in selection of play materials. Toys that may be appropriate developmentally may present dangers to a child who is strong enough to break them or use them incorrectly.

Communication. Verbal skills are often delayed more than other physical skills. Speech requires hearing and interpretation (receptive skills) and facial muscle coordination (expressive skills). Both may be impaired in mentally retarded children. These children should have frequent audiometric testing and be fitted with hearing aids

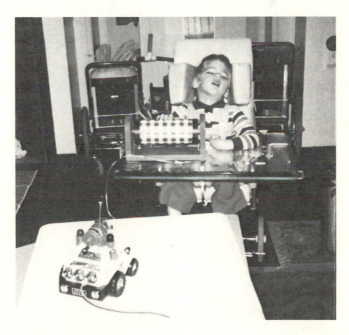

FIG. 17-4

A barrel switch allows a retarded child to play with a battery-operated truck.

if needed. In addition, they may need help in learning to control their facial muscles. For example, in children with Down syndrome the large protruding tongue often interferes with speech. These children may need tongue exercises to correct the tongue thrust or gentle reminders to keep the lips closed.

Nonverbal communication may be appropriate for

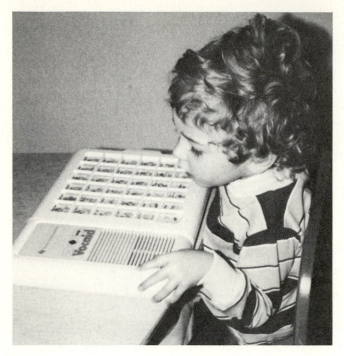

FIG. 17-5
The Vocaid is a communication board with a voice synthesizer. The child pushes the picture he wants and that word or phrase is spoken. Manufactured by Texas Instruments, Dallas, Tex.

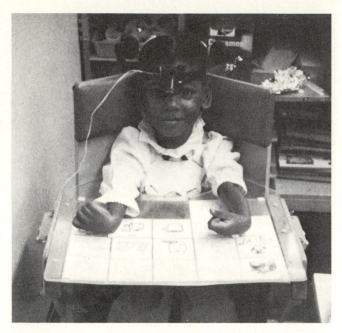

FIG. 17-6
A child with physical impairments can use a communication board by pointing with an optical head pointer.

some of these children and various devices are available. For the child without associated physical disabilities, a talking picture board is helpful (Fig. 17-5). For children with physical handicaps any number of adaptations or types of communication devices are available to facilitate selection of the appropriate picture or word (Fig. 17-6).* Some children may be taught a special method of communication called *Blissymbols*. These graphic symbols are composed from a relatively small number of forms or elements that when used in various combinations represent thousands of meanings. The symbols are not self explanatory and if the child communicates with them the nurse needs to be familiar with them.

Discipline.   Discipline must begin early. For the retarded child, limit-setting measures must be simple, consistent, and appropriate for his age. Control measures are based on teaching a specific behavior—not on understanding the reasons behind it. Stressing moral lessons are of little value to a child who lacks the cognitive skills to learn from self-criticism or from a lesson based on previous

wrongdoing. Behavior modification is an excellent technique for limit setting.

Socialization.   Parents are encouraged early to teach their child socially acceptable behavior, such as waving good-bye, saying hello and thank you, responding to his name, greeting visitors but not being overly affectionate, and sitting modestly. The greatest teaching method is being a role model combined with giving gentle, consistent reminders to perform the behavior.

Dressing and grooming are also important aspects of socialization. A child who is dressed in appropriate-age clothing and well-groomed is much more likely to be accepted and to develop good self-esteem. Clothes should be clean, up-to-date, and well-fitted. Many attractive outfits can be adapted with Velcro fasteners and elastic openings to facilitate self-dressing.*

Children of all ages need peer relationships and retarded children are no exception. Prior to preschool age the parents should contact the nearest day-training center or special school. Not only do these centers provide appropriate education and training, they also offer an opportunity for social experiences among the children.

As the child grows older, he should have peer expe-

---

*A resource for information about communication devices is by Vanderheiden, G.C., editor: Non-vocal communication resource book, Baltimore, 1978, University Park Press.

*A helpful book is Hotte, E: Self-help clothing, available from The National Easter Seal Society, 2023 W. Odgen Avenue, Chicago, IL 60612.

riences similar to those of normal children, including group outings, sports, and organized activity, such as Boy Scouts, Girl Scouts, or Special Olympics for retarded children. He should be encouraged to form a close relationship with a best friend.

Adolescence may be a particularly difficult time for parents, especially in terms of the child's sexual behavior, possibility of pregnancy, future plans to marry, and ability to be independent. Frequently little anticipatory guidance has been offered parents to prepare the child for physical and sexual maturation. The nurse can help in this area by providing parents with information about sex education that is geared to the child's developmental level. For example, the adolescent female needs a *simple* explanation of menstruation and instructions on personal hygiene during the menstrual cycle.*

The question of contraceptive protection for female retarded adolescents is often a parental concern. Of the available methods, the intrauterine device (IUD) or birth control pills are the most satisfactory. However, both have their disadvantages. The IUD requires regular checking of the string's placement and can cause menorrhagia. Birth control pills must be used regularly; their effectiveness can be maximized by devising reminder charts or by using dated pill dispensers. Sterilization as a form of contraception is a special dilemma because of moral and ethical questions as well as psychologic effects on the adolescent. The decision regarding sterilization of minors and incompetent adults is a legal one; if parents consider permanent sterilization for their mentally retarded daughter, she should be included in the decision according to her level of understanding.

Because of the embarrassment some parents feel regarding sexual information, many concerns may go unmentioned. The nurse can be instrumental in discussing topics such as contraception or advisability of marriage with them and the adolescent. In this way plans can be made early and potential problems avoided.

Help families adjust to future care

Not all families are able to cope with home care of a retarded child, especially one who is severely or profoundly retarded and/or multihandicapped. Older parents may not be able to assume care responsibilities once they reach retirement or old age. For these parents, the decision regarding residential placement is a difficult one.

There are a number of alternatives to living at home. For children under age 18 years, these include (1) foster homes (private homes with a full-time family-type care program for less than five children), (2) group foster homes (full-time family-type homes for five to eight children); (3) child-welfare institutions, (4) boarding homes (homes for one to four children who need a place to live while attending a specialized school program), and (5) temporary-care homes (short-term care for one to four children to relieve the family or to provide emergency housing while plans are made for more permanent living arrangements).

For persons over 18 years there are additional types of residential programs. The nurse working with a family should help them investigate and evaluate various programs, in addition to assisting them in their adjustment to the decision for placement.

Caring for hospitalized retarded children

Caring for retarded children during hospitalization is a special challenge to nurses. Frequently nurses are unfamiliar with retarded children and cope with their feelings of insecurity and fear by ignoring or isolating the retarded child. Not only is this approach nonsupportive, it may also be destructive for the child's sense of self-esteem and optimum development and in terms of the parents' ability to cope with the stress of the experience. One method successfully avoiding this nontherapeutic approach is to use the mutual participation model in planning the child's care. Parents should be encouraged to room with their child but should not be made to feel as if the responsibility is totally theirs.

When the child is admitted, a detailed history is taken (see Chapter 18), especially in terms of all self-help activity. During the interview the nurse simultaneously assesses the child's developmental age. It is best to avoid directly asking about IQ levels, since this may make the parents uncomfortable and often tells little about the child's actual abilities. Questions are approached positively. For example, rather than asking, ''Is he toilet trained yet?'' the nurse may state, ''Tell me about his toileting habits.'' The assessment should also focus on any special devices the child uses, effective measures of limit setting, unusual or favorite routines, and any behaviors that may require intervention. For example, if the parent states that the child engages in self-stimulatory activities, the nurse inquires about events that precipitate them and techniques that the parents use to manage them.

The child's functional level of eating and playing, his ability to express verbally his needs, his progress in toilet training, and his relationship with objects, toys, and other children are also assessed. He is encouraged to be as independent as possible, even though he is in a hospital setting. If the child has already accomplished self-help skills

*A helpful book on this subject is Pattulio, A.: Puberty in the girl who is retarded, available from the National Association of Retarded Citizens, 2709 Avenue E East, P.O. Box 6109, Arlington, TX 76011.

in eating, he should continue to eat with a spoon or a fork. He is also encouraged to be independent in his toileting functions and to make his needs known.

Realizing that the child may be lonely in the hospital, the nurse makes certain that he has toys and other activities to entertain him, is included in group activities on the ward, and sets time aside each day to talk to or play with him. He is placed in a room with other children of approximate developmental age, preferably an area with two beds, to avoid overstimulation. The nurse discusses with the other parents the retarded child's abilities and introduces the parents and children to each other. By the nurse's example of treating the retarded child with dignity and respect, others who may be fearful of what they do not understand are encouraged to accept the child.

Procedures are explained to the child using methods of communication that are at his cognitive level. Generally explanations should be simple, short, and concrete, emphasizing what the child will experience *physically*. Demonstration either through actual practice or with visual aids is always preferable to verbal explanation. The nurse repeats instructions often and evaluates the child's understanding by asking questions such as, "What did I say it will feel like?" "What will the doctor look like?" "Show me how you must lie." "Where will the dressing be?" and so on. Parents are included in preprocedural teaching for their own learning and to help the nurse learn effective methods of communicating with the child.

During hospitalization the nurse should also focus on growth-promoting experiences for the child. For example, hospitalization may be an excellent opportunity to emphasize to parents abilities that the child does have but has not had the opportunity to practice, such as self-dressing. It may also be an opportunity for social experiences with peers, group play, or new educational/recreational activities. For example, one child who had the habit of screaming and kicking demonstrated a definite decrease in those behaviors after he learned to pound pegs and use a punching bag. Through social services the parents may become aware of specialized programs for the child. Nutritional counseling is available if the child is overweight or has evidence of specific deficiencies, such as iron deficiency. Hospitalization may also offer parents a respite from everyday care responsibilities and an opportunity to discuss their feelings with a concerned professional.

DOWN SYNDROME

Down syndrome is the most common chromosomal abnormality of a generalized syndrome, occurring once in every 600 to 650 live births. It owes its once common but unacceptable name, *mongolism,* to the particular facial characteristics, which resemble those of the Mongol race.

Etiology

About 95% of all cases of Down syndrome are attributable to an extra chromosome 21 (group G), hence the name *trisomy 21*. Trisomy 21 is associated with advanced maternal age, particularly over 35 years of age. Recent evidence is demonstrating that paternal aging is also responsible for some cases of Down syndrome. About 4% of the cases may be caused by *translocation* of chromosomes 15 and 21 or 22. This type of genetic aberration is usually hereditary and is not associated with maternal age. A small percentage of persons with this disorder are called *mosaics,* because their cells show both normal and abnormal chromosomes on analysis. As a rule mosaicism is associated with significantly higher intellectual potential and fewer physical difficulties than the other two types.

For a more detailed study of genetic transmission, see Chapter 3.

Clinical manifestations

Down syndrome can usually be diagnosed by the clinical manifestations alone, but a chromosomal analysis should be done to confirm the genetic abnormality if the parents are young or if the diagnosis is doubtful, as in mosaic transmission. The principal physical findings include (see also Fig. 17-7):

- a small rounded skull with a flat occiput
- inner epicanthal folds and oblique palpebral fissures (upward, outward slant of the eyes)
- speckling of the iris (Brushfield's spots)
- small nose with a depressed bridge (saddle nose)
- a protruding, sometimes fissured, tongue
- small, sometimes low-set ears
- short, thick neck
- hypotonic musculature (protuding abdomen, umbilical hernia)
- hyperflexible and lax joints
- simian line (transverse crease on the palmar side of the hand; see Fig. 5-11, *B*)
- broad, short, and stubby hands and feet
- delayed or incomplete sexual development (menstruation usually occurs at the average age; affected women have had offspring and the majority of them were born with some type of abnormality; men with Down syndrome are infertile)

Several physical problems are associated with Down syndrome. Many of these children have congenital heart malformations, the most common being septal defects. Respiratory infections are very prevalent and account for the high morbidity in these children. When combined with cardiac anomalies, it is the chief cause of death, particularly during the first year of life. Hypotonicity of chest and abdominal muscles probably predisposes to the development of respiratory infection.

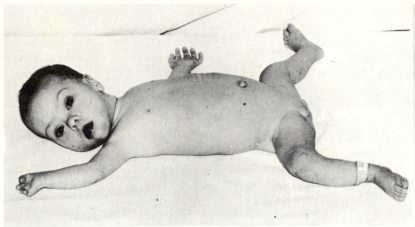
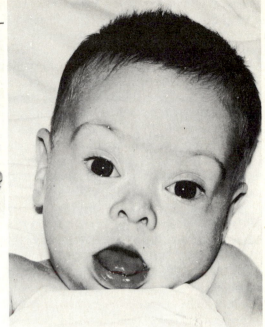

FIG. 17-7

Down syndrome in newborn. **A,** *Floppy, hypotonic newborn.* **B,** *Small, square head with mongoloid slant to the eyes, flat nasal bridge, and protruding tongue. (From Reisman, L.E., and Matheny, A.P.: Genetics and counseling in medical practice, St. Louis, 1969, The C.V. Mosby Co.)*

Structural defects such as renal agenesis, duodenal atresia, aganglionic megacolon (Hirschsprung's disease), and tracheoesophageal fistula are common. The incidence of different types of leukemia is about 15 times more frequent. Visual defects include strabismus, myopia, nystagmus, or cataracts. Inflammation of the conjunctiva and lids occurs frequently. There is a high incidence of hearing loss, principally of the conductive type.

The most significant feature of Down syndrome is mental retardation. Degrees of mental retardation differ, but the IQ is generally within the trainable range.

Nursing considerations

Caring for the child with Down syndrome involves several short- and long-term goals. Support for parents from health professionals, especially nurses, is increasingly more important with the present trend to rear these children at home. This discussion focuses on supporting parents at the time of diagnosis and preventing physical problems in the child. Long-term interventions for the child with mental retardation are discussed later in this chapter.

Support parents at time of diagnosis. Because of the unique physical characteristics, the infant with Down syndrome is usually diagnosed at birth. However, parents are not always informed of the diagnosis at this time. This presents special difficulties for those caring for the postpartal mother, since she or the father may notice differences in the child and question others about their concern.

Generally parents wish to know the diagnosis as soon

as possible. This approach prevents such dilemmas as telling others that the child has Down syndrome after indicating that he was fine and experiencing unconfirmed doubt over the child's development. Most parents prefer that both of them be present during the informing interview because it is a problem that both of them will have to face, they can emotionally support one another, and it eliminates the difficult task of revealing the diagnosis to the other partner. They appreciate receiving reading material about the syndrome* and being referred to others for help or advice, such as parent groups or professional counseling.

Once parents are aware of the diagnosis, they are confronted with the crisis of losing a perfect or dream child and grieving for and accepting their reality child. Consequently, the parents' responses to the child may greatly influence decisions regarding future care. Whereas some families willingly wish to take the child home, others consider immediate institutionalization. The nurse must carefully answer questions regarding developmental potential and institutionalization, since the responses may influence the parents' decision. It is important to stress to parents that a decision regarding placement will affect all of their lives and need not be made at the time of diagnosis.

Assist parents in preventing physical problems. Many of the physical characteristics of Down syndrome present nursing problems. The hypotonicity of muscles and hyperextensibility of joints complicate posi-

---

*Several books are available. One that is written very positively in terms of home care and includes a list of other references is Pitt, D.: Your Down syndrome child, available from the National Association for Retarded Citizens.

tioning. The limp, flaccid extremities resemble the posture of a rag doll; as a result, holding the infant is difficult and cumbersome. Sometimes parents perceive this lack of molding to their bodies as evidence of inadequate parenting. The extended body position promotes heat loss because more surface area is exposed to the environment. Parents are encouraged to swaddle or wrap the infant tightly in a blanket before picking him up to provide security and warmth. The nurse also discusses with parents their feelings concerning attachment to the child, emphasizing that the child's lack of clinging or molding is a physical characteristic, not a sign of detachment or rejection.

Decreased muscle tone compromises respiratory expansion. In addition, the underdeveloped nasal bone causes a chronic problem of inadequate drainage of mucus. The constant stuffy nose forces the child to breathe by mouth, which dries the oropharyngeal membranes, increasing the susceptibility to upper respiratory infections. Measures to lessen these problems include clearing the nose with a bulb-type syringe, rinsing the mouth with water after feedings, using a cool-mist vaporizer to keep the mucous membranes moist and the secretions liquefied, changing the child's position frequently, and performing postural drainage and percussion. If antibiotics are ordered, the importance of completing the full course of therapy for successful eradication of the infection and prevention of growth of resistant organisms is stressed.

Inadequate drainage and pooling of mucus in the nose also interfere with feeding. Because the child breathes by mouth, he is unable to suck for any length of time as a result of his need for air. When eating solids, he may gag on the food because of mucus in the oropharynx. Parents are advised to clear the nose before each feeding, give small, frequent feedings, and allow opportunities for rest at mealtime.

The large, protruding tongue also interferes with feeding, especially of solid foods. Parents need to know that the tongue thrust is not an indication of refusal to feed, but a physiologic response. Parents are advised to use a small but long, straight-handled spoon to push the food toward the back and side of the mouth. If food is thrust out, it is refed.

Dietary intake needs supervision. Decreased muscle tone affects gastric motility, predisposing the child to constipation. Dietary measures such as increased residue and fluid promote evacuation. The child's eating habits may need careful scrutiny to prevent obesity. Height and weight measurements should be obtained on a serial basis, especially during infancy, since excessive weight gain can impede motor development. The child should receive calories in accordance with his height and weight, not his chronologic age.

During infancy the child's skin is pliable and soft.

However, it gradually becomes rough and dry and is prone to cracking and infection. Skin care involves the use of minimum soap and application of lubricants. Lip balm is applied to the lips, especially when the child is outdoors, to prevent excessive chapping.

Prevention. There is no cure for Down syndrome. However, through amniocentesis, chromosomal analysis of fetal cells can detect the presence of trisomy or translocation. The nurse has a role in genetic counseling of those parents of advanced age or who have a family history of the disorder to discuss the possibility of amniocentesis. If the fetus is affected, the nurse must allow the parents to express their feelings concerning elective abortion and support their decision either to terminate or proceed with the pregnancy.

SENSORY IMPAIRMENTS

Sensory impairments pose special threats to a child's developmental potential. Deprived of visual or auditory cues, the child must rely more heavily on other sensory experiences to learn about and relate to his environment. Without assistance and rehabilitation, these children are vulnerable to the lifelong disadvantages of being a handicapped individual. However, with assistance they can lead essentially normal and productive lives.

HEARING IMPAIRMENT

Hearing impairment is the most frequent handicap in the United States. It is estimated that 3 million children have some degree of hearing loss. The number of school-age children with subnormal hearing is approximately 5%. Such figures support the need for nurses' knowledge of and intervention in hearing disorders.

Classification of hearing defects

Hearing defects may be classified according to etiology, pathology, or symptom severity. Each is important in terms of treatment, possible prevention, and rehabilitation.

Etiology. Hearing loss may be caused by a number of prenatal and postnatal conditions. These include a family history of childhood hearing impairment, anatomic malformations of the head or neck, low birth weight, severe perinatal asphyxia, perinatal infection (cytomegalovirus, rubella, herpes, syphilis, toxoplasmosis, and bacterial meningitis), chronic ear infection, cerebral palsy, Down syndrome, or administration of ototoxic drugs.

Another significant potential cause is excessive expo-

SUMMARY OF NURSING CARE OF THE CHILD WITH DOWN SYNDROME

GOALS	RESPONSIBILITIES
Assist with diagnosis	Observe for physical characteristics Observe for signs of structural defects
Support parents at time of diagnosis	Accompany parents at informing conference Give the parents written information about syndrome Discuss with the parents benefits of home care vs institutionalization; allow them opportunities to investigate all residential alternatives before making a decision Encourage the parents to meet other families with Down children Refrain from giving definitive answers about the degree of retardation; stress the potential learning abilities of retarded children, especially with early stimulation Demonstrate acceptance of infant through own example Emphasize normal characteristics of child
Prevent physical problems associated with syndrome Respiratory infections	Teach the parents postural drainage and percussion Stress importance of changing child's position frequently, especially sitting posture Encourage use of cool-mist vaporizer Teach suctioning of nares Stress importance of good mouth care (follow feedings with clear water)
Feeding difficulties	Suction nares before each feeding Schedule small frequent feedings; allow the child to rest during feedings Feed solid food by pushing it to back and side of mouth; use long, straight-handled infant spoon Point out to the parents that tongue thrust does not indicate refusal of food Calculate caloric needs to meet energy requirements; base intake on height and weight, not chronologic age Monitor height and weight at regular intervals Provide sufficient bulk and fluids to prevent constipation
Skin breakdown	Keep skin well lubricated with topical creams or lotions Use soap sparingly Apply lip balm when the child is outdoors
Promote optimum development	Involve the child and parents in an early infant stimulation program Assess the child's developmental progress at regular intervals; keep detailed records to distinguish subtle changes in functioning Help the parents set realistic goals for the child Encourage learning of self-care skills as soon as child achieves readiness Encourage the parents to investigate special daycare programs and education classes as soon as possible; point out that toilet training may be a prerequisite to eligibility Emphasize child's needs for play, discipline, social interaction Before adolescence, counsel the child and parents regarding physical maturation, sexual behavior, marriage, and family Encourage optimum vocational training
Help family prepare for future care of child	As the child grows older, discuss with the parents options to home care, especially as the parents near retirement or old age Help the family investigate residential settings other than institutionalization Encourage the family to include retarded member in planning and to continue meaningful relationships with him after placement
Prevent Down syndrome	Discuss with high-risk women risks of giving birth to child with Down syndrome Encourage all pregnant women at risk (age over 35 years, family history of Down syndrome, or previous birth of child with Down syndrome) to consider amniocentesis during twelfth to sixteenth week of pregnancy to rule out Down syndrome in fetus Discuss option of elective abortion with women who are carrying an affected fetus Discuss with parents of adolescent children with Down syndrome the possibility of conception in a female and the need for contraceptive methods

TABLE 17-1. INTENSITY OF SOUNDS EXPRESSED IN DECIBELS

DECIBELS (dB)	REPRESENTATIVE SOUND
0	Softest sound normal ear can hear
10	Heartbeat, rustling of leaves
20	Whisper at 1.8 M (5 feet)
30-45	Normal conversation
60	Noise in average restaurant
70-80	Street noises
80	Loud radio in home
90-100	Train
120	Thunder, rock music
140	Jet airplane during departure
>140	Pain threshold

TABLE 17-2. CLASSIFICATION OF HEARING LOSS BASED ON SYMPTOM SEVERITY

HEARING LEVEL (dB)	EFFECT
Slight—<30 (hard of hearing)	Has difficulty in hearing faint or distant speech Usually is unaware of hearing difficulty Likely to achieve in school but may have problems No speech defects
Mild—30-55 (hard of hearing)	Understands conversational speech at 3 to 5 feet but has difficulty if speech faint or not facing speaker May have speech difficulties
Moderate—55-70 (hard of hearing)	Unable to understand conversational speech unless loud Considerable difficulty with group or classroom discussion Requires special speech training
Severe—70-90 (deaf)	May hear a loud voice if nearby May be able to identify loud environmental noises Can distinguish vowels but not most consonants Requires speech training
Profound—>90 (deaf)	May hear only loud sounds Requires extensive speech training

sure to high noise levels. This may occur from urban living, loud rock music, model airplanes, snowmobiles, sport shooting, motorcycle and sport racing, or heavy machinery.

In addition, high-risk neonates who are surviving formerly fatal prenatal or perinatal conditions may be susceptible to hearing loss from the disorder or its treatment. For example, sensorineural hearing loss may be the result of continuous humming noises or high noise levels associated with incubators, oxygen hoods, or intensive care units, especially when combined with the use of potentially ototoxic antibiotics.

Pathology. Disorders of hearing are divided according to location of the defect. *Conductive* or middle-ear hearing loss results from interference of transmission of sound to the middle ear. It is the most common of all types of hearing loss and most frequently is a result of recurrent serous otitis media. Conductive hearing impairment mainly involves interference with loudness of sound. Consequently, hearing is improved with the use of a hearing aid to amplify sound.

Sensorineural hearing loss, also called perceptive or nerve deafness, involves damage to the inner ear structures and/or the auditory nerve. The most common causes are congenital defects of inner ear structures or consequences of acquired conditions, such as kernicterus, infection, administration of ototoxic drugs, or exposure to excessive noise.

Sensorineural hearing loss results in distortion of sound and problems in discrimination. Although the child hears some of everything going on around him, the sounds are distorted, severely affecting discrimination and comprehension. Since the defect is not one of intensity of sound, hearing aids are of little value in improving discrimination, since they merely amplify distorted sounds.

Mixed conductive-sensorineural hearing loss results from interference with transmission of sound in the middle ear and along neural pathways. It frequently results from recurrent otitis media and its complications.

Central auditory imperception includes all hearing losses that do not demonstrate defects in the conductive or sensorineural structures. They are usually divided into organic or functional losses. In the organic type of central auditory imperception, the defect involves the reception of auditory stimuli along the central pathways and the expression of the message into meaningful communication. Examples are *aphasia,* an inability to express ideas in any form, either written or verbally; *agnosia,* the inability to interpret sound correctly; and *dysacusis,* difficulty in processing details or discrimination among sounds.

In the functional type there is no organic lesion to explain a central auditory loss. Examples of functional hearing loss are conversion hysteria (an unconscious withdrawal from hearing to block remembrance of a traumatic event), infantile autism, and childhood schizophrenia.

Symptom severity. Hearing impairment is expressed in decibels (dB), a unit of loudness (Table 17-1).

Hearing impairment can be classified according to hearing-threshold level (the measurement of an individual's hearing threshold by means of an audiometer) and the degree of symptom severity as it affects speech (Table 17-2). These classifications offer general guidelines regarding the effect of the impairment on any individual child, since children differ greatly in their ability to use residual hearing.

NURSING CONSIDERATIONS WITH HEARING-IMPAIRED CHILDREN

Nursing intervention with hearing-impaired children is often a specialized area, requiring additional training in hearing assessment and rehabilitation. However, general nursing goals that focus on prevention, detection, and rehabilitation of the child with a hearing impairment are every nurse's responsibility. In addition, nurses may have to care for a hearing-impaired child who is hospitalized and must know how to best meet the child and family's special needs.

Prevention

The primary nursing role is prevention of hearing loss. Since the most common cause of impaired hearing is chronic otitis media, it is essential that appropriate measures be instituted to treat existing infections and prevent recurrences (see Chapter 12). Children with a history of other conditions known to increase the risk of hearing impairment should receive periodic auditory testing.

Detection

Aside from prevention, the most important nursing responsibility is detection. Discovery of a hearing impairment within the first 6 to 12 months of life is essential to prevent social, physical, and psychologic damage to the child. Detection involves (1) isolating those children who by virtue of their history are at risk, (2) observing for behaviors that indicate a hearing loss, and (3) screening all children for auditory function. This discussion focuses on developmental/behavioral indices associated with hearing impairment. Tests for assessing hearing are included in Chapter 5.

Infancy. At birth the nurse can observe the neonate's response to auditory stimuli as evidenced by the startle reflex, head turning, eye blinking, and cessation of body movement. The infant may vary in the intensity of his response, depending on his state of alertness. However, a consistent absence of a reaction should lead to suspicion of hearing loss. Other danger signals suggesting hearing problems in the developing infant include the following:

1. Persistence of the Moro reflex beyond age 4 months
2. Failure to be awakened or disturbed by loud environmental sounds during the first 4 months
3. Failure to turn the face toward a source of sound by age 6 months
4. Absence of babbling or voice inflection by age 7 months
5. Inability to understand words or short phrases by age 12 months
6. Consistent use of gestures rather than verbalization to indicate wants after age 15 months

Childhood. The profoundly deaf child is much more likely to be diagnosed during infancy than the less severely affected one. If the defect is not detected during early childhood, the likelihood is that it will surface during entry to school, when the child has difficulty in learning. Unfortunately some of these children are erroneously placed in special classes for the learning disabled or the mentally retarded. Therefore, it is essential that the nurse suspect a hearing impairment in any child who demonstrates the following behaviors:

1. Shows less interest than his peers in casual conversation
2. Is often inattentive unless the environment is quiet and the speaker is close to the child
3. Is more responsive to movement than to sound
4. Observes the speaker's face intently, responding more to facial expression than verbalization
5. Often asks to have statements repeated
6. May not follow directions exactly
7. Tends to be shy, withdrawn, timid, and dreamy
8. Talks in a very loud or very soft voice
9. Does not respond when called from another room
10. Turns the same ear toward sounds
11. Tends to avoid social interaction with other children
12. In response to the frustration of not being able to make others understand him, may develop temper tantrums, yelling, head banging, or other behavioral patterns

Of primary importance is the effect of hearing impairment on speech development. A child with a mild conductive hearing loss may speak fairly clearly but in a loud voice. A child with a sensorineural defect usually has difficulty in articulation. For example, inability to hear higher frequencies may result in the word ''spoon'' being pronounced ''poon.'' Children with articulation problems need to have their hearing tested.

Since exposure to excessive noise pollution is a cause of sensorineural hearing loss, the nurse should routinely assess the possibility of environmental noise pollution and advise children and parents of the potential danger. Signals suggesting exposure to excessive noise are ringing or buzzing in the ears and/or perceiving sounds as muffled or dull after leaving the source of the noise. When individuals engage in activities associated with high-intensity noise, such as flying model airplanes, target shooting, or snow-

SUMMARY OF NURSING CARE OF THE HEARING-IMPAIRED CHILD

GOALS	RESPONSIBILITIES
Prevention	
Prenatal	Identify pregnant women at risk
	Counsel pregnant women regarding risk of ingesting ototoxic medications
	Isolate pregnant women from exposure to rubella if their immune titers are low
	Encourage immunization of all females against rubella
Childhood	Participate in immunization programs for children
	Assess hearing ability of children who are receiving ototoxic antibiotics
	Promote compliance with treatment regimens for otitis media
	Discuss with parents measures to prevent otitis media
	Evaluate auditory ability of children prone to chronic ear or respiratory problems
	Assess sources of excessive noise in child's environment; institute appropriate measures to decrease sound levels (turn music lower, use ear protection)
Detection	
Infancy	At birth assess the neonate's response to a loud noise; observe for signs associated with congenital deafness
	At each well-baby visit assess orientation responses; as early as possible administer hearing tests and refer for audiometry
Childhood	Listen carefully to the parents' concerns regarding hearing loss
	Take a thorough history regarding factors that support an auditory impairment
	Evaluate speech development
	Observe for behaviors that may suggest a hearing impairment
Rehabilitation	
Assist the family in adjusting to child's loss of hearing	Anticipate the usual grief reaction to loss
	Help the parents deal with any guilt feelings regarding previous responses to the child when true nature of the problem was unknown
	Help the parents realize extent of the child's disability and its tremendous influence on speech and language development
	Discuss advantages and limitations of amplifying devices with different types of hearing loss
	Encourage formal rehabilitation as soon as possible
Promote parent-child attachment	Help parents identify clues other than verbal ones that signify infant's communication with them
	Encourage the parents to stimulate the child with visual and tactile cues; stress importance of continuing to talk to the child even though he may not hear their voice
	Encourage the parents to discuss their feelings regarding attachment process
Promote communication process	Encourage both parents to attend the rehabilitation program in order to continue learning in the home; encourage them to learn sign language
	Teach language that serves a useful purpose
	Encourage use of language and books in the home
	Encourage spontaneous language but correct speech impairments
Facilitate lipreading	Attract the child's attention before speaking
	Speak clearly and distinctly; do not exaggerate pronunciation or rhythm of words
	Stand at eye level with the child
	Face the child directly; do not turn away to show him something while talking or move back and forth
	Ensure that the speaker's face is well illuminated
	Stand close to the child while speaking, but do not shout
	Test the child for visual problems that may interfere with learning to lip-read or use sign language

SUMMARY OF NURSING CARE OF THE HEARING-IMPAIRED CHILD—cont'd

GOALS	RESPONSIBILITIES
Maximize residual hearing	Help the family investigate reliable hearing aid dealers Discuss types of hearing aids and their proper care Teach the child how to regulate hearing aid for maximum benefit Help the child focus on all sounds in his environment and talk to him about them For the older child discuss methods of camouflaging the aid to make it less conspicuous
Promote independence and development	Help the family apply normal childrearing practices to this child Emphasize importance of attaining independence in self-care Provide the child with devices that foster independence (hearing ear dog, special signaling aids for telephone or door bell) Discuss importance of discipline and limit setting
Provide opportunities for play and socialization	Guide the parents in selection of toys that maximize visual and tactile senses, as well as residual hearing Encourage the child to participate in group activities; help him follow group discussion by pointing out the speaker and arranging the group in a semicircle Help him develop friendships among hearing and deaf peers Help him achieve a sense of security in his ability to compete with his peers
Encourage education within a regular classroom	Discuss with the teacher ways of communicating effectively with the child (such as through facilitating lipreading) Promote socialization with his classmates
Provide emotional support	Be available to the family for assistance Encourage family members to discuss their feelings regarding the disability Stress the child's abilities rather than disability to promote self-esteem If following the family on a longitudinal basis, become familiar with techniques used for communication Refer the family to appropriate community agencies for medical, psychiatric, educational, vocational, or financial assistance Involve the parents in a local parent group for deaf children

mobiling, they should wear ear protection such as earmuffs or earplugs (not ordinary dry cotton).

Rehabilitation

Once the diagnosis of hearing impairment is made, parents need extensive support to adjust to the shock of learning about their child's disability and an opportunity to realize the extent of the hearing loss. The nurse's initial role in rehabilitation is to help the family accept the defect and participate in an auditory training program.* Rehabilitation training consists of using a hearing aid and learning lipreading (speech reading), sign language, and verbal communication.

Hearing aids. The nurse should be familiar with the types of hearing aids. These include ones worn in or behind the ear, models incorporated into an eyeglass frame, or types that are worn on the body with a wire connection to the ear. Several sources of information are available, such as the National Hearing Aid Society† and the American Speech-Language-Hearing Association.‡

Lipreading. Even though the child may become expert at lipreading, only about 40% of the spoken word is understood, and less if the speaker has an accent, mustache, or beard. Exaggerating pronunciation or speaking in an altered rhythm further lessens comprehension.

Sign language. The child who is severely or profoundly deaf is usually taught sign language and is encouraged to supplement talking with his mouth with "talking" using his hands. Family members are encouraged to learn sign language.

---

*Home training correspondence programs are sponsored by the John T. Tracy Clinic, 806 West Adams Blvd., Los Angeles, CA 90007. Another source of information on several aspects of hearing loss and on the International Parents' Organization is the Alexander Graham Bell Association for the Deaf, 3417 Volta Place, Washington, DC 20007.

---

†20361 Middlebelt, Livonia, MI 48152.
‡10801 Rockville Pike, Rockville, MD 20852.

Speech therapy. The most formidable task in the education of a deaf child is learning to speak. Speech is learned through a multisensory approach, using visual, tactile, kinesthetic, and auditory stimulation. Since the usual mechanism for learning language (imitation and reinforcement) is not available to the deaf child systematic formal education is required. Parents are encouraged to participate fully in the learning process.

Additional aids. Everyday activities present problems to the older child. For example, he may not be able to hear the telephone, doorbell, or alarm clock. Several commercial devices are available to help the deaf person adjust to these dilemmas. Flashing lights can be attached to a telephone or doorbell to signal its ringing. Recently trained hearing ear dogs have provided great assistance to deaf individuals because they alert the person to sounds, such as someone approaching, a moving car, a signal to wake up, and a child's cry. Special teletypewriters help deaf people communicate with each other over the telephone because the typed message is conveyed via the telephone lines.

Any audiovisual medium presents dilemmas to the child because while he can see the picture, he cannot hear the message. However, *closed captioning* is one solution. Through a special decoding device the audio portion of a television program is translated into captions (subtitles) that appear on the screen.*

As the deaf child learns to compensate for his lack of hearing, he becomes extremely perceptive to visual and vibratory changes. He often knows when another person wishes to talk to him because the person will walk close by him but not pass. He learns to be alert to other people approaching him by seeing their shadows or feeling the vibrations of their footsteps. He is acutely aware of facial expressions and may comprehend the unspoken word more quickly than the spoken word.

Socialization. The child with a hearing impairment may need special help in school or social activities. Since lipreading is the main mode of receptive communication, the environment should facilitate visualization of the speaker's face, such as good lighting, favorable seating close to the speaker, and as much eye contact as possible. Since many of these children are able to attend regular classes, the teacher may need assistance in adapting methods of teaching for the child's benefit, such as speaking while facing the class, standing still rather than walking back and forth, and refraining from speaking when turning away from the group.

When the child is in a group setting, it is helpful for the other members to sit in a semicircle in front of him so that he can see their faces. Since one of the difficulties in following a group discussion is that the deaf child is unaware of who speaks next, it helps to have someone point out each speaker. This can inconspicuously be accomplished by giving each speaker a number or using his name and marking this down as that person talks. If one person writes down the main topic of the discussion, the child is able to follow lipreading more closely. Such suggestions can increase the child's ability to participate in sports, clubs such as Boy or Girl Scouts, and group projects.

Caring for hospitalized deaf children

The needs of the hospitalized deaf child are the same as those of any other child, but his disability presents special challenges to the nurse. For example, verbal explanations as the primary method of preparation for admission or procedures must be supplemented with tactile and visual aids, such as books or actual demonstration and practice. The child's understanding of the explanation needs to be constantly reassessed. If the child's verbal skills are poorly developed, he can answer questions through drawing, writing, or gesturing. For example, if the nurse is attempting to clarify where a spinal tap is done, the child is asked to point to where the doctor will insert the needle. Since deaf children often need more time to grasp the full meaning of an explanation, the nurse is careful not to judge the slowness as a sign of retardation and to allow ample time for understanding.

When communicating with the child, the same principles are used as those that are outlined for facilitating lipreading. Ideally, nurses without foreign accents should be assigned to the child. The child's hearing aid is checked to assure that it is working properly. If it is necessary to awaken the child at night, the nurse gently shakes him to signal his or her presence or turns on the hearing aid before arousing the child and always makes sure that the child can see him or her before any procedures, even routine ones such as changing a diaper or regulating an infusion, are performed. It is important to remember that the child may not be aware of one's presence until alerted through visual or tactile cues.

Ideally parents are encouraged to room with the child. However, it must be conveyed to them that this is not to serve as a convenience to the nurse but as a benefit to the child. Although the parents' aid can be enlisted in familiarizing the child with the hospital and explaining procedures, the nurse also talks directly to him, encouraging expression of his feelings about the experience. If there is difficulty in understanding the child's speech, an effort is made to become familiar with his pronunciation of words. Parents often can be helpful by explaining the child's usual speech habits.

---

*Additional information is available from the National Captioning Institute, Inc., 5203 Leesburg Pike, Falls Church, VA 22041.

The nurse honestly admits if the child cannot be understood, and encourages him to write his statements. However, at no time is it implied that the child's speech is imperfect. Rather let the child know that it will take some time to become familiar with his words and that in the meantime he can help by using gestures or written messages. Expressing an interest in learning sign language, especially useful words, such as yes, no, water, and toilet, not only improves communication efforts but greatly strengthens the nurse-child-parent relationship. Nonvocal communication devices are also available that employ pictures or words that the child can point to (see Fig. 17-5). Such boards can also be made up by drawing pictures or writing the words of common needs on cardboard, such as parent, food, water, or toilet.

The nurse has a special role as child advocate with the deaf and is in a strategic position to alert other health team members and other patients to the child's special needs regarding communication. For example, the nurse should accompany the physician on visits to the child's room to ensure that the physician speaks to the child and that the child understands what was said. Not infrequently caregivers forget that the child has the abilities to perceive and learn despite a hearing loss and consequently communicate only with the parents. As a result, the child's needs and feelings remain unrecognized and unmet.

Since deaf children often have difficulty in forming social relationships with other children the child is introduced to his roommates and encouraged to engage in play activities. The hospital setting can provide growth-promoting opportunities for social relationships. With the assistance of a child life specialist, the child can learn new recreational activities, experiment with group games, and engage in therapeutic play. The use of puppets, dollhouses, role playing with dress-up clothes, building with a hammer and nails, finger painting, needle play, and water play can help the deaf child express feelings that previously were suppressed.

VISUAL IMPAIRMENT

Serious visual impairments occur in approximately one of every 1000 school-age children. There are nearly 70,000 visually impaired children from birth to 19 years of age. These figures do not take into account the number of children with refractory errors that require corrective lenses. It is estimated that about 7½ million school children have some type of visual difficulty, yet only one fourth will demonstrate symptoms. The other three fourths require specific testing to identify the problem. The nurse's role is clearly one of detection, referral, and in some instances rehabilitation.

Classification of visual defects

Visual defects are legally classified as *blind,* a corrected vision of 20/200 or less or peripheral vision (tunnel vision) of less than 20 degrees in the better eye, and *partially seeing,* corrected vision between 20/200 and 20/70. Visual defects are also divided into congenital and acquired types. Any child who suffers a loss of vision before the age of 5 or 6 years is classified for educational purposes as a child with a congenital visual defect. Children who lose their sight after the age of 6 years are considered to have acquired blindness. The impact of vision loss after the age of 5 years has different implications, both for the child emotionally as well as for the provision of educational services. The child who is newly blinded may retain the basic process of reading and transfer this to new learning of the braille system.

Causes

Visual impairment can be caused by a number of genetic and prenatal or postnatal conditions. These include Tay-Sachs disease, perinatal infections (herpes, chlamydia, gonococci, rubella, syphilis, or toxoplasmosis), retrolental fibroplasia, trauma, postnatal infections (meningitis), and disorders such as sickle cell disease, juvenile rheumatoid arthritis, and retinoblastoma. The following discussion focuses on the most common types of visual disorders in children.

Refractive errors. The term *refraction* means bending and refers to the bending of light rays as they pass through the lens of the eye. Normally light rays enter the lens and fall directly on the retina. However, in refractive disorders the light rays either fall in front of the retina (myopia) or beyond it (hyperopia).

Children are normally hyperopic until 5 to 6 years of age, at which time their visual acuity approaches 20/20. This is an important fact to remember when screening children for refractive errors, since hyperopia in children in this age-group does not require correction.

Myopia. Myopia or nearsightedness refers to the ability to see objects clearly at close range but not at a distance. In most instances it results from an eyeball that is too long, causing the image to fall in front of the retina. Correction involves the use of biconcave lenses, which permits the lens of the myopic eye to focus the two rays on the retina.

Hyperopia (hypermetropia). Hyperopia or farsightedness is the reverse of myopia. The eyeball is too short in length; as a result, rays of light are theoretically focused behind the retina. These children can see objects clearly at a distance and, because of their accommodative ability, can usually see objects at close range. However, the continual muscular effort produces eyestrain and may result in strabismus. Correction involves the use of convex lenses that bend the light rays so that the lens of the eye can focus them on the retina.

Astigmatism. The refractive surfaces of the eye are rarely perfectly spherical. Normally the imperfection is so slight that it does not interfere with refraction or vision. In astigmatism there are unequal curvatures in the cornea or lens so that light rays are bent into different directions, producing a blurred image. Correction involves the use of specially ground lenses that compensate for the errors in refraction. Astigmatism may occur with or without other refractive disorders.

Strabismus. Strabismus, which literally means squinting, refers to malalignment of the eyes (Fig. 17-8). Normally the two eyes work as a unit (binocular vision). Images of an object are focused on the retina of each eye and passed to the brain so that the images are seen as one (fusion). When the eyes are malaligned, each retina receives two different images, resulting in diplopia (double vision). The brain accommodates for the visual confusion by suppressing the less intense image.

If the malalignment is not corrected, the weaker or "lazy" eye eventually becomes blind from nonuse. This results in a condition called *amblyopia ex anopsia.* Early recognition of strabismus to prevent amblyopia cannot be overemphasized. The optimum time for correction of amblyopia is during early childhood, particularly before age 4 to 6 years.

The goal in treating strabismus is preservation of vision, binocularity, and improvement in cosmetic appearance. Treatment consists of patching the good eye so that the child will be forced to use the weaker eye. If refractive errors are present, corrective lenses are worn. When strabismus is caused by muscle imbalance, treatment is surgical.

Cataracts. A cataract is an opacity of the crystalline lens. Since the lens is normally transparent to allow light rays to enter the eye and refract them for a clear image on the retina, a cataract interferes with both of these functions. Cataracts may be congenital, such as those caused by maternal rubella during the first trimester, or acquired, most commonly as a result of penetrating injuries.

Glaucoma. Glaucoma refers to a condition in which intraocular pressure is increased, causing pressure on the optic nerve and, eventually, atrophy and blindness. *Congenital glaucoma* results from defective development of the structures of the eye in the region of the anterior chamber angle (outflow tracts for aqueous humor). Consequently there is obstruction to the flow of fluid, resulting in increased intraocular pressure.

Trauma. Trauma is the most common cause of blindness in children over 2 years of age. Injuries to the eyeball and adnexa (supporting or accessory structures,

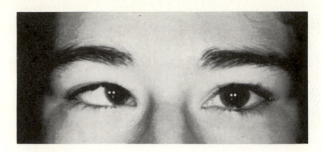

FIG. 17-8
Strabismus. Note the obvious malalignment of the eyes. The light reflections are centered in the left cornea and to the side of the right cornea. (From Havener, W.H., Saunders, W.H., Keith, C.F., and Prescott, A.W.: Nursing care in eye, ear, nose, and throat disorders, ed. 3, St. Louis, 1974, The C.V. Mosby Co.)

such as eyelids, conjunctiva, lacrimal glands, and so on) can be classified as penetrating or nonpenetrating. Penetrating wounds are most often the result of sharp instruments, such as knives or scissors; propulsive objects, such as firecrackers, guns, bows and arrows, or slingshots; and a powerful contusion by a blunt object, which may occur during a fight or from a serious car accident. Nonpenetrating injuries may be the result of foreign objects in the eyes, lacerations, a blow from a blunt object such as a fist, and thermal or chemical burns.

Treatment is aimed at preventing further ocular damage and is primarily the responsibility of the ophthalmologist. It involves adequate examination of the injured eye (with the child sedated or anesthetized in severe injuries), appropriate immediate intervention such as removal of the foreign body or suturing of the laceration, and prevention of complications, such as administration of antibiotics or steroids and complete bed rest to allow the eye to heal and blood to reabsorb. Prognosis varies according to the type of injury. It is usually guarded in all cases of penetrating wounds because of the high risk of serious complications.

Infections. Infections of the adnexa and the structures of the eyeball or globe are not infrequent in children. The most common eye disease is conjunctivitis (see Chapter 12). Treatment is usually ophthalmic antibiotics. Severe infections may require systemic antibiotic therapy. Steroids are used cautiously because they exacerbate viral infections such as herpes simplex, increasing the risk of damage to the involved structures.

NURSING CONSIDERATIONS WITH VISUALLY IMPAIRED CHILDREN

Nursing intervention with visually impaired children is often a specialized area, requiring additional training in vi-

SUMMARY OF NURSING CARE OF THE VISUALLY IMPAIRED CHILD

GOALS	RESPONSIBILITIES
Prevention	
Before occurrence of ocular problems	Identify pregnant women at risk
	Encourage adequate prenatal care to decrease likelihood of premature delivery or low-birth-weight infant
	Administer oxygen cautiously to neonate
	Periodically screen all children from birth through adolescence for visual impairment
	Participate in immunization programs for children
	Teach safety regarding common accidental causes of eye injuries
	Stress importance of good eye care—use of proper lighting, avoidance of excessive close work, proper rest and nutrition, and yearly eye examinations
Following detection and/or diagnosis of eye disorders	Encourage compliance with corrective therapies
Strabismus	Discuss with the school-age child necessity of patch in preserving vision
	Allow him to verbalize feelings regarding altered facial appearance
	Help him overcome visual difficulties imposed by seeing with weaker eye (favorable seating in school, large-print books, and additional time to complete assignments)
	Teach the parents correct procedures for instilling anticholinesterase drugs
Refractive errors	For secure fit of glasses, use ones with rounded temporal pieces or attach elastic strap to handles and around back of head
	Include older child in selection of frames
	Encourage the parents to compare value of more expensive attractive frames and inducement for wearing them against cost
	If glasses are recommended for continuous wearing, discuss possibility of temporary removal for special occasions
	Encourage use of protective shields during contact sports
	Stress improvement in visual acuity as reason for wearing glasses
	Discuss feasibility of contact lenses with selected families
	Know procedures for care, insertion, and removal of lens; teach these to parents and older children
Infections	Teach the parent correct procedure for instilling ophthalmic preparations (always in conjunctival cul-de-sac)
	Ensure proper dosage by holding dropper vertically, slowly closing the lids, and having child rotate the eyeball for even distribution
	Wipe excess medication from inner canthus outward to prevent contamination of contralateral eye
	Emphasize regular administration of drug for entire time of therapy to completely eradicate infection
Trauma	Prevent further injury by instituting appropriate emergency care
	Obtain history of incident; avoid any implication of guilt
	Reassure the parent and child; avoid giving false reassurance; apprise them of each step of treatment, especially if therapy interferes with vision (patching eyes)
Detection	
Infancy	At birth assess the neonate's response to a bright, shiny object; observe for signs associated with congenital blindness
	After 4 months of age, check for strabismus (lack of binocularity); refer to ophthalmologist for evaluation
	Listen to parents' concerns regarding visual loss
	Assist with testing (brainstem auditory-evoked response)

Continued.

SUMMARY OF NURSING CARE OF THE VISUALLY IMPAIRED CHILD—cont'd

GOALS	RESPONSIBILITIES
Childhood	Test for visual acuity as soon as the child is cooperative (sometimes by age 2 years)
	Advise the parents of Home Eye Test for Preschoolers, which is available from National Society to Prevent Blindness
	Observe for signs or behaviors indicative of eye problems (Table 17-3); specifically include questions regarding behavioral indications of vision impairment in health histories
	As school nurse, assume responsibility for follow-up care of children who require corrective lenses or other types of treatments, such as patching
	Stress to parents importance of continued periodic eye examinations, since the child's eyesight may change significantly in a short time
Rehabilitation Assist family in adjusting to child's loss of sight	Anticipate the usual grief reactions to loss
	Stress to parents (and older child) that such feelings are normal and that grief takes time to resolve
	Help the parents gain a realistic concept of the child's handicap and abilities
	Encourage formal rehabilitation as soon as realistically feasible
	Assist the parents in orienting newly blind child to his environment and in making immediate surroundings safe to encourage ambulation
Promote parent-child attachment	Help the parents identify clues other than eye contact from the infant that signify his communication with them
	Encourage the parents to discuss their feeling regarding lack of visual contact or smiling from the child
	Stress that lack of such responses is not an indication of the child's rejection or dislike of his parents
	Demonstrate by own example acceptance of the child
	Emphasize positive abilities or attributes
	Encourage the parents in their attempts to promote child's development
Promote development and independence	Provide visual-motor activities for infant (sitting in chair or swing, holding head up, standing, crawling, grasping for objects and so on)
	Provide an environment that fosters familiarity and security, arrange furniture to allow safe ambulation; place identifying markers to denote steps or other dangerous areas
	Enroll the child in special programs for the blind as soon as possible to learn independent skills, braille reading and writing, and navigational skills (cane method, sighted guide, or dog guide)
	Encourage participation in active play
	Discuss need for experimenting with active play in safe environment and with other children
Provide opportunities for play/socialization	Always talk to the child about his environment
	Guide the parents to selection of play material that encourages motor development and stimulates the sense of hearing and touch
	Discuss with the parents how play for blind children differs from that of sighted children
	Encourage parents to initiate play activities and teach the child how to use toys
	If blindisms are present, assess adequacy of environmental stimulation
	Discuss importance of consistent limit setting in helping the child learn acceptable behavior and tolerate frustration
Provide emotional support	Be available to family for assistance
	Encourage the parents, child, and siblings to discuss their feelings regarding the disability
	Stress the child's abilities rather than disability to promote self-esteem
	Refer families to appropriate community agencies for medical, psychiatric, vocational, or financial assistance

sion assessment and rehabilitation. However, general nursing goals that focus on prevention, detection, and rehabilitation are every nurse's responsibility. In addition, nurses may have to care for a visually impaired child who is hospitalized and must know how to best meet the child's and family's special needs.

Prevention

The primary nursing objective is to prevent visual impairment. This involves many of the same interventions discussed under hearing impairments, namely (1) prenatal screening for pregnant women at risk, such as those with rubella or syphilis infection and family histories of genetic disorders associated with visual loss, (2) adequate prenatal and perinatal care to prevent prematurity and iatrogenic damage from excessive administration of oxygen, (3) periodic screening of all children, especially newborns through preschoolers, for congenital blindness and visual impairments caused by refractive errors, strabismus, and so on, (4) rubella immunization of all children, and (5) safety counseling regarding the common causes of ocular trauma.

Following detection of eye problems, the nurse has a responsibility to prevent further ocular damage by ensuring that corrective treatment is employed. For the child with strabismus, this often necessitates occlusion patching of the stronger eye. Compliance with the procedure is greatest during the early preschool years. It is more difficult to encourage school-age children to wear the occlusive patch because the poor visual acuity of the uncovered weaker eye interferes with schoolwork and the patch sets them apart from their peers. In school they benefit from being positioned favorably (closer to the blackboard) and allowed extra time to read or complete an assignment.

For the child with refractive errors, the nurse helps the child adjust to wearing glasses. Young children who often pull glasses off benefit from temporal pieces that wrap around the ears or an elastic strap attached to the frames and around the back of the head to hold them on securely. Once a child appreciates the value of clear vision, he is more likely to wear the corrective lenses.

Glasses should not interfere with any activity. Special protective guards are available during contact sports to prevent accidental injury and all corrective lenses should be made from safety glass, which is shatterproof. Often corrective lenses improve visual acuity so dramatically that children are able to compete more effectively in sports. This in itself is a tremendous inducement to continue wearing glasses.

Contact lenses have been gaining in popularity and usage during the past several years. The three main types are hard lenses, soft lenses, and extended wear lenses. Contact lenses offer several advantages over conventional

spectacles, namely, greater visual acuity, total corrected field of vision, and optimum cosmetic benefit. Unfortunately they are quite costly, require much more care than glasses, and involve considerable practice in learning techniques for insertion and removal. If they are prescribed, the nurse can be very helpful in teaching parents or older children how to care for the lenses.

If treatment of the eye disorder requires instillation of ophthalmic medication, parents are taught the correct procedure (see Chapter 19). If the child is not cooperative it may be necessary to have two people perform the procedure: one to properly position the lids and the other to instill the drug.

Since trauma is the leading cause of blindness, the nurse has the major responsibility of preventing further eye injury until the physician orders specific treatment. The major principles to follow when caring for eye emergencies are:

1. Reassure the child and parents—everyone with an eye injury fears blindness.
2. Test visual acuity.
3. Never apply a patch on a penetrated eye (an eye patch will exert more pressure, causing further structural damage); instead, use a Fox shield (a small, metal shield shaped like an eye that has tiny perforations).
4. Never try to remove a foreign body that has penetrated the eye.
5. Do not apply medication unless specifically ordered.

In the event of a hematoma (black eye), the eye is checked with a flashlight for gross hyphema (visible fluid meniscus across the iris). It is more easily seen in light-colored than in brown eyes. If no hyphema is present, ice is applied for first 24 hours to reduce swelling, followed by heat to absorb the extravasated blood. If a hyphema is present, the child is examined by an ophthalmologist.

Detection

Equally important as prevention is early detection of eye problems. As has already been pointed out, detection and treatment of many ocular defects, such as strabismus, often prevent any permanent visual impairment. Every child from birth onward should receive periodic visual screening. Chapter 5 includes tests for visual acuity in children in various age-groups. Table 17-3 summarizes the usual signs and symptoms associated with ocular disorders.

Rehabilitation

Rehabilitation is a continuous process that relates to every area of the child's life. Nursing goals include (1) helping the family and child adjust to the diagnosis, (2) promoting parent-child attachment, (3) fostering optimum develop-

TABLE 17-3. DETECTION OF VISUAL IMPAIRMENT

CAUSE	BEHAVIOR	SIGNS/SYMPTOMS
Congenital blindness	Does not follow a moving light; no orientation response to visual stimuli Does not initiate eye-to-eye contact with caregiver	Constant nystagmus Fixed pupils Marked strabismus Slow lateral movements
Refractive errors	Rubs eyes excessively Tilts head or thrusts head forward Has difficulty in reading or other close work Holds books close to eyes Writes or colors with head close to table Clumsy; walks into objects Blinks more than usual or is irritable when doing close work Is unable to see objects clearly Does poorly in school, especially in subjects that require demonstration, such as arithmetic	Dizziness Headache Nausea following close work
Strabismus	Squints eyelids together or frowns Has difficulty in focusing from one distance to another Inaccurate judgment in picking up objects Unable to see print or moving objects clearly Closes one eye to see Tilts head to one side If combined with refractive errors, may see any of the above	Diplopia Photophobia Dizziness Headache Cross-eye
Glaucoma	Mostly seen in acquired types—loses peripheral vision May bump into objects that are not directly in front of him Sees halos around objects May complain of mild pain or discomfort (severe pain, nausea, and vomiting if sudden rise in pressure)	Redness Excessive tearing (epiphora) Photophobia Spasmatic winking (blepharospasm) Corneal haziness Enlargement of the eyeball (buphthalmos)
Cataract	Gradually less able to see objects clearly May lose peripheral vision	Nystagmus (with complete blindness) Gray opacities of lens Strabismus

ment and independence, (4) providing for play/socialization, and (5) being aware of educational facilities.

Adjusting to diagnosis. The shock of learning that their child is blind or partially sighted is an immense crisis for parents. Of all types of disabilities, many people fear loss of sight the most. Certainly it is one of the senses that is involved in almost every activity of daily living. However, every effort is made to assist parents in forming a positive image of blindness and blind people. Most blind individuals who do not have additional handicaps lead full, productive lives.

Parents need support during the initial phase of learning about the diagnosis and help to gain a realistic understanding of their child's abilities. The family is encouraged to investigate appropriate stimulation and educational programs for their child as soon as possible. Sources of information include state commissions for the blind, local schools for the blind, the National Federation of the Blind (an organization of blind people),* and the American Foundation for the Blind.†

When blindness is not congenital but acquired, the

---

*1800 Johnson Street, Baltimore, MD 21230; an excellent publication is by Willoughby, D.: A resource guide for parents and educators of blind children.
†15 W. 16th Street, New York, NY 10011.

newly blind child needs a great deal of support to help him adjust to the handicap. He is usually frightened and confused by the sudden or progressive loss of sight and benefits from an environment that provides security and familiarity. This is especially important to remember when he is hospitalized.

Parent-child attachment. A crucial time in the life of the blind infant is when he and his parents are getting acquainted with each other. Pleasurable patterns of interaction between the infant and his parents may be lacking if there is not enough reciprocity. For example, if the parent gazes fondly at the infant's face and seeks eye contact but the infant fails to respond because he cannot see the parent, a troubled cycle of responses may occur. The nurse can help parents learn to look for other cues that indicate the infant is responding to them, such as if his eyelids blink, whether his activity level accelerates or slows, if respiratory patterns change, such as if he breathes faster or slower when they come near, and whether the infant makes throaty sounds when they speak to him. In time parents learn that the infant has his own unique way of relating to them. They are encouraged to show affection using nonvisual methods, such as talking or reading, cuddling, and walking the child.

Development and independence. Motor development is almost as dependent on sight as verbal communication is on hearing. From earliest infancy parents are encouraged to expose the infant to as many visual-motor experiences as possible, such as sitting supported in an infant seat or swing and given opportunities for holding up his head, sitting unsupported, reaching for objects, crawling, and so on. Ideally the child should be enrolled in an educational stimulation program for blind infants to develop age-appropriate motor skills.

Despite visual impairment the child can become independent in all aspects of self-care. The same principles used for promoting independence in sighted children apply with additional emphasis on nonvisual cues. For example, the child learns self-feeding as a normal child would. If he is given a deep bowl and a lightweight spoon, he is able to scoop food more easily and can determine the quantity by the increased weight of the utensil. During the preschool years the child is encouraged to develop table manners. Parents need to realize that without the assistance of imitation they must explain verbally the importance of manners and gently remind the child to practice them.

Play and socialization. The blind child does not learn to play automatically. Because he cannot imitate others or actively explore his environment as sighted children do, he depends much more on others to stimulate and teach him how to play. Parents need help in selecting appropriate play material, especially those that encourage fine and gross motor development and stimulate the senses of hearing, touch, and smell. Toys are selected that are fun without being frustrating. For example, construction sets with interlocking pieces are preferable to those that are stackable and fall apart easily when bumped.

To compensate for lack of stimulation, blind or partially seeing children may develop self-stimulatory habits called *blindisms,* such as eye rubbing, body rocking, finger flicking before the eyes, sniffing and smelling, arm twirling, or repetitive vocal tics. Since such habits retard socially acceptable behavior, the child's environment is assessed for clues to when they occur and how parents manage them. Suitable substitute stimulation within an appropriate social context, such as a play group of peers or within the family setting, is suggested.

The blind child has the same needs for socialization as normal children. Since he has little difficulty in learning verbal skills, he is able to communicate with age-mates and participate in suitable activities. The nurse discusses with parents opportunities for socialization outside of the home, especially regular nursery schools. The trend is to include these children with sighted children to help them adjust to the outside world for eventual independence.

Education. The main obstacle to learning is the child's total dependence on nonvisual cues. Although the child can learn via verbal lecturing, he is unable to read the written word or to write without special education. Therefore, he must rely on *braille,* a system that uses raised dots to represent letters and numbers. The child can then read the braille with his fingers and can write a message using a braille writer. However, unless others read braille this type of communication is not useful for communicating with others. A more portable system for written communication is the use of a braille slate and stylus (Fig. 17-9) or a microcassette tape recorder. A recorder is especially helpful for leaving messages for others and for note-taking during classroom lecturing. Both the braille slate and stylus and the tape recorder are as important to a blind person as paper and pencil are to a sighted individual. For mathematical calculations portable calculators with voice synthesizers are available.*

Records and tapes are significant sources of reading material other than braille books, which are large and cumbersome. The Library of Congress has talking books, braille books, and a special records program, which are available at many local libraries, state libraries, and directly from the Library of Congress. The talking book machine and tape player are provided at no cost to families and there is no postage fee for returning the materials. Recording for the Blind, Inc.† also provides texts and tapes of books, which are very helpful for secondary and college students who are blind.

---

*A catalog of numerous products for people with vision problems is available from the American Foundation for the Blind.
†725 Park Avenue, New York, NY 10021.

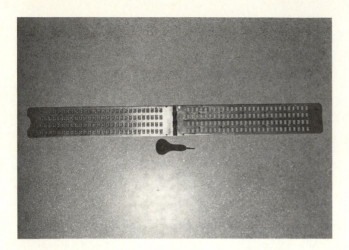

FIG. 17-9

Braille slate and stylus. The hinged slate consists of a series of open rectangles on one side and standard braille cells on the other. The paper is clamped or sandwiched between these two metal bars and the appropriate dots are punched with the stylus.

Learning to use a regular typewriter is another form of writing but has the disadvantage of the blind person being unable to check the accuracy of the typing. Recent developments with the use of computers for the disabled have eliminated this drawback. A home computer with a voice synthesizer can be adapted to speak each letter or word that has been typed.

The partially sighted child benefits from specialized visual aids, which produce a magnified retinal image. The basic devices are accommodation, such as bringing the object closer, special plus lenses, hand-held and stand magnifiers, telescopes, video projection systems, and large print. Children with low vision often prefer to do close work without their glasses and compensate by bringing the object very near to their eyes. This should be allowed. The exception is the child with vision in only one eye, who should always wear glasses for protection. Information about services for the partially sighted is available from the National Association for Visually Handicapped.*

Touch is a principal medium for learning. Touch becomes extremely important in gaining some idea of "appearance." For example, using the fingers to touch someone's face helps the child learn distinguishing marks for each individual. Blind children are frequently able to decipher a person's emotional mood from facial muscle tenseness, positioning of the lips, cheeks, and eyes, and other subtle body language. However, facial touching can make others feel very uncomfortable and should be reserved for individuals the child knows well.

*305 East 24th Street, New York, NY 10010.

The blind child also must learn to become independent in navigational skills. The two main techniques are the *tapping method* (use of a cane to survey the environment for direction and to avoid obstacles) and *guides,* such as a human sighted guide or a dog guide, such as a Seeing Eye dog. Both afford the blind person sufficient mobility to travel in unfamiliar surroundings using public transportation.

Caring for hospitalized children with temporary loss of vision

Children may be hospitalized for ocular surgery that requires temporary patching, such as strabismus or some types of cataract removal, or because of trauma and temporary loss of vision resulting from the injury or treatment. The nursing care objectives in either situation are to (1) reassure the child and family throughout every phase of treatment, (2) orient the child to his surroundings, (3) provide a safe environment, and (4) encourage independence. Whenever possible the same nurse should care for the child to assure consistency in the approach. These same principles also apply to a blind child who requires hospitalization.

When a sighted child temporarily loses his vision, almost every aspect of his environment becomes bewildering and frightening. He is forced to rely on nonvisual senses for help in adjusting to the blindness without the benefit of any special training. Nurses have a major role in minimizing the effects of temporary loss of vision. They talk to the child about everything they are doing, emphasizing aspects of procedures that are felt or heard. They approach the child by always identifying themselves as soon as they enter the room. Since unfamiliar sounds are especially frightening to the child, these are explained. Parents are encouraged to room with him and participate in his care. Familiar objects, such as a teddy bear or doll, should be brought from home to help lessen the strangeness of the hospital. As soon as the child is able to be out of bed, he is oriented to his immediate surroundings. If the child is able to see on admission, this opportunity is taken to point out significant aspects of his room and he is encouraged to practice ambulating with his eyes closed to accustom him to this experience.

The room is arranged with safety in mind. For example, a stool or chair is placed next to the bed to help the child climb in and out of bed. The furniture is always placed in the same position to prevent accidental collisions. Cleaning personnel are reminded of the need to keep the room in order. If the child has difficulty navigating by feeling the walls, a rope can be attached from the bed to the point of destination, such as the bathroom. Attention to details such as well-fitting slippers or robes that do not hang on the floor is important in preventing tripping.

The child is encouraged to be independent in self-care activities, especially if the visual loss may be prolonged or potentially permanent. For example, during bathing the nurse sets up all the equipment and encourages the child to participate. At mealtime the nurse explains where each food item is on the tray, opens any special containers, prepares cereal or toast, but encourages the child to feed himself. Since manipulating utensils may be difficult, favorite finger foods, such as sandwiches, hamburgers, hot dogs, or pizza, are selected. The nurse encourages the child to use a straw to drink soups or fluids, rather than feeding him. If he has accidental spills, these are quickly cleaned up, with no emphasis placed on them. Instead he is praised for efforts at being cooperative and independent, and any improvements he makes in self-care, no matter how small, are stressed.

Appropriate recreational activities are provided for the child. If a child life specialist is available, such planning is done jointly. Since the child with temporary blindness has a wide variety of play experiences to draw on, he is encouraged to select activities. For example, if he liked to read, he may enjoy being read to. If he preferred manual activity, he may appreciate playing with clay or building blocks or feeling different textures and naming them. If he needs an outlet for aggression, activities such as pounding or banging on a drum can be helpful. Simple board and card games can be played if the child has a ''seeing partner'' or if the opponent helps him with the game. He should have familiar toys from home to play with, since they are more easily manipulated than new ones. If parents wish to bring him presents, they should be things that stimulate hearing and touch, such as a radio, music box, or stuffed animal.

Occasionally children who are blind come to the hospital for procedures to restore their vision. Although this is an extremely happy time, it also requires intervention to help the child adjust to sight. The child needs an opportunity to take in all that he sees. He should not be bombarded with visual stimuli. He may need to concentrate on people's faces or his own to accustom himself to this experience. He often has the need to talk about what he sees and to compare the visual image with his mental one. The child may also go through a period of depression as he begins to realize all that he had lost. This depression must be respected and supported. The nurse or parents should refrain from statements, such as, ''How can you be so sad when you can see again?'' Instead the child should be encouraged to discuss how it feels to see, especially in terms of seeing himself.

The child also needs time in adjusting to his ability to engage in activities that were impossible before. For example, he may prefer to use braille to read, rather than learning a new ''visual approach'' because of his familiarity with the touch system. Eventually, as he learns to recognize letters and numbers, he will integrate these new skills into reading and writing. However, parents and teachers must be careful not to push the child before he is ready. This applies to social relationships and physical activities as well as learning situations.

DEAF-BLIND CHILDREN

The most traumatic sensory impairment is loss of sight and hearing. Obviously, auditory and visual handicaps have profound effects on the child's development. They interfere with the normal sequence of physical, intellectual, and psychosocial growth. Although the child often achieves the usual motor milestones, they are more slowly developed. Children only learn communication with specialized training. Some deaf-blind children, especially those with residual hearing or sight, can learn to speak. Whenever possible, speech is encouraged, since it allows communication with other individuals.

The future prospects for deaf-blind children are at best unpredictable. Not infrequently congenital blindness and/or deafness is accompanied by other physical or neurologic handicaps, which further lessen the child's learning potential. The most favorable prognosis is often for children who have acquired deaf blindness and have few, if any, associated disabilities. Their learning capacity is greatly potentiated by their previous developmental progress prior to the sensory impairments. Although total independence, including gainful vocational training, is the goal, some deaf-blind children are unable to develop to this level. They may require lifelong parental or residential care. The nurse working with such families helps them deal with future goals for the child, including possible alternatives to home care during the parents' advancing years.

RETINOBLASTOMA

Retinoblastoma is a relatively rare congenital malignant tumor arising from the retina. It may be present at birth or may arise in the retina during the first 2 years of life. Retinoblastoma may be hereditary or nonhereditary and unilateral or bilateral. Hereditary retinoblastomas are transmitted as an autosomal-dominant trait with incomplete penetrance.

Clinical manifestations

Retinoblastoma has few grossly obvious signs. Typically it is the parent who first observes a whitish ''glow'' in the pupil. The white reflex known as the *cat's eye reflex* represents visualization of the tumor as the light momentarily falls on the mass (Fig. 17-10). The next most common

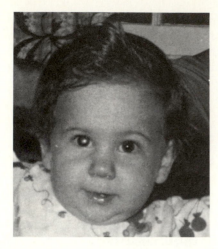

FIG. 17-10

Cat's eye reflex. Whitish appearance of lens is produced as light falls on tumor mass in right eye.

sign is strabismus resulting from poor fixation of the visually impaired eye, particularly if the tumor develops in the macula, the area of sharpest visual acuity. Another presenting sign is a red, painful eye, often accompanied with glaucoma. Blindness is usually a late sign, but it frequently is not obvious unless the parent consciously observes for behaviors indicative of loss of sight, such as bumping into objects, slowed motor development, or turning of the head to see objects lateral to the affected eye.

Diagnostic evaluation

The first step in diagnosis is carefully listening to and recognizing the significance of reports from family members regarding suspected abnormalities within the eye. Since the cat's eye reflex is a momentary sign visualized only under specific conditions, the physician or nurse must attempt to duplicate those conditions necessary to observe the tumor. Children suspected of having this disorder are referred to an ophthalmologist. Definitive diagnosis is usually based on indirect ophthalmoscopy, which is done under general anesthesia with maximum dilation of the pupils.

Therapeutic management

Treatment of retinoblastoma depends chiefly on the stage of the tumor at diagnosis. In general, early stage unilateral retinoblastomas are treated with irradiation or other techniques, such as cryotherapy, which freezes the tumor. Radiotherapy is avoided whenever possible because of the risk of secondary malignancies, especially osteogenic sarcoma, in patients with bilateral tumors. The aim of therapy

is to preserve useful vision in the affected eye and eradicate the tumor.

With advanced tumor growth, especially optic nerve involvement, enucleation of the affected eye is the treatment of choice. When confirmed clinical metastatic disease is present, chemotherapy, particularly the use of vincristine, cyclophosphamide, and adriamycin, can provide palliation but not cure.

With bilateral disease, every attempt is made to preserve useful vision in the least affected eye with enucleation of the severely diseased eye. Irradiation (or other techniques) of the preserved eye, sometimes combined with chemotherapy, is used to eradicate the tumor and prevent metastatic spread.

The overall prognosis for retinoblastoma is very favorable, with a survival rate of approximately 90% and bilateral tumors may not be associated with increased mortality.

Nursing considerations

Since the tumor is usually diagnosed in infants or very young children, most of the preparation for diagnostic tests and treatment involves parents. After indirect ophthalmoscopy, the child may not see very clearly or his eyes may be sensitive to light because of pupillary dilation. Parents are made aware of these normal reactions prior to the procedure. They also are informed that a battery of screening tests, such as bone surveys, bone marrow aspiration, and so on, may be performed to detect metastasis.

Once the disease is staged, the physician confers with the parents regarding treatment. Unless the diagnosis is made very early, an enucleation is performed. Parents are told about the procedure as well as about the positive benefits of a prosthesis. Showing them pictures of another child with an artificial eye may be very helpful in their adjusting to the thought of disfigurement (Fig. 17-11). Although the idea of blindness is a very distressing one, most parents seem to realize that there is no alternative. The fact that the unaffected eye retains normal vision is particularly helpful in their accepting the imposed handicap and should be emphasized.

After surgery the parents are prepared for the child's facial appearance. An eye patch is in place, and the child's face may be edematous or ecchymotic. Parents often fear seeing the surgical site because they imagine a cavity in the skull. On the contrary, the lids are usually closed and the area does not appear sunken because a surgically implanted sphere maintains the shape of the eyeball. The implant is covered with conjunctiva, and when the lids are open the exposed area resembles the mucosal lining of the mouth. Once the child is fitted for a prosthesis, usually within 3 weeks, the facial appearance returns to normal.

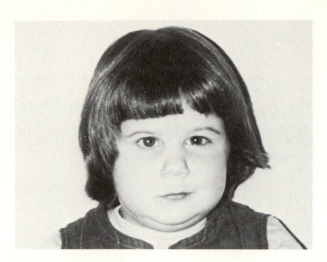

FIG. 17-11
Preschooler with right prosthetic eye.

Initial instructions for care of the prosthesis are given by the ocularist, who fits and manufactures the device.

Care of the socket is minimal and easily accomplished. The wound itself is clean and has little or no drainage. If an antibiotic ointment is prescribed, it is applied in a thin line on the surface of the tissues of the socket. To cleanse the site, an irrigating solution may be ordered and is instilled daily or more frequently if necessary, *before* application of the antibiotic ointment. The dressing consists of an eye pad taped over the surgical site with nonirritating tape; it is changed daily. Once the socket has healed completely, a dressing is no longer necessary, although it is a preventive measure against infection.

A long-term consideration is the survivor's ability to transmit the defective gene to his offspring. Parents are encouraged to seek genetic counseling for themselves and for the child after he reaches puberty.

Emotional support. Families with a history of the disorder may feel great guilt for transmitting the defect to their offspring. In families with no history of retinoblastoma, the discovery of the diagnosis is a shock, frequently complicated by guilt for not having found it sooner. Since parents frequently are the first to observe the cat's eye reflex, they may feel angry at themselves or others, especially physicians, for delaying a more thorough examination. The nurse assesses each of these variables in planning care based on understanding the parents' emotional reactions and adjustment (see Chapter 16).

REFERENCES

Grossman, H.J.: Manual on terminology and classification in mental retardation, American Association on Mental Deficiency, Baltimore, 1977, Garamond Pridemark Press.

Whaley, L., and Wong, D.: Nursing care of infants and children, St. Louis, 1983, The C.V. Mosby Co.

BIBLIOGRAPHY
Mental retardation

Bean, N.R., and Bell, B.J.: Nursing intervention in the care of the physically handicapped, severely retarded child, Nurs. Clin. North Am. **10**(2):353-359, 1975.

Blackwell, M.W., and Roy, S.A.: Surgical "routines" for profoundly retarded patients, Am. J. Nurs. **78**(3):402-404, 1978.

Bowness, S., and Zadik, T.D.: Implementing the nursing process at a unit for mentally handicapped children, Nurs. Times **77**(16):695-696, 1981.

Cranston, J.A.: A Down's baby, Nurs. Times **75**(42):1792-1794, 1979.

Curry, J.B., and Peppe, K.K., editors: Mental retardation: nursing approaches to care, St. Louis, 1978, The C.V. Mosby Co.

Del Campo, E., and Josephson, D.: Accommodating the severely retarded child in our schools, Am. J. Maternal Child Nurs. **3**(1):34-37, 1978.

Eddington, C., and Lee, T.: Sensory-motor stimulation for slow-to-develop children: a home-centered program for parents, Am. J. Nurs. **75**(1):59-62, 1975.

Erickson, M.L.: Care approaches to the child with mental retardation in a hospital setting, Clin. Pediatr. **17**(7):539-547, 1978.

Erickson, M.L.: Talking with fathers of young children with Down's syndrome, Child. Today **3**(6):22-25, 1974.

Godfrey, A.: Sensory-motor stimulation for slow-to-develop children, Am. J. Nurs. **75**(1):56-59, 1975.

Kluss, K.: Training the mentally retarded child in self-help skills. In Brandt, P.A., Chinn, P.L., and Smith, M.E.: Current practice in pediatric nursing, vol. 1, St. Louis, 1976, The C.V. Mosby Co.

Koch, R.: Down's syndrome: pediatric care, Feelings Med. Signif. **22**(1):1-6, 1980.

Lepler, M.: Having a handicapped child, Am. J. Maternal Child Nurs. **3**(1):32-33, 1978.

Long, A.: Down's syndrome, Nurs. Times **76**:814-819, May 1980.

Pipes, P.L.: Nutrition and feeding of children with developmental delays and related problems. In Pipes, P.L.: Nutrition in infancy and childhood, ed. 2, St. Louis, 1981, The C.V. Mosby Co.

Pipes, P.L., and Holm, V.A.: Feeding children with Down's syndrome, J. Am. Diet. Assoc. **77**:277-282, Sept. 1980.

Roberts, M.J., and Canfield, M.: Behavior modification with a mentally retarded child, Am. J. Nurs. **80**(4):679, 1980.

Roberts, S.E., Coffin, G., and Dunn, M.J.: Feeding techniques for the physically impaired child, Pediatr. Basics **21**:4-7, 1978.

Tudor, M.: Nursing intervention with developmentally disabled children, Am. J. Maternal Child Nurs. **3**(1):25-31, 1978.

Wasch, S.W.: Hospitalization of profoundly and severely mentally retarded children, Child Health Care **9**:126-131, 1981.

Williams, J.K.: Reproductive decisions: adolescents with Down syndrome, Pediatr. Nurs. **9**(1):43-44, 1983.

Williams, R.: A community nursing service for mentally handicapped children, Nurs. Times **76**:2011-2012, Nov. 1980.

Hearing impairment

American Academy of Pediatrics, Joint Committee on Infant Hearing, Position Statement 1982, Pediatrics **70**(3):496-497, 1982.

Davis, H., and Silverman, S.R.: Hearing and deafness, ed. 4, New York, 1978, Holt, Rinehart & Winston, Inc.

Downs, M.P.: Hearing development during infancy: children are different: behavioral development monograph series: No. 6, Ohio, 1983, Ross Laboratories.

Holder, L.: Hearing aids: handle with care, Nursing 82 **82**(4):64-67, 1982.

Holm, C.: Deafness: common misunderstandings, Am. J. Nurs. **78**(11):1910-1912, 1978.

McRae, M.J.: Bonding in a sea of silence, Am. J. Maternal Child Nurs. **4**(1):29-34, 1979.

Morgan, R.H.: Breaking through the sound barrier, Nursing 83 **13**(2):112-113, 1983.

Northern, J., and Downs, M.: Hearing in children, ed. 4, Baltimore, 1984, Williams & Wilkins.

Peltzman, P., and Lipson, E.: Infant hearing assessment: a new approach, Pediatr. Basics **28**:11-14, Jan. 1981.

Sataloff, R.: Pediatric hearing loss, Pediatr. Nurs. **6**(5):16-18, 1980.

Smith, M.P., and Cloonan, P.A.: Meeting the special needs of the hearing-impaired child, Issues Compr. Pediatr. Nurs. **3**(6):21-34, 1979.

Wright, J.: Deaf but not mute, Am. J. Nurs. **76**(5):795-799, 1976.

Visual impairment

Bischoff, R.W.: Early childhood development of the visually handicapped, Issues Compr. Pediatr. Nurs. **3**(6):36-49, 1979.

Bumbalo, J., and Seidel, M.: Identifying and serving a multiple handicapped population, Nurs. Clin. North Am. **10**(2):341-352, 1975.

Dupont, J.: What to do for common eye emergencies, Nursing 76 **6**(5):17-19, 1976.

Fenwick, A., and others: Traumatic blindness: a flexible approach for helping a blind adolescent, Nursing 79 **9**(1):36-41, 1979.

Fochtman, D., and Foley, G.V., editors: Nursing care of the child with cancer, Boston, l982, Little, Brown, & Co.

Herget, M.: For visually impaired diabetics, Am. J. Nurs. **83**(11):1557-1560, 1983.

Hiles, D.A.: Strabismus, Am. J. Nurs. **4**(6):1082-1089, 1974.

Kahn, H.: Visual dysfunctions, Nursing 74 **4**(10):26-27, 1974.

McNeer, K.W.: Pediatric ophthalmology, Pediatr. Nurs. **5**(6):47-49, 1979.

Pugh, R.: Effects of visual impairment on children: development in sight, Nurs. Mirror **150**(21):303-32, 1980.

Severtsen, B.M.: Sensory impairment: its effect on the family. In Hymovich, D.P., and Barnard, M.U., editors: Family health care, New York, 1979, McGraw-Hill Book Co.

Wong, D.L., and Dornan, L.R.: Nursing care in childhood cancer: retinoblastoma, Am. J. Nurs. **82**(3):425-431, 1982.

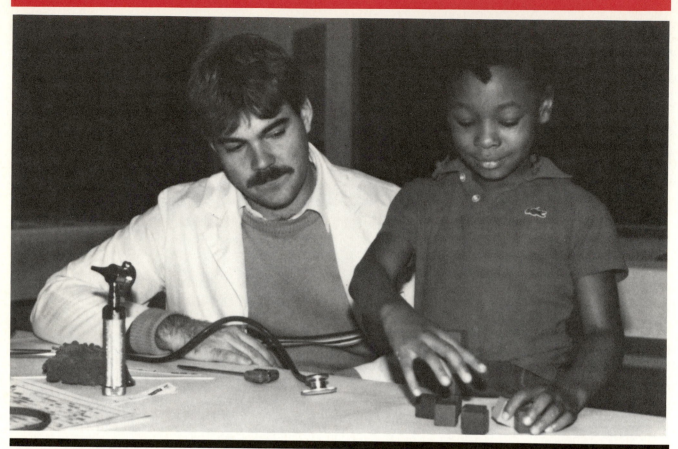

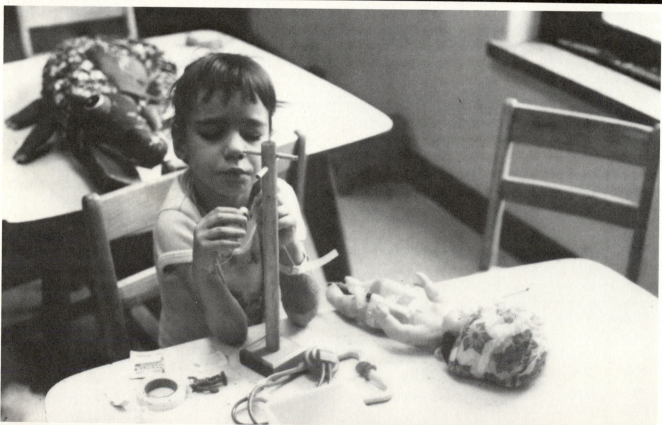

UNIT 8

THE HOSPITALIZED CHILD

When illness requires hospitalization, it creates a crisis for the child. Depending on his age, the child must deal with separation from familiar caregivers and environment, exposure to painful experiences, loss of independence, and disruption of nearly every aspect of his usual life-style. Often the reason necessitating hospitalization is of much less concern to the child than the consequences of confinement. Emergency admissions pose an even greater threat because of the lack of time to prepare the child for this event.

Chapter 18, *The Child's Reaction to Illness and Hospitalization,* is concerned with the child's age-related reactions to illness and hospitalization and with interventions that lessen the psychologic trauma of the experience, particularly parent participation and preparation for admission to the hospital. Chapter 19, *Pediatric Variations of Nursing Intervention,* deals with pediatric variations of nursing procedures and with preparation of the child for various procedures. It is not designed to present a detailed description of how to perform specific procedures but rather how to safely implement them with children.

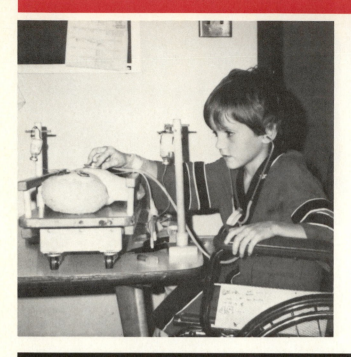

18

THE CHILD'S REACTION TO ILLNESS AND HOSPITALIZATION

OBJECTIVES

On completion of this chapter the reader will be able to:

- Identify the stressors of illness and hospitalization for children during each developmental stage

- Outline nursing interventions that prevent or minimize the stress of separation during hospitalization

- Outline nursing interventions that minimize the stress of loss of control during hospitalization

- Outline nursing interventions that minimize the fear of bodily injury during hospitalization

- Describe methods of assessing and managing pain in children

- Outline nursing interventions that support parents and siblings during a child's illness and hospitalization

- List the admission procedures for a child on admission to the hospital

- Describe nursing interventions when children are admitted to special units

NURSING DIAGNOSES

Nursing diagnoses identified for the child who is ill or hospitalized include, but are not restricted to, the following:

Health perception-health management pattern

- Infection, potential for, related to environmental hazards

Nutritional-metabolic pattern

- Nutrition, alterations in: potential for more or less than body requirements, related to (1) loss of appetite; (2) altered feeding habits

Elimination pattern

- Bowel elimination, alteration in: potential for related to altered toileting habits

Activity-exercise pattern

■ Activity intolerance, potential for, related to illness (specify)

■ Diversional activity deficit, potential for, related to hospitalization

■ Mobility, impaired physical, related to (1) illness (specify); (2) limitations imposed by environment

■ Self-care deficit (specify level: feeding, bathing/hygiene, dressing/grooming, toileting) related to developmental level

Sleep-rest pattern

■ Sleep-pattern disturbance, related to altered schedules

Cognitive-perceptual pattern

■ Comfort, alteration in: pain related to illness (specify)

■ Knowledge deficit, related to unfamiliarity with environment

■ Sensory-perceptual alterations, related to (1) isolation; (2) environmental stimuli

Self-perception—self-concept pattern

■ Anxiety, related to actual or perceived threat of bodily injury

■ Fear, related to unfamiliar environment

■ Powerlessness, related to dependency of patient role

Role-relationship pattern

■ Grieving, anticipatory, related to outcome of illness

■ Parenting, alteration in, potential: related to separation

■ Social isolation, related to hospitalization

Coping-stress tolerance pattern

■ Coping, family: potential for growth related to successful coping

Value-belief pattern

■ Spiritual distress, related to separation from religious/cultural ties

For children illness and hospitalization constitute a major life crisis. Children are particularly vulnerable to the crises of illness and hospitalization because (1) stress represents a change from the usual state of health and environmental routine and (2) children have a limited number of coping mechanisms to resolve the stressful events. Children's reactions to these crisis are influenced by (1) their developmental age, (2) previous experience with illness, separation, or hospitalization, (3) available support system, and (4) the seriousness of the illness and threat of hospitalization.

It is the purpose of this chapter to acquaint nurses with the various aspects of illness and hospitalization in children and to assist them in providing the kind of care that promotes optimum resolution of the crisis and positive growth from the experience.

STRESSORS AND REACTIONS RELATED TO DEVELOPMENTAL STAGE

Children's understanding of, reaction to, and method of coping with illness or hospitalization are influenced by the significance of individual *stressors* (those events that produce stress) during each developmental phase. The major stressors are separation, loss of control, and bodily injury. Table 18-1 summarizes the principal behavioral responses to each stressor during the developmental periods of childhood and the appropriate nursing interventions for each.

Infancy

Although infancy is generally regarded as the period from birth to the completion of 1 year of age, to understand the reactions of infants to illness and hospitalization it is more relevant to divide this age span into (1) preattachment to the significant caregiver and (2) postattachment. Before the recognition and attachment of young children to their parents, the major reactions of infants to illness or hospitalization are to pain, immobilization, and changes in the usual caring activities of bathing, dressing, and feeding.

By the end of the first 4 to 6 months of life, infants selectively recognize their parents, are strongly attached to them, and protest furiously if separated from them. Reactions to the stress of pain, illness, or hospitalization occur mostly from separation of child and parent. The behaviors typically seen during separation are discussed in the section on toddlerhood. If separation is avoided, infants seem to have a tremendous capacity for withstanding any type of stress.

Pain.   Behavioral reactions to pain correlate with age. Neonates' degree of perception of pain is controversial. Many health professionals believe that infants are relatively insensitive to pain and often perform painful procedures such as cut-downs or circumcision with no anesthetic. However, there are no data to support this view. Analysis of crying, oxygen utilization, and palm sweating indicate that they feel pain. The general reaction is total body movement associated with brief loud crying that ceases on distraction.

By the end of the first month, there is a noticeable decrease in the generalized response to pain. Somewhere between 3 and 10 months of age, infants localize the pain. For example, they react to an injection by withdrawing the leg.

By 4 to 6 months of age infants no longer react solely to the painful stimulation, but to a complex range of perceptual cues from their environment and demonstrate memory of previous painful experiences. They react intensely with physical resistance and uncooperativeness. They may refuse to lie still, attempt to push the person away, or try to escape with whatever motor activity they have achieved. Distraction does little to lessen their immediate reaction to pain, and anticipatory preparation, such as showing them the equipment, tends to increase their fear and resistance.

Toddlerhood

Toddlers' primary source of stress is separation. In addition, their reactions to stress are compounded by the developmental striving for autonomy. The main threats to the achievement of this goal are (1) loss of control from physical restriction, altered routine or rituals, and dependency and (2) bodily injury and pain. Their principal responses to these stressors are physical resistance, aggression, negativism, and regression.

Separation anxiety.   The major stress from latter infancy throughout the preschool years is separation anxiety. Three distinct phases are evident in the crisis of separation.

During the phase of *protest*, the child cries loudly, screams for his parent, refuses the attention of anyone else, and is inconsolable in his grief. The child may continue this behavior for a few hours or for several days. Some children may protest continuously, ceasing only from physical exhaustion. If a stranger approaches the child, he will initially protest even louder.

During the phase of *despair*, the crying subsides. The child is much less active, is disinterested in play or food, and withdraws from others. The child looks sad, lonely, isolated, and apathetic (Fig. 18-1). The major behavioral characteristic is depression, which results from increasing hopelessness, grief, and mourning.

During the third phase of *detachment* (also called denial), it appears superficially that the child has finally adjusted to the loss. He becomes more interested in his surroundings, plays with others, and seems to form new

TABLE 18-1. CHILDREN'S REACTIONS TO STRESS

AGE	DEVELOPMENTAL ACHIEVEMENT AND MAJOR FEARS	BEHAVIOR REACTIONS	INTERVENTIONS*
Infant	Trust vs mistrust Separation	Protest—cries, screams, searches for parent with eyes; clings to parent; avoids and rejects contact with strangers Despair—inactive, withdrawn, depressed, disinterested in environment Detachment—resignation; superficial "adjustment," that is, appears interested in surroundings, happy, friendly	Meet physical needs promptly Allow unrestricted visiting by parents Interview parents to determine their customary means for comforting the child and meeting his needs; apply this knowledge in the role of surrogate parent Provide consistency in personnel to allow for continuity of care
	Pain	Neonate—total body reaction, easily distracted Later infancy—localized reaction, uncooperative, offers physical resistance	Encourage parents to stay with infant and assist with care Employ pain reduction techniques, including medication Employ comfort measures
Toddler	Autonomy vs shame and doubt Separation	Protest—verbal cries for parent; verbal attack on others; physical fighting, that is, kicks, bites, hits, pinches; tries to escape to find parent, clings to parent and physically tries to force parent to stay Despair—passive, depressed, disinterested in environment, uncommunicative; loss of newly learned skills Detachment—similar to infants; less regressive behaviors	Allow child to express feelings of protest Accept regressive behaviors without comment Encourage child to talk about parents and/or others in his life Encourage parents to room-in if possible Encourage parents to leave comfort objects, for example, a favorite blanket and favorite toy Interpret child's behaviors to the parent(s)
	Loss of control—physical restriction, loss of routine and rituals, dependency Bodily injury and pain	Regression Negativisim Temper tantrums Resistance Physical aggression Verbal uncooperativeness	Incorporate home routines important to the child in his care as much as possible, for example, bedtime and bath rituals Allow child as much mobility as possible Employ pain reduction techniques, including medication Employ comfort measures
Preschool	Initiative vs guilt Separation	Protest—less direct and aggressive than toddler may displace feelings on others Despair ⎫ Detachment ⎭ similar to toddler	Allow child to express protest and anger Encourage the child to discuss home and family Accept regressive behaviors

*Many interventions are appropriate for each age, although they are not repeated for each section.

Continued.

TABLE 18-1. CHILDREN'S REACTIONS TO STRESS—cont'd

AGE	DEVELOPMENTAL ACHIEVEMENT AND MAJOR FEARS	BEHAVIOR REACTIONS	INTERVENTIONS*
Preschool—cont'd	Loss of control—sense of own power Bodily injury and pain—intrusive procedures, mutilation, castration	Aggression—physical and verbal Regression—dependency; withdrawal; feelings of fear, anxiety, guilt, shame; physiologic responses; immature behavior	Assist child in moving from regressive responses to behaviors appropriate to his age as he is ready Provide play and diversional activities Encourage child to "play out" feelings and fears Allow as much mobility as possible Encourage parents to visit often Encourage rooming-in if available Encourage parents to leave the child's favorite toy and some tangible evidence of their love Acknowledge the child's fears and anxieties Avoid intrusive procedures when possible
School-age	Industry vs inferiority Separation (parents as well as peers) Loss of control—enforced dependency, altered family roles Bodily injury and pain—fear of illness itself, disability, and death; intrusive procedures in genital area	Usually do not see stage behavior of protest, despair, or detachment Any of following may indicate separation as well as other fears—loneliness, boredom, isolation, withdrawal, depression, displaced anger, hostility, frustration, excessive sleeping or TV watching Seeks information Passively accepts pain Groans or whines Holds rigidly still Tries to act brave Communicates about pain May try to postpone an event	Allow expression of feelings, both verbally and nonverbally Acknowledge child's fears and concerns; encourage discussion of these fears and concerns Involve child in activities appropriate to his developmental level and condition Provide the child with in-ward or unit activities Employ appropriate interventions to alleviate pain Encourage parents to visit or room-in where possible Encourage peer contacts Continue with schooling Provide individualized recreation
Adolescent	Identity vs role diffusion Loss of control—loss of identity, enforced dependency Bodily injury and pain—mutilation, sexual changes Separation (especially peer group)	Rejection Uncooperativeness Withdrawal Self-assertion Self-control Cooperativeness Fear, anxiety Overconfidence May capitalize on gains from pain Depression Loneliness Withdrawal Boredom	Explore feelings regarding the hospital and the significance his specific illness might have on his relationships, identity formation, and future plans Help to adjust to new authority figures Explain procedures, therapies, and routines Help develop positive coping mechanisms Encourage maintaining contact with peer group Provide privacy Provide individualized schooling and recreation

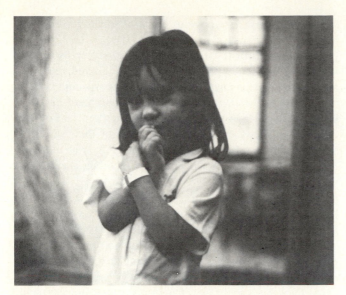

FIG. 18-1

Separation from parents during hospitalization constitutes a major stress for the young child.

relationships. However, this behavior is the result of resignation and is not a sign of contentment. He detaches from his parent in an effort to escape the emotional pain of desiring her presence. The child copes by forming shallow relationships with others, becoming increasingly self-centered, and attaching primary importance to material objects.

Without an understanding of the meaning of each stage of behavior, health team members may erroneously label the behaviors as positive or negative. In the stage of protest, they may view the loud crying as "bad" behavior. Since the protesting increases if a stranger approaches, they may interpret the reaction as evidence of their need to stay away. During the quiet, withdrawn phase of despair, they regard the child as finally "settling in" to his new surroundings and the detachment behaviors as proof of a "good adjustment." The faster a child reaches this stage, the more likely he will be regarded as the "ideal patient."

Since children seem to react "negatively" to visits by their parents, uninformed observers feel justified in restricting parental visiting privileges. For example, during the protest stage, children outwardly do not appear happy to see their parents. Instead, they may cry louder than before their visit, have temper tantrums, refuse to comply with the usual routines of mealtime, bedtime, or toileting, or regress to more primitive levels of development. If they are depressed, they may reject their parents or begin to protest once more. Often they cling to their parents in an effort to assure their continued presence. Consequently such behavior reactions may be regarded as "disturbing"

the child's adjustment to his surroundings. If the separation has progressed to the phase of detachment, children will respond no differently to their parents than to any other strange or familiar person.

Such reactions are equally distressing to parents, who are unaware of their meaning. If health team members regard parents as intruders, parents will view their absence as "beneficial" to the child's adjustment and recovery. They may respond to the child's behavior by staying for short periods of time, decreasing the frequency of visits, or lying to the child when it is time to leave. Consequently a *destructive* cycle of misunderstanding and unmet needs results.

Loss of control.   Any restriction or limitation on toddlers' newly gained motor skills results in an immediate threat to their sense of security and is met with physical resistance. Toddlers' need for freedom of movement is so essential that the attempt to place toddlers on their back can cause resistance and noncompliance.

Loss of control also results from altered routines and rituals. Toddlers rely on the consistency and familiarity of daily rituals to provide a measure of stability and control in their complex world of growing and developing. The experience of hospitalization or illness severely limits their sense of expectation and predictability, because practically every detail of the hospital environment differs from that of the home.

Toddlers' main areas for rituals include eating, sleeping, bathing, toileting, and play. When the routines are disrupted, one can expect difficulties in any or all of these areas. The principal reaction to such change is regression. For example, when mealtime and food choices differ from those at home, toddlers often refuse to eat, demand a bottle, or request that others feed them. Although regression to earlier forms of behavior may seem to increase toddlers' security and comfort, it is very threatening for them to relinquish their most recently acquired achievements.

Toddlers' striving for autonomy is evident in most of their behaviors. Play, interpersonal relationships, activities of daily living, and communication focus on their desires and needs. When their egocentric pleasures are not met, toddlers react with negativism, especially temper tantrums. Enforced dependency, a chief characteristic of the sick role, accounts for the numerous instances of toddler negativism. For example, rigid schedules, altered caregiving activities, unfamiliar surroundings, separation from parents, and medical procedures usurp toddlers' control over their world. Although most toddlers initially react negatively and aggressively to such dependency, prolonged loss of autonomy may result in passive withdrawal from interpersonal relationships and regression in all areas of development. Therefore the effects of the sick role are most severe in instances of chronic, long-term illnesses or in those families in which the sick role is fostered despite the child's improved state of health.

Bodily injury and pain. Toddlers' concept of body image, particularly the definition of body boundaries, is poorly developed. Intrusive experiences, such as examining the ears or mouth or taking a rectal temperature, are very anxiety producing. Toddlers may react to such painless procedures as intensely as they do to painful ones.

Toddlers' reactions to pain are similar to those seen during late infancy, except that the number of variables influencing the individual response is highly complex and varied. Memory, physical restraint, parent separation, emotional reactions of others, and lack of preparation partially determine the intensity of the behavioral response. In general, children in this age-group continue to react with intense emotional upset and physical resistance to any actual or perceived painful experience. Behaviors indicative of pain include grimacing, clenching their teeth/lips, rocking, rubbing, opening their eyes wide, restlessness, and aggressiveness, such as biting, kicking, hitting, or running away.

By the end of the age period toddlers are usually able to verbally communicate about their pain. Although they have not developed the ability to describe the type or intensity of the pain, they usually are able to localize it. For example, they may tell their parents that their ear or belly hurts. Such complaints should be taken seriously because children in this age-group rarely imagine or fake discomfort.

Preschool years

Preschoolers have advanced dramatically since infancy. They appear quite mature and self-sufficient in usual activities of daily living. They begin to assume increasing responsibility. However, under the stress of illness and hospitalization, preschoolers exhibit many of the same needs as toddlers.

Separation. Preschoolers are much more secure interpersonally. Not only can they tolerate brief periods of separation from their parents, but they also are able to develop substitute trust in other significant adults. However, the stress of illness usually renders them less able to cope with separation; as a result they manifest many of the stage behaviors of separation anxiety.

In general, the protest behaviors are more subtle and passive than those seen in younger children. Preschoolers may demonstrate separation anxiety through refusing to eat, difficulty in sleeping, crying quietly for their parents, continually asking when they will visit, or withdrawing from others. They may express anger indirectly by breaking their toys, hitting other children, or refusing to cooperate during usual self-care activities. Nurses need to be

sensitive to these less obvious signs of separation anxiety in order to intervene appropriately.

Loss of control. Preschoolers also suffer from loss of control caused by physical restriction, altered routines, and enforced dependency. However, their specific cognitive abilities, which make them feel omnipotent and all-powerful, also have the effect of making them feel out of control. This loss of control as a result of their sense of self-power is a critical influencing factor in their perception of and reaction to separation, pain, illness, and hospitalization.

Preschoolers' egocentric and magical thinking limits their ability to understand events because they view all experiences from their own self-referenced perspective. Without adequate preparation for unfamiliar settings or experiences, preschoolers' fantasy explanation for such events are usually more exaggerated, bizarre, and frightening than the actual facts. One typical fantasy to explain the reason for illness or hospitalization is that it represents punishment for real or imagined misdeeds. The response to such thinking is usually feelings of shame, guilt, and fear.

Bodily injury and pain. The psychosexual conflicts of children in this age-group make them very vulnerable to threats of bodily injury. Intrusive procedures, whether painful or painless, are threatening to preschoolers, whose concept of body integrity is still poorly developed. It is not uncommon for preschoolers to react to an injection with as much concern for withdrawal of the needle as for the actual pain. They fear that the intrusion or puncture will not reclose and that their "insides" will leak out.

Concerns of mutilation are paramount during this age period. Loss of any body part is threatening, but preschoolers' fears of castration complicate their understanding of surgical or medical procedures associated with the genital area, such as circumcision, repair of hypospadias or epispadias, cystoscopy, or catheterization. Their limited comprehension of body functioning also increases their difficulty in understanding how or why body parts are "fixed." For example, telling preschoolers that their tonsils are to be removed may be interpreted as "taking out their voice," or having the penis "fixed" may be understood as cutting it off. Although in general it is best to use the term "fixed" rather than removed, it is also important to explain what will be done to them as concretely as possible.

Reactions to pain change during this age period. By the end of the fourth year, many preschoolers exhibit an increasing degree of self-control while experiencing pain. Cultural expectations are also evident in these children. The stereotyped sex role of "brave men don't cry" is often seen in young boys who attempt to be courageous and, if they fail, feel guilty and ashamed.

The potential gains from the sick role also become obvious to preschoolers, and psychosomatic pain may surface at this time. Recurrent abdominal pain is the most common somatic complaint in children and may first occur in preschoolers who are facing the crisis of entering kindergarten.

Preschoolers' reactions to the stress of pain and fear are aggression, verbal expression, and dependency. *Aggression* in preschoolers is more specific and goal directed than in younger children and is geared toward fight or flight. Instead of total body resistance, preschoolers may push the person away, try to secure the equipment, or attempt to lock themselves in a safe place. Much more thought is evident in their plan of attack or escape.

Verbal expression in particular demonstrates their advanced development in response to stress. They may verbally abuse the attacker by stating, "Get out of here" or "I hate you." They may also use a more cunning approach of trying to persuade the person to give up the intended activity. A common plea expressed by preschoolers is, "Please don't give me that shot; I'll be good." Some statements are not only attempts to avoid the event but also evidence of children's perceptions about the experience.

Although language helps them communicate more fully, their ability to use concrete thinking rather than abstraction makes it necessary for others to interpret the words in light of the behavior. For example, the child who exclaims, "I hate you," may really be expressing his fear of strange, unfamiliar sights and sounds. The nurse who interprets that statement as personal rejection cannot meet the underlying need expressed by the child.

Dependency very often represents regression to more stable and comforting modes of behavior. Anxiety related to uncertainty, fear, pain, or separation may be expressed through behaviors such as clinging to a parent, refusing to play with other children, reverting to nonverbal means of communication, wanting to be held, or refusing to be left alone. A common expression denoting the need for dependency is, "Help me." It is important to recognize such requests as the need for support from others during a time of stress. Admonishing children to act grown-up or encouraging them to do things by stating, "I know you can do it yourself," deprives them of the support they are requesting and increases their own feelings of guilt and shame.

School-age years

The period of school-age includes children from 6 years of age to the end of preadolescence. Since this is a fairly large age span, it is more relevant to view this period as three separate but overlapping groups: (1) late preschool–early school-age, (2) middle school-age, and (3) late school-age–preadolescence. Many of the fears and reactions of children in this age-group are carried over from the preschool years, whereas others begin during preadolescence.

Separation.   Although school-age children are better able to cope with separation in general, the stress imposed by illness or hospitalization may increase their need for parental security and guidance. This is particularly true for young school-age children who have only recently left the safety of the home and are struggling with the crisis of school adjustment. These youngsters may still require the presence of their parents during hospitalization because the usual response of regression to stress may leave them with the same needs as preschoolers.

Middle and late school-age children may react more to the separation from their usual activities and social attachments than to absence of their parents. Their high level of physical and mental activity frequently finds no suitable outlets in the hospital environment. Even when they dislike school, they admit to missing its routine and associated activities. Feelings of loneliness, boredom, isolation, and depression are common. It is important to recognize that such reactions may occur more as a result of separation than from concern over the illness, treatment, or hospital setting.

School-age children may need and desire parental guidance or support from other adult figures but be unable or unwilling to ask for it. Because the goal of attaining independence is so important to them, they are reluctant to seek help directly for fear that they will appear weak, childish, or dependent. Cultural expectations to "act like a man" or to "be brave and strong" bear heavily on these children, especially males, who tend to react to stress with stoicism, withdrawal, or passive acceptance. Often the need to express hostile, angry, or other negative feelings finds outlets in alternate ways, such as irritability and aggression toward parents, withdrawal from hospital personnel, inability to relate to peers, rejection of siblings, or subsequent behavioral problems in school.

Loss of control.   Because they are striving for independence and productivity, school-age children are particularly vulnerable to events that may lessen their feeling of control and power. In particular, altered family roles, physical disability, fears of death, abandonment, or permanent injury, loss of peer acceptance, lack of productivity, and inability to cope with stress according to perceived cultural expectation may result in loss of control.

Because of the nature of the patient role, many routine hospital activities usurp individual power and identity. For these children, dependent activities such as enforced bed rest, use of a bedpan, inability to choose a menu, lack of privacy, help with a bed bath, or transport by use of a wheelchair or stretcher can be a direct threat to their security. Although all of these usual hospital procedures seem routine and inconsequential, nurses must remember that to children who want to "act grown-up," these activities allow no freedom of choice. However, when children are allowed to exert a measure of control, regardless of how limited it may be, they generally respond very well to any procedure. For example, some of the most cooperative, satisfied, and contented patients are those school-age children who help make their beds, choose their schedule of activities, assist in procedures, and help the nurses care for the younger children. An increased sense of control is usually an outcome of a feeling of usefulness and productivity.

Besides the hospital environment, illness may also cause a feeling of loss of control. One of the most significant problems of children in this age-group centers on boredom. When physical or enforced limitations curtail their usual abilities to care for themselves or to engage in favorite activities, school-age children generally respond with depression, hostility, or frustration. Keeping a normally active child on bed rest is no small challenge. However, emphasizing areas of control and capitalizing on quiet activities, particularly hobbies such as building models or collecting specific objects, promote their adjustment to physical restriction. Nursing judgment regarding selection of a roommate is one of the most important contributing factors to their overall adjustment to illness and hospitalization.

Bodily injury and pain. Fears of the physical nature of the illness surface at this time. There may be less concern with actual pain than there is for disability, uncertain recovery, or possible death. Because of their developing cognitive abilities, school-age children are aware of the significance of different illnesses, the indispensability of certain body parts, the potential hazards in treatments, the lifelong consequences of permanent injury or loss of function, and the meaning of death. They generally take a very active interest in their health or illness. Even those children who rarely ask questions usually reveal detailed knowledge of their condition by listening attentively to all that is said around them. They request factual information and quickly perceive lies or half-truths. Seeking information tends to be one way of their maintaining a sense of control despite the stress and uncertainty of illness.

School-age children begin to show concern for the potential beneficial and hazardous effects of procedures. Besides wanting to know if a procedure will hurt, they want to know what it is for, how it will make them better, and what injury or harm could result. For example, these children fear the actual procedure of anesthesia. Unlike preschoolers who fear the mask and the strange surroundings, school-age children fear what may happen while they are asleep, if they will wake up, and if they may die. Pread-

olescents also worry about the operation itself, particularly one that will result in visible changes in body image.

Intrusive procedures of a nonsexual nature, such as routine physical examination of the ears, nose, mouth, and throat, are generally well tolerated. However, concerns for privacy become evident and increasingly significant. Although school-age children may be cooperative during examination of, or procedures that are performed on, the genital area, it is usually very stressful for them, especially for preadolescents who are beginning pubertal changes. Nurses who respect children's need for privacy provide them with much assurance and support. Since the parents' presence may or may not be wanted by children during such procedures, nurses should also assess the child's individual preference. It may also be necessary to explain to parents why children prefer to be alone. Many parents forget the special needs of children in this age-group and believe that concerns for privacy surface only during adolescence.

By the age of 9 or 10 years most school-age children show little fright or overt resistance to pain. They generally have learned passive methods of dealing with discomfort, such as holding rigidly still, clenching their fists or teeth, or trying to act brave by the "grin and bear it" routine. If they do display signs of overt resistance, such as biting, kicking, pulling away, trying to escape, crying, or plea bargaining, they tend to deny such reactions later, especially to their peers for fear of losing status within the group.

School-age children verbally communicate about their pain in respect to its location, intensity, and description. They may also use words as a means of controlling their reactions to pain. For example, these children may ask the nurse to talk to them during a procedure. Some prefer to participate in a procedure, whereas others choose to distance themselves by not looking at what is happening. Most appreciate an explanation of the procedure and seem less fearful when they know what to expect. Others try to gain control by attempting to postpone the event. A typical request is, "Give me the shot when I am finished with this." Although the ability to make decisions does increase their sense of control, unlimited procrastination results in heightened anxiety. When choices are allowed, such as selection of the injection site, it is best to structure the number of possible sites and to limit the number of "procrastination" techniques.

Similar to their more passive acceptance of pain is their nondirective request for support or help. School-age children will rarely initiate a conversation about their feelings or request that someone stay with them during a lonely or stressful period. In fact, their visible composure, calmness, and acceptance often belie their inner longing for support. It is especially important to be aware of nonverbal clues, such as a serious facial expression, a halfhearted reply of, ''I am fine,'' silence, lack of activity, or social isolation, as signs of the need for help. Usually when someone identifies the unspoken messages and offers support, they readily accept it.

Adolescence

Of all periods during childhood, adolescents have the most well-developed coping mechanisms to deal with stress. They have a widely developed support system, the ability to think abstractly as well as concretely, the communication powers to make all their needs known, the physical stability to withstand bodily injury and stress, and previous life experiences to guide them through the present and future. Yet, with all these strengths, they are one of the most vulnerable groups to succumb to the stress of illness and hospitalization. The main threats are loss of control, especially in terms of loss of identity; fear of altered body image; and separation, primarily from members of their peer group.

Separation. Separation from home and parents may be a welcomed and appreciated event. However, loss of peer group contact may be a severe emotional threat because of loss of group status, inability to exert group control or leadership, and loss of group acceptance. Deviations within peer groups are poorly tolerated, and, although members may express concern for the adolescent's illness or need for hospitalization, they continue their group activities, quickly filling the gap of the absent member. During the temporary separation from their usual group, ill adolescents may benefit from group associations of other hospitalized age-mates.

Loss of control. Adolescents' struggle for independence, self-assertion, and liberation centers on the quest for personal identity. Anything that interferes with this poses a threat to their sense of identity and results in a loss of control. Illness, which limits their physical abilities, and hospitalization, which separates them from usual support systems, constitute major situational crises.

The patient role fosters dependency and depersonalization. In addition, hospitalization imposes on the adolescent a new set of authority figures. Adolescents may react with rejection, uncooperativeness, or withdrawal. They may respond to depersonalization with self-assertion, anger, or frustration. Regardless of which response they manifest, hospital personnel generally tend to regard them as difficult, unmanageable patients. Parents may not be a source of help because these behaviors serve to further isolate them from understanding the adolescent. Although peers may visit, they may not be able to offer the kind of support and guidance needed. Sick adolescents often voluntarily isolate themselves from age-mates until they feel they can compete on equal bases and meet group expectations. As a result ill adolescents are left with virtually no support systems.

Loss of control also occurs for many of the reasons discussed under school-age children. However, adolescents are more sensitive to potential instances of loss of control and dependency than younger children. For example, both groups seek information about their physical status and rely heavily on anticipatory preparation to decrease fear and anxiety. However, adolescents react not only to the kinds of information supplied them but also to the means by which it is conveyed. They may feel very threatened by others who relate facts in a derogatory manner. Adolescents want to know that others can relate to them on their own level. This necessitates a careful assessment of their intellectual abilities, previous knowledge, and present needs. It may also require a willingness on the part of the nurse to learn the language of the adolescent.

Bodily injury and pain. Although body image begins at birth, its significance is paramount during adolescence. Injury, pain, disability, and death are viewed primarily in terms of how each affects the adolescent's view of himself in the present. Any change that differentiates the adolescent from his peers is regarded as a major tragedy. For example, diseases such as diabetes mellitus often present a more difficult adjustment period for children in this age-group than for younger children because of the necessary changes in the adolescent's life-style. Conversely, serious, even life-threatening illnesses that entail no visible body changes or physical restrictions may have less immediate significance for the adolescent. Therefore, the nature of bodily injury may be more important in terms of adolescents' perception of the illness than its actual degree of severity.

Adolescents' rapidly changing body image during pubertal development often makes them feel insecure about their bodies. Illness, medical or surgical intervention, and hospitalization increase their existing concerns for normalcy. They may respond to such events by asking numerous questions, withdrawing, rejecting others, or questioning the adequacy of care. Frequently their fear for loss of control and body image change is demonstrated as overconfidence, conceit, or a ''know-it-all'' attitude.

Because of the sexual changes that take place at this time, adolescents are very concerned about privacy. Lack of respect for this need can cause greater stress than physical pain. In addition, adolescents look for signs that indicate that they are developing normally and according to acceptable standards. When illness occurs, they fear that growth may be retarded, leaving them behind their peers. Although they may not voice this concern, they may demonstrate it by carefully observing others' reactions to them during physical examinations or procedures.

Adolescents generally react to pain with self-control. Physical resistance and aggression are unusual at this age, unless an adolescent is totally unprepared for a procedure. However, the social gains from playing the sick role are clearly evident. Psychosomatic complaints are frequent and most often disclose an underlying psychosocial problem. Complaints of fatigue, abdominal pain, headache, or backache may indicate problems in the home, school, or peer group. Effective intervention involves a careful assessment of adolescents' environment, not only an investigation of organic problems. Inquiring about sexual activity is an area of prime significance. Psychosomatic complaints may follow initial sexual relationships because of associated guilt, shame, or confusion.

NURSES' ROLE: MINIMIZE STRESS OF ILLNESS AND HOSPITALIZATION

Although children in each developmental age-group respond differently to the stressors of separation, loss of control, and bodily injury and pain, it is evident that intervention in each of these areas is essential for optimum adjustment to illness and/or hospitalization. The challenge of nursing is to realize the stressors of each age period, to accept the behavioral reactions, and to provide the support and assistance needed for successful coping.

Prevent or minimize separation

The primary nursing goal is preventing or minimizing the effects of separation, particularly in children under 5 years of age. Ideally parents should stay with their child and if desired, participate in the care. Since the mother tends to be the usual family caregiver, she spends more time in the hospital than the father. However, not all mothers feel equally comfortable in assuming responsibility for their child's care. Some may be under such great emotional stress that they need a temporary reprieve from total participation in caregiving activities. Others may feel insecure in participating in specialized areas of care, such as bathing the child after surgery. Individual assessment of each parent's preferred involvement is necessary in order to prevent the effects of separation while supporting the parent in his or her needs as well.

With life-styles and sexual roles changing, it is conceivable that some fathers may assume all or some of the usual mothering roles in the household. In this case it may be the father-child relationship that requires preservation. Since the majority of nurses are women, it is necessary for them to include fathers in the plan of care and respect the parental role of that person. It is equally important to support the mother's role as family provider or part-time housekeeper in order to meet the needs of each parent. In single-parent families the caregiver may not be a parent but an extended family member, such as a grandparent or aunt.

One of the potential problems with continuous parent visiting is neglect of the parent's need for sleep, nutrition, and relaxation. Often the sleeping accommodations are limited to a chair and sleep is disrupted by nursing procedures. After a few days parents can become exhausted, but feel obligated to stay. Encouraging them to leave for brief periods, arranging for sleeping quarters on the unit but outside the child's room, and planning a schedule of alternating visiting with the other parent or family member can minimize the stresses for the parent.

Although prevention of separation is the ideal goal, often this is not possible. Therefore, minimization of the effects of separation becomes the substitute objective. This is best accomplished by assigning a primary nurse to care for the child (Fig. 18-2) and by identifying the child's established daily routine by taking a nursing admission history (see p. 524). Usual daily activities such as food preparation and the method of feeding help establish a complementary schedule of caregiving practices. It also helps the parent feel as if he or she is participating in the child's care.

The nurse who is caring for the child must have an appreciation of separation behaviors. As discussed earlier, the phases of protest and despair are normal. The child is allowed to cry. Even if he rejects strangers, the nurse provides support through physical presence in the room. Saying to the child, "I know you are unhappy because you miss your mommy and daddy. It's all right to cry. I will sit here for awhile so you are not alone," reinforces to the child the nurse's awareness of his feelings without abandoning him. The child's contact with his parents is maintained by frequently talking about them, encouraging him to remember them, and stressing the significance of their visits, telephone calls, or letters.

Separation may be equally as difficult for parents, especially when they do not understand the behaviors of separation anxiety. To avoid the immediate protest, parents may sneak out or lie to the child about leaving. As a result the child does not learn that absence is associated with a guaranteed return but that absence means loss of parents. Helping parents realize the necessity and value of telling the child when they will leave assists the child in adjusting to the temporary separation. When parents openly admit their good-byes, children learn that such behavior is eventually met with a "hello."

Explaining to parents how the child reacts after they leave may also be helpful. Many parents imagine that the child cries for hours after they leave, whereas in reality he may cry for a few minutes but settle down when comforted by someone else.

Toddlers and preschoolers have a very limited concept

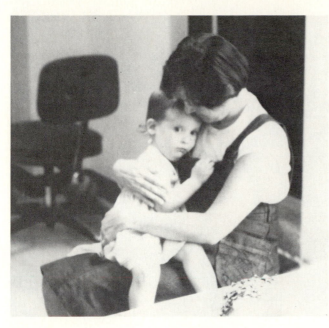

FIG. 18-2

A primary nurse can help overcome some of the stress imposed by separation.

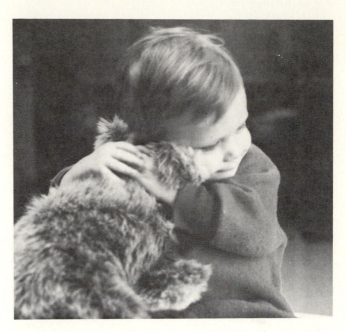

FIG. 18-3

A favorite "friend" can help a child feel more secure in the strange environment of the hospital.

of time. The young child's question of, "Will my mommy come yesterday?" symbolizes a lack of understanding for usual measurements of time, such as days, hours, weeks, and so on. Time is measured in associations, such as, "Eating dinner when daddy comes home." Therefore, when helping parents with their fears of separation, nurses need to suggest ways of explaining leaving and returning. For example, if parents must leave to go to work or to make meals for the other family members, they should tell the hospitalized child the reason for leaving. They also need to convey the expected time of return in terms of anticipated events. For example, if the parents return in the morning, they can tell the child that they will see him "After the sun comes up," or "When [a favorite program] is on television."

If parents leave after the child is asleep, they still need to communicate their absence. The parents of a 5-year-old boy solved this problem by devising a sign; on one side they drew a picture of a telephone and on the other they drew a hamburger. Before they left, they turned the sign to the appropriate side to tell the child when he awoke that they were out on the telephone or eating.

For older children who know how to tell time, it is helpful to give them a clock or watch. However, these children have the same needs for honesty from their parents regarding visiting schedules. Because peer groups are also important, adolescents often appreciate planning visiting hours with their parents to provide them with some private time for friends.

Familiar surroundings also increase the child's adjustment to separation. If parents cannot room-in, they should leave favorite home articles, such as a blanket, toy, bottle, feeding utensil, or article of clothing, with the child. Since young children associate such inanimate objects with significant people, they gain comfort and reassurance from such possessions (Fig. 18-3). They make the association that if the parent left this, the parent will surely return. Placing an identification band on the toy lessens the chances of its being misplaced.

Photographs of family members and tape recordings of the parent's voice, such as reading a story, singing a song, saying prayers before bedtime, or relating events at home, can help the child feel closer to his loved ones. The tapes are played at lonely times, such as on awakening or before sleeping.

Older children also appreciate familiar articles from home, particularly photographs, a radio, a favorite toy or game, and pajamas. Often the importance of treasured objects to school-age children is overlooked or criticized. However, many school-age children have a special object to which they formed an attachment in early childhood and this is a normal and healthy phenomenon. Therefore such treasured or transitional objects can help even older children feel more comfortable in a strange environment. Helping them to maintain their usual contacts outside the home by continuing school lessons during the period of illness and confinement, visiting with friends either directly or through letter writing, telephone calls, and so on, and participating in extracurricular projects whenever possible minimizes the effects of separation imposed by hospitalization.

Minimize loss of control

Feelings of loss of control result from separation, physical restriction, altered routines, enforced dependency, and magical thinking. Although some of these, such as separation from parents, can be prevented, all of them can be minimized through individualized planning of nursing care.

Physical restriction. Younger children react most strenuously to any type of physical restriction or immobilization. Although some restraint, such as immobilizing an extremity for maintenance of an intravenous line, is frequently necessary, much physical restriction can be prevented if the child's cooperation is gained.

For young children, particularly infants and toddlers, preserving parent-child contact is the best means of decreasing the need for or the stress of restraint. For example, almost the entire physical examination can be done in a parent's lap, with the parent hugging the child for procedures such as otoscopy or rectal temperatures. For painful procedures the parents' preferences for assisting, observing, or waiting outside the room are assessed. Parents may not wish to participate in restraining the child either because of their own fear or because they do not want the child to associate them with the event. In this case the parents can be readily available to console the child immediately following the procedure. Older children may or may not wish their parents' presence, particularly if privacy is a concern.

Most children feel more in control when they know what to expect because the element of fear is reduced. Anticipatory preparation and information giving are significant methods of lessening stress and often result in little need for physical restraint.

Environmental factors also influence the need for physical restraint. Keeping children in cribs or playpens may not represent immobilization in a concrete sense, but it certainly limits sensory stimulation. Increasing mobility by transporting children in carriages, wheelchairs, carts, wagons, or on stretchers or beds provides them with mechanical freedom (Fig.18-4).

The choice of a transporting conveyance should be guided by the child's age, physical condition, and destination. In general, the sitting position is preferred to the horizontal position, regardless of age. However, sometimes a stretcher or bed is required, such as when the child is in traction or has a spica cast. Young children feel more secure in proportionately smaller conveyances, such as wagons, carriages, or narrow wheelchairs. Older children prefer wheelchairs because they can move and guide them

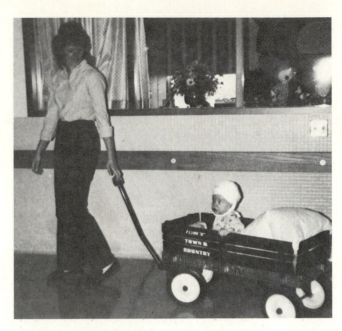

FIG. 18-4
Riding in a sided-wagon, this young child is able to leave the confines of his hospital room.

without assistance, thus increasing their independence. There is also the novelty of riding in a wheelchair and the adventure of races (Fig. 18-5). Safety is also a prime factor, especially when children are left in supervised group areas. For example, toddlers may satisfactorily be transported in any sitting-type conveyance, but a carriage with a restraining belt may provide the most protection.

In some cases physical restraint is necessary for promotion of recovery, such as using elbow restraints on children with eczema. Whenever possible, restraints should be removed to allow the child some period of supervised freedom, such as during the bath or when parents visit. In those instances when restraints cannot be moved, such as in severe burns, nurses can manipulate the environment to increase sensory freedom. For example, moving the bed toward the door or window, providing musical, visual, or tactile toys, and increasing interpersonal contact can substitute mental mobility for the limitations of physical movement.

Altered routines. Altered daily schedules and loss of rituals are particularly stressful for infants and young children and may increase the stress of separation. As has been discussed previously, the nursing admission history provides a baseline for planning care around the child's usual home activities.

Children's response to loss of routine and ritualism is often demonstrated in problems with activities such as feeding, sleeping, dressing, bathing, toileting, and social interaction. Although some regression is to be expected in

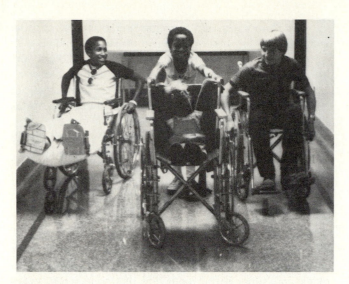

FIG. 18-5
Riding in wheelchairs is more than a means of transportation—it is also fun!

all of these areas, sensitivity to the special needs of children can minimize the negative effects. For example, loss of appetite and marked food preferences are common in ill or hospitalized children. In addition, the food selections on hospital menus may differ greatly from preferred cultural or ethnic food preparation. Encouraging children to eat while avoiding conflicts is a difficult yet essential nursing responsibility (see Chapter 19).

Because most children cope with the stress of illness and/or hospitalization by regressing to a more dependent and secure level of functioning, hospitalization is generally regarded as a poor time to introduce children to new skills. For example, young children who do not feed themselves should continue to be fed during this time. Expecting them to use a spoon "because they are old enough" does not respect their present level of functioning or their need for increased or maintained dependency.

Although regression is expected and normal, nurses also have the responsibility of fostering children's optimum growth and development. There are instances during which hospitalization becomes a significant opportunity for learning and advancing. For example, extended hospitalization for long-term chronic illness or situations of failure to thrive, abuse, or neglect represent instances in which regression must be seen as one adjustment period, to be followed by plans for promoting appropriate developmental skills.

One of the aspects of altered routines that is frequently neglected is the change in the child's daily activities. A nonhospitalized child's day, especially during the school years, is structured with specific times for eating, dressing, going to school, playing, and sleeping. However, this time structure vanishes when the child is hospitalized. One technique that can minimize the disruption in the child's routine is *time structuring*, which involves scheduling the child's day to include all those activities that are important to the nurse and child, such as treatment procedures, school work, exercise, television, playroom, and hobbies (Volz, 1981). Together, the nurse, parent, and child then plan a daily schedule with time and activity recorded in the nursing care plan.

Enforced dependency.   The dependent role of the hospitalized patient engenders tremendous feelings of loss of control on older children. The principal nursing interventions focus on demonstrating respect for the child and providing the opportunity for control through activities such as jointly planning care, time structuring, wearing street clothes, making choices in food selections and bedtime, continuing school activities, and rooming with an appropriate age-mate. For example, although school-age children may enjoy the responsibility of caring for a toddler or preschooler in their room, adolescents generally prefer quarters that are separate from the pediatric unit. Because their self-concept depends on outside influences, they are sensitive to even slight associations with childish "stigma," such as cartoons painted on their walls. They need surroundings and individuals who enhance their identity as adolescents. Nurses who call them by name, take an interest in them personally, and talk to them on their level usually are most supportive of adolescents' needs for control and self-identity.

Decrease bodily injury and pain

Beyond early infancy, all children fear bodily injury either from fears of mutilation, bodily intrusion, body image change, disability, or death. In general, preparation of children for painful procedures decreases their fears (see Chapter 19). Selecting alternative techniques also minimizes fear of bodily injury. For example, since toddlers and young preschoolers are traumatized by insertion of a rectal thermometer, axillary temperatures or electronic temperature probes can effectively be substituted. Whenever procedures are required, the most supportive intervention is to perform them as quickly as possible and to maintain parent-child contact.

Children also need permission to express pain. Telling these children that it is all right to say "ouch," scream, or cry allows them to express their feelings in an atmosphere of support and acceptance.

Because of young children's poorly defined body boundaries, the use of bandages may be particularly significant. For example, telling them that the bleeding will stop after the needle is removed does little to relieve their fears, whereas applying a small Band-Aid usually provides reassurance. The size of bandages is also significant to children in this age-group. The larger the bandage, the more importance is attached to the wound. Using successively smaller surgical dressings is one way of their measuring healing and improvement. Prematurely removing a dressing may cause them considerable concern for their well-being.

Children also benefit from recognition of their courage, such as "hero badge" or an "ICU diploma," which are positive mementos of an otherwise stressful experience. Giving them a choice in color or design also provides them with an opportunity for control.

Of particular importance in decreasing fear is ensuring that discussions are held where the child cannot overhear them. It is very easy to forget that the patient is listening and make remarks that are misunderstood. Usually a quiet reminder of how frightened the child can become from listening to these discussions is sufficient. If bedside conferences are necessary, the nurse interprets them for family members in language they can comprehend.

Pain assessment. Pain assessment is a critical component of the nursing process. Unfortunately nurses tend to underestimate the existence of pain in children. One of the principal reasons is a lack of understanding of what pain is—a personal phenomenon that *cannot* be experienced by any other individual. Therefore defining pain in terms of another's perceptions is inappropriate and inaccurate. McCaffery (1979) offers an operational definition that is useful in clinical practice: *pain is whatever the experiencing person says it is, existing whenever he says it does.* This definition implies a very important attitude toward the patient—*that he is believed.* It is meant to encompass both verbal and nonverbal expressions of pain.

Recognition of the existence and evaluation of the severity of pain is facilitated by an understanding of the response to pain of children in each age-group, as well as the influence of factors such as cultural or ethnic background, previous experience with pain, and response from others to the pain (as discussed in the previous section). Assessment of pain involves 3 areas: observation, questioning, and measurement tools.

Observe the child. The most important tool in assessing pain is observation of behavioral changes and physiologic responses. *Behavioral changes* are the most common indications of pain in children, particularly in preverbal youngsters and in those children with mental retardation or sensory/communication deficits. Behavioral changes include irritability, lethargy, loss of appetite, unusual quietness, disturbed sleep patterns, voluntary resting, increased restless movement or rigid posturing, flat affect, or anger. Specific reactions often indicate discomfort in localized body regions, such as rolling the head from side to side or pulling the ears for an earache, lying on the side with legs flexed on the abdomen for abdominal pain, or favoring a body part during usual activity.

The child's response to medication is another valuable indicator of pain. For example, in preverbal children who communicate a wide variety of emotions through behavior, obvious change in behavior following administration of an analgesic is evidence of existing pain. This knowledge can help to determine the cause of behaviors that suggest pain, such as crying or restlessness. If behavior changes, such as cessation of crying or restlessness, after administering one dose of an analgesic, this confirms the cause as pain, which requires continued relief.

Physiologic responses include flushed skin, increased sweating, blood pressure, pulse, and respiration, restlessness, and dilation of the pupils. However, these signs are seen in acute pain from stimulation of the sympathetic nervous system. If pain persists, body adaptation produces a decrease in these responses. If nurses rely on these physiologic indicators before believing that pain exists, many instances of pain will be unrecognized.

Question the child and parent. Children and parents can be excellent sources of information about pain. Although verbal indicators are much less common in children than in adults, children can describe pain if asked the right questions. Children, even those up to preadolescence, do not necessarily understand the meaning of terms like "pain" and "discomfort" and have very limited use of descriptive words, such as "burning," "cramping," "severe," or "excruciating." Children may globally describe pain as, "I hurt," or "I don't feel good." Using a variety of words that may be associated with pain, such as "bad," "funny," "hot," "pushing," or "banging," may help them describe the sensation. Other suggestions for describing pain are discussed on p. 77. Asking children to point to where it hurts or having them mark or color the area on a drawing, such as those on p. 537, is also helpful.

Children may deny that pain exists for fear of injectable pain medication or of not behaving appropriately. Such verbal negations of pain must be correlated with observations that indicate discomfort, such as lying rigidly. Sometimes telling a child that the momentary discomfort of an injection will take away the bigger pain results in a child's more honest appraisal of his pain.

Parents know their child and are sensitive to changes in his behavior. Frequently, they are aware that the behavior signals pain based on the child's previous response to painful events. Children will often reveal how they feel to parents because the parents are regarded as safe and trusted. It is not unusual for a child who has been quiet to start crying when the parent visits and complain that he hurts. Nurses sometimes erroneously judge this behavior as seeking attention, when it reflects the child's true feelings. The best intervention is to talk with the parent and child and *believe* that the child hurts.

Use a pain rating scale. Numerous investigators have developed measurement tools or scales that use nu-

FIG. 18-6
''Faces'' pain rating scale.

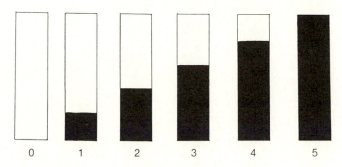

FIG. 18-7
''Glasses'' pain rating scale.

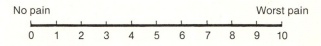

FIG. 18-8
Numeric pain rating scale.

meric values (usually from 0 to 5 or 10) to provide a more quantitative measure of pain. Tools that may be used with children include the following.

The *faces scale* uses six faces; the first picture is a very happy smiling face, the last is a sad, tearful face, and pictures in between show varying degrees of happiness and sadness (Fig. 18-6). The child chooses which face is most like him during the painful procedure.

The *chips scale* uses five plastic chips. These chips are compared to pieces of hurt: one chip is a ''little hurt'' and five chips are the ''most hurt.'' The child chooses the number of chips he feels equals his pain (Hester, 1979).

In the *glasses scale* a picture of six ''glasses'' or cylinders is presented to the child. The first glass is empty to represent ''no pain'' and the other five are filled with increasing amounts of black to represent increasing levels of pain (Fig. 18-7). The child chooses the glass with the amount of pain he feels.

The *numeric scale* uses a straight line with the end points identified as ''no pain'' and ''worst pain'' and divisions along the line marked in units from 0 to 10 (Fig.18-8). The child chooses the number that he thinks describes the intensity of his pain. This tool is useful in school-age and older children; the other three scales have been used successfully with children as young as 4 years of age.

Pain management. The reason for assessing pain is to relieve it. Comfort must be regarded as a basic need

of all children, yet nurses and physicians are often reluctant to order analgesics for children. The two reasons cited most often for this are: (1) the child is not in pain and (2) narcotics are dangerous—they depress respirations and cause addiction.

The first reason should not exist if one assesses pain appropriately and believes the patient. The second reason is an unwarranted fear. Narcotics given in safe dosages rarely cause respiratory depression because pain is a physiologic antidote to side effects, such as respiratory depression. In addition, as tolerance to the narcotic occurs, it also develops against the side effects. Fears of addiction typically stem from confusion between what addiction is and what occurs physiologically when patients take narcotics for extended periods. Addiction is a *voluntary psychologic dependence* on drugs. Studies on hundreds of terminally ill patients receiving narcotics daily for long periods show that psychologic dependence is virtually nonexistent. Although drug tolerance and physical dependence may occur, these are *involuntary physiologic events* and in no way are synonymous with addiction. Even when patients require greatly increased amounts of a drug over its recommended dosage, there are relatively few side effects and a dose remains that can continue to relieve pain.

Effective pain management requires that nurses be willing to try a number of interventions. Basically, methods to relieve pain can be grouped into two categories: nonpharmacologic and pharmacologic (see the boxed material on p. 514). Whenever possible, both of these should be used; however, nonpharmacologic measures should not be viewed as substitutes for analgesics.

Nonpharmacologic management. A number of nonpharmacologic techniques exist for reducing the perception of pain. These include (1) preparation for the painful

---

SUGGESTIONS FOR MANAGING PAIN IN CHILDREN

1. Prepare children in advance of potentially painful procedures but avoid "planting" the idea of pain. For example, instead of saying, "This is going to (or may) hurt," say "Sometimes this feels like pushing, sticking, or pinching, and sometimes it doesn't bother people. You tell me what it feels like to you." This allows for variation in sensory perception, avoids suggesting pain, and gives the child control in describing his reactions.

2. Avoid evaluative statements or descriptions, such as, "This is a terrible procedure," or "It really will hurt a lot."

3. Stay and/or invite the parents to stay with the child during a painful procedure; parents are often a neglected source of support for the child and can be involved in distracting him.

4. Use the power of positive suggestion by saying, "I am giving you a medicine that *will* take the hurt away."

5. Reinforce the effect of the analgesic by telling the child that he will begin to feel better in _____ amount of time (according to drug use). A clock or timer can be used to measure the onset of relief with the child. By reinforcing the cause and effect of pain and analgesic, the child becomes conditioned to *expecting* relief.

6. Avoid saying, "I'm going to give you a shot for pain," since this adds one pain to an existing pain; if the child refuses the shot, explain that the little hurt from the shot will take away the bigger hurt for a long time.

7. Give the child control whenever possible, for example, choosing which leg for a shot, taking bandages off, holding the tape or other equipment.

8. For long-term pain control give the child a doll that becomes "his patient" and allow him to do everything to the doll that is done to him. Pain control can be emphasized through the doll by stating, "Dolly feels better after her medicine."

9. Use distraction as much as possible (involve the parent and child in identifying strong distractions).
   a. Involve the child in play, use a radio, tape recorder, record player, or have him sing or use rhythmic breathing.
   b. Have the child concentrate on yelling or saying "ouch" by focusing on "yelling loud or soft as you feel it hurt; that way I know what's happening."

10. Use relaxation techniques. Teaching the child to relax may decrease painful stimuli (e.g., release tension on abdominal incision) or may act as distraction.
    a. Ask the child to take a deep breath and "go limp as a rag doll" as he exhales slowly. Then ask the child to yawn.
    b. Help the child assume a comfortable position (e.g., place a pillow under neck and knees).

11. Use cutaneous stimulation, such as simple rhythmic rubbing; use of pressure, use of electric vibrator; massage with hand lotion, powder, or menthol cream; application of heat or cold, such as ice cube on site before giving injection. Stimulation is most effective if rhythmic or constant and moderate in intensity.

---

event, (2) distraction, (3) relaxation, and (4) cutaneous stimulation. These techniques can lessen the perception of pain, and when used with analgesics, can enhance their effectiveness.

Pharmacologic management. Numerous nonnarcotic and narcotic analgesics exist; it is not the pupose of this discussion to describe individual drugs but to present general guidelines in selecting and administering analgesics. Two basic principles govern successful pharmacologic pain control:

1. Schedule the medication for *prevention* of pain
2. Titrate the dosage for maximum comfort

If pain is continuous, the goal is to relieve pain while maintaining maximum mental functioning. Administration of medications as needed (PRN) does not meet this goal. Rather, scheduled medication times that are individualized for each child are necessary. The nurse plans a *preventive* schedule by assuming that pain will be continuous, such as after certain procedures, or by recording for at least one

24-hour period the times of day when the child needs pain medication. For example, if the child complains of pain at 4- to 6-hour intervals, pain medication is given before the times the child would ask for it.

Successful manipulation of pain medication requires use of a *pain flow chart* to record the time the medication was administered, the medication given, and an assessment or rating of pain at the time the drug is given and every hour thereafter until the next dose of analgesic. This documentation provides evidence of the drug's effectiveness and facilitates collaboration with the physician regarding changes in medication orders.

Whenever possible the oral or suppository form of the safest drug is used. For example, the use of oral nonnarcotic analgesics may eliminate the need for injectable narcotics. More severe pain is controlled by the combination of a narcotic with a nonnarcotic analgesic the two drugs attack pain at different physiologic levels—the central nervous system (narcotics) and the peripheral nervous system (nonnarcotics). By adding a nonnarcotic, analgesia may be significantly increased without increasing the narcotic dose. When combining narcotics and nonnarcotics, the maximum dose of the nonnarcotic is used before increasing the dose of the narcotic. This also avoids the undesirable effects of narcotics.

Morphine sulfate (0.1 to 0.2 mg/kg of body weight) is the narcotic of choice for severe pain; it is superior to meperidine (Demerol), which has a very short duration of 2 to 4 hours and the potential for toxicity from repeated use. When large doses of morphine are required for intractable pain, continuous morphine infusion is effective. Oral methadone may be used for chronic pain and has the advantage of longer duration (6 to 8 hours) than most other narcotics.

When parenteral narcotics are required, every effort is made to switch to the oral route as soon as possible. However, conversion from parenteral to oral medication *must* be based on the equianalgesic doses for the drug. For example, if the child is receiving 5 mg of morphine by injection, he needs to receive 30 mg orally to achieve the same amount of analgesia.

Use of play to minimize stress

Play is one of the most important aspects of a child's life and one of the most effective tools for managing stress. Illness and hospitalization constitute crises in the life of a child and are often fraught with overwhelming stresses; allowing children to play out their fears and anxieties provides a way in which they can cope with these stresses.

Play is the "work" of children. It is essential to their mental, emotional, and social well-being, and, like their developmental needs, the need for play does not stop when children are ill or when they enter the hospital. On the contrary, play serves many functions while in the hospital:

> Provides diversion and brings about relaxation
> Helps the child feel more secure in a strange environment
> Helps to lessen the stress of separation and the feelings of being homesick
> Provides a means for release of tension and expression of feelings
> Encourages interaction and development of positive attitudes toward others
> Provides an expressive outlet for creative ideas and interests
> Provides a means for accomplishing therapeutic goals

The playroom does more to alleviate the stressors of hospitalization than any other hospital facility. Here children temporarily distance themselves from the fears of separation, loss of control, and bodily injury. They can work through their feelings in a nonthreatening, comfortable atmosphere and in the manner that is most natural for them. They also know that within the boundaries of this room they are safe from intrusive or painful procedures, strange faces, and probing questions. The playroom be-

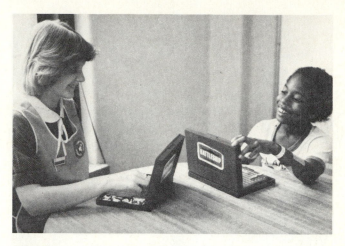

FIG. 18-9
Games are a popular play activity for hospitalized children.

comes a sanctuary of peace and safety in an otherwise frightening environment.

Diversional activities. Almost any form of play can be used for diversion and recreation; the following offers only a few of the numerous activities that are possible.* The activity is selected on the basis of the child's age, interests, and limitations. Children do not necessarily need special direction for using play materials. All they require is the raw materials with which to work, adult approval, and supervision to help keep their natural enthusiasm or expression of feelings from getting out of control. Small children enjoy a variety of small, colorful toys that they can play with in bed or in their room or more elaborate play equipment, such as playhouses, sandboxes, rhythm instruments, and large boxes and blocks, that may be a part of the hospital playroom.

Games that can be played alone or with another child or an adult are popular with older children (Fig. 18-9). Other activities that are enjoyed by children include puzzles, reading material, quiet individual activities such as sewing, stringing beads, and weaving, and Tinker-Toys, Lego blocks, and other building materials. Assembling models is an excellent pasttime, but it is a good idea to make certain that all pieces and necessary materials are included in the package. It is disappointing to the child to be ready to begin a project only to find that an essential item, such as glue, is missing from the set.

Well-selected books are of infinite value to the child. Children never tire of stories. To have someone read aloud provides endless hours of pleasure and is of special value to the child who has limited energy to expend in play. A

---

*An additional resource is *Ideas for Activities with Hospitalized Children*, available from the Association for the Care of Children's Health, 3615 Wisconsin Avenue, N.W., Washington, DC 20016.

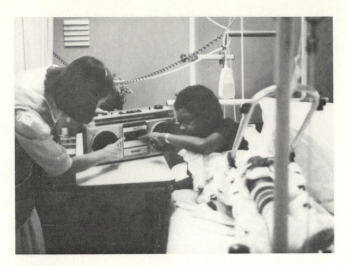

FIG. 18-10

A tape recorder provides the bedfast child with hours of enjoyment.

television set, a part of most hospital room equipment, is a useful tool for entertaining a child, but parents and nurses should monitor program selection and it should not be used as a substitute for social interaction or therapeutic play. Music is loved by all children. A tape recorder combines the pleasure of listening to music with the ability to hear a message from home or send one to special friends (Fig. 18-10).

When supervising play for ill or convalescent children, it is best to select activities that are simpler than would be chosen according to the developmental level of the child. These children usually do not have the energy to cope with more challenging activities. Other limitations also influence the type of activities. Special consideration must be given to the child who is confined in terms of movement, has an extremity restricted, or is isolated. Toys for isolated children must be disposable or capable of being disinfected after use.

Toys. Parents of hospitalized children often ask nurses about the types of toys that would be best to bring for their child who is hospitalized. Most want to bring new ones to cheer and comfort the child and assuage their own guilt feelings regarding the child's need for hospitalization. It is wise to assure the parents that, although it is natural to want to provide these things for their child, it is often better to wait awhile to bring new things, especially in the case of younger children. Small children need the comfort and reassurance of familiar things, such as the stuffed animal the child hugs for comfort and takes with him to bed at night. These are a link with home and the world outside the hospital.

Large numbers of toys often confuse and frustrate a small child. A few small, well-chosen toys are usually preferred to one large expensive one. Children who are hospitalized for an extended time benefit from changes. Rather than a confusing accumulation of toys, older toys are replaced periodically as interest wanes. A helpful suggestion is to have parents provide the child with a shoe box, a child's small suitcase, or knapsack to attach to the bed for an easy storage receptacle to prevent small items from becoming lost in the sheets or under the bed. Children love putting things in and taking things out of a larger container. Many simple items, such as a small magnifying glass, a magnet, grooming aids, a small mirror, crayons and coloring books, colorful paper with scissors and paste, a magic slate, small dolls or toy soldiers, small cars, and beads to string, afford endless hours of amusement. It is the responsibility of the nurse to assess the safety of the toys brought to the child.

A highly successful diversion for a child who is hospitalized for a length of time and whose parents are unable to visit frequently is for them to bring a box with seven small, inexpensive, and brightly wrapped items with a different day of the week printed on the outside. The child will eagerly anticipate the time for opening each one. When the parents know when their next visit will be, they can provide the number of packages that corresponds to the days between visits. In this way the child knows that the diminishing packages also represent the anticipated visit from the parent.

Expressive activities. Play provides one of the best opportunities for encouraging emotional expression, including the safe release of anger and hostility. Nondirective play that allows children freedom for expression can be tremendously therapeutic. Therapeutic play, however, should not be confused with the psychologic technique of play therapy. *Play therapy* is reserved for use by trained and qualified therapists who use the technique as an interpretative method with emotionally disturbed children. *Therapeutic play,* on the other hand, is a very effective nondirective modality for helping children deal with their concerns and fears, whereas at the same time it often helps the nurse to gain insights into their needs and feelings.

Tension release can be facilitated through almost any activity. Large-muscle activity such as use of tricycles and wagons is especially beneficial with younger ambulatory children. A great deal of aggression can be safely directed into pounding and throwing games and activities (Fig. 18-11). Bean bags are often thrown at a target or open receptacle with surprising vigor and hostility. A pounding board is employed with enthusiasm by young children; clay and Play-Doh are marvelous media for use at any age. It is not uncommon to see an angry child of 9 or 10 years of age attacking a mound of clay with the same intensity

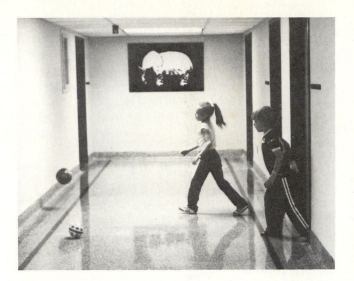

FIG. 18-11
Playing kickball in an empty hospital corridor helps children release tension.

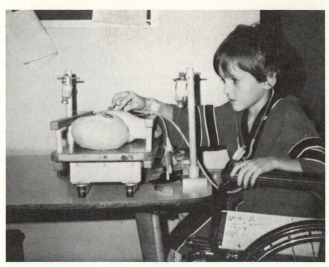

FIG. 18-12
Child playing with miniature hospital furniture.

that is observed in his 3- or 4-year-old counterpart.

Creative expression. Drawing and painting are excellent media for expression. The child need only be supplied with the raw materials, such as crayons and paper; plots of bright poster color, large brushes, and an ample supply of newsprint supported on easels; or materials for finger painting. Children usually require little direction for self-expression; however, older children may be given some direction in what to paint or draw. For example, they may be asked to draw the hospital room, draw what they like about the hospital, or draw what they do not like about the hospital. Groups of children can enjoy this creative activity either working individually or, with older children, collaborating on a group project such as a mural painted on a long piece of butcher paper. For children confined to bed, an old sheet (acquired from the laundry) spread over the bed and a large gown that extends down over the bedclothes to cover their own gown provide protection to clean linen.

Holidays provide stimulus and direction for unlimited creative projects. The children can participate in decorating the pediatric unit, and making pictures and decorations for their rooms gives the children a sense of pride and accomplishment. This is especially beneficial for immobilized and isolated children. Making gifts for someone at home helps to maintain interpersonal ties.

Dramatic play. Dramatic play is a well-recognized technique for emotional release, as children reenact frightening or puzzling hospital experiences. Through use of puppets, replicas of hospital equipment, or some actual hospital equipment, children can play out the situations that are a part of their hospital experience. Dramatic play

enables children to learn about procedures and events that will concern them and to assume the roles of the adults in the hospital environment (Fig. 18-12).

Puppets are universally effective for communicating with children. Most children view them as peers and readily relate to the puppet feelings that they hesitate to express to adults. Puppets can share children's own experiences and help them to find solutions to their problems. Puppets dressed to represent figures in the child's environment, for example, a physician, nurse, or therapist and members of the child's own family, are especially useful. Small, appropriately attired dolls are equally effective in encouraging the child to play out situations, although puppets are usually best for direct conversation.

In planning any play activities for the hospitalized child, the nurse must not lose sight of the fact that the reason for the child's hospitalization always takes precedence over other considerations, including the need for play. Play is scheduled around medical needs and any limitations imposed by the child's condition. For example, it is not uncommon for small children to eat paste and other creative media; therefore, a child who is allergic to wheat should not be given finger paint made from wallpaper paste or play dough made with flour. A child on a restricted salt intake should not play with modeling dough, since salt is one of its major constituents. Treatment schedules and the rules and policies of the institution are also considered. At home the play program should be planned around the therapy regimen. However, play can be incorporated satisfactorily into the child's care, if the nurse and others involved allow some flexibility and use creativity in planning for play.

SUMMARY OF NURSING CARE TO MINIMIZE STRESS OF THE HOSPITALIZED CHILD

GOALS	RESPONSIBILITIES
Help the child to feel safe in a strange environment	Provide consistency of nursing personnel as much as possible; assign a primary nurse Provide an atmosphere of warmth and acceptance for both child and parents Determine from parents or other caregiver the child's customary routine and manner of handling (see nursing admission history, p. 524) Attempt to maintain routine similar to the one the child is accustomed to at home Attempt to place the child in a nonthreatening environment Allow the child to retain as many attachments to home as permissable Encourage parents to leave some tangible symbol of continuing love Minimize hospital-like environment as much as possible, for example, allowing the child to sit at a table to eat meals, wear own pajamas, and so on Use terms familiar to the child, such as those for body functions Implement appropriate limit setting
Reduce or alleviate fear of the unknown	Help parents to prepare the child for elective hospitalization Explain routines, items, procedures, and events in a language appropriate to the child's developmental level; use simple language Reassure the child and repeat reassurance as necessary Absolve the child from any guilt he might feel regarding his hospitalization Allow the parent(s) to participate in the child's care Allow the child to handle items that he may perceive as strange and/or threatening Allow the child some control over his environment; encourage him to help plan his activities
Allow expression of feelings	Accept expression of feelings Provide an atmosphere that encourages free expression of feelings Provide opportunities to verbalize, "play out," or otherwise express feelings without fear of punishment
Help the child to feel he is cared for as a person	Maintain the child's identity Address the child by his name or usual nickname Avoid assigning a nickname to the child or converting a given name to its counterpart in another language, such as Joe instead of José Avoid communicating any signals of rejection, distaste, or other negative feelings to the child Criticize or communicate disapproval of unacceptable *behavior,* not disapproval of the *child* Communicate (verbally and nonverbally) to the child that he is a valued person
Provide for love and affection	Protect family interpersonal relationships Encourage parents to room-in whenever possible Encourage parents and others to cuddle, fondle, and otherwise demonstrate affection for the child Arrange work load and schedule to allow personal contact with the child Assign "foster grandparent" to the child if available

SUMMARY OF NURSING CARE TO MINIMIZE STRESS OF THE HOSPITALIZED CHILD—cont'd

GOALS	RESPONSIBILITIES
Minimize separation	Recognize the child's separation behaviors as normal
	Allow the child to cry
	Provide support through physical presence
	Maintain the child's contact with his parents
	Talk about his parents frequently
	Encourage the child to talk about and remember them
	Stress the significance of the parents' visits, telephone calls, or letters
	Help the parents understand the behaviors of separation anxiety and suggest ways of supporting the child
	Explain to the child when they leave and will return
	Tell the hospitalized child the reason for leaving
	Convey the expected time of return in terms of anticipated events. For example, if the parents return in the morning, they can tell the child that they will see him, "After the sun comes up," or, "When [a favorite program] is on television"
	Visit for short but frequent times rather than one long time; encourage parents and relatives to take turns visiting
	Allow siblings to visit
	Leave favorite home articles, such as a blanket, toy, bottle, feeding utensil, or article of clothing, with the child
	Provide photographs of family members and tape recordings of the parents' voices, such as reading a story, singing a song, saying prayers before bedtime, or relating events at home
	Leave small gifts for the child to open each day; if parents know when their next visit will be, have them leave the number of packages that corresponds to the days between visits
Establish a trusting relationship with the child	Be positive in approach to the child
	Be honest with the child
	Provide explanations of unfamiliar objects and happenings
	Convey to the child behaviors expected of him
	Be consistent in expectations and in relationships with the child
	Treat the child fairly and help him to feel that he is being treated fairly
	Encourage parents to maintain a truthful relationship with the child
Allow for regression during periods of illness	Recognize that regressive behavior is a feature of illness
	Accept regressive behavior and help the child with his dependency
	Assist the child in reconquering the negative counterpart of the psychosocial stage to which he has regressed, for example, overcome mistrust; facilitate development of trust
Provide opportunity for play	Allow ample time for play
	Make play materials available to the child
	Encourage play activities and diversions appropriate to the child's age, condition, and capabilities
	Use play as a teaching strategy and an anxiety-reducing technique
	Provide diversional activities
	Encourage interaction with other children

NURSES' ROLE: MAXIMIZING GROWTH POTENTIAL OF ILLNESS AND HOSPITALIZATION

Thus far the stressors of illness and hospitalization have been viewed as crisis situations that are capable of producing negative adjustments in children. However, the experience of illness and hospitalization can lead to positive changes. Therefore, nurses' roles must focus on both minimizing the stress and maximizing the growth potential of either experience.

Support parent-child relationships

The crisis of illness and/or hospitalization can mobilize parents into more acute awareness of their child's needs and can provide opportunities for parents to learn more about their child's growth and development. When nurses help parents understand their child's usual reactions to stress, such as regression or aggression, parents are not only better able to support the child through the hospital experience but may also extend their insights into child-rearing practices following discharge.

Difficulties in parent-child relationships that may result in feeding problems, negative behavior, and enuresis may decrease during hospitalization. The temporary cessation of such problems sometimes alerts parents to the role they may play in reinforcing the negative behavior. With assistance from health professionals, parents can restructure ways of relating to their children to foster more positive behavior.

Hospitalization may also represent a temporary reprieve or refuge from a disturbed home. Typically, abused or neglected children's dramatic physical and social improvement during hospitalization is proof of the growth potential of this experience. Hospitalized children temporarily are able to seek support, reassurance, and security from new relationships, particularly with nurses, hospitalized peers, and others.

Provide educational opportunities

Illness and hospitalization represent excellent opportunities for children and other family members to learn more about their bodies, each other, and the health professions (Fig. 18-13). For example, during a hospital admission for a diabetic crisis, the child may learn about his disease, the parents may learn about the child's needs for independence, normalcy, and appropriate limits, and each of them may find a new support system in the hospital staff. Older children may consider a health-related career based on their hospital experience.

Since nurses are in an optimum position to institute health teaching, they can often help people of different cultures understand the goals and philosophy of modern

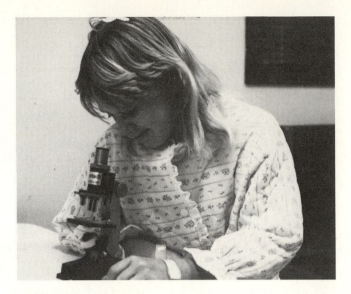

FIG. 18-13
The hospitalized youngster has the opportunity to learn more about herself, her body, and her disease.

medicine and, thereby, help them adhere to prescribed treatment plans.

Promote self-mastery

The experience of facing a crisis such as illness or hospitalization, coping successfully with it, and maturing as a result of it constitutes an opportunity for self-mastery. Younger children have the chance to test out fantasy vs reality fears. They realize that they were not abandoned, multilated, castrated, or punished. In fact, they were loved, cared for, and treated with respect for their individual concerns. It is not unusual to hear children who have undergone hospitalization or surgery tell others of how "it was nothing" or proudly display their scars or bandages.

For older children hospitalization may represent an opportunity to demonstrate decision making, independence, and self-reliance. They are proud of having survived the experience and may expect their parents to treat them as more "grown-up" following discharge. School nurses can capitalize on the school-age child's hospital experience by encouraging the child to discuss it with his classmates. In this way the child feels important as a result of having faced the crisis, and the other children learn about hospitalization.

Provide socialization

Hospitalization may offer to children a special opportunity for social acceptance. Lonely, asocial, sometimes delin-

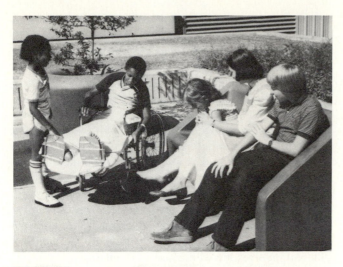

FIG. 18-14

The hospital environment can present a unique opportunity for forming new friendships and an accepting peer group.

quent children find a sympathetic environment in the hospital. Children who are physically deformed or in some other way ''different'' from their age-mates may find an accepting social peer group (Fig. 18-14). Although this does not always occur spontaneously, nurses can structure the environment to foster a supportive child group.

Parents may also encounter a new social group in other parents who have similar problems. The waiting room or hallway ''self-help'' groups are inherent to every institution. Nurses can capitalize on this informal gathering by encouraging parents to collectively discuss their concerns and feelings. They can also refer parents to organized parent groups or can use the help and support of recovered hospitalized patients.

FAMILIES OF ILL CHILDREN

The crisis of childhood illness and hospitalization affects every member of the nuclear family and, to various degrees, members of the extended family. Because a family is a system of interdependent parts, a change in any one member of the system causes a corresponding change in every other member. Under normal circumstances the parents are the dominant force in the family. However, when illness occurs, the child often becomes the principal force and, as such, causes major responses in each of the other family members.

Parents' reactions

Parents' reactions to illness in their child depend on a variety of influencing factors, but in many instances they are quite similar. Initially parents may react with *denial* and *disbelief*. For example, if a child complains of severe abdominal pain, parents initially may ascribe it little meaning. Even when the diagnosis of appendicitis is confirmed, parents may question the immediate need for surgery.

Following the realization of illness, parents react with *anger, guilt,* or both. To return to the above example, parents may direct the anger at the child for not having complained sooner or at themselves for not having realized the severity of the condition.

Guilt is almost a universal response. Even in the mildest of illnesses, parents question their adequacy as caregivers and review any actions or omissions that could have prevented or caused the illness. When hospitalization is indicated, parental guilt is intensified because they feel helpless in alleviating the child's physical and emotional pain. Guilt is especially prominent when children are admitted with accidental injuries. Parents feel responsible and are concerned that health professionals will view them as ''poor'' or negligent parents.

Fear, anxiety, and *frustration* are common feelings expressed by parents. Fear and anxiety may be related to the seriousness of the illness and the type of medical procedures involved. Often a great deal of anxiety is related to the trauma and pain inflicted on the child because of the various procedures.

Parents' anxieties regarding their child's hospitalization also fuel their feelings of frustration. Mothers often report that lack of information about procedures and treatment causes them the greatest concern. Frustration and a feeling of loss of control also occur as a result of uncertainty regarding hospital rules and regulations, a sense of unwelcomeness from the staff, or fear of asking questions. It is obvious that much frustration can be alleviated in a pediatric unit in which parents participate in their child's care and are regarded as the most significant contributors to the child's total health. Parents need to be informed of hospital policies regarding what they are permitted to do and where they can go on the unit.

Parents eventually react with some degree of *depression*. The depression usually occurs when the acute crisis is over, such as following hospital discharge or complete recovery. Mothers often comment on their feeling of physical and mental exhaustion after all the other family members have resumed their usual activities. Both parents may express concern for the financial burden incurred from the hospitalization.

Siblings' reactions

Siblings' reactions to a sister's or brother's illness or hospitalization are anger, resentment, jealousy, and guilt.

Guilt is usually a result of repressing the other feelings and occurs more commonly in older children.

Siblings' ability to cope is determined primarily by their developmental age but is also influenced by the strength of the family system, previous or concurrent experiences with stress, and usual coping mechanisms. For example, young children may have more difficulty in adjusting to the stress imposed by the separation from the parents. Older children who use verbal communication as a coping mechanism may have less difficulty adjusting, provided they are given adequate information. Children who are experiencing concurrent stresses, such as entry into school, may have increased difficulty in coping, regardless of their age.

Nursing considerations

Because dealing with a crisis involves a feeling of loss of control when previous coping mechanisms fail, parents' and siblings' principal need is a reestablishment of control. Nurses' main mode of intervention is supportive, which involves (1) fostering family relationships, (2) providing support, and (3) supplying information.

Foster family relationships. The nurse's role is to counsel parents regarding the effects of illness on the family. Parents should keep the family well informed and communicating as much as possible. They should treat all the children as equally and as normally as before the illness occurred. Discipline, which initially may be modified for the ill child, needs to be continued to provide a measure of security and predictability. When ill children know that their parents expect certain standards of conduct from them, they feel certain that they will recover. Conversely, when all limits are removed, they fear that something catastrophic will happen.

Parents are helped to understand and accept the meaning of posthospitalization behaviors in the child. Young children who have been separated from their parents during hospitalization may continue to show regressive behavior, such as emotional dependence, food finickiness, resistance to going to bed, and regression in self-toileting, for a month or longer. Older children may express posthospitalization behaviors such as anger, jealousy, and emotional coldness, followed by intense, demanding dependence on the parent. Other negative behaviors include new fears, nightmares, insomnia, withdrawal and shyness, hyperactivity, temper tantrums, attachment to blanket or toy, and tics or other nervous mannerisms. Younger children tend to exhibit more of these behaviors for longer periods of time. Parents who do not expect such reactions may misinterpret them as evidence of the child's "being spoiled" and expect him to conform to behavioral standards at a time when he is still reacting to the stress of illness and hospitalization. If these behaviors, especially the demand

for attention, are dealt with in a supportive manner, accompanied with reasonable limits on and expectations for acceptable behavior, most children are able to relinquish them in a short time.

Parents are also forewarned of the possible reactions of siblings to the ill child, particularly anger, jealousy, and resentment. Older siblings may deny such reactions because they provoke feelings of guilt. However, everyone needs outlets for emotions, and repressed feelings may surface as problems in school or with age-mates, as psychosomatic illnesses, or as delinquent behavior.

Provide support. The term "family-centered care" defines the focus of pediatric care because nursing of children cannot be performed optimally unless each family member is designated the "patient" or "client." Support involves the willingness to listen to parents' verbal and nonverbal messages. Sometimes the support is not given directly. For example, the nurse may offer to stay with the child to allow the parents time alone for them to support each other. The nurse may discuss with other family members the parents' need for extra relief. Often, relatives and friends want to help but do not know how. Suggesting ways such as baby-sitting, preparing meals, tending the garden or home, doing laundry, or transporting the siblings to school lessens the responsibilities that burden parents.

Parents with deep religious beliefs may appreciate the counsel of a clergy member, but because of their stress may not have sufficient energy to initiate the contact. Nurses can be supportive by arranging for clergy to visit, acknowledging parents' religious beliefs, and respecting their individual meaning and significance.

Support involves an acceptance of cultural, socioeconomic, and ethnic values. For example, health and illness are defined differently by various ethnic groups. For some, disorders that have few outward manifestations of illness, such as diabetes, hypertension, or cardiac problems, are not viewed as a sickness. Consequently, following a prescribed treatment may be seen as unnecessary. When one understands this, it is possible to point out signs of the disease that may have gone unnoticed or unappreciated.

Supply information. The term *information* involves much more than relaying facts. It is guidance through (1) knowledge of the disease, its treatment, and prognosis; (2) awareness of the child's emotional, as well as physical, reaction to illness and hospitalization; and (3) anticipation of the probable emotional reactions of the parents and siblings to the crisis.

Conveying information about the child's illness involves assessing the parents' present level of understanding and desire for additional knowledge. Because parental anxiety decreases their perception of information and leads to misinterpretation, nurses need to assess repeatedly the level of understanding. Often this prerequisite for effective intervention is ignored, resulting in information overload or omission of significant facts.

Probably one of the most neglected areas involves giving information to siblings. Children in every age-group deserve some explanation for the sibling's illness or hospitalization, especially regarding the following concerns: (1) "Will I get sick and have to go to the hospital?" (2) "Did I cause the illness?" (for actual or imagined reasons), and (3) "Will my parents abandon me if my brother or sister doesn't recover?" If parents or nurses address the explanations to these three questions, the siblings' own fears of illness, guilt, and abandonment are minimized.*

HOSPITAL ADMISSION: NURSING CONSIDERATIONS

The preparation that children require on the day of admission depends on the kind of prehospital counseling they have received.† The prepared child will usually know what to expect in terms of initial medical procedures, inpatient facilities, and nursing staff. However, prehospital counseling does not preclude the need for support during procedures such as drawing blood, x-ray tests, or the physical examination. For example, undressing young children before they feel comfortable in their new surroundings can be very upsetting. In addition, spending this time with the child gives the nurse an opportunity to evaluate his understanding of subsequent procedures, such as surgery.

When children have not had the benefit of prehospital counseling, the day of admission is critical. However, before beginning any preparation, nurses must assess the needs of the child. Sample questions that nurses can use to plan their care for further hospital preparation are listed in the admission history on p. 524. Guidelines for preparing the child for procedures are discussed on p. 533.

In addition to the admission responsibilities outlined in the box (right), a primary nurse is assigned whenever possible. The value of a consistent nurse during the child's entire hospitalization allows for individualized care and offers a substitute support system when stressors such as separation cannot be prevented.

Placing the child. Room assignments are usually made before the child is admitted to the pediatric unit. The minimum considerations for room assignment are the child's age and the nature of the illness. Ideally, however, room selection should be based on a variety of developmental and psychobiologic needs. Determining compatible

---

*A helpful book about siblings' needs is *Becky's Story: A Book to Share* by Donna Baznik available from the Association for the Care of Children's Health.
†Suggested resources for preparing children are listed at the end of this chapter.

OUTLINE OF ADMISSION PROCEDURES

Preadmission
1. Assign a room based on child's developmental age, seriousness of diagnosis, and projected length of stay.
2. Prepare the roommate or roommates for the arrival of a new patient (where children are too young to benefit from this consideration, prepare the parents).
3. Have the room ready for the child, with admission forms and equipment nearby to eliminate any need to leave the child.

Admission
1. Introduce the primary nurse to the child and parents.
2. Orient the family to inpatient facilities, especially in own room (call light, emergency bell, lights, bed controls, bathroom, telephone, and television [where applicable]). Emphasize positive areas of the pediatric unit such as the playroom, dining room, or other areas.
3. Introduce the family to the roommate and his or her parents.
4. Apply the identification band to the child's wrist, ankle, or both.
5. Explain hospital regulations for visiting hours (give written information if available).
6. Perform a nursing history.
7. Take the vital signs, blood pressure, height, and weight. Obtain a urine sample.
8. Support the child and assist the physician with the physical examination (for purposes of nursing assessment).

---

roommates, both for the children and rooming-in parents, greatly influences the growth potential from the hospital experience.

Although there are no absolute rules to govern room selection, in general, placing children of the same age-group and with similar types of illness in the same room is both psychologically and medically advantageous. However, there are many exceptions. For example, a school-age child may thrive on the responsibility of caring for a younger child. A child in traction may be very therapeutic for another child confined to bed because of a serious illness, such as rheumatic fever. An adolescent may find social acceptance from a peer of the opposite sex who is in a neighboring room. A child who is very independent despite handicaps may help another child with similar or different physical limitations and his parents achieve deeper insight and acceptance of the disability.

Nursing admission history. One of the most important nursing goals is to develop a trusting relationship with the child and parents. The nurse introduces himself or herself to the family and should begin an admission history. An admission history elicits baseline data on the child's usual habits and helps establish a greater similarity

NURSING ADMISSION HISTORY

Family data

1. Child's favorite name or nickname
2. Other members of immediate family, others who live in home (relatives, pets)
3. Usual caregiver (other than parent), baby-sitter, relative
4. Experiences with and reactions to temporary separation or absence of parent
5. Parents' occupations
6. Special considerations (adoption, foster child, stepparent or siblings, divorce, single parent)

Preparation for hospitalization

1. What does the child know about this hospitalization?
   a. Ask the child why he came to the hospital.
   b. If the answer is, "For an operation," ask the child to tell you about what will happen before, during, and after the operation.
   c. Is there anything the parents do not want the child to know? If so, inquire as to the reason.
2. Has the child ever been in the hospital before?
   a. Did anything unpleasant or traumatic occur in an earlier hospitalization that could have been avoided?
   b. Has anyone close to the child died in a hospital?
3. Are there any current illnesses or disabilities other than those for which the child is now admitted that limit his activity or require special care?
4. Have any major changes in the family occurred lately (death, divorce, separation, birth of a sibling, loss of a job, financial strain, mother beginning a career)? If so, explain the child's reaction.
5. How does the child act when he is upset or annoyed? What do the parents usually do?
6. Does the child have any fears (places, objects, animals, people, situations)? If so, what do the parents do?

Activities of daily living

1. Eating
   a. Usual mealtimes (with other family members or alone)
   b. Favorite foods, snacks, and beverages; average amounts
   c. Way in which food is served (warmed, cold, one item at a time)
   d. Food and beverage dislikes
   e. Feeding habits (cup, spoon, bottle, eats by self, needs assistance)
   f. Description of usual appetite
   g. Any problems (spitting up, ruminating)
   h. Remedies for problems
   i. Special cultural habits
   j. Any known or suspected food allergies

Activities of daily living—cont'd

2. Sleeping
   a. Usual hour of sleep and awakening
   b. Schedule for naps
   c. Routine before sleeping (bottle, drink of water, bedtime story, night-light, favorite blanket or toy, prayers)
   d. Type of bed
   e. Sleeps alone or with others (siblings, parents, other relatives)
   f. Favorite sleeping position
   g. Any problems (waking during night, nightmares, sleepwalking)
   h. Remedies for problems

3. Elimination
   a. Toilet trained (day and/or night, use of word to communicate urination or defecation, potty-chair, diapers, other routines)
   b. Usual pattern of elimination (bowel movements)
   c. Any problems (bed-wetting, constipation, diarrhea)
   d. Remedies for problems

4. Hygiene
   a. Usual habits for bathing (daily bath in tub or shower, sponge bath, usual schedule for shampoo)
   b. Dental habits
   c. Dressing
   d. Degree of assistance needed for above
   e. Any problems (refusal to wash or brush teeth, disliking having hair washed)
   f. Remedies for problems
   g. Care of special prostheses (glasses, contact lenses, hearing aid, orthodontic appliances, dentures, artificial elimination appliances, orthopedic devices)

5. Play
   a. Schedule during day (nursery, daycare center, regular school [grade in school], extracurricular activites)
   b. Preferred play companions (peer groups, alone, adults, younger or older children)
   c. Favorite activities or toys (both active and quiet interests)
   d. "Security" objects (pacifier, bottle, blanket, thumb, doll)
   e. Any favorite objects with him in hospital
   f. Any television restrictions, favorite programs; usual television hours at home

6. Spiritual habits
   a. Prayers before meals or at bedtime
   b. Attendance at services, prayer group, or other

between home and hospital environment (see the boxed material, opposite).

When a hospital admission is urgent a lengthy admission interview may not be feasible. However, several items are essential: (1) the child's name is ascertained and he is called by that name—terms such as "honey" or "dear" often confuse children; (2) the child's age is determined and some judgment made about developmental age (if the child is of school age, asking about his grade level will offer some evidence for concurrent intellectual ability); (3) the child's general state of health, any problems that may interfere with medical treatment, such as sensitivity to medication, and previous experience with hospital facilities are ascertained; and (4) the chief complaint is focused on, from both the parents' and the child's viewpoints.

Physical assessment. Although physical examinations by physicians are a required part of the admission, nurses should also use this valuable information in planning care. Subjecting children to two separate examinations is unnecessary if the nurse and physician cooperate. For example, when the nurse is present to psychologically support the child, the opportunity can also be used to observe the child's body for any bruises, rash, signs of neglect, deformities, or physical limitations.

The nurse should also listen to the heart and lungs as baseline data. For example, it is impossible to evaluate improvement in respiratory function in a child admitted with pulmonary disease unless there is data with which to compare subsequent findings.

SPECIAL HOSPITAL SITUATIONS: NURSING CONSIDERATIONS

In addition to elective, overnight hospital admission, children may be admitted to a day hospital, through an emergency department, to an isolation room, or to an intensive care unit. These admissions require special preparation based on an awareness of the child's needs.

Day hospital

The purpose of a day hospital or outpatient unit is to provide needed medical services for the child while eliminating the necessity of overnight admission. Among the benefits of a day hospital are (1) minimization of the stressors of hospitalization, especially separation from the family, (2) reduced chance of infection, and (3) economic saving. Typically admission to the day hospital is for minor operative or diagnostic procedures such as insertion of tympanostomy tubes, hernia repair, cystoscopy, or bronchoscopy.

Because of the limited contact with the child, nursing admission procedures are extremely important. Ideally, each child and family should receive preadmission counseling, including a tour of the facility and a review of the day's expected procedures. However, when it is not possible, surgery should be scheduled to allow some time for children to become acquainted with their surroundings and nurses to assess, plan, and complement appropriate teaching.

Emergency admission

One of the most traumatic hospital experiences for the child and parents is an emergency admission. The sudden onset of an illness or an accident leaves little time for preparation and explanation. Sometimes the emergency admission is compounded by admission to an intensive care unit or the need for immediate surgery. However, even in instances requiring treatment as an outpatient, the child is exposed to a strange, frightening environment and to people who often inflict pain. Therefore, every medical emergency requires psychologic intervention to reduce the fear and anxiety so frequently associated with the experience.

Unless an emergency is life threatening, children need to participate in their care to maintain a sense of control. Because emergency units are frequently hectic, there is a tendency to rush through procedures. However, the extra few minutes needed to allow children to participate may save many more minutes of useless resistance and uncooperativeness during subsequent procedures.

Isolation

Admission to an isolation room increases many of the stressors typically associated with hospitalization. There is further separation from familiar persons, additional loss of control, and added environmental changes such as sensory deprivation. These stressors are compounded by children's limited understanding of isolation. Preschool children, who may view isolation as a further punishment, are unable to comprehend the cause-and-effect relationship between germs and illness. Older children understand the causality better but still require factual information to decrease fantasizing or misinterpretation.

When a child is placed in isolation, preparation is essential for the child to feel in control. With young children the best approach is a simple explanation, such as, "You need to be in this room to help you get better. This is a special place to make all the germs go away. The germs made you sick and you could not help that." If the child is in protective isolation, one can emphasize that other people's germs can make him sick and this is a special place that keeps the germs from coming in.

With older children and parents the explanation can be based more on the cause-and-effect relationship, including how germs enter another's body, such as "by breathing them in." Family members are more likely to practice good handwashing, toileting hygiene, and so on if they are aware of their value.

All children, but especially younger ones, need preparation in terms of what they will see, hear, or feel in isolation. Therefore, they are shown the mask, gloves, and gown and are encouraged to "dress up" in them. Playing with the strange apparel lessens the fear of seeing "ghostlike" people walk into the room.

Before entering the room, nurses and other health personnel should introduce themselves and let the child see their face before donning a mask. In this way he associates them with significant experiences and gains a sense of familiarity in an otherwise strange and lonely environment.

When the child's condition improves, appropriate play activities are provided to minimize the boredom. Rather than dwelling on the negative aspects of isolation, the child can be encouraged to view this experience as challenging and positive. For example, the nurse can help the child look at isolation as a method of keeping others out and letting only special people in. Children often think of intriguing signs for their doors, such as, "Enter at your own risk" or "Many have entered but few have left." These signs also encourage people "on the outside" to enter and talk with the child about the ominous greetings.

Intensive care unit

Admission to an intensive care unit (ICU) can be a particularly traumatic event for both the child and the parents. Whenever possible the child and family should be prepared beforehand. However, even with preparation numerous stressors are present. Obviously the nature and severity of the illness are major factors, especially for parents. In addition, the physical appearance of the ICU can be awesome, frightening, and intimidating. Lights are on constantly, and there are strange, loud, and monotonous noises. Unfamiliar people speak *about* the child but rarely *to* him. The atmosphere is often charged with a sense of urgency over which the child has little control and no means of escape.

Extensive monitoring makes a usual day-night cycle difficult in an ICU. However, some schedule should be established that maintains a similarity to daily events in the child's life. These include organizing care during normal waking hours, keeping regular bedtime schedules, including quiet times when televisions and radios are lowered or turned off, closing and opening drapes as appropriate, dimming lights, placing a curtain around the bed for privacy and decreased stimulation, and having clocks or calendars in easy view for older children. When numerous procedures are required they should be scheduled to allow for 90 minutes of uninterrupted sleep to provide complete

sleep cycles. In particular staff members must be cognizant of the need for quiet and refrain from loud talking or laughing. Such measures can reduce the sleep deprivation commonly associated with ICU admissions.

Despite the stresses of the ICU, a type of security develops in being a patient in such a unit. Children and parents feel comforted by the quality of medical and nursing care, and the constant close, personal supervision they receive can make the transfer from ICU to the regular unit difficult for the family. Therefore, planning for transition to the regular unit is essential. It should include (1) assignment of a primary nurse on the regular unit who visits before the transfer, (2) continued visits by the ICU staff to assess the child's and parents' adjustment and to act as a temporary liaison with the nursing staff, (3) explanation of the differences between the two units and the rationale for the change to less intense monitoring of the child's physical condition, and (4) selection of an appropriate room and roommate.

Selecting a room that is close to the nursing station can help lessen the initial insecurity of being away from constant nursing supervision of the ICU. A roommate can overcome some of the feelings of separation the child experiences once he is no longer surrounded by familiar nursing staff.

DISCHARGE AND HOME CARE

Ideally preparation for hospital discharge and home care begins during the admission assessment. Specifically the establishment of short- and long-term goals determines discharge planning. General long-term goals can be summarized as: (1) evaluating improvement in physical status and (2) evaluating the child's subsequent psychologic adjustment to the hospital experience. It is important for nurses to consider the obvious short-term goals and the more subtle, but equally significant, long-range objectives.

Discharge planning also focuses on those procedures that parents or children are expected to continue at home. In planning for such goals, nurses need to assess (1) the actual and perceived complexity of the skill, (2) the parents' or child's willingness to assume the responsibility, and (3) the parents' or child's previous or present experience with such procedures. One example is the very common expectation of continuing antibiotic medication following discharge.

Rooming-in automatically facilitates preparing parents for home procedures, because they are available to observe and participate in the child's care. However, even though multiple opportunities exist for teaching, nurses should establish a specific plan that incorporates levels of learning, such as observing, participating with assistance, and, finally, acting without help or guidance. In those situations in which parents visit during scheduled times, such plans must be carefully determined to allow sufficient time for observation, participation, and evaluation.

It is also advisable to include more than one family member in discharge planning. Although the most consistent caregiver is the prime learner, at least one other member should be prepared, in order to allow the other person occasional respite from the responsibility.

Referral

Establishing appropriate referrals also stems from short- or long-term goals. This may be formal, such as referring to the visiting nursing service, or informal, such as introducing parents to another family with similar experiences. It may be initiated by the nurse or by the family. Regardless of which method is used, nurses need to assess the specific needs of the family and their probable reactions to the referral. The latter is particularly significant, because, although the needs may be quite evident, the family may reject the offered help. Preparing the family for the referral is as important as informing the referral service of the family's needs.

Some of the more usual referrals following hospital discharge include visiting nurse agency, private nurse practitioner, private physician, school tutor, physical therapist, mental health counselor, social worker, or other specialist. Sharing the important issues surrounding the child's hospitalization is essential. Referral summaries should be concise, specific, and factual. For example, if part of the referral to the visiting nurse focuses on the parent-child relationship, it is more effective to state observations supporting the reason for the referral, rather than judgmental statements. In this way visiting nurses have actual areas designated to help them form a plan of care.

REFERENCES

Hester, N.: The preoperational child's reaction to immunization, Nurs. Res. **28**(4):250-255, 1979.

McCaffery, M.: Nursing management of the patient with pain, ed. 2, Philadelphia, 1979, J.B. Lippincott Co.

Volz, D.D.: Time structuring for hospitalized school-aged children, Issues Compr. Pediatr. Nurs. **5**:205-210, 1981.

BIBLIOGRAPHY

Association for the Care of Children's Health: Preparing children and families for health care encounters, Washington, D.C., 1980, The Association.

Bellack, J.P., and Fore, C.V.: The young children in the critical care unit, Crit. Care Update **8**:26-38, May 1981.

Berner, C.: Assessing the child's ability to cope with stresses of hospitalization. In Brandt, P.A., Chinn, P.L., and Smith, M.E., editors: Current practice in pediatric nursing, St. Louis, 1976, The C.V. Mosby Co.

Birchfield, M.E.: Nursing care for hospitalized children based on different stages of illness, Am. J. Maternal Child Nurs. **6**(1):46-52, 1981.

Calkin, J.: Are hospitalized toddlers adapting to the experience as well as we think? Am. J. Maternal Child Nurs. **4**(1):18-23, 1979.

Canright, P., and Campbell, M.J.: Nursing care of the child and his family in the emergency department, Pediatr. Nurs. **3**(4):43-45, 1977.

Carty, R.: Observed behaviors of preschoolers to intensive care, Pediatr. Nurs. **6**(4):21-25, 1980.

Chinn, P.L.: Activities of daily living for the hospitalized child. In Brandt, P., Chinn, P.L., and Smith, M.E., editors: Current practice in pediatric nursing, vol. II, St. Louis, 1978, The C.V. Mosby Co.

Clark, D.: Parents' meeting in a pediatric unit: helping parents cope with their child's hospitalization, J. Assoc. Care Child. Hosp. **8**(2):32-35, 1979.

Coucouvanis, J.A., and Solomons, H.C.: Handling complicated visitation problems of hospitalized children, Am. J. Maternal Child Nurs. **8**(2):131, 1983.

Droske, S.: Children's behavioral changes following hospitalization—have we prepared the parents? J. Assoc. Care Child. Hosp. **7**(2):3-7, 1978.

Eland, J.M., and Anderson, J.E.: The experience of pain in children. In Jacox, A. editor: Pain: a source book for nurses and other health professionals, Boston, 1977, Little, Brown & Co.

Facteau, L.M.: Self-care concepts and the care of the hospitalized child, Nurs. Clin. North Am. **15**(1):145-155, 1980.

Fletcher, B.: Psychological upset in posthospitalized children: a review of the literature, Maternal Child Nurs. J. **10**(3):185-195, 1981.

Fore, C.V., and Holmes, S.S.: A care-by-parent unit revisited, Am. J. Maternal Child Nurs. **8**(6):408-410, 1983.

Gerbing, D.D.: Putting play to work in pediatrics, Am. J. Maternal Child Nurs. **2**(6):387, 1977.

Gohsman, B.: The hospitalized child and the need for mastery, Issues Compr. Pediatr. Nurs. **5**:67-76, 1981.

Gohsman, B., and Yunck, M.: Dealing with the threats of hospitalization, Pediatr. Nurs. **5**(5):32-35, 1979.

Green, M.: Parent care in the intensive care unit, Am. J. Dis. Child. **133**:1119-1120, 1979.

Hagemann, V.: Night sleep of children in a hospital. Part 1. Sleep duration, Maternal Child Nurs. J. **10**:1-13, 1981.

Hedenkamp, E.A.: Humanizing the intensive care unit for children, Crit. Care Quart. **3**(1):63-73, 1980.

Hill, C.: The mother on the pediatric ward: insider or outlawed, Pediatr. Nurs. **4**(5):26-29, 1978.

Huth, M.M.: Guidelines for conducting hospital tours with early school-age children, Pediatr. Nurs. **9**(6):414-415, 1983.

Knafl, K.A., and Dixon, D.M.: The role of siblings during pediatric hospitalization, Issues Compr. Pediatr. Nurs. **6**:13-22, 1983.

Koss, T., and Teter, M.: Welcoming a family when a child is hospitalized, Am. J. Maternal Child Nurs. **5**(1):51-54, 1980.

Lamb, J.M., and Rodgers, D.R.: Assisting the hostile, hospitalized child, Am. J. Maternal Child Nurs. **8**(5):336-339, 1983.

Lewandowski, L.A.: Psychosocial aspects of pediatric critical care. In Hazinski, M.F.: Nursing care of the critically ill child, St. Louis, 1984, The C.V. Mosby Co.

Lybarger, P.M.: The intensive care environment: its effect on the child and parents, Issues Compr. Pediatr. Nurs. **3**(6):50-57, 1979.

McCaffery, M.: Pain relief for the child: problem areas and selected nonpharmacological methods, Pediatr. Nurs. **3**(4):11-16, 1977.

McCain, G.C., and Bies, D.C.: Television viewing and the hospitalized child, Pediatr. Nurs. **9**(1):33-35, 1983.

McGuire, L., and Dizard, S.: Managing pain...in the young patient, Nursing 82 **12**(8):52-57, 1982.

McGuire, M., Shepherd, R., and Greco, A.: Hospitalized children in confinement, Pediatr. Nurs. **4**(6):31-35, 1978.

McLellan, C.L.: Hero badges mean more than courage, Pediatr. Nurs. **2**(3):7, 1976.

Miles, M.S., and Carter, M.C.: Assessing parental stress in intensive care units, Am. J. Maternal Child Nurs. **8**(5):354-359, 1983.

Miles, M.S.: Impact of the intensive care unit on parents, Issues Compr. Pediatr. Nurs. **3**(7):72-90, 1979.

Nelson, M.: Identifying the emotional needs of the hospitalized child, Am. J. Maternal Child Nurs. **6**(3):181-183, 1981.

Norberta, S.: Caring for children with the help of puppets, Am. J. Maternal Child Nurs. **1**(1):22-26, 1976.

Petrillo, M., and Sanger, S.: Emotional care of hospitalized children, ed. 2, Philadelphia, 1980, J.B. Lippincott Co.

Pomarico, C., Marsh, K., and Doubrava, P.: Hospital orientation for children, AORN J. **29**(5):864-875, 1979.

Stevens, K.R.: Humanistic nursing care for critically ill children, Nurs. Clin. North Am. **16**(4):611-622, 1981.

Tesler, M., and Savedra, M.: Coping with hospitalization: a study of school-age children, Pediatr. Nurs. **7**(2):35-40, 1981.

White, J.E.: Special nursing needs of hospitalized children with learning disabilities, Am. J. Maternal Child Nurs. **8**(3):209-212, 1983.

Wong, D.L.: Childhood trauma: its developmental aspects and nursing interventions, Crit. Care Quarterly **5**(3):47-60, 1982.

Wood, S.P.: School aged children's perceptions of the causes of illness, Pediatr. Nurs. **9**(2):101-104, 1983.

RESOURCES FOR CHILDREN AND PARENTS ABOUT HOSPITALIZATION

The following publications are available from the Association for the Care of Children's Health (ACCH), 3615 Wisconsin Avenue, N.W., Washington, DC 20016. ACCH is an international, multidisciplinary organization that promotes the emotional and psychosocial well-being of children and their families in all health care settings.

Caring for your child in the emergency room
Caring for your hospitalized baby
A child goes to the hospital
For teenagers: your stay in the hospital
Preparing your child for the hospital: a checklist
Preparing your child for repeated or extended hospitalizations
Selected books for children and teenagers about hospitalization, illness, and handicapping conditions
When you visit the ICU

An annotated list of books on various aspects of illness and hospitalization are in Fassler, J.: Helping children cope: mastering stress through books and stories, New York, 1978, The Free Press.

Bibliographies for children about health and illness are available from Pediatric Projects, Inc., P.O. Box 1880, Santa Monica, CA 90406.

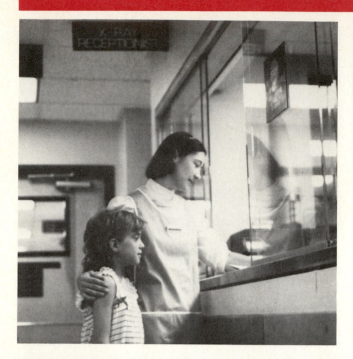

PEDIATRIC VARIATIONS
OF NURSING INTERVENTION

OBJECTIVES

On completion of this chapter the reader will be able to:

- Identify those instances in which informed consent is required and in which minors may be considered emancipated

- Formulate general guidelines for preparing children for procedures, including surgery

- Implement uses of play in therapeutic procedures

- Outline general hygiene and care procedures for hospitalized children

- Implement feeding techniques that encourage food and fluid intake

- Describe methods of reducing temperature in a febrile child

- Describe safe methods of administering oral, parenteral, rectal, optic, otic, and nasal medications to children

- Identify nursing responsibilities in maintaining fluid balance

- Demonstrate the correct procedures for postural drainage and tracheostomy care

- Describe the procedures involved in providing nutrition via gavage, gastrostomy, and hyperalimentation

- Describe the procedures involved in administering an enema and ostomy care to children

NURSING DIAGNOSES

Nursing diagnoses identified for the pediatric patient undergoing various procedures include, but are not restricted to, the following:

Health perception-health management pattern

- Infection, potential for, related to specific procedures

- Injury, potential for (poisoning, trauma), related to incorrect implementation of procedure

- Noncompliance, potential for, related to knowledge deficit

Nutritional-metabolic pattern

- Fluid volume deficit, potential or actual, related to intravenous therapy

- Nutrition, alterations in: potential for, more or less than body requirements related to alternative feeding techniques

- Skin integrity, impairment of: potential for, related to restraints

Elimination pattern

- Bowel elimination, alterations in: related to ostomy

Activity-exercise pattern

- Airway clearance, ineffective, related to thick excess secretions

- Diversional activity deficit related to use of restraints

- Home maintenance management, impaired, potential for, related to (1) knowledge deficit; (2) inadequate support system

- Self-care deficit (specify level: feeding, bathing/hygiene, dressing/grooming, toileting) related to developmental level

Sleep-rest pattern

- Sleep-pattern disturbance, potential for, related to schedule of procedures

Cognitive-perceptual pattern

- Comfort, alterations in: pain related to procedures

- Knowledge deficit related to inability to use materials or resources

- Sensory-perceptual alteration related to use of restraints

Self-perception—self-concept pattern

- Anxiety related to actual or perceived threat of bodily injury

- Fear related to (1) intrusive procedures; (2) anesthesia; (3) surgery and its outcome; (4) pain

Role-relationship pattern

- Parenting, alterations in: potential for, as related to lack of knowledge

Coping-stress tolerance pattern

- Coping, family: potential for growth related to successful coping

Children are not simply small adults. They differ from their older counterparts in the areas of biologic, cognitive, and emotional function and response. Consequently, many of the standard techniques employed in nursing practice must be altered to meet the special needs of this small but important group of patients.

INFORMED CONSENT

Informed consent has various legal meanings throughout the United States, but basically it means that the patient clearly, fully, and completely understands the medical treatment to be performed and he understands all the risks, consequences, or results that may or may not occur from the medical treatment. The patient must also be informed of alternative treatments that could be offered, including their risks, consequences, benefits, and other positive or negative factors.

Because of the numerous variations of the laws within different regions of the United States, the following discussion of informed consent is presented in general terms and is not to be interpreted as legal advice. Rather the purpose is to acquaint the reader with an overview of this highly important and complex subject and to encourage nurses to keep current on legal aspects of practice within their community.

When informed consent is required

Written informed consent of the parent or legal guardian is usually required for medical or surgical treatment, including many diagnostic procedures. One blanket consent is not sufficient. Separate informed permissions must be obtained for each surgical or diagnostic procedure, including:

1. Major surgery
2. Minor surgery, for example, cutdown, biopsy, dental extraction, suturing a laceration (especially one that may have a cosmetic effect), removal of a cyst, and closed reduction of a fracture
3. Diagnostic tests with an element of risk, for example, bronchoscopy, needle biopsy, angiography, electroencephalogram, lumbar puncture, cardiac catheterization, ventriculography, and bone-marrow aspiration
4. Medical treatments with an element of risk, for example, blood transfusion, thoracocentesis or paracentesis, radiation therapy, and shock therapies

In addition, there are certain situations, such as the following, that are not directly related to medical treatment but that require parental consent:

1. Taking photographs for medical, educational, or other public use

2. Removal of the child from the hospital against the advice of the physician
3. Post mortem examinations except in unexplained deaths, such as sudden infant death, violent death, or suspected suicide
4. Examination of medical records by unauthorized persons, such as attorneys, insurance representatives, and so on

Who may give informed consent

In most situations the parents or legal guardian gives informed consent. However, problems may arise when parents are not available to give informed consent, the child is a borderline or emancipated minor, or the parents neglect or refuse care for their minor children. Although it is the physician's duty to explain the procedure, treatment, alternatives, risks, consequences, and possible results to the parents or guardian, the nurse is often the person responsible for making certain that such informed consent is a part of the child's record.

Informed consent of parents or legal guardian. Parents have been considered to have full responsibility for the care and rearing of their minor children, including legal control over them. Therefore, as long as a child remains classified as a minor, the parent or the person designated as legal guardian for the child is required to give informed consent before medical treatment is implemented or any procedure is performed on the child.

Informed consent of persons other than parents or legal guardian. In the absence of the parents or legal guardian, a person in charge of the child is usually allowed to give informed consent for treatment. Depending on state law, this person, *in loco parentis,* may be a relative or other person who is caring for the child while the parents are away.

Temporary caregivers, such as baby-sitters, should know the location of the parents and the child's home address and have written permission from the parents for treatment in the event of an emergency. Special forms are available in many hospitals to authorize emergency care to minors.

Oral informed consent. When the parent is not immediately available to sign a consent form, informed oral consent may be obtained. This may be a telephone consent or an oral consent from a parent who is for some reason unable to sign, such as because of an injury following an accident. When verbal informed consent is being secured, it is wise to have a witness, such as another nurse, on a telephone extension. Both nurses can record that informed consent was given and the name, address, and relationship of the person giving consent, together with their signatures indicating that they witnessed the consent. Another alternative to obtaining verbal informed consent is to record the telephone call, making certain that the recording includes the identity of the individuals and the permission to record. As in any other situation, the nurse must be aware of state laws governing oral informed consent.

Informed consent of mature and emancipated minors. One of the areas in which modifications have been made in the usual view of parental obligation is in regard to borderline minors, that is, youngsters who are legally minors but who are considered to possess the maturity to give consent for their own medical care. Most states have enacted legislation that permits emancipated minors to give consent for their medical and surgical treatment.

An *emancipated minor* is one who is legally underage but is recognized as having the legal capacity of an adult under circumstances prescribed by state law. Minors may become emancipated by pregnancy, marriage, judicial decree, military service, consent of the parent(s), failure by parents to meet legal responsibilities, or living apart from the parents and being self-supported. A minor of any age can consent to treatment for venereal disease and has the right of privacy in obtaining contraception. Although state laws vary, the Supreme Court has held that when parents do not give permission for an abortion, the pregnant minor must have legal remedy available in the courts to prove that she is mature enough to consent to the abortion or that an abortion would be in her best interests. The majority of states provide a specific statutory age (usually 15 or 16 years) at which a minor may consent to medical or surgical treatment without parental consent. In this case the child is known as a *mature minor* even though he is not considered emancipated (Leiken, 1983).

State laws differ in their interpretation of when a child attains the age of majority. Even within the same state a child may be considered an adult in certain situations, for instance, in being responsible for necessities of life (food, clothing, and shelter) but may not be considered an adult in other situations. Many states now consider a child, male or female, an adult upon their 18th birthday. However, this may vary; some states may even differentiate between the sexes on attainment of maturity. Because the age of majority and other changes vary within jurisdictions, nurses need to be aware of the way in which the law functions in their state regarding medical care to children.

Treatment without parental consent. An exception to the general rule that parental consent is obtained before medical treatment of minor children occurs in situations in which children need prompt medical or surgical treatment and a parent is not readily available to give consent. Many states recognize this exception and permit treatment if the life or health of such a minor is in jeopardy or if delayed treatment would create a risk to the health of the minor. When surgical intervention is indicated in such situations, the procedure is usually begun only after consultation with another physician.

Parental negligence. The state is able to intervene in situations that jeopardize the health and welfare of children. Children may need protection from their parents in cases in which parents neglect or impose excessive or improper punishment on a child. In most communities there are procedures by which custody of the child can be transferred to a governmental or a private agency when parental neglect can be proved. In many cases the state interferes with the parental rights in the interest and protection of minor children.

PREPARING CHILDREN FOR HOSPITAL PROCEDURES

Children, regardless of their age, require preparation for procedures. With appropriate preparation the fear and discomfort is minimized and the child is helped to feel success and mastery from a potentially traumatic experience. However, nurses must be aware that a child's responses are strongly influenced by developmental characteristics such as physical and cognitive abilities; environmental factors, including past experiences with hospitalization, procedures, and health personnel; and his perception of the present situation. The child's general disposition and behavior patterns should be assessed, as well as his condition and the degree of regression he has experienced as a result of his illness. All of these areas are considered in planning an approach best suited to the child as an individual.

Provide psychological preparation

The principles governing preparation for hospital procedures, such as diagnostic tests, medical treatments, surgery, physical therapy, and so on, are similar and include the following:

1. Determine the details of the exact procedure to be performed.
2. Review the parents' and child's present level of understanding.
3. Plan the actual teaching based on the child's developmental age and existing level of knowledge.
4. Incorporate parents in the teaching if they desire and especially if they plan to participate in the care.
5. While preparing the child, allow for ample discussion to prevent information overload and ensure adequate feedback.

The exact timing of the preparation for a procedure varies with the child's age and type of procedure. In general, the younger the child, the closer the explanation should be to the actual procedure to prevent undue fantasizing and worrying. With complex procedures more time may be needed for assimilation of information, especially with older children. For example, the explanation for an

TABLE 19-1. GUIDELINES FOR PREPARING CHILDREN FOR PROCEDURES

DEVELOPMENTAL CHARACTERISTICS	RESPONSIBILITIES
Infancy: developing trust	
Attachment to parent	Involve the parent in procedure if desired Keep the parent in the infant's line of vision If the parent is unable to be with the infant, place a familiar object with the infant, such as stuffed toy
Stranger anxiety	Have usual caregivers perform or assist with procedure Make advances slowly and in nonthreatening manner Limit the number of strangers from entering room during procedure
Sensorimotor phase of learning	During procedure use sensory soothing measures, such as stroking skin, talking softly, giving pacifier Use analgesics, such as local anesthetic, sedation, to control discomfort Cuddle and hug the child after procedure; encourage the parent to comfort the child
Increased muscle control	Expect older infants to resist Restrain adequately Keep harmful objects out of reach
Memory for past experiences	Realize that older infants associate objects or persons with prior painful experiences Keep in mind that older infants will cry and resist at sight of objects or persons that inflict pain Keep frightening objects out of view Perform painful procedures in a separate room, not in crib
Imitation of gestures	Model desired behavior, for example, opening month
Toddler: developing autonomy	Use same approaches as above in addition to the following
Egocentric	Explain procedure in relation to what the child will see, hear, taste, smell, and feel Emphasize those aspects of procedure that require cooperation, such lying still Tell the child he can cry, yell, or use other means to verbally express discomfort
Negative behavior	Expect treatments to be resisted; the child may try to run away Use firm, direct approach Ignore temper tantrums Use distraction techniques Restrain adequately
Limited language skills	Communicate using behaviors Use few and simple terms that are familiar to the child Give one direction at a time, such as "Lie down," and then, "Hold my hand" Use small replicas of equipment; allow the child to handle equipment Use play; demonstrate on doll but avoid the child's favorite doll as he may think doll is really "feeling" the procedure Prepare the parents separately to avoid the child's misinterpreting words
Limited concept of time	Prepare the child shortly or immediately before procedure Keep teaching sessions short (about 5 to 10 minutes) Have preparations completed before involving the child in procedure Have extra equipment nearby, such as alcohol swabs, new needle, or Band-Aids to avoid delays Tell the child when procedure is completed
Striving for independence	Allow choices whenever possible but realize that the child may still be resistant and negative Allow the child to participate in care and to help whenever possible, for example, drink medicine from a cup, hold a dressing

TABLE 19-1. GUIDELINES FOR PREPARING CHILDREN FOR PROCEDURES—cont'd

DEVELOPMENTAL CHARACTERISTICS	RESPONSIBILITIES
Preschooler: developing initiative	
Preoperational thought; egocentric	Explain procedure in simple terms and in relationship to how it affects the child (as with toddler, stress sensory aspects)
	Demonstrate use of equipment
	Allow the child to play with miniature or actual equipment
	Encourage ''playing out'' experience on a doll both before and after procedure to clarify misconceptions
	Use neutral words to describe the procedure, such as ''make better'' or ''fixed'' instead of ''cut out'' or ''taken out'' and ''discomfort'' rather than ''pain''
Increased language skills	Use verbal explanation but avoid overestimating the child's comprehension of words
	Encourage the child to verbalize ideas and feelings
Concept of time and frustration tolerance still limited	Implement same approaches as for toddler but may plan longer teaching session (10 to 15 minutes); may divide information into more than one session
Illness and hospitalization often viewed as punishment	Clarify why all procedures are performed, such as, ''This medicine will make you feel better''
	Ask the child his thoughts regarding why a procedure is performed
	State directly that procedures are never a form of punishment
Fears of bodily harm, intrusion, and castration	Point out on drawing, doll, or child where the procedure is performed
	Emphasize that no other body part will be involved
	Use nonintrusive procedures whenever possible, such as axillary temperatures, oral medication
	Apply a Band-Aid over the puncture site
	Realize that procedures involving the genitals provoke anxiety
	Allow the child to wear underpants with his gown
	Explain unfamiliar situations, especially noises or lights
Striving for initiative	Involve the child in care whenever possible, for example, hold equipment, remove dressing
	Give choices whenever possible but avoid excessive delays
	Praise the child for helping and cooperating; never shame the child for lack of cooperation
School-age: developing industry	
Increased language skills; interest in acquiring knowledge	Explain procedures using correct scientific/medical terminology
	Explain the reason for procedure using simple diagrams of anatomy and physiology
	Explain functioning and the mechanism of equipment in concrete terms
	Allow the child to manipulate equipment; use doll or another person as model to practice using equipment whenever possible (doll play may be considered ''childish'' by older school-age child)
	Allow time before and after procedure for questions and discussion
Improved concept of time	Plan for longer teaching sessions (about 20 minutes)
	Prepare in advance of procedure
Increased self-control	Gain the child's cooperation
	Tell the child what is expected
	Suggest ways of maintaining control such as deep breathing, relaxation, counting
Striving for industry	Allow responsibility for simple tasks, such as collecting specimens
	Include in decision making, such as time of day to perform procedure, preferred site
	Encourage active participation, such as removing dressings, handling equipment, opening packages
Developing relationships with peers	May prepare two or more children for same procedure or encourage one to help prepare another peer
	Provide privacy from peers during procedure to maintain self-esteem

Continued.

TABLE 19-1. GUIDELINES FOR PREPARING CHILDREN FOR PROCEDURES—cont'd

DEVELOPMENTAL CHARACTERISTICS	RESPONSIBILITIES
Adolescents: developing identity	
Increasingly capable of abstract thought and reasoning	Supplement explanations with reasons why procedure is necessary or beneficial
	Explain long-term consequences of procedures
	Realize that adolescent may fear death, disability, or other potential risks
	Encourage questioning regarding fears, options, and alternatives
Conscious of appearance	Provide privacy
	Discuss how procedure may affect appearance, such as scar, and what can be done to minimize it
	Emphasize any physical benefits of procedure
Concerned more with present than future	Realize that immediate effects of procedure are more significant than future benefits
Striving for independence	Involve in decision making and planning, for example, choice of time, place, individuals present during procedure (such as parents), clothing to wear
	Impose as few restrictions as possible
	Suggest methods of maintaining control
	Accept regression to more childish methods of coping
	Realize that adolescent may have difficulty in accepting new authority figures and may resist complying with procedures
Developing peer relationships and group identity	Same as for school-age child but assumes even greater significance

injection can immediately precede the procedure for all ages, but preparation for surgery may begin the day before for young children and a few days before for older children.

In addition to these general principles, certain guidelines apply to the actual preparation process. Specific suggestions for each age group are included in Table 19-1.

Establish trust and provide support. The nurse who has spent time with and who has established a positive relationship with a child will usually find it easy to gain his cooperation. If the relationship is based on trust, the child will associate the nurse with caregiving activities that give him comfort and pleasure most of the time and not as someone who brings discomfort and stress. If the nurse does not know the child, it is best if she is introduced by another staff person whom the child trusts. The first visit with the child should avoid any painful procedure and ideally should focus on the child first, then on the explanation of the procedure. When talking with the child, the nurse uses the same guidelines for communicating with children that are discussed in Chapter 4.

Children need support during procedures, and for young children the greatest sources of support are the parents. However, controversy exists regarding the role parents should assume during the procedure, especially if discomfort is involved. The child may view the parent's participation as complicity and then blame the parent for allowing such indignities or pain to be inflicted on him. Children normally associate parents with a comforting, "make it better" role; therefore, parents should be a source of comfort and security to the child. Conversely, not allowing the parents to participate inflicts the additional stress of separation on the child and deprives him of his parents' support. While no definitive answer is available, it is suggested that parents and older children be given the choice of parental participation. Most parents choose to participate, are not disruptive of the procedure, and even when they find the experience difficult and stressful, support their children.

Provide an explanation. Children need an explanation for anything that involves them directly. Before performing a procedure, the nurse explains to the child what is to be done and what is expected of him. The explanation should be short, simple, and appropriate to the child's level of comprehension. Long explanations are not necessary and may only increase anxiety in a small child. This is especially true regarding painful procedures. When explaining the procedure to parents with the child present, the nurse uses language appropriate to the child because unfamiliar words can be misunderstood. If the parents

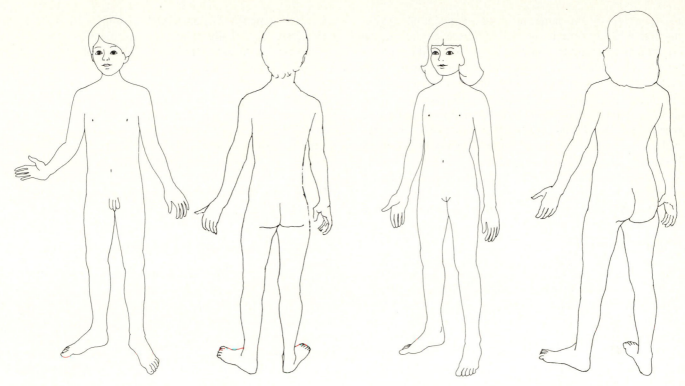

FIG. 19-1
Examples of line drawings to be used in preparing children for procedures.

need additional preparation, this is done in an area away from the child. Teaching sessions are planned at times most conducive to the child's learning, for example, after a rest period, and for the usual span of attention.

Special equipment is not necessary for preparing a child, but for young children who cannot yet think in concepts, using objects to supplement verbal explanation is important. Allowing children to handle actual items that will be used in their care, such as a stethoscope, sphygmomanometer, or oxygen mask, helps them to develop familiarity with these items and to reduce the threat often associated with their use. Miniature versions of hospital items, such as gurneys and x-ray and intravenous equipment, can be used to explain what the children can expect and permit them to experience safely the situations that are unfamiliar and potentially frightening.

Although the precise words used to describe a procedure will vary for children in each age-group and for each specific event, several important considerations apply to any situation:

1. Use concrete, not abstract, terms and visual aids to describe the procedure. For example, use a simple line drawing of a boy or girl (Fig. 19-1), and mark the body part that will be involved in the procedure.
2. Emphasize that no other body part will be involved.

3. Use words appropriate to the child's level of understanding and clarify all words, such as ''anesthesia is a *special* sleep.''
4. Allow the child to practice those procedures that will require his cooperation, such as turning, coughing, deep breathing, using a blow bottle or mask, or breathing on an intermittent positive pressure (IPPB) machine.
5. If the body part is associated with a specific function, stress the change or noninvolvement of that ability, for example, following tonsillectomy, the child can still speak.
6. Introduce anxiety-laden information last, such as the preoperative injection.
7. Be honest with the child about the unpleasant aspects of a procedure but avoid creating undue concern. When discussing that a procedure may be uncomfortable, state that it feels differently to different people and the child can tell you how it felt.
8. Emphasize the end of the procedure and any pleasurable events afterward, such as going home or seeing the parent. Stress the positive benefits of the procedure, for example, ''After your tonsils are fixed, you won't have as many sore throats.''

Perform the procedure

Supportive care continues during the procedure and can be a major factor in a child's ability to cooperate and achieve mastery. Ideally the same nurse who explains the procedure should perform it or assist. Before beginning, all equipment is assembled and the room is readied to prevent unnecessary delays and interruptions that only serve to increase the child's anxiety. If at all possible, procedures should be performed in a special treatment room rather than the child's bedroom. Procedures should never be performed in "safe" areas, such as the playroom. If the procedure is lengthy, conversation that could be misinterpreted by the child is avoided. As the procedure is nearing completion the nurse informs the child that it is almost over.

Expect success. Nurses who approach children with confidence and who convey the impression that they expect to be successful are less likely to encounter difficulty. It is best to approach a child as though he is expected to cooperate. Children sense anxiety in another and will respond to a perceived threat by striking out or with active resistance. Although it is not possible to eliminate such behavior in every child, a firm approach with a positive attitude on the part of the nurse tends to convey a feeling of security to most children.

Involve the child. As in any other aspect of care, involving children helps to gain their cooperation. Permitting them to make choices gives them some measure of control. However, a choice is given only in situations in which one is available to him. To ask a child, "Do you want to take your medicine now?" or "I'm going to give you a shot now, okay?" leads him to believe that there is an option and provides him with the opportunity legitimately to refuse or delay the medication. This places the nurse in an awkward, if not impossible, position. It is much better to state firmly, "It's time to drink your medicine now." Children usually like to make choices, but the choice must be one that they do indeed have, for example, "It's time for your medicine. Do you want to drink it plain or with a little water?"

Many children respond to tactics that appeal to their maturity or courage. This also gives them a sense of participation and achievement. For example, preschool children will be proud that they can hold the the dressing during the procedure or remove the tape. The same is true for the school-age child who cooperates with a minimum of resistance.

Provide distraction. When a child is occupied with some activity that interests him, he is less likely to focus on the procedure. For example, when an injection is given, it is helpful to give the child something to do or something on which to focus his attention. For example, asking the child to point the toes inward and wiggle them not only helps relax the gluteal muscles but provides a diversion. Other strategies for diverting attention are to have the child tightly squeeze the hands of a parent or an

assistant, count aloud, sing a familiar song such as a nursery rhyme, or verbally express his discomfort.

Allow expression of feelings. The child should be allowed to express feelings of anger, anxiety, fear, frustration, or any emotion he feels. It is natural for children to strike out in frustration or to try to avoid stress-provoking situations. The child needs to know that it is all right to cry. Whatever the response, it is important that the nurse accept the behavior for what it is. Telling a child with limited verbal skills, such as a toddler, to stop kicking, biting, or otherwise expressing his frustration conveys to him that he is not being understood. Behavior is his primary means of communication and coping.

Provide postprocedural support

After the procedure the child continues to need reassurance that he performed well and is accepted and loved. If the parents did not participate, the child is united with them as soon as possible so that they can comfort him.

Encourage expression of feelings. Some planned activity after the procedure is helpful in encouraging expression of feelings in a constructive way. Infants and young children are given opportunity for gross motor movement. Even older children are able to vent their anger and frustration in acceptable pounding or throwing activities. Play-Doh is a remarkably versatile medium for pounding and shaping. Dramatic play provides an outlet for anger and places the child in a position of control, in contrast to his position of helplessness in the real situation. One of the most effective activities for reducing the stress of injections is to permit the child to give a "shot" to a doll or stuffed toy.

Praise the child. The child needs to hear from others that they know that he did the best he could in the situation—no matter how he behaved. It is important for the child to know that his worth is not being judged on the basis of his behavior in a stressful situation. Although bribes are seldom effective over an extended period, some reward systems, for example, saving the empty medicine cup as evidence of achievement, are often helpful. Children who require distasteful medications, such as prednisone, or shots over a period of time can look with pride on a series of stars or stickers on a calendar, especially if an accumulated number represents a special privilege or reward.

Returning to the child a short while after the procedure helps the nurse to strengthen a positive relationship with the child. Relating with the child during a relaxed and nonstressful time allows him to see the nurse not only as someone associated with stressful situations but as someone with whom to share pleasurable experiences as well.

USING PLAY IN PROCEDURES

The use of play is an integral part of relationshps with children, and, as such, its value in specific situations is discussed throughout this book. Many institutions have very elaborate and well-organized play areas and programs under the direction of child life specialists. Some institutions have limited facilities, and others have no designated play area. No matter what the institution provides for the children, nurses can still include play activities as part of nursing care. Play can be used to teach, for expression of feelings, or as a method to achieve a therapeutic goal. Consequently, it should be included in preparing children for and encouraging their cooperation during procedures. The following is a discussion of some of the ways play can facilitate therapeutic interventions.

Fluid intake. Sometimes it is difficult to persuade children to drink an adequate amount of fluid. They may not feel well, their throat or mouth may hurt, or the unfamiliar hospital environment and the strangers who inhabit it may be deterrents. However, children are more likely to take fluid if drinking is part of a game or other fun activity. Incorporating the drinking into a story is a useful ploy, for example, taking a drink each time the page is turned. A drink can be part of the child's "turn" in a game or in "Simon Says," and children love to drink from interesting containers such as small decorated cups, glasses, or other containers. Children will often drink a great deal when fluid is served at a tea party at which they can pour drinks from a toy teapot, pitcher, or coffee pot into toy cups or glasses (Fig. 19-2). A child may enjoy filling a syringe with water and squirting it directly into his mouth or using

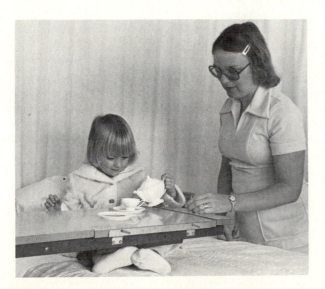

FIG. 19-2
Children enjoy drinking from interesting utensils, such as a toy teacup filled from a toy teapot.

it to fill a small cup. A medicine cup is a convenient size for this purpose, but it should be decorated or otherwise modified so that the intake of fluid is not associated with taking medicine.

Deep breathing. There are a number of devices and activities that can be used effectively to encourage a child to breathe deeply. There are several devices manufactured specifically for this purpose; however, when these are unavailable, a number of play activities serve as practical substitutes or supplemental exercises. Blowing soap bubbles appeals to many children, and blowing up balloons is an excellent measure for increasing end-expiratory pressure. Interesting balloons can be fashioned from surgical gloves, which the child can also decorate with felt pens. Blow bottles designed to force liquid from one container to another can be constructed with discarded bottles, stoppers, and tubing and are more enticing when the water is colored with food coloring. Other activities that stimulate lung expansion are blowing feathers, whistle toys (such as those used for parties), musical instruments where the environment permits, and blowing cotton balls around the table through a straw.

Range of motion and use of extremities. There are a variety of ways to provide range of motion exercises for children that combine fun with therapy. Any kind of throwing activity provides movement for the shoulder, elbow, and wrist. The game Twister encourages movement of all parts of the body. Wadded-up paper or bean bags can be thrown into a wastebasket, a box, or a target such as a hole cut into a large box. Toys attached to the end of a pulley are fun to manipulate. Activities that involve imaginative movement encourage exercising the extremities, for example, pretending to be bird, a butterfly, or a wild horse. A tricycle, where permitted, requires knee, hip, and ankle movement. Positioning the bed so that the child must turn to view the television or the doorway encourages him to assume different positions.

Injections. One of the most threatening procedures and a familiar one to all children is the hypodermic injection. Hospital play involving this stress-provoking equipment can be very revealing as well as therapeutic. Children respond in various ways to play with syringes. Usually children approach the syringe with respect and caution as though it were a dangerous weapon. Many hesitate to handle the equipment and require some time to muster the courage to touch the feared object. Once the initial hesitancy is overcome, however, children cannot resist handling the syringe and are willing to "give a shot" to a doll or stuffed animal (Fig. 19-3). Some handle the syringe gingerly and carefully imitate the ritual they have observed in their role models, that is, wiping the area with an alcohol sponge before and after injecting the solution and placing a Band-Aid over the puncture site. Others repeatedly

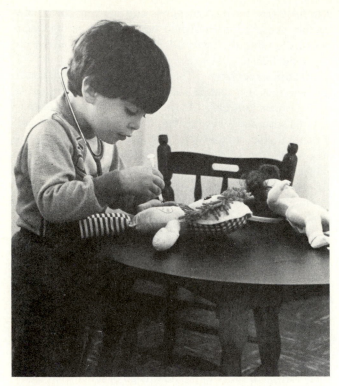

FIG. 19-3
Giving a shot to a doll requires intense concentration.

ram the needle into the doll with surprising vigor and expression of hostility.

Children who are exposed to needle play are often able to tolerate the procedure with less apparent distress. Although they still protest when they must receive an injection, the overt manifestations are less violent and last for a shorter period of time.

GENERAL HYGIENE AND CARE

Hygienic care is continued throughout the child's hospital stay and is essentially no different from that provided to persons of any age. The primary differences are those related to the size of the patient. Grooming aids and attractive attire are important adjuncts to hygienic care. Children are delighted with anything that makes them feel more attractive.

Certain caregiving activities present special challenges, especially feeding the sick child. In addition, children often have high fevers, which require attention and interventions, such as cooling baths. Any of these activities present excellent opportunities for health teaching.

Bathing

Unless contraindicated, most infants and children can be bathed in a tub at the bedside, on the bed, or in a standard bathtub located on the unit, which is often conveniently adapted for pediatric use.

Infants and small children are *never* left unattended in a bathtub, and infants who are unable to sit alone are held securely with one hand during the bath. The infant's head is supported securely with one hand or the farther arm is firmly grasped in the nurse's hand while the head rests comfortably on the wrist. This provides secure control of the infant while the other hand is free to wash the infant's body (Fig. 19-4). Infants or children who are able to sit without assistance need only close supervision and a pad placed in the bottom of the tub to prevent slipping and loss of balance, which could result in a bump on the head or submersion of the face.

Older children may enjoy a shower if it is available. School-age children may be reluctant to bathe and many are not accustomed to a daily bath. However, most children who feel well require little encouragement to participate in their daily care. Nurses will need to use judgment regarding the amount of supervision the child requires. Some children can be trusted to assume this responsibility unaided, whereas others will need someone in constant attendance. Retarded children, those with physical limitations such as severe anemia or leg deformities, and suicidal or psychotic children (who may commit bodily harm) require close supervision.

Areas that require special attention during bed baths and for children performing their own care are the ears, between skin folds, the neck, the back, and the genital area. The genital area is carefully cleaned and dried with particular care to skin folds, and in uncircumcised boys the foreskin is gently retracted, the exposed surfaces cleaned, and the foreskin replaced. Older children have the tendency to avoid these areas; therefore they may need a gentle reminder.

Children who are ill or debilitated will need more extensive assistance with bathing and other aspects of hygienic care, but they should be encouraged to perform as much as they are capable of without overtaxing their energies. Increasing involvement can be expected with improved strength and endurance. Children who are limited in the capacity for self-help and who have no other contraindications benefit a great deal from tub baths. They can be transported to the tub and, with the aid of lifting devices and/or an appropriate number of persons to assist, gain the advantages of a tub bath.

Mouth care

Mouth care is an integral part of daily hygiene and is continued in the hospital. Infants and debilitated children will require the nurse to perform mouth care. Although small children can manage a toothbrush and are encouraged to use it, most will need assistance to perform a satisfactory

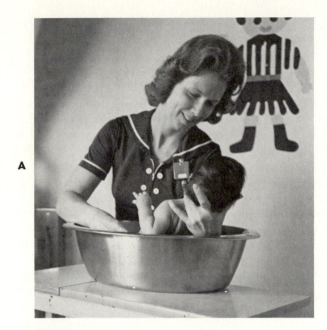
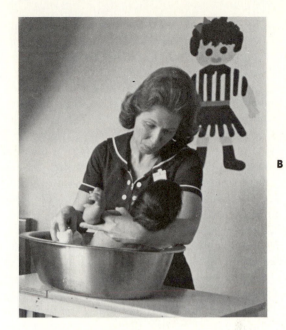

FIG. 19-4

Proper method for holding an infant for tub bath. **A,** *Supporting the neck.* **B,** *Neck supported on the wrist.*

job. Older children, although capable of brushing without assistance, often need to be reminded that this is a part of their hygienic care. Most hospitals have equipment available for those children who do not have toothbrush or toothpaste of their own. (See pp. 304 and 384 for specific oral hygiene techniques.)

Hair care

Brushing and combing hair are a part of the daily care for all persons in the hospital, including infants and children. If the child does not have a brush or comb, many hospitals provide one as part of the usual admission kit. If not, the parents should be asked to bring hair care equipment for the child's use. Both boys and girls are helped to comb or brush their hair, or it is done for them, at least once daily. There is no special hairstyle that is prescribed for hospitalized children. The hair should be styled for comfort and in a manner pleasing to the child and parents. The hair is not cut without parental permission, although shaving hair to provide access to a scalp vein for intravenous needle insertion is frequently carried out without permission.

Infants require little extra attention. The hair is washed daily as part of the bath in the newborn period and less often in later infancy. It is usually sufficient for most children to wash the hair and scalp once or twice weekly, but if there is any indication otherwise in children of any age, it is washed more frequently. Some hospitals have shampoo basins, but almost any child can be conveniently transported by a gurney to an accessible sink or washbasin

for shampooing. Those who are unable to be transported can receive a shampoo in their beds with adequate protection and/or specially adapted equipment or positioning.

Teenagers, with their normally increased oily sebaceous secretions, are particularly in need of frequent hair care and usually require more frequent shampoos. Commercial "dry shampoo" products may also prove useful on a short-term basis. If a commercial variety is not available, talcum powder placed on the hair will absorb oils and can be removed by vigorous brushing.

Black children require special hair care, and this need is frequently neglected or inadequately managed. For the black child with kinky hair, most standard combs are inadequate and may cause hair breakage and discomfort to the child. If a special comb with widely spaced teeth is not available on the unit, the parent can be reminded to bring a comb, if possible, for the child's use. This type of hair also requires a special hair dressing or pomade, which usually has a coconut oil base. The preparation is rubbed on the hands and then transferred to the hair to make it more pliable and manageable. The child's parents should be consulted regarding the preparation they wish to be used on their child's hair and asked if they can provide some for use during the child's hospitalization. Vaseline or petroleum jelly should *not* be used.

Feeding the sick child

Loss of appetite is a symptom common to most childhood illnesses. It is frequently the initial evidence of illness, preceding fever and other overt signs of infection. In most cases the child can be permitted to determine his own need for food. Since an acute illness is usually short, the nutritional state is seldom compromised. In fact, urging foods on the sick child may precipitate nausea and vomiting and in some cases even cause an aversion to the feeding situation that can extend into the convalescent period and beyond.

Refusing to eat may also be one way children can exert power and control in an otherwise helpless situation. For young children, loss of appetite may be related to the depression of separation from their parents and their natural tendency toward negativism.

Parents' concern with eating can intensify the problem. Forcing a child to eat only meets with rebellion and reinforces the behavior as a control mechanism. Parents are encouraged to relax any pressure during the period of acute illness. Although it is best to encourage high-quality nutritious foods, the child may desire foods and liquids that contain mostly calories. Some well-tolerated foods include gelatin, clear soups, carbonated drinks, popsicles, dry toast, crackers, and hard candy. Even though these substances are not nutritious, they can provide necessary fluid and calories.

Dehydration is always a hazard when children are febrile or refusing food, especially when these conditions are accompanied by vomiting or diarrhea. An adequate fluid intake should be encouraged by offering small amounts of favored fluids at frequent intervals and salty foods if allowed. High-calorie liquids such as colas, fruit juices, water flavored and sweetened with corn syrup, or similar drinks help prevent catabolism and dehydration. Fluids should not be forced, and the child should not be wakened from his rest to take fluids. Forcing fluids may create the same difficulties as urging unwanted food.

A variety of techniques can be employed to encourage an intake of food and fluid. Several suggestions are offered in the box on the facing page Using play techniques (see p. 539) can also be very effective.

Recording the amount of foods and fluids consumed is an important nursing responsibility. Descriptions need to be detailed and accurate, such as ''4 ounces of orange juice, one pancake, no bacon, and 8 ounces of milk.'' Comments such as ''ate well'' or ''ate poorly'' are inadequate. If parents are involved in the child's care, they are encouraged to keep a list of everything eaten. Using a premeasured cup for fluids ensures a more accurate estimate of intake. A comparison of the intake at each meal can isolate food deficiencies, such as insufficient intake of meat or vegetables. Behaviors associated with mealtime also identify possible factors influencing appetite. For example, the observation that, ''Child eats well when with other children but plays with food if left alone in room,''

helps the nurse plan mealtime activities that stimulate the appetite.

Control of fever

Fever is probably the most common symptom of disease in children. It is a great source of concern to parents and is frequently overtreated, which may lead to serious problems, such as salicylate overdose. Most fevers in children are of viral origin, of relatively brief duration, and with limited consequences. In addition, there is some evidence that fever may play a role in enhancing body defenses and/or reducing the growth of infecting organisms. A disadvantage in treating fever is the masking of other signs of the illness and less effective monitoring of the disease and its treatment.

Fever is defined as a temperature over 37.8° C (100° F) orally or 38° C (100.5° F) rectally. With the exception of children who are prone to febrile seizures, treatment with antipyretic medication is indicated if the temperature is above 39° C (102° F) and sponging is recommended if the temperature is higher than 40° C (104° F). Low-grade fever does not require treatment other than light clothing and additional fluids to prevent dehydration.

Pharmacologic management. Aspirin and acetaminophen are the preferred drugs for management of fever, although aspirin should not be given to children possibly infected with influenza virus or chickenpox because of the risk of Reye syndrome (American Academy of Pediatrics, 1982). The recommended dosage of aspirin and acetaminophen are given in Tables 19-2 and 19-3. Aspirin should not be given more often than every 4 hours, since there is risk of toxic effects from accumulation. In most cases the temperature decreases at night; therefore, three to four doses in 24 hours are usually sufficient to control most fevers. The temperature is retaken 15 to 30 minutes after administering the antipyretic and repeated as often as necessary.

The oral route is the usual method of administration, either in tablet or liquid preparations. Older children are able to swallow the tablet; younger ones chew the flavored variety or can be given the tablet crushed and mixed in syrup or jelly. The tablet must be crushed well in order to avoid chunks that might be aspirated into the larynx or trachea. Sometimes the rectal route, using aspirin or acetaminophen suppositories, is easier, especially with infants or children with sore, swollen throats. However, unless the suppository contains the exact dose, the oral route is used. Some children respond well to aspirin incorporated into a chewing gum (Aspergum), although the dosage must be carefully calculated.

Environmental management. Cool, moist applications to the skin help to reduce the core temperature.

SUGGESTIONS FOR FEEDING THE SICK CHILD

Take a dietary history (see p. 524) and use the information to make eating time as much like home as possible.

Encourage parents or other family members to feed the child or to be present at mealtimes.

Have children eat at tables in groups; bring nonambulatory children to the eating area in wheelchairs, beds, strollers, gurneys, or wagons.

Use familiar eating utensils, such as a favorite plate, cup, or bottle for small children.

Make mealtimes pleasant; avoid any procedures immediately before or after eating; make sure the child is rested and pain-free.

Have a nurse present at mealtimes to offer assistance, prevent disruptions, and praise children for their eating.

Serve small, frequent meals rather than 3 large meals or serve 3 meals and nutritious between-meal snacks.

Bring in foods from home, especially if food preparation is markedly different from the hospital; consider cultural differences.

Provide finger foods for young children.

Involve children in food selection and preparation whenever possible.

Serve small portions, and serve each course separately, such as soup first, followed by meat, potatoes, and vegetables, and ending with dessert; with young children camouflage the size of food by cutting meat thicker so less appears on the plate or folding a cheese slice in half; offer second helpings; ensure a variety of foods, textures, and colors.

Provide food selections that are favorites of most children, such as peanut butter/jelly sandwiches, hot dogs, hamburgers, macaroni and cheese, pizza, spaghetti, tacos, fried chicken, and corn on the cob.

Avoid foods that are highly-seasoned, have strong odors, are served hot, or are all mixed together, unless typical of cultural practices.

Provide fluid selections that are favorites of most children, such as fruit punch, cola, ginger ale, sweetened tea, ice pops, sherbet, ice cream, milk and milk shakes, eggnog, pudding, gelatin, clear broth, or creamed soups.

Offer nutritious snacks, such as frozen yogurt or pudding, ice cream, oatmeal or peanut butter cookies, hot cocoa, cheese slices or ''kisses,'' pieces of raw vegetable or fruit, and dried fruit or cereal.

Make food attractive and different, for example:
Serve a ''picnic lunch'' in a paper bag.
Put a ''face'' or a ''flower'' on a hamburger or sandwich with pieces of vegetable.
Use a cookie-cutter to shape a sandwich.
Serve pudding, yogurt, or juice frozen as a popsicle; make slurpies or snowcones by pouring flavored syrup over crushed ice; add vegetable coloring to water or milk.
Serve fluids through brightly colored or unusually shaped straws.
Do *not* punish children for not eating by removing their dessert or putting them to bed; instead, accept refusals, offer choices, distract the child, and offer food again.

TABLE 19-2. RECOMMENDED DOSAGE OF ASPIRIN (1¼-GRAIN TABLETS) FOR CHILDREN BY AGE AND WEIGHT*

AGE (years)	WEIGHT (pounds)	DOSAGE (tablets)
Under 2	Below 27	As directed by physician
2-3	27-35	2
4-5	36-45	3
6-8	46-64	4
9-10	66-76	5
11	77-83	6
12+	84+	8

Modified from Done, A., and others: J. Pediatr. **95**(4):617-629, 1979.
*If child's weight falls outside the range for his age, give dosage according to weight, not age. Aspirin may be given every 4 hours, but not to exceed five times a day unless prescribed by a physician.

TABLE 19-3. DOSAGE RECOMMENDATIONS FOR ACETAMINOPHEN (Tylenol)*

AGE	WEIGHT (pounds)	DOSE (mg)
Under 3 months	6-11	40
4-11 months	12-17	80
12-23 months	18-23	120
2-3 years	24-35	160
4-5 years	36-47	240
6-8 years	48-59	320
9-10 years	60-71	400
11 years	72-95	480
12-14 years	96+	640

*Doses should be administered four or five times daily, but not to exceed five doses in 24 hours.

Cooled blood from the skin surface is conducted to inner organs and tissues, and warm blood is circulated to the surface where it is cooled and recirculated. The surface blood vessels dilate as the body attempts to dissipate heat to the environment and facilitate this cooling process.

Tepid tub baths are fast, simple, and effective for reducing an elevated temperature in a child. When using the tub, it is usually best to start with warm water and gradually add cool water until the desired water temperature of 37° C (98.6° F) is reached. In this way the child becomes more easily accustomed to the lower water temperature. The child is placed directly into the tub of tepid water for 20 to 30 minutes while water is gently squeezed from a washcloth over his back and chest or gently sprayed over his body from a sprayer. The bath is even more effective if the child can tolerate lying down in the water with his head supported on the nurse's arm or a padded support. This is more easily accomplished with a small infant or an older child. Small children dislike lying down and often resist any efforts to force them into the horizontal position. For conscious children a floating toy or other distraction can be employed during the bath. The child is never left alone in the tub.

The cooling bath can also be given in the bed or crib. The child is completely undressed and placed on an absorbent blanket or towel spread over the bed. He is covered with a large towel or lightweight, absorbent cotton blanket. A cool washcloth or ice pack is placed on the child's forehead and changed as it warms. One area of the body is exposed at a time and sponged with a washcloth soaked in tepid water. Special care is taken where two body surfaces touch. The sponge bath is continued for approximately 30 minutes.

A safe, easy, and effective alternate method, and the one most often employed, is the *towel method*. The child is undressed and placed on an absorbent towel or blanket, and a cool cloth or ice bag is applied to the forehead. Each extremity is wrapped in a towel moistened in tepid water, one is placed under the back, and another covers the neck and torso. Special care is taken to make certain that opposing body surfaces, such as the groin and lateral torso between the arms and chest, are covered. The towels are changed as they warm. This is continued for approximately 30 minutes.

After the tub or sponge bath, the child is dried and dressed in lightweight pajamas, nightgown, or diaper and placed in a dry bed. The temperature is retaken 30 minutes after the tub bath or sponge bath and repeated as often as indicated. The child is observed carefully during any of these procedures, and if he shows signs of chilling, the cool treatment is discontinued immediately. The child is dried by gently rubbing the skin surface with a towel to stimulate circulation. The tub or sponge bath should not be continued or restarted until the skin surface is warm. Chilling causes vasoconstriction, which defeats the purpose of the cool applications, as little blood is carried to the skin surface but remains primarily in the viscera to become heated. In addition, the process of shivering generates additional heat. Therefore cool tub or sponge baths should never be continued if the child shows evidence of chilling.

In addition, the feverish child should wear light clothing and have minimal or no bedclothes. Blankets should not be used until the temperature returns to normal. The room should be well ventilated with good circulation of air. A small fan is sometimes helpful to keep the air moving to help dissipate heat by convection, but it is used with care to avoid chilling.

Health teaching

Nurses have a unique opportunity for teaching and reinforcing good hygienic care while the child is hospitalized. Although most children have learned self-care and hygiene in the home or at school, many have not. For some young children this is their first introduction to the use of a toothbrush. A great deal of health teaching can be accomplished even when the child is hospitalized for only a short time. The daily bath, handwashing before meals and after bowel and bladder evacuation, and conscientious dental hygiene are taught by example during routine care. Clean hair, nails, and clothing as well as good grooming are emphasized as essential to a pleasing appearance. Positive reinforcement of good hygiene practices helps to create a positive body image, promote the development of self-esteem, and prevent health problems, for example, teaching girls to wipe the genital area from front to back after toileting.

SAFETY

Since small children are separated from their usual environment and since they do not possess the capacity for abstract thinking and reasoning, it is the responsibility of everyone who comes in contact with them to maintain protective measures throughout their hospital stay. Nurses need a good understanding of the age level at which each child is operating and should plan for safety accordingly.

Name bands, a part of hospital safety practices, are particularly important for children in the pediatric age-group. Infants and unconscious patients are unable to tell or respond to their names. Toddlers may answer to any name or to a nickname only. It is not uncommon for older children to exchange places, give an erroneous name, or choose not to respond to their own names as a form of joke, unaware of the hazards of such practices.

Environmental factors

All the environmental safety measures in operation for the protection of adults apply to children as well, such as good illumination, floors clear of fluid or other objects that might contribute to falls, and nonskid surfaces in showers and tubs; electrical equipment that is maintained in good working order, is used only by personnel familiar with its use, and is not in contact with moisture or near tubs where it could prove to be a shock hazard; beds of ambulatory patients locked in place and at a height that allows easy access to the floor; proper care and disposal of small breakable items such as thermometers, bottles, and so on; and a well-organized fire plan known to all staff members. Medical asepsis and isolation techniques differ very little from those in any other hospital unit and should be strictly adhered to by personnel, since infants and small children are highly susceptible to cross-infection.

All windows should be securely screened, and elevators and stairways should be made safe. Ideally, electrical outlets should be provided with covers to prevent burns in small children whose exploratory activities may extend to inserting objects into the small openings. Bath water should be carefully checked by the nurse before placing the child in the bath, and children should never be left alone in a bathtub. Infants are helpless in water, and small children (and some older children) may turn on the hot water faucet and be severely burned.

Furniture is safest when it is scaled to the child's proportions, sturdy, and well balanced to prevent tipping over. Infants and small children must be securely strapped into infant seats, feeding chairs, and strollers. Infants and small, agitated, or mentally retarded children should not be left unattended on treatment tables, on scales, or in treatment areas. Even tiny premature infants are capable of surprising mobility; therefore portholes in Isolettes must be securely fastened when not in use.

Crib sides should be kept up and fastened securely unless an adult is at the bedside. The crib sides should be left up even when the crib is unoccupied to remove the temptation for the child to climb in. Anyone attending an infant or small child in a crib that has the sides down should never turn away without maintaining hand contact with the child, that is, one hand should be kept on the child's back or abdomen to protect him from rolling, crawling, or jumping from the open crib (Fig 19-5). A child who is apt to or who has demonstrated the inclination to climb over the sides of the crib is safest when placed in a specially constructed crib with a cover or one that has a safety net placed over the top. If the net is used it must be tied to the frame in such a manner that there is ready access to the child in case of emergency. Nets are never tied to the movable crib sides, and the knots should be tied in a manner that permits quick release. Cribs are not placed

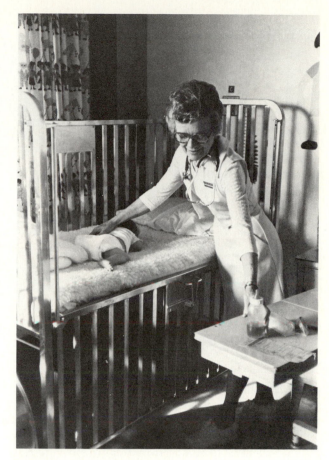

FIG. 19-5
The nurse maintains hand contact when her back is turned.

within reach of heating units, appliances, dangling cords, or other objects that can be reached by curious hands.

Toys. Toys play a vital role in the everyday life of children, and they are no less important in the hospital setting. However, it is up to nurses to assess the safety of toys brought to the hospital by well-meaning parents and friends. Toys should be appropriate to the child's age and condition and inspected to make certain that they are allergy-free, washable, and unbreakable and that they have no small, removable parts that can be aspirated or swallowed or that can in other ways inflict injury to a child.

Limit setting

Setting limits is essential to a child's safety. Children must understand where they are permitted to go and what they are permitted to do in the hospital. These limitations are made clear to them, consistently enforced, and repeated as frequently as necessary to make certain that they are un-

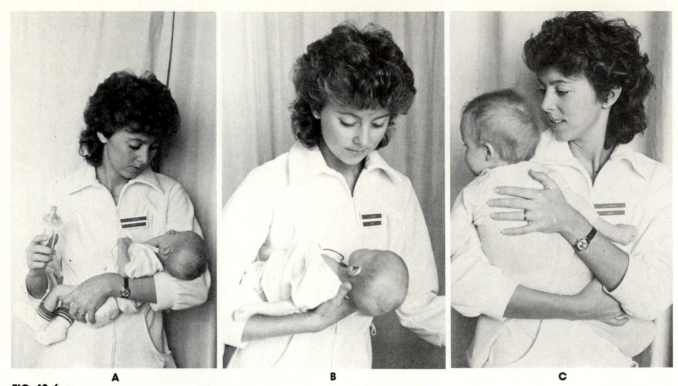

FIG. 19-6

Transporting infants. **A,** *The infant's thigh is firmly grasped in the nurse's hand.* **B,** *Football hold.* **C,** *Back supported.*

derstood. The nurse is responsible for where children are at all times. Children can easily wander off unnoticed.

Older children often become restless when their activity is restricted and may resort to pillow fights, water fights, and other rough play that might endanger the safety of the involved children or of bystanders (other children, staff, and visitors). Children in the hospital require surveillance, and appropriate tension-reducing activities can be planned and supervised by nurses and/or by the child life specialist.

Transporting infants and children

In the course of a hospital stay, infants and children usually need to be transported within the unit and to areas outside the pediatric unit. It is ordinarily safe to carry infants and small children for short distances within the unit, but for more extended trips the child should be securely transported in a suitable conveyance.

Small infants can be held or carried in the horizontal position with the back supported and the thigh grasped firmly by the carrying arm (Fig. 19-6, *A*). In the football hold the infant is supported on the nurse's arm with the head supported by the hand and the body held securely between the nurse's body and her elbow (Fig. 19-6, *B*).

Both of these holds leave the nurse's other arm free for activity. The infant can be held in the upright position with the buttocks on the nurse's forearm and the front of the body resting against the nurse's chest. The infant's head and shoulders are supported by the nurse's other arm to allow for any sudden movement by the infant (Fig. 19-6, *C*).

Infants can be transported to other areas, such as the x-ray department, in their bassinet or crib. Baby buggies are sometimes used for infants who are not likely to stand up. Strollers and wheeled feeding chairs or tables are also convenient transporters in some situations, such as trips to the playroom or nurse's station.

The method of transporting children is determined by their age, condition, and destination. Most older children are safe in wheelchairs or in gurneys. Younger children can be transported in their crib, on a gurney, in a wagon with raised sides, or in a wheelchair with a safety belt. Gurneys should be equipped with high sides and a safety belt, both of which are kept in place during transport.

Restraints

Frequently some method of restraint is needed for a child's safety or comfort, to facilitate examination, or to carry out

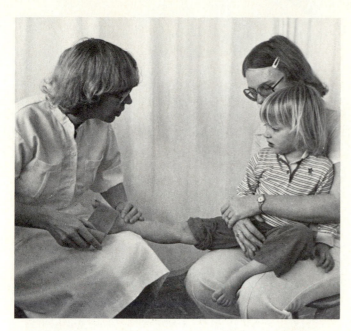

FIG. 19-7
An assistant supplies comfort and security while the nurse carries out the procedure.

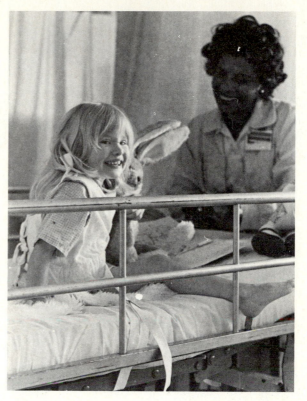

FIG. 19-8
Jacket restraint.

diagnostic and therapeutic procedures. Restraint can be accomplished with the hand or with physical devices. Restraining the child with the hand provides an element of human contact that is lacking in restraint by mechanical means. For example, a large infant or small child can be effectively restrained by having him sit astride the lap facing an assistant. The assistant hugs him close against the body to provide both comfort and restraint while the nurse safely carries out the necessary procedure (Fig. 19-7).

Mechanical restraints are never used as a punishment or as a substitute for observation. When a child must be restrained, he and his parents need a simple explanation, and, if the restraint is applied for an extended period of time, the explanation must be repeated often to gain his cooperation and to help him understand that it is not a punishment. Restraining devices are not without risk and must be checked frequently to make certain that they are accomplishing the purpose for which they are intended, that they are applied correctly, and that they do not impair circulation.

Parents need to know the purpose of restraints, how to remove and reapply them, and the signs of complications from their use. Parents are sometimes upset when their child must be restrained and need to understand how they can help to assure the maximum benefit and minimize the stress related to their use. Children, too, should be prepared for both the procedure or the circumstance for which the restraint is required.

Removing restraints whenever possible (at least every

2 hours) is an essential part of nursing care of children who are restrained for treatments or other purposes. Alternate methods may be devised to replace the need for passive restraints. Holding the child for periods is a pleasant alternative, as is restraining him in a highchair where he can observe the activities around him. If feasible, distraction techniques such as play and reading to the child are employed to gain the child's cooperation without resorting to restraints. Parental participation is always encouraged in these efforts.

Jacket restraint. A jacket restraint is sometimes used as an alternative to the crib net to prevent the child from climbing out of the crib or to keep the child safe in various kinds of chairs. The jacket is put on the child with the ties in back so that the child is unable to manipulate them, and the long tapes, secured to the understructure of the crib, keep the child inside the crib (Fig. 19-8). The jacket restraint is also useful as a means to maintain the child in a desired horizontal position. A Posey belt scaled to fit the child is an alternative device.

Mummy restraint. When an infant or small child requires short-term restraint for examination or treatment that involves the head and neck, such as venipuncture, throat examination, gavage feeding, and so on, the mummy device effectively controls the child's movements.

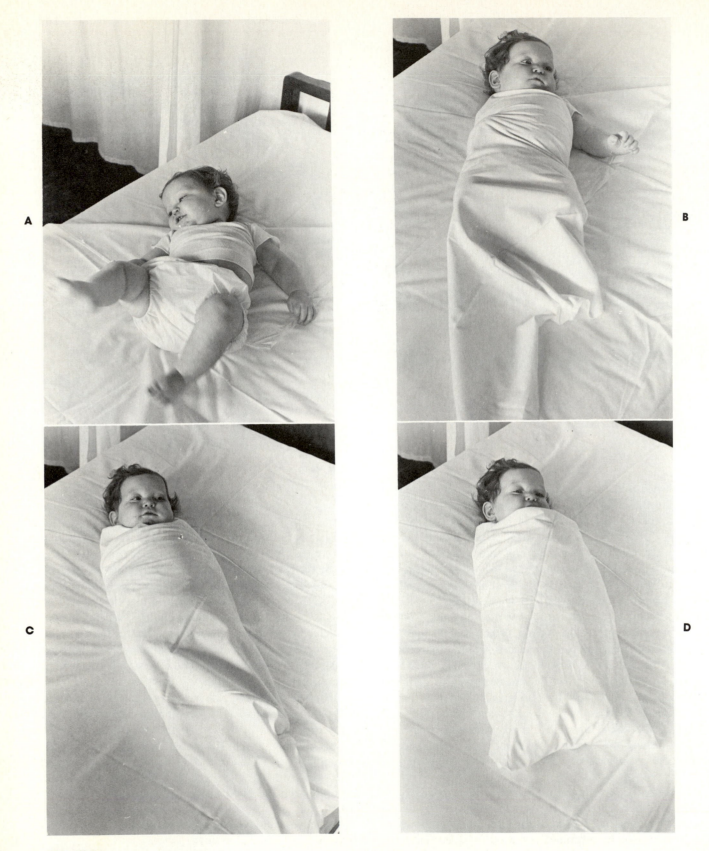

FIG. 19-9

Application of a mummy restraint. **A,** *The infant is placed on a folded corner of the blanket.* **B,** *One corner of the blanket is brought across the infant and secured beneath the body.* **C,** *The second corner is brought across the body and secured.* **D,** *The lower corner is folded and tucked or pinned in place.*

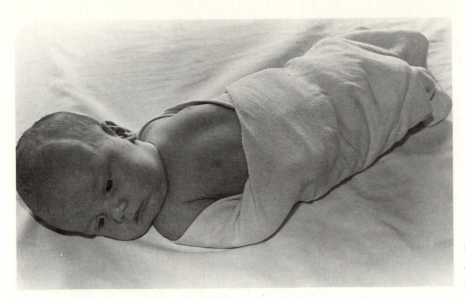

FIG. 19-10
Modified mummy restraint with the chest uncovered.

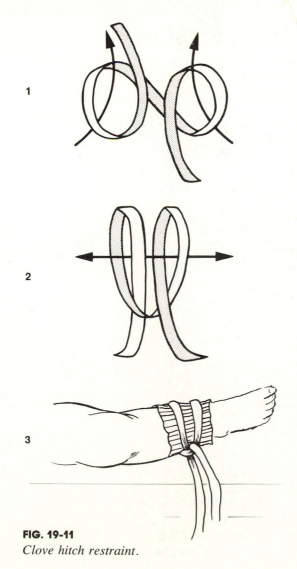

FIG. 19-11
Clove hitch restraint.

A blanket or sheet is opened on the bed or crib with one corner folded to the center. The infant is placed on the blanket with his shoulders at the fold and his feet toward the opposite corner (Fig. 19-9, *A*). With the infant's right arm straight down against his body, the right side of the blanket is pulled firmly across the infant's right shoulder and chest and secured beneath the left side of his body (Fig. 19-9, *B*). The left arm is placed straight against his side, and the left side of the blanket is brought across the shoulder and chest and locked beneath the child's body on the right side (Fig. 19-9, *C*). The lower corner is folded and brought over the body and tucked or fastened securely with safety pins. Safety pins can be used to fasten the blanket in place at any step in the process.

To modify the mummy restraint for chest examination, the folded edge of the blanket is brought over each arm and under the back, after which the loose edge is folded over and secured at a point below the chest to allow visualization and access to the chest (Fig. 19-10).

Arm and leg restraints. Occasionally one or more extremities must be restrained or limited in motion. A number of commercial restraining devices are available, or a restraint can be fashioned from gauze tape, muslin strips, or a length of narrow stockinette. When this type of restraint is used, it must be appropriate to the size of the child, it must be padded to prevent undue pressure, constriction, or tissue injury, and the extremity must be observed frequently for signs of irritation and/or impairment of circulation.

The *clove hitch* restraint is fashioned from a length of gauze or muslin tape. When properly applied, the restraint should provide a snug fit with minimum danger of pulling too tightly. See Fig. 19-11 for the method of tying and applying a clove hitch restraint.

The ends of the restraints are never tied to the crib rails, since lowering of the rail will disturb the extremity, frequently with a jerk, which may hurt or injure the child. Restraints can and should be released periodically to allow the child to move the restrained extremities. The child can remain unrestrained when someone can be with him to achieve the desired restraints on his movements.

Elbow restraint. Sometimes it is important to prevent the child from reaching his head or face, for example, after lip surgery, when a scalp vein infusion is in place, or to prevent scratching in skin disorders. For this purpose, elbow restraints fashioned from a variety of materials

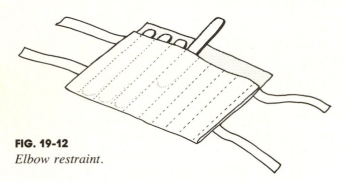

FIG. 19-12
Elbow restraint.

function very well. The most common form of elbow restraint consists of a piece of muslin long enough to reach comfortably from just below the axilla to the wrist with a number of vertical pockets into which tongue depressors are inserted (Fig. 19-12). The restraint is wrapped around the arm and secured with tapes or pins. Sometimes it is necessary to pin the tops to the child's undershirt to prevent the restraint from slipping.

Similar restraints can be made from padded large-diameter towel rollers or appropriate sized plastic containers from which the tops and bottoms have been removed. Both types need to be padded and to have some means to prevent the restraint from slipping from the extremity.

Positioning for procedures

Infants and small children are unable to cooperate for many procedures; therefore the nurse is responsible for minimizing their movement and discomfort with proper positioning. Older children usually need only minimal, if any, restraint. Careful explanation and preparation beforehand and support and simple guidance during the procedure are ordinarily adequate.

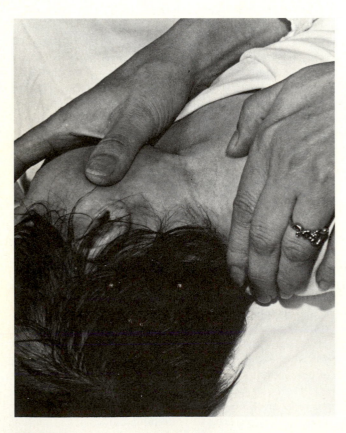

FIG. 19-13
Restraining the child for jugular vein puncture.

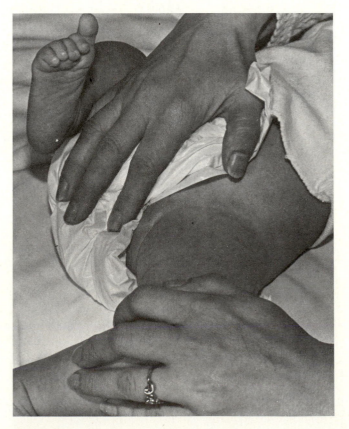

FIG. 19-14
Restraining the child for femoral vein puncture.

Jugular venipuncture. The large, superficial external jugular vein is frequently used to obtain blood specimens from infants and young children. For easy access to the vein, the child is first placed in a mummy restraint in which the top edge of the restraint is low enough to allow sufficient exposure to permit access to the vein. The child is placed so that his head and shoulders extend over the edge of a table or a small pillow with his neck extended and his head turned sharply to the side (Fig. 19-13). One alternate method for restraining the child is with the nurse restraining the child's arms and legs with his or her arms at the same time as the head is restrained and positioned. It is important for the nurse holding the infant to maintain control of the infant's head without interfering with the operator's approach to the vein. The infant's crying during the procedure increases intravenous pressure, which facilitates visualization of the vein. Following venipuncture, digital pressure is applied to the site with a dry gauze square for 3 to 5 minutes or until the bleeding has been stopped. Care must be taken not to apply excessive pressure that might compromise circulation or breathing during or following the procedure.

Femoral venipuncture. Other commonly used sites for venipuncture are the large femoral veins. The nurse restrains the infant by placing him supine with his legs in a frog position to provide extensive exposure of the groin area. Both the arms and legs of the infant can be effectively controlled by the nurse's forearms and hands (Fig. 19-14). Only the side used for the venipuncture is uncovered so that the operator is protected if the child should urinate during the procedure. Pressure is applied to the site after the withdrawal of blood to prevent oozing from the site.

Extremity venipuncture. The most common sites of venipuncture are the veins of the extremities, especially the arm and hand. A convenient position for restraint is having one person on either side of the bed. The child's outstretched arm is partially stabilized by the technician drawing the blood. The other person leans across the child's upper body, preventing its movement, and uses an arm to immobilize the venipuncture site. This type of restraint also comforts the child because of the close body contact and allows each person to maintain eye contact with her (Fig. 19-15).

Lumbar puncture. The technique for lumbar puncture in infants and children is similar to that in the adult. Pediatric lumbar puncture sets contain smaller spinal needles, but sometimes the operator will specify a particular size or type of needle that the nurse should make certain is placed on the tray.

Children are usually controlled best in the side-lying position, with the head flexed and the knees drawn up toward the chest. Even cooperative children need to be restrained to prevent possible trauma from unexpected, involuntary movement. They can be reassured that, although they are trusted, the restraint will serve as a reminder to maintain the desired position. It also provides a measure of support and reassurance to them.

The child is placed on his side with his back close to the edge of the examining table on the side from which the operator is working. The nurse maintains the child's spine in a flexed position by holding the child with one arm behind his neck and the other behind his thighs. The position can be effectively stabilized if the nurse's hands are clasped in front of the child's abdomen (Fig. 19-16, *A*). The flexed position enlarges the spaces between the lumbar vertebral spines, which facilitates access to the spinal fluid space. It is helpful to wrap the legs before positioning to decrease leg movement.

An alternate position used with small infants and some older children is the sitting position. The child is placed with the buttocks at the edge of the table and with the neck flexed so that the chin rests on the chest. The infant's arms and legs are immobilized by the nurse's hands (Fig. 19-16, *B*). Since this position may interfere with chest expansion and diaphragm excursion, the child is observed for difficulty in breathing. In addition, the soft, pliable trachea of the infant is subject to collapse. Specimens and spinal fluid pressure are obtained, measured, and sent for analysis

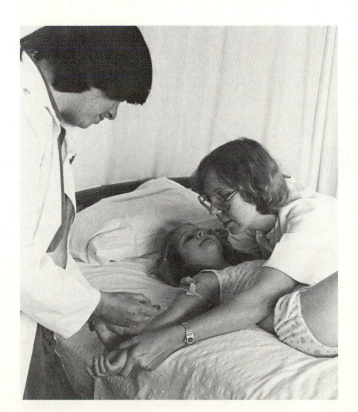

FIG. 19-15
Restraining the child for extremity vein puncture.

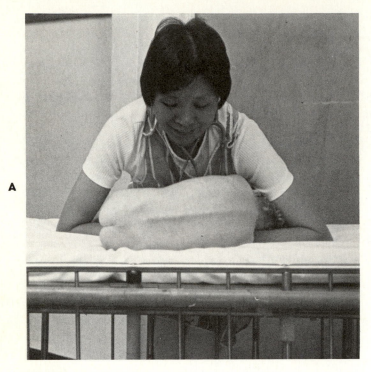

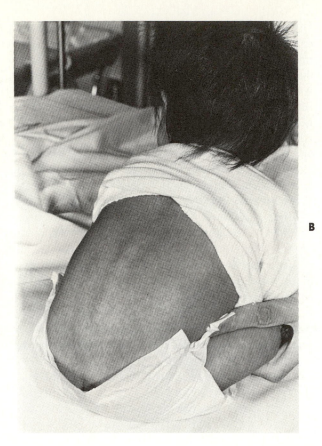

FIG. 19-16
Position for lumbar puncture. **A,** *Lying on side.* **B,** *Sitting.*

in the same manner as for the adult patient. It is advisable for the child to lie quietly for an hour following the procedure to decrease the likelihood of headache, and he is offered fluids to drink. Vital signs are taken as ordered, and the child is observed for any changes in level of consciousness, motor activity, or other neurologic signs.

Other. For subdural puncture through a fontanel or burr hole, the infant is wrapped in a mummy restraint and placed in the supine position with the head accessible to the examiner. The head is controlled with a firm hold on each side by the nurse. Procedures for immobilizing the head for examining the ears, nose, or throat are discussed in Chapter 5.

COLLECTION OF SPECIMENS

Many of the specimens needed for diagnostic examination of children are collected in much the same way as they are for adults, and older children are able to cooperate if given proper instruction regarding what is expected from them. Infants and small children, however, are unable to follow directions or control body functions sufficiently to help in collecting some specimens.

Urine specimens

All children admitted to the hospital and most clinic or office visits require a urine specimen as a routine diagnostic procedure. Older children and adolescents will readily use the bedpan or urinal or can be trusted to follow directions for collection in the bathroom. Self-conscious adolescents who may be reluctant to carry a specimen bottle through a hallway or waiting room can be provided with a paper bag or other means for disguising the container. The presence of menses is sometimes an embarrassment to teenage girls; therefore, it is a good idea to ask them if it might be that particular time of the month and make adjustments as necessary. The specimen can be delayed or a notation made on the laboratory slip to explain the presence of red blood cells.

School-age children are cooperative but curious. They are concerned about the reasons behind things and are likely to ask questions regarding the disposition of their specimen and what one expects to discover from it.

Preschoolers and toddlers are less cooperative primarily because they are usually unable to void on request. It is often best to offer them water or other liquids that they enjoy and wait about 30 minutes until they are ready to void voluntarily or set a timer to alert the child that he

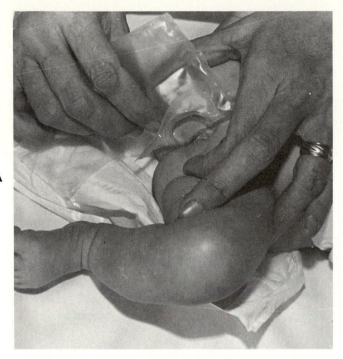

A

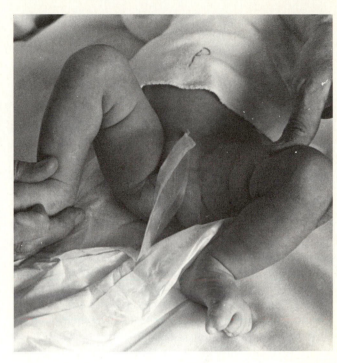

B

FIG. 19-17

Application of a urine collection bag. **A,** *On little girls the adhesive portion is applied to the exposed and dried perineum first.* **B,** *The bag adheres firmly around the perineal area to prevent urine leakage.*

needs to void shortly. The child will better understand what is expected if the nurse uses his terms for the function, such as ''pee-pee'' or ''tinkle.'' Some will have difficulty voiding in an unfamiliar receptacle. Potty-chairs or a bedpan placed on the toilet will ordinarily prove satisfactory. Toddlers who have recently acquired bladder control may be especially reluctant, since they undoubtedly have been admonished for ''going'' in places other than those approved by parents. A useful approach is to enlist the help of a parent; the parent is likely to be successful, and this helps them to feel a part of the child's care.

For infants and toddlers who are not toilet trained, special urine collection devices are used. These devices are clear plastic single-use bags with self-adhering material around the opening at the point of attachment. To prepare the infant, the genitalia, perineum, and surrounding skin are washed and dried thoroughly, since the adhesive will not adhere to a moist, powdered, or oily skin surface. The collection bag is easiest to apply if attached first to the perineum, progressing to the symphysis (Fig. 19-17). With little girls the perineum is stretched taut during application to that area to assure a leak-proof fit. With small boys the penis and scrotum are placed inside the bag. The adhesive portion of the bag must be firmly adhered to the skin all around the genital area to avoid possible leakage. The diaper is carefully replaced. The bag is checked frequently and removed as soon as the specimen is available, since the moist bag may become loosened on an active child. For some types of urine testing, such as checking specific gravity, urine can be aspirated directly from the diaper.

Clean-catch specimens. Older children can be instructed in the proper cleaning technique, but the nurse performs the cleaning procedure on infants and young children. The perineum is cleansed with a soap- or an antiseptic-soaked sterile pad, wiping from front to back only once with each pad. This is repeated at least two times. The area is then wiped with sterile water to prevent accidental contamination of the urine with a solution that may destroy the pathogens, although minute amounts of antiseptic such as iodine do not alter bacterial counts.

To collect the urine, the nurse holds the infant over a sterile container or applies a sterile plastic collecting bag. The infant can be encouraged to void by applying pressure over the suprapubic area or by stroking the paraspinal muscles to elicit a Perez reflex. This reflex, which usually disappears by 4 to 6 months of age, results in crying, extension of the back, flexion of the arms and legs, and urination.

When voiding has occurred, the bag is removed immediately. Urine that has been allowed to remain at room temperature is unacceptable because the number of bacteria doubles every 20 to 30 minutes. If the urine is not tested within 30 minutes, the specimen is refrigerated. If the child has not voided within 45 minutes, the bag is removed and the cleansing procedure repeated.

24-hour collection. Collection of urine voided over a 24-hour period creates some special problems in infants and children. Collection bags and sometimes restraining methods are required to collect specimens from infants and small children. Older children require special instruction about notifying someone when they need to void or have a bowel movement so that urine can be collected separately and not discarded. Some older school-age children and adolescents can be trusted to take responsibility for collection of their own 24-hour specimens. They can keep output records and transfer each voiding to the 24-hour collection container if this is permitted.

As in any 24-hour urine collection, the collection period always starts and ends with an empty bladder. At the time the collection begins the child is instructed to void and the specimen is discarded. All urine voided in the subsequent 24 hours is saved in a refrigerated container. Twenty-four hours from the time the precollection specimen was discarded, the child is again instructed to void, the specimen is added to the container, and the entire collection is taken to the laboratory for examination.

Infants and small children who are prepared for 24-hour urine collection will require a special collection bag; frequent removal and replacement of adhesive collection devices can produce skin irritation. A thin coating of tincture of benzoin applied to the skin helps to protect it and aids adhesion. Plastic collection bags with collection tubes attached are ideal when the container must be left in place for a time. These can be connected to a collecting device or emptied periodically by aspiration with a syringe. When such devices are not available, a regular bag with a feeding tube inserted through a puncture hole at the top of the bag serves as a satisfactory substitute. However, care must be taken to empty the bag as soon as the infant urinates to prevent leakage and loss of contents.

Special techniques. *Catheterized* or *suprapubic aspiration* is employed when a specimen is urgently needed or when the child is unable to void or otherwise provide an adequate specimen. Catheterization is most often used when urethral obstruction or anuria caused by renal failure is believed to be the cause of the child's failure to void. Suprapubic aspiration is useful in clarifying the diagnosis of suspected urinary tract infection in acutely ill infants.

Catheterizing a child requires aseptic technique, good light, and gentle, thorough cleansing of the vulva or glans penis. Most children, including female infants, accommodate a size 8 or 10 French catheter, but in male infants or when the larger catheters cannot be passed, a smaller, soft plastic feeding tube may be needed. Most children are frightened of this procedure, and few small children are entirely cooperative; therefore, even when the procedure is adequately explained, the presence of an assistant is needed to help restrain and reassure the child. Special care must be exercised when catheterizing young males to avoid trauma that might result in sterility from damage to the ductal and glandular openings into the urethra.

Suprapubic aspiration, which is performed by the physician, involves aspirating bladder contents by inserting a 20- or 21-gauge needle in the midline approximately 1 cm above the symphysis and directed vertically downward. The skin is prepared as for any needle insertion, but the bladder should contain an adequate volume of urine. This can be assumed if the infant has not voided for at least 1 hour, or if the bladder can be palpated above the symphysis. This technique is especially useful for obtaining clean specimens from young infants. The bladder is an abdominal organ at this time and is easily accessible.

Blood specimens

Most blood specimens are obtained by the laboratory staff or physicians. However, nurses are often responsible for making certain that specimens, such as serial examinations and fasting specimens, are collected on time and that the proper equipment, such as correct collection tubes and ice for blood gas samples, is available. However, in some areas, such as intensive care units, nurses routinely collect specimens that are needed frequently.

Venous blood samples can be obtained by venipuncture or by aspiration from an intravenous infusion site. When using an intravenous infusion site for specimen collection, it is important to consider the type of fluid being infused. For example, a specimen collected for glucose determination would be inaccurate if removed from a catheter through which glucose-containing solution is being administered.

No matter how or by whom the specimen is collected, nurses should be aware that children fear the loss of their blood. This is particularly true for children whose condition requires frequent blood specimens. Ignorant about the process of hemopoiesis, they mistakenly believe that blood removed from their bodies is a threat to their lives. Explaining to them that their blood is continually being produced by their bodies provides them with a measure of reassurance regarding this aspect of the stress-provoking procedure. When the blood is drawn, a simple comment, such as, "Just look how red it is. You're really making a lot of nice red blood," confirms this information and affords them an opportunity to express their concern. A Band-Aid gives them added assurance that the vital fluids will not leak out through the puncture site.

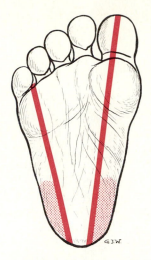

FIG. 19-18
Puncture site (red stippled area) on sole of infant's foot.

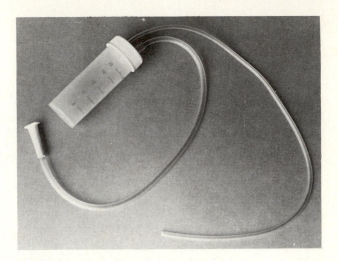

FIG. 19-19
Device for collecting sputum specimens.

Capillary blood samples from children are taken by finger or earlobe stick methods, just as in the adult patient. The best method for taking peripheral blood samples from infants is by a heel stick. Before taking the blood sample, the heel is warmed with warm, moist compresses for 5 to 10 minutes in order to dilate the vessels in the area. The area is cleaned with alcohol, and with the infant's foot firmly restrained with the free hand, the heel is punctured with a Bard-Parker No. 11 or Redi-Lance blade. The needed specimens are quickly collected and pressure applied to the puncture site with a dry gauze square until the bleeding stops. The site is then covered with a Band-Aid. Applying warm compresses to ecchymotic areas increases circulation, helps remove extravasated blood, and decreases pain.

The most serious complication of infant heel puncture is necrotizing osteochondritis from lancet penetration of the underlying calcaneus bone. To avoid this, the puncture should be no deeper than 2.4 mm and should be made at the outer aspects of the heel. The boundaries of the calcaneus can be marked by an imaginary line extending posteriorly from a point between the fourth and fifth toes and running parallel to the lateral aspect of the heel and another line extending posteriorly from the middle of the great toe and running parallel to the medial aspect of the heel (Fig. 19-18).

Sputum specimens

Older children and adolescents are able to cough as directed and supply sputum specimens when given proper directions. It must be made clear to them that a coughed specimen, not what is cleared from the throat, is needed. It is helpful to demonstrate a deep cough so that commu-

nication is clear. Infants and small children are unable to follow directions to cough and will swallow any sputum produced when they do; therefore, gastric washings (lavage) may be used to collect a specimen. Sometimes it is possible to get a satisfactory specimen by using a suction device such as a mucous trap if the catheter is inserted into the trachea and the cough reflex elicited. A catheter that is inserted into the back of the throat is not sufficient. For children with a tracheostomy, a specimen is easily aspirated from the trachea or major bronchi by attaching a collecting device to the suction apparatus (Fig. 19-19).

ADMINISTRATION OF MEDICATIONS

The administration of medications to children presents a number of problems that are not encountered in giving medication to adult patients. Children vary widely in age, weight, surface area, and the ability to absorb, metabolize, and excrete medications. Nurses must be particularly alert when computing and administering drugs to infants and children.

Determining drug dosage

It is the physician's responsibility to prescribe drugs in the correct dosage to achieve the desired effect without endangering the health of the child. However, nurses must have an understanding of the safe dosage of medications they administer to children as well as the expected action, possible side effects, and signs of toxicity. Unlike adult medications, there are no standardized dosage ranges for children in the pediatric age-groups; therefore, drugs are often prepared and packaged in average adult-dosage strengths.

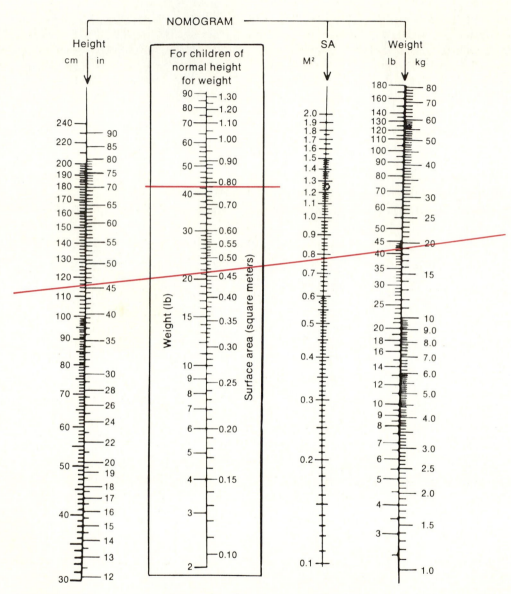

FIG. 19-20

West nomogram (for estimation of surface areas). The surface area is indicated where a straight line connecting the height and weight intersects the surface area (SA) column or, if the patient is roughly of normal proportion, from the weight alone (enclosed area). Red line illustrates surface area determination (0.78 m²) for a child 115 cm tall who weighs 19 kg. (Nomogram modified from data of E. Boyd by C.D. West; Berman, R.E., and Vaughan, V.C., editors: Nelson textbook of pediatrics, ed. 12, Philadelphia, 1983, W.B. Saunders Co.)

Various formulas involving age, weight, and body surface area (BSA) as the basis for calculations have been devised to determine children's drug dosage from a standard adult dose. Since the administration of medication is a nursing responsibility, nurses need not only a knowledge of drug action and patient responses but also some resources for estimating safe dosages for children.

Body surface area as a basis for determining drug dosage. The most reliable method for determining children's dosage is to calculate the proportional amount of body surface area to body weight. The ratio of body surface area to weight varies inversely to length; therefore, the infant who is shorter and weighs less than an older child or adult has relatively more surface area than would be expected from his weight.

The usual determination of surface area requires the use of a nomogram. Body surface area is estimated from height and weight of the child, and then this information is applied to a formula for dosage. To obtain the surface area, a line is drawn with a straight edge, such as a ruler, from points that represent the child's height and weight on the appropriate scale. The surface area in square meters (m^2) is indicated by the point at which the line bisects the surface area scale (Fig. 19-20).

One formula that will obtain the appropriate fraction of the adult dose is:

$$\frac{\text{Body surface area of child}}{\text{Body surface area of adult}} \times \text{Adult dose} = \frac{\text{Estimated}}{\text{child's dose}}$$

Preparation for administering medications

Unit dose packaging, which is gaining wide usage in hospital pharmacies, does not always extend to pediatric medications. Therefore, the ability to calculate fractional doses from larger dosages is absolutely essential. In addition, measuring doses, identifying patients, and gaining their cooperation create problems not usually encountered in giving medications to adults.

Checking dosage. Administering the correct dosage of a drug is a shared responsibility between the physician who orders the drug and the nurse who carries out that order. Children react with unexpected severity to some drugs, and ill children are especially sensitive to drugs. Therefore, checking the dose if there is any doubt about the accuracy of the dose ordered is a valuable habit to acquire. When a dose is ordered that is outside the usual range or if there is some question regarding the preparation ordered or the route of administration, this should always be checked with the physician before proceeding with the administration, since the nurse is legally liable for any drug administered.

Administering some medications requires added safeguards. Even when it has been determined that the dosage is correct for a particular child, there are many drugs that are potentially hazardous or lethal. Most hospital units or other facilities where medications are given to children have regulations requiring that specified drugs be double-checked by another nurse before they are given to the child. Among those drugs that require such safeguards are digoxin, heparin, and insulin. Others that are frequently included are epinephrine, narcotics, and sedatives. Even if this precaution is not mandatory, nurses would be wise to take such precautions for their own sense of security.

Identification. No matter what route is used to administer a medication, the child must be correctly identified. As mentioned previously, children are not totally reliable in giving correct names on request. An infant is unable to give his name, a toddler or preschooler may admit to any name, and a school-age child may deny his identity in an attempt to avoid the medication. Children sometimes exchange beds for awhile. Parents may be present to identify their child, but the only safe method for identifying children is to check their hospital identification bands with the medication card.

Parents. Parents can be useful sources of information regarding the child and his capabilities. Nearly all parents have given some kind of medication to their child and can describe the approaches that they have found to be successful. They can also provide information regarding the child's reaction to similar experiences if the child has been hospitalized before or if he has been given medication in a physician's office or clinic. In some cases it is less traumatic for the child if a parent gives the medication to the child, provided the nurse prepares the medication and supervises its administration and the practice is consistent with hospital or ward policy. Children being given daily medications at home are accustomed to the parent functioning in this capacity and are less apt to fuss than they would if the medication is administered by a stranger.

Oral administration

The oral route is preferred for administering medications to children whenever possible and, because of the ease of administration of oral medications, most are dissolved or suspended in liquid preparations. Although some children are able to swallow or chew solid medications at an early age, solid preparations are not recommended for children under 5 years of age. There is danger of aspiration in any oral preparation, but solid forms (pills, tablets, and capsules) are especially hazardous if their administration causes marked resistance or crying.

Most pediatric medications come in palatable and colorful preparations for added ease of administration. Some have a slightly unpleasant aftertaste, but the majority of children will swallow these liquids with little if any resistance. Many oral medications are more readily swallowed

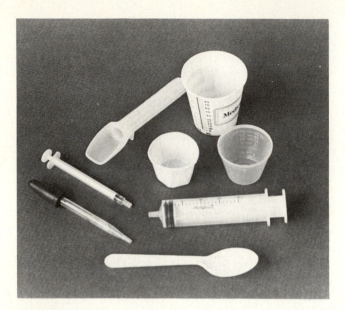

FIG. 19-21
Devices for administration of medications to pediatric patients.

if they are diluted with a small amount of water and followed by a "chaser" of water, juice, a soft drink, or a popsicle or frozen juice bar. Large quantities of water should not be used for dilution, since the child may refuse to drink the entire amount and thus would receive only a partial dose of the medication. Carbonated beverages poured over finely crushed ice given before or immediately after a medication are an excellent means to prevent or allay nausea.

The nurse should taste a minute amount of an oral preparation to ascertain if it palatable or bitter. In this way legitimate signs of dislike from the child can be accepted and the taste camouflaged whenever possible. Most pediatric units have preparations available for this purpose. Sweet-tasting substances that are suitable include honey, flavored syrups, jam, and some fruit purees. Syrups are ideal for mixing with medicines that do not dissolve in water and for powdered drugs or pulverized tablets. When drugs are mixed, only a small amount of liquid or food is used, since the child may refuse to take the entire amount and thus receive only a partial dose of the medication. When selecting a substance to mix with a medication, *essential food items,* such as milk, cereal, and orange juice, are avoided. If they are used, children may become conditioned against them and refuse these foods in their diet.

Preparation. Selecting a vehicle to measure and administer a medication requires careful consideration. The devices available to measure medicines are not always sufficiently accurate for measuring the small amounts needed in pediatric nursing practice (Fig. 19-21). Standard medicine glasses have been replaced by disposable plastic

or paper cups. Although the carefully molded plastic cups offer reasonable accuracy in measuring moderate or large doses of liquids, the paper cups are likely to have irregularly shaped or crumpled bottoms. Calibrations on the cups (especially the teaspoon mark) and the personal equation or interpretation of a given measure are highly variable. Measures less than a teaspoon are impossible to determine accurately with a cup.

Many liquid preparations are prescribed in measurements of teaspoons. However, the teaspoon (and other household measures) is an inaccurate measuring device and is subject to error from a number of variables. For example, household teaspoons vary greatly in capacity, and different persons using the same spoon will pour different amounts. This variability is also influenced by the adequacy of available light, the color of the liquid, and the size of the bottle from which it is poured. Therefore, a drug ordered in teaspoons should be measured in milliliters. The American Standards Institute has established 5 ml as the standard teaspoon measurement; this is also the volume accepted by the United States Pharmacopeia (U.S.P.).

Another device that is not reliable for measuring liquids is the drop, which varies to a greater extent than the teaspoon or measuring cup. Droppers are available in numerous sizes but, even with the standard U.S.P. dropper, the volume of a drop will vary according to the viscosity of the liquid measured. Viscid fluids produce much larger drops than thin liquids. Many medications are supplied with caps or droppers designed for measuring each specific preparation. These are accurate when used to measure that specific medication but are not reliable for measuring other liquids. Emptying dropper contents into a medicine cup invites additional error. Since some of the liquid clings to the sides of the cup, a significant amount of the drug can be lost.

The most accurate means for measuring small amounts of medication is the syringe, and, for volumes less than 1 ml, the tuberculin syringe offers even greater accuracy. Not only does the syringe provide a reliable measure, but it also serves as a convenient means for transporting and administering the medication. The medication can be placed directly into the child's mouth from the syringe. However, only the disposable plastic syringes are safe for placing in children's mouths to avoid the possibility that they may be cut by broken glass if they should clench their teeth on the syringe. For added safety, a short length of flexible tubing can be placed on the tip of the syringe to prevent injury to the mouth.

Small children and some older children as well have difficulty in swallowing tablets or pills. Since a number of drugs are not available in pediatric preparations, the tablet will need to be crushed before it can be given to these children. To minimize loss of the drug, the tablet can be crushed between two spoons or placed between two small paper soufflé cups and crushed in a mortar and then mixed with syrup or juice for the child to swallow. The nurse must make certain that the bits of pulverized medication that tend to cling to the sides of the medicine cup or spoon are not lost.

Not all drugs can be crushed, for example, medication with an enteric or protective coating or those formulated for slow release. For some children it may be possible to encourage swallowing the tablet or capsule by using a special glass designed with a shelf that holds the drug.* The child drinks normally and the tablet is carried to the back of the throat.

Preparing dosage. Since pediatric doses often require dividing adult preparations of medication, the nurse may be faced with the dilemma of accurate dosage. With tablets, only those that are scored can be halved or quartered. If the medication is soluble, the tablet or contents of a capsule can be mixed in a small premeasured amount of liquid and the appropriate portion given. For example, if half a dose is required, the tablet is dissolved in 5 ml of water and 2.5 ml is administered.

Medications that are not scored cannot be divided accurately. For example, suppositories cannot be divided into equal halves. In addition the manufacturer does not guarantee that the drug is evenly dispersed throughout the petrolatum base.

Administration. Administering liquids to infants is relatively easy, but care must be observed to prevent aspiration. With the infant held in a semireclining position (Fig. 19-22), the medication is placed in his mouth from a spoon, plastic cup, plastic dropper, or plastic syringe (without the needle). The dropper or syringe is best placed along the side of the infant's tongue and administered slowly to avoid causing him to choke. Because of the natural outward tongue thrust in infancy, medications may need to be retrieved from lips or chin and refed. Allowing the infant to suck the medication that has been placed in any empty nipple or inserting the syringe or dropper into the side of the mouth, parallel to the nipple while the infant nurses are other convenient methods for giving liquid medications to infants. Medicine cups can be used effectively for older infants who are able to drink from a cup. Medication is not added to the infant's formula feeding.

The small child who refuses to cooperate or resists consistently despite explanation and encouragement may require mild physical coercion. If so, it is carried out quickly and carefully. Every effort should be made to determine why the child resists, and the reasons for this alternative should be explained to the child in such a way that he will know that it is being carried out for his well-being and is not a form of punishment. There is always a

*Manufactured by Apex Medical Corp, Bloomington, MN 55420.

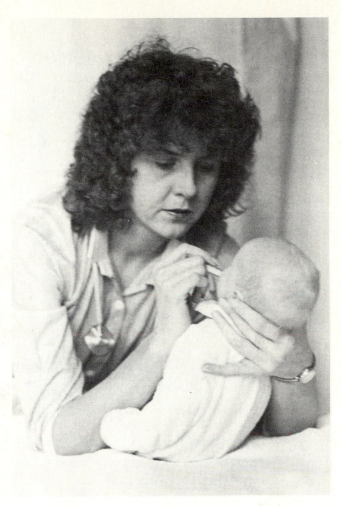

FIG. 19-22
Administering oral medication to an infant.

risk in using even mild forceful techniques. A crying child can aspirate a medication, particularly when he is lying on his back. If the nurse holds the child in the lap with the child's right arm behind the nurse, the left hand firmly grasped by the nurse's left hand, and the head securely restrained between the nurse's arm and body, the medication can be slowly poured into the mouth (Fig. 19-23).

Intramuscular administration

Injections constitute some of the most traumatic health-related experiences for children. No one likes a "shot," especially young children who may associate the procedure with body mutilation and punishment. At times it can be no less stressful to the nurse who must inflict the distress. Because of this characteristic, children are given injections only when the drug cannot be given by any other acceptable route.

Selecting syringe and needle. The volume of

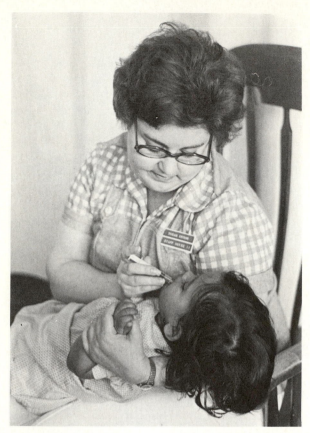

FIG. 19-23

The nurse partially restrains the child for easy and comfortable administration of medication.

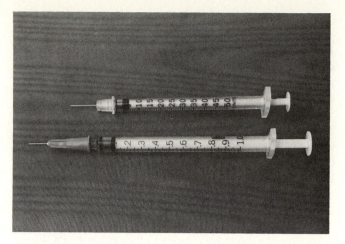

FIG. 19-24

Top, *Low-dose (0.5-ml), and* bottom, *standard tuberculin (1.0 ml) syringes.*

medication prescribed for small children and the small amount of tissue for injection require that a syringe be selected that can measure very small amounts of solution. For volumes less than 1 ml the tuberculin syringe, calibrated in one-hundredth increments, is appropriate. Very minute doses may require the use of a 0.5-ml, low-dose syringe (Fig. 19-24). These syringes with specially constructed needles minimize the possibility of inadvertently administering incorrect amounts of a drug because of dead space, which allows fluid to remain in the syringe and needle after the plunger is pushed completely forward. A minimum of 0.2 ml of solution remains in a standard needle hub; therefore, when very small amounts of two drugs, such as atropine and meperidine or mixtures of insulin, are combined in the syringe, the ratio of the two drugs can be altered significantly.

Dead space is also a significant factor to consider when injecting medication, since flushing the syringe with an air bubble or parenteral fluid adds an additional amount of medication to the prescribed dose. This can be hazardous when very small amounts of a drug are given. Consequently flushing is not advisable, especially when less than

1 ml of medication is given. Flushing may be necessary when the entire contents of a vial are to be administered in order to completely expel the fluid that remains in the needle.

The needle length must be sufficient to penetrate through the subcutaneous tissue and deposit the medication well in the body of the muscle. One method of estimating this distance is grasping the vastus lateralis or deltoid muscle and measuring half the distance between the thumb and index finger, which is the approximate needle length required to penetrate that muscle. With the ventrogluteal or dorsogluteal site, only the subcutaneous tissue is grasped and half this distance is the *minimal* needle length needed to reach the muscle. Additional length is required to penetrate the muscle. In both instances needle length must also allow for a small portion of the needle to be exposed at the skin surface as a precaution if the needle should break off from the hub. The most satisfactory needles for intramuscular injections in children are the 25- to 27-gauge needles with a length of ½ to 1 inch. Regular intramuscular needles are too large in both length and gauge for pediatric use, except for very large, obese children.

Determining site. Factors that are considered when selecting a site for an intramuscular injection on an infant or child include:

The amount and character of the medication injected
The amount and general condition of the muscle mass
The frequency or number of injections given during the course of treatment
The type of medication being given
Factors that may impede access to or cause contamination of the site
The ability of the child to assume the required position safely

Ordinarily older children and adolescents pose few problems in selecting a suitable site for intramuscular injections, but infants with their small and underdeveloped muscles have fewer available sites. It is sometimes difficult to assess the amount of fluid that can be safely injected into a single site. Usually 1 ml is the maximum volume that should be administered in a single site to small children and older infants. The muscles of small infants may not tolerate more than 0.5 ml. As the child approaches adult size, volumes approaching those given to adults may be used. However, the larger the amount of solution, the larger must be the muscle into which it is injected.

Injections must be placed in muscles large enough to accommodate the medication, and major nerves and blood vessels are avoided. There is no universal agreement regarding the best intramuscular injection site for children. The preferred site for infants is the vastus lateralis, although the ventrogluteal muscle can also be used. In older children and adolescents the preferred sites are much the same as in the adult.

Table 19-4 summarizes the 4 major injection sites and illustrates their anatomic location for children.

Administration. Although injections that are executed with care seldom produce trauma to the child, there have been reports of serious disability related to intramuscular injections. Repeated use of a single site has been associated with fibrosis of the muscle with subsequent muscle contracture, and injections in the neighborhood of large nerves, such as the sciatic nerve, have been responsible for permanent disability, especially when potentially neurotoxic drugs are administered. Therefore careful attention to detail is essential.

The box on p. 564 summarizes administration techniques that maximize safety and minimize the discomfort often associated with injections.

Most children are unpredictable, and few are totally cooperative when receiving an injection. Even children who appear to be relaxed and constrained can lose control under the stress of the procedure. It is advisable to have someone available to help restrain the child if needed. Since children often jerk or pull away unexpectedly, it is a good idea to carry an extra needle to exchange for a contaminated one so that there is a minimum of delay. The child, even a small one, is told that he is getting an injection, and then the procedure is carried out as quickly and skillfully as possible to avoid prolonging the stressful experience. Delay caused by lengthy explanations, attempts to hide the syringe from sight, or efforts to soothe the child will only serve to increase his anxiety. It must be kept in mind that intrusive procedures such as injections are especially anxiety provoking in preschool children and that small children usually associate any assault to the ''behind'' area with punishment.

Small infants offer little resistance to injections. Although they squirm and may be difficult to hold in position, they can usually be restrained without assistance. The muscle mass of the thigh to be injected is firmly grasped in one hand to stabilize the limb and compress the muscle mass for injection with the other hand. The body of a larger infant can be securely restrained between the nurse's elbow and body (Fig. 19-25).

If medication is given around the clock, the nurse must be certain to wake the child before giving the injection. Although it may seem easier to surprise the sleeping child and get it over with as quickly as possible, performing the procedure in this way can cause the child to fear going back to sleep. If he is awakened first, the child will know that nothing will be done to him unless he is forewarned.

Intravenous administration

Use of the intravenous route for administering medications has gained widespread use in pediatric therapy. For some important drugs it is the only effective route of administration. This method is used for giving drugs to children who have poor absorption as a result of diarrhea, dehydration, or peripheral vascular collapse; children who need a high serum concentration of a drug; and children with resistant infections that require parenteral medication over an extended time.

Insertion sites and observation of the intravenous infusion are discussed on p. 569. However, there are a number of factors to be considered and nursing responsibilities related to intravenous medication. When a drug is administered intravenously, the effect is almost instantaneous and further control is limited. Most drugs for intravenous administration require a specified minimum dilution and/or rate of flow, and many are highly irritating or toxic to tissues outside the vascular system. In addition to the precautions and nursing observations related to intravenous therapy, factors that are considered when preparing and administering drugs to infants and children by way of the intravenous route include:

1. Amount of drug to be administered
2. Minimum dilution of drug
3. Type of solution in which drug can be diluted
4. Length of time over which drug can be safely administered
5. Rate of infusion that child and his vessels can tolerate safely
6. Time that this or another drug is to be administered
7. Compatibility of all drugs that child is receiving intravenously

Before any intravenous infusion the site of insertion is checked for patency. Medications are never administered by way of blood products.

TABLE 19-4. INTRAMUSCULAR INJECTION SITES IN CHILDREN

SITE	DISCUSSION
Vastus lateralis 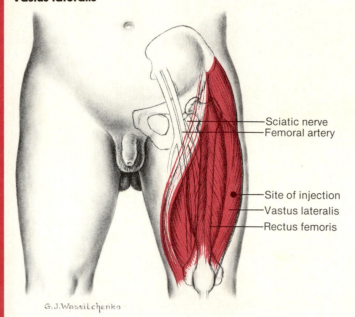 G.J.Wassilchenko Intramuscular injection (vastus lateralis)	**Location** Palpate to find greater trochanter and measure hand's width below this point and hand's width above knee; inject within these boundaries (middle two thirds of thigh) on anterolateral aspect of thigh. **Needle insertion** Insert needle at 45° angle toward knee or needle perpendicular to thigh or slightly angled toward anterior thigh. **Advantages** Large, well-developed muscle that can tolerate larger quantities of fluid No important nerves or blood vessels in this location Easily accessible if child is prone, supine, side-lying, or sitting A tourniquet can be applied above injection site to delay drug hypersensitivity reaction if necessary **Disadvantages** Thrombosis of femoral artery from injection in midthigh area Sciatic nerve damage from long needle injected posteriorly and medially into small extremity
Ventro gluteal 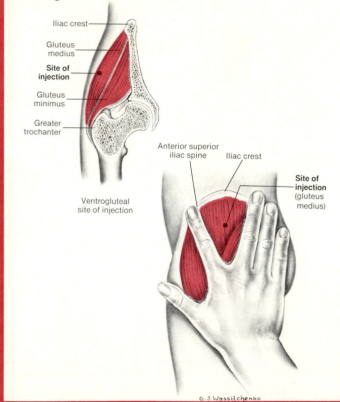 G.J.Wassilchenko	**Location** Palpate to locate greater trochanter, anterior superior iliac tubercle (found by flexing thigh at hip and measuring up to 1 to 2 cm. above crease formed in groin), and posterior iliac crest; place palm of hand over greater trochanter, index finger over anterior superior iliac tubercle, and middle finger along crest of ilium posteriorly as far as possible; inject into center of V formed by fingers. **Needle insertion** Insert needle perpendicular to site but angled slightly toward iliac crest. **Advantages** Free of important nerves and vascular structures Easily identified by prominent bony landmarks Thinner layer of subcutaneous tissue than in dorsogluteal site, thus less chance of depositing drug subcutaneously rather than intramuscularly Easily accessible if child is supine, prone, or side-lying Less painful than vastus lateralis **Disadvantages** Health professionals' unfamiliarity with site Not suitable for use of a tourniquet

TABLE 19-4. INTRAMUSCULAR INJECTION SITES IN CHILDREN—cont'd

SITE	DISCUSSION

Dorsogluteal

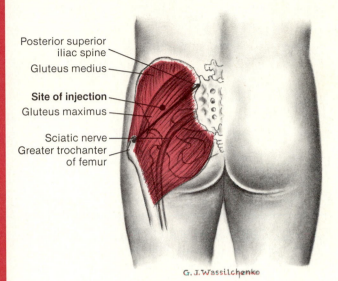

Posterior superior iliac spine
Gluteus medius
Site of injection
Gluteus maximus
Sciatic nerve
Greater trochanter of femur

G. J. Wassilchenko

Intramuscular injection (gluteus maximus)

Location

Locate greater trochanter and posterior superior iliac spine; draw imaginary line between these two points and inject lateral and superior to line into gluteus muscle.

Needle insertion

Insert needle perpendicular to surface on which child is lying when prone.

Advantages

In older child large muscle mass; well-developed muscle can tolerate greater volume of fluid

Child does not see needle and syringe

Easily accessible if child is prone or side-lying

Disadvantages

Contraindicated in children who have not been walking for at least 1 year

Danger of injury to sciatic nerve

Thick, subcutaneous fat, predisposing to deposition of drug subcutaneously rather than intramuscularly

Not suitable for use of a tourniquet

Inaccessible if child is supine

Exposure of site may cause embarrassment in older child

Deltoid

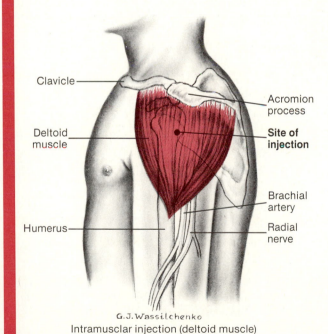

Clavicle
Acromion process
Deltoid muscle
Site of injection
Humerus
Brachial artery
Radial nerve

G. J. Wassilchenko

Intramusclar injection (deltoid muscle)

Location

Locate acromion process; inject only into upper third of muscle that begins about 2 finger-breadths below acromion.

Needle insertion

Insert needle perpendicular to site but angled slightly toward shoulder.

Advantages

Faster absorption rates than gluteal sites

Tourniquet can be applied above injection site

Easily accessible with minimal removal of clothing

Disadvantages

Small muscle mass; only limited amounts of drug can be injected

Small margins of safety with possible damage to radial nerve

Pain with repeated injections

ADMINISTRATION OF INTRAMUSCULAR INJECTIONS

Expose injection area for unobstructed view of landmarks.

Select a site where the skin is free of irritation and danger of infection; palpate for and avoid sensitive or hardened areas.

Place the child in a lying or sitting position; the child is not allowed to stand because:
1. Landmarks are more difficult to assess.
2. Restraint is more difficult.
3. The child may faint and fall.

Use a new sharp needle with the smallest diameter that permits free flow of the medication.

Grasp the muscle firmly between the thumb and other fingers to isolate and stabilize the muscle for deposition of the drug in its deepest part; in obese children spread the skin with the thumb and index finger to displace subcutaneous and grasp the muscle deeply on each side.

Allow the skin preparation to dry completely before the skin is penetrated.

Have the medication near room temperature.

Decrease the perception of pain:
1. Distract the child with conversation.
2. Give the child something on which to concentrate, such as squeezing a hand or bed rail, pinching his own nose, humming, or yelling ''ouch''.
3. Place a cold compress or wrapped ice cube on the site a few minutes before the injection.

Insert the needle quickly.

Inject into a relaxed muscle:
1. Dorsogluteal—place child on abdomen with his legs and toes rotated inward.
2. Ventrogluteal—place child on side with the upper leg flexed and placed in front of the lower leg.

Avoid tracking any medication through superficial tissues:
1. Replace needle after withdrawing medication or wipe medication from needle with sterile gauze.
2. If withdrawing medication from an ampule, use a needle equipped with a filter that removes glass particles and use a second needle for injection.
3. Use the Z-track and/or air bubble technique as indicated.
4. Avoid any depression of the plunger during insertion of needle.

Aspirate to be sure the needle is not in a blood vessel; if it is, begin again with a new needle and syringe.

Inject the medication slowly.

Remove the needle quickly; hold a gauze sponge firmly against the skin near the needle when removing it to avoid the needle's pulling on the tissue.

Apply firm pressure to the site after injection; massage the site to hasten absorption unless contraindicated.

Place a small Band-Aid on the puncture site; with young children decorate Band-Aid by drawing a smiling face or other symbol of acceptance.

Hold and cuddle young child and encourage parents to comfort him; praise older child.

When a drug with poor stability, such as ampicillin, is being administered, not only must the Soluset (or similar container) be emptied of the drug-containing solution, but the tubing from the Soluset to the insertion site must also be emptied. The child does not receive the full dose of the drug until the 10 ml or more of solution within the tubing has also been infused. This is a significant consideration when drugs are given in small amounts of fluid. For example, if a drug is added to 10 ml of fluid in the Soluset, it does not reach the bloodstream until all of the fluid in the tubing is absorbed.

As a general rule, all antibiotics administered via Soluset should infuse within 1 hour. Only one antibiotic should be administered at a time. If the intravenous solution contains other medications such as some electrolytes or vitamins, antibiotics are not added to this preparation because the other drugs may inactivate the antibiotic. In this situation another bottle of intravenous solution is hung and attached via a stopcock to the main infusion line. This ''piggyback'' setup allows antibiotics to be infused without mixing with the other solution.

Other methods of intravenous infusion are via retro-

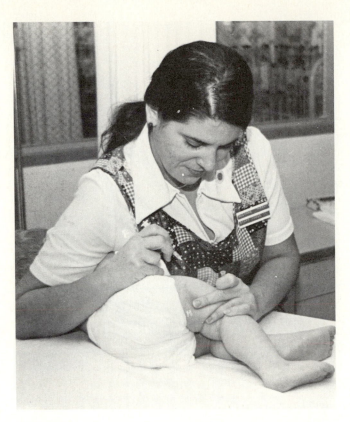

FIG. 19-25
Restraining a small child for intramuscular injection. Note how the nurse grasps and stabilizes the muscle. ⊕

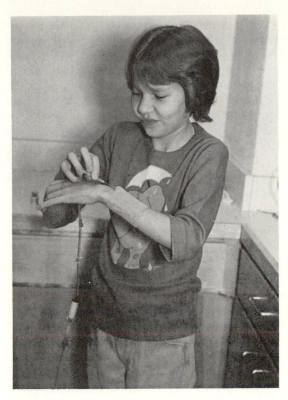

FIG. 19-26
Child injecting medication by way of heparin lock.

grade injection, a heparin lock (intermittent infusion), or Broviac catheter, which is discussed in relation to hyperalimentation (p. 583), although it can also be used for drug administration, blood withdrawal and infusion, and central venous monitoring. In the *retrograde technique*, the medication is injected directly into the intravenous tubing at the site of the Y connection. However, the drug is injected *back* toward the Soluset while the tubing is pinched between the Y connection and the venipuncture site. After the drug is injected, the tubing is no longer pinched and the intravenous infusion is allowed to infuse. This allows for slower administration of the drug and greater dilution in the fluid than if it were placed in the open tubing toward the vein. It is advantageous in administering medication when fluid intake is limited, such as in infants with congestive heart failure.

The *heparin lock* is used as an alternative for a keep-open infusion when long-term access to a vein is required without the need for fluid. It is most frequently employed for intermittent infusion of medication, as well as for repeated collection of blood samples or peripheral alimentation. A short, flexible catheter or scalp vein needle is inserted into a site where there will be minimal movement, such as the forearm. The needle is secured in the same

manner as any intravenous infusion device, but the needle hub is occluded with a stopper. The needle remains in place and is flushed with heparin at regular intervals to prevent blood from clotting in the needle between infusions. To infuse medication the plastic cap is removed, the rubber diaphragm is wiped with alcohol, and the drug is injected through the diaphragm either directly from a syringe or via a Soluset (Fig. 19-26). Children and/or parents are often taught to administer medications by this route.

Rectal administration

The rectal route for administration is less reliable but sometimes used when the oral route is difficult or contraindicated. Some of the drugs available in suppository form are aspirin, sedatives, analgesics (morphine), and antiemetics. The difficulty in using the rectal route is that, unless the rectal ampulla is empty at the time of insertion, the absorption of the drug may be delayed, diminished, or prevented by the presence of feces. Sometimes the drug is later evacuated, securely surrounded by stool. However, the rectal route is used most frequently in children who are unable to take anything by mouth and who are unlikely to have large amounts of stool. It is also used when oral preparations are unsuitable to control vomiting.

The wrapping on the suppository is removed. Using a glove or finger cot, the suppository is quickly but gently inserted into the rectum, making certain that it is placed beyond both of the rectal sphincters. The buttocks are then held or taped together firmly to relieve pressure on the anal sphincter until the urge to expel the suppository has passed—5 to 10 minutes. Sometimes the amount of drug ordered is less than the dosage available. The irregular shape of most suppositories makes the process of dividing them into a desired dose difficult if not dangerous. If it must be halved, it should be cut lengthwise.

The same procedure is used to administer medication in a retention enema. Drugs given by enema are diluted in the smallest amount of solution possible to minimize the likelihood of being evacuated.

Optic, otic, and nasal administration

There are few differences in administering eye, ear, and nose medication to children than to adults. The major difficulty is in gaining their cooperation or employing restraining techniques. The infant or young child's head can be immobilized in the same manner as described in Fig. 5-25. Older children need only explanation and direction. For greater comfort medications stored in the refrigerator should be warmed to room temperature before instillation. For example, cold solutions striking the tympanic membrane may produce pain or vertigo.

To administer eye medication the child is placed supine or sitting with the head extended and the child is asked to look up. One hand is used to pull the lower lid downward; the hand that holds the dropper rests on the head (Fig. 19-27). In this way the hand moves synchronously with the child's head and reduces the possibility of trauma to a struggling child or dropping medication on the face. As the lower lid is pulled down, a small conjunctival sac is formed; the solution or ointment is applied to this area, never directly on the eyeball. Another effective technique is to pull the lower lid down and out to form a cup, into which the medication is dropped.

The lids are gently closed to prevent expression of the medication, and the child is asked to look in all directions to enhance even distribution of the preparation. Excess medication is wiped from the inner canthus outward to prevent contamination to the contralateral eye. Applying finger pressure to the lacrimal punctate at the inner aspect of the lid for 1 minute prevents drainage of medication to the nasopharynx and eliminates the unpleasant "tasting" of the drug.

Instilling eye medications in infants can be most dif-

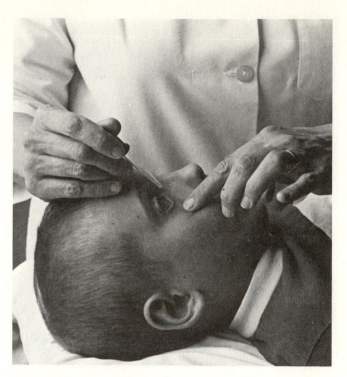

FIG. 19-27
Administering eye drops.

ficult as they often clench the lids tightly closed. One approach is to place the drops in the nasal corner where the lids meet. The medication pools in this area and when the child opens the lids the medication flows onto the conjunctiva. For young children playing a game can be helpful. Instruct the child to keep the eyes closed until the count of three, then to open them at which time the drops are quickly instilled. Ointment can be applied when the child is sleeping by gently pulling down the lower lid and placing the ointment in the lower conjunctival sac.

Ear drops are instilled with the child restrained in the supine position and the head turned to the appropriate side. For children younger than 3 years of age, the external auditory canal is straightened by gently pulling the pinna downward and straight back. The pinna is pulled upward and back in children older than 3 years of age (see Fig. 5-21). After instillation, the child should remain lying on the unaffected side for a few minutes. Gentle massage of the area immediately anterior to the ear facilitates the entry of drops into the ear canal. The use of cotton pledgets prevents medication from flowing out of the external canal. However, they should be loose enough to allow any discharge to exit from the ear.

Nose drops are instilled in the same manner as in the adult patient. Unpleasant sensations associated with medicated nose drops are minimized when care is taken to po-

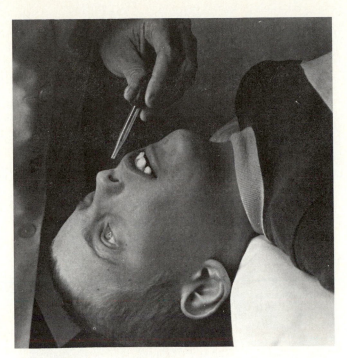

FIG. 19-28
Proper position for instilling nose drops.

sition the child with the head extended well over the edge of the bed or a pillow (Fig. 19-28). Strangling sensations are caused by medication trickling into the throat rather than up into the nasal passages. Following instillation of the drops, the child should remain in position for 1 minute to allow the drops to come in contact with the nasal surfaces.

Plain saline or vasoconstricting nose drops are sometimes prescribed for infants with "stuffy noses" caused by upper respiratory infections. Since these children naturally breathe by nose, nasal congestion interferes with feeding; therefore, drops are instilled before feedings to clear nasal passages and reduce congestion. Depending on the size of the infant, he can be positioned in the football hold (p. 546), in the nurse's arm with the head extended and stabilized between the nurse's body and elbow and the arms and hands immobilized with the nurse's hands, or with the head extended over the edge of the bed or a pillow.

Teaching parents

It is usually the nurse who assumes the responsibility for preparing parents to administer medications at home. The parents need an understanding of why the child is receiving the medication and the effects that might be expected, as well as the amount, frequency, and length of time the drug is to be administered. Instructions are carried out in an unhurried, relaxed manner, preferably in an area away from busy ward or office routine.

Some persons have difficulty in understanding or interpreting terminology from the pharmacy, and just because they nod or otherwise indicate an understanding, it cannot be assumed that the message is clear. It is important to ascertain their interpretation of, for example, a teaspoon—is it rounded, level, or scant? If the drug is packaged with a dropper in the cap, the nurse should show the point on the dropper that indicates the prescribed dose and demonstrate how the dose is drawn up and measured and the bubbles eliminated. If there is any doubt about the parent's ability to administer the correct dose, it is wise to have him or her give a return demonstration. This is especially important when the drug has potentially serious consequences from incorrect dosage, such as insulin or digitalis, and with administration of injectable or optic medication. Teaching a parent to give an injection usually requires instruction and practice over 2 or 3 days.

The time that the drug is to be administered is clarified with the parent. For instance, when a drug is prescribed in association with meals, the number of meals that the family is accustomed to eat influences the amount of drug the child receives. Do they have meals twice a day or five times a day? When a drug is to be given several times during the day, together the nurse and parents can work out a schedule that accommodates the family routine. This is particularly significant if the drug must be given at equal intervals throughout a 24-hour period. For example, telling them that the child needs 1 teaspoon of medicine four times a day is not necessarily adequate, since parents may routinely schedule the doses at incorrect times. Instead, a preplanned schedule based on 6-hour intervals should be set up with the number of days required for therapeutic dosage listed. For most mild infections the optimum administration schedule can be altered to conform with the family's routine provided on interval exceeds 10 to 12 hours. Following is an example of home care instructions:

Schedule for home administration of antibiotic medication
General instructions:
   Give the child 1 teaspoon ampicillin four times a day.
Specific instructions:
   1. Use medicine dropper and fill with liquid to 5-ml mark.
   2. Give *1 hour* before meals.
   3. Avoid giving acidic fruit juices with drug.
   4. Refrigerate bottle and *shake well* before using.
   5. Use for each day listed below, or until all the medication is taken.
   6. Cross off appropriate time and date each time child is given medicine.

Date*		Times		
5/21	Discharge	12:00 PM	5:00 PM	10:00 PM
5/22	6:30 AM	12:00 PM	5:00 PM	10:00 PM
5/23	6:30 AM	12:00 PM	5:00 PM	10:00 PM
5/24	6:30 AM	12:00 PM	Discard any remaining drug	

PROCEDURES RELATED TO MAINTAINING FLUID BALANCE

Nursing observation and intervention are essential to the detection and therapeutic management of changes in the fluid and electrolyte balance. Nurses need to be comfortable with equipment used to deliver fluids to infants and children and the knowledge and techniques for assessment.

Intake and output (I & O) measurement

One of the most important roles of the nurse in maintaining fluid balance is accurate measurements of fluid balance. Although the physician usually indicates when intake and output are to be recorded, it is a nursing responsibility to keep an accurate intake and output record on patients in the following situations:

  Children receiving intravenous therapy
  Children with severe thermal burns or injuries
  Children with renal disease or damage
  Children with congestive heart failure
  Children with dehydration (vomiting and diarrhea)
  Children with diabetes mellitus
  Children with oliguria
  Children receiving diuretic therapy
  Children receiving corticosteroid therapy
  After major surgery

Infants or small children who are unable to use a bedpan or those who have bowel movements with every voiding will require the application of a collecting device (p. 553). If collecting bags are not used, wet diapers or pads are carefully weighed to ascertain the amount of fluid lost. This includes liquid stool, vomitus, and other losses. The volume of fluid in milliliters is equivalent to the weight of the fluid measured in grams. The specific gravity as a measure of osmolality is determined with a urinometer or a refractometer and assists in assessing the degree of hydration (Fig. 19-29).

It is important to measure and record all intake, oral and parenteral, and output from all sources, including

*Based on number of days for administration of drug after discharge.

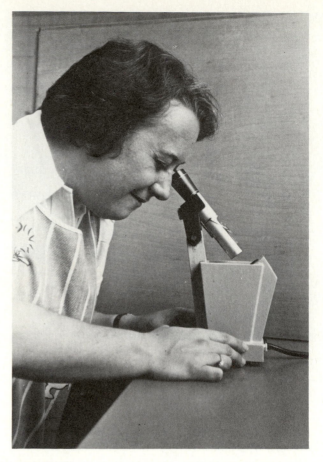

FIG. 19-29
The nurse measures the specific gravity of a drop of urine by means of a refractometer.

urine, stool, emesis, drainage tubes, fistulas, and wounds from which appreciable amounts of fluid are lost.

Special needs

Infants or children who are unable to take fluids by mouth will require special mouth care. Oral hygiene, a part of routine hygienic care, is especially important when fluids are restricted or withheld. To meet the need to suck, the infant is provided with a pacifier, either with a commercial variety or with one constructed from a nipple stuffed with gauze and/or taped to a rolled washcloth.

To prevent imbalances resulting from the inadvertent substitution of salt for sugar in infant or nasogastric formulas, great care should be exerted in their preparation. Children, especially infants, are quickly subject to life-threatening hypernatremic dehydration from this rare but conceivable accident. It is important to stress to parents and others responsible for mixing formula feedings the

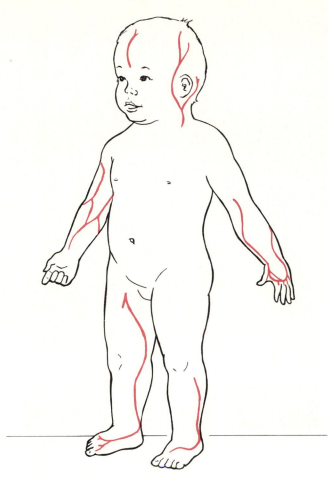

FIG. 19-30

Superficial veins are used most often for intravenous infusion. (From Kempe, C.H., Silver, H.K., and O'Brien, D.: Current pediatric diagnosis and treatment, ed. 8, Los Altos, Calif., 1984, Lange Medical Publications.)

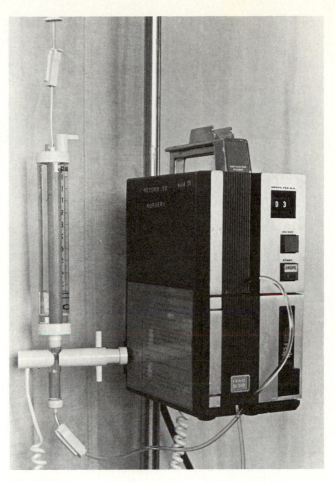

FIG. 19-31

Gravity drainage apparatus attached to an infusion pump for administration of intravenous fluids (IVAC Corp.).

harm that excessive sodium intake can cause and the simple modes of prevention.

Parenteral fluid therapy

Since most hospitalized infants and children with serious disturbance of fluid and electrolyte balance are almost always maintained on intravenous fluids, monitoring intravenous fluid replacement is a major nursing responsibility. Most of the general principles of intravenous therapy apply to infants and children, but with a number of important variations.

Site. The site selected for intravenous infusion depends on accessibility and convenience. In older children any accessible vein may be used. In small infants a scalp vein or a superficial vein of the wrist, hand, foot, or arm is usually most convenient and most easily stabilized (Fig. 19-30). Since superficial veins of the scalp have no valves, they can be infused in either direction and are used frequently for intravenous therapy in infants.

Equipment. There are several modifications in equipment used for intravenous infusion for children. A gravity drainage apparatus used for children is much the same as that for adults except that it is designed to deliver a reduced drop size (60 drops/ml) and contains a calibrated volume control chamber that limits the maximum amount of fluid that can be infused. A microdropper greatly facilitates calculation of flow rate because a prescribed *number of milliliters per hour equals the number of drops per minute*. For example, if the solution is to infuse at a rate of 30 ml/hour, the infusion is regulated to deliver 30 drops per minute. A variety of types are available, but all have

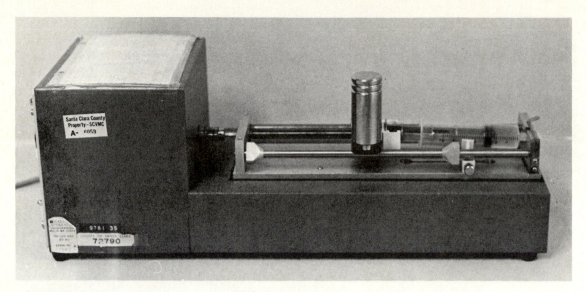

FIG. 19-32

Syringe (Harvard) pump for infusion of a very small amount of fluid over a specified period of time.

a limited capacity, refillable from the bottle above, to minimize the possibility of overloading the circulation. When using this device it is important that the tubing between the bottle and the chamber is firmly clamped to prevent additional fluid from dripping into the chamber. When sets with collapsible chambers and rigid cylinders with an automatic shutoff valve are employed, the infusion stops automatically when the chamber is empty. It is an important nursing responsibility to calculate the amount to be infused in a given length of time, set the infusion rate, and monitor the apparatus frequently to make certain that the desired rate is maintained and that the infusion does not stop.

To facilitate a more precise flow rate, mechanical infusion pumps are used extensively for pediatric intravenous fluid administration (Fig. 19-31). Most of these devices pump a given amount of fluid by peristaltic action on the tubing, governed by a flow rate setting, and regulated by a drop sensor that activates an alarm when no drops are formed. For administering a very small amount of fluid over a specific period of time, precision-controlled syringe pumps may be preferable (Fig. 19-32). These devices, although convenient and efficient, are not without attendant risks. Overreliance on the accuracy of the machine can cause either too much or too little fluid to be infused. Excess pressure can build up if the machine is set at a rate faster than the vein is able to accommodate (or continues to pump when the needle is out of the lumen). This is especially true in very small infants and when circumstances necessitate the use of a capillary. No matter

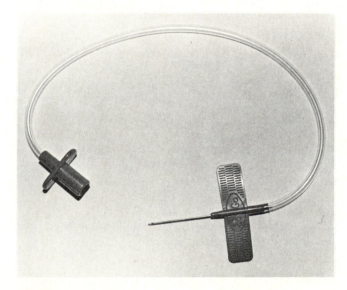

FIG. 19-33

Scalp vein needle.

what device is used, a thorough understanding of the apparatus and careful periodic assessment of the infusion are essential for safe fluid administration.

For most intravenous infusions in children, a scalp-vein needle size 21 or 23 is used with flexible winged tabs that are easily secured to the skin (Fig. 19-33). In situations in which fluids are urgently needed and there is difficulty in entering a vein, a polyethylene tube inserted by the surgical cutdown procedure may be necessary. The

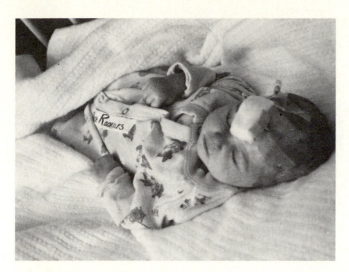

FIG. 19-34
Scalp vein infusion.

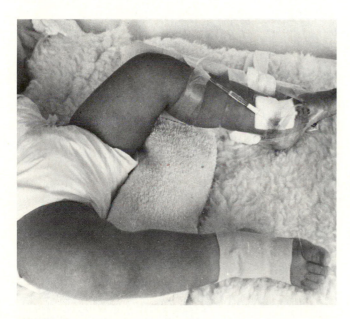

FIG. 19-35
Extremity immobilized with a board and firmly secured to bedding with pins. Note sheepskin, which protects bony prominences.

vein of choice for this alternative is the internal saphenous vein located just anterior to the medial malleolus of the tibia. For long-term intravenous therapy a number of other techniques may be used, including a flexible plastic catheter, a heparin lock (p. 565), or a Broviac catheter (p. 583).

Selection of a scalp vein as the venipuncture site requires shaving the area around the site to better visualize the vein and provide a smooth surface on which to tape the tubing (Fig. 19-34). A rubber band slipped onto the head from brow to occiput will usually suffice as a tourniquet. Shaving off a portion of the infant's hair is very upsetting to parents; therefore, they should be told what to expect and reassured that the hair will grow in again rapidly.

Special precautions. To maintain the integrity of the intravenous site, the child will require adequate restraint. The needle is secured firmly at the puncture site with nonallergenic tape and protected from becoming dislodged by immobilization of the extremity. A plastic cup applied directly over the needle site will further protect the infusion. The head can be immobilized with covered sandbags. A sandbag or a small board, well padded with plastic foam and a cloth or stockinette cover, provides a suitable means for immobilization (Fig. 19-35). Some form of resilient padding is required to prevent areas of pressure necrosis over bony prominences, such as the ankle. To prevent trauma to the skin from removal of tape, the nurse can place some gauze between the skin and adhesive.

Older children who are alert and cooperative can usually be trusted to protect the intravenous site. Infants, small children, and uncooperative children require restraint. A board used to stabilize a joint is secured to the bed, and the remaining extremities that might be used to dislodge the needle are restrained as described previously (p. 549). This includes feet as well as hands, since most infants will attempt to brush away the offending attachment by rubbing it against another extremity or body part. Range of motion exercises are employed on infants and children who are too ill or unable to move their extremities, but others should be encouraged to move their arms and legs in response to a natural stimulus. Most infants or small children will instinctively move their extremities when released. If not, a toy or other stimulus can be provided for an incentive.

The same precautions regarding maintenance of asepsis, prevention of infection, and observation for infiltration are carried out with patients of any age. However, infiltration is more difficult to detect in infants and small children than it is in adults. The increased amount of subcutaneous fat and the amount of tape used to secure the needle often obscure the signs of early infiltration. When the usual assessment techniques fail to detect the problem, it may be necessary to remove carefully some of the tape and other material that obscures a clear view of the venipuncture site. Dependent areas, such as the palm and undersides of the extremity or the occiput and behind the ears, with a scalp vein infusion, are examined for signs of extravasation.

PROCEDURES RELATED TO MAINTAINING RESPIRATORY FUNCTION

Procedures to improve ventilation are employed with increasing frequency in the prevention and management of pulmonary dysfunction. Most of these involve the nurse in the hospital or the home situation.

Inhalation therapy

The term ''inhalation therapy'' is an all-inclusive term that encompasses a variety of therapies that involve changing the composition, volume, or pressure of inspired gases. This includes primarily increasing the oxygen concentration of inspired gas (oxygen therapy), increasing the water vapor content of inspired gas (humidification), addition of airborne particles with beneficial properties (aerosol therapy), and various means for controlling or assisting respiration (artificial ventilation, intermittent positive pressure breathing).

Oxygen therapy.   Oxygen therapy is almost always carried out in the hospital. Oxygen delivered to the infant Isolette is satisfactory when lower levels are adequate to prevent cyanosis, but the highest concentration (almost 100%) is supplied by way of a plastic hood (Fig. 19-36). The gas should not be allowed to blow directly into the infant's face, and the hood should not rub against the infant's neck, chin, or shoulder. Older cooperative children can use a nasal cannula or prongs, which can supply a concentration of about 50%. A nasal catheter or a mask is not well tolerated by children.

For most children beyond early infancy the oxygen tent, or canopy, is the most satisfactory means for administration of oxygen (Fig. 19-37). A tent does not require any device to come into direct contact with the face, but the concentration of oxygen within the tent is difficult to control and to maintain above about 40%. The comfort to the child makes it the method of choice except in cases of marked respiratory distress. A major difficulty with the use of the tent is keeping the tent closed so that oxygen concentration is maintained. To reduce oxygen loss, nursing care should be planned carefully so that the tent is opened as little as possible. Since oxygen is heavier than air, loss will be greater at the bottom of the tent; therefore the tent should be tucked in snugly without open edges. The bottom of the tent should be examined more often when the child is restless and fussy and liable to pull the covers loose. Some tents are even open at the top. Because of the rapid diffusing qualities of carbon dioxide, the levels of the gas do not build up within these enclosures.

After the tent has been opened for an extended period of time, it is flushed with oxygen by increasing the flow meter for a few minutes to quickly raise the oxygen and mist concentration. The flow meter is then reset to the prescribed number of liters.

The enclosed tent becomes very warm; therefore, some type of cooling mechanism is provided. The temperature inside the tent must be checked periodically to be certain that it is maintained at the desired temperature. It is important to make certain that the child is kept warm and dry. Mist is usually prescribed in conjunction with oxygen therapy, and the moisture condenses on the tent walls. The child's bedding and clothing are examined periodically and changed as needed to prevent chilling.

The reactions of children to the oxygen tent are variable. Some, especially older children, feel comfortable in the tent and like the cozy, close privacy it affords. Others,

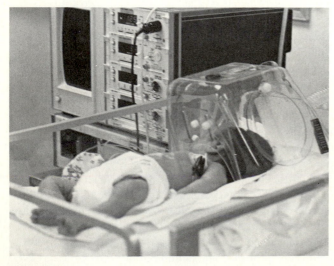

FIG. 19-36
Oxygen administered to an infant by a plastic hood.

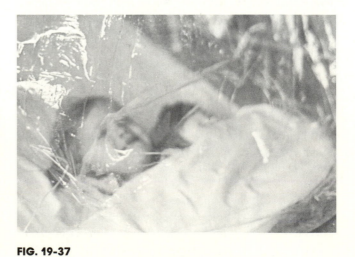

FIG. 19-37
The tent provides a comfortable method for oxygen administration but may be frightening to a small child, even when shared by a familiar ''friend.''

more often younger children, may be frightened by the forced enclosure. The plastic walls distort their view of the world and constitute a barrier between them and their source of comfort, their mother. Their distress can be minimized if they are able to see someone nearby and are reassured that they will not be left alone. A favorite toy or object can accompany the child inside the tent. However, all toys should be inspected for safety and suitability. The high oxygen environment makes any source of sparks (such as some mechanical toys) a potential fire hazard. Other familiar items can be placed at the foot of the bed or otherwise in view.

No matter what method is used to administer the oxygen, the child's color and respiratory status are monitored frequently and evaluated in terms of efficacy of treatment. The oxygen content within the device is analyzed periodically (always at a point near the child's head) to determine the rate of flow needed to maintain the desired concentration. The equipment is changed and/or cleaned at regular intervals (at least once weekly) to prevent bacterial growth when the child requires oxygen over an extended period.

In most instances the child can be removed from the oxygen tent for activities such as feeding and bathing, whereas in other cases the child is placed in the tent only during periods of rest. Still others may require oxygen continuously and can be removed from the tent or Isolette only if an oxygen source is held close to the child's face. Any change in color, increased respiratory effort, or restlessness is an indication to return the child to the oxygen tent.

Oxygen toxicity. Oxygen is essential to life and a valuable therapeutic aid. However, prolonged exposure to high oxygen tensions can be damaging to some body tissues and functions. The organs most vulnerable to the adverse effects of excessive oxygenation are the retina of the premature infant and the lungs of persons at any age.

Oxygen-induced carbon dioxide narcosis is a physiologic hazard of oxygen therapy that may occur in persons with chronic pulmonary disease. It is seldom encountered in children except those with cystic fibrosis. These children have chronic alveolar hypoventilation with a concomitant chronic carbon dioxide retention and hypoxemia. In these patients the respiratory center has adapted to the continuously higher PCO_2 levels, and, therefore, hypoxia becomes the more powerful stimulus to respiration. When the PO_2 is elevated during oxygen administration, the hypoxic drive is removed, causing increasing hypoventilation and increased PCO_2 levels, and the child rapidly becomes unconscious.

Aerosol therapy. The inhalation and subsequent deposition of airborne water particles within the airway is the function of aerosol therapy. Saline may be used to help moisten the airway and help liquefy secretions, or the particles may contain mucolytic, bronchodilating, decongestant, or antimicrobial agents.

For continuous aerosol therapy a misting device is attached to or incorporated into the mist tent. Distilled water is used most commonly, although propylene glycol in aqueous solution is often employed, especially in jet-type nebulizers. For intermittent administration of small quantities of an agent with specific pharmacologic action, a small nebulizer can be used powered by a small electric motor or in association with a positive pressure breathing apparatus.

Aerosol therapy is widely used in treatment of both upper and lower respiratory tract disease and of conditions in which there is weakness of the muscles of respiration. In some instances aerosol therapy is employed prophylactically (for example, cystic fibrosis) to prevent complicating pulmonary problems. There is a decided relationship between aerosol therapy and bronchial drainage. Drainage is much more effective immediately after aerosol therapy.

Aerosol therapy is usually performed under the guidance of a respiratory therapist, although nurses may assume this responsibility in the home or in association with the therapist. Nurses need to know how the apparatus works and to recognize when it is functioning improperly. Because of the danger of bacterial growth, the equipment is thoroughly cleaned daily.

Bronchial (postural) drainage

Bronchial drainage is indicated whenever excessive fluid or mucus in the bronchi is not being removed by normal ciliary activity and cough. The techniques of segmental drainage, percussion, and vibration assist the normal cleansing mechanisms of the lung. Positioning the child to take maximum advantage of gravity further facilitates removal of secretions.

Postural drainage is carried out three to four times daily or as often as every 2 hours and is more effective when it follows other respiratory therapy, such as bronchodilator and/or nebulization medication. Bronchial drainage is generally performed before meals (or 1 to 1½ hours after meals) to minimize the chance of vomiting and at bedtime. The length and duration of treatment depend on the child's condition and tolerance level—usually 20 to 30 minutes. Different positions are used to facilitate drainage from all major lung segments (Fig. 19-38), but all positions are not employed at each session. Children will usually cooperate for four to six positions, but more than six tend to exceed their limits of tolerance. In older children longer periods can be reasonably expected. In the hospital an older child can be positioned over the elevated knee rest. Small children and infants can be positioned with pillows (Fig. 19-39) or on the therapist's lap and legs (Fig. 19-40). Special modifications of the techniques are

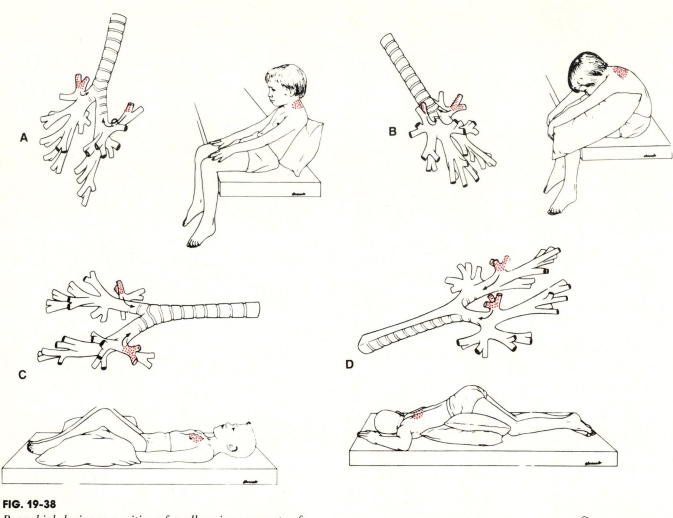

FIG. 19-38

*Bronchial drainage positions for all major segments of child. For each position, model of tracheobronchial tree is projected beside child in order to show segmental bronchus (striped) being drained and pathway (arrow) of secretions out of bronchus. Drainage platform is horizontal unless otherwise noted. Striped area on child's chest indicates area to be cupped or vibrated by therapist. (From Kendig, E.L., Jr., editor: Disorders of the respiratory tract in children, ed. 2, Philadelphia, 1977, W.B. Saunders Co.) **A,** Apical segment of right upper lobe and apical subsegment of apical-posterior segment of left upper lobe; **B,** posterior segment of right upper lobe and posterior subsegment of apical-posterior segment of left upper lobe; **C,** anterior segments of both upper lobes; child should be rotated slightly away from side being drained.*

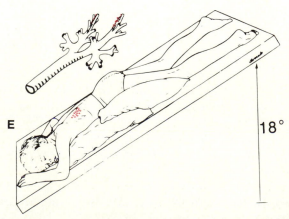

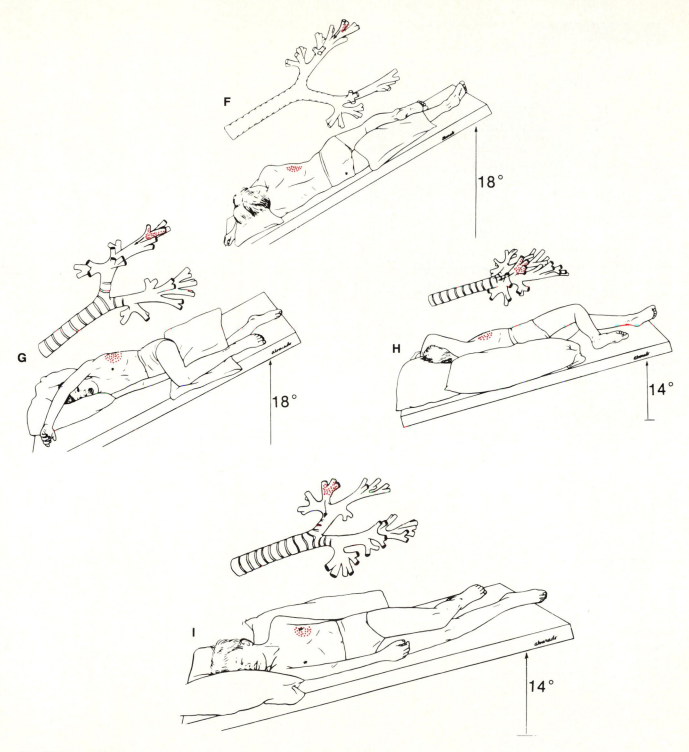

FIG. 19-38, cont'd

D, *Superior segments of both lower lobes;* **E,** *posterior basal segments of both lower lobes.* **F,** *Lateral segments of right lower lobe, left lateral basal segment would be drained by mirror image of this position (right side down).* **G,** *Anterior basal segment of left lower lobe; right anterior basal segment would be drained by mirror image of this position (left side down);* **H,** *medial and lateral segments of right middle lobe;* **I,** *lingular segments (superior and inferior) of left upper lobe (homologue of right middle lobe).*

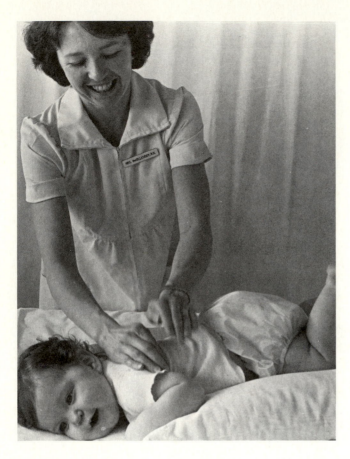

FIG. 19-39
Child positioned for postural drainage.

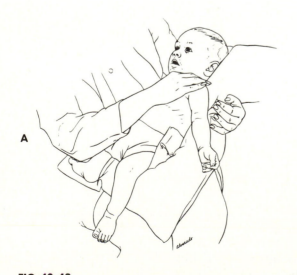

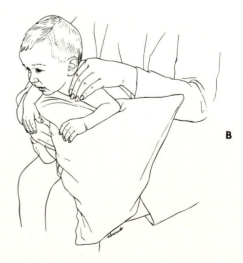

FIG. 19-40
Bronchial drainage positions for major segments of all lobes in infant. Procedure is most easily carried out in therapist's lap. Therapist's hand on chest indicates area to be cupped or vibrated. **A,** *Apical segment of left upper lobe;* **B,** *posterior segment of left upper lobe;*

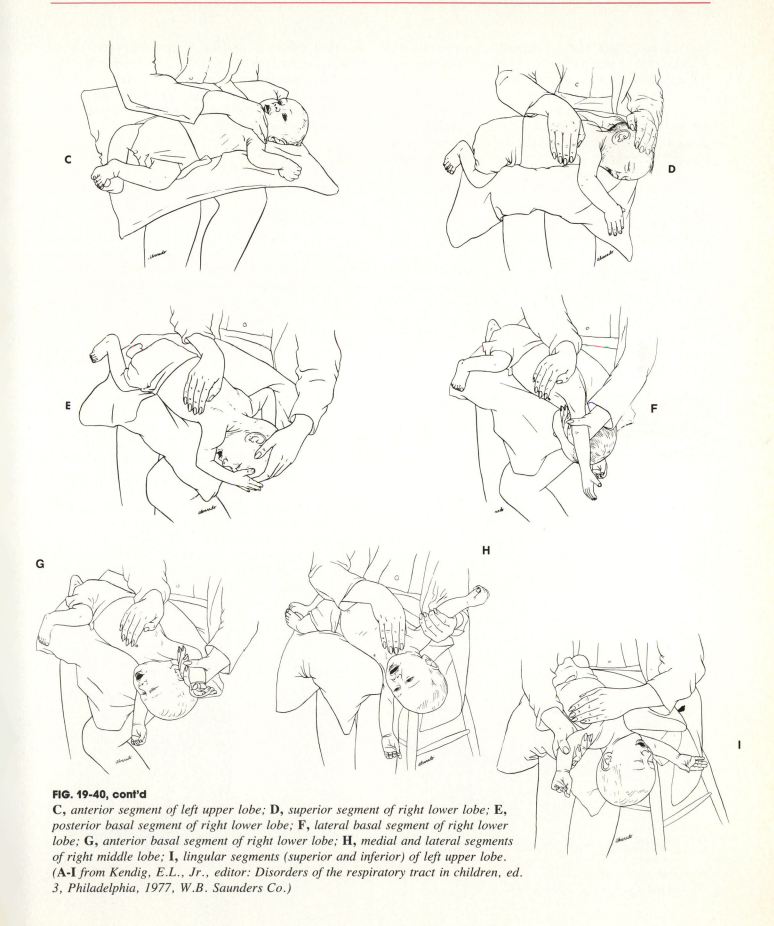

FIG. 19-40, cont'd
C, *anterior segment of left upper lobe;* **D,** *superior segment of right lower lobe;* **E,** *posterior basal segment of right lower lobe;* **F,** *lateral basal segment of right lower lobe;* **G,** *anterior basal segment of right lower lobe;* **H,** *medial and lateral segments of right middle lobe;* **I,** *lingular segments (superior and inferior) of left upper lobe. (A-I from Kendig, E.L., Jr., editor: Disorders of the respiratory tract in children, ed. 3, Philadelphia, 1977, W.B. Saunders Co.)*

required in children whose conditions contraindicate the standard positioning, such as head injuries, some types of surgical incisions or burns, and casts or traction. At home small children can be positioned on a padded ironing board. Children who require postural drainage over a period of months or years may benefit from specially constructed tables padded and adjusted to their individual needs. The position used and the frequency and duration of treatment are individualized.

Since viscid secretions may not drain by gravity alone, various maneuvers, including deep breathing, reinforced cough, "cupping," or "clapping," and vibration, are performed in association with drainage to assist in their removal.

Percussion. Percussion—clapping or cupping—is performed intermittently during postural drainage. The operator's hands are held in the cupped position (Fig. 19-41) and vigorously and repeatedly strike the chest wall under which the specific lung segment to be drained is situated. The simile used to illustrate this concept is that of a freshly opened catsup bottle. Even inverted, the catsup will not flow until it is loosened and ejected by repeated blows to the bottom of the bottle. Performed properly, percussion is painless. The operator's hand should not strike the bare skin. A light cotton undershirt or gown is an appropriate covering to protect the skin from possible irritation. The hand does not slap but conforms to the contour of the chest wall, the entire circumference of the cupped hand touching the chest wall at the same instant. When correctly applied the clapping emits a loud, hollow sound. Care is exerted to clap over the *rib cage only*.

For an infant whose chest is too small for conventional hand percussion, a small face mask is substituted for the operator's hand (see Fig. 7-17).

Vibration. Vibration, a more difficult procedure, is performed only during the exhalation phase of breathing. The child is instructed to take a deep breath and exhale slowly through pursed lips. The operator places one hand on top of the other over the target lung segment and, as the child exhales, transmits a rapid vibratory impulse through the chest wall by a tensing contraction of the forearm flexor and extensor muscles. After full expiration, pressure is released. In infants whose respirations are rapid, the padded handle of an electric toothbrush serves as an excellent mechanical vibrator.

Artificial ventilation

The regulation and maintenance of mechanical ventilators are the responsibility of respiratory therapists. However, nurses should understand the function of the ventilator in use and be able to detect signs of malfunction and deviations from the desired settings. The nurse also promotes the effectiveness of ventilation by suctioning, positioning, and providing support and reassurance to the child receiving mechanical respiration. See p. 198 for assisted and controlled respiration in the neonate.

Artificial airways. An artificial airway is usually used in association with artificial ventilation and in children with upper airway obstruction. Endotracheal intubation can be accomplished by the nasal (nasotracheal), oral (orotracheal), or direct tracheal (tracheostomy) routes. Although it is more difficult to place technically, nasotracheal intubation is preferred to orotracheal intubation because it facilitates oral hygiene and provides more stable fixation, which reduces the complication of tracheal erosion and the danger of accidental extubation. Endotracheal tubes may be cuffed, to provide an airtight seal, or uncuffed. Cuffed tubes are used when high-inflation pressures are needed, they are inflated to the minimum volume, and the pressure cuff must be deflated hourly for 2 to 5 minutes to minimize the possibility of pressure necrosis. However, pressure cuffs are rarely used in children

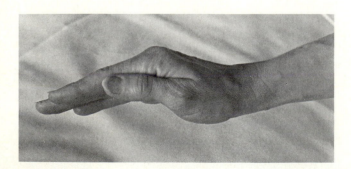

FIG. 19-41
Cupped hand position for percussion.

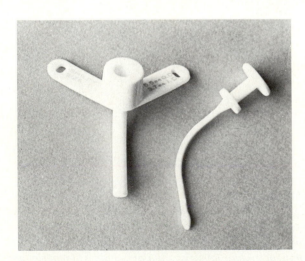

FIG. 19-42
Silastic pediatric tracheostomy tube and obturator.

younger than 10 years of age. Air or gas delivered directly to the trachea must be humidified as in tracheostomy. Although newborn infants have been successfully maintained on nasotracheal tubes for longer periods, in older children who require intubation beyond a week, a tracheostomy is usually performed.

Tracheostomy. Tracheostomy can be a lifesaving procedure. It is an emergency or an elective procedure and may be combined with mechanical ventilation.

Plastic and silastic have largely replaced silver as the preferred material for tracheostomy tubes, especially for pediatric use (Fig. 19-42). These materials can be constructed with a more acute angle and, since they soften at room temperature, are better able to conform to the contours of the airway. The flexibility of the material resists kinking, and the smooth surface reduces crust formation; therefore, most tubes are constructed without an inner cannula. The tube is held in place by appropriate length of sturdy cloth tape around the child's neck. Umbilical cord tape is ideal. A better fit can be achieved if the child's head is flexed, rather than extended, while the tape is fixed. If the cord is too loose the tube may be coughed out. The ties should fit snugly enough that one finger can be inserted with difficulty between the tape and the child's neck (Fig. 19-43). New ties are attached before the old ones are removed to reduce the possibility of the tracheostomy tube becoming dislodged. The obturator is kept in a sterile package taped to the head of the bed.

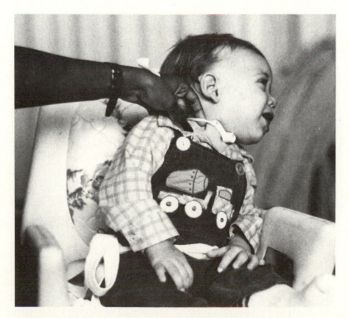

FIG. 19-43
Tracheostomy ties are snug but allow one finger to be inserted.

Since the normal warming, wetting, and filtering functions of the upper airway are inoperative, air entering the tracheostomy opening is humidified by placing the child in a mist tent, by attaching a special tracheostomy mask or "collar" to deliver humidified gas directly to the tracheostomy opening, or by direct attachment to a mechanical ventilator. The humid gas helps to loosen mucus and reduce the chances of crust formation and a mucous plug. Moisture from the humidified gas tends to accumulate on the inner surface of the flexible plastic tubing and must be eliminated periodically to prevent occlusion of the tube and/or accidental aspiration. The tubing is disconnected at the collar or tracheostomy tube and drained into a container. It is not allowed to flow back into the humidifying receptacle.

The airway must remain patent, and it requires frequent suctioning during the first few hours posttracheostomy to remove mucous plugs and excess secretions. A small amount of sterile isotonic saline injected into the tube helps to loosen the secretions and crusts for easier aspiration. The amount of saline used (0.5 to 2 ml) depends on the size of the child. The suction catheter is one with a side hole or Y connector so that the catheter can be introduced without suction and removed while simultaneously applying intermittent suction. This reduces the likelihood of mucosal damage from the catheter. The catheter is inserted gently, never jabbing up and down, and the minimal amount of negative pressure is used. The entire process should take no longer than 15 to 30 seconds. A convenient method used by many nurses to estimate the length of time the tube is occluded is to hold their own breath during the procedure. Hyperventilation of the child with 100% oxygen before and after suctioning may also be performed to prevent hypoxia. Suctioning is carried out at frequent intervals to avoid buildup of crusts and as often as needed for signs of mucus in the airway, such as bubbling, noisy breathing, or coughing. The cough, although noisy, is ineffectual because the glottis, which normally closes and releases suddenly to effect a cough, is bypassed by the tracheostomy. The child is allowed to rest after each aspiration, then the process is repeated until the trachea is clear.

Aseptic technique is essential during care of the tracheostomy. Secondary infection is a major concern, since the air entering the lower airway bypasses the natural defenses of the upper airway. One or two sterile gloves are worn during the aspiration procedure. Many institutions are using the two-glove procedure to protect the nurse from infections, such as herpetic whitlow, a painful infection of the finger from direct contact with herpes simplex virus (Lucey and Baroni, 1984). A new tube and gloves are used each time. Aseptic technique is used to clean and dress the site. Sterile saline solution that is used to moisten and clean the tube is discarded after each use. A duplicate tracheostomy tube and equipment needed for its insertion are kept at the bedside in the event that the tube becomes dislodged and needs to be replaced. If the tube inadvertently becomes dislodged, the attending nurse should maintain the patency of the incision by spreading the edges with a sterile clamp until the tube can be replaced. Children with tracheostomies that must remain in place for months or years require a weekly tube change.

A child with a tracheostomy requires continuous nursing attendance. Vital signs are monitored regularly, and the patency of the tube is maintained. The child is observed closely for any signs of distress or complications. Nursing observation is vital to the child who is unable to verbally signal for help. Signs of impending difficulty include restlessness, dyspnea, pallor or cyanosis, changes in pulse or blood pressure, overt bleeding from the trachea or around the incision site, retractions, and noisy respirations.

Some children may be discharged from the hospital with tracheostomy tubes. Before discharge the parents will need careful instruction and practice in the care and management of the tracheostomy. During hospitalization the parents should be involved in the child's care as soon as possible in anticipation of this eventuality. The more comfortable they are with all the aspects of tracheostomy care, the more confident and less anxious they will be when faced with total care of the child at home. It sometimes requires weeks before they feel comfortable with suctioning, cleaning, and changing the tube. Instructions should be detailed and explicit. To facilitate their adjustment, supplies identical to the ones they are accustomed to should be available to the parents. Parents often become anxious when they encounter even small differences from the familiar. In the event of substitution, they need to be reassured that the unfamiliar equipment is safe to use on their child.

PROCEDURES RELATED TO ALTERNATIVE FEEDING TECHNIQUES

Children who are unable to take nourishment by mouth because of anomalies of the throat or esophagus, impaired swallowing capacity, severe debilitation, respiratory distress, or unconsciousness are frequently fed by way of a tube inserted directly into the stomach (gastrostomy) or by gavage. Premature infants who are either unable to suck or who become exhausted from bottle-feeding are fed by gavage. Children unable to tolerate feedings in the gastrointestinal tract are fed by hyperalimentation.

Gavage feeding

Infants and children can be fed simply and safely by a tube passed into the stomach through either the nares or the mouth. The tube can be left in place or inserted and removed with each feeding. In older children it has usually been found to be less traumatic to tape the tube securely in place between feedings. When this alternative is used, the tube should be removed and replaced with a new tube once every 24 to 72 hours, depending on hospital policy or specific orders. Meticulous handwashing should be practiced during the procedure to prevent bacterial contamination of the feeding, especially during continuous drip feedings.

Preparation. The equipment needed for gavage feeding includes:

A silicone, polyurethrane, rubber, or polyvinyl feeding tube selected according to the size of the child and the viscosity of the solution being fed; for infants a 15-inch French catheter or feeding tube size 5 to 8 is appropriate. In larger children longer catheters with a larger diameter, usually sizes 10 to 14 French, are needed.

A receptacle for the fluid; for small amounts a 10- to 30-ml syringe barrel or Asepto syringe is satisfactory; for larger amounts a 50-ml syringe with a catheter tip is more convenient.

A syringe to aspirate stomach contents and/or to inject air after the tube has been placed

Water to lubricate the tube; sterile water is used for infants

Paper or nonallergenic tape to mark the tube and to attach the tube to the infant's or child's cheek

A stethoscope to determine the correct placement in the stomach

The solution for feeding

Procedure. Infants will be easier to control if they are first wrapped in a mummy restraint (p. 548). Even tiny infants with random movements can grasp and remove the tube. Premature infants do not ordinarily require restraint, but if they do, a small towel folded across the chest and secured beneath the shoulders is usually sufficient. Care must be taken so that breathing is not compromised.

Gavage feeding is usually carried out with the infant or child lying on the back or toward the right side and the head and chest elevated slightly. A folded blanket under the head and shoulders is satisfactory for infants, and a pillow is useful for small children. The head of the bed is raised for larger children. The feeding tube can be passed through either the nose or the mouth. Since young infants are obligatory nose breathers, insertion through the mouth causes less distress to the infant and helps to stimulate sucking. A tube passed through one of the nares in older infants and children seems quite satisfactory once the tube is in place. An indwelling tube is almost always placed through the nose; the tube is alternated between nares with each insertion to minimize irritation, chance of infection, and possible breakdown of mucous membranes from pressure that occurs over a period of time.

The procedure for gavage feeding is carried out as follows:

1. Measure the tube for correct length of insertion and mark the point with a small piece of tape. Correct length can be determined by one of two methods: (a) measuring from the bridge of the nose to the umbilicus or (b) measuring from the tip of the nose to the earlobe (or vice versa) and then to the tip of the xiphoid process (ensiform cartilage) of the sternum (Fig. 19-44). However, the tube may need to be advanced a few centimeters farther for correct placement as verified by aspiration of stomach contents in step 3.

2. Insert the tube, which has been lubricated with sterile water or water-soluble lubricant, through either the mouth or one of the nares to the predetermined mark. Since the esophagus is situated behind the trachea, the tube is more easily inserted when the child's head is hyperflexed. This reduces the chance of the tube entering the trachea. When using the nose, the tube is slipped along the base of the nose and directed straight back toward the occiput; when entering through the mouth the tube is directed toward the back of the throat (Fig. 19-45, A). The tube is passed quickly and, if the child is able to swallow, synchronized with swallowing.

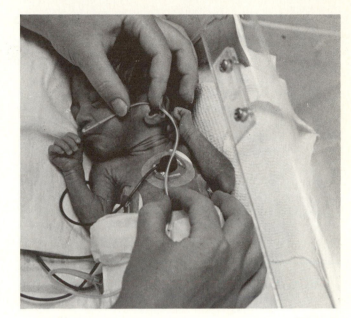

FIG. 19-44
Measuring tube for gavage feeding. From tip of nose to earlobe and to tip of sternum.

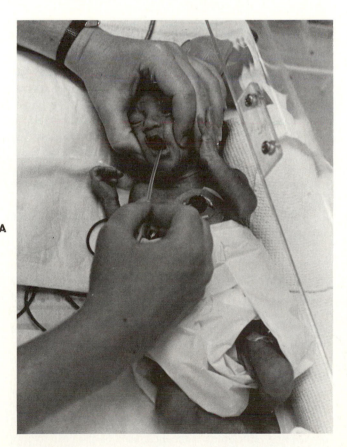

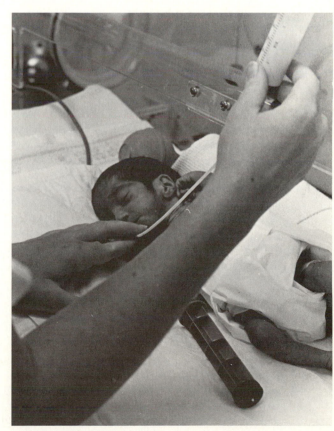

FIG. 19-45
Gavage feeding. **A,** *Insertion of tube.* **B,** *Formula flowing into tube by gravity.*

3. Check the position of the tube by using one or both of the following:
   a. The syringe is attached to the feeding tube and gentle negative pressure is applied. Aspiration of stomach contents indicates proper placement. The amount and character of any fluid aspirated is noted and returned to the stomach. Absence of fluid is not necessarily evidence of improper placement. The stomach may be empty or the tube may not be in contact with stomach contents.
   b. With the syringe, inject a small amount of air into the tube while simultaneously listening with a stethoscope over the stomach area. Sounds of gurgling or growling will be heard if the tube is properly situated in the stomach. The air is then withdrawn. The amount of air injected is determined by the size of the child: 0.5 to 1 ml in premature or very small infants to 5 ml in larger children. This method is not recommended with small-bore tubes because they may inadvertently be passed into a bronchus during insertion.
4. Stabilize the tube by holding or taping it in place to maintain correct placement. When taped, the tube is secured to the cheek, not to the forehead because of possible damage to the nostril.
5. Feed the formula, which has been warmed to room temperature. Formula is poured into the barrel of the syringe attached to the feeding tube (Fig. 19-45, *B*). To start the flow a gentle push with the plunger may be required, but the plunger should then be removed and the fluid allowed to flow into the stomach by gravity. The rate of flow should not exceed 5 ml every 5 to 10 minutes in premature and very small infants and 10 ml/minute in older infants and children to prevent nausea and regurgitation. The rate is determined by the diameter of the tubing and the height of the reservoir containing the feeding and is regulated by adjusting the height of the syringe. A usual feeding requires 15 to 30 minutes to complete.
6. Flush the tube with sterile water (1 or 2 ml for small tubes to 5 ml or more for large ones) to clear it of formula. Indwelling catheters are capped or clamped to prevent loss of feeding and entry of air into stomach.
7. If the tube is to be remove first pinch it firmly to prevent escape of fluid as the tube is withdrawn. Withdraw the tube quickly.
8. Position the child on the right side or abdomen for at least 1 hour in the same manner as following any infant feeding to minimize the possibility of regurgitation and aspiration. If the child's condition permits, he can be bubbled after the feeding.
9. Record the feeding, including the type and amount of residual, the type and amount of formula, and the manner in which it was tolerated. For most infant feedings any amount of residual fluid aspirated from the stomach is refed and the amount subtracted from the prescribed amount of feeding. For example, if the infant is to receive 30 ml and 3 ml is aspirated from the stomach

before the feeding, the 3 ml of aspirated stomach contents is refed plus 27 ml of feeding.
10. Provide emotional care. Give the infant a pacifier during feeding time and hold or cuddle if his condition permits. If the child is bedfast, spend time talking or reading with him during feeding. Encourage parents to participate in the care.

Gastrostomy feeding

Feeding via gastrostomy tube is a variation of tube feeding that is often used for children in whom passage of a tube through the mouth, pharynx, esophagus, and cardiac sphincter of the stomach is contraindicated or impossible or to avoid the constant irritation of a nasogastric tube in children who require tube feeding over an extended period. Placement of a gastrostomy tube is an operative procedure usually performed under general anesthesia. The tube is inserted through the abdominal wall into the stomach about midway along the greater curvature and secured by a purse-string suture. The stomach is anchored to the peritoneum at the operative site. The tube used can be a Foley, wing-tip, or mushroom catheter. Immediately after surgery the catheter is left open and attached to gravity drainage for 24 hours or more. Postoperative care of the wound site is directed toward prevention of infection and irritation. The area is cleansed and covered with a sterile dressing daily or as often as needed to keep the area dry. After healing takes place meticulous care is needed to keep the area surrounding the tube clean and dry to prevent excoriation and infection. Daily applications of antiobiotic ointment or other preparations may be prescribed to aid in healing and prevention of irritation. Care is exercised to prevent excessive pull on the catheter that might cause widening of the opening and subsequent leakage of highly irritating gastric juices. Sliding the tube through a sterile disposable nipple whose tip is cut off and whose base is then taped to the abdomen keeps the tube from rotating and causing erosion and enlargement of the skin opening.

Positioning and feeding of water, formula, or pureed foods are carried out in the same manner and rate as gavage feeding. However, residual may not be aspirated and is measured as the amount of feeding left in the tube and syringe. After feedings the infant or child is positioned on the right side or in Fowler's position, and the tube may be left open and suspended or clamped between feedings, depending on the child's condition (Fig. 19-46). A clamped tube allows more mobility, but is only appropriate if the child can tolerate intermittent feedings without vomiting or prolonged backup of feeding into the tube. Sometimes a Y tube is used to allow for simultaneous decompression during feeding. If a Foley catheter is used as the gastrostomy tube, very slight tension is applied to ascertain that the balloon is at the gastrostomy opening. The tube is then

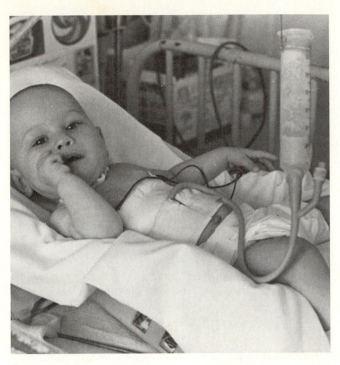

FIG. 19-46
Gastrostomy feeding. Syringe barrel suspended to allow thick formula to enter stomach by gravity.

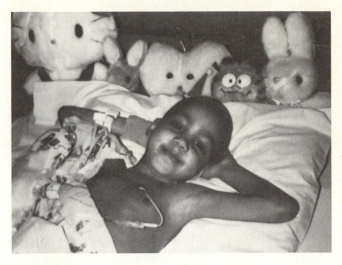

FIG. 19-47
Child with a Broviac catheter (dressing removed) for hyperalimentation.

securely taped into place to prevent the possibility that the balloon might move toward the pyloric sphincter and occlude the stomach outlet. As a precaution the length of the tube should be measured postoperatively and then remeasured each shift to be sure it has not slipped. When the gastrostomy is no longer needed, the skin opening ordinarily closes spontaneously by contracture after removal.

Intravenous hyperalimentation

A significant advance in nutritional therapy is total parenteral nutrition (TPN), also known as intravenous alimentation, which provides for the total nutritional needs of infants or children whose lives are threatened because feeding by way of the gastrointestinal tract is impossible, inadequate, or hazardous.

Hyperalimentation therapy involves intravenous infusion of highly concentrated solutions of protein, glucose, and other nutrients. The hyperalimentation solution is infused through conventional tubing with a millipore filter attached to remove particulate matter or microorganisms that may have contaminated the solution. The highly concentrated solutions require infusion into a vessel with sufficient volume and turbulence to allow for rapid dilution. The wide-diameter vessels selected are the superior vena cava and innominate or intrathoracic subclavian veins approached by way of the external or internal jugular veins.

For long-term alimentation a Broviac silastic catheter (similar to Hickman catheter in adults) may be inserted by tunneling it under the subcutaneous tissue from the chest or abdominal wall to a centrally located superficial vein into the superior or inferior vena cava (Fig. 19-47). The distal end of the Broviac catheter has a luer-lock connector to enable snug insertion of intravenous tubing and to allow secure screw capping of the catheter when not in use. Its superiority over regular catheters facilitates home hyperalimentation.

The highly irritating nature of concentrated glucose precludes the use of the small peripheral veins in most instances. However, amino acid-glucose solutions and fat emulsions (lipids) can be infused into peripheral veins and are sometimes used in patients who are able to tolerate the fluid load. Since emulsified fat cannot be mixed with the glucose solutions and must bypass the millipore filter, it requires administration through a separate bottle and tubing that enters the circuit near the venous entry site through a Y-type of injection adaptor. Special administration sets are available for the simultaneous infusion of these products.

Nursing responsibilities. The major nursing responsibilities are the same as for any intravenous therapy: control of sepsis, monitoring of infusion rate, and continuous observations.

The total parenteral nutrition solution must be prepared under rigid aseptic conditions best accomplished in the pharmacy under a laminar air flow hood by specially trained technicians. The solution and tubing are changed and the infusion site redressed by the specially trained intravenous team, using meticulous aseptic precautions. In some institutions this may be a nursing responsibility. If so, the procedure is carried out according to hospital protocol.

The infusion is maintained at a slow uniform rate to ensure the proper use of glucose and amino acids, usually by means of a constant infusion pump. This requires accurate calculation of the rate required to deliver a measured amount in a given length of time. Since alterations in flow rate are relatively common, the drip should be checked frequently to ensure an even, continuous infusion. If for some reason the infusion rate slows, the rate should not be increased to compensate for the uninfused amount.

General assessments such as vital signs, intake and output measurements, and checking results of laboratory tests facilitate early detection of infection or fluid and electrolyte imbalance. Additional amounts of potassium and sodium chloride are often required in hyperalimentation; therefore, observation for signs of potassium or sodium deficit or excess is part of nursing care. This is rarely a problem except in children with reduced renal function or metabolic defects. Hyperglycemia may occur during the first day or two, as the child adapts to the high-glucose load of the hyperalimentation solution. The addition of insulin may be required to assist the body's adjustment to the hyperglycemia. Nursing responsibilities include blood glucose testing to monitor the effectiveness of the insulin therapy. To prevent hypoglycemia at the time the hyperalimentation is disconnected, the rate of the infusion and the amount of insulin are decreased gradually.

Home hyperalimentation. Some children require total parenteral nutrition over an extended period, often weeks or months. Home total parenteral nutrition (HTPN) may be selected for children as an alternative to long-term hospitalization. Before a home care program can be implemented, a thorough assessment is made of the family and the home situation. Then the parent (or parents) and/or child are tutored by a specially trained nurse as they learn to carry out the procedure under his or her supervision. The family eventually assumes full responsibility for the child's total care, with help readily available if needed.

The emotional and economic benefits of this approach are readily apparent. The familiar environment and the atmosphere of normality are enormously therapeutic and the stress of separation is avoided. With support from health professionals, a home care program can be the ideal alternative to hospitalization for a capable, motivated family of a child who requires total parenteral nutrition.

PROCEDURES RELATED TO ELIMINATION

Children seldom have problems with elimination, but in cases of severe constipation or when an empty rectum is needed before surgery or diagnostic procedures, an enema may be administered to stimulate rectal emptying. A number of conditions in the newborn and childhood period also require formation of an ostomy for purposes of elimination.

Enema

The procedure for giving an enema to an infant or child does not differ essentially from that for an adult. A French catheter size 10 to 12 is inserted approximately 2 to 4 inches into the ampulla of the rectum. An isotonic solution is used in children; if prepared saline is not available, it can be made from 1 tsp table salt in 500 ml (1 pint) of tap water. Plain water is rarely used in children because, being hypotonic, it can cause rapid fluid shift and fluid overload. The Fleet enema is not advised for children because of the harsh action of its ingredients (sodium biphosphate and sodium phosphate).

The amount of solution to be administered varies with the size of the child. Suggested amounts are:

Age	Amount (ml)
Infant	150-250
Small child	250-350
Large child	300-500
Adolescent	500-750

Infants and small children are unable to retain the solution after it is administered; therefore the buttocks must be held together for a short time if fluid is to be retained. The enema is administered and expelled while the child is lying with the buttocks over the bedpan and his head and back supported with pillows. Older children are ordinarily able to hold the solution if they understand what to do and if they are not expected to hold it for too long a period. It is well to have the bedpan handy or, for the ambulatory child, to make certain that the bathroom is clear and available before beginning the procedure. An enema is an intrusive procedure and thus threatening to the preschool child; therefore, a careful explanation is especially important to ease possible distress.

Ostomies

Children may require stomas for various health problems. The most frequent causes are necrotizing enterocolitis and imperforate anus in the infant and, less often, Hirschsprung's disease. In the older child the most frequent causes are inflammatory bowel disease, congenital defects (such as Hirschsprung's disease and familial colon polyps), and ureterostomies for distal ureter or bladder defects.

Care and management of ostomies in the older child differ little from the care of ostomies in the adult patient. The major emphasis in pediatric care is the preparation of the child for the procedure and teaching care of the ostomy to the child and his family. The basic principles of prepa-

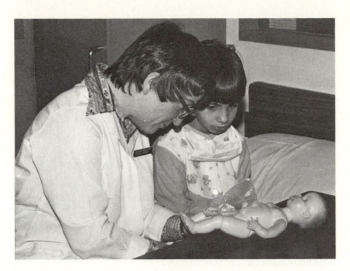

FIG. 19-48
Preparing the child for colostomy. Note the use of a urine-collecting bag as part of colostomy equipment.

ration are the same as for any procedure (p. 533). Simple, straightforward language is most effective together with the use of illustrations and a replica model; for example, drawing a picture of a child with a stoma on the abdomen and explaining it as "another opening where bowel movements (or any other term the child uses) will come out." At another time the nurse can draw a bag over the opening to demonstrate how the contents are collected. Using a doll to demonstrate the process is an excellent teaching strategy (Fig. 19-48) and special books are available.*

Because the stoma is edematous after surgery, an appliance is usually not fitted for several days. Once an appliance is in place, drainage is directly measured from the collecting bag. In order to accurately measure colostomy drainage before a collecting appliance is applied, the nurse weighs the dry dressing and reweighs it when wet. The difference in weight is calculated as fluid because 1 g equals 1 ml. If formed stool is passed, it is not weighed and calculated as part of fluid loss.

Ostomies performed on infants create special problems. The fragile nature of the skin increases the risk of breakdown, and the small surface area of the abdomen is ill-suited to the standard appliances. Regardless of the type of stoma (ileostomy or colostomy), initially most infants are left with merely a gauze dressing over the stoma and secured to the opening by Kerlix or similar expansible wrap. The dressing may or may not be saturated with petroleum jelly or other protective material. The skin is cleansed well after each bowel movement, and a nonpo-

Chris has an ostomy available from United Ostomy Association, Inc., 2001 W. Beverly Boulevard, Los Angeles, CA 90057.

rous substance, such as zinc oxide ointment, aluminum paste, or karaya products, is applied.

A variety of inexpensive techniques have been devised to absorb drainage around the stoma. Squares of tissue paper, facial tissue, or gauze with openings cut to fit the stoma are gently pressed against the layer of protective substance on the area around the stoma. They can be kept in place with a diaper or Montgomery straps and are replaced after each bowel movement. As a rule, if a sigmoid colostomy is to be performed on an infant, a colostomy appliance is usually not used because the stools are formed and less likely to irritate the skin. Usually only diapers and a nonporous ointment such as zinc oxide around the stoma are used.

When the stoma is healed and the infant has grown to a size that permits their use, appropriate infant-sized stoma bags are introduced. Until then, sometimes the small urine collection bags prove to be sufficient, although they require frequent changes. When either stoma bags or urine collection bags are used, the skin is prepared with tincture of benzoin and karaya powder, paste, or gum to prevent breakdown and to facilitate adherence.

To prepare for the child's discharge, the parents are involved in his care as early as possible during hospitalization. They are carefully instructed in the application of the device, care of the skin, and instructions regarding appropriate action in case skin problems develop. Early evidence of breakdown should be brought to the attention of the physician, the nurse, or the stoma specialist.

In teaching parents, it is best not to assume that they understand a verbal explanation of a colostomy. Using simple language and demonstrations with frequent repetition is the best approach. Drawing a picture or using the doll is excellent for parents as well as children. They need to know why the procedure is performed, what they can expect, and that they will not be expected to care for the stoma until they are prepared to do so.

PROCEDURES RELATED TO SURGERY

Some of the most traumatic procedures for children involve surgery. Both the psychologic and physical aspects of care are significant in the child's adjustment and recovery. Although procedures related to surgery differ according to the type of surgery, the following is an overview of general nursing interventions.

Psychologic preparation

In general, psychologic preparation is similar to that discussed earlier in the chapter for any procedure. However, there are some important differences. Even though children are asleep for the actual surgical intervention, they

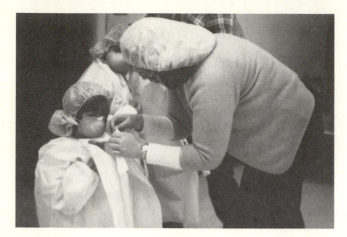

FIG. 19-49

"Dressing up" for surgery and touring an operating room can help alleviate children's fear of the unknown.

are subjected to numerous preoperative and postoperative procedures, which require a series of preparatory sessions to prevent overstressing the child with too much information. Five events before and after surgery have been identified as being significant in terms of causing stress and needing psychologic preparation: (1) admission, (2) the blood test, (3) preoperative medication, (4) transport to the operating room, and (5) return from the recovery room.

In addition, more than one nurse is often responsible for different aspects of care. Although the same supportive nurse should remain with the child through as many of the procedures as possible, this is not always possible, especially when children return to special care units postoperatively. However, joint planning of care between the various nursing staffs, such as in pediatrics and the recovery room, can overcome some of the disadvantages of unfamiliar nurses caring for the child. Many hospitals have surgical tours for children and parents to familiarize them with the strange environment and to introduce them to other individuals who will be involved in their care (Fig. 19-49).

Special fears are often associated with surgery that are not present with other procedures. One special fear is of anesthesia. Children under 5 years of age primarily worry about what will happen when they wake up, such as where they will be and who will be with them. Showing youngsters the recovery room whenever possible, telling them where their parents will visit them after surgery, and encouraging the parents to be with the children as soon as possible after surgery decreases these fears. School-age children fear the anesthesia itself. Seeing the mask and learning how the "gas" or "medicine" works helps minimize their concerns. Children about age 9 years and older fear the anesthesia, the operation itself, and possible death. They may ask, "Will I wake up?" or "What happens if I

don't wake up?" Adolescents share these concerns with a special anxiety for change in body image. They fear the loss of control while under anesthesia, both in terms of their behavior and for their body integrity. Reassuring them that only what is supposed to be done will be performed is essential.

Because anesthesia is a type of sleep, children often supply their own definitions to this concept. Children worry about whether they will awaken during the procedure and how the doctor knows when to awaken them. Stressing that anesthesia is a "special sleep," caused by the mask, gas, and so on, that is controlled by a special person, called the anesthesiologist, is important in minimizing children's fear-provoking fantasies.

Because children are often restless when coming out of anesthesia, it is best to have the parents with them or, if this is not possible, to have a favorite possession or person, such as the primary nurse, greet them on gaining consciousness. This helps decrease the disorienting effect of anesthesia.

Physical preparation

Besides psychologic preparation, children usually require various types of physical preparation for surgery (see summary that follows). Although these preparations are routine, nurses should keep in mind that they can be anxiety provoking for children and parents. For example, seeing their infant's scalp shaved for a craniotomy can intensify parents' fears of the actual surgical procedure. For preschoolers, having to wear a loose-fitting hospital gown without the security of underpants or pajama bottoms can be traumatic. Explaining the reason for each preoperative procedure and altering it whenever possible to meet the needs of various children and parents combines physical care with effective psychologic support.

Postsurgical care

After surgical procedures, various physical interventions and observations are required to prevent or minimize possible untoward effects (see summary that follows). Although most of these interventions are prescribed by physicians, it is the nurse's responsibility to exercise judgment in their implementation. For example, vital signs are taken as frequently as necessary until they are stable. Simply recording temperature, pulse, respiration, and blood pressure without comparing the present readings to previous ones is a useless technical function. Each value is evaluated in terms of side effects from anesthesia and signs of impending shock. Pain is assessed and the child given analgesics as needed to provide comfort and facilitate his cooperation in postoperative procedures, such as ambulating, coughing, and deep breathing.

SUMMARY OF NURSING CARE DURING PREOPERATIVE AND POSTOPERATIVE CARE OF THE CHILD

GOALS	RESPONSIBILITIES
Preoperative	
Assure legal authorization	Check chart for signed consent form
	Obtain informed consent
	Contact the physician to determine if the parents have been informed of procedure (informed consent is the physician's responsibility)
	Obtain and/or witness signature
Provide information needed	Make certain the following procedures have been performed and evidence is in the chart: urinalysis; blood work such as blood count, bleeding and clotting times, and type and cross-match, if ordered; radiographs; electrocardiograph; note by anesthesiologist
Prevent complications	Be certain any allergies are clearly indicated on chart
	Check laboratory values for any sign of systemic abnormality
	Infection (increased white blood cells)
	Anemia (decreased hemoglobin and/or hematocrit)
	Bleeding tendencies (reduced platelets or prolonged bleeding or clotting time)
	Maintain the child NPO (nothing by mouth) usually 12 hours before surgery (prevents aspiration from vomiting during anesthesia [gag reflex is depressed]; last feeding indicated by physician)
	Hydrate the child well before NPO begins
	If oral medication is ordinarily given, consult with the physician for appropriate change in schedule or route of administration
	Take and record vital signs
	Report any deviations from admission readings, especially elevated temperature, which may indicate infection
	Have the child void before preoperative medication is administered
	If unable to void, record time of last voiding
Attend to hygienic preparation	Bathe the child
	Cleanse the site according to prescribed method, if ordered
	Special cleansing and shave may not be done in children, but operative area should be cleansed during regular bath
	Attire the child appropriately
	Special operating room gown may be needed
	Privacy may be a concern; if possible, allow the child to wear underwear or pajama bottoms
	Mark personal articles of clothing with name
	Remove any makeup and/or nail polish (to observe for cyanosis)
	Remove jewelery and/or prosthetic devices (such as mouth retainers)
	Check for loose teeth
	Inform anesthesiologist if detected
Achieve optimum relaxation and sedation before the child arrives in operating room	Administer preoperative sedation 20 minutes before surgery, as ordered
	Place the child in quiet room with minimal distraction
	Encourage the parents to stay with the child as long as permitted
Increase the child's sense of security	Encourage the parents to accompany the child as far as possible
	Explain where the parents will be while the child is in operating room
	Explain nature and function of recovery room
	Allow for significant objects to accompany the child if possible, such as a favorite toy
	Some cultures wear objects for religious or other reasons; to respect these traditions, fasten objects securely to gown or body part
	Orient the child to strange surroundings and decrease anxiety

Continued.

SUMMARY OF NURSING CARE DURING PREOPERATIVE AND POSTOPERATIVE CARE OF THE CHILD—cont'd

GOALS	RESPONSIBILITIES
Ensure safety	Ascertain that identification band is securely fastened Check identification band with surgical personnel Fasten side rails of bed or crib Use restraints during transport by use of stretcher (or other conveyance) Do not leave the child unattended Explain what is happening, unless the child is asleep
Postoperative Assess physiologic status	Monitor vital signs as ordered; for example, every 15 minutes for 1 hour, every 30 minutes for 1 hour, then every hour until stable Record more frequently if any value fluctuates; blood pressure cuff kept in place, deflated in order to lessen the amount of disturbance to the child Evaluate vital signs for signs of shock: increased weak, thready pulse; increased weak, shallow respirations; decreased temperature; decreased blood pressure; cool, clammy, pale skin Evaluate the effects of postanesthesia: hyperthermia, decreased blood pressure, respiratory depression Report any deviations from normal

Assess operative site	Check dressing if present
	    Note presence of dark or fresh blood noted immediately after surgery; circle area with pen to assess any further drainage
	    Observe areas below surgical site for blood that may have drained toward bed
	    Reinforce, but do not remove, loose dressing
	Assess for bleeding and other symptoms in areas not covered with a dressing, such as throat following tonsillectomy, external auditory meatus after ear procedures
	Notify the physician of any irregularities

Prevent complications	Encourage the child to turn, cough, and deep breathe Splint the operative site with hand or pillow if possible before coughing Dangle and ambulate as soon as feasible according to the physician's orders

Provide for hydration	Monitor intravenous infusion at prescribed rate
	    Attach pediatric intravenous apparatus if not done in operating room
	Maintain the child NPO until fully awake
	    Start with small sips of water and advance as tolerated
	    Avoid brown- or red-colored fluids (to distinguish old and fresh blood from oral fluids) in oral or abdominal surgery
	    For gastrointestinal procedures listen for bowel sounds before and after beginning fluids

Provide for nutrition	Monitor bowel sounds in abdominal surgery Feed diet as ordered Advance as appropriate

Assess elimination	Encourage the child to void when awake
	    Offer bedpan
	    Boys may be allowed to stand at bedside
	Notify physician if unable to void

Relieve discomfort	Position for comfort (see "Pain assessment," p. 512) Administer pain medication as prescribed Administer medication for nausea as ordered

During the recovery period some time should be spent with the child to assess his perception of surgery. Play, drawing, and story telling are excellent methods of discovering the child's thoughts. With such information the nurse can support or correct his perceptions and assist the child in achieving mastery for having endured a stressful procedure.

REFERENCES

American Academy of Pediatrics, Committee on Infectious Diseases: Aspirin and Reye syndrome, Pediatrics **69**:810, 1982.

Leikin, S.L.: Minors' assent or dissent to medical treatment, J. Pediatr. **102**(2):169-176, 1983.

Lucey, J., and Baroni, M.: Herpetic whitlow, Am. J. Nurs. **84**(1):60-61, 1984.

BIBLIOGRAPHY
Consent

Dunn, L.J.: Legal aspects of communication with and about the pediatric patient, Issues Compr. Pediatr. Nurs. **4**:13-18, 1980.

Elsea, S.J., and Miya, P.A.: Refusal of blood—an ethical issue, Am. J. Maternal Child Nurs. **6**(6):379-387, 1981.

Gargaro, W.J.: Informed consent. Part I. A good thing for patients: a better thing for doctors and nurses, Cancer Nurs. **1**(1):81-82, 1978.

Gargaro, W.J.: Informed consent. Part II. How much to tell the patient, Cancer Nurs. **1**(2):167-168, 1978.

Gargaro, W.J.: Informed consent. Part III. The nurse's right to inform, Cancer Nurs. **1**(3):249-250, 1978.

Preparing for hospital procedures and surgery/use of play

Beckemeyer, P., and Bahr, J.E.: Helping toddlers and preschoolers cope while suturing their minor lacerations, Am. J. Maternal Child Nurs. **5**(5):326-330, 1980.

Crawford, C., Finke, L., and Henning, M.A.: Nursing management of the postoperative pediatric patient, Issues Compr. Pediatr. Nurs. **6**:157-165, 1983.

Droske, S.C., and Francis, S.A.: Pediatric diagnostic procedures: with guidelines for preparing children for clinical tests, New York, 1981, John Wiley & Sons, Inc.

Hansen, B.D., and Evans, M.L.: Preparing a child for procedures, Am. J. Maternal Child Nurs. **6**(6):392-397, 1981.

Johnson, J.E., Kerchhoff, K.T., and Endress, M.P.: Easing children's fright during health care procedures, Am. J. Maternal Child Nurs. **1**(4):206-210, 1976.

Knudsen, K.: Play therapy: preparing the young child for surgery, Nurs. Clin. North Am. **10**:679-686, 1975.

Luciano, K., and Shumsky, C.J.: Pediatric procedures, Nursing 75 **5**(1):49-52, 1975.

Norberta, Sr. M.: Caring for children with the help of puppets, Am. J. Maternal Child Nurs. **1**(1):22-25, 1976.

Petrillo, M., and Sanger, S.: Emotional care of hospitalized children, ed. 2, Philadelphia, 1980, J.B. Lippincott Co.

Ritchie, J.A.: Preparation of toddlers and preschool children for hospital procedures, Can. Nurse **75**(11):30-32, 1979.

Robinson, S.J.: A nurse's role in preparing children for surgery, AORN J. **30**(4):619-621, 1979.

Savedra, M.: Parental responses to a painful procedure performed on their child. In Azarnoff, P., and Hardgrove, C., editors: The family in child health care, New York, 1981, John Wiley & Sons, Inc.

Safety/collection of specimens

Mason, G.: Bottle type restraints, Am. J. Nurs. **76**:1258, 1976.

Misik, I.: About using restraints—with restraint, Nursing 81 **11**(8):50-55, 1981.

Strohbach, M.E., and Kratina, S.H.: Diaper versus bag specimens: a comparison of urine specific gravity values, Am. J. Maternal Child Nurs. **7**:198-201, 1982.

General care and hygiene

Bishop, B.: How to cool a feverish child, Pediatr. Nurs. **4**(1):19-20, 1978.

Brown, B., and Younger, J.: Facts about fever, Children's Nurse **2**(3):1-3, 1984.

Dininny, J.B.: Food rummy, the game of nutrition, Am. J. Maternal Child Nurs. **2**(2):90-91, 1977.

Farrell, E., Sr., and McKiernan, B.: A positive approach to nutrition for hospitalized children, Am. J. Maternal Child Nurs. **2**(2):113-117, 1977.

Grier, M.E.: Hair care for the black patient, Am. J. Nurs. **76**:1781, 1976.

Mandelbaum, J.: The food square: helping people of different cultures understand balanced diets, Pediatr. Nurs. **9**(1):20-21, 1983.

Reynolds, J.: How to take a temperature, Pediatr. Nurs. **4**(6):67-68, 1978.

Snell, B., and McClellan, C.: Whetting hospitalized preschooler's appetites, Am. J. Nurs. **76**:413-415, 1976.

Administration of medications

Brandt, P.A., and others: IM injections in children, Am. J. Nurs. **72**:1402-1406, 1972.

Eland, J.M.: Minimizing pain associated with prekindergarten intramuscular injections, Issues Compr. Pediatr. Nurs. **5**:361-372, 1981.

Evans, M.L., and Hansen, B.D.: Administering injections to different-aged children, Am. J. Maternal Child Nurs. **6**(3):194-199, 1981.

Hanson, R.L.: Heparin-lock or keep-open I.V.? Am. J. Nurs. **76**:1102-1103, 1976.

Hays, D.: Do it yourself the Z-track way, Am. J. Nurs. **74**(6):1070-1071, 1974.

Jerrett, M.D.: Taking the ouch out of injections, Can. Nurse. **79**(1):24-27, 1983.

Lang, S., Zawacki, A., and Johnson, J.: Reducing discomfort from IM injections, Am. J. Nurs. **76**(5):800-801, 1976.

Lenz, C.L.: Make your needle selection right to the point, Nursing 83 **13**(2):50-51, 1983.

McConnell, E.A.: The subtle art of really good injections, RN **45**(2):24-34, 1982

Mitchell, J.F., and Liadis, M.: Oral solid dosage forms that should not be crushed prior to administration, Hosp. Pharm. **17**:148-156, 1982.

Ormond, E.A.R., and Caulfield, C.: A practical guide to giving oral medications to young children, Am. J. Maternal Child Nurs. **1**:320-325, 1976.

Perez, S.: Reducing injection pain, Am. J. Nurs. **84**(5):645, 1984.

Rettig, F.M., and Southby, J.R.: Using different body positions to reduce discomfort from dorsogluteal injection, Nurs. Res. **31**(4):219-221, 1982.

Rimar, J.M.: Guidelines for the intravenous administration of medications used in pediatrics, Am. J. Maternal Child Nurs. **7**(3):184-197, 1982.

Sbravati, E.C., and Fischer, R.G.: What medication do parents need to get up and give their child at night? Pediatr. Nurs. **8**(2):126, 1982

Weeks, H.F.: Administering medication to children, Am. J. Maternal Child Nurs. **5**(1):63, 1980.

Wertsching, J.H.: Reconstituting parenteral antibiotics for children, Am. J. Maternal Child Nurs. **7**(2):128-133, 1982.

Wong, D.L.: Significance of dead space in syringes, Am. J. Nurs. **82** (8):1237, 1982.

Procedures related to maintaining fluid balance (IV therapy)

Gruber, D.: Helping the child accept I.V. therapy, Am. J. I.V. Ther. **4**:50-55, 1977.

Guhlow, L., and Kolb, J.: Pediatric I.V.s, RN **42**:40-51, 1979.

Huey, F.L.: Using the machines: setting up and troubleshooting, Am. J. Nurs. **83**(7):1026-1028, 1983.

Huey, F.L.: What's on the market? a nurse's guide, Am. J. Nurs. **83**(6):902-909, 1983.

McGrath, B.J.: Fluids, electrolytes, and replacement therapy in pediatric nursing, Am. J. Maternal Child Nurs. **5**:58-62, 1980.

Piercy, S.: Children on long-term I.V. therapy, Nursing 81 **11**(9):66-69, 1981.

Programmed instruction: Fundamentals of I.V. maintenance, Am. J. Nurs. **79**:1274-1287, 1979.

Steel, J.: Too fast or too slow: the erratic IV, Am. J. Nurs. **83**(6):898-910, 1983.

Wittig, P., and Semmler-Bertanzi, D.J.: Pumps and controllers—an assessment guide, Am. J. Nurs. **83**(7):1022-1025, 1983.

Procedures related to respiratory function

Aradine, C.E.: Home care for young children with long-term tracheostomies, Am. J. Maternal Child Nurs. **5**:121-125, 1980.

Bishop, B.: How to make a home croup tent, Pediatr. Nurs. **4**(2):37-38, 1978.

Fuchs, P.L.: Understanding continuous mechanical ventilation, Nursing 79 **9**(12):26-33, 1979.

Glassanos, M.R.: Infants who are oxygen dependent—sending them home, Am. J. Maternal Child Nurs. **5**:42-45, 1980.

Kaler, J., and Kaler, H.: Michael has a tracheostomy, Am. J. Nurs. **74**:852-855, 1974.

Kennedy, A.H., Johnson, W.G., and Sturdevant, E.W.: An educational program for families of children with tracheostomies, Am. J. Maternal Child Nurs. **7**(1):42-49, 1982.

McFadden, R.: Decreasing respiratory compromise during infant suctioning, Am. J. Nurs. **81**:2158-2161, 1981.

Nielson, L.: Potential problems of mechanical ventilation, Am. J. Nurs. **80**:2206-2213, 1980.

Nielson, L.: Pulmonary oxygen toxicity and other hazards of oxygen therapy, Am. J. Nurs. **80**:2213-2215, 1980.

Nielson, L.: Ventilators and how they work, Am. J. Nurs. **80**:2201-2205, 1980.

Nielson, L.: Weaning patients from mechanical ventilation, Am. J. Nurs. **80**:2214-2217, 1980.

O'Donnell, B.: How to change tracheostomy ties—easily and safely, Nursing 78 **8**(3):66-69, 1978.

Sandham, G., and Reid, B.: Some Q's and A's about suctioning, Nursing 77 **7**(10):60-65, 1977.

Schraeder, B.D.: A creative approach to caring for the ventilator-dependent child, Am. J. Maternal Child Nurs. **4**:165-170, 1979.

Smith, A.E.: Endotracheal suctioning ''are we harming our patients?'' Crit. Care Update **10**:29-31, 1983.

Waterson, M.L.: Teaching your patients postural drainage, Nursing 78 **8**(3):51-53, 1978.

Procedures related to alternative feeding techniques/elimination

Bayer, L.M., Scholl, D.E., and Ford, E.G.: Tube feeding at home, Am. J. Nurs. **83**(9):1321-1325, 1983.

Bishop, W.S., and Head, J.J.: Care of the infant with a stoma, Am. J. Maternal Child Nurs. **1:**315-319, 1976.

Bjeletich, J., and Hickman, R.O.: The Hickman indwelling catheter, Am. J. Nurs. **80**(1):62-65, 1980.

Broadwell, D.C., and Jackson, B.S., editors: Principles of ostomy care, St. Louis, 1982, The C. V. Mosby Co.

Colley, R., and Wilson, J.: Meeting patients' nutritional needs with hyperalimentation: providing hyperalimentation for infants and children, Nursing 79 **9**(7):50-53, 1979.

Konstantinides, N.N., and Shronts, E.: Tube feeding: managing the basics, Am. J. Nurs. **83**(9):1312-1320, 1983.

Parfitt, D.M., and Thompson, V.D.: Pediatric home hyperalimentation: educating the family, Am. J. Maternal Child Nurs. **5:**196-195, 1980.

Perry, S., Johnson, S., and Trump, D.: Gastrostomy and the neonate, Am. J. Nurs. **83**(7):1030-1033, 1983.

Wink, D.M.: The physical and emotional care of infants with gastrostomy tubes, Issues Compr. Pediatr. Nurs. **6:**195-203, 1983.

Ziemer, M., and Carroll, J.S.: Infant gavage feeding, Am. J. Nurs. **78:**1543-1544, 1978.

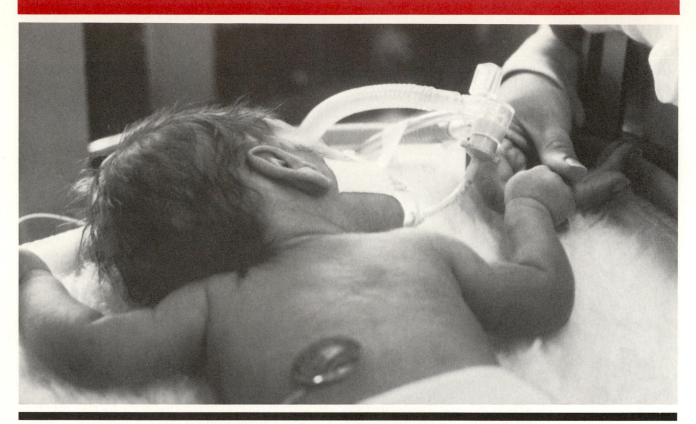

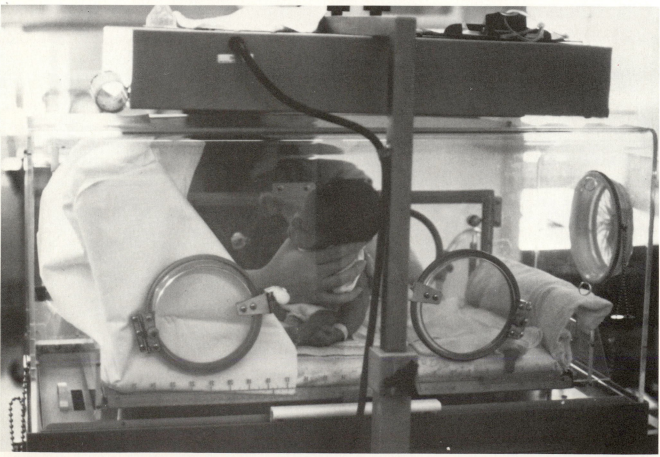

unit 9

THE CHILD WITH PROBLEMS RELATED TO THE TRANSFER OF OXYGEN AND NUTRIENTS

The survival of an individual depends on a continuous supply of energy for maintaining the function of all the cells in the body. This energy is obtained through oxygen and nutrients, which are incorporated by the body and converted to energy by the process of oxygenation-reduction. Any circumstance or condition that requires an increase in energy requires a concomitant increase in the materials that the body converts into energy.

The need for oxygen is most acute, and without this vital substance the body is unable to survive more than a few minutes without permanent damage to vital structures or death. Therefore, oxygen must be supplied constantly. Nutrients and water, on the other hand, can be stored within the body for use at times of increased need or diminished supply.

Alterations in the ability to supply oxygen or nutrients are some of the most common health problems of childhood. Interference with respiratory and gastrointestinal function is encountered at all ages, but very young children are especially vulnerable to dysfunctions in these systems. Respiratory and gastrointestinal disorders are encountered most frequently and the effects are more serious in children in the younger age-groups. Chapter 20, *The Child with Respiratory Dysfunction*, describes the more common conditions that impair the exchange of oxygen and carbon dioxide. Chapter 21, *The Child with Gastrointestinal Dysfunction*, is concerned with factors that interfere with digestion or absorption of body nutrients. There are other situations in which there are disturbances in the availability of oxygen and nutrients for energy, for example, diabetes mellitus and disorders of fluid and electrolyte balance, but these are more appropriately discussed elsewhere.

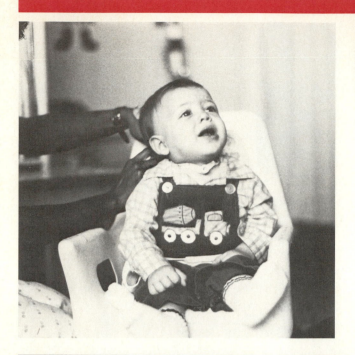

THE CHILD WITH RESPIRATORY DYSFUNCTION

OBJECTIVES

On completion of this chapter the reader will be able to:

■ Identify the significant differences between the respiratory tract of the infant or young child and that of the adult

■ Contrast the effects of various respiratory infections observed in infants and children

■ Outline a nursing care plan for a child with an upper respiratory tract infection

■ Outline a nursing care plan for a child with a lower respiratory tract infection

■ Demonstrate an understanding of the ways in which inhalation of noninfectious irritants produce pulmonary dysfunction

■ Describe the ways in which the various therapeutic measures relieve the symptoms of asthma

■ Outline a plan for teaching home care for the child with bronchial asthma

■ Describe the physiologic effects of cystic fibrosis on the gastrointestinal and pulmonary systems

■ Outline a plan of care for the child with cystic fibrosis

■ List the major signs of respiratory distress in infants and children

NURSING DIAGNOSES

Nursing diagnoses identified for the child with respiratory dysfunction include, but are not restricted to, the following:

Health perception-health management pattern

■ Infection, potential for, related to (1) aspiration of foreign substances; (2) presence of secretions; (3) presence of infectious organisms

■ Injury, potential for, related to (1) injudicious application of therapies; (2) presence of foreign substances

Nutritional-metabolic pattern

■ Fluid volume deficit, potential related to abnormal losses from lungs and skin

■ Nutrition, alteration in: less than body requirements related to inability to eat (rapid respirations)

■ Skin integrity, impairment of: potential related to irritation from appliances (endotracheal tube, tracheostomy, etc.) or secretions

Activity-exercise pattern

- Activity intolerance related to (1) altered breathing pattern; (2) fatigue

- Airway clearance, ineffective, related to (1) excess thick secretions; (2) fatigue; (3) poor positioning

- Diversional activity deficit related to environmental restriction (e.g., mist tent, bed rest), ventilatory appliances

- Self-care deficit, related to (specify level: feeding, bathing/hygiene, dressing/grooming, toileting) (1) developmental level; (2) discomfort

Sleep-rest pattern

- Sleep pattern disturbance related to (1) difficulty breathing; (2) sensory overload; (3) discomfort

Cognitive-perceptual pattern

- Comfort, alteration in: pain related to physical position

- Sensory-perceptual alterations related to (1) mechanical appliances; (2) environment (e.g., intensive care unit); (3) isolation

Self-perception—self-concept pattern

- Anxiety related to (1) strange environment; (2) perception of impending event (specify); (3) separation; (4) anticipated discomfort; (5) knowledge deficit; (6) discomfort; (7) difficulty breathing; (8) feelings of powerlessness

- Self-concept, disturbance in, related to (1) perceived effect of chronic disease; (2) unrealistic self-expectations (chronic disease)

Role-relationship pattern

- Communication, impaired verbal, related to presence of therapeutic devices

- Family process, alteration in, related to situational crisis

- Parenting, alteration in: potential, related to family stress

- Social isolation related to (1) impaired mobility; (2) hospitalization

Coping-stress tolerance pattern

- Coping, family: potential for growth

Some of the most common problems in the pediatric age-group are related to disturbed respiratory function, and respiratory failure is the chief cause of morbidity in the newborn period. Respiratory illness can be caused by disease, trauma, or physical anomalies, or it can be seen as a manifestation of a disturbance in another organ or system, such as neurologic disorders involving the respiratory center or innervation to the respiratory musculature. Most communicable diseases have respiratory symptoms. The type and pattern of respiratory disturbances also vary tremendously according to the age of the child. There are differences in susceptibility to infections and in response to various organisms and conditions at various ages. Moreover, manifestations of illness vary according to the age of the child and may involve different organ systems.

This chapter is concerned primarily with infectious, allergic, and mechanical disturbances.

ANATOMIC DEFECTS

Thoracic cage and skeletal deformities are rare but, when present, significantly impair respiration. Diaphragmatic and hiatal hernias interfere with lung expansion when abdominal contents protrude through openings in the diaphragm. Tracheoesophageal fistulas pose a hazard to breathing by allowing saliva, mucus, and ingested material to enter the lungs (see Chapter 21). The most common nasal abnormality is choanal atresia.

CHOANAL ATRESIA

Choanal atresia is a rare congenital deformity that consists of a bony or membranous septum between the nose and the pharynx. It can be bilateral or unilateral and frequently appears in association with other congenital abnormalities. It is observed twice as often in girls as in boys.

When the disorder is unilateral the infant displays few symptoms and its presence may be unidentified for an indefinite period. Bilateral atresia can be life-threatening in the obligatory nose-breathing neonates who make vigorous attempts to inspire by sucking in their lips and who develop respiratory distress, cyanosis and, sometimes, apnea. These infants are at risk of suffocation until they can learn mouth breathing.

The diagnosis is made when a firm catheter cannot pass through each nostril 3 to 4 cm into the nasopharynx. Treatment consists of establishing an oral airway and gavage feeding until the infant learns to both eat and breathe without the airway, usually in 2 to 3 weeks. Some sur-

geons prefer immediate correction of the defect, others delay repair until months, or even years, in infants who adapt well to the obstruction.

Nursing care is directed first toward detection of possible obstruction in newborn infants who have difficulty feeding or who show evidence of respiratory distress. Attempting to pass a firm catheter has become a routine procedure in the initial assessment of the newborn; therefore, atresia is usually identified early and appropriate measures instituted to ensure an adequate airway. Management of an artificial airway and gavage feeding are discussed elsewhere. Parents will need to be taught to continue these procedures at home if surgical correction is delayed, and they should be involved in the child's care as soon as possible.

ACUTE INFECTIONS OF THE RESPIRATORY TRACT

Acute infection of the respiratory tract is the most common cause of illness in infancy and childhood. Young children ordinarily have four or five such infections each year that manifest a wide range of severity from trivial to severe or even fatal illness. They are seldom localized to a single anatomic structure or area but tend to spread to a variable extent as a result of the continuous nature of the mucous membrane lining the respiratory tract. Consequently infections of the respiratory tract generally involve several areas rather than a single structure, although the effect on one may predominate in any given illness.

Acute infections of the respiratory tract will be discussed according to the general areas of involvement in the more common infections: the *upper respiratory tract* or upper airway, which consists primarily of the nose and pharynx; the *middle respiratory tract,* consisting of the structurally stable portion of the airway, which includes the epiglottis and larynx; the *lower respiratory tract,* composed of the rigid trachea and the bronchi and bronchioles, whose smooth muscle content has the ability to constrict; and the *primary respiratory unit,* the lungs.

GENERAL ASPECTS OF ACUTE RESPIRATORY TRACT INFECTIONS IN CHILDREN

The respiratory tract has several anatomic and biochemical characteristics (such as the cough, tracheobronchial secretions and cilia, lymphoid tissues, and the epiglottis) that provide natural defenses against the multitude of agents that can damage respiratory tissues. Effective as these are, they are frequently impaired by conditions that predispose to infection such as chronic illness, malnutrition, or continual exposure to substances that break down defenses.

Influencing factors

The type of illness and the physical response are also related to a variety of factors, including:

1. *The nature of the infectious agent*. The respiratory tract is subject to a wide variety of infectious agents.
2. *The size and frequency of the dose*. The larger the dose and the more frequent the exposure, the greater the likelihood of a significant infection.
3. *The age of the child*. Nursery and grade school children are more often exposed to infectious agents; infants have less resistance to infections.
4. *The size of the child*. Airways are smaller in young children and are subject to considerable narrowing from edema.
5. *The ability to resist invading organisms*. School-age children have greater resistance to infection than infants and young children.
6. *The presence of general conditions*. Malnutrition, anemia, fatigue, chilling of the body, and immune deficiencies decrease normal resistance to infection.
7. *The presence of disorders that affect the respiratory tract*. Allergies, cardiac abnormalities, and cystic fibrosis of the pancreas weaken respiratory defense mechanisms.

Etiology

The respiratory tract is subject to a wide variety of infective organisms, but the largest percentage of infections is caused by viruses, particularly in the upper respiratory passages. Other organisms that may be involved in primary or secondary invasion are group A β-hemolytic *Streptococcus*, *Staphylococcus aureus*, *Hemophilus influenzae*, and pneumococci. Of special significance is the β-hemolytic *Streptococcus* because of the relationship between respiratory infection with this organism and the incidence of subsequent nephritis or rheumatic fever.

General manifestations of acute respiratory tract infections in children

Infants and young children react more severely to acute respiratory tract infection than older children, and they appear to be much more ill than their local manifestations would indicate. This is especially true regarding children between 6 months and 3 years of age. Young children display a number of generalized signs and symptoms as well as local manifestations that differ from those seen in older children and adults. An infant or child may display any or all of the following signs and symptoms:

1. *Cough*. Coughing is a common manifestation of a respiratory infection. A cough may be described as dry, moist, hacking, barking, brassy, croupy, productive, or nonproductive.
2. *Nasal blockage*. The small nasal passages of the infant are easily blocked by mucosal swelling and exudation. Infants have difficulty breathing through their mouths; therefore, this occlusion can interfere with respiration and feeding.
3. *Fever*. Most children manifest a fever with respiratory infections. In children 6 months to 3 years, the temperature may reach 39.5° to 40.5° C (103° to 105° F), even with mild infections.
4. *Febrile seizures*. In some small children a sudden temperature rise to 40° C (104° F) or higher will precipitate febrile convulsions (p. 846).
5. *Anorexia*. Loss of appetite is a symptom common to most childhood illnesses, and it almost invariably accompanies acute infections in small children.
6. *Vomiting*. Small children vomit readily with illness, and vomiting occurs so frequently at the onset of infection that its appearance for no obvious reason is a clue to the advent of infection.
7. *Meningism*. Signs associated with meningitis but without actual inflammation of the meninges include headache, stiffness in the back and neck, and positive Kernig's and Brudzinski's signs.
8. *Diarrhea*. Mild transient diarrhea often accompanies respiratory infections in small children, particularly viral infections.
9. *Abdominal pain*. Abdominal pain, sometimes indistinguishable from the pain of appendicitis, is a common complaint in small children with acute respiratory infections.

ACUTE INFECTIONS OF THE UPPER CONDUCTING AIRWAYS

The upper conducting airways consist of the nose, nasopharynx, and pharynx. The tonsils, which are situated within the upper passages, are also included in this category but are not discussed here (see p. 341). Acute pharyngitis and nasopharyngitis (the equivalent of the "common cold" in adults; also called *acute rhinitis* or *coryza*) are extremely common in pediatric age-groups. These disorders can be merely a part of a generalized upper respiratory infection, or they may be the dominant feature of an infection. The organisms usually responsible are the viruses. Those infections of bacterial origin are caused predominantly by group A β-hemolytic *Streptococcus*. In general, viral infections have a gradual onset, as contrasted with the abrupt onset seen with bacterial infections, they

TABLE 20-1. COMPARISON OF COMMON UPPER RESPIRATORY INFECTIONS*

	NASOPHARYNGITIS	PHARYNGITIS
Anatomic site	Nose and pharynx	Principal involvement is throat, including tonsils
Etiology	Viral, principally rhinoviruses	Viral, group A β-hemolytic *Streptococcus*
Epidemiology	Occurs throughout the year Most common respiratory infection	Uncommon in children under age 1 year Peak incidence between ages 4 and 7 years Prevalent throughout childhood

Manifestations	Younger child
	  Fever
	  Irritability, restlessness
	  Sneezing
	  Vomiting and/or diarrhea,
	    sometimes
	Older child
	  Dryness and irritation of nose
	    and throat
	  Sneezing, chilly sensation
	  Muscular aches
	  Cough, sometimes
		Younger child
		  Fever
		  General malaise
		  Anorexia
		  Moderate sore throat
		  Headache
		Older child
		  Fever (may reach 40° C)
		  Headache
		  Anorexia
		  Dysphagia
		  Abdominal pain
		  Vomiting

Pathology	Edema and vasodilation of mucosa	Younger child
		  Mild to moderate hyperemia
		  May or may not exhibit follicular exudate; if so, limited to posterior wall
		  Cervical lymph nodes not enlarged or only slightly enlarged
		Older child
		  Mild to fiery red, edematous pharynx
		  Hyperemia of tonsils and pharynx; may extend to soft palate and uvula
		  Often abundant follicular exudate that spreads and coalesces to form pseudomembrane on tonsils
		  Cervical glands enlarged and tender
		  Polymorphonuclear leukocytosis

Complications	Infant
	  Otitis media
	  Lower tract infection
	Older child
	  Sinusitis
		Infant
		  Usually causes no complications
		  Otitis media, sometimes
		Older child
		  May cause otitis media
		  Acute cervical adenitis
		  Retropharyngeal abscess
		  Downward invasion of respiratory tract
		  May be followed by nephritis or rheumatic fever

*Tonsilitis and otitis media are discussed on pp. 341 and 345.

produce a shorter and milder illness with less intense inflammation, and they cause fewer complications.

Differentiation on the basis of symptoms is often difficult. Diagnosis is confirmed by throat culture, although many children harbor streptococci as part of their normal flora. See Table 20-1 for comparison of common upper respiratory infections.

Therapeutic management

Children with upper respiratory infections are treated at home unless there are serious complications. Treatment is important, however, to prevent or minimize complications. The usual recommendations are (1) have the child rest in bed until he is free of fever for at least 1 day, (2) encourage liquids, and (3) control fever.

Most physicians prescribe antipyretic drugs for oral temperatures exceeding 38° C (100.5° F) or rectal temperatures exceeding 38.4° C (101° F). Acetylsalicylic acid (aspirin) or acetaminophen (Tylenol) are usually prescribed. (For an extensive discussion of fever and administration of antipyretics see p. 542.)

Local measures may be advised, including nose drops to shrink congested membranes, throat irrigations (in older cooperative children), hot or cold applications, and carefully managed moist air administration. Nose drops are helpful in relieving nasal stuffiness (see p. 566 for administration of nose drops). Medication instilled into the nose should not be continued more than 4 to 5 days. Beyond this time the medication may cause a chemical irritation that produces nasal congestion indistinguishable from that of the original illness.

Oral decongestants are sometimes prescribed to reduce the swelling of nasal mucosa, but there is little evidence that they are effective in the majority of cases. Potent antitussives to depress the cough reflex are contraindicated where nasal discharge is profuse because of the increased risk of aspirating the secretions.

Although 80% to 90% of all cases of acute pharyngitis are viral, a throat culture should be done to rule out group A β-hemolytic *Streptococcus* infection. If streptococcal sore throat infection is present, penicillin is administered in doses sufficient to control the acute local manifestations and to maintain an adequate level for at least 10 days to eliminate any organisms that might remain to initiate kidney or rheumatic symptoms.

Nursing considerations

Since the majority of children with upper respiratory tract infections are treated at home, most of the nursing care is directed toward education and guidance of parents in caring for their child and serving as resources for problem solving. If the physician has given the parents written instructions, these can be explained and reinforced as appropriate. If written instructions have not been furnished, the nurse should provide the parents with written guidelines and, in some cases, outlines of procedures to be employed.

Rest. Any child who has an acute febrile illness should be placed on bed rest. This is usually not difficult while the temperature is elevated but may be difficult when the child feels fairly well, particularly in young children. When parents take the advice seriously and consistently keep the child in bed, most children learn to cooperate during illness. A number of entertainment devices can be employed to keep the child quiet, based on the child's individual interests.

Every endeavor should be made to remove the child from contact with other children. Ideally the ill child should be isolated in a separate bedroom at the first sign of illness. This is seldom a problem with an only child but is often difficult when living arrangements are crowded and there are several children in the family. If the child has no bedroom of his own, sometimes another child can sleep on a couch or cot or with relatives or friends. Well children can be taught to stay away from the ill child if the living conditions allow for segregation and if the rule is rigidly enforced.

Nutrition. Anorexia is characteristic of acute infections in children, and, in most cases, the child can be permitted to determine his own need for food. Many children show no decrease in appetite, and others respond well to certain foods such as gelatin, soup, and puddings. Since the illness is relatively short, the nutritional state is seldom compromised. Sometimes reducing the milk intake of formula-fed infants is helpful during the initial phase of an acute respiratory infection.

Dehydration is always a hazard when children are febrile or anorexic, especially when vomiting or diarrhea also occur. An adequate fluid intake should be encouraged by offering small amounts of favored fluids at frequent intervals. High-calorie liquids such as colas, fruit juices, water flavored and sweetened with corn syrup, or similar drinks help prevent catabolism and dehydration. Fluids should not be forced, and the child should not be wakened from his rest to take fluids.

Control fever. If the child has a significantly elevated temperature, controlling the fever becomes a major nursing task. The parent should know how to take the child's temperature and read the thermometer accurately. Most parents are able to do this, but nurses cannot make this assumption. Those who cannot will require instruction in use of the thermometer. The reader is referred to Chapter 19 for an extensive discussion of fever, its assessment, and its management. Cool liquids are encouraged to help reduce the temperature and to minimize the chances of dehydration.

Local measures. Older children are usually able to manage nasal secretions with little difficulty. They should be taught to use a tissue or their hand to cover their nose and mouth when they cough or sneeze and to dispose of the tissues properly. The parents are instructed concerning the correct administration of nose drops and throat irrigations, if ordered. For very young infants, who normally breathe through their noses, an infant nasal aspirator or a rubber ear syringe is helpful in removing nasal secretions before feeding. This, followed by instillation of saline nose drops, often clears nasal passages and facilitates feeding.

For older infants and children who can better tolerate decongestants, phenylephrine nose drops may be administered 15 to 20 minutes before feeding and at bedtime. Two drops are instilled, and, since this shrinks only the anterior mucous membranes, 2 more drops are instilled 5 to 10

SUMMARY OF NURSING CARE OF THE CHILD WITH AN ACUTE INFECTION OF THE UPPER RESPIRATORY TRACT

GOALS	RESPONSIBILITIES
Provide rest	Keep the child in bed until free of fever for 1 full day Provide entertainment and quiet diversional activities appropriate to age and interest of the child
Reduce fever	Reduce environmental temperature Place the child in lightweight clothing and bed linen Administer antipyretic drugs (aspirin, acetaminophen) in prescribed dosage Administer tepid sponges or baths Encourage cool liquids

Prevent spread of infection	Isolate the child from other family members as much as possible
	    Separate bedroom if possible
	    Avoid close contact between well persons and the ill child
	    Discourage parents and others from lying down with the ill child
	Keep others from using the child's eating and drinking utensils
	Use separate washcloth and towel for the ill child
	Teach the child proper behavior when coughing or sneezing and proper disposal of tissues

Facilitate respirations and promote comfort	Provide moist air: shower, humidifier Administer nose drops as prescribed Remove secretions with suction apparatus, nasal aspirator, or ear syringe Administer throat irrigations (older children) Administer hot or cold compresses
Prevent dehydration	Offer high-calorie liquids Encourage fluid intake Keep track of number of times and amount of voiding Observe the child for signs of dehydration
Rule out streptococcal sore throat	Assess nature of throat manifestation Obtain throat culture
If bacterial infection, eradicate organisms	Administer antibiotics as ordered

minutes later. Older cooperative children often prefer nasal sprays. They are taught to compress the plastic container at the moment of inspiration to gain relief. Spray bottles and bottles of nose drops should be used for one child only and only for one illness, since they become easily contaminated with bacteria.

Hot or cold applications sometimes provide relief to older children with painful cervical adenitis. An ice bag or heating pad applied to the neck may decrease the discomfort, but safety precautions must be observed in order to prevent burns. The ice bag or heating device must be covered, and the heating pad should not be set at the high ranges.

Warm or cool mist has been a common therapeutic measure for symptomatic relief of respiratory discomfort.

The moisture soothes inflamed membranes and seems especially beneficial when there is hoarseness or any laryngeal involvement. Mist tents and hoods are frequently employed in the hospital for liquefying secretions and relieving discomfort. However, moisturizing air by use of steam vaporizers in the home is not advised and should be discouraged because of the hazards related to their use and the little evidence to support their efficacy (Colombo, Hopkins, and Waring, 1981). Alternate suggestions are available, such as humidification systems and cool mist vaporizers. Shallow pans with wide surface areas for evaporation increase humidity but should be placed where they do not pose a safety hazard. A large, wet beach towel hung with one end in shallow water in the bathtub will increase humidity if the bathroom door remains open.

A time-honored method of producing steam is the shower. Running the shower of hot water into the empty bathtub or open shower stall with the bathroom door closed produces a quick source of steam. Ten to fifteen minutes in this environment offers the same advantages as the croup tent without the fear and restraint often associated with the confines of a tent. A small child can be held on the lap of a parent or other adult. Older children can sit in the bathroom under the supervision of an adult.

Medication.   In addition to antipyretics and nose drops, the child may require antibiotic therapy if the infection is caused by group A β-hemolytic *Streptococcus*. The nurse is often the one who collects the throat-culture specimens, administers medication, and instructs the parents regarding continuing the medication. Parents of children who are sent home with oral antibiotics need to understand the importance of regular administration and of continuing the drug for the prescribed length of time, regardless of whether the child appears ill (see p. 567 for teaching parents to administer medications).

ACUTE INFECTIONS OF THE MIDDLE AIRWAYS

Infections of the middle conducting airways involve all areas to some extent. Infections involving primarily the epiglottis, the glottis, and the larynx are described by some authorities as upper respiratory tract infections; others consider them as lower respiratory tract infections. For the convenience of this discussion they are considered as middle airway infections. The general term "croup" is applied to a symptom complex involving these structures and characterized by hoarseness, a resonant cough described as "barking" or "brassy" (croupy), inspiratory stridor, and varying degrees of respiratory distress resulting from swelling of the airway. Table 20-2 compares and contrasts the major types of middle airway infections.

Epiglottitis is a serious obstructive inflammatory disorder. It is one of the most dramatic diseases of childhood. It must be recognized early and treated vigorously to avoid a fatal outcome. The causative organism is almost always *Hemophilus influenzae*, and the onset is very rapid in a previously healthy child.

Acute subglottic infections are of greater importance in infants and small children than they are in older children in part because of the increased incidence in children in this age-group and partly because of the smaller diameter of the airway, which renders it subject to significantly greater narrowing with the same degree of inflammation.

Laryngitis, laryngotracheitis, and *laryngotracheobronchitis (LTB)* are all considered together because of their similarity in manifestations and therapy. The principal etiologic agents in croup are viruses, except in those cases associated with diphtheria, pertussis, and acute epiglottitis. In most children the disease is relatively mild with cough, stridor, and mild retractions and gradual improvement to recovery in 3 to 7 days. However, complications of viral croup occur in a number of children, the most common of which are extensions of the infection to other areas of the respiratory tract to cause otitis media, bronchiolitis, and pneumonia. The most serious complication, and the one responsible for most deaths from croup, is laryngeal obstruction. Complications of tracheostomy are another hazard related to these disorders.

Therapeutic management

The major objective in medical management of infectious croup is maintaining an airway and providing for adequate respiratory exchange. Afebrile children with mild laryngitis and a croupy cough are usually managed at home with symptomatic treatment. Bed rest and humidified air during sleep may be helpful.

Children with spasmodic croup are managed at home. Mist inhalation as described for upper respiratory infection is recommended, especially the quick vaporization that is afforded by steam from hot running water in a closed bathroom (a shower is recommended if available). This quick and easy treatment usually provides almost immediate relief of acute laryngeal spasm and respiratory distress. Sometimes the spasm is relieved by sudden exposure to cold air (as when the child is taken out into the night air for medical care). Parents are usually advised to have the child sleep with either warm or cool humidified air until the cough has subsided so that, hopefully, subsequent episodes will be prevented.

Although many children with croup and significantly elevated temperatures above 39° C (102.2° F) can be managed at home, hospitalization is often advised. Those for whom hospitalization is indicated are children with:

Presence or suspicion of epiglottitis, progressive stridor, and respiratory distress (especially during the daytime)
Presence of hypoxia, restlessness, cyanosis, pallor, and/or depressed sensorium
A high temperature and toxic appearance

Facilities and equipment for tracheostomy, as well as reliable observation, are readily available in the hospital setting. If the hospital does not provide close, skilled observation, the child may be safer at home where the parents can maintain vigilance.

In cases of suspected epiglottitis, attempts to visualize the epiglottis directly with a tongue depressor may precipitate sudden laryngospasm, complete obstruction, and death. Therefore, the nurse does not attempt examination

TABLE 20-2. COMPARISON OF COMMON INFECTIONS OF THE MIDDLE AIRWAY

ACUTE EPIGLOTTITIS (supraglottitis)	**ACUTE LARYNGITIS, LARYNGOTRACHEITIS, LARYNGOTRACHEOBRONCHITIS**	**ACUTE SPASMODIC LARYNGITIS (spasmodic croup)**
Description Severe rapidly, progressive infection of the epiglottis and surrounding area	Most common form of croup May be localized or one manifestation of a variety of conditions	Distinct clinical entity characterized by sudden paroxysmal attacks of laryngeal obstruction that occur chiefly at night
Age-group affected Chiefly ages 3 to 7 years May occur in younger children	Most common at ages 3 months to 3 years	Usually affects small children ages 1 to 3 years
Etiologic agent Generally *Hemophilus influenzae,* type B	Viral agents, especially parainfluenza viruses	Viral agents In some cases, allergy and psychogenic factors have been implicated Certain children appear to be predisposed
Manifestations Usually in good health before onset May be preceded by upper respiratory tract infection Abrupt onset; rapidly progressive High fever Appears ill Sore throat Difficulty or inability to swallow Drooling of saliva Retching Difficulty in breathing progressing to severe respiratory distress in minutes or hours Child will sit upright, leaning forward, with chin thrust out and mouth open—tripod position Thick, muffled voice Croaking, "froglike" sound on inspiration Anxious and frightened expression Suprasternal and substernal retractions may be visible Seldom struggle to breathe; breathing slowly and quietly provides better air exchange Sallow color of mild hypoxia to frank cyanosis Throat red, inflamed Distinctive large, cherry-red, edematous epiglottis	Preceded by upper respiratory tract infection Wide range of manifestations from few symptoms to severe obstructive laryngitis Infection rapidly descends, with first laryngeal symptoms—hoarseness, brassy cough, stridor, respiratory distress Fever and prostration increase Respiratory distress, especially inspiratory dyspnea with substernal and suprasternal retractions Bronchi involvement becomes evident with increased dyspnea Expiratory difficulty with labored and prolonged expirations Scattered rales of various types; rhonchi Diminished breath sounds bilaterally Pallor or cyanosis Irritability and restlessness	Usually preceded by mild to moderate nasopharyngitis or slight laryngitis Child suddenly wakens with characteristic barking, metallic cough, hoarseness, noisy inspirations, and restlessness; child appears anxious, frightened, and prostrated Accessory muscles of respiration used and inspiratory retractions sometimes evident Dyspnea aggravated by excitement May be some cyanosis Attack wears off in a few hours and child appears well the following day except for some hoarseness and cough May be repeated 1 or 2 nights in succession

TABLE 20-2. COMPARISON OF COMMON INFECTIONS OF THE MIDDLE AIRWAY—cont'd

ACUTE EPIGLOTTITIS (supraglottitis)	ACUTE LARYNGITIS, LARYNGOTRACHEITIS, LARYNGOTRACHEOBRONCHITIS	ACUTE SPASMODIC LARYNGITIS (spasmodic croup)
Treatment		
Minimize disturbance	If mild, treated at home	High-humidity atmosphere
Avoid visualization of epiglottis without skilled personnel	If severe, hospitalized	Induction of expectoration with single dose of ipecac (1 drop per month of age up to 2 years; 2-5 ml for older children)
Establishment of an airway is urgent—endotracheal tube or tracheostomy often necessary	High-humidity therapy with high-oxygen concentration	Mild sedation with phenobarbital
Humidification with oxygen	Tracheostomy set at bedside	Reassure parents
Vigorous antibiotic therapy intravenously	Rest; disturb as little as possible; reduce need to talk or cry	
Nasopharyngeal culture	Adequate fluid intake; intravenous fluids to save strength and decrease possibility of vomiting; less severely affected—oral fluids	
Blood culture		
Rest		

of the throat. Examination is made by a trained practitioner with intubation or tracheostomy equipment at hand.

Children with croup, whether treated at home or in the hospital, require close observation for signs of respiratory obstruction. They are placed in high humidity, preferably in a mist tent or Croupette with cool mist vapor. Since a rapidly rising heart rate is an early signal of hypoxia and impending airway obstruction, regular monitoring of cardiac rate is instituted, preferably using a cardiac monitor. Oxygen therapy is also indicated to alleviate hypoxia and reduce apprehension.

Fluid by the intravenous route is indicated to lessen physical exertion and to reduce the likelihood of vomiting with the attendant risk of aspiration. Infants with rapid respirations may aspirate feedings.

Medications. Children with suspected bacterial epiglottitis are given ampicillin intravenously. The use of corticosteroids for reducing edema has not been determined to be of benefit. Expectorants, bronchodilators, and antihistamines are rarely helpful in croup, and sedatives are contraindicated because of their depressant effect on the respiratory center. Dramatic relief of laryngeal stridor has been achieved in treatment of croup with the use of racemic epinephrine (Vaponefrin) in nebulized mist or intermittent positive-pressure breathing.

Nursing considerations

The most important nursing function in the care of children with croup is vigilant observation for signs of respiratory embarrassment and relief of laryngeal obstruction. The child is placed in a cool high-humidity environment with oxygen, usually administered by way of a mist tent or Croupette, and with skilled nursing personnel in attendance to observe for any indications of respiratory distress. Vital signs are monitored frequently, and the child's appearance and behavior are observed to detect early signs of impending airway obstruction, such as increased pulse and respiratory rate, substernal, suprasternal, and intercostal retractions, flaring nares, and increased restlessness. Equipment for performing a tracheostomy or endotracheal intubation should be at hand in case an artificial airway must be supplied immediately and is left there until respiratory difficulty has subsided completely. *Any child with laryngeal stridor requires constant surveillance.* Laryngeal stridor is a shrill, harsh respiratory sound, often described as a "crowing" sound, that is particularly marked during inspiration.

As distress increases, the child becomes increasingly restless and anxious. He dozes, wakens startled, and makes visible efforts to draw in air. Tracheostomy or endotracheal intubation is usually performed at this stage of distress. If not, the inspiratory stridor and retractions progress until he becomes markedly pale or ashen, his skin is cold and clammy, and all his attention and effort are focused on fighting for air. He becomes increasingly agitated, thrashes about, and tries to climb the sides of the Croupette in his efforts to breathe. His status is critical. An artificial airway is mandatory for survival. The child may or may not be cyanotic; he is often pale to ashen and looks very ill. Cyanosis is often a late sign.

Fortunately only a small percentage of children with croup require intubation or tracheostomy. Immediately after the procedure the child becomes more relaxed as a re-

SUMMARY OF NURSING CARE OF THE CHILD HOSPITALIZED WITH LOWER RESPIRATORY TRACT INFECTION (CROUP)

GOALS	RESPONSIBILITIES

Assess respiratory status and detect impending airway obstruction	Monitor respirations for rate, depth, pattern, presence of retractions, and flaring nares
	Auscultate lungs
	  Evaluation of breath sounds
	  Detection of presence of rales or rhonchi
	Observe color of skin and mucous membranes for pallor, and cyanosis
	Observe the child for presence of hoarseness, stridor, and cough
	Monitor heart rate and regularity
	Observe the child's behavior
	  Restlessness
	  Irritability
	  Apprehension
	Report and record significant observations

Ease respiratory efforts	Provide high-humidity environment Place the child in a mist tent or Croupette with cool vapor Promote rest Implement measures to reduce anxiety and apprehension Provide oxygen as prescribed Give nothing by mouth to prevent aspiration of fluids
Conserve energy	Promote rest Implement measures to reduce apprehension Disturb the child as little as possible
Prevent dehydration	Administer fluids as prescribed Monitor intravenous infusion during acute phase Administer oral fluids when tolerated Keep accurate records of intake and output Measure urine specific gravity to assess state of hydration
Be prepared to assist with tracheostomy	Have tracheostomy equipment at bedside Obtain parental permission for procedure
Reduce apprehension	Remain in constant attendance Hold and cuddle the child whenever possible—preferably by parent or familiar person Provide comforting devices such as familiar toy, blanket, and so on Encourage parental attendance and, when possible, involvement in the child's care
Provide nutrition	Administer intravenous glucose during acute phase, as ordered Encourage high-calorie liquids when no longer danger of aspiration Progress to regular diet as condition improves
Reduce parental anxiety	Recognize parental concern and need for information and support Explain therapy and the child's behavior Provide support as needed Encourage the parents to become involved in the child's care
Educate the parents	Prepare the parents for the child's discharge Refer to appropriate health agency as indicated

Keep the child calm	Do nothing to make the child more anxious than he already is
	  Maintain a relaxed manner
	  Establish rapport with the child and parents
	Instill confidence in both parents and child
	Try to avoid any intrusive procedures

sult of the relief from laryngeal obstruction, breathing becomes regular, and he usually falls asleep from exhaustion. Later he may become frightened to discover that he is unable to speak or to cry. One of the greatest fears is that he will be unable to call someone to his side. He will need continued emotional support as well as physical vigilance required in tracheostomy care. The tracheostomy is usually left in place only as long as needed to relieve respiratory distress.

To conserve energy, the child is given every opportunity to rest. Fluids are administered intravenously during the acute phase of illness, and other measures are implemented to promote rest and to reduce anxiety. An infant or small child finds that being enclosed within the mist tent, coughing, laryngeal spasms, and restraint for intravenous therapy are additional sources of distress. He needs the security of the parent's or the nurse's presence. When his condition allows, a small child can be removed for short periods for comfort and reassurance, especially to reduce apprehension during coughing spells.

The rapid progression of croup and epiglottitis, the alarming sound of the cough or stridor, and the child's apprehensive behavior and ill appearance combine to create a very frightening experience for the parents. They need reassurance regarding the child's progress and an explanation of treatments. They may feel guilty for not having suspected the seriousness of the condition sooner, especially if an artificial airway is needed. The nurse can provide them with an opportunity to express their feelings, thus minimizing any blame or guilt. Fortunately, as the crisis subsides and as the child responds to therapy, his breathing becomes easier and recovery is generally prompt.

ACUTE INFECTIONS OF THE LOWER AIRWAYS

The lower portion of the respiratory passages includes the trachea, bronchi, and bronchioles. Infectious disorders of these structures are diverse in nature and etiology and primarily involve the bronchioles. Bronchial inflammation is usually seen as tracheobronchitis or laryngotracheobronchitis. Tracheitis is now recognized as a cause of subglottic obstructive airway disease in children.

Tracheitis is a serious disease characterized by fever, toxicity, and stridor. The child has difficulty breathing because of copious, thick, purulent tracheal secretions. It must be recognized early in order to prevent life-threatening airway obstruction.

In *asthmatic bronchitis* the predominant pathology is bronchospasm with increased mucus production. It is often confused with bronchiolitis and represents a peculiar response to a variety of upper respiratory tract infections. The affected children are seldom ill, but wheezing, pro-

ductive cough, and signs of moderate emphysema are apparent. There is usually a history of attacks associated with upper respiratory infections.

Bronchitis, an isolated condition that is unusual in childhood, may be associated with either upper or lower respiratory tract conditions. A variety of etiologic agents may initiate the dry, hacking, and nonproductive cough. Noxious chemicals in urban air pollution are becoming an important cause.

Bronchiolitis is represented by severe infectious and mechanical changes in the bronchioles. Bronchiole mucosa is swollen, and lumina are filled with mucus and exudate, the walls of the bronchi and bronchioles are infiltrated with inflammatory cells, and peribronchiolar interstitial pneumonitis is usually present. The variable degrees of obstruction produced in small air passages by these changes lead to hyperinflation, obstructive emphysema resulting from partial obstruction, and patchy areas of atelectasis.

Table 20-3 compares the major characteristics of tracheal, bronchial, and bronchiolar infections.

Therapeutic management

Tracheitis is managed by antibiotic therapy, frequent tracheal suctioning to remove copious secretions, and endotracheal intubation is often required to ensure an adequate airway. Humidified oxygen is provided by appropriate means.

Asthmatic bronchitis is effectively treated with bronchodilators and expectorants. Immediate relief of dyspnea and wheezing is obtained by subcutaneous administration of epinephrine, and the effect is maintained with oral administration of an ephedrine preparation (pseudoephedrine [Sudafed], triprolidine [Actifed]). The stimulant effect of these drugs is offset or counterbalanced by small doses of phenobarbital. A high-humidity environment is provided and an expectorant is given to help liquefy and remove bronchial secretions. Since the majority of attacks are triggered by viral infections, antimicrobials are rarely indicated.

There is no specific treatment for viral bronchitis, and the treatment is, therefore, symptomatic. Expectorants are sometimes used, but their value is questioned. Cough suppressants are contraindicated since coughing is necessary to bring up secretions. High humidity or mist helps liquefy secretions and provides symptomatic relief, and percussion and postural drainage promote the mobilization of secretions.

Bronchiolitis is treated with an atmosphere of high humidity, an adequate fluid intake, and rest. Hospitalization is usually recommended, and the child is placed in a mist tent or Croupette to help loosen tenacious secretions and minimize fluid loss from the lungs. Mist therapy is gener-

TABLE 20-3. COMPARISON OF INFECTIONS OF THE LOWER AIRWAYS

TRACHEITIS	ASTHMATIC BRONCHITIS	BRONCHITIS	BRONCHIOLITIS
Description			
Begins with signs and symptoms similar to croup A serious cause of airway obstruction in children May be a complication of LTB	Exaggerated response of bronchi to upper respiratory tract infection, with spasm and exudation similar to those of older children with asthma	Seldom occurs as an isolated entity in childhood Acute tracheobronchitis commonly found in association with upper respiratory tract infection	One of more common infectious diseases of lower respiratory tract, with maximal obstructive impact at bronchiolar level; consists of hypersecretion, edema, and inflammatory reaction confined to smaller bronchioles
Age-group affected			
1 month to 6 years	Late infancy and early childhood	Affects children in first 4 years of life Highest incidence in September and October	Usually children between ages 2 and 12 months; number 3 cause of death in children in this age-group Rare after age 2 years Peak incidence at approximately age 6 months of age Increased incidence in children born prematurely
Etiologic agent			
Bacterial—majority *Staphylococcus aureus, Hemophilus influenzae*	Response to variety of infections, most commonly viral infections of upper respiratory tract	Usually viral agents—same as those responsible for croup syndrome; other agents, such as bacteria, fungus, allergic disorders, and airborne irritants, may trigger symptoms	Viral; predominantly respiratory syncytial (RS) virus; also, adenoviruses, parainfluenza viruses, and *Mycoplasma pneumoniae*
Manifestations			
Follows previous upper respiratory infection Croupy cough, stridor, unaffected by position Copious purulent secretions—may be severe enough to cause respiratory arrest High fever, toxicity No response to LTB therapy	Previous upper respiratory tract infection Wheezing Productive cough Moderate signs of emphysema	Abrupt onset with upper respiratory tract infection Persistent dry, hacking nonproductive cough that is worse at night and becomes productive in 2-3 days Audible and palpable rhonchi May be low-grade fever	Begins as simple upper respiratory tract infection with serous nasal discharge May be accompanied by moderate temperature elevation Gradually develops increasing respiratory distress, paroxysmal cough, dyspnea, and irritability Tachypnea with flaring nares and intercostal and subcostal retractions Emphysema with barrel chest and palpable liver and spleen from depressed diaphragm Shallow respiratory excursion Fine rales and prolonged expiratory phase; diminished breath sounds, hyperresonance, and scattered consolidation May be wheezing

TABLE 20-3. COMPARISON OF INFECTIONS OF THE LOWER AIRWAYS—cont'd

TRACHEITIS	ASTHMATIC BRONCHITIS	BRONCHITIS	BRONCHIOLITIS
Treatment Humidified oxygen Tracheal suctioning Antibiotics Often requires artificial airway (endotracheal tube)	Bronchodilators, such as epinephrine, ephedrine Sedatives, such as phenobarbital Expectorants, principally saturated solution of potassium iodide (SSKI) High-humidity atmosphere	No specific therapy Symptomatic and supportive therapy	Rest High-humidity atmosphere Oxygen in moderate to severe cases Adequate hydration

ally combined with oxygen in concentrations sufficient to alleviate dyspnea and hypoxia, after which mist alone is continued for mild dyspnea. Fluids by mouth may be contraindicated because of tachypnea, weakness, and fatigue; therefore, intravenous fluids are preferred until the crisis of the disease has passed.

Most authorities use the conservative approach regarding medications. Antibiotics are not routinely employed, bronchodilators are ineffectual since bronchospasm is not part of the pathology, corticosteroids have not been proved to be of universal value, cough suppressants and expectorants have not been found useful, and sedatives are contraindicated. The disease lasts about 7 to 10 days, and the prognosis is generally good.

ACUTE INFECTIONS OF THE LUNGS (PNEUMONIA)

Pneumonia, inflammation of the pulmonary parenchyma, is common throughout childhood but occurs more frequently in infancy and early childhood. Pneumonia can be classified according to its morphology, etiology, and clinical form. Clinically, pneumonia may occur as either a primary disease or as a complication of some other illness. Morphologically, pneumonias are recognized as: (1) *lobar pneumonia,* involving all or a large segment of one or more pulmonary lobes; (2) *bronchopneumonia or lobular pneumonia,* involving the terminal bronchioles and nearby lobules; and, (3) *interstitial pneumonia,* involving the alveolar walls (interstitium) and the peribronchial and interlobular tissues.

The most useful classification of pneumonia is based on the etiologic agent. In general, pneumonia is caused by four processes: viruses, bacteria, mycoplasmas, and aspiration of foreign substances. Less often pneumonia may be caused by histomycosis, coccidioidomycosis, and other fungi. The causative agent is identified largely from the clinical history, the child's age, his general health history, the physical examination, radiographs, and the laboratory examination.

Viral pneumonia

Viral pneumonias occur more frequently than bacterial pneumonias and are seen in children of all age-groups. They are often associated with viral upper respiratory infections, and the respiratory syncytial virus (RSV) accounts for the largest percentage. Others are the influenza virus, parainfluenza virus, psittacosis, rhinovirus, and adenovirus. There are few clinical symptoms to distinguish between the responsible organisms, and differentiations between viruses can be made only by laboratory examination.

The onset may be acute or insidious, and symptoms are variable, ranging from mild fever, slight cough, and malaise to high fever, severe cough, and prostration. Early in the course of the illness the cough is likely to be unproductive or productive of small amounts of whitish sputum. There is often evidence of obstructive emphysema as bronchi become plugged by necrotic material from ulceration and necrosis of tracheal and bronchial mucosa. The alveoli are generally free of fluid. Chest physical signs are noncontributory but may include a few rhonchi or fine crepitant rales. Radiographs reveal diffuse or patchy infiltration with a peribronchial distribution.

The prognosis is generally good, although viral infections of the respiratory tract render the affected child more susceptible to secondary bacterial invasion, especially when there is denuded bronchial mucosa. Treatment is usually given symptomatically. Although some recommend antimicrobial therapy in hope of reducing or preventing secondary bacterial infection, it is usually reserved for cases in which the presence of such infection is demonstrated by appropriate cultures.

Primary atypical pneumonia

Approximately 10% to 20% of hospital admissions of children with pneumonia are caused by *Mycoplasma pneumoniae*. It occurs principally in the fall and winter months and is more prevalent where there are crowded living conditions. The onset may be sudden or insidious and is usually manifest first by general systemic symptoms including fever, chills (in older children), headache, malaise, anorexia, and muscle pain (myalgia). These are followed by rhinitis, sore throat, and a dry, hacking cough. The cough, initially nonproductive, becomes productive of seromucoid sputum that later becomes mucopurulent or blood streaked. The duration and degree of fever vary widely and may last from several days to 2 weeks. Dyspnea is uncommon.

Radiographic examination reveals evidence of pneumonia before physical signs are apparent. There may be fine crepitant rales over various areas of the lung fields, but consolidation is usually not demonstrated.

Most affected persons recover from acute illness in 7 to 10 days with symptomatic treatment followed by a week of convalescence. Hospitalization is rarely necessary.

Bacterial pneumonia

In children beyond the neonatal period, bacterial pneumonias display distinct clinical patterns that facilitate their differentiation from other forms of pneumonia, and each individual microorganism produces a distinct clinical picture. The largest percentage of bacterial pneumonias in childhood is caused by pneumococci. Onset is abrupt and is generally preceded by a viral infection that disturbs the natural defense mechanisms of the upper respiratory tract and allows the pathogenic bacteria normally harbored in the upper passages to increase in number.

Children with bacterial pneumonia appear ill and exhibit both general and localized physical findings. Symptoms and signs include fever, malaise, rapid and shallow respirations, cough, and chest pain that is often exaggerated by deep breathing. The pain may be referred to the abdomen and confused with appendicitis. Chills frequently

occur, and meningeal symptoms (meningism) are also common. Pleural reactions and effusions often accompany the disease, and the consolidation process usually proceeds rapidly.

The majority of older children with pneumococcal pneumonia can be treated at home, especially if the condition is recognized and treatment initiated early. Antibiotic therapy, bed rest, liberal oral intake of fluid, and administration of aspirin for fever constitute the principal therapeutic measures. Hospitalization is indicated when pleural effusion or empyema accompanies the disease and is mandatory for children with staphylococcal pneumonia. Pneumonia in the infant or young child is best treated in the hospital since the course of illness is more variable and complications are more common in very young patients. Also, fluids are usually given intravenously, and oxygen administration greatly reduces the restlessness associated with respiratory distress.

At the present time the classic features and clinical course of pneumonia are rarely seen because of early and vigorous antibiotic and supportive therapy. However, a large number of children, especially infants, with staphylococcal pneumonia develop empyema, pyopneumothorax, or tension pneumothorax. Pleural effusion is not uncommon in children with lobar (pneumococcal) pneumonia. A diagnostic thoracentesis is performed if there is suspected fluid in the pleural cavity. Nonpurulent effusions, such as occur in pneumococcal pneumonia, do not require surgical drainage. Continuous closed chest drainage is instituted when purulent fluid is aspirated, a frequent finding in staphylococcal infections.

The prognosis for pneumococcal infections is generally good, with rapid recovery when they are recognized and treated early. Streptococcal infections vary in duration but usually resolve spontaneously. The course of staphylococcal pneumonia is generally prolonged. The prognosis varies with the length of illness prior to treatment, although early recognition and treatment are usually effective. Complications of bacterial pneumonia include pleural effusion, empyema, and tension pneumothorax. The major bacterial pneumonias are compared in Table 20-4.

A newly developed vaccine for pneumococcal pneumonia is promising but is not yet available for widespread use. It is not recommended for mass immunization but rather for children over age 2 years who are debilitated and children with diseases that predispose to pneumonia, such as cystic fibrosis.

Nursing considerations

Nursing care of the child with an infection of the air passages is primarily supportive and symptomatic to meet each child's needs. The child is assigned a bed away from others, frequently in a small, segregated ward used only for children who have respiratory infections. Ideally, the same nurses should be assigned to these children and have responsibility for the care of no other children. It has been shown that many respiratory viruses, especially respiratory syncytial virus (RSV), are readily transmitted to personnel, families, and other children by both direct contact (especially cuddling) and fomites (especially hard smooth surfaces). Therefore, infection control should stress hand-washing for all persons caring for affected children and wearing of gowns while in the room. Masks appear to have limited if any value. Children with staphylococcal infections are isolated to prevent cross-contamination.

Rest and conservation of energy are encouraged by relief of physical and psychologic stresses. The child is disturbed as little as possible. Since rapid improvement is the rule in most types of pneumonia, feedings may be omitted, especially when the respiration is rapid, in order

TABLE 20-4. COMPARISON OF THE THREE MAJOR BACTERIAL PNEUMONIAS

PNEUMOCOCCAL PNEUMONIA	STAPHYLOCOCCAL PNEUMONIA	STREPTOCOCCAL PNEUMONIA
Epidemiology		
Most common agent in lobar pneumonia	Most common agent in bronchopneumonia	Less common than other bacterial pneumonias
Occurs most often in late winter and early spring	Greatest incidence in first 2 years of life	Usually occurs as complication of influenza or measles
Highest attack rate during the first 4 years and declines with increasing age	Occurs most often in winter months	
Uncommon in infants less than 1 year of age	Usually contracted as primary infection	
	Cross-contamination common in hospitals	
Pathology		
Usually lobar but may be lobular	Localized abscesses in older children; more diffuse in infants	Interstitial bronchopneumonia
Untreated cases progress through four stages:	Exotoxin causes necrosis and sloughing of bronchial mucous membranes	Spreads via lymphatics
Engorgement	Formation of peribronchial abscesses	Although usually lobular, areas of consolidation may coalesce to become lobar
Red heparinization	Pneumatocele formation	
Gray heparinization		
Resolution		
Clinical manifestations		
Infants	Usually in infants less than age 1 year, often with history of staphylococcal skin lesion	May appear without evidence of illness
Fretfulness and diminished appetite followed by abrupt onset of fever	Abrupt onset of fever, listlessness and lethargy when undisturbed, irritability on arousal, anorexia, nasal discharge, cough; grunting respirations, progressively severe dyspnea that may include subcostal and sternal retractions and cyanosis	Symptoms similar to those of pneumococcal pneumonia
May be accompanied by convulsions		Onset sudden
Restlessness, apprehension, respiratory distress, appears acutely ill, flushed cheeks, circumoral cyanosis	Shocklike state may be present	High temperature
Decreased breath sounds and crackling rales; exaggerated breath sounds on opposite side; pleural friction rub may be heard	Symptoms of complications, for example, pneumothorax, empyema, septicemia, and so on	Chills
Older children	Some infants have gastrointestinal disturbances, for example, vomiting, diarrhea, and sometimes abdominal distention	Signs of respiratory distress
Usually follows an upper respiratory tract infection	Rapid progression of symptoms characteristic	At times, extreme prostration
Shaking chill followed by high fever, chest pain, tachypnea		Occasionally, only mild symptoms
Drowsiness with intermittent periods of restlessness, anxiety		Tachypnea, usually mild
Occasionally, delirium		Rales generally unilateral and exaggerated by deep inspiration

Continued.

TABLE 20-4. COMPARISON OF THE THREE MAJOR BACTERIAL PNEUMONIAS—cont'd

PNEUMOCOCCAL PNEUMONIA	STAPHYLOCOCCAL PNEUMONIA	STREPTOCOCCAL PNEUMONIA
Clinical manifestations		
Circumoral cyanosis	Chest—early, diminished breath sounds, rales, and rhonchi with effusion or pneumothorax; dullness on percussion; respiratory lag on affected side; exaggerated excursion on opposite side	
Hacking, unproductive cough (initially)		
Splinting of side caused by pleurisy pain		
Chest—dullness; diminished breath sounds, tactile and vocal fremitus; consolidation on second or third day evidenced by dullness, increased fremitus, tubular breath sounds, and disappearance of rales		
With resolution—moist rales; productive cough with large amounts of blood-tinged mucus		
Antibiotic therapy		
Pneumococcus highly susceptible to penicillin G and therefore the preferred drug	Methicillin parenterally	Penicillin G (IV or IM) is highly effective
Alternate drugs—ampicillin, tetracycline, chloramphenicol, erythromycin, and sulfonamides	Equally effective are oxacillin, cloxacillin, dicloxacillin, or nafcillin	
Resolution begins about 24 hours after initiation of therapy	For penicillin-sensitive organisms, penicillin G may be given	
	Duration of treatment usually 3 weeks	

to prevent possible aspiration. To prevent dehydration, fluids are frequently administered intravenously during the acute phase. Oral fluids, if allowed, are given cautiously to avoid aspiration and to decrease the possibility of aggravating a fatiguing cough.

The child is placed in a mist tent with oxygen. Cool mist moistens the airways, helps mobilize secretions, reduces bronchial edema, and provides a cool atmosphere that aids in temperature reduction. The child often requires frequent clothing and linen changes to prevent chilling in the damp atmosphere. He is usually more comfortable in a semi-erect position but should be allowed to determine his position of comfort. Lying on the affected side (if pneumonia is unilateral) splints the chest on that side and reduces the pleural rubbing that often causes discomfort.

Fever is usually controlled by the cool environment and administration of antipyretic drugs as prescribed. Temperature is monitored regularly to detect a rapid rise that might trigger a febrile seizure.

Vital signs and chest sounds are monitored to assess the progress of the disease and to detect early signs of complications. Children with ineffectual cough or those with difficulty in handling secretions, especially infants, will require suctioning to maintain a patent airway. A simple bulb syringe is usually sufficient for clearing the nares and nasopharynx of infants, but a suction machine should be readily available if needed. Older children can usually handle secretions without assistance. Percussion, vibration, and suctioning or drainage are generally prescribed every 4 hours or more often depending on the child's condition.

The child in the hospital is apprehensive, and many of the treatments and tests are frightening and stress producing. Reducing anxiety and apprehension not only reduces psychologic distress in the child but, when the child is more relaxed, the respiratory efforts are lessened. Easing respiratory efforts makes the child less apprehensive, and encouraging the presence of the caregiver provides the child with his customary source of comfort and support.

PULMONARY DYSFUNCTION CAUSED BY NONINFECTIOUS IRRITANTS

Inflammation of lung tissue can occur occasionally as the result of irritation from foreign material. Aspiration of

SUMMARY OF NURSING CARE OF THE CHILD WITH PNEUMONIA

GOALS	RESPONSIBILITIES
Promote rest	Maintain rest in bed Organize nursing care to disturb as little as possible Remove or minimize sources of anxiety Administer sedatives as indicated if ordered for restlessness and pain Avoid stimulating excessive coughing
Maintain patent airway	Administer nothing by mouth during acute stage of dyspnea Promote drainage of secretions from airway Suction secretions as needed Carry out percussion, vibration, and drainage and/or suctioning Prevent aspiration of secretions
Ease respiratory efforts	Promote rest Maintain patent airway Provide high-humidity atmosphere Position for comfort Administer oxygen as needed Reduce anxiety Organize activities to allow for minimal expenditure of energy
Control fever	Provide cool environment Administer antipyretics as indicated Monitor temperature to detect status of temperature

Prevent dehydration	Administer intravenous fluid as prescribed
	   Monitor intravenous infusion for patency
	   Regulate intravenous infusion rate
	Observe for signs of dehydration
	Monitor intake, output, urine specific gravity, and daily weight
	Encourage fluids when tolerated

Determine causative organisms	Collect specimens, as needed Assist with diagnostic procedures
Control causative organisms	Administer antimicrobial medications if prescribed Support body's natural defenses
Provide nutrition	Encourage high-calorie fluids when tolerated, then progress to diet as tolerated

Monitor respiratory status	Observe respiratory rate and pattern
	Auscultate to determine
	   Breath sounds
	   Presence of rales, rhonchi, wheezing
	   Areas of consolidation
	Assess
	   Skin color
	   Presence or absence of retractions, nasal flaring

Reduce anxiety and apprehension	Provide constant attendance during acute phase of illness Encourage presence of the parents Provide comfort and cuddling when possible Remove restraining devices when and as often as possible Provide quiet diversion appropriate to the child's age and condition

Detect complications early	Carry out periodic assessment of respiratory status
	Change position every 2 hours
	Observe for signs of
	   Chest pain
	   Abdominal pain
	   Dyspnea
	   Pallor or cyanosis

food, oral secretions, smoke or other substances by otherwise healthy infants or children can set up an inflammatory response or chemical pneumonia. Young children are especially prone to aspiration of foreign substances, and weak and debilitated children are subject to aspiration of food or secretions. The major problems associated with aspiration in children are asphyxia or respiratory tract inflammation as the result of inhaling foreign material. Medical and nursing care of a subsequent pneumonitis and/or bronchitis are similar to that for lower respiratory tract inflammation resulting from infectious agents.

FOREIGN BODY (FB) IN THE NARES

Foreign bodies, such as pebbles, erasers, beads, lentils, and wads of paper, are frequently placed in the nose by children. The initial symptoms are usually sneezing, mild discomfort, and local obstruction followed by irritation from mucosal swelling. Objects that absorb moisture, such as beans, swell and increase obstruction and discomfort. Succeeding infection causes a purulent, malodorous, or bloody discharge. If the discharge and obstruction are unilateral, a foreign body should be suspected.

Treatment is early removal to prevent aspiration or damage to mucosal tissues. The object is ordinarily situated anteriorly but attempts at removal by unskilled persons may force it deeper into the nasal passages. Infection usually clears promptly following removal and requires no further treatment. Therefore, the nurse should refer the family to a physician for removal of any suspected foreign object in the nose.

FOREIGN BODY (FB) ASPIRATION

Small children characteristically explore matter with their mouths and are, therefore, particularly prone to aspirate a foreign body into the air passages. Aspiration of a foreign object can occur at any age but is seen most commonly in children between 6 months and 5 years of age. The signs and changes produced depend on the degree of obstruction and the nature of the object. For example, dry vegetable matter, such as a seed, nut, or piece of carrot or popcorn, that does not dissolve and may swell when wet creates a particularly difficult problem (fun foods are the worst offenders). A food that has caused several deaths is the hot dog. Because its diameter, shape, and consistency allow for complete occlusion of the airway, when offered to children it should be cut into small pieces—not served whole. Balloons, portions of balloons, and bubble gum pose serious threats. A sharp or irritating object produces irritation and edema. A small object may cause little if any pathologic changes, whereas an object of sufficient size to ob-

struct a passage can produce various changes, including atelectasis, emphysema, inflammation, and abscess.

Clinical manifestations

Initially a foreign body in the air passages produces choking, gagging, wheezing, or coughing. After the initial period there is often an interval of hours, days, or even weeks without symptoms. Secondary symptoms are related to the anatomic area in which the object is lodged and are usually caused by a persistent respiratory infection focused distal to the obstruction. A foreign body is always a possibility in acute or chronic pulmonary lesions.

The most common symptoms of laryngotracheal obstruction are dyspnea, cough, and inspiratory stridor. When the object is lodged in the larynx there is inability to speak. An object in the bronchi produces cough, decreased airway entry, wheezing, and dyspnea. A nonobstructive, nonirritating object may cause few symptoms; an obstructive object quickly produces pathologic changes; a slight obstruction may only be evidenced by a wheeze.

Diagnostic evaluation

The diagnosis of foreign body aspiration is usually suspected on the basis of history and physical signs. Radiographic examination reveals opaque foreign bodies but may be of limited use in localizing vegetable matter. Bronchoscopy is usually required for definitive diagnosis of an object in the larynx and trachea. Fluoroscopic examination is a valuable aid in detecting and localizing an object in the bronchi.

Therapeutic management

A foreign body is rarely coughed up spontaneously; therefore, it must be removed instrumentally by direct laryngoscopy or bronchoscopy. This should be carried out as soon as possible since the progressive local inflammatory process triggered by the foreign material hampers removal, a chemical pneumonia soon develops, and vegetable matter begins to macerate within a few days, causing it to be even more difficult to remove. Some advocate removal with a Foley catheter inserted to a point beyond the object, inflated, and used to draw the object into the bronchoscope or withdrawn simultaneously with the scope. After removal of the object, the child is placed in a high-humidity atmosphere and any secondary infection is treated with appropriate antibiotics.

Nursing considerations

The primary treatment for aspiration of foreign substances is prevention. Small children should not be allowed access to enticing small objects that they might place in their mouth. Children younger than 2½ years of age should not be allowed whole hot dogs, nuts, popcorn, or whole-kernel corn. Proper feeding techniques should be carried out for weak, debilitated, and uncooperative children and preventive measures used to prevent aspiration of any material that might enter the nasopharynx. Solid foods are not introduced until the child is old enough to handle them and has teeth for proper chewing. Thorough chewing, not talking while chewing, and cutting solid food into bite-size pieces should be emphasized. Children should not be permitted to eat or place small items in their mouths while lying on the floor or while they are overactive. Oily nose drops and oil-based vitamin preparations are not appropriate for infants and small children. Solvents, lighter fluid, and other hydrocarbon substances should be kept away from older infants and small children who are apt to put anything in their mouths and who may be attracted by their slightly sweet taste. (see p. 630 for management of choking.)

Prevention

Nurses, as child advocates, are in a position to teach prevention in a variety of settings. They can educate parents, singly or in groups, about hazards of aspiration in relation to the developmental level of their children and encourage them to teach their children safety. Parents teach by example; therefore, they should be cautioned about behaviors that their children might imitate, for example, holding foreign objects, such as pins, nails, toothpicks, and so on, in their lips or mouths. Infants and debilitated children should be positioned on the abdomen or the right side after feedings to minimize the possibility of aspirating vomitus or regurgitated feeding. Nurses are major forces in education for accident prevention (see the segments on accident prevention in Chapters 8, 10, 11, 13, and 14).

ASPIRATION PNEUMONIA

Aspiration of fluid or food substances is a particular hazard in the child who has difficulty with or is unable to swallow because of paralysis, weakness, debility, congenital anomalies such as cleft palate or tracheoesophageal fistula, absent cough reflex (unconscious), or who is force fed, especially while crying or breathing rapidly. The newborn may develop a severe pneumonia from aspirating amniotic fluid and debris during the birth process. Rarely aspiration causes immediate death from asphyxia; more often the irritated mucous membrane becomes a site for secondary bacterial infection. In addition to fluids, food, vomitus, and nasopharyngeal secretions, other substances that cause pneumonia when aspirated are hydrocarbons, lipids, or powder (rare).

Hydrocarbon pneumonia

Children frequently develop pneumonia secondary to the ingestion of various forms of hydrocarbons, such as kerosene, gasoline, solvents, and lighter fluid. Coughing and vomiting occur almost immediately after ingestion and probably contribute to aspiration. Central nervous system symptoms may consist of agitation and restlessness, confusion, drowsiness, or coma. The temperature is elevated.

Inducing the child to vomit is contraindicated because of the renewed danger of aspiration. Bronchitis or pneumonia usually develop early (within the first 24 hours) but may be delayed. Recovery from pulmonary involvement occurs in most instances despite a severe clinical course. Death, if it occurs, is generally the result of hepatic failure complicated by pulmonary factors. Treatment is the same as for any lower respiratory tract inflammation and consists of high humidity, oxygen, hydration, and treatment of any secondary infection.

Lipid pneumonia

Oily substances aspirated into the respiratory passages cause inflammation of the lung tissues. There are no characteristic manifestations. Cough is usually present, and dyspnea is seen in severe cases. Secondary bronchopneumonia infections are common. The outcome depends on the extent of pulmonary damage, the general condition of the infant, and discontinuance of the oily inhalation. There is no specific treatment.

Powder

Although the use of powder has been discouraged for infants, a significant number of infants still suffer talcum powder aspiration. The true incidence is unknown but in those children with respiratory distress serious enough to require medical attention, the mortality is high. Treatment is symptomatic.

Nursing considerations

Since inhalation of foreign substances produces an inflammation of lung and airway tissues, nursing care is essentially the same as for any child with pneumonia.

NEAR DROWNING

Drowning is not an uncommon accident in childhood. Of accidental deaths from drowning, the majority are children between ages 10 and 19 years but a significant number are infants under 3 years of age. Most are accidental, usually involving children who are helpless in water, such as inadequately attended children in or near swimming pools or infants in bathtubs; small children who fall into ponds, streams, and flooded excavations, usually near home; occupants of pleasure boats who fail to wear life preservers; diving accidents; and children who are able to swim but overestimate their endurance. With expeditious treatment many children can and are being saved. To clarify this discussion, two terms need clarification

> **drowning** death from asphyxia while submerged, regardless of whether fluid has entered the lungs
>
> **near drowning** survival at least 24 hours after submersion in a fluid medium

Pathophysiology

The changes that occur in drowning are directly related to the length of submersion (regardless of the type and amount of fluid aspirated), the physiologic response of the victim, and the development and degree of immersion hypothermia. The major difficulty is acute ventilatory insufficiency. Approximately 10% of drowning victims die without aspirating fluid but succumb from acute asphyxia as a result of prolonged reflex laryngospasm. Simple asphyxia is the primary cause of death when fluid is aspirated.

Resistance to asphyxia and anoxia appears to be age-related; the younger the child, the better he can tolerate hypoxia. Perhaps more important is the drowning, or diving, reflex that is triggered by immersion of the face in cold water. Blood is shunted away from the periphery and viscera, and the flow is concentrated to the brain and heart predominantly. Consequently, although it may appear to be severely damaged, the brain has the potential for recovery.

Immersion in cold water produces a significant and slow fall in body temperature, which slows metabolism and decreases the body's need for oxygen. The most common reaction to immersion in cold water is the development of hypothermia and loss of consciousness. Infants and children, with their relatively large surface develop hypothermia very rapidly.

Older children are sometimes victims of hypoxia before aspiration of fluid as a result of shallow-water blackout or holding their breath while diving. For example, older children and teenagers blackout when they attempt to swim long distances (several lengths of the pool) underwater. Before entering the water, the youngster hyperventilates, which reduces respiratory stimulation from carbon dioxide accumulation and stretch receptors in the lung. The cerebral hypoxia causes the youngster to lose consciousness before he has the desire to surface for air. Often these youngsters are found dead at the bottom of a lake or pool.

Therapeutic management

Resuscitative measures should begin at the scene of the near drowning and the victim transported to the hospital with maximum support. If the victim is one of the 10% who does not aspirate water, is rescued and resuscitated before circulatory arrest, and does not suffer damage to the central nervous system, recovery should be complete. Many need care for some time after aspiration of fluid. In the hospital, intensive pulmonary care is implemented and continued according to the needs of the patient. A spontaneously breathing child will do well in an oxygen-enriched atmosphere, whereas the more severely affected child will require endotracheal intubation and mechanical ventilation. Blood gases and pH are monitored frequently as a guide to oxygen, fluid, and electrolyte therapies.

Salvaging cerebral function is one of the primary goals of therapy and takes priority over treatment of other body systems. In the unconscious patient the intracranial pressure is monitored and the fever that commonly follows near drowning is reduced by hypothermia to reduce total oxygen requirements. Sedatives are administered to protect the brain from any movements, grunting, and straining that often accompany acute brain damage and which tend to raise intracranial pressure (see Chapter 25 for care of the child with cerebral damage).

Because of the frequency of complications after near drowning, any patient should be hospitalized for 48 hours for observation. Aspiration pneumonia is a frequent complication that occurs about 48 to 72 hours after the episode. The child who suffers from prolonged hypoxia is in danger of irreversible central nervous system damage, which then becomes a neurologic problem after recovery from pulmonary disturbances.

Nursing considerations

Nursing intervention depends on whether the child is a near drowning or a drowning victim. If he survives, he may need intensive respiratory nursing care with attention to vital signs, mechanical ventilation and/or tracheostomy, intracranial pressure monitoring, blood gas determination, chest therapy, and intravenous infusion. In some instances the child is comatose for an indefinite period of time and requires the same care as an unconscious child (p. 816).

If the child dies, the principal intervention is emotional support of the family. The sudden, unexpected nature of the death and the particular circumstances of the accident, especially in terms of guilt for not preventing it, compound the grief for these individuals (see Chapter 16).

Prevention

Every child should be taught to swim. Even very young children can learn to handle themselves in the water sufficiently to avoid panic and to propel themselves to safety until they can be removed from the water. Water safety and survival training should be required for all school-age children, and nurses can be active advocates in their communities. Nurses are also in a position to emphasize the importance of adequate adult supervision when children are in the water. Young children should never be left unattended when in the water.

INHALATION INJURY

A number of noxious substances that may be inhaled are toxic to humans. They are primarily products of incomplete combustion and are believed to cause more deaths from fires than flame injuries. The severity of the injury depends on the nature of the substances generated by the material being burned and whether the victim is confined in a closed space. Inhaled substances produce injuries in two ways: (1) some noxious gases and particles cause irritation, inflammation, and damage to pulmonary tissues, and (2) others produce their effect systemically.

Noxious irritants

A wide variety of gases may be generated during the combustion of materials such as clothing, furniture, and floor coverings. The synthetic materials are especially toxic. Irritant gases such as nitrous oxide or carbon dioxide combine with water in the lungs to form corrosive acids; aldehydes cause denaturation of proteins, cellular damage, and edema of pulmonary tissues.

Possible inhalation injury is suspected when there is a history of flames in a closed space whether burns are present or not. Sooty material around the nose or in the sputum, singed nasal hairs, or mucosal burns of the nose, lips, mouth, or throat are all signs that the affected person demands observation for possible pulmonary injury from inhalants. A hoarse voice and cough, inspiratory and expiratory stridor, and signs of respiratory distress are further evidence of airway involvement.

Passive inhalation. There is increasing evidence that children in families with cigarette smokers ''passively'' inhale sufficient smoke to adversely affect their health. Children living in these families (especially in families where the mother smokes) show lower performance of pulmonary function tests, have an increased number of respiratory infections, and develop symptoms of rhinitis and asthma at an earlier age than children in nonsmoking households. It may be a factor in the development of chronic lung disease in later life. Therefore, it is important that nurses and other health workers continue to include anti-smoking efforts as part of health education of parents and children.

Carbon monoxide

Carbon monoxide is an extremely dangerous gas and is responsible for more than half of all fatal poisonings in the United States. It is a colorless, odorless gas with an affinity for hemoglobin 230 times greater than that of oxygen. Carbon monoxide combines readily with hemoglobin to form carboxyhemoglobin (COHb), but is released less readily. Therefore, tissue hypoxia reaches dangerous levels before oxygen is available to meet tissue needs.

Accidental poisoning is most often the result of exposure to fumes of heaters or smoke from structural fires, although poorly ventilated recreational vehicles with improperly operated or maintained gas lamps or stoves and cooking in underventilated areas with charcoal grills or hibachis are also frequent causes. Carbon monoxide is produced by incomplete combustion of carbon or carbonaceous material such as wood or charcoal.

The signs and symptoms of carbon monoxide poisoning are secondary to tissue hypoxia and vary with the level of carboxyhemoglobin. Mild manifestations may produce headache, visual disturbances, irritability, and nausea, whereas more severe intoxication causes confusion, hallucinations, ataxia, and coma. The bright, cherry-red lips and skin often described are less often observed; pallor and cyanosis are seen more frequently.

Therapeutic management

When inhalation injury is suspected, the patient is given humidified 100% oxygen by mask until carboxyhemoglobin levels fall to the nontoxic range, and artificial ventilation may be implemented in selected cases. Where a hyperbaric oxygen chamber is available, the breakdown of the carbon monoxide-hemoglobin bond is greatly accelerated.

Respiratory distress may occur early in the course of smoke inhalation as a result of hypoxia, or patients who are breathing well on admission may later develop sudden respiratory distress. Therefore, intubation and/or tracheostomy equipment should be available at the bedside. There is a good deal of controversy regarding tracheostomy, but many prefer this procedure when the obstruction is proximal to the larynx and reserve nasotracheal intubation for lower tract involvement.

Use of corticosteroids, although controversial, may be of value in reducing edema, and bronchodilators (usually isoproterenol) are often given intravenously or by nebulizer. A broad-spectrum antibiotic is sometimes administered prophylactically but this too is controversial.

Nursing considerations

Nursing care of the child with inhalation injury is the same as that for any child with respiratory distress. Vital signs and other respiratory assessments are performed frequently, and the pulmonary status is carefully observed and maintained. Pulmonary physical therapy is usually part of the therapeutic program, and mechanical ventilation or periodic intermittent positive-pressure breathing with bronchodilators is employed.

In addition to the observation and management of the physical aspects of inhalation injury, the nurse also deals with the psychologic needs of a frightened child and distraught parents. As with any accidental injury, the parents feel overwhelming guilt, even when the accident occurred through no fault of their own. More often, however, the accident could have been prevented, which compounds their guilt feelings. They need a great deal of support and reassurance, as well as information regarding the child's condition, treatment, and progress.

LONG-TERM RESPIRATORY PROBLEMS

There are some respiratory disorders that, although they may have acute episodes, are primarily long-term conditions. Children and families must adjust to the effects of these disorders including the way in which they can alter the lifestyle of the families. The most common of these long-term respiratory disorders are bronchial asthma and cystic fibrosis.

BRONCHIAL ASTHMA

Bronchial asthma is a reversible obstructive process characterized by an increased responsiveness of the airway, especially the lower respiratory tract. It is manifest by labored breathing, bilateral wheezing, prolonged expiration, and an irritative tight cough caused by a reduction in the diameter of the airway. The symptoms can vary from a mild cough to severe respiratory distress with hypoxemia, retention of carbon dioxide, and respiratory acidosis that may result in prostration and even fatal asphyxia.

Asthma is a common disorder and one of the leading causes of chronic illness in childhood. It is believed by many to be the single most important cause of morbidity in childhood.

Etiology

The usual cause of the asthmatic manifestations is an allergic hypersensitivity to foreign substances, usually those carried in the air, such as plant pollens. However, in some instances no allergic process can be detected. Most asthma in children is caused by an allergic reaction in the bronchi, but there may be nonallergic causes such as bronchial compression from external pressure, a foreign body in the airway, a diffuse endobronchial inflammation, or postexercise bronchial constriction.

There is a heritable tendency in asthma. In approximately 75% of children with asthma there is a positive family history with an immediate family member manifesting some form of allergy. Usually the child has other manifestations of allergy such as nasal allergy (hay fever), eczema, or urticaria. Frequently there is a history of eczema in early childhood.

Pathophysiology

There is general agreement that heightened airway reactivity is characteristic of children with asthma. The reasons for this are less clear, and most theories do not explain all types and causes of asthma. However, the mechanisms responsible for the obstructive symptoms of asthma are (Fig. 20-1):

1. Edema of the mucous membranes
2. Accumulation of tenacious secretions from mucous glands
3. Spasm of the smooth muscle of the bronchi and bronchioles, which decreases the caliber of the bronchioles

The role that each of these mechanisms plays varies from patient to patient, and during the course of the disease in a given patient. In some patients, smooth muscle contraction is the major factor early in the episode, followed by mucosal edema and increased mucous secretion. In others the sequence of the responses is reversed.

Many of the stimuli that provoke asthmatic episodes may do so by being directly toxic or irritative, such as smoke, fumes, odors, or infection, by eliciting the immune response, or by a combination of mechanisms. Other factors that contribute to the responses are rapid changes in environmental temperature (especially cold), physical stress (fatigue, exertion), psychologic stress (tension, fear, anxiety), or infections in the respiratory tract or nearby structures (such as the ears or sinuses).

Bronchial constriction is a normal reaction to foreign stimuli, but in the asthmatic child it is abnormally severe, producing impaired respiratory function. The smooth muscle, arranged in spiral bundles around the airway, causes narrowing and shortening of the airway, which significantly increases airway resistance to airflow. Since the bronchi normally dilate and elongate during inspiration and contract and shorten on expiration, the respiratory difficulty is more pronounced during the expiratory phase of respiration.

Increased resistance in the airway causes forced expi-

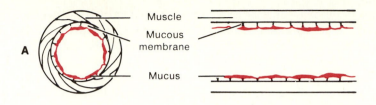

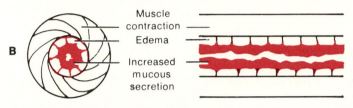

FIG. 20-1

Mechanisms of obstruction in asthma. **A,** *Normal bronchus.* **B,** *Asthmatic bronchus.*

ration through the narrowed lumen. The volume of air trapped in the lungs increases as airways are functionally closed at a point between the alveoli and the lobar bronchi by the combined mechanisms just described. This trapping of gas forces the individual to breathe at a higher and higher lung volume. Consequently the person with asthma fights to inspire sufficient air. This expenditure of effort for breathing causes fatigue, decreased respiratory effectiveness, and increased oxygen consumption. Also, the inspiration occurring at higher lung volumes hyperinflates the alveoli and reduces the effectiveness of the cough. The child becomes progressively dyspneic, cyanotic, and tachypneic. As the severity of obstruction increases, there is a reduced alveolar ventilation with carbon dioxide retention, hypoxemia, respiratory acidosis, and, eventually, respiratory failure.

Clinical manifestations

Children with bronchial asthma may show signs and experience symptoms that range from acute episodes of shortness of breath, wheezing, and cough followed by a quiet period to a relatively continuous pattern of chronic symptoms that fluctuate in severity. The onset of an attack may develop gradually or appear abruptly and may be preceded by an upper respiratory infection. The age of the child is often a significant factor, since the onset of most cases occurs between ages 3 and 8 years. In infancy an attack usually follows respiratory infection.

An asthmatic episode usually begins with a hacking, paroxysmal, irritative, and nonproductive cough caused by bronchial edema. Accumulated secretions, acting as a foreign body, stimulate the cough. As the secretions become more profuse, the cough becomes rattling and productive of frothy, clear, gelatinous sputum. Bronchial spasm and mucosal edema reduce the size of the bronchial lumen, which is, as a result, more easily occluded by mucous plugs.

The child appears short of breath, he tries to breathe more deeply, and the expiratory phase becomes prolonged and is accompanied by an audible wheezing. He often appears pale but may have a malar flush and red ears. His lips assume a deep, dark red color that may progress to cyanosis observed in the nail beds and skin, especially around the mouth. The child is restless and apprehensive, and his facial expression is anxious. Sweating may be prominent as the attack progresses. Older children have a tendency to sit upright with shoulders in a hunched-over position, hands on the bed or chair, and arms braced to facilitate the use of accessory muscles of respiration. The child speaks with short, panting, broken phrases. Infants and small children are restless, irritable, and difficult to make comfortable.

Examination of the chest reveals hyperresonance on percussion. Breath sounds are course and loud, with sonorous rales throughout the lung fields. Expiration is prolonged. Coarse rhonchi, as well as generalized inspiratory and expiratory wheezing that becomes more high pitched as obstruction progresses, can be heard. With minimal obstruction, wheezing may be only slight or even absent, but it can be accentuated by rapid, deep breathing.

With severe spasm or obstruction, breath sounds and rales may become almost audible. Cough is ineffective despite repeated, hacking maneuvers. This represents lack of air movement and may be misinterpreted as improvement by unknowing examiners. Shallow or irregular respirations and a sudden rise in the rate of respiration are ominous signs indicating ventilatory failure and imminent asphyxia.

With repeated episodes the thoracic cavity becomes fixed in a hyperventilated state (barrel chest) with depressed diaphragm, elevated shoulders, and use of accessory muscles of respiration. The child's face takes on a typical appearance with flattened malar bones, circles beneath the eyes, narrow nose, and prominent upper teeth.

Diagnostic evaluation

The diagnosis is determined on the basis of clinical manifestations, history, physical examination, and, to a lesser extent, laboratory tests. Radiographic examinations are used primarily to rule out other diseases and to evaluate coexisting disease. Sputum examination shows large numbers of eosinophils and colorless crystalloid fragments representing degenerations of eosinophils—Charcot-Leyden crystals, a unique feature of asthma.

Therapeutic management: acute

Acute attacks of asthma are a medical emergency. The goal is to control the acute attack; therefore, early recognition and treatment at the onset are most important. Rapid relief of the bronchospasm reduces the need for drastic measures and increases the likelihood that relief will be complete. Objectives of therapy for an acute asthmatic attack are to relieve bronchial obstruction by dilating the bronchi, reducing the mucosal edema, and removing excess bronchial secretions. Supportive measures include maintenance of adequate hydration, prevention and relief of fatigue, and treatment of coexisting bacterial infection.

Relieve bronchial obstruction. Rapid-acting bronchodilators are the major therapeutic tools for the relief of bronchospasm. The most important of these are described here.

Epinephrine (Adrenalin) is probably the most important drug in treatment of an acute severe attack. Subcutaneous administration of 0.01 ml/kg/dose (maximum 0.5 ml) of 1:1000 aqueous solution rapidly relieves most cases of acute bronchospasm. Duration of action is short; therefore, if there is no relief, the dose is repeated in 20 minutes two or four times. If there is no relief after three to four doses, the drug is discontinued. Since the drug is readily destroyed by light, only preparations that are stored in dark glass vials should be used. Brownish discoloration or the formation of sediment is an indication of deterioration. The side effects of epinephrine are tachycardia, elevated blood pressure, pallor, weakness, tremors, and nausea. An aerosol form is available for use in nebulizers but is not generally recommended for children because of the overdependency it produces.

Sus-Phrine, also given subcutaneously, is composed of 50% epinephrine for immediate effect and 80% crystalline epinephrine, which is released slowly over 4 to 8 hours to prolong the immediate effect. The dose is 0.05 to 0.3 ml of 1:200 solution.

Isoproterenol (Isuprel) gives rapid relief when administered by intermittent positive-pressure breathing to relieve severe asthma in the hospital. Isoproterenol potentiates the side effects of epinephrine and should not be given within 1 hour after administration of epinephrine or Sus-Phrine.

Ephedrine is an effective, but less potent, bronchodilator with a more prolonged action than epinephrine; therefore, it is better suited to preventing a mild episode from progressing to a severe attack. It is usually administered orally, often combined with phenobarbital to minimize the side effects. It is also combined with theophylline.

Isoetharine (Bronkosol-2) is used for administration by intermittent positive-pressure breathing, 0.5 ml in 2 ml normal saline every 4 hours.

Theophylline and *aminophylline* are probably the most effective and versatile asthmatic drugs. They are prepared for intravenous, intramuscular, oral, or rectal administration. *Theophylline* is given in doses of 5 mg/kg every 6 hours and then increased slowly, if needed, to maximum tolerance. *Aminophylline* is 85% theophylline and is given in corresponding doses. Use of the intravenous route is recommended for hospitalized children only.

Reduce mucosal edema. The principal agents for reducing edema are the corticosteroids; their antiinflammatory effect diminishes the inflammatory component of asthma and thereby reduces the airway obstruction. The drugs can be given intravenously, orally, or topically by aerosol. Results may not be apparent for up to 6 hours.

Although corticosteroids are useful drugs, there are dangers of steroid dependency and undesirable side effects, including cushingoid changes, increased susceptibility to infection, and growth suppression. When steroids are used over a long period of time, they are gradually reduced to the smallest possible maintenance dose, then discontinued as soon as possible. *Hydrocortisone (Solu-Cortef)* and *methylprednisolone (Solu-Medrol)* are the preferred intravenous preparations, and *prednisone,* which is short acting in terms of suppression of adrenal function, is the preferred oral preparation. Long-acting varieties are *triamcinolone, betamethasone,* and *dexamethasone.*

Remove excess bronchial secretions. An important aspect of asthma therapy is the use of expectorants. Oral administration of *saturated solution of potassium iodide (SSKI)* (1 drop per year of age in water or juice, three times a day); *guaifenesin (glyceryl guaiacolate [Robitussin])* usually given in syrup form, (5 ml, three times a day); or *ipecac syrup* (in subemetic dosage) is frequently helpful for mobilizing mucous secretions. Mucolytic agents such as *acetylcysteine (Mucomyst)* may be administered in conjunction with nebulization.

Other drugs are used in treatment of asthma in addition to those that affect the bronchial tree directly. Infection is frequently the triggering mechanism in cases of bronchial asthma in children; therefore, antibiotic therapy is an important part of overall management. Mild sedatives such as *phenobarbital* and *chloral hydrate* orally or rectally or the tranquilizer *hydroxyzine (Vistaril, Atarax)* is frequently employed to reduce anxiety and provide relaxation.

Status asthmaticus.   Children who continue to display respiratory distress despite vigorous therapeutic measures, especially injections of epinephrine, are considered to be in status asthmaticus. The condition may develop gradually or rapidly, often with complicating conditions such as pneumonia that can influence the duration and treatment of the attack. These children are acutely ill and require hospitalization, preferably where intensive care is available. They need continuous nursing attendance with frequent monitoring and observation.

Therapy of status asthmaticus is directed toward correction of dehydration and acidosis, improvement of ventilation, and treatment of any concurrent infection. The child is given intravenous fluids and nothing by mouth except liquids if his condition permits. The intravenous infusion provides a means for hydration, liquefying secretions, and administering medications. Humidified oxygen is administered by tent, face mask, or cannula, according to the individual needs of the child. Antibiotics and mild sedatives are also given as needed.

As the attack subsides, fluids and medication are given orally and postural drainage and breathing exercises are done to help remove secretions. Administration of steroids is discontinued as rapidly as possible.

Therapeutic management: long range

The long-range goal in management of asthma in children is to assist the child to live as normal and happy a life as possible. To accomplish this, efforts are extended to determine the cause of the attacks, prevent or control the attacks, and help the child to deal constructively with the disease. Basic to any therapeutic plan is an evaluation of the child's general health and an assessment of the specific allergenic factors and the nonspecific factors that precipitate symptoms. Specific allergens are identified with protein-allergen extracts, usually by direct skin tests using the scratch or intradermal technique.

Allergen control.   Once the specific allergens are identified and confirmed, steps are taken to eliminate or avoid the offending allergens. Often simply removing environmental factors will provide protection from attacks,

for example, removal of a dog or cat from the home of a child sensitive to dogs or cats. Allergenic foods are eliminated from the diet. Nonspecific factors that may trigger an attack, such as extremes of temperature, are sometimes controlled by humidifiers or air conditioners, and the child can be helped to develop a tolerance to temperature fluctuations by gradual or systematic exposure to temperature differences.

Medications.   Most children do not require medication continuously. Parents and older asthmatic children are taught to implement therapy at the onset of symptoms or when they will be exposed to symptom-provoking situations. Bronchodilators such as *metaproterenol* or *terbutaline* in aerosol sprays provide quick relief and are effective in controlling an attack at the onset, but the child and the parents need careful instruction in their use. Oral administration, although somewhat slower, is a safer mode of administration, especially in younger children.

Children with persistent and continuous asthma receive bronchodilators around the clock, usually theophylline, prescribed alone or combined with an expectorant to be taken three times daily and at bedtime. Corticosteroids are given to the majority of children with chronic asthma, administered on intermittent days to minimize the undesirable side effects.

A relatively recent drug used in asthma treatment is *cromolyn sodium*. Neither a bronchodilator nor an antiinflammatory agent, cromolyn sodium acts superficially to inhibit the release of chemical mediators, especially histamine, in the human lung. The action is essentially prophylactic and is of no value when administered after the allergic reaction. Its chief value is to prevent an attack, and it is especially useful in preventing exercise-induced bronchospasm.

Physical therapy.   Physical therapy is one of the standard adjuncts to treatment of chronic asthma. This includes chest physical therapy, breathing exercises, physical training, and inhalation therapy. These therapies help to produce physical and mental relaxation, improve posture, strengthen respiratory musculature, and develop more efficient patterns of breathing. Postural drainage, which includes percussion, vibration, deep breathing, and assisted coughing, helps to clear mucus from the bronchial tree. For the motivated child, breathing exercises and controlled breathing are of value in preventing overinflation and in improving the strength of respiratory muscles and the efficiency of the cough. Stretch exercises sometimes help to increase the flexibility of the ribs. Sit-ups and leg exercises strengthen abdominal muscles and aid expiration.

Exercise.   Vigorous physical activity is frequently followed by an asthmatic attack; therefore, many children choose a sedentary existence. This can seriously hamper peer interaction. It has been found that moderate exercise is advantageous for children with asthma. Selection of activities that do not overtax the respiratory mechanism and use of inhalant bronchodilators prior to activity allow the asthmatic child to participate in a variety of sports and activities. Asthmatic children can tolerate exercise that involves stopping and starting activities, such as baseball, skiing, and short sprints, but that they do not tolerate activities that involve endurance exercise, such as running, basketball, or soccer, and strenuous sports, such as wrestling. Swimming, even long-distance swimming, is well tolerated by children with asthma.

Asthma camps have become popular in recent years as a means of encouraging physical activity in a more homogenous, controlled, and less competitive environment. Not all persons subscribe to this practice. There are those who support the positive benefits, which are primarily that the denominator of asthma is removed as a factor. Everyone at the camp has asthma; therefore, no child is different from the others. On the other hand, many believe that such segregation from family and peers serves only to reinforce the sick role.

Psychologic aspects of childhood asthma

Emotional factors are known to be associated with childhood asthma; however, it is not known whether emotional disturbance is present before the onset of asthma and is a probable causative factor in its development or whether it occurs as a result of the asthma. Although no decisive evidence is available regarding the relative importance of all etiologic factors, the consensus accepts a multicausal etiology for childhood asthma in which hereditary, allergic, infectious, and psychologic factors assume importance independently or, more often, in combination.

Behavioral problems are apt to occur in asthmatic children whose attacks commenced before age 2 years and those with continuing asthma and symptoms that are more severe and prolonged. It is unclear whether the emotional disturbances are peculiar to children with asthma or are similar to those that may occur in children with other chronic diseases. Children with any chronic condition are at higher risk to develop adjustment problems than are healthy children.

Both short- and long-term adaptation of the asthmatic child to his disease depends to a great extent on the family's acceptance of his disorder. The task of living day-to-day with an asthmatic child involves the family continually. There are periodic crises and the ever-present threat of a crisis, requiring parental vigilance, sleepless nights, frequent emergency trips to the hospital, and often overwhelming medical expenses. Throughout these stresses the parents are expected and encouraged to promote as normal a life as possible for the asthmatic child without neglecting the needs of the siblings.

Where family relationships are determined to produce an adverse effect on the asthmatic child, psychiatric help is recommended and, where disturbances are marked, foster placement or respite care in a residential facility for asthmatic children is advised. When a child repeatedly improves during separation from family members, it is strongly suspected that emotional and family interactional factors are contributing to the course of the disease.

Prognosis

The outlook for children with asthma varies widely. An impressive number of children lose their symptoms at puberty. The prognosis for control of symptoms or disappearance of symptoms will differ from children who have rare and infrequent attacks to those who are constantly wheezing or some who are subject to status asthmaticus. In general there is a poorer prognosis for improvement in the child with more severe and numerous symptoms, who has symptoms present for a longer period of time, and with a family history of allergy. However, it is impossible to predict which children will outgrow their symptoms of childhood asthma. Many who outgrow them are subject to exercise-induced asthma as adults, and the associated pathologic conditions, such as growth impairment, chest deformity, and airway obstruction, are maintained throughout life.

Nursing considerations

Nursing care of children with asthma involves both acute and long-term care. Children who are admitted to the hospital with acute asthma are ill, anxious, and uncomfortable. In most instances the child is admitted as an emergency with status asthmaticus and is in acute distress. An intravenous infusion is begun immediately, and medication, usually corticosteroids and aminophylline, is administered to relieve bronchospasm. The child is monitored closely and continuously during aminophylline administration for relief of respiratory distress and signs of side effects or toxicity. The pulse, respiration, and blood pressure are taken and recorded every 5 minutes during rapid infusion and every 15 minutes for at least an hour after the drug has been absorbed. If there is a drop in blood pressure, no further medication is infused and the physician is immediately notified. Other signs of toxicity include fever, restlessness, nausea, vomiting, hypotension, and abdominal discomfort that may progress to convulsions and coma. Some of the signs of toxicity are easily confused with worsening of the asthma.

The child usually prefers the high-Fowler's position, although he may be more comfortable sitting upright and leaning slightly forward. Since oxygen is indicated, he is placed in a mist tent for relief of dyspnea and cyanosis.

An older child may prefer a nasal cannula. Oxygen is not administered indiscriminately but regulated according to the blood gas analysis and objective observation of color, respiratory effort, and sensorium. Associated treatments such as intermittent positive-pressure breathing or postural drainage, and tests, such as blood gases or pulmonary function tests, are often performed by specialized personnel, or they may be the nurse's responsibility.

The child with status asthmaticus is apprehensive and anxious. Moreover, he is usually tired from his respiratory efforts and loss of sleep. The calm, efficient presence of a nurse helps to reassure him that he is safe and will be cared for during this stressful period. It is important to assure the child that he will not be left alone and that his parents are near and available when he needs them.

Parents need reassurance too. They want to be informed of their child's condition and of the therapies being employed. They are upset, apprehensive regarding the child's condition, and feeling guilty. Often they feel that they may have in some way contributed to the child's condition or could have prevented the attack. They may even feel, consciously or unconsciously, anger toward the child for continuing to display symptoms despite their efforts to prevent or control the attack. Reassurance regarding their efforts expended on the child's behalf and their parenting capabilities can help alleviate their stress. All efforts to reduce the parental apprehension will, in turn, help reduce the child's distress. Anxiety is easily communicated to the child from parents and members of the staff.

Long-term support

Nurses who are involved with asthmatic children in the home, clinic, or physician's office play an important role in helping the children and their families learn to live with the condition.* The disease can be tolerated if it does not interfere with family life, physical activity, or school attendance or if it does not require hospitalization.

Parents need to know the nature of the disease and, when the allergens are determined, how they can avoid and/or relieve asthmatic attacks. The nurse assists the mother in planning and carrying out an elimination diet to detect foods that may precipitate symptoms. When the allergen or allergens are identified, nurses can provide valuable assistance to the parents in modifying the environment to reduce contact with the offending allergen(s).

The parents are cautioned to avoid exposing the child to excessive cold, wind, or other extremes of weather and to smoke, sprays, or other irritants. Foods known to provoke symptoms should be eliminated from the diet. The foods most frequently allergenic are eggs, milk, grains, and chocolate. Parents should be advised to read labels on prepared foods and snacks to determine the presence of allergens. For example, a tremendous number of foods contain sodium caseinate or dried milk products.

The parents and the older child need to learn how to use the medications prescribed to relieve bronchospasm. They are taught to recognize early signs and symptoms of an impending attack so that it can be controlled before symptoms become distressful. Many children are given theophylline or other medication, and parents should understand the importance of taking the drugs as prescribed. Older children who use a nebulizer or aerosol device to deliver adrenergic drugs need to be taught how to use the device. The child and parents also need to be cautioned about the adverse effects of the drugs and the dangers of overuse. They should know that it is important to use them when needed but not indiscriminately or as a substitute for avoiding the symptom-provoking allergen.

The child should be protected from a respiratory infection that can trigger an attack or aggravate the asthmatic state, especially in young children. Their airways are mechanically smaller and more reactive; therefore, edema from infection causes wheezing and other signs of respiratory obstruction. Also, the equipment used for the child, such as nebulizers, must be kept absolutely clean to decrease the chances of contamination with bacteria and fungi.

Breathing exercises and controlled breathing are taught and encouraged for the motivated youngster, and the nurse can help him select activities suitable to his capacity.* Play techniques can be employed for younger children that extend their expiratory time and increase expiratory pressure, for example, blowing cotton balls or a ping-pong ball on a table, blowing a pinwheel, or preventing a tissue from falling by blowing it against the wall. Anything that promotes proper diaphragmatic breathing, side expansion, and generally improved mobility of the chest wall is encouraged. If the child requires segmental drainage and percussion, someone in the family must assume responsibility of carrying out the procedure. It is the responsibility of the physical therapist or the nurse to teach the parent the proper technique.

Children with emotional overtones associated with their asthma create additional problems. In these children an attack can be triggered by emotional experiences. Even some respiratory behaviors (such as crying, laughing, coughing, and hyperventilation) that accompany strong emotions may trigger a mechanical or reflex narrowing of the airway.

---

*A helpful book written for children is Parcel, G., and others: Teaching myself about asthma, St. Louis, 1979, The C.V. Mosby Co.

*A comic book explaining breathing exercises for asthmatic children, "Captain Wonderlung," is available from the American Academy of Pediatrics, P.O. Box 927, Elk Grove Village, IL 60007.

SUMMARY OF NURSING CARE OF THE CHILD WITH BRONCHIAL ASTHMA

GOALS	RESPONSIBILITIES

Determine causative factor(s)	Take a careful history to identify possible precipitating factor(s) including
	    Contact with allergens
	    History of allergic reaction(s) (such as eczema in infancy)
	    Exercise
	Assist with sensitivity testing
	Supervise elimination diet
	Assess environment for presence of possible allergic factors
	Explore parent-child relationships

Determine extent of respiratory involvement	Assist with diagnostic procedures such as
	    Pulmonary function tests
	    Radiographs
	    Blood work

Detect status of respiratory distress	Assess skin color for cyanosis Assess character of respirations for depth, rate, presence of retractions or nasal flaring, effort (inspiratory and expiratory), and lung sounds Collect or assist in collection of blood gases if indicated
Relieve dyspnea	Position for maximum ventilatory efficiency such as high Fowler or sitting leaning forward Administer appropriate bronchodilator
Reduce mucosal edema	Administer corticosteroids as ordered Provide cool mist
Promote expectoration of mucous secretions	Administer mucolytic agents Administer expectorants Provide adequate fluid intake Remove accumulated mucus Perform percussion, vibration, and postural drainage Provide cool mist inhalation

Increase oxygen supply to lungs	Position for maximum ventilation
	Administer oxygen
	    Mist tent
	    Mask, cannula, hood
	    Intermittent positive-pressure breathing apparatus

Reduce anxiety and apprehension during attack	Remain with the child and assure him that he will not be left alone Provide reassurance with calm words and manner Encourage the parents to remain near the child Administer appropriate medication, oxygen, and/or other therapies without delay
Avoid sedentary habits	Encourage activities appropriate to the age, interests, and capabilities of the child Encourage physical exercise involving stop-and-start activity that does not overtax the respiratory mechanism

Improve ventilatory capacity	Assist with physical therapy, chest physical therapy (p. 573)
	Instruct and/or supervise
	    Breathing exercises
	    Controlled breathing
	Assist the child and family to select physical exercises appropriate to the child's capabilities
	Encourage regular exercise

SUMMARY OF NURSING CARE OF THE CHILD WITH BRONCHIAL ASTHMA—cont'd

GOALS	RESPONSIBILITIES
Use medications judiciously	Teach the child and family to recognize early signs and symptoms so that an impending attack can be controlled before it becomes distressful Teach the child to understand how equipment works Teach the child correct use of inhalators
Prevent acute attack	Educate the parents and child 　Avoid contact with offending allergens 　Avoid extremes of environmental temperature 　Avoid undue excitement and/or physical exertion 　Use prophylactic medication(s) according to instructions 　Recognize early symptoms of impending attack 　Implement therapeutic measures at earliest symptoms
Promote positive adaptation to disease	Foster positive family relationships Encourage the child to participate in normal childhood activities commensurate with his capabilities Encourage and reinforce age-appropriate behaviors, experiences, and socialization with peers Discourage physical inactivity Use every opportunity to increase the parent's and child's understanding of the disease and its therapies Encourage the child to discuss his feelings about his disease Be alert to signs of parental rejection or overprotection Be alert to signs that the child may be using his symptoms to manipulate his interpersonal environment Intervene appropriately if evidence of maladaptation Collaborate with school nurse to assure continuity of care plan Refer the parents and child to agencies or groups in the community where special assistance is available (American Lung Association, Special Child Health Services, and so on)
Support, assist, and reassure families	Be available to the parents Allow for expression of feelings Explain procedures, therapies, and the child's symptoms to the parents Support and emphasize strengths and abilities of the parents Discuss age-appropriate behaviors and activities for the child Help the parents to establish and/or maintain a nonstressful environment for the child Refer to other agencies and persons for additional interpersonal support Refer to agencies for financial support
Reduce anxiety during diagnostic procedures	Explain unfamiliar procedures and equipment to the child Remain with the child during procedures Employ calm, reassuring manner
Reduce parental anxiety during an attack	Provide support and reassurance to the parents Explain therapies and the child's behavior
Determine effectiveness of therapy	Take vital signs frequently (every 1 to 2 hours) Observe 　Type and rate of respirations 　Color 　Apprehensiveness

Continued.

SUMMARY OF NURSING CARE OF THE CHILD WITH BRONCHIAL ASTHMA—cont'd

GOALS	RESPONSIBILITIES
Promote physical comfort	Improve ventilatory capacity Position the child for comfort
Promote rest and reduce fatigue	Implement measures to improve ventilation Administer sedation as ordered Organize care to allow for maximum rest Disturb as little as possible when resting or asleep
Promote adequate hydration	Maintain intravenous infusion if part of therapy Measure intake and output Assess urine for concentration and specific gravity Encourage fluids as prescribed Assure adequate humidification of environment Assess for objective signs of adequate hydration

Long term management
Maintain optimum health
	Encourage sound health practices
	    Balanced, nutritious diet
	    Adequate rest
	    Hygiene
	    Appropriate exercise
	    Avoid exposure to infection

Control allergens	Assist the parents to eliminate or avoid allergens that trigger attack, such as
	    Meal planning to eliminate allergenic foods
	    Removal of pets
	    Modification of environment ("allergy proof" the home)
	Assist the parents to obtain and/or install device to control environment (humidifier, air conditioner, electronic air filter)

Prevent infection	Encourage sound health practices Employ meticulous care of equipment to avoid bacterial and/or fungal growth Administer prophylactic antibiotics, if ordered

The interactions of members of the family need careful assessment to identify maladaptive behaviors and precipitating factors. Sometimes it is necessary to remove the child from the family for short-term respite care and provide the family with crisis therapy. In severe cases long-term respite care is the only satisfactory solution. The children live in one of the residential treatment centers throughout the country in which the needs of the child are met by professionals. There is also Camp Bronco Junction which offers a short-term practical program for holistic management of asthmatic children.* Several organizations provide education and services for health professionals and families of asthmatic children.†

---

*Allergy Rehabilitation Foundation, 810 Atlas Building, Charleston, WV 25168.

†American Lung Association, 1740 Broadway, New York, NY 10019; Asthma and Allergy Foundation of America, 19 West 44th Street, New York, NY 10036; National Asthma Center, 3800 E. Colfax Ave., Denver, CO 80206; The National Foundation for Asthma, P.O. Box 42195, Tucson, AZ 85733.

CYSTIC FIBROSIS (CF)

Cystic fibrosis of the pancreas, fibrocystic disease of the pancreas, and mucoviscidosis are all terms that are or have been applied to this most common inherited disease of children. Cystic fibrosis is a generalized dysfunction of the exocrine (especially mucous-producing) glands and is one of the most serious chronic diseases that affect white children. It accounts for a large percentage of lung disease in children; however, the disease affects multiple organ systems in varying degrees of severity, which presents some problems with early recognition.

Etiology

Cystic fibrosis is believed by most authorities to be inherited as an autosomal-recessive trait, and, as such, the affected child inherits the defective genes from both parents with an overall incidence of 1 in 4 (see inheritance patterns, p. 49). However, there are some who suggest that

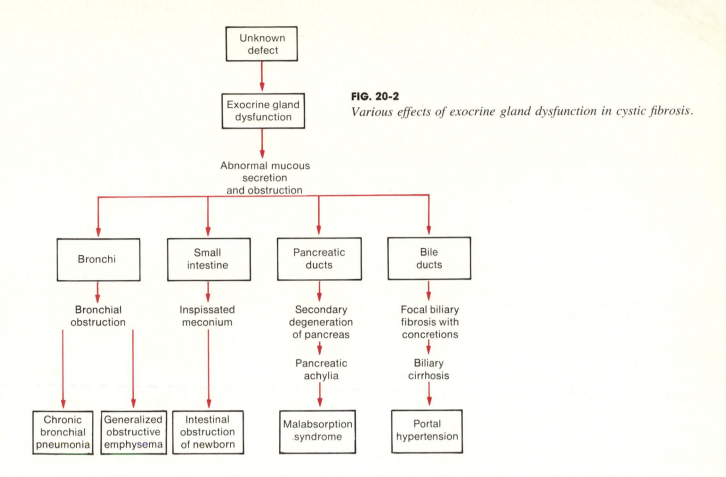

FIG. 20-2

Various effects of exocrine gland dysfunction in cystic fibrosis.

the disease may be a symptom complex caused by more than one gene. The incidence of the disease is estimated at 1 in 1500 to 2000 births in predominantly white populations.

Pathophysiology

The basic biochemical defect in cystic fibrosis is unknown. It is believed to be caused by alteration in a protein, probably an enzyme. The defect gives rise to several apparently unrelated clinical features—increased viscosity of mucous gland secretions, a striking elevation of sweat electrolytes, an increase in several organic and enzymatic constituents of saliva, and possible abnormalities in autonomic nervous system function.

The primary factor, and the one that is responsible for the multiple clinical manifestations of the disease, is mechanical obstruction caused by the increased viscosity of mucous gland secretions (Fig. 20-2). Instead of forming a thin, freely flowing secretion, the mucous glands produce a thick, inspissated mucoprotein that accumulates and dilates them. Small passages in organs such as the pancreas and bronchioles become obstructed as secretions precipitate or coagulate to form concretions in glands and ducts.

In the pancreas the thick secretions block the ducts.

This blockage (1) leads to cystic dilations of the acini (small lobes of the gland), which then undergo degeneration and progressive diffuse fibrosis, and (2) prevents essential pancreatic enzymes from reaching the duodenum, which causes marked impairment in the digestion and absorption of nutrients. The islands of Langerhans remain unaffected but may decrease in number as pancreatic fibrosis progresses and, in the liver, localized biliary obstruction and fibrosis are common and become more extensive with time.

Pulmonary complications are present in almost all children with cystic fibrosis and constitute the most serious threat to life. Bronchial and bronchiolar obstruction by the abnormally thick, tenacious mucus causes patchy atelectasis with hyperinflation. The child is unable to expectorate the mucus because of its increased viscosity. This retained mucus serves as an excellent medium for any bacterial growth. Reduced oxygen–carbon dioxide exchange causes variable degrees of hypoxia, hypercapnia, and acidosis.

Clinical manifestations

The earliest manifestation of cystic fibrosis is *meconium ileus* in the newborn. The lumen of the small intestine is blocked with thick puttylike, tenacious, mucilaginous meconium, which gives rise to signs of intestinal obstruction, including abdominal distention, vomiting, failure to pass stools, and rapid development of dehydration with associated electrolyte imbalance.

As the disease progresses, obstruction of pancreatic ducts and the absence of enzymes (trypsin, amylase, and lipase) in the duodenum prevent conversion of ingested food into compounds that can be absorbed by the intestinal mucosa. Consequently, the nondigested food is excreted as large, bulky, loose stools. As solid foods are added to the diet, the excessively large stools become frothy and extremely foul smelling.

Because so little is absorbed from the intestine, the child compensates with a voracious appetite; however, since he is unable to compensate for the fecal wastage, he loses weight with marked wasting of tissues and failure to grow. The abdomen is distended and the extremities are thin, and the sallow skin droops from wasted buttocks. The impaired ability to absorb fats results in a deficiency of the fat-soluble vitamins A, D, E, and K, and anemia is a common complication.

The most common gastrointestinal complication associated with cystic fibrosis is *prolapse of the rectum*, which occurs most often in infancy and childhood. Affected children of all ages are subject to intestinal obstruction from inspissated or impacted feces.

Pulmonary problems are present in almost all children with cystic fibrosis, but the time of appearance is variable. The majority of children show evidence before 1 year of age; others may not develop symptoms for weeks, months, or years. Initial manifestations are often wheezy respirations and a dry, nonproductive cough. Eventually diffuse bronchial and bronchiolar obstruction lead to irregular aeration with progressive pulmonary disturbance. Dyspnea increases, the cough often becomes paroxysmal, and the mucoid impactions within the small air passages cause a generalized obstructive emphysema and patchy areas of atelectasis.

Progressive pulmonary involvement with hyperaeration of functioning alveoli produces the overinflated, barrel-shaped chest in which the anteroposterior diameter approaches the lateral diameter. When ventilation is significantly impaired, there is cyanosis and clubbing of fingers and toes. The child suffers repeated episodes of bronchitis and bronchopneumonia.

Diagnostic evaluation

The consistent finding of abnormally high sodium and chloride concentrations in the sweat is a unique characteristic of cystic fibrosis. Mothers frequently observe that their infants taste "salty" when they kiss them. For diagnostic purposes the quantitative test is performed on sweat

usually obtained by electrophoresis of pilocarpine. Normally the sweat chloride content is less than 40 mEq/liter; a chloride concentration greater than 60 mEq/liter is diagnostic of cystic fibrosis.

Measurements of duodenal trypsin activity may be made to confirm a diagnosis. Only trypsin and chymotrypsin are measured. Trypsin is absent in over 80% of patients with the disease. Sometimes fat-absorption is measured by a 5-day stool collection and calculated as a percentage of intake.

Therapeutic management

Wherever possible the goals of care are aimed at promoting a normal life for the affected child. This includes maintaining good nutrition, preventing and controlling pulmonary infections, and promoting a satisfactory psychologic adjustment to the disease and all of its ramifications.

Diet. The impaired intestinal absorption in cystic fibrosis necessitates a diet significantly higher in calories and protein than is normally required in a child of similar size. Fat content is reduced, although opinions vary regarding the quantities allowed. Fat supplies twice the calories of carbohydrate but may interfere with absorption of other nutrients. High-protein formulas with low-curd tension are recommended during the first weeks of life, followed by low-fat or skim milk and homogenized milk in older children, if they are able to tolerate it. Medium-chain triglycerides (MCT) are more readily absorbed than longer chain fats and are sometimes given to the infant as a dietary supplement.

Water-miscible preparations of vitamins A, D, and E are provided daily in twice the usual recommended dosage. Vitamin K is indicated if hypoprothrombinemia is present as a result of accompanying liver involvement. Supplementary iron is also prescribed, and diet supplements (such as Carnation Instant Breakfast, Ensure or Ensure Plus, Sustacal, or Sustacal pudding) are frequently given to provide additional protein, vitamins, and calories.

Pancreatic enzyme replacement is given in conjunction with meals and snacks and is regulated in order to obtain normal bowel movements, nutrition, and growth. A variety of preparations are available but the preferred preparation consists of enteric-coated microspheres contained in a capsule (Cotazym-S, Pancrease). The enteric coating delays release of the enzyme and its destruction in the acid environment of the stomach. The capsules may be swallowed intact or broken apart and the contents sprinkled on soft foods, which do not require chewing, such as applesauce or pudding. Other preparations that are used for some children are pancreatin (Panteric and Viokase) and pancrelipase (Cotazym). Sometimes antacids (such as

Maalox) or cimetidine (Tagamet) are administered with the enzymes to lower the gastric acidity.

Since salt depletion through sweating is a hazard, children are allowed to use salt generously. Most children are able to adjust this to their needs, and older children often exhibit a preference for salty foods. Additional salt should be taken during hot weather or febrile periods.

Pulmonary therapy. Pulmonary therapy to improve pulmonary function and loosen and eliminate bronchial secretions is probably the most important aspect of treatment. Postural drainage through positioning, clapping, and vibration (see p. 573) is carried out to encourage coughing and to assist in removal of mucus and exudate. The procedure should be carried out several times daily prophylactically and, during infections, as often as the child is able to tolerate it without undue fatigue. Chest physiotherapy should not be performed before or immediately after meals, therefore activities should be planned so that they do not coincide with meals.

Breathing exercises are recommended for the majority of children with cystic fibrosis, even for those with minimal pulmonary involvement. The exercises are usually performed twice daily, and they are preceded by postural drainage. Exercises to improve posture and mobilize the thorax are included, such as swinging the arms and bending and twisting the trunk. Children are encouraged to increase physical activity and participate in sports. The ultimate aim of these exercises and activities is to establish a good habitual breathing pattern.

Moisture-laden air that is provided by intermittent inhalation therapy moistens bronchial secretions and assists in their evacuation. The recommended schedule for intermittent, or interrupted, therapy is carried out at least twice daily (morning and evening) and more often if needed. Intermittent therapy consists of three steps:

1. Postural drainage for 5 to 10 minutes
2. Nebulization with appropriate solution
3. Postural drainage for 10 to 20 minutes

Nebulization following postural drainage permits deeper penetration of the droplet particles.

Mist-tent therapy is controversial in treatment of cystic fibrosis; it is most often used during hospitalization for acute episodes of the disease. For some children it may be recommended for home use, usually when the child is asleep. Oxygen therapy is usually recommended for children during acute episodes, and, when lung involvement becomes extensive, it may be needed with nebulization and at night for comfort and to prevent hypoxia.

Expectorants, particularly the iodides, which are believed to make bronchial secretions thinner, are used frequently. During acute exacerbations of pulmonary disease, intensive antibiotics are employed to control pulmonary in-

fection. Many physicians prefer to use antibiotics only when there is evidence of infection, whereas others prescribe their use as a prophylactic measure. When used therapeutically, it is important that the drugs be given over a long enough period of time and in sufficient dosage to be effective.

Other complications are treated symptomatically. Meconium ileus usually responds to administration of diatrizoate methylglucamine (Gastrografin) or acetylcysteine (Mucomyst) enemas. Rectal prolapse is reduced by gently pressing against the everted rectum with a gloved, lubricated finger while the child is in the knee-chest position. The buttocks are then strapped together with tape for 20 to 30 minutes.

Prognosis

It is the pulmonary involvement that determines the ultimate outcome of the disease. Pancreatic enzyme deficiency is less of a problem if adequate nutrition is assured. Hemorrhage from liver cirrhosis and massive salt depletion in hot weather are occasional hazards. With early diagnosis and improved therapeutic measures, the life expectancy has improved. Many more children are reaching adulthood; however, the variation in severity of the disease is an important factor in determining the ultimate outcome.

Nursing considerations

The nurse's contact with an affected child usually begins when the child is brought to the hospital or clinic for confirmation of the diagnosis. Perhaps the reason for hospitalization is failure to thrive or recurrent respiratory infections. Later, during recurrent admission to the hospital or during ongoing follow-up in the clinic or at home, the nurse and the child develop a sustained relationship.

On the initial contact, frequently in the hospital setting, nurses are involved in performing or assisting with diagnostic tests and obtaining sweat for laboratory analysis of chloride content and, occasionally, of stool specimens for trypsin and fat. The child, usually an infant, needs comfort during these procedures; young children need distraction while they are confined during collection of sweat for testing.

The shock associated with the diagnosis is overwhelming to parents. They must face the impact of the chronic, life-threatening nature of the disease and the prospect of intensive treatment, for which they must assume a major part of the responsibility and for which they are ill prepared. They often fear that they will be unable to provide the care the child needs. One of the most difficult aspects of the diagnosis is the implications inherent in its cause, that is, the recognition that each parent contributed the gene responsible for the defect in their child. They need patient and careful explanations of the disease, how it might affect their particular family, and what they can do to provide the best possible care for their child.

Hospital care. When the child is hospitalized for confirmation of the diagnosis or for pulmonary complications, aerosol therapy is instituted or continued. The child may or may not be placed in a mist tent, but nebulization is almost always central to hospital management. Respiratory therapy is usually initiated and supervised by a trained respiratory therapist or physiotherapist. In institutions with large support staffs, they may provide all treatments. If not, it becomes the responsibility of the nurse to perform the prescribed nebulization, postural drainage, percussion, and vibration and to teach supervised breathing exercises. (See Chapter 19 for care of the child in a mist tent.)

The hazard of oxygen narcosis is a constant threat in children with long-standing disease who receive oxygen. Intensive aerosol therapy may cause large volumes of sputum to be thinned suddenly in the early hours of treatment; therefore, the child requires close observation to assist him with expectoration and to prevent deeper aspiration. Expectorant drugs are administered orally, which further facilitates the expectoration of mucus.

A diet is implemented for the newly diagnosed child or continued for the child who is hospitalized for pulmonary disease. Enzymes are supplied for each meal or snack, and adequate salt is provided, especially for febrile children. Unless the child is ill, his appetite is usually satisfactory. An ample supply of food should be made available to satisfy the voracious appetite characteristic of many of these children. However, some younger children may object to the extra fluids that are encouraged to promote thinning of mucous secretions.

Special efforts are made to protect the child from further infection, even though a respiratory infection is probably the reason for hospitalization. These children are particularly vulnerable to cross-contamination; therefore, reverse isolation may be implemented for the child's protection.

The child will need support for the many treatments and tests that are a necessary part of the hospital therapy. Intravenous fluids, intramuscular injections, and blood tests are almost always a part of the treatment, and the child soon associates hospitalization with these stress-provoking procedures. These children are usually quite thin with little muscle mass, which requires careful selection of injection sites.

Support to both the child and family is a vital part of nursing care. The progressive nature of the disease makes each illness requiring hospitalization a potentially life-threatening event. Skilled nursing care and sympathetic attention to the emotional needs of the child and family help them cope with the stresses associated with repeated respiratory infections and hospitalization.

Home care. After the diagnosis is confirmed and a treatment program determined, parents will need help in finding inhalation equipment available for home use that best meets their needs. They will need opportunities to learn about and practice the use of the equipment as well as some of the problems they may encounter.

Parents need to learn about the preferred diet of nutritious meals with limited fat and ample protein and carbohydrate and the administration of pancreatic enzymes. They need to be taught to perform percussion, vibration, and drainage. For those children and families who are selected to administer antibiotics by the intravenous route at home, the nurse will be responsible for teaching the technique. The nurse can assist the family to contact resources that provide help to families with affected children. The various crippled children's services, many local clinics, private agencies, service clubs, and other community groups often offer equipment and medications either free or at reduced rates. The Cystic Fibrosis Foundation* has chapters throughout the country to provide education and services to families and professionals.

Emotional support. One of the most important and difficult aspects in providing care for the family of a child with cystic fibrosis is coping with the emotional needs of the child and family. The diagnosis, treatment, and prognosis are fraught with a multiplicity of problems, frustrations, and feelings. The diagnosis with all its implications evokes feelings of guilt and self-recrimination in the parents. These feelings may be particularly marked if the newly diagnosed child is the second affected child in the family and if the parents had been counseled regarding the one in four risk of such an event occurring.

The long-range problems are those encountered in the care of a child with a chronic illness (Chapter 16). The child and the family must both make many adjustments, the success of which depends on their ability to cope and on the quality and quantity of support they receive from sources outside the family.

For the family the illness means modification of numerous family activities. Meals require planning in order not to place too many restrictions on the affected child or deprive the other members of the family. Limits on mobility restrict family recreational activities, especially when the child's therapy includes respiratory equipment that is not transportable. Postural drainage must be continued wherever the child may be. Also, members of the family hesitate to take the child too far from familiar and trusted medical care. The illness even determines the family's place of residence and employment, as the child's condi-

---

*6000 Executive Blvd., Suite 309, Rockville, MD 20852.

SUMMARY OF NURSING CARE OF THE CHILD WITH CYSTIC FIBROSIS

GOALS	RESPONSIBILITIES

Assist in diagnosis	Perform nursing assessment of the child
	Take the family history and health history
	Encourage medical evaluation for any child who displays suggestive signs of the disease
	Prepare the child for diagnostic tests
	Assist with diagnostic procedures
	    Collect stool specimens
	    Perform sweat test
	    Assist with radiographs

Maintain nutrition	Provide diet high in carbohydrate and protein Discourage use of foods high in fat; provide appropriate fat if recommended by the physician Assure adequate intake of salt Administer pancreatic enzyme replacement with meals and snacks Administer water-miscible vitamins and iron supplement
Assist the patient to expectorate sputum	Perform postural drainage as prescribed Teach and/or supervise breathing exercises Provide nebulization with appropriate solution equipment as prescribed Place the child in mist tent as ordered; make certain compressor or ultrasonic mechanism provides very small droplets in ample supply Administer expectorants Administer bronchodilators, if ordered
Prevent infection	Restrict contact with persons who have respiratory tract infections, including family, other children, friends, and members of staff Administer antibiotics as prescribed Manage respiratory infections as in pneumonia
Conserve energy	Provide or encourage activities appropriate to the child's developmental level and physical capacity
Improve aeration	Perform postural drainage Supervise breathing exercises Administer medications that promote breathing (bronchodilators, expectorants) Administer oxygen, if indicated and prescribed Provide nebulization Prevent and treat respiratory tract infections Encourage good posture and active exercises suitable to the child's needs, capabilities, and preferences

Teach the child about disease and treatment	Teach the child to assist in his own care
	    Food selection
	    Use of pancreatic enzymes
	    Use of equipment
	    How he can cooperate during treatments and tests

Promote growth and development	Provide or encourage nutritious diet Encourage the child to maintain usual activities Arrange for continued family contacts during hospitalization Arrange for continued schooling while hospitalized Encourage relationships with peers Promote development of a positive self-image

Continued.

SUMMARY OF NURSING CARE OF THE CHILD WITH CYSTIC FIBROSIS—cont'd

GOALS	RESPONSIBILITIES
Provide material support to the child and family	Guide to available resources equipped to deal with their special needs Provide counseling services Collaborate with the family and health team in assessing family needs and coping mechanisms
Administer optimal home care	Assess home situation Help devise individualized regimen based on assessment Teach the family home care Help the family acquire needed drugs and equipment Arrange for regular follow-up care to reassess effectiveness of home management Assist the family in problem solving

Educate the family	Provide accurate information at a rate the family can absorb
	Teach the family members physical care of the child
	    Use of equipment
	    Exercises and procedures
	    Diet and administration of pancreatic enzymes
	    Administration of drugs
	    Protection from infection
	Provide or arrange for genetic counseling regarding inherited aspects of the disease

Emotionally support the family	Listen to family members—singly or collectively Act on cues that indicate a family member's reaction to the child Help the family to gain confidence in their ability to cope with the child, disability, and its impact on other family members Encourage interaction with other families who have a similarly affected child Help the family face the possibility of the child's death
Participate in community education	Educate community groups regarding disorder Support research efforts Become actively involved in fund raising for cystic fibrosis research and treatment

tion dictates that he should remain near medical care facilities that offer the specialized care he needs.

A constant source of anxiety for both parents and child is the ever-present fear of death. The expected life span, although significantly increased during the past years, offers only limited encouragement regarding prognosis. The future is always uncertain. These families need all the support and skill the nurse can offer to cope with the guarded prognosis (see Chapter 16).

RESPIRATORY EMERGENCY

Nurses must be prepared to deal effectively with respiratory emergencies. Although the interventions are similar to those used for adults, there are some variations for infants and children. The most common respiratory emergencies are choking and respiratory failure.

CHOKING

All persons working with children should be prepared to deal effectively with a choking emergency. Choking on food or other material should not be fatal. Very simple procedures, which can be used both by health professionals and lay persons, save children's lives. It is the obligation of nurses to learn the techniques and to teach it to parents and other groups.

To aid a child who is choking, nurses need to recognize when he is indeed in distress. Not every child who gags or coughs while eating is truly choking. The child in distress *cannot speak, becomes cyanotic,* and *collapses.* These three signs indicate that the child is truly choking and requires immediate and quick action to save his life. He can die within 4 minutes.

When a child is obviously choking, the initial step is to open his mouth and reach in and try to remove the obstruction *without forcing it further down.* If this fails, any or all of the following should be attempted. At present no clear consensus has been reached regarding which proce-

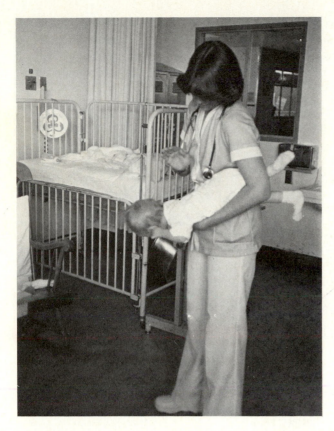

FIG. 20-3
Infant positioned for back blows.

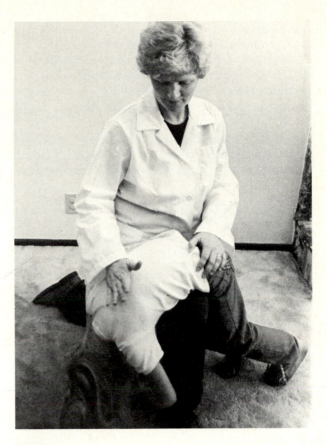

FIG. 20-4
Child positioned over knee for back blows.

dure best accomplishes the purpose without damage to the chest and/or abdomen. It is believed that the best chance for survival from choking from a foreign body is back blows combined with manual thrusts—either chest or abdominal.

Back blows and chest thrusts

A choking infant is placed over the rescuer's arm with his head lower than his trunk and his head supported (Fig. 20-3). Additional support can be achieved if the rescuer rests his arm on his thigh. Four quick, sharp, back blows are delivered between the infant's shoulder blades with the heel of the rescuer's hand. Less force is required than would be applied to an adult. Following delivery of the back blows, the rescuer's free hand is placed flat on the infant's back so that the infant is "sandwiched" between the two hands, making certain the neck and chin are well supported. While the rescuer maintains support with the infant's head lower than his trunk, the infant is turned and placed supine on the rescuer's thigh, where four chest thrusts are applied in rapid succession in the same manner as external chest compressions described on p. 633.

Children who are too large to straddle the rescuer's

forearm can be draped across the rescuer's thighs with the rescuer kneeling on the floor (Fig. 20-4). The head is maintained at a level lower than the trunk, as described for the infant. Greater force can be applied for the back thrusts than those used in the infant. The child is positioned supine on the floor for external chest compression.

It is neither necessary nor desirable to squeeze or compress the arms during the procedure. The child may vomit after relief of the obstruction and is positioned to prevent aspiration. After breathing is restored, the child should receive medical attention so that he can be assessed for complications.

Abdominal thrusts

Abdominal compression to relieve obstruction employs the *Heimlich maneuver,* which is carried out in the same fashion in children as in adults:

1. The fisted hand is placed, thumb side in, against the child's abdomen at a point just below the rib cage and slightly above the navel. The fist is firmly grasped with the other hand.
2. The fist is pressed into the abdomen with a quick upward thrust.
3. The thrust is repeated if needed.

The operator stands or kneels behind the child, with his or her arms around the child's waist and hands correctly placed, and carries out the procedure as described. If the child is sitting, the operator's arms are wrapped around both chair and child. For a child who is lying on his back, the operator takes a position facing the child from above, places the *heel* of the bottom hand at the proper location on the abdomen, and administers the quick inward and upward thrust.

The technique is applied to infants in the following manner:

1. The infant is placed on the lap in a sitting position and facing forward. The index and middle fingers of both hands are placed against the infant's abdomen in a position above the naval and below the lower ribs.
2. Three quick upward thrusts are delivered.

The Heimlich maneuver is not a punch or a bear hug. The child may vomit after relief of the obstruction and should be positioned to prevent aspiration. After breathing is restored, the child should receive medical attention so that he can be assessed for complications.

The success of the technique is primarily a result of the fact that obstruction takes place at the end of a maximum respiration. The victim is most likely to choke on food during inspiration; therefore, the tidal volume plus expiratory reserve volume are present in the lungs. When pressure is exerted on the diaphragm by the maneuver, the food bolus is ejected with considerable force by this trapped air.

RESPIRATORY FAILURE

Respiratory insufficiency is the general term applied to two conditions: (1) children with increased work of breathing while preserving gas exchange function near normal, and (2) children who are unable to maintain normal blood gas tensions and develop hypoxemia and acidosis secondary to carbon dioxide retention. *Respiratory failure* is defined as the inability of the respiratory apparatus to maintain adequate oxygenation of the blood, with or without carbon dioxide retention.

Respiratory arrest is the cessation of respiration.

Effective pulmonary gas exchange requires clear airways, normal lungs and chest wall, and adequate pulmonary circulation. Anything that affects these functions or their relationships can compromise the respiration.

Recognition

Respiratory failure that occurs as the result of acute obstruction of a major airway or cardiac arrest is sudden and readily apparent. Gradual and more covert development of

signs and symptoms is less easily recognized. Therefore, nursing observation and judgment are vital to the recognition and early management of respiratory failure. Nurses must be able to assess a situation and initiate appropriate action within moments.

The cardinal symptoms of respiratory failure are:

- Restlessness
- Tachycardia
- Tachypnea
- Diaphoresis

Early signs that are less obvious include:

Mood changes, such as euphoria or depression
Headache
Altered depth and pattern of respirations (deep, shallow, apnea, irregular)
Exertional dyspnea
Anorexia
Increased cardiac output and renal output
Cyanosis, peripheral or central (may or may not be evident until later)
Central nervous system symptoms, such as decreased efficiency, impaired judgment, anxiety, confusion, restlessness, and irritability
Flaring nares
Chest wall retractions
Expiratory grunt
Wheezing and/or prolonged expiration

Management

The interventions used in the management of respiratory failure are often dramatic, requiring special skills, and are often emergency procedures. Some of the techniques employed to assist ventilation include artificial ventilation, artificial airway, and cardiopulmonary resuscitation.

Artificial ventilation. There are a variety of methods for controlling or assisting ventilation. Temporary assistance can be provided by a hand-operated self-inflating ventilation bag with mask and a nonreturnable valve to prevent rebreathing (AMBU bag). With the mask placed on the child's nose and mouth (an open airway is established by correct positioning with the chin forward and the neck extended to the "sniffing" position), the bag is rhythmically compressed, forcing the gas from the bag into the patient's lungs.

For more prolonged assistance, mechanical ventilation is employed to replace the bellows function of the diaphragm and thoracic wall muscles. The lungs are inflated by the application of either positive or negative pressure. The positive-pressure machine inflates the lung by increasing airway pressure above atmospheric pressure, and a negative-pressure ventilator creates a subatmospheric pressure around the chest wall, whereas airway pressure remains atmospheric. Application of positive pressure by mechanical means usually improves the distribution of gas within the lung and often reinflates partially collapsed lung segments. The overall effect is the improvement of gas exchange.

Cardiopulmonary resuscitation. Complete apnea signals the need for rapid and vigorous action to prevent cardiac arrest. In such situations nurses must be prepared to initiate action immediately. In anticipation, emergency equipment should be readily available in areas in which respiratory arrest might take place, and the status of this resuscitation equipment should be checked regularly (at least once daily). Regardless of the cause of the arrest, some very basic procedures are carried out, modified somewhat according to the size of the child.

The initial step after cessation of respiration is to palpate peripheral pulses and quickly check the heartbeat. Absence of carotid or temporal pulse is considered sufficient indication to begin external cardiac massage. Feeling a pulse in an infant poses some difficulties. The very short, and often fat, neck of the infant renders the carotid pulse (ordinarily used in the adult) difficult to palpate. Therefore, it is preferable to use the brachial pulse, located on the inner side of the upper arm midway between the elbow and shoulder.

After rapid ascertainment and restoration of a patent airway by removal of foreign material and secretions (if indicated), cardiac massage is initiated with simultaneous ventilation of the lungs. To ventilate the lungs in the infant and small child, the mouth of the operator is placed in such a way that both the mouth and the nostrils are in-cluded. Older children are ventilated through the mouth while the nostrils are firmly pinched for airtight contact.

Two essential elements determine the safety and efficacy of external cardiac massage: (1) the patient's spine must be supported during compression of the sternum and (2) sternal pressure must be forceful but not traumatic.

Sternal compression to infants is applied with two or three fingers on the midsternum exerting a sharp downward thrust (Fig. 20-5, *A*). For children age 1 to 8 years pressure is applied with the heel of one or both hands at the junction of the middle and lower two-thirds of the sternum (Fig. 20-5, *B*). The depth of compression is also adapted to the size of the child—infants, ½ to 1 inch; young children, 1 to 1½ inches; and older children, 1½ to 2 inches. The location, rate, and depth for adolescents are the same as for adults (Standards for CPR and ECC, 1980).

External massage is administered at a rate of 100 to 120 times/minute in the newborn and 60 to 80 times/minute in older children. Breathing rates for children are more rapid than those applied to adults. For the infant the prescribed rate is one every 3 seconds, or 20 times/minute; for the child, once every 4 seconds, or 15 times/minute is recommended. Cardiac compression should be interspersed with ventilation, administered by the mouth-to-mouth method or artificial ventilator, at a ratio of one breath for five to eight compressions. Massage is continued until there are signs of recovery as evidenced by palpable peripheral pulses, return of pupils to normal size, and the disappearance of mottling and cyanosis.

FIG. 20-5

A, *Closed chest massage in infant, with two fingers over midsternum.* **B,** *Closed chest massage in older child, with heel of hand over midsternum. (From Wong, D.L., and Whaley, L.F.: Clinical handbook of pediatric nursing, St. Louis, 1981, The C.V. Mosby Co.)*

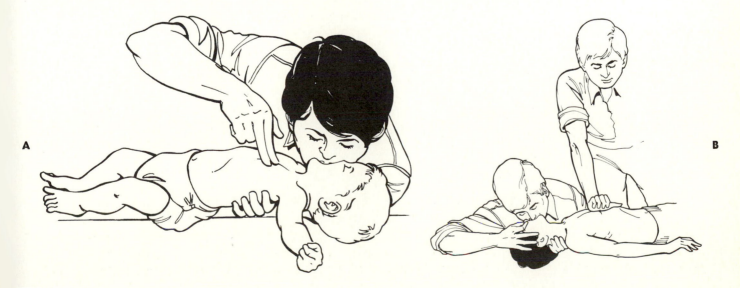

REFERENCES

Bean, B.: Survival of influenza viruses on environmental surfaces, J. Infect. Dis. **146**:47-51, 1982.

Bennett, R.M.: Drowning and near-drowning, etiology and pathophysiology, Am. J. Nurs. **76**:919-921, 1976.

Colombo, J.L., Hopkins, R.L., and Waring, W.W.: Steam vaporizer injuries, Pediatrics **67**:661-663, 1981.

Standards for CPR and ECC. Part III. Basic life support in infants and children, J.A.M.A. **244**:472-478, 1980.

BIBLIOGRAPHY
Cardiopulmonary resuscitation

Basic life support in infants and children, J.A.M.A. **244**(5):472-478, 1980.

Hoops, E.J.: Cardiopulmonary resuscitation in children, Nurs. Clin. North Am. **16**:623-634, 1981.

Longo, A.: Teaching parents CPR, Pediatr. Nurs. **9**:445-447, 1983.

Melker, R.: CPR in neonates, infants and children, Crit. Care Q. **1**(4):49-65, May 1978.

Pfister, S.: Respiratory arrest. Are you prepared? Nursing 82, **12**(9):34-41, 1982.

Taylor, P., and Gideon, M.: Cardiac arrest: a crisis for all people, Nursing 80 **10**(9):42-45, 1980.

Acute respiratory infection

Bishop, B.: How to cool a feverish child, Pediatr. Nurs. **4**(1):19-20, 1978.

Bridgewater, S.C., and Voignier, R.R.: A teaching-learning guide for parents, Pediatr. Nurs. **5**(5):55-58, 1979.

Cormier, J.F., and Bryant, B.G.: Treating the common cold, Pediatr. Nurs. **4**(1):7-13, 1978.

Eade, N.R., Taussig, L.M., and Marks, M.I.: Hydrocarbon pneumonitis, Pediatrics **54**:351, 1974.

Fathers, B.: Micoplasma pneumonia, Nurs. Times **77**:1661-1664, 1981.

Fried, W.: Acute epiglottitis, Issues. Compr. Pediatr. Nurs. **4**:29-36, 1980.

Pantell, R.H., and others: Fever in the first six months of life, Clin. Pediatr. **19**:77-82, 1980.

Ryan, A.M.: Pneumonia: aggressive treatment is the key, RN **45**(8):44-50, 1982.

Shaw, E.B.: Acute epiglottitis, Am. J. Dis. Child. **130**:782-784, 1976.

Aspiration

Banks, W., and Potsic, W.P.: Elusive unsuspected foreign bodies in the tracheobronchial tree, Clin. Pediatr. **16**:31-35, 1977.

Blazer, S., Naveh, Y., and Friedman, A.: Foreign body in the airway, Am. J. Dis. Child. **134**:68-71, 1980.

Sumner, S.M., and Grau, P.E.: Emergency! First aid for choking, Nursing 82, **12**(7):40-49, 1982.

Thompson, S.W.: How to use the Heimlich maneuver on choking infants and children, Pediatr. Nurs. **9**:13-16, 1983.

Wagner, T.J., and Hindi-Alexander, M.: Hazards of baby powder? Pediatr. Nurs. **10**:124-125, 1984.

Near-drowning

Bennett, R.M.: Drowning and near-drowning, etiology and pathophysiology, Am. J. Nurs. **76**:919-920, 1976.

Caudle, J.T.: Emergency nursing of near-drowning victims, Am. J. Nurs. **76**:922-923, 1976.

Donahue, A.: Beware of the obvious with near-drowning victims, RN, **45**(6):41-44, 1982.

Emergency steps in near-drowning, Nurs. Update **7**(7):10-14, 1976.

Molyneux-Luick, M.: Water-sports injuries: the old and the new, Nursing 78 **8**(8):51-55, 1978.

Stickler, J.F.:, and Shawman, T.: A child drowns: a nursing perspective, Am. J. Maternal Child Nurs. **6**:324-328, 1981.

Wolf, D.: Near drowning, Crit. Care Update **7**(6):31-35, 1980.

Inhalation injury

Arena, J.M.: The treatment of poisoning, Clin. Symp. **30**(2):3-47, 1978.

Brandeburg, J.: Inhalation injury: carbon monoxide poisoning, Am. J. Nurs. **80**:98-100, 1980.

Burton, J.: Carbon monoxide poisoning, Crit. Care Update! **10**(2):19-21, 1983.

Gaston, S.F., and Schuman, L.L: Inhalation injury: smoke inhalation, Am. J. Nurs. **80**:94-97, 1980.

Bronchial asthma

Bergner, M., and Hutelmyer, C.: Teaching kids how to live with their allergies, Nursing 76 **6**(8):11-12, 1976.

Burton, J.: Drug therapy for severe asthma. Part III. Crit. Care Update **5**(5):24-27, 1978.

Burton, J.: Extrinsic allergic alveolitis, Crit. Care Update **10**(1):33-37, 1983.

Cotton, E.K.: Status asthmaticus, Respir. Care **22**:1077-1083, 1977.

Dyer, B.: Asthmatic kids—independence. One giant step, Pediatr. Nurs. **3**(2):16-23, 1977.

Foster, S.D.: Theophylline, Am. J. Maternal Child Nurs. **5**:136, 1981.

Gever, L.N.: Theophylline: know how to handle this potent bronchodilator, Nursing 80 **10**(11):50-53, 1980.

Hawkins-Walsh, E., and Pettrone, C.R.: Drugs used in the treatment of pediatric allergy and asthma, Pediatr. Nurs. **3**(2):12-15, 1977.

Hill, M.: Asthmatic child or asthma expert? Pediatr. Nurs. **3**(2):25-26, 1977.

Hudgel, D.W., and Madsen, L.A.: Acute and chronic asthma: a guide to intervention, Am. J. Nurs. **80**:1791-1795, 1980.

Jennings, C.: Controlling the home environment of the allergic child, Am. J. Maternal Child Nurs. **7**:376-381, 1982.

Kirilloff, L.H., and Tibbals, S.C.: Drugs for asthma. A complete guide, Am. J. Nurs. **83**:55-61, 1983.

Lough, M.D., Bolek, J., and Stern, R.C.: Ten year's experience with a camp for children with pulmonary disease, Respir. Care **22**:828-831, 1977.

McCaully, H.E.: Breathing exercises as play for asthmatic children, Am. J. Maternal Child Nurs. **5**:340-344, 1980.

Nicholson, D.P.: A problem in clinical research: asthma and cromolyn sodium, Heart Lung **5**:71-76, Jan./Feb. 1976.

Nursing Grand Rounds: Fighting the frustrations of status asthmaticus, Nursing 82, **12**(3):58-63, 1982.

Webber-Jones, J.E., and Bryant, M.K.: Over-the-counter bronchodilators, Nursing 80 **10**(1):34-39, 1980.

Weeks, H.F.: The xanthines, Am. J. Nurs. **5**:206, 1980.

Wolf, S.I.: Exercise and the asthmatic child and PL 94-142, Pediatr. Nurs. **6**(6)21-23, 1980.

Cystic fibrosis

Burnette, B.A.: Family adjustment to cystic fibrosis, Am. J. Nurs. **75**:1986-1988, 1975.

Burns, W.T., and others: Test strip meconium screening for cystic fibrosis, Am. J. Dis. Child. **131**:71-73, 1977.

Johnson, M.P.: Self-instruction for the family of a child with cystic fibrosis, Am. J. Maternal Child Nurs. **5**:345-348, 1980.

Pumariega, A.J.: The adolescent with cystic fibrosis: developmental issues, Children's Health Care **11**:78-81, 1982.

Selekman, J.: Cystic fibrosis, Pediatr. Nurs. **3**(2):32-35, 1977.

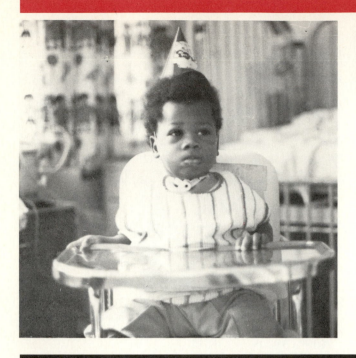

THE CHILD WITH GASTRO-INTESTINAL DYSFUNCTION

OBJECTIVES

On completion of this chapter the reader will be able to:

■ Describe the characteristics of infants that affect their ability to adapt to fluid loss or gain

■ Outline a plan of care for the infant with acute diarrhea

■ Discuss the management and nursing care of a child who ingests a foreign substance

■ Discuss the nursing care of the child and family with a pinworm infection

■ Outline a plan for teaching the parents pre- and postoperative care of a child with a cleft lip and/or palate

■ Compare the pre- and postoperative care of an infant with a structural defect of the gastrointestinal tract

■ Plan the diet for a child with a malabsorption syndrome

■ Outline a plan of care for a child with an obstructive disorder

■ Compare and contrast the inflammatory diseases of the gastrointestinal tract

■ Discuss the cause, prevention, and nursing care of the child with hepatitis

NURSING DIAGNOSES

Nursing diagnoses identified for the child with gastrointestinal dysfunction include, but are not restricted to, the following:

Health perception-health management pattern

■ Infection, potential for, related to (1) presence of infectious organisms; (2) damaged tissues

Nutritional-metabolic pattern

■ Fluid volume deficit related to excessive fluid losses

■ Nutrition, alteration in; less than body requirements, deficit related to loss of appetite

■ Skin integrity, impairment of: potential related to irritation from body secretions

Elimination pattern

■ Bowel elimination, alteration in: constipation

■ Bowel elimination, alteration in: diarrhea

Activity-exercise pattern

- Activity intolerance related to decreased energy

- Home maintenance management, impaired, related to knowledge deficit

- Self-care deficit (specify level: feeding, bathing/hygiene, dressing/grooming, toileting) related to (1) developmental level; (2) discomfort

Sleep-rest pattern

- Sleep pattern disturbance related to (1) physical discomfort; (2) schedule therapies

Cognitive-perceptual pattern

- Comfort, alterations in: pain related to (1) alterations in bowel motility; (2) bowel distention

Self-perception—self-concept pattern

- Anxiety related to (1) strange environment; (2) perception of impending events; (3) separation; (4) anticipated discomfort; (5) knowledge deficit; (6) pain

- Self-concept, disturbance in, related to perception of physical defect or disease

Role-relationship pattern

- Communication, impaired verbal, related to (1) ineffective use of abnormal structures; (2) physical defect

- Family process, alterations in, related to (1) hospitalization; (2) skill deficit; (3) family stress

- Social isolation related to (1) physical isolation; (2) body image disturbance

Coping-stress tolerance pattern

- Coping, family: potential for growth

Disorders of the gastrointestinal tract are very common and constitute one of the largest categories of illnesses that occur in infancy and childhood. Vomiting and diarrhea occur as isolated disturbances and are among the symptoms most often associated with a variety of childhood illnesses. Structural and obstructive defects interfere with the ingestion and transport of ingested foodstuffs, and inflammatory, malabsorptive, and maldigestive disturbances impair the functional integrity of the gastrointestinal tract. Furthermore, in most of the disorders the primary defect can produce additional complications. For example, loss of gastrointestinal contents causes significant alterations in fluid and electrolytes, and obstructive or inflammatory conditions affect digestion and absorption because bowel motility, mucosal functioning, enzymatic activity, and bacterial flora are altered. This chapter is concerned with those conditions that in some way interfere with normal digestion and absorption of nutrients.

THE GASTROINTESTINAL SYSTEM

The gastrointestinal (GI) system serves to process and absorb nutrients necessary to maintain metabolic processes and to support growth and development. All actions of the gastrointestinal tract are subject to a variety of outside influences at all ages. They are sensitive to tensions and anxieties, and many diseases and disorders are reflected in altered gastrointestinal function.

Most biochemical and physiologic functions of the gastrointestinal tract are established at the time of birth. However, the mechanical functions of digestion are relatively immature. Sucking and swallowing are present prenatally but do not become fully developed until after birth. Swallowing is an automatic reflex action for the first 3 months, but the normal infant begins to exert voluntary control at approximately 6 weeks of age. By 6 months the infant is capable of swallowing, holding food in the mouth, or spitting it out at will.

Sucking is also a reflex activity in the newborn. The muscular action of the tongue has a typical forward thrust highly efficient for sucking but ineffectual for spoon feeding. With neural and muscular development, the infant gradually acquires the ability to perform the coordinated muscular action typical of the adult type of swallowing. The chewing function is facilitated by eruption of the primary teeth, and the timing of the infant's dietary changes closely parallels these progressive capabilities. First, the infant diet consists of foods that require merely swallowing, then those that need no mastication, and, finally, those that require biting and chewing.

The size and configuration of the stomach also changes with age. The stomach is round and situated horizontally until approximately 2 years of age, which influences positioning practices during and after feeding in infancy (p. 159). It gradually elongates until it assumes the shape and anatomic position of the adult at about 7 years of age. At birth, capacity of the stomach is only about 10 to 20 ml, but, a distensible organ, the stomach rapidly expands to triple its capacity in 3 weeks and to reach five to ten times its original birth capacity at the age of 1 month.

The immaturity of the digestive system in the infant is demonstrated by the rapidity with which swallowed food is propelled through the length of the gastrointestinal tract. For example, the emptying time of the stomach increases from 2½ to 3 hours in the newborn to 3 to 6 hours in older infants and children. The small stomach capacity with a rapid transit time has implications for determining the amount and frequency of feedings during this period of growth. The frequency and character of stools are also affected by the rate of peristalsis and the nature of ingested food. For example, the frequent, yellow stools of the neonate gradually assume a more adult regularity and character as the infant develops and the composition of his diet changes. In addition, peristalsis is more rapid in infancy than at other periods of life, and it is not uncommon for peristaltic waves to reverse and cause spitting up or, if vigorous, vomiting of stomach contents. An immature, relaxed cardiac sphincter in infancy and early childhood contributes to this ease of regurgitation.

The length of the intestine in infants is six times the body length and is proportionately greater than that of the full-grown individual, which is four to five times the body length. There are two periods of accelerated growth of the intestine that correlate with nutritional and physiologic changes that are taking place—the first, between 1 and 3 years of age, during a period of diet transition, and the second, between 10 and 15 years of age, which coincides with the adolescent growth spurt.

Water balance in infants

Because of several characteristics, infants and young children have a greater need for water and are more vulnerable to alterations in fluid and electrolyte balance. Compared to older children and adults, they have a greater fluid intake and output relative to size, water and electrolyte disturbances occur more frequently and more rapidly, and they adjust less promptly to these alterations.

The fluid compartments in the infant vary significantly from those in the adult primarily because of an expanded extracellular compartment. The extracellular fluid compartment comprises over half of the total body water at birth and, accompanying this, a greater relative content of extracellular sodium and chloride. This neonatal "excess" extracellular fluid is largely lost in the first 10 days of life through insensible perspiration that amounts to up to 10%

of the infant's birth weight. The infant maintains a larger amount of extracellular fluid than the adult until about 2 years of age, which contributes to greater and more rapid water loss and poorer adjustment during this age period (see Fig. 2-5, p. 31).

Surface area. The infant's relatively greater surface area allows larger quantities of fluid to be lost in insensible perspiration through the skin. It is estimated that the body surface area of the premature infant is five times as great, and that of the newborn is two to three times as great, as that of the older child or adult. The proportionately longer gastrointestinal tract (sometimes considered to be an extension of the body surface area) in infancy is a source of relatively greater loss, especially from diarrhea. Also, the daily volume of secretions into the gastrointestinal tract is much higher in infants than in children.

Metabolic rate. The rate of metabolism in infancy is significantly higher because of the larger surface area in relation to the mass of active tissue. Consequently there is a greater production of metabolic wastes that must be excreted by the kidneys. Any condition that increases metabolism causes greater heat production, with its concomitant insensible fluid loss and an increased need for water for excretion.

Kidney function. The kidneys of the infant are functionally immature at birth and are, therefore, inefficient in excreting waste products of metabolism. Of particular importance for fluid balance is the inability of the infant's kidneys to concentrate or dilute urine, to conserve or excrete sodium, and to acidify urine. Therefore, the infant is less able to handle large quantities of solute-free water than the older child.

Fluid requirements. As a result of these characteristics, infants ingest and excrete a greater amount of fluid per kilogram of body weight than older children. Since electrolytes are excreted with water and the infant has limited ability for conservation, maintenance requirements include both water and electrolytes. The daily exchange of extracellular fluid in the infant is greatly increased over that of older children, which leaves them little fluid volume reserve in dehydrated states.

The child with abdominal surgery

Surgical procedures are common in gastrointestinal disorders. They may be as simple as an appendectomy or as complex as colostomy construction or repair of congenital malformations. In any procedure the general preparation and management of both children and their parents are similar and the reader is referred to Chapters 18 and 19 for all aspects of hospitalization. The summary on pp. 653 and 654 outlines both general and specific care of children with disorders that require abdominal surgery.

DISORDERS OF MOTILITY

Acute attacks of vomiting and diarrhea are so common in the pediatric age-group that they can almost be regarded as part of the normal way of life. However, the nature of the anatomic and physiologic structure of the infant and small child renders them particularly vulnerable to fluid and electrolyte imbalances when pathologic changes affect the fluid compartments. Most illnesses create some disturbance in body fluids and/or electrolytes, and, in vomiting and diarrhea, these disturbances are more threatening than the primary pathology.

VOMITING

Vomiting, a very common symptom in childhood, is usually of little concern. Often it is of a minor and temporary nature, but when vomiting is persistent and prolonged, the consequences to the infant or child can be rapid and serious. Vomiting in childhood can be caused by numerous intrinsic and extrinsic factors but is usually the result of readily detectable infections or psychologic causes.

Vomiting is the forcible ejection of stomach contents and is ordinarily accompanied by nausea. It is one of the most primitive protective functions and involves a complex reflex that is associated with widespread autonomic discharge that causes salivation, pallor, sweating, and tachycardia. In *projectile vomiting* vomitus is forcefully ejected as far as 2 to 4 feet (0.6 to 1.2 m) from the child. Projectile vomiting is not associated with nausea. Spitting up and regurgitation, characteristics of infants, are described on p. 268.

Therapeutic management

Medical management is directed toward detection and treatment of the cause of the vomiting and prevention of complications from the loss of fluid. Fluids are administered in the same manner and in a similar electrolyte composition to those administered in diarrhea (p. 646). Although most children respond well to these measures, centrally acting antiemetic drugs such as promethazine (Phenergan), diphenidol (Vontrol), or trimethobenzamide hydrochloride (Tigan) may be recommended. For children who are prone to motion sickness, it is often helpful to administer an appropriate dose of dimenhydrinate (Dramamine) before a journey.

Nursing considerations

The major emphasis of nursing care of the vomiting infant or child is on observation and reporting of vomiting behavior and associated symptoms and the implementation of measures to reduce the vomiting. Accurate assessment of the type of vomiting, the appearance of the vomitus, and the child's behavior associated with the vomiting greatly aids in establishing a diagnosis of disorders that have vomiting as a clinical feature.

Nursing interventions are determined by the cause of the vomiting. When the vomiting is identified as a manifestation of improper feeding methods, establishing proper techniques through teaching and example will ordinarily correct the situation. If the vomiting is assessed as a probable sign of a gastrointestinal obstruction, food is usually withheld or special feeding techniques are implemented. In situations in which vomiting is related to concurrent infection, dietary indiscretion, or emotional factors, efforts are directed toward maintaining hydration or preventing dehydration.

The thirst mechanism is the most sensitive guide to fluid needs, and ad libitum administration of a glucose-electrolyte solution to an alert child will restore water and electrolytes satisfactorily. It is important to include carbohydrate to spare body protein and to avoid ketosis resulting from exhaustion of glycogen stores. Once vomiting has abated, more liberal amounts can be offered, followed by simple foods such as gelatin, crackers, clear broth, and buttered toast in small portions, when the child desires, followed by gradual resumption of the regular diet.

GASTROESOPHAGEAL REFLUX (GER, CHALASIA)

Gastroesophageal reflux (chalasia, cardiochalasia) is relaxation or incompetence of the lower esophageal sphincter, which results in frequent return of stomach contents into the esophagus. In newborns this is considered a normal phenomenon because of immature neuromuscular control of the gastroesophageal sphincter. However, in a small percentage of infants reflux continues, producing symptoms that warrant investigation. The exact cause is not known, although it is thought to result from delayed maturation of lower esophageal neuromuscular function or impaired local hormonal control mechanisms.

Clinical manifestations

The most common manifestations of GER are vomiting, weight loss, respiratory problems, and bleeding. Vomiting is the most prominent symptom and in infants can be quite forceful—sometimes so severe that there is sufficient loss of calories to cause weight loss and failure to thrive.

Reflux of stomach contents to the pharynx predisposes to aspiration and the development of respiratory symptoms, particularly pneumonia. Repeated irritation of the esophageal lining with gastric acid can lead to esophagitis

and subsequent bleeding. Blood loss produces anemia and is seen as hematemesis or melena (blood in stools). Heartburn is also a frequent symptom in older children who are able to describe it but which may go unrecognized in infants.

Diagnostic evaluation

In addition to a history, several tests are available to establish the presence of reflux: fluoroscopic observation of reflux following a barium swallow, manometry, which measures esophageal sphincter pressure, direct measurement of the pH of the distal esophagus, and scintigraphy, which detects radioactive substances in the esophagus after a feeding of the compound.

Therapeutic management

Medical management of GER involves (1) positioning the child prone with the head elevated at about a 30-degree angle (Fig. 21-1) for 24 hours a day, (2) thickened formula, and (3) small-volume feedings every 2 to 3 hours. Length of time to recovery is variable but is observed initially by 2 weeks. By 6 weeks a normal physiologic barrier to reflux usually develops. Once symptoms are controlled for 4 to 6 weeks, prolonged positioning is reduced. For example, the child can be removed from the prescribed position for short periods *before* the next feeding.

Surgical intervention is selected for those children with severe complications, such as respiratory distress (choking, aspiration, recurrent apnea), esophagitis, or esophageal stricture. A commonly used surgical procedure

FIG. 21-1

Five-week-old infant positioned in harness (From Orenstein, S.R., and Whitington, P.F.: Positioning for prevention of infant gastroesophageal reflux, J. Pediatr. **103:** *534-537, 1983).*

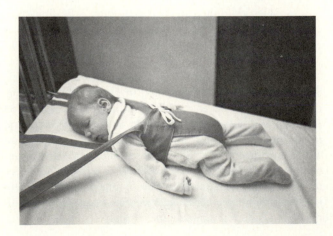

is one that creates a valve mechanism at the distal esophagus.

Nursing considerations

Nursing care is directed toward (1) identifying children with symptoms that suggest GER, (2) helping parents with positioning and feeding at home, and (3) if appropriate, providing care for the child undergoing surgical repair.

The greatest challenge lies in maintaining the desired position for the child and adhering to a frequent feeding schedule. The 30 degree angle can be provided by elevating the head of the infant's crib with extra bedding, a wood or metal frame, or a wedge constructed from a cardboard box. An alternative is a specially constructed frame that can be moved about to allow the child a change of environment with minimum disturbance. The child is suspended from the head of the crib or frame in a prepared or improvised harness. When the infant is older and more mobile, maintaining correct positioning becomes increasingly difficult. An alternative frame has been described that consists of a cradle bed, bassinet, or board with a firm wooden base and a wooden spindle or large dowel that protrudes through the center of the mattress. The infant is positioned prone with his legs straddling the well-padded spindle and secured to the mattress with a harness or folded diaper across his back and pinned to the mattress. To prevent undue pressure on areas such as the infant's knees and elbows the mattress is covered with a sheepskin or egg-crate pad.

Early in the treatment program both parents and other available family members should be encouraged to participate in the feeding regimen, especially with alternate night shifts. Nurses need to be sensitive to the demands placed on the family and recognize those situations when hospitalization may be required to ensure continued treatment.

DIARRHEA

Diarrhea is defined as an increase in the number of stools or a decrease in their consistency as a major clinical manifestation of alterations of water and electrolyte transport by the alimentary tract. It is a symptom of diverse origin and results from disorders involving digestive, absorptive, and secretory functions. However, a precise definition and identification of what constitutes diarrhea pose a problem in terms of number or consistency of stools, since there are wide variations in colonic function between individuals. For example, one infant may have one firm stool every second or third day, whereas another normally passes from five to eight small, soft stools daily. Therefore, more important are (1) a noticeable or sudden increase in number

of stools, (2) a reduction in their consistency with an increase in fluid content, and (3) a tendency for the stools to be greenish in color.

Diarrhea may be acute or chronic, and the physiologic consequences vary considerably in relation to its severity, duration, associated symptoms, the age of the child, and the child's nutritional status before the onset of diarrhea.

Etiology

Diarrhea can be attributed to a large number of specific causes, mechanisms, and predisposing factors. Factors that predispose a child to diarrhea and its physiologic consequences include: (1) the younger the child, the more susceptible he is to diarrhea and the more severe the diarrhea is likely to be; (2) children who are malnourished or debilitated from disease are more susceptible to diarrhea; (3) warm climates (and warm weather) where sanitation and refrigeration are a problem; (4) crowded and substandard environment with poor facilities for preparation and refrigeration of food.

Specific causes. A variety of factors can produce diarrhea in the infant or child either as the presenting symptom or as an associated symptom. Often a specific etiologic diagnosis is lacking. *Acute* diarrhea, a sudden change in frequency and consistency of stools, is more often caused by an inflammatory process of infectious origin but may also be the result of a toxic reaction to ingestion of poisons, dietary indiscretions, or associated with infection outside the alimentary tract, for example, communicable diseases, infections of the respiratory or urinary tracts, and emotional tension. Most are self-limited and will ultimately subside without specific treatment if consequent dehydration does not create a serious complication.

Chronic diarrhea, the passage of loose stools with increased frequency of more than 2 weeks' duration, is more apt to be associated with disorders of malabsorption, anatomic defects, abnormal bowel motility, hypersensitivity (allergic) reaction, or an inflammatory response.

Diarrheal disturbances can involve the stomach and intestine (*gastroenteritis*), the small intestine (*enteritis*), the colon (*colitis*), or the colon and intestine (*enterocolitis*). *Dysentery* is a term that describes intestinal inflammation, especially of the colon, that is accompanied by cramping abdominal pain, tenesmus, and watery stools, containing blood and mucus.

Enteropathologic organisms. There are many organisms that can cause diarrheal disturbances in children, especially in infants. These can be enteric pathogens primarily, such as *Campylobacter jejuni* and the *Shigella* and *Salmonella* groups of bacteria. Other organisms have the potential to produce diarrhea under favorable circumstances, such as *Staphylococcus aureus*. Most infectious organisms are transmitted through contaminated feedings or by infected "carriers," including animal reservoirs.

Organisms that are considered "normal flora" in most situations are enteropathic under certain conditions and in susceptible children, particularly newborns and young infants. These include certain strains of *Escherichia coli* and *Staphylococcus aureus*. Some strains of *E. coli* produce diarrhea by invasion of the intestinal mucosa and others by elaboration of enterotoxins. *S. aureus* can cause diarrhea by (1) food poisoning from contamination (especially milk or egg products) with exotoxin production, (2) enteritis as a result of prolonged broad-spectrum antibiotic therapy that destroys and eliminates enteric organisms that normally control staphylococcal invasion, (3) enteritis as a complication of staphylococcal infection elsewhere (skin or lungs), and (4) primary staphylococcal infection in newborn infants who have not yet established competing enteric flora. Other bacteria may cause diarrhea but are less likely to do so. The enteropathic bacteria are briefly outlined in Table 21-1.

Viral diarrheas are probably quite common, but, with the possible implication of the enteroviruses and adenoviruses, no specific etiologic agents have been identified. Other agents such as *Pseudomonas, Klebsiella,* and *Proteus* organisms may cause diarrhea but do not ordinarily have a tendency to do so. Amebic dysentery seldom occurs in infants.

In addition to such dietary indiscretions as eating green apples or, in some children, dried or fresh fruits in large amounts it has been found recently that sorbitol, the sweetener used in most "sugar free" gum and other products, is poorly absorbed in the gastrointestinal tract and may produce osmotic diarrhea if ingested in large amounts.

TABLE 21-1. ENTEROPATHOLOGIC CAUSES OF BACTERIAL DIARRHEA

ORGANISM	CHARACTERISTICS	COMMENTS
Pathogenic *Escherichia coli*	Variable clinical manifestations Most—green, watery diarrhea with mucus Afebrile Symptoms generally subside in 3-7 days Relapse rate approximately 20%	Usually interpersonal transmission but may transmit via inanimate objects A cause of nursery epidemics
Salmonella groups (nontyphoidal)—gram-negative, nonencapsulated, nonsporulating	Variable symptoms—mild to severe Nausea, vomiting, and colicky abdominal pain followed by diarrhea, occasionally with blood and mucus Chills not uncommon Hyperactive peristalsis and mild abdominal tenderness Symptoms usually subside within 5 days May have high fever, headache, and cerebral manifestations, for example, drowsiness, confusion, meningismus, or seizures	Two thirds of patients are less than 20 years of age; highest incidence in children under age 9 years, especially infants Highest incidence occurs July through October, lowest from January through April Transmission primarily via contaminated food and drink—most from animal sources, including fowl, mammals, reptiles, and insects Most common sources are poultry and eggs; in children—pets, especially pet turtles Communicable as long as organisms are excreted
Salmonella typhi	Variable in infants Older children—irregular fever, headache, malaise, lethargy Diarrhea occurs in 50% at early stage Cough is common In a few days, fever rises and is consistent; fatigue, cough, abdominal pain, anorexia, and weight loss develop; diarrhea begins	Same as above

Pathophysiology

Invasion of the gastrointestinal tract by pathogens produces diarrhea by (1) production of enterotoxins that stimulate secretion of water and electrolytes, (2) direct invasion and destruction of intestinal epithelial cells, and (3) local inflammation and systemic invasion by the organisms. However, the most serious and immediate physiologic disturbances associated with severe diarrheal disease are (1) dehydration, (2) acid-base derangements with acidosis, and (3) shock that occurs when dehydration progresses to the point that circulatory status is seriously disturbed.

Types of dehydration. Dehydration can be classified as three general types according to the compositional changes in the plasma: (1) isotonic, isonatremic, or isosmotic, (2) hypotonic, hyponatremic, or hyposmotic, and (3) hypertonic, hyponatremic, or hyperosmotic.

Isotonic (isonatremic) dehydration occurs in conditions in which the electrolyte and water deficits are present in approximately balanced proportion. Shock is the greatest threat to life in isotonic dehydration, and the child displays the symptoms characteristic of hypovolemic shock. Plasma sodium remains within normal limits, between 130 and 150 mEq/liter.

Hypotonic (hyponatremic) dehydration occurs when the electrolyte deficit exceeds the water deficit, leaving the serum hypotonic. Since intracellular fluid is more concentrated than extracellular fluid in hypotonic dehydration, water moves from the extracellular to the intracellular fluid to establish osmotic equilibrium. Therefore, this further increases the extracellular fluid volume loss, and shock is a frequent finding. Since there is a greater proportional loss of extracellular fluid in hypotonic dehydration, the physical signs tend to be more severe with smaller fluid losses

TABLE 21-1. ENTEROPATHOLOGIC CAUSES OF BACTERIAL DIARRHEA—cont'd

ORGANISM	CHARACTERISTICS	COMMENTS
Shigella groups—gram-negative, nonmotile, anaerobic bacilli	Onset variable but usually abrupt Fever and cramping abdominal pain initially Fever—may reach 40.5° C (105° F) Convulsions in about 10%—usually associated with fever Patient appears sick Headache, nuchal rigidity, delirium Watery diarrhea with mucus and pus starts about 12-48 hours after onset Stools preceded by abdominal cramps; tenesmus and straining follow Symptoms usually subside in 5-10 days	Approximately 60% of cases in children under age 9 years with more than one third between ages 1 and 4 years Peak incidence late summer Transmitted directly or indirectly from infected persons Communicable for 1-4 weeks
Campylobacter jejuni	Fever and cramping periumbilical pain, which may be quite severe, followed by watery, profuse, foul-smelling diarrhea Most stools become blood-streaked	Epidemiology not well understood Person-to-person transmission Food (chicken) and waterborne—especially untreated surface water Illness generally lasts a week Relapses have been reported Recovery spontaneous but erythromycin shortens the duration of symptoms
Vibrio cholerae (cholera) groups	Sudden onset of profuse, watery diarrhea without cramping, tenesmus, or anal irritation, although children may complain of cramping Stools are intermittent at first then almost continuous Stools are whitish, almost clear, with flecks of mucus "rice water stools"	Rare in infants less than 1 year old Mortality rate high in both treated and untreated infants and small children Transmitted via contaminated food and water Endemic in Bengal Attack confers immunity

than isotonic or hypertonic dehydration. Plasma sodium concentration is less than 130 mEq/liter.

Hypertonic (hypernatremic) dehydration results from water loss in excess of electrolyte loss and is usually caused by either a proportionately larger loss of water and/ or a larger intake of electrolytes. This sometimes occurs in infants with diarrhea who are given fluids by mouth that contain large amounts of solute or in children receiving high-protein nasogastric tube feedings that place an excessive solute load on the kidneys. In hypertonic dehydration fluid shifts from the lesser concentration of the intracellular to the extracellular fluid. Plasma sodium concentration is greater than 150 mEq/liter. Since the extra-cellular fluid volume is proportionately larger, hypertonic dehydration has a larger degree of water loss for the same intensity of physical signs. Shock is less apparent in hypertonic dehydration. However, neurologic disturbances, such as seizures, are more likely to occur. Cerebral changes are serious and may result in permanent damage.

Intractable diarrhea of infancy. The term "intractable diarrhea" has been used only recently to describe infants whose diarrhea is not caused by recognized pathogens and does not respond to treatment. It is classified as either primary, which is identified as nonspecific enterocolitis, or secondary, associated with disease entities such as allergy, bowel anomalies, or a variety of congenital diseases. The age of onset ranges from 4 days to 3 months of age. Dehydration is always present, and a prominent feature is malnutrition with hypoproteinemia and hypoalbuminemia.

The primary form may be the result of such trivial events as an infection or feeding difficulties. The diarrhea rapidly becomes self-perpetuating through a combination of secondary consequences—malnutrition deprives the infant of the elements protein, vitamins, calcium, and magnesium needed for mucosal regeneration; the villi of the small intestine atrophy; the bowel wall becomes inflamed and irritated by undigested foodstuffs or microorganisms; and secondary digestive and absorptive disorders develop as a result of malnutrition, various patterns of motility, and overgrowth of bacteria caused by the infant's debilitated state (Fig. 21-2).

Clinical manifestations

Mild diarrhea is described as a few loose stools each day without other evidence of illness that terminates in a few days. With moderate diarrhea, the child is sicker, may have a fever, vomits, appears fretful and irritable, and passes several loose or watery stools daily. Although the child may not gain weight or may even show a slight loss, signs of dehydration are usually absent. If the diarrhea persists, if the child loses weight, if there is blood in the stools, or if the child develops associated signs such as

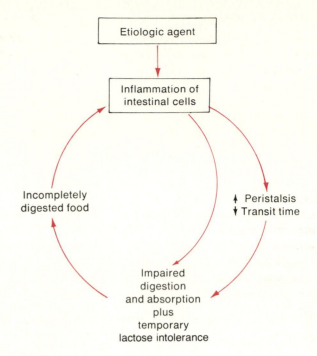

FIG. 21-2
Vicious pathologic cycle in diarrhea plus temporary lactose intolerance.

deep breathing, listlessness, or reduced urinary output that may signal complications, the child should be seen by the physician.

Degree of dehydration. The most serious consequence of diarrhea is dehydration, especially in infants. In infants, isotonic dehydration is usually described as 5% (mild), 10% (moderate), and 15% (severe). Older children and adolescents, with proportionately less total body water, display smaller proportional losses; therefore, the estimates of 3%, 6%, and 9% more nearly describe mild, moderate, and severe dehydration, respectively, in these age-groups.

Shock is a common feature of severe depletion of extracellular fluid volume with tachycardia and low blood pressure. Peripheral circulation is poor as a result of reduced blood volume; therefore, the skin is cool and mottled, with poor capillary filling after blanching. Impaired kidney circulation often leads to oliguria and prerenal azotemia. Skin and mucous membranes are dry, skin turgor is poor, and, in infants, the anterior fontanel is depressed. At the opposite extreme, a mild degree of dehydration is associated with barely discernible physical signs and absence of shock (Table 21-2).

Diagnostic evaluation

The history provides valuable information regarding exposure to infectious agents, personal contact, travel, or

TABLE 21-2. INTENSITY OF CLINICAL SIGNS ASSOCIATED WITH VARYING DEGREES OF ISOTONIC DEHYDRATION IN INFANTS

	DEGREE OF DEHYDRATION		
	MILD	**MODERATE**	**SEVERE**
Body weight	Up to 5%	5%-9%	10%-15%
Skin color	Pale	Gray	Mottled
Skin turgor	Decreased	Poor	Very poor
Mucous membranes	Dry	Very dry	Parched
Urine output	Decreased	Oliguria	Marked oliguria and azotemia
Blood pressure	Normal	Normal or lowered	Lowered
Pulse	Normal or increased	Increased	Rapid and thready

probable contact with contaminated foods. Allergic and dietary history may indicate food allergies.

The age of the child provides clues to the cause of diarrheal disturbances. For example, with the exception of nursery epidemics, infectious enteritis is uncommon during the first days of life. *E. coli* disease is the usual agent after the first week of life, with a peak incidence from 1 to 3 months of age in bottle-fed infants; it is uncommon after 1 year of age. In breast-fed infants the time sequence is later. Shigellosis is most common from ages 2 to 4 years, but the most severe form is more apt to occur in children over 5 years of age. *Campylobacter* enteritis is a disorder associated with children over 10 years of age. Although *Salmonella* infection is encountered in children in any age-group, it appears to be most prevalent in children under age 2 years, as are the so-called viral diarrheas of unknown etiology. It is characteristic that multiple cases in a household are usually shigellosis, whereas a single case is more typical of enteropathogenic *E. coli*. Likewise, milk allergy or intolerance of other formula constituents is suspected in early infancy. In later infancy new foods added to the diet are frequent offenders. Parenteral infections are very common causes of diarrhea in infancy.

Most acute, inflammatory diarrheas are infectious, and the type of stools and symptoms associated with diarrhea provide clues to the organism. Fever is not a symptom of *E. coli* disease until late, whereas it is a common early feature even in mild cases of shigellosis. Abdominal cramps are common in shigellosis. Explosive onset of diarrhea accompanied by or preceded by vomiting suggests food poisoning. Although vomiting may occur in all infectious diarrheas, it is not a major feature.

The magnitude of fluid loss is best ascertained by a comparison of preillness weight with the current weight, since any weight loss is substantially equivalent to the amount of water lost. If preillness weight is unknown, the degree of dehydration is estimated by assessing the intensity of clinical signs.

Laboratory examination. Stools are examined for pH, blood, and evidence of bacterial invasion. The stool specimen obtained from evacuated stool should include mucus or tissue shreds, if present. The specimen is examined with indicator paper for pH and a Clinitest tablet will detect the acid stool containing sugar that is characteristic of disaccharide intolerance. Bulky stools containing fat suggest malabsorption diarrhea.

The specimen is also examined for the presence of red blood cells. Rectal swabs for culture are indicated whenever a bacterial agent is suspected. Examination of the stool for leukocytes often differentiates between some bacteria. No leukocytes appear in normal stools or in diarrheal disease of viral or enterotoxin-producing bacteria, but many leukocytes or clumps of pus cells are seen in infections caused by enteroinvasive organisms.

Serum electrolyte values are obtained in the young infant who is hospitalized with diarrhea because of the likelihood of complicating dehydration and associated electrolyte imbalances, particularly in relation to sodium and potassium alterations. Dehydrated infants will have an elevated hematocrit as a result of volume loss, and an elevated blood urea nitrogen will be found in the presence of reduced renal circulation.

Therapeutic management

Mild or moderate diarrhea is usually managed by simple measures and seldom requires hospitalization. When the moderate diarrhea becomes worse or does not respond to simple measures, hospitalization is indicated.

Severe diarrhea. Severe diarrhea is largely a problem of infants and very young children, and, regardless of the cause, successful management relies primarily on appropriate treatment of physiologic disturbances and is only secondarily concerned with specific treatment of the causative agent. Severe diarrhea warrants hospitalization, comprehensive evaluation, and parenteral fluid therapy.

Fluid therapy is directed toward replacement of (1) the fluid deficit as determined by weight loss and clinical signs, (2) ongoing normal losses from urine, lungs, and sweat, and (3) continued abnormal gastrointestinal losses.

The initial intravenous fluids are administered rapidly to correct the dehydration and restore circulation. The fluid is usually a dextrose solution with appropriate electrolytes added. As the initial losses are replaced, the fluid administration is adjusted to meet maintenance needs and to replace gastrointestinal losses. Potassium is added when renal function is established.

Once the child is well hydrated, oral feedings of a glucose-electrolyte solution are begun unless anorexia, vomiting, or nervous system disturbances prevent the use of this route. In this event, parenteral feedings are continued. A number of commercially prepared fluids are available, or a solution can be made with simple ingredients. Milk feedings (diluted) are not resumed until at least the end of 24 hours.

Reintroduction of milk feedings is conducted slowly. Ordinarily about one fifth the usual daily intake of milk is recommended for the initial reintroduction, with the remainder provided by the glucose-electrolyte solution already employed. The amount of milk is gradually increased each day until the former diet is resumed. The possibility of a secondary lactase deficiency (especially in severely affected infants) makes a nonlactose-containing formula the feeding of choice. A normal nutritional regimen is usually resumed by the end of the fourth or fifth day.

Once the severe effects of dehydration are under control, specific diagnostic and therapeutic measures are instigated to detect and treat the cause of the diarrhea. This includes mild sedation, antimicrobial therapy where indicated, and treatment of secondary effects of the illness or its therapy. For example, secondary bacterial growth may be countered with a short course of nonabsorbable antibiotics and/or the oral administration of lactobacilli to recolonize the normal flora of the gastrointestinal tract.

Nursing considerations

The infant or child admitted to the hospital with diarrhea is always isolated from other children, and appropriate precautions are implemented to prevent possible spread to other children and personnel. Each hospital has a policy regarding isolation and enteric precautions.

The child is weighed on admission and frequently during the emergency phase of rapid hydration. Accurate intake and output measurement is imperative, and a urine collection bag is placed to determine the volume of output, to measure specific gravity, and as an indication that renal blood flow is sufficient to permit administration of potassium. Unless urine is separated from stool, this essential information cannot be obtained.

Children who are sufficiently ill to require hospitalization are almost always placed on parenteral fluid therapy with nothing by mouth for 12 to 24 hours. Monitoring the intravenous infusion is a primary nursing function, with careful attention to ascertain that the correct fluid and electrolyte concentration is infused, the flow rate is adjusted to deliver the desired volume in a given period of time, and the intravenous site is maintained. Restraint of some type is needed with infants and small children, whose purposeful or random movements might disturb the needle placement.

The nurse is responsible for examination of stools and the collection of specimens for laboratory examination. Care is exerted in obtaining and transporting stools to prevent possible spread of infection. Stool specimens are transported to the laboratory in appropriate containers and media according to hospital policy. A clean tongue depressor can be used to obtain specimens for laboratory examination when a larger volume is needed or as an applicator for transfer to a culture medium. Tests for pH, blood, and sugar can be done without removing the stool from the diaper.

Since diarrheal stools are highly irritating to the skin, extra care is needed to protect the skin of the diaper region from becoming excoriated. Exposing the reddened areas to heat and light is an effective method to facilitate healing. An excellent way to provide dry heat to the area is by means of a goose-necked lamp, but the lamp must be placed at a distance sufficient that the child is unable to reach any part of it. The heat source should be no closer than 18 inches. The child will require close observation during treatment, and the length of each application should not exceed 20 minutes.

Oral feedings are begun according to the physician's orders. Although the amount and frequency vary according to individual philosophy, the initial oral fluids are water, usually with some added electrolytes, such as the commercial electrolyte solutions Pedialyte or Lytren. When the diet is advanced to clear liquids, diluted fruit juice, liquid or solid Jell-O, sweetened tea, Popsicles, and decarbonated cola or ginger ale are well tolerated. Broth or other high-sodium liquids are used with caution to avoid the possibility of hypernatremia.

Soft foods are gradually added when liquids are well tolerated, as evidenced by no vomiting and an increased consistency and decrease in number of stools. Appropriate soft foods include gelatin desserts, soups (not creamed), bananas, applesauce, strained carrots, crackers (including pretzels), rice, and toast with jelly. Milk and lactose-containing formulas are usually withheld for at least a week in children with severe diarrhea. Soybean formulas (such as Isomil and ProSobee) or hydrolyzed protein formulas with nonlactose sugar (such as Nutramigen or Pregestimil) are substituted until the gastrointestinal tract is again able to tolerate milk and milk products.

SUMMARY OF NURSING CARE OF THE CHILD WITH ACUTE DIARRHEAL DISTURBANCES

GOALS	RESPONSIBILITIES

Assess status of diarrhea	Record fecal output: number, volume, characteristics
	Observe and record presence of associated signs: tenesmus, cramping, vomiting
	Collect specimens as needed
	Assist with specimen collection when indicated
	Make appropriate diagnostic tests
	    Stools: pH, blood, sugar
	    Urine: pH, specific gravity

Prevent spread of hospital infection	Isolate the affected child from contact with others
	Implement protective techniques as dictated by hospital policy, including
	    Disposal of excreta and laundry
	    Appropriate handling of specimens
	Maintain careful handwashing
	Apply diaper snugly to reduce likelihood of fecal spread
	Instruct others (parents, members of staff) in protective procedures
	Teach affected children protective methods to prevent spread of infection, for example, remaining in restricted area, handwashing, handling genital area, care after using bedpan or toilet, and so on
	Endeavor to keep infants and small children from placing hand and objects in contaminated areas
	Assess home situation and implement protective measures as feasible in individual circumstances

Observe for signs of complications	Assess frequently
	    Vital signs—temperature, pulse, respiration, and blood pressure
	    Skin characteristics
	    Sensory response
	    Neurologic signs
	    Behavior

Prevent skin breakdown	Change diaper after each soiling; disposable diapers absorb poorly, cloth diapers are preferred May need to apply rubber pants or thick cotton panties to keep stool contained in diaper Cleanse buttocks and genital area well Apply protective lotion or ointment Expose reddened area to heat and air where feasible (risk of contamination great in explosive diarrhea)
Prevent dehydration	Administer fluids as prescribed and as tolerated
Prevent interference with therapeutic regimen	Apply appropriate restraining methods where indicated
Prevent complications from restraining devices	Remove restraints from extremities as often as possible Change position at least every 2 hours Observe frequently circulation, position, and pressure points

Continued.

SUMMARY OF NURSING CARE OF THE CHILD WITH ACUTE DIARRHEAL DISTURBANCES—cont'd

GOALS	RESPONSIBILITIES

Rehydrate child	Administer fluids as ordered
	    Intravenous
	        Administer correct fluid
	        Maintain desired drip rate
	        Add appropriate electrolytes as prescribed
	        Maintain integrity of infusion site
	    Oral
	        Feed electrolyte and glucose-containing solutions as prescribed
	        Observe response to feedings
	        Describe feeding behavior
	Maintain accurate record of intake

Assess progress of hydration	Weigh the child daily or as ordered Assess all parameters, for example, vital signs, skin characteristics Apply urine collection device when indicated Measure urine volume and specific gravity Collect specimens as needed
Provide comfort measures	Administer special mouth care while fluids by mouth are restricted Provide pacifier for infants who are receiving nothing by mouth Bubble the child periodically to help expel swallowed air Hold the infant or child when this does not interfere with therapy Touch, talk, and otherwise comfort the child who is unable to be held Provide sensory stimulation and diversion appropriate to the child's level of development Encourage the parents to visit and allow them to comfort and care for the child to the extent possible
Eradicate infectious agent	Administer antimicrobial medications as prescribed Administer other medications as prescribed
Reestablish diet appropriate for age	Gradually reintroduce foods as prescribed
Detect source of infection	Examine other members of household and refer for treatment where indicated Collect stool specimens from household members where indicated

Support parents	Reassure parents, especially the mother
	Explain therapeutic measures that may be distressing to parents
	    Nothing by mouth
	    Parenteral fluids
	    Restraints necessary
	    Shaving of the infant's head for intravenous therapy
	    Isolation from other children
	    Need for precautions that parents must observe
	Help parents provide comfort and support for child

Educate parents	Instruct the parents in diet planning Help the caregiver plan diet to meet needs of the affected child in relation to family diet pattern Instruct in preparation and storage of food, based on assessment of individual family needs and facilities Instruct in care and disposal of waste materials Teach and emphasize importance of good hygiene and sanitation
Arrange for follow-up care	Emphasize importance of posthospitalization health assessment Refer to community health agency for care and instruction when indicated

CONSTIPATION

Constipation is the regular passage of firm or hard stools or of small, hard masses at longer intervals. The apparent difficulty in passing stools is not a reliable sign, especially in infancy. The development and course of constipation can be influenced by a number of familial, cultural, and social factors. Psychologic factors play an important role in bowel habits as well as toilet-training techniques, diet, overuse of laxatives, and enemas. Physical and mental disorders are often associated with defecation problems, for example, neurologic or anatomic disorders, mental retardation, hypothyroidism, and hypercalcemia.

Newborn

Normally the newborn infant passes a first meconium stool within 24 to 36 hours of birth. Any infant who does not do so should be assessed for evidence of intestinal atresia or stenosis, congenital aganglionic megacolon (50% of cases), hypothyroidism, meconium plugs, or meconium ileus. Meconium plugs are caused by meconium that has reduced water content and are usually evacuated following digital examination but may require irrigations of normal saline or the iodinated contrast medium *diatrizoate meglumine (Gastrografin)*.

Meconium ileus, the initial manifestation of cystic fibrosis, is the presence of thick, mucilagenous meconium that clings to the abdominal wall making it difficult, if not impossible, to pass. Treatment is the same as for a meconium plug. Rarely, surgical intervention may be necessary.

Infancy

Medical causes such as Hirschsprung disease, hypothyroidism, and strictures must be ruled out in chronic cases of constipation. However, the most frequent cause in infancy is dietary mismanagement. It is almost unknown in breast-fed infants and rare in bottle-fed infants who receive an adequate diet. The infant's behavior during passage of stools is often misinterpreted by parents as having difficulty. He grunts and appears to be straining while his face turns red and he draws his legs up on his abdomen. Artificially fed infants may develop constipation if they do not receive a sufficient amount of food or fluid.

Simple measures ordinarily correct the problem, such as increasing the amount of fluid or sugar in the formula in the very young infant or adding or increasing the amount of cereal, vegetables, and fruit in the diet of the older infant. Enemas or suppositories may be used as a temporary measure.

Childhood

Older children who have fewer than three bowel movements a week are considered to be outside the normal range but not necessarily constipated. The character of the stools and the difficulty in expelling the stools, blood-streaked stools, and abdominal discomfort are more significant. If there are associated manifestations, such as vomiting, abdominal distention, or pain, and evidence of growth failure, the condition merits further investigation. Constipation may result from some medications, such as iron preparations, diuretics, antacids, and anticholinergic agents.

The management of simple constipation is primarily dietary. Increasing the intake of fluids plus high-fiber foods, prune juice, prunes, and bran is advised, and sometimes a stool softener such as dioctyl sodium sulfosuccinate (Colace) is of benefit. Cathartics are not usually recommended because of their tendency to produce dependency.

Nursing considerations

Constipation, unfortunately, tends to be self-perpetuating. If the child has difficulty or discomfort when attempting to evacuate his bowels he has a tendency to retain the bowel contents, and thus begins a vicious cycle. Nursing assessment begins with an accurate history of bowel habits, diet, events that may be associated with the onset of constipation, drugs or other substances that the child may be taking, and the consistency, color, frequency, and other characteristics of the stool. If there is no evidence of a pathologic condition that requires further investigation, the major task of the nurse is to educate the parents regarding normal stool patterns and to relieve the cause of the constipation.

Infants and children may need to increase their fluid intake, and solid foods introduced too soon to infants should be discontinued until constipation is no longer evident. Simply increasing the carbohydrate (sugar or corn syrup) in an infant formula will often relieve the problem. Parents will benefit from guidance in dietary planning especially regarding foods that facilitate bowel movements (see Table 21-3). They will need reassurance concerning the benign nature of the condition. It is also important to discuss with them their attitudes and expectations regarding toilet habits and to discourage the use of stool softeners, laxatives, and enemas. If they have been prescribed by a physician they should understand that these are merely temporary measures and not to be continued beyond the current need.

HIRSCHSPRUNG DISEASE (CONGENITAL AGANGLIONIC MEGACOLON)

Hirschsprung disease is a mechanical obstruction caused by inadequate motility in part of the intestine. It accounts for about one fourth of all cases of neonatal obstruction, although it may not be diagnosed until later in infancy or childhood. It is four times more common in males than females, follows a familial pattern in a small number of cases, and is considerably more common in children with Down syndrome. Depending on its presentation, it may be an acute, life-threatening condition or a chronic disorder.

Pathophysiology

The term "congenital aganglionic megacolon" describes the pathology. The primary defect is absence of parasympathetic ganglion cells in one segment of colon. The functional defect as a result of lack of innervation is absence of propulsive movements (peristalsis), causing accumulation of intestinal contents and distention of the bowel proximal to the defect, hence the term "megacolon," or large colon. In addition there is failure of the internal rectal sphincter to relax, which prevents evacuation of solids, liquids, and gas and, thus, contributes to the manifestations of obstruction (Fig. 21-3).

Clinical manifestations

Clinical manifestations vary according to the age when symptoms are first recognized and the presence of complications, such as enterocolitis. In the newborn the chief signs and symptoms are failure to pass meconium within 24 to 48 hours after birth, reluctance to ingest fluids, bile-stained vomitus, and abdominal distention. During infancy aganglionic megacolon manifests as failure to thrive, constipation, abdominal distention, and episodes of diarrhea and vomiting. Explosive, watery diarrhea, fever, and severe prostration are ominous signs that often signify the presence of enterocolitis, which greatly increases the risk of fatality.

During childhood the symptoms are more chronic and include constipation, passage of ribbonlike, foul-smelling stools, abdominal distention, and visible peristalsis. Fecal masses are easily palpable. The child is usually poorly nourished, anemic, and hypoproteinemic from malabsorption of nutrients.

Diagnostic evaluation

In the neonate diagnosis is usually made based on clinical signs of intestinal obstruction and failure to pass meconium. Roentgenograms, barium enema, and anorectal manometric examinations assist in the differential diagnosis, which is then confirmed by histologic examination of a full-thickness rectal biopsy demonstrating absence of ganglia.

Therapeutic management

Treatment may be symptomatic in a child with chronic, but not severe, symptoms of megacolon and consists of isotonic (saline) enemas, stool softeners, and low-residue diet that decreases the bulk of the stool and reduces irritation to the bowel.

Corrective therapy is the surgical removal of the aganglionic portion of the bowel in order to permit normal bowel motility and establish continence by improved functioning of the internal anal sphincter. In most cases this is accomplished in two stages. First, a temporary colostomy

FIG. 21-3
Hirschsprung disease.

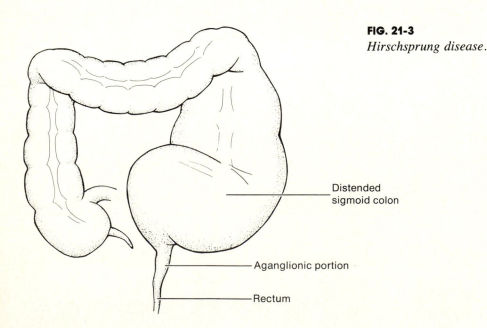

Distended
sigmoid colon

Aganglionic portion

Rectum

of the sigmoid or transverse colon is performed to allow the normal bowel a period of time to rest and resume its normal caliber and tonicity.

Complete correction with a pull-through anastomosis of the bowel may be done at the time of performing the colostomy or later, especially in those infants or children with preoperative complications. The type of surgical procedure for reanastomosis involves "pulling" the end of functioning ganglionated bowel down to a point near the rectum from which it can propel stool through the anus. In many cases a sphincterotomy of the internal sphincter is performed to improve anal control. Closure of the colostomy depends on the physician's evaluation of the child's postoperative progress but is usually performed within a few months to a year.

Nursing considerations

Many of the nursing concerns depend on the child's age and the type of treatment. If the disorder is diagnosed during the neonatal period, the main objectives are: (1) to help the parents adjust to a congenital defect in their child, (2) to foster infant-parent bonding, (3) to prepare them for the medical/surgical intervention, and (4) to assist them in colostomy care after discharge.

If the regimen of enemas, stool softeners, and low-residue diet is used, parents need detailed explanation regarding each procedure. The nurse demonstrates proper administration of an isotonic enema and has the parent perform at least one return demonstration.

Explanation of the low-residue diet includes the reason for its use and a list of foods to avoid (Table 21-3). Since eating difficulties are characteristic of children with Hirschsprung's disease, a dietary history regarding general food habits is essential before planning to alter the diet.

Preoperative care. Much of the child's preoperative care depends on his age and clinical condition. If the child is malnourished, he may not be able to withstand surgery until his physical status improves. Often this involves symptomatic treatment with enemas, a low-residue, high-calorie and high-protein diet, and, in severe situations, the use of parenteral alimentation.

Physical preoperative preparation entails the same measures that are common to any surgery (p. 585). In the newborn, whose bowel is sterile, no additional preparation is necessary. However, in other children emptying the bowel with repeated saline enemas and decreasing bacterial flora with systemic antibiotics and colonic irrigations using antibiotic solution are usually ordered. A nasogastric tube is sometimes inserted to prevent abdominal distention, and antibiotic solution may be instilled through the tube to further prepare the gastrointestinal tract. The nurse records all intake and output of irrigant and drainage, noting particularly any marked discrepancy in retention or loss of fluid.

Since progressive distention of the abdomen is a serious sign, the nurse measures abdominal circumference with a paper tape measure at the level of the umbilicus. The point of measurement is marked with a pen to assure reliability of subsequent measurements. In order to reduce any stress to the acutely ill child when frequent measurements are needed, the tape measure can be left in place beneath the child, rather than removed each time. As a rule of thumb, abdominal measurement can be performed at the same time that vital signs are taken and recorded in serial order so that a change will be readily apparent.

The age of the child dictates the type and extent of psychologic preparation. Since a colostomy is usually performed, the child of at least preschool age is told about the procedure in concrete terms and visual aids (see p. 584

TABLE 21-3. HIGH-FIBER FOODS

FOOD GROUP	SELECTIONS
Bread, grains	Whole-grain bread or rolls Whole-grain cereals Most prepared cereals, except corn-flakes, Rice Krispies, puffed wheat or rice, and some cooked cereals Pancakes and waffles Muffins with fruit or bran Unrefined (brown) rice
Dairy products	Highly flavored cheeses Ice cream or yogurt with fruits or nuts Fried eggs
Meats	Fatty or tough meats such as pork Fried or highly spiced meat, rich meat gravy
Vegetables	Raw or whole cooked vegetables, except vegetables such as beets, spinach, peas, or squash that must be cooked and strained Fried vegetables such as French fries or potato chips
Fruits	Raw fruits, especially those with skins or seeds, other than ripe banana or avocado Raisins, prunes, or other dried fruits Jams, preserves, or marmalade
Miscellaneous	Nuts, spices, highly spiced condiments, vinegar, olives, popcorn

for preparing a child for a colostomy). It is important to space explanations to prevent anxiety and confusion from too much information.

It is important to stress to parents and older children that the colostomy for Hirschsprung disease is temporary, unless so much bowel is involved that a permanent ileostomy must be performed. In most instances the physician is fairly certain of the extent of bowel resection prior to surgery, although the nurse should be aware of those instances when there is doubt concerning repair. The nurse should also keep in mind that, although a temporary colostomy is favorable in terms of future health and adjustment, it also necessitates additional surgery, which may be very stressful to parents and children.

Parents also need preparation prior to surgery. Since a colostomy represents a change in body function and appearance, the nurse should investigate parents' previous knowledge of this procedure. It is not uncommon for parents to have previous knowledge of a colostomy. For example, one mother related that a friend's father had a permanent colostomy because of cancer. As soon as the mother heard that her child needed this procedure, she was convinced that the mass in her child's abdomen was a cancerous tumor.

Postoperative care. Physical postoperative care usually includes (1) nothing by mouth until bowel sounds return and the colostomy and/or anastomosed bowel are ready for feedings, (2) intravenous fluid to maintain hydration and replace lost electrolytes, (3) nasogastric suctioning to prevent abdominal distention, (4) frequent stomal dressing changes, and (5) perineal dressing changes, especially if a pull-through procedure was performed.

The postoperative care is the same as for any child or infant with abdominal surgery (p. 653). When a colostomy is part of the corrective procedure, stomal care becomes a major nursing problem (p. 584). To prevent contamination of the abdominal wound with urine in the infant, the diaper should be pinned below the dressing. Sometimes a Foley catheter is used in the immediate postoperative period to divert the flow of urine away from the abdomen.

The nurse emphasizes the expected changes in the appearance of the stoma, which initially is large, protruding, red, and raw looking. Since the stomal site appears painful, it is also important to stress that bowel mucosa is nonsensitive but that the surrounding abdominal skin must be protected. During the early postoperative period, including parents and the older child in dressing changes can enhance teaching of colostomy care when an appliance is fitted and promotion of gradual acceptance of the body change.

Discharge care. Postoperatively parents need in-

struction concerning colostomy care. Even a preschooler can be included in the care by handing articles to the parent, rolling up the colostomy bag after emptying, or applying cream to the surrounding skin. Since these children may have had difficulties with bowel training before surgery because of constipation and erratic stool patterns, the period during the temporary colostomy can relieve the pressures previously associated with bowel control. Although diagnosis of Hirschsprung disease is less frequent in school-age children or adolescents, if discovered in older children, they should be involved in colostomy care to the point of total responsibility.

Referral to a public health nurse establishes continuity of care, especially in relation to colostomy care and dietary management. The community nurse can also assist parents and children in anticipating subsequent surgery. Sometimes families require financial assistance and additional psychologic support. Therefore, a referral to a social worker or other service agency may be necessary.

INGESTION OF FOREIGN SUBSTANCES

Children are prone to place their hands and any attractive object or substance into their mouths, particularly infants and small children who explore items with their mouths instinctively. Older children often place items in their mouths and accidentally swallow them. Rarely, a child deliberately swallows unusual objects or substances. Hands come into contact with dirt and contaminated objects that contain ova or larvae of a variety of parasites.

PICA

Pica is the Latin word for magpie, a bird of voracious and indiscriminate appetite. The use of the term today refers to the habitual, purposeful, and compulsive ingestion of nonfood substances in the environment. The list of ingested substances is practically endless but most commonly includes clay, dirt, ashes, paint chips, laundry starch, cornstarch, paper, pencils, erasers, crayons, cigarette butts, and matches. Most children have a particular craving for a few items, which is largely determined by the availability of the substance.

It is believed by some that certain forms of pica are manifestations of a deficiency in the diet, especially of minerals. For example, clay-eating has been related to zinc deficiency and eating chalk to calcium deficiency. In most instances pica is relatively harmless but if the substance ingested contains a harmful ingredient, such as lead in

SUMMARY OF NURSING CARE OF THE CHILD REQUIRING ABDOMINAL SURGERY

GOALS	RESPONSIBILITIES
Preoperative Prepare the child and parent for expected surgical procedure and postoperative care	Obtain or make certain there is written parental consent
	Explain reason for surgery; if bowel diversion is to be performed, explain basic principle of ostomy and brief outline of bowel care
	Explain all preoperative procedures, such as blood work, nasogastric tube, bowel preparation, and any other laboratory test
	Collect specimens as indicated, for example, urine, CBC
	Order and/or assist with special tests such as radiographs
	Prepare for postoperative procedures, as indicated, such as nasogastric tube, intravenous fluids, nothing by mouth, dressing changes, and wound drains if necessary
	In emergency situation, explain most essential components of surgery, such as where the child will be before and after surgery, anesthesia, and dressing on abdomen; accept behavioral reactions of the parents and child
	See also preoperative preparation, p. 585
Assist in preparing bowel for surgery (if indicated)	Administer colonic enemas as ordered, using only saline solution
	Administer antibiotics as ordered, observing for known side effects (neomycin and kanamycin can cause auditory and renal damage)
Observe for complications Shock	Monitor vital signs and blood pressure
Intestinal obstruction	Observe for decreased or absent bowel sounds, increasing abdominal distention, vomiting, absence of stools, pain
Perforation and peritonitis	Observe for sudden relief from pain followed by increased diffuse abdominal pain, absence of bowel sounds, tachycardia, pallor, high temperature, abdominal splinting, and rapid, shallow respirations
Prevent and observe for abdominal distention	Give the child nothing by mouth as ordered
	Maintain patency of nasogastric tube, if present
	Check functioning of suction machine
	Irrigate tube if no drainage is obtained but the child vomits around tube
	Check proper placement of tube
	Secure tube by taping to nose or upper lip (not forehead) to maintain proper stomach placement
	Keep the child in semi-Fowler's position or as ordered to facilitate drainage of abdominal contents and to promote respiratory expansion
	Measure abdominal circumference at widest point (mark with pen, usually at umbilicus); record measurements on graph or in sequence to detect changes
	Check often for bowel sounds
Prevent dehydration	Record all output (urinary, stool, vomiting, nasogastric) and input (intravenous, oral if allowed, and nasogastric irrigant); notify physician of marked discrepancies
	Monitor intravenous infusion, if present
	Take temperature frequently; notify physician of elevations
Postoperative Assess general status	Monitor vital signs as ordered
	Check dressings for bleeding or other abnormalities
	Assess level of consciousness
	Assess for evidence of discomfort
	Place in position of comfort in accordance with surgeon's orders
	Check bowel sounds

Continued.

SUMMARY OF NURSING CARE OF THE CHILD REQUIRING ABDOMINAL SURGERY—cont'd

GOALS	RESPONSIBILITIES
Provide nutrition and hydration	Monitor intravenous infusion until discontinued Administer oral fluids when indicated by patient's condition and surgeon's orders Provide diet as prescribed
Provide wound care	Assess wound for signs of complications, unless ordered not to remove dressing Change dressings as prescribed by surgeon Report any unusual appearance or drainage Carry out special wound care as prescribed: irrigation, drain care, etc.
Prevent infection	Change dressings (abdominal and/or perineal), if indicated, whenever soiled; carefully dispose of soiled dressings Pin diapers below abdominal dressing to prevent contamination Maintain respiratory hygiene with coughing, deep breathing, and turning; suction secretions if needed Use proper hand washing techniques, especially if wound drainage is present Administer antibiotics as prescribed

Detect early signs of complications	Observe for signs of
	    Shock
	    Abdominal distention
	    Wound infection
	    Other infections

Prevent skin breakdown	If dressings require frequent change, use Montgomery straps Provide appropriate care to special procedures and equipment such as ostomy, drains, etc.
Provide comfort measures	Administer mouth care Lubricate nostril to decrease irritation from nasogastric tube, if present Allow the child position of comfort if not contraindicated (usually side-lying or prone with legs flexed on chest) Perform procedures (for example, dressing change, deep breathing, and so on) after administering analgesics
Prevent respiratory complications	Administer pain medication as prescribed Assist to turn, cough, deep breath Stimulate the infant to cry Assist with use of spirometer or blow bottle Perform percussion and vibration, if indicated
Observe for elimination	Observe and record first voiding Report if not voided within 8 to 12 hours after surgery Observe and record first bowel movement
Prepare for discharge Wound care	If dressing changes are required at home, teach parent sterile or aseptic procedures; provide written list of necessary equipment and instructions
Administration of medications	Instruct the parents regarding administration of medications (p. 567)
Special procedures	Instruct the parents in care and management of special procedures such as ostomy care, irrigations
Support and reassure parents and child	Explain all procedures Keep informed of progress Encourage expression of feelings If emergency procedure, review the child's memory of previous events Refer to public health nurse if necessary Refer to appropriate agency for specific help

paint, the practice becomes a serious matter. If the eating of a specific substance persists it should probably be evaluated. Certainly if pica involves a potentially harmful substance it should be removed from the environment or the child denied access to it.

FOREIGN BODIES (FB)

Most ingested foreign bodies, such as marbles, coins, beads, and small safety pins, pass through the alimentary tract without difficulty once they reach the stomach. Larger items and straight or sharp objects, such as bobby pins, hairpins, needles, and large safety pins, become lodged in the duodenal loop.

Once an ingested object passes the pylorus, its progress is followed by radiograms, and the stools are examined for its presence. The child is fed his customary diet. If serial radiographs indicate that the object remains stationary, it is removed by a magnetized nasogastric tube or laparotomy.

Foreign bodies, such as coins, that become lodged in the esophagus require immediate attention since they may adhere to the esophageal wall where they cause erosion of the epithelium. Of particular concern is the increasing incidence of ingestion of ''button'' batteries commonly found in watches, hearing aids, cameras, and calculators. Some have been found to leak their alkaline electrolytes and other corrosive substances or have been acted upon by stomach and intestinal secretions. The most difficulty arises from the larger diameter batteries, which become impacted in the esophagus. At the present time there is no established protocol for treating battery ingestions, but it is recommended that the presence of the battery in the esophagus should be confirmed by radiographic examination then removed before corrosive damage can occur. The object is removed by esophagoscopy. Sometimes a blunt object can be removed by introduction of a Foley catheter into the esophagus to a point beyond the object, the bulb inflated, and the catheter and foreign object gently removed together.

HELMINTHIC INFECTIONS

Parasitic diseases constitute the most frequent infections in the world, and although many are concentrated in the tropical regions, others are not. A number of these infections are encountered with relative frequency in the United States and are of importance in children in the pediatric age-groups. Of the various species capable of infecting man, the helminths (worms), arthropods (spiders, insects), and protozoa are seen most frequently. Since arthropod infestations are not ingested and are considered later in re-

lation to disorders affecting the skin (p. 912), only helminthic infections will be discussed here.

Most infections result from ingestion of parasite eggs that hatch within the environment of the host. Light infections may be asymptomatic, but all infections produce symptoms and pathology when present in large numbers. In general, parasitic worms do not multiply in the host; therefore, the number of worms in the body depends on the intensity (especially the first) and the frequency of exposure. Parasitic helminthic infections of humans include those caused by nematodes (roundworms), cestodes (tapeworms), and trematodes (flukes). Tapeworm and fluke infections are rare in North America; therefore, the discussion will be limited to those caused by the more common nematodes. Table 21-4 describes the outstanding features of these parasitic infections, including treatment.

Nursing considerations

Nursing responsibilities related to parasitic worm infections are directed toward (1) identification of the parasite, (2) treatment of the infection, and (3) prevention of initial infection or reinfection. Identification of the organism is accomplished by laboratory examination of substances containing the worm, its larvae, or embryonated ova. Most are identified by examining fecal smears from the stools of persons suspected of harboring the parasite. Stool specimens should be large enough to get an ample sampling, not merely a fecal fragment. Fresh specimens are best for revealing parasites or larvae; therefore, collected specimens should be taken directly to the laboratory for examination.

Pinworm specimens are collected in the morning before the child has a bowel movement or bathes, usually before he gets out of bed. A loop of transparent tape, sticky side out, is placed around the end of a tongue depressor, which is then firmly pressed to the child's perianal area, first one side, then the other, to attach eggs to both sides. A convenient commercially prepared tape can be given to the parents. If the parents collect the specimen, they should be instructed to place the tongue blade in a glass jar or loosely in a plastic bag so that it can be brought in for microscopic examination. For specimens collected in the hospital, physician's office, or clinic, the tape is placed smoothly on a glass slide, sticky side down, for examination.

In most worm infections examination of other family members, especially children, may be carried out to identify those who are similarly affected. (With pinworm infections, rather than performing clear tape tests on all members, the entire family is often treated.) Nurses frequently assume the responsibility for directing and instructing the families in the collection and disposition of specimens. The treatment regimen may need further expla-

TABLE 21-4. COMMON HELMINTHIC INFECTIONS

INFECTION AND ORGANISM	CLINICAL MANIFESTATIONS	TRANSMISSION AND PREVENTION	TREATMENT	COMMENTS
Trichuriasis—*Trichuris trichiura* (whipworm)	Light infections: asymptomatic. Heavy infections: abdominal pain and distention; diarrhea. Ova in fecal smears	Transmitted from contaminated soil, vegetables, toys, and other objects	Mebendazole (Vermox) for 3 days	Most frequent in warm, moist climates. Occurs most often in undernourished children living in unsanitary conditions
Hookworm disease—*Nectator americanus*	Light infections in well-nourished individuals: no problems. Heavier infections: mild to severe anemia, malnutrition. May be itching and burning ("ground itch") followed by erythema and a papular eruption in anal area. Ova in fecal smears; positive occult blood in heavier infections	Humans initiate extrinsic phase by discharging eggs on the soil and, in turn, pick up infection from direct skin contact with contaminated soil. Prevention: proper sanitary disposal of human excreta	Bephenium hydroxynaphthoate (Alcopara), single dose. Tetrachloroethylene, single dose. Pyrantel pamoate, single dose	Wearing shoes is helpful, although children playing in contaminated soil expose many skin surfaces
Strongyloidiasis—*Strongyloides stercoralis* (threadworm)	Light infection: asymptomatic. Heavy infection: respiratory signs and symptoms; abdominal pain, distention, nausea and vomiting, diarrhea—large pale stools, often with mucus. Larvae in feces and duodenal aspirate; sometimes in sputum	Same as above except autoinfection common	Thiabendazole (Mintezol) for 2 days	Older children and adults affected more often than young children. Severe infections may lead to severe nutritional deficiency
Trichinosis—*Trichinella spiralis*	Nonspecific and generalized: gastroenteritis during invasive phase; later myositis, periorbital edema, dyspnea, fever, enlarged lymph nodes, eosinophilia. History of eating poorly cooked pork. Diagnosis by muscle biopsy	Transmitted from flesh of infected animals (pork). Prevention: thorough cooking of pork	Corticosteroids for symptoms. Thiabendazole kills worm in intestines; no effect on larvae in muscles. No treatment for muscle involvement	Seldom affects infants and young children. More common in Europe and North America
Ascariasis*—*Ascaris lumbricoides* (common roundworm)	Light infections: asymptomatic. Heavy infections: anorexia, irritability, nervousness, enlarged abdomen, weight loss, fever, intestinal colic	Transferred to mouth by way of contaminated food, fingers, toys, etc.	Pyrantel pamoate (Antiminth), single dose. Piperazine citrate (numerous preparations) for 2 days	Affects principally young children 1-4 years of age. Prevalent in warm climates

Disease	Clinical manifestations / Diagnosis	Comments / Prevention	Therapy	Remarks
	Severe infections: intestinal obstruction, appendicitis, perforation of intestine with peritonitis, obstructive jaundice, lung involvement—pneumonitis Microscopic examination of stool for ova and parasites	Prevention: community sanitation	Mebendazole (Vermox) for 3 days	Reinfection is the rule
Enterobiasis (oxyuriasis)*—*Enterobius vermicularis* (pinworm, seatworm)	Intense itching of perianal area; no systemic reaction In females, adult may migrate to vagina to produce perivaginal itching Rarely, appendicitis Microscopic examination of perianal swabbings: sticky surface of Cellulose tape is firmly pressed against perianal folds, then placed, sticky side down, on a slide, which is subsequently examined under a microscope	Transferred to mouth by fingers from scratching or from soiled night clothes, underclothes, bed linens, or other contaminated objects; may breathe in and ingest airborne eggs Prevention: hygienic measures	Pyrvinium pamoate (Povan), single dose Piperazine citrate for 8 days Pyrantel pamoate (Antiminth) Mebendazole	Sometimes other family members are treated as well as affected child Povan stains clothing, vomitus, and stool; parents may mistake for blood
Giardiasis—*Giardia lamblia*	Acute: explosive, watery, foul-smelling diarrhea; marked abdominal distention, foul gas and belching, nausea, anorexia, vomiting, fatigue, epigastric cramps Chronic: periodic brief episodes of loose, foul-smelling stools, failure to thrive, fatigue Examine stool for parasites: zinc-sulfate flotation test, duodenal fluid examination	Primarily waterborne Requires high levels of chlorine to destroy; filtration is best method of purification of water In high-risk situations water should be boiled 10 minutes or purified	Quinacrine hydrochloride (Atabrine) for 7 days Metronidazole (Flagyl) for 7-10 days Furazolidone (Furoxone) for 7 days	Increasingly important source of disease
Visceral larva migrans*—*Toxocara canis* (dogs) Intestinal toxocariasis *Toxocara cati* (cats)	Depends on reactivity of infected individual May be asymptomatic except for eosinophilia Specific diagnosis difficult Difficult to detect in humans; organ biopsy Suspected by eosinophilia and elevated isoagglutinin titers	Transmitted by direct contamination of hands from contact with dog, cat, or objects or ingestion of soil Periodic deworming of diagnosed dogs and cats Control of dog population See comments, also	No specific therapy known	Dogs and cats should be kept away from areas where children play; sandboxes especially important transmission areas Continued education and laws needed to prevent indiscriminate canine defecation; personal hygiene

*Diseases caused by nematodes (roundworms).

nation and reinforcement, especially when it involves other members of the household and care of clothing and bed linen. When other members are treated, the family needs to understand the nature of transmission and that, in many cases, the medication is repeated in 2 weeks to 1 month to kill organisms that have been hatched or reintroduced since the initial treatment.

The child with pinworm infection is especially prone to continual reinfection, particularly via the anal-oral route. Pinworm eggs persist in the home to contaminate anything they contact, such as hands, bed linen, underwear, and food. They may float in the air. Parents are instructed to wash all bedding immediately after treatment. The child should wear a clean pair of long pajamas to sleep in each night and underclothing that fits snugly and is changed daily. All underwear and bed linen are washed in hot water to kill any adherent eggs, and pajamas are ironed with a hot iron. The child's fingernails should be cut short to minimize the chance of ova collecting under the nails. The movement of the worms on skin and mucous membrane surfaces causes intense itching that promotes scratching and contributes to reinfection and secondary infection and sometimes aids in the diagnosis. In both home and hospital, bed linen and clothing should be handled carefully to avoid scattering eggs into the air and onto the floor.

The nurse's most important function in relation to these parasites is preventive education of children and families regarding good hygiene and health habits. The importance of careful hand washing before eating or handling food, after using the toilet, or before placing fingers in the mouth should be emphasized. Children and parents need to be advised about washing foods that have been in or near the soil, such as raw fruits and vegetables, or food that has fallen on the floor. Children need to be discouraged from biting their nails or scratching the bare anal area and taught to wear shoes when they are outside. Contaminated soil can be carried long distances on feet into houses or conveyances.

STRUCTURAL DEFECTS

There are numerous congenital abnormalities that involve any segment of the gastrointestinal tract. They are attributed to defective development during cell division and organ formation in the embryo. Most are apparent at birth or shortly after and are anomalies in which normal growth ceased at a crucial stage of development, leaving the structure in an embryonic form or only partially completed.

Some structural defects are considered elsewhere, for example, obstructive disorders and hereditary defects in which gastrointestinal symptoms are part of a symptom complex.

CLEFT LIP AND/OR CLEFT PALATE (CL/P)

Clefts of the lip and palate are facial malformations that are common to all human populations and constitute a severe handicap to the affected individual. The incidence of cleft lip and/or cleft palate shows a wide variation in races: it occurs in about one in 1000 live births in whites, and less than half as many in American blacks. The incidence of cleft palate is about one in 2500. Affected males outnumber females with cleft lip with or without cleft palate, particularly in the more severe defects.

Etiology

In the majority of cases, cleft lip and/or palate appears to have a mixed genetic and environmental cause. There is an increased incidence in relatives, and identical twins are more apt to share the disorder than fraternal twins. Many recognized syndromes include these defects as a feature.

Pathophysiology

Cleft lip and/or palate results from failure of the maxillary and premaxillary processes to come in contact during early embryonic life. Although often appearing together, cleft lip and cleft palate are distinct malformations embryologically, occurring at different times during the developmental process. Merging of the upper lip at the midline is completed between the seventh and eighth weeks of gestation. Fusion of the secondary palate (hard and soft palate) takes place later in development, between the seventh and twelfth weeks of gestation.

Clinical manifestations

The cleft that involves the lip with or without cleft palate is readily apparent at birth and is one of the defects that elicits the most severe emotional reactions in parents. Clefts of the lip may be unilateral or bilateral and may range from a notch in the vermilion border of the lip to complete separation extending to the floor of the nose (Fig. 21-4). Varying degrees of nasal distortion usually accompany cleft lip with or without cleft palate, and the defect frequently involves supernumerary, deformed, or absent teeth.

Clefts of the palate may occur as an isolated defect or in association with cleft lip. Less obvious than cleft lip,

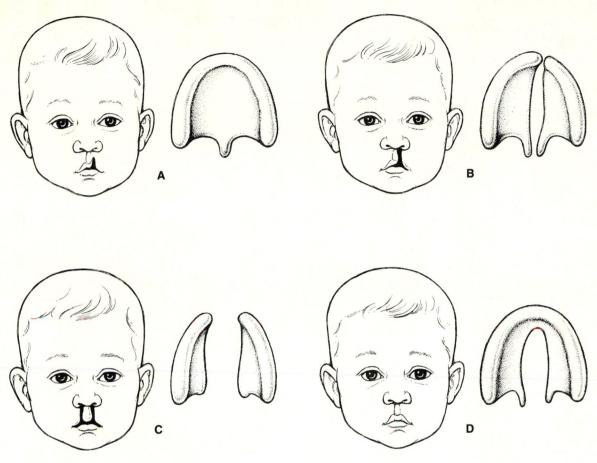

FIG. 21-4

Variations in clefts of the lip and palate at birth. **A,** *Notch in vermilion border.*
B, *Unilateral cleft lip and palate.* **C,** *Bilateral cleft lip and palate.* **D,** *Cleft palate.*

the defect may not be detected without a thorough assessment of the mouth. The deformity can be identified by placing the examiner's fingers directly on the palate. Clefts of the hard palate form a continuous opening between the mouth and the nasal cavity. This creates special feeding problems. The infant is unable to develop suction because of the defect and has difficulty in swallowing. The open pathway must be closed in order to provide sufficient pressure for the swallowing sequence.

Therapeutic management

Treatment of the child with cleft lip and palate involves the cooperative efforts of a number of specialists—pediatrician, nurses, plastic surgeon, orthodontist, prosthodontist, otolaryngologist, speech therapist, and, sometimes, a psychiatrist. Medical management is directed toward closure of the cleft(s), prevention of complications, habilitation, and facilitation of normal growth and development of the child.

Surgical correction.   Closure of the lip defect precedes that of the palate, although the optimum times for surgery are still being debated. Those who favor immediate repair of the lip argue that it makes the infant more acceptable to the parents before discharge from the hospital, thereby improving establishment of satisfactory parent-child relationships. Others prefer to wait until the infant shows a steady weight gain and a hemoglobin level of at least 10 g/100 ml, usually at 6 to 12 weeks of age. They believe that the delay helps the infant better withstand the surgery.

Immediately after surgery the suture line is protected from tension by a thin, arched metal device (the Logan bow) (Fig. 21-5) taped to the cheeks or a butterfly-type adhesive restraint, and the arms are restrained at the elbows to prevent the infant from rubbing the incision with his hands. In the absence of infection or trauma, healing takes place with little scar formation.

Cleft palate repair is generally postponed until later in order to take advantage of palatal changes that take place

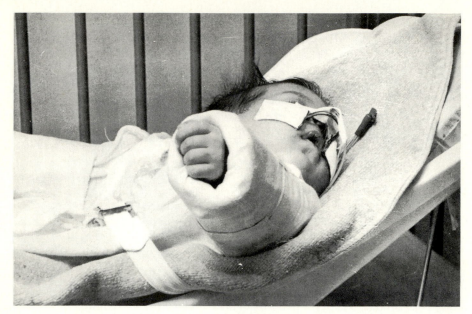

FIG. 21-5

Infant with Logan bow in place to prevent tension on suture line. Note elbow restraints. (Courtesy Children's Health Center, San Diego, Calif. From Ingalls, A.J., and Salerno, M.C.: Maternal and child health nursing, ed. 4, St. Louis, 1983, The C.V. Mosby Co.)

with normal growth, sometime between the ages of 6 months and 5 years. Most surgeons prefer to close the cleft between 1 and 2 years of age, before the child develops faulty speech habits.

Long-term problems. Even with good anatomic closure, the majority of children with cleft lip and/or cleft palate have some degree of speech impairment, which requires speech therapy. Physical problems result from inefficient functioning of the muscles of the soft palate and nasopharynx, improper tooth alignment, and varying degrees of hearing loss. Improper drainage of the middle ear, as the result of inefficient function of the eustachian tube, contributes to recurrent otitis media with scarring of the tympanic membrane, which leads to hearing impairment in a large proportion of children with palatal clefts. Upper respiratory infections require immediate and meticulous attention, and extensive orthodontics and prosthodontics are needed to correct problems of malposition of teeth and maxillary arches.

Nursing considerations

The immediate nursing problems in the care of an infant with cleft lip and palate deformities are related to feeding the infant and dealing with the severe parental reaction to the defect. A cleft lip is the most disfiguring of the visible defects and one that generates strong negative responses in both nurses and parents. It is especially important for nurses to emphasize the positive aspects of the infant's physical appearance and optimism regarding surgical correction. Sometimes showing parents a photograph of the possible cosmetic improvement as a result of surgery does

much to relieve their anxiety. The manner of the nurse in handling the infant should convey to the parents that the infant is indeed a precious, although incompletely formed, human being. (See Chapter 16 for interventions in assisting parents to accept a birth defect.)

Throughout the course of therapy parents need an explanation of the immediate and long-range problems frequently associated with cleft palate. Often they are unaware that more is involved than merely repairing the defect. Whenever possible, they should be referred to a comprehensive cleft palate team.

Feeding. Feeding the infant offers a special challenge to nurses. Clefts of lip or palate reduce the infant's ability to suck, which interferes with compression of the areola and renders breast-feeding almost impossible and makes bottle-feeding difficult. Liquid taken into the mouth has a tendency to escape via the cleft through the nose. Feeding is usually best accomplished with the infant's head in an upright position, either held in the caregiver's hand or cradled in the arm. Normal nipples are unsuitable for these infants, who are unable to generate the suction required; therefore, special nipples or other feeding devices are needed. A variety of special "cleft palate" nipples have been devised and used with some success. However, large, soft nipples with large holes, Nursettes, or the long, soft lamb's nipples appear to offer the best means for nipple feeding (Fig. 21-6). The newer "gravity flow" nipple* attached to a squeezable plastic bottle allows formula to be deposited directly into the pharynx in much the same manner as a bulb syringe. Success has also been

---

*Ross Laboratories, Columbus, OH 43216.

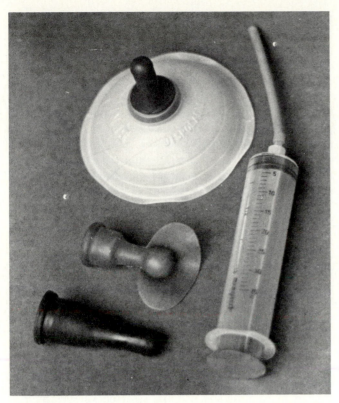

FIG. 21-6
Some devices used to feed an infant with a cleft palate.
Clockwise, *Lamb's nipple, flanged nipple, special nurser,
and syringe with rubber tubing (Breck feeder).*

achieved by the modification of a standard nipple. A single
small slit or crosscut is made in the end of the nipple with
a sharp surgical blade or a pair of scissors with sharp, thin
blades. This allows the infant to express the formula readily. The size of the slit is adjusted to the needs of the
infant.

Using these various types of nipples for feeding also
has the advantage of helping to meet the infant's sucking
needs and, when placed in the normal sucking position
(not through the cleft), encourage use of the sucking muscles. Muscle development is especially important for later
development of speech. The nipple should be positioned
in such a way that it is compressed by the infant's tongue
and existing palate. If a single-slit nipple is used, the slit
should be placed vertically so that the infant will be able
to produce and stop a flow of milk by alternately opening
and closing the opening. No matter which type of nipple
is used, gentle, steady pressure on the base of the bottle
reduces the chance of choking or coughing, and the person
feeding should resist the temptation to remove the nipple
frequently because of the noise the infant makes or for fear
that he will choke. Since these infants have a tendency to

swallow excessive amounts of air, they require frequent
bubbling.

When the infant has trouble with nipple feeding, a
rubber-tipped medicine dropper, Asepto syringe, or
"Breck feeder" often provides an efficient, safe feeding
device. The rubber extension should be sufficiently long to
extend well back into the mouth to reduce the likelihood
of regurgitation through the nose. The formula is deposited
on the back of the tongue and the flow controlled by bulb
compression that is adjusted to the infant's capacity to
handle it. With some infants, spoon feeding works best,
especially if the formula is slightly thickened with cereal.
After feeding the infant is given water to rinse the mouth.

The mother should begin to feed the infant as soon as
possible, preferably after the initial nursery feeding. In this
way she is able to help determine the method best suited
to her and the infant and to become adept in the technique
before they are discharged from the hospital.

Preoperative care. In preparation for surgical repair, the mother is frequently instructed to accustom the
infant to some of the needs of the early postoperative period, particularly if surgery is delayed several months.
Since it is mandatory for the infant to be positioned on the
back postoperatively, it is helpful to train him to lie in this
position a great deal of the time to reduce the irritability
and resistance associated with any change in routine. It is
also helpful to place the infant or child in arm restraints
periodically prior to admission and, after admission, to
feed him with a rubber-tipped Asepto syringe or other device in the manner to be used postoperatively. No special
formula is required, and the infant is usually allowed to
eat up to about 6 hours preoperatively. Preoperative preparation, including medication, is determined by the surgeon and anesthesiologist.

Postoperative care: cleft lip. The major efforts
in the postoperative period are directed toward protecting
the operative site. Before the infant leaves the operating
room the metal appliance is securely taped to the cheeks
to relax the operative site and prevent tension on the suture
line caused by crying or other facial movement. Arm restraints are needed to prevent the infant from rubbing or
otherwise disturbing the suture line and are ready at the
bedside for immediate application on his arrival at the unit.
It is advisable to pin the cuff of the restraints to the infant's clothing or bed to prevent rubbing the face with the
upper arms. The older infant who is able to roll over will
require a jacket restraint in addition to restricting arm
movement to prevent his rolling on the abdomen and rubbing his face on the sheet, especially if the repair involves
the lip. It is important to remove the restraints periodically
to exercise the arms, to provide relief from restrictions,
and to observe the skin for signs of irritation. It is advisable to release the restraints one at a time, especially in a

very vigorous, active infant. Removing restraints also offers an opportunity for cuddling and body contact. Sitting him in an infant seat provides a change of position and a different perspective of the environment. Sedation is sometimes needed for a very restless, anxious infant. Rooming-in is always encouraged because preserving parent contact greatly increases the child's comfort.

Feeding is essentially the same as before surgery. It is safe to offer clear liquids when the infant has fully recovered from the anesthesia, and formula feeding is usually resumed when tolerated. Asepto-syringe feeding is preferred in most cases. Care is taken to slip the rubber tip in from the side of the mouth to avoid the operative area and to prevent the infant from sucking on the tubing. This method is continued until the lip is well healed, after which bottle-feeding can be resumed if this has been the infant's mode of feeding. The mouth should be rinsed with water after each feeding. The suture site is carefully cleansed of formula or serosanguineous drainage as needed with a gauze- or cotton-tipped swab dipped in saline or hydrogen peroxide. Meticulous care of the suture line is a nursing responsibility since inflammation or sloughing will interfere with optimum healing and the ultimate cosmetic effect of the surgical repair.

Gentle aspiration of mouth and nasopharynx secretions may be necessary to prevent aspiration and respiratory complications. A side-lying or partial side-lying position is helpful for the infant in the immediate postoperative period and for one who has difficulty in handling secretions. As with any infant, the child with cleft palate repair is placed on the right side after feedings to reduce the chance of aspirating regurgitated formula.

Postoperative care: cleft palate. The child with a cleft palate repair is allowed to lie on the abdomen, especially immediately postoperatively. The nurse avoids the use of suction or other objects in the mouth, such as a tongue depressor when the suture lines are being checked or straws when the child is given liquids. Fluids are best taken from a cup. Young children are not given a pacifier and children old enough to understand are cautioned against rubbing their tongue against the roof of the mouth. Spoons should not be allowed in the mouth. The child with a cleft palate repair may be fed with a wide-bowl spoon (such as a soup spoon) that cannot enter the mouth.

As with cleft lip repair the elbows are immobilized to keep the hands away from the mouth, and the parents are instructed to continue this precaution at home until the palate is healed. They are instructed to remove the restraints (usually one at a time) at frequent intervals to allow the child to exercise the arms. It is important to stress that the child should be closely supervised during this time.

The child is generally discharged on a soft diet, which parents are instructed to continue until the surgeon directs them otherwise. They are cautioned against allowing the child to eat hard items such as toast, hard cookies, and potato chips, which could damage the newly repaired palate. The nurse might suggest that the parents not offer the child any food harder than mashed potatoes.

Occasionally the child will have difficulty in breathing following surgery, especially the child with cleft palate repair who must alter an established pattern of breathing and adjust to breathing through the nose. This is frustrating but seldom requires more than positioning and support. Sometimes the infant or child is placed in a mist tent for a short period after surgery.

Long-term care. Children with cleft lip and/or palate often require a variety of services during the process of habilitation. Families of these children need support and encouragement by health professionals and guidance in activities that facilitate the most normal outcome for their children. With the combined efforts of family and the health team the majority of these children achieve a satisfactory habilitation. Parents need to understand the function of therapy and the purpose and care of any appliance and of establishing good mouth care and proper brushing habits. Throughout the child's habilitation many local areas have Cleft Palate Parents groups who offer help and support to parents, and national associations such as the American Cleft Palate Association,* Special Child Health Services,† and the National Institute of Dental Research‡ provide education and services for parents and health professionals.

ESOPHAGEAL ATRESIA WITH TRACHEOESOPHAGEAL FISTULA (TEF)

Congenital atresia of the esophagus and tracheoesophageal (T-E) fistula are rare malformations that represent a failure of the esophagus to develop as a continuous passage. These defects may occur as separate entities or in combination (Fig. 21-7) and, without early diagnosis and treatment, are rapidly fatal.

Etiology

The cause of esophageal atresia and tracheoesophageal fistula is not known. The incidence has been estimated to be from one in 800 to one in 5000 live births. There appear to be no sex differences, but the birth weight of most affected infants is significantly lower than average and there is an unusually high percentage of prematurity.

---

*331 Salk Hall, University of Pittsburgh, Pittsburgh, PA 15261.
†2023 W. Ogden Ave., Chicago, IL 60612.
‡Westwood Building, 5333 Westbard Ave., Bethesda, MD 20205.

SUMMARY OF POSTOPERATIVE HOSPITAL NURSING CARE OF THE CHILD WITH CLEFT LIP AND/OR PALATE

GOALS	RESPONSIBILITIES
Prevent trauma to suture line	Position on back or side (on abdomen for cleft palate) Maintain lip protective device or other closure Use nontraumatic feeding techniques Restrain arms to prevent access to operative site Use jacket restraints on older infant
Prevent tissue infection and breakdown	Cleanse suture line gently after feeding and as necessary in manner ordered by surgeon Keep suture line dry Rinse mouth after each feeding Avoid placing objects in the mouth following cleft palate repair (suction catheter, tongue depressor, straw, pacifier, small spoon)
Facilitate breathing	Position to allow for mucous drainage (partial side-lying position)

Provide adequate nutritional intake	Administer diet appropriate for age
	Modify feeding techniques to adjust to defect
	    Feed in sitting position
	    Use special appliances
	    Encourage frequent bubbling

Provide comfort measures	Remove restraints periodically Provide cuddling and tactile stimulation Involve parents in infant's care
Facilitate parents' acceptance of infant	Allow expression of feelings Convey attitude of acceptance of infant and parents Indicate by conduct that child is a valuable human being
Educate parents	Involve parents in determining best feeding methods Teach feeding and suctioning techniques Teach cleansing and restraining procedures especially when infant will be discharged before suture removal
Meet parents' concerns about recurrence in future children	Refer to genetic counseling services
Provide for continued support	Refer to public health agency for continuity of care Refer to social service Refer to Special Child Health Services for financial assistance Refer to local cleft palate parent group

Pathophysiology

The most commonly encountered form of esophageal atresia and tracheoesophageal fistula (80% to 95% of cases) is one in which the proximal esophageal segment terminates in a blind pouch and the distal segment is connected to the trachea or primary bronchus by a short fistula at or near the bifurcation (Fig. 21-7, *C*). The second most common variety (5% to 8%) consists of a blind pouch at each end, widely separated and with no communication to the trachea (Fig. 21-7, *A*). Less frequently an otherwise normal trachea and esophagus are connected by a common fistula (Fig. 21-7, *E*). Extremely rare anomalies involve a fistula from the trachea to the upper esophageal segment (Fig. 21-7, *B*) or to both the upper and lower segments (Fig. 21-7 *D*).

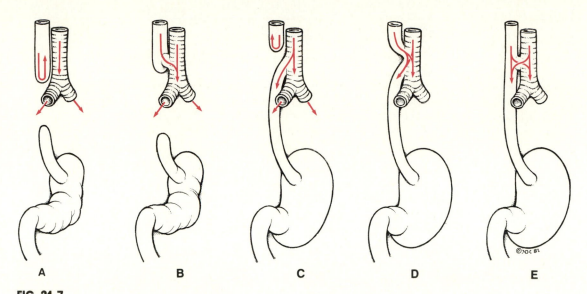

FIG. 21-7

The five most common types of esophageal atresia and tracheoesophageal fistula.

Clinical manifestations

The presence of esophageal atresia is suspected in an infant with excessive salivation and drooling that is frequently accompanied by choking, coughing, and sneezing. If fed, the infant swallows normally but suddenly coughs and struggles and the fluid returns through the nose and mouth. He becomes cyanotic and may stop breathing as the overflow of fluid from the blind pouch is aspirated into the trachea or bronchus. The cyanosis is the result of laryngospasm, the protective mechanism that operates to prevent aspiration into the trachea.

Diagnostic evaluation

To rule out esophageal atresia a catheter is gently passed into the esophagus. It will meet with resistance if the lumen is blocked but will pass unobstructed if the lumen is patent. A moderately stiff catheter is used to avoid coiling in the esophageal pouch. Aspiration of stomach contents or auscultation over the stomach as air is introduced through the catheter confirms a patent esophagus. Radiopaque fluid carefully instilled in the esophagus under fluoroscopy will readily establish the diagnosis. Sometimes fistulas are not patent, which makes their presence more difficult to diagnose.

Therapeutic management

The treatment of esophageal atresia and tracheoesophageal fistula includes prevention of pneumonia and surgical repair of the anomaly. Since type C anomaly is the most common, the discussion will be directed primarily toward that defect.

When a tracheoesophageal fistula is suspected, the infant is immediately deprived of oral intake, started on intravenous fluids, and placed in the most advantageous position to decrease the likelihood of aspiration. Accumulated secretions are suctioned frequently from the mouth and pharynx. A catheter is placed into the upper esophageal pouch and the infant's head is kept in an upright position, so that fluid collected in the pouch is easily removed. A gastrostomy is usually performed to decompress the stomach and prevent further aspiration of gastric contents by way of the fistula. Since aspiration pneumonia is almost inevitable and appears early, broad-spectrum antibiotic therapy is instituted.

Surgical correction consists of a thoracotomy with division and ligation of the tracheoesophageal fistula and an end-to-end anastomosis of the esophagus. For infants who are premature, have multiple anomalies, or are in very poor condition, a staged operation is preferred that involves palliative measures including gastrostomy, ligation of the tracheoesophageal fistula, and provision of constant drainage of the esophageal pouch.

There are rare instances in which a primary anastomosis cannot be accomplished because of insufficient length of the two segments of esophagus. In these cases the defect must be bridged with a segment of intestine. This esophageal replacement is usually deferred until the child is 18 to 24 months old. In the meantime the fistula is closed and the child fed directly by gastrostomy, whereas the upper esophageal segment is drained by means of a cervical esophagostomy.

Nursing considerations

Nursing responsibility for detection of this serious malformation begins *immediately* after birth. Nurses should suspect any infant who has an excessive amount of mucus or difficulty with secretions and unexplained episodes of cyanosis. Ideally the condition is diagnosed before the initial feeding, but often it is not. For this reason it is customary for the nurse to give the infant the first feeding of glucose water in order to observe his reactions.

Cyanosis is usually the result of laryngospasm caused by overflow of saliva into the larynx from the proximal esophageal pouch, and it normally clears after removal of the secretions from the oropharynx by suctioning. These two signs, excessive mucus and unexplained episodes of cyanosis, should alert nursery nurses to the possibility of a tracheoesophageal fistula or esophageal atresia. Any such suspicion is reported to the physician immediately.

The infant is placed in an Isolette or under a radiant warmer, and oxygen is administered to help relieve respiratory distress. Positive pressure is contraindicated since it may add to air pressure in the stomach.

Preoperative care. The infant's mouth and nasopharynx are carefully suctioned. The most desirable position for a newborn who is suspected of having a tracheoesophageal fistula is supine with the head elevated on an inclined plane of at least 30 degrees. This positioning serves to minimize the reflux of gastric secretions up the distal esophagus into the trachea and bronchi, especially when intraabdominal pressure is elevated during crying.

It is imperative that the source of aspiration be removed at once. Until surgery the blind pouch is kept empty by intermittent or continuous suction through an indwelling nasal catheter that extends to the end of the pouch. The catheter needs attention since it has a tendency to become clogged with mucus. It is usually replaced daily by the physician. On diagnosis the gastrostomy tube is inserted and left open so that air entering the stomach through the fistula can escape, thus minimizing the danger that gastric contents will be regurgitated into the trachea. The tube empties by gravity drainage. Feedings through the gastrostomy tube are contraindicated prior to surgery. The intravenous infusion is carefully monitored and the infant is observed for adequate hydration.

Postoperative care. Postoperative care for these infants is essentially the same as the care of any high-risk newborn (see p. 173). The infant is returned to the warm, high-humidity atmosphere of the Isolette, and the gastrostomy tube is returned to gravity drainage until the infant can tolerate feedings, usually the second or third postoperative day. At this time the tube is elevated and secured at a point above the level of the stomach. This allows gastric secretions to pass to the duodenum, whereas swallowed air can escape through the open tube. If tolerated,

gastrostomy feedings are continued until the esophageal anastomosis is healed, about the tenth to fourteenth day, after which oral feedings are initiated.

The initial attempt at oral feeding must be carefully observed to make certain that the infant is able to swallow without choking. Oral feedings are begun with glucose water followed by frequent, small feedings of formula. Until the infant is able to take a sufficient amount by mouth, oral intake may need to be supplemented by gastrostomy feedings. Ordinarily the infant is not discharged until he is taking oral fluids well and the gastrostomy tube has been removed. However, the infant who has undergone palliative surgery will be discharged with the gastrostomy tube in place. The nurse is responsible for making certain that the caregiver is educated and practiced in the care of the gastrostomy (p. 582).

Special problems. Upper respiratory complications are a threat to life in both the preoperative and postoperative period. In addition to pneumonia, there is a constant danger of respiratory embarrassment resulting from atelectasis, pneumothorax, and laryngeal edema. Any persistent respiratory difficulty after removal of secretions is reported to the surgeon immediately.

In the infant awaiting esophageal replacement surgery, the catheter is removed and the upper esophageal segment is drained by means of an artificial opening in the neck (cervical esophagostomy), which allows escape of the swallowed saliva. This is a source of annoyance as the skin may become irritated by moisture from the continual discharge of saliva. Frequent removal of drainage and application of a thin layer of protective ointment are usually sufficient treatment.

Meeting the oral needs of infants who are unable to suck on a bottle should not be overlooked. A pacifier offered periodically is an acceptable substitute until oral feedings are instituted. The child who has corrective surgery delayed until 18 to 24 months of age may have a different problem. Some children who have not been able to go through the processes of eating in the normal manner have difficulty with this new task and require patient, firm guidance in learning the techniques of taking food into the mouth and swallowing.

As with any congenital anomaly parents need much support in adjusting to the child (see Chapter 16). One of the difficulties in tracheoesophageal fistula is the immediate and sometimes lengthy transfer of the sick newborn to the intensive care unit. The attachment process needs to be facilitated by encouraging parents to visit the infant, participate in his care where appropriate, and express their feelings regarding his defect. The nurse in the intensive care unit or on the postpartal floor should assume responsibility for ensuring that the parents are kept fully informed of the infant's progress.

SUMMARY OF NURSING CARE OF THE INFANT WITH ESOPHAGEAL ATRESIA AND TRACHEOESOPHAGEAL FISTULA

GOALS	RESPONSIBILITIES
Preoperative	
Maintain patent airway and lung expansion	Remove accumulated secretions from oropharynx
	Position for patent airway, lung expansion, and prevention of aspiration of saliva or stomach contents
	Observe for signs of respiratory distress
Recognize defect early	Be alert to danger signs
	Excess salivation
	Three C's—choking, coughing, and cyanosis
	Acute gastric distention
	Assist with diagnostic procedures
Prevent aspiration pneumonia	Administer nothing by mouth
	Position advantageously; usually supine with head elevated at 30-degree incline
	Change position every 2 hours
	Aspirate secretions from oropharynx and esophageal pouch
	Facilitate drainage from gastrostomy
Postoperative	
Prevent infection at operative sites	Administer judicious care of operative site
	Observe for signs of inflammation, bleeding, and/or other drainage
	Cleanse and apply dressings as ordered
Maintain fluid and electrolyte balance	Record accurate measurement of intake and output
	Regulate intravenous fluids carefully
	Measure and record gastrostomy drainage
	Record weight daily
	Measure specific gravity of urine
Facilitate ventilation	Maintain patent airway
	Suction secretions as needed
	Maintain care of chest tubes and drainage apparatus
	Position for optimum ventilation
	Administer oxygen as indicated
	Prevent aspiration of feedings

HERNIAS

A hernia is a protrusion of a portion of an organ or organs through an abnormal opening. The danger from herniation arises when the organ protruding through the opening is constricted to the extent that circulation is impaired or when the protruding organs encroach upon and impair the function of other structures. The herniations of concern are those that protrude through the diaphragm, the abdominal wall, or the inguinal canal (see p. 802).

Diaphragmatic hernia

In congenital herniations through a large diaphragmatic defect on the left side, it is not unusual to find most of the abdominal organs (stomach, small intestine, spleen, left lobe of liver, left kidney, and all but the descending colon) in the thorax. Ineffective motion of the leaf of the diaphragm on the affected side interferes with the normal diaphragmatic breathing of the neonate. Respiration is further compromised by atelectasis of the lung on the affected side and by the stomach and intestine (generally found within the chest), which rapidly become distended with swallowed air as the result of crying. Moreover, this increased volume in the chest cavity displaces the mediastinum to the unaffected side to produce a partial collapse of the opposite lung. The infant is positioned on the affected side to take advantage of gravity (which facilitates expansion of the unaffected lung) and provided with respiratory sup-

SUMMARY OF NURSING CARE OF THE INFANT WITH ESOPHAGEAL ATRESIA AND TRACHEOESOPHAGEAL FISTULA—cont'd

GOALS	RESPONSIBILITIES
Administer postoperative nutrition	Administer gastrostomy feedings when tolerated Progress to oral feedings as prescribed according to the child's condition
Control pneumonia	Administer antibiotics as ordered Administer oxygen as needed Suction secretions Position for optimum ventilation
Administer comfort measures	Provide tactile stimulation Position comfortably postoperatively Avoid restraints where possible Administer mouth care Offer pacifier frequently
Support parents	Facilitate attachment process Encourage frequent visiting to intensive care unit Encourage participation in infant's care Encourage expression of feelings
Educate parents in home care	Teach parents Positioning Signs of respiratory distress Signs of contracture—refusal to eat, dysphagia, increased coughing Care of gastrostomy and esophagostomy when the infant has staged surgery including techniques such as suctioning, care of operative site and/or ostomies, dressing changes, and so on Assist in acquiring needed equipment and services
Administer oral feedings	Teach to take feedings orally after repair Introduce foods one at a time Provide foods with various textures and flavors Begin with slightly liquid feedings and progress to more solid food
Maintain contact with family	Refer to appropriate clinics and/or agencies for needed services Continue nursing follow-up care

port, which includes administration of oxygen, nasogastric suction for decompression of the stomach, and conscientious efforts to prevent the infant from crying. Negative thoracic pressure from crying tends to pull the intestines into the chest and further distend those already there.

When the abdominal viscera are replaced in the abdomen and the defect repaired, the infant recovers with the usual postoperative care and management. Fatalities are usually the consequence of pulmonary insufficiency caused by the compressed and often hypoplastic lung on the affected side.

Nursing considerations. Nursing care is directed toward teaching parents correct feeding techniques, including holding the infant upright during and propping him

after feeding, thickened formula, and frequent burping. If surgery is performed, nursing care is similar to that for any type of abdominal operation.

Hiatal hernia

Congenital herniations through the normal esophageal hiatus in the newborn are usually of the sliding type. Because the muscular ring of the hiatus is not snug, it permits the cardiac end of the stomach to slide above the diaphragm and back into the abdomen. This produces the symptoms seen with associated incompetent or relaxed cardiac sphincter (*chalasia*), with reflux of gastric contents into the esophagus and subsequent regurgitation. When conservative management such as upright posture and feeding modification is disappointing, the defect is repaired surgically.

Nursing care is the same as for diaphragmatic hernia.

Umbilical hernia

Ordinarily the umbilical ring, through which the umbilical blood vessels provide essential elements to the developing fetus, undergoes spontaneous, gradual closure after birth. Incomplete closure of this fascial ring results in the protrusion of portions of omentum and intestine through the opening. The size of the defect varies from less than 1 cm to 4 or 5 cm. The hernias are seen as soft swellings or protrusions covered by skin that are readily reducible with the finger, and small defects usually close spontaneously by 1 or 2 years of age. Very large hernias often persist and those that have not disappeared by school age require surgical closure. Strangulation or incarceration of herniated bowel is rare but requires immediate surgical intervention.

Nursing considerations. Because the sight of an umbilical hernia is very disconcerting to parents, they need reassurance regarding the innocuous nature of the defect. Taping or strapping appears to be of no value in expediting closure and may even cause troublesome skin irritation.

Omphalocele

Omphalocele is a serious congenital malformation in which a variable amount of the abdominal contents protrudes into the base of the umbilical cord. In contrast to an umbilical hernia, the omphalocele is covered only by a translucent sac of amnion to which the umbilical cord inserts. The sac may contain only a small loop of bowel or most of the bowel, and other abdominal viscera. If the sac ruptures, the abdominal contents eviscerate through the opening in the abdominal wall. The abdomen is smaller than usual, making replacement of the bowel more difficult.

The treatment is immediate surgical repair before infection or tissue damage takes place. When the abdomen is too small to accommodate the extruded contents, a protective sac of Silastic or other synthetic material is constructed to contain the omphalocele to aid in reduction of the viscera until surgical closure is attempted. The defect is often associated with other malformations.

Nursing considerations. Special nursing care consists of careful positioning and handling to prevent infection or rupture of the sac. The infant is kept supine and the omphalocele is covered immediately and kept moist until the infant is taken to the operating room.

Because of the obviousness of the defect and the need for immediate repair, the attachment process can be hindered. Parents of these children require the same interventions as that discussed for tracheoesophageal fistula (p. 665).

Gastroschisis

Gastroschisis is herniation through a defect in the abdominal wall that permits extrusion of abdominal contents without involving the umbilical cord. The defect is always located to the right of the intact umbilicus and is not encased in a protective sac. If the evisceration takes place early in fetal life, the abdominal cavity will be small and the protruding bowel is thickened from poor blood supply and irritation. When evisceration takes place just before birth the bowel is almost normal and the abdominal cavity has achieved adequate size to accommodate the viscera.

Treatment is directed toward preventing infection, providing nutrition, and closing the defect surgically. When the abdomen is too small to accommodate the extruded contents, a Silastic pouch is placed over the herniated viscera to contain the bowel and, with the aid of gravity, to return it to the abdominal cavity. The return may take a few hours to a few days after which the defect is closed.

Nursing considerations. Nursing care of the infant with gastroschisis is the same as for any high-risk infant and similar to that for the infant with omphalocele.

MALABSORPTION SYNDROMES

The term ''malabsorption syndrome'' is applied to a long list of disorders associated with some degree of impaired digestion and/or absorption. Most are classified according to the locations of the supposed anatomic and/or biochemical defect.

GENERAL CLASSIFICATION

Digestive defects mainly include those conditions in which the enzymes necessary for digestion are diminished or absent, such as (1) cystic fibrosis, in which pancreatic enzymes are absent, (2) biliary or liver disease, in which bile production is affected, or (3) lactase deficiency, in which there is congenital or secondary lactose intolerance.

Absorptive defects include those conditions in which the intestinal mucosal transport system is impaired. It may be because of a primary defect (such as in celiac disease) or secondary to inflammatory disease of the bowel that results in impaired absorption because bowel motility is accelerated (such as ulcerative colitis). Obstructive disorders (such as Hirschsprung disease) can also cause secondary malabsorption from enterocolitis.

Anatomic defects, such as extensive resection of the bowel or ''short bowel syndrome,'' affect digestion by decreasing the transit time of substances with the digestive juices and affects absorption by severely compromising the absorptive surface.

Emotional factors

There are also several disorders that result in malabsorption but for which no specific organic cause can be found. One of the classic examples is nonorganic failure to thrive, in which malnutrition results despite adequately functioning body systems and is reversed by a program of emotional stimulation rather than medical intervention.

Celiac syndrome

"Celiac syndrome" and "malabsorption syndrome" are terms used to describe a symptom complex associated with several different diseases that have four characteristics in common: (1) steatorrhea (fat, foul, frothy, bulky stools), (2) general malnutrition, (3) abdominal distention, and (4) secondary vitamin deficiencies. Celiac disease and cystic fibrosis are the two most common malabsorptive disorders in children. Presently celiac disease refers to a specific condition, called gluten enteropathy. In adults this same condition is often referred to as nontropical sprue.

CELIAC DISEASE (CD)

Celiac disease, also known as gluten-induced enteropathy, gluten-sensitive enteropathy (GSE), and celiac sprue, is second only to cystic fibrosis as a cause of malabsorption in children. The incidence is variously reported as one in 300 to one in 4000, and appears to be declining—possibly related to the current practice of delayed introduction of solid food. It is seen more frequently in Europe than in America and is rarely reported in Orientals or blacks. The exact cause of celiac disease and mode of transmission are not known, but there is a tendency for the disease to occur in several members of the same family.

Pathophysiology

The disease is characterized by an intolerance for gluten, one of the proteins found in wheat, barley, rye, and oats. Gluten consists of two fractions, glutenin and gliadin. Although the pathologic process is still obscure, susceptible individuals are unable to digest the gliadin faction, resulting in an accumulation of a toxic substance that is damaging to the mucosal cells (Fig. 21-8). Eventually villi atrophy, reducing the absorptive surface of the small intestine.

Clinical manifestations

Symptoms of celiac disease are first noted about 3 to 6 months following the introduction of gluten-containing grains into the diet, typically at 9 to 12 months of age, although it may not be evident until early childhood. The clinical manifestations are usually insidious and chronic. The first evidence of the disease may be failure to regain weight or appetite after a bout of diarrhea.

In the early stages of celiac disease fat absorption is primarily affected, which results in the frequent passage of excessively large, pale, oily, frothy stools with an exceedingly foul odor (steatorrhea). Impaired absorption of nutrients results in malnutrition, with muscle wasting (especially prominent in legs and buttocks), and anemia. Behavioral changes, such as irritability, fretfulness, uncooperativeness, or apathy, are common. As the disease progresses, signs of general wasting become evident. Abdominal distention is common and vomiting may be a dominant feature in very young infants.

Although usually insidious, the onset of celiac disease in very young children is sometimes characterized by acute, severe episodes of profuse watery diarrhea and vomiting, the so-called *celiac crisis*, which may be precipitated by infections (especially gastrointestinal), prolonged fluid and electrolyte depletion, an emotional disturbance, or anticholinergic drugs, such as the preanesthetic agents atropine or scopolamine.

Diagnostic evaluation

A definitive diagnosis is based on a peroral jejunal biopsy, which demonstrates the atrophic changes in the architecture of the mucosal wall. This procedure is performed by passing a polyethylene tube through the mouth along the alimentary tract to the jejunum of the small bowel.

The other essential criterion of diagnosis is dramatic clinical improvement after adherence to a gluten-restricted diet. Within a day or two after instituting the diet, most children with celiac disease demonstrate a favorable personality change. Weight gain, improved appetite, and disappearance of diarrhea and steatorrhea usually do not occur for several days or weeks.

Therapeutic management

Treatment of chronic celiac disease is primarily dietary management. Although the diet is called "gluten free" it is in reality low in gluten, since it is impossible to remove every source of this protein. Also, studies demonstrate that most patients are able to tolerate restricted amounts of gluten. Because gluten is found primarily in the grains of wheat and rye, but also in smaller quantities in barley and oats, these four foods are eliminated. Corn and rice become substitute grain foods.

In children with severe malnutrition, specific deficiencies may be treated with supplemental vitamins, iron, and calories and, because absorption of fat-soluble vitamins is impaired, these are supplied in a water-miscible form.

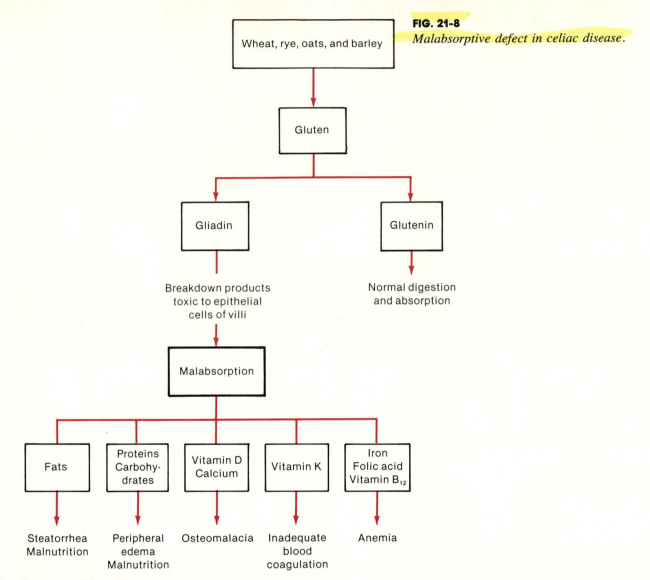

FIG. 21-8
Malabsorptive defect in celiac disease.

Nursing considerations

The main nursing consideration is helping the parents and child adhere to the prescribed diet. A considerable amount of time is involved explaining the disease process, the specific role of gluten in aggravating the pathology, and those foods that must be restricted. Although the chief source of grain is cereal and baked goods, grains are frequently added to processed foods as thickeners or fillers. To add to the difficulty, gluten is added to many foods but obscurely listed on the label as "hydrolyzed vegetable protein." The nurse must advise parents of the need to carefully read all ingredients on labels in order to avoid hidden sources of gluten. Many of the gluten-containing products can be eliminated from the infant's or young child's diet fairly easily, but monitoring the diet of a school-age child or adolescent is a much more difficult situation. Many "favorite" foods, such as hot dogs, pizza, and spaghetti, are chief offenders. Luncheon preparation away from home is particularly difficult, since bread, luncheon meats, and instant soups are not allowed.

In addition to restricting gluten, other dietary alterations may also be necessary in the beginning. For example, in some children who have more severe mucosal damage, the digestion of disaccharides is impaired, especially in relation to lactose. Therefore, these children often need a temporary lactose-free diet, which necessitates eliminating all milk products.

Generally management includes a diet high in calories and proteins, with simple carbohydrates, such as fruits and vegetables but low in fats. Since the bowel is usually inflamed as a result of the pathologic processes in absorption, coarse, rough foods with high residue, such as nuts, raisins, raw vegetables, and raw fruits with skin, are avoided until inflammation has subsided.

It is the recommendation that the child continue the diet indefinitely. This is especially difficult for parents and children to understand when there have been no symptoms of the disease for an extended period of time and occasional dietary indiscretions, probably the result of increased tolerance to glutens, have not caused untoward ef-

SUMMARY OF NURSING CARE FOR THE CHILD WITH CELIAC DISEASE (CELIAC SPRUE, GLUTEN-INDUCED ENTEROPATHY)

GOALS	RESPONSIBILITIES
Recognize early signs of celiac disease	Following introduction of cereal in the diet be alert to signs in an older infant or a child
Assist with diagnosis	Collect stool specimens for 3-day fat analysis Order or collect blood for hematologic studies Order and assist with radiographic examinations Assist with glucose tolerance test Assist with jejunal biopsy Prepare the child for and assist the child during above tests in manner appropriate to his age
Provide adequate nutritional intake	Provide gluten-free diet tailored to child's appetite and capacity to absorb Arrange conference with dietitian to help select foods compatible with diet and the child's preferences Administer supplemental water-miscible vitamins and minerals as ordered Monitor peripheral parenteral nutrition line when employed
Prevent celiac crisis	Teach the parents specifics of dietary control, especially dangers of prolonged fasting Stress importance of good health in preventing infection and need to avoid known sources of infection Notify other treating physicians of celiac disorder and risk of anticholinergic drugs
Prevent complications from celiac crisis	Monitor intravenous fluids closely Give mouth care during period when nothing is given by mouth Observe the child closely for signs of metabolic acidosis (weakness, irritability, decreasing level of consciousness, irregular heartbeat, poor muscular control) Observe the child closely for signs of dehydration Monitor nasogastric suctioning and record drainage Observe for signs of shock Administer corticosteroids if ordered; when discontinued by decreasing doses, observe for return of signs suggestive of celiac disease
Teach the parents dietary control	Explain reason for eliminating gluten from diet Give written list of common food sources of wheat, rye, barley, and oats Emphasize suitable substitutes, especially rice and corn Stress importance of reading labels of prepared food for hidden sources of gluten In addition to gluten-restricted diet, emphasize a balanced diet and vitamin supplements Make referral to public health nurse and nutritionist for continued dietary counseling after hospital discharge
Help the parents and child adjust to life-long adherence to dietary restriction	Allow parents and child opportunity to express discouragement or personal doubt in terms of necessity of diet, especially after symptom-free course Stress positive benefits of diet: remarkable clinical improvement, prevention of crises and complications
Promote normal life for the child	Help the child adjust by focusing on ways he can be normal rather than solely on restrictions that make him feel different Encourage the parents to treat the child no differently than other siblings; stress need for appropriate limit setting Introduce the child to another peer with celiac disease, which may be helpful to all family members Promote positive self-concept; encourage attractive, age-appropriate grooming

fects. However, evidence demonstrates that the majority of individuals who relax their diet will experience a relapse of their disease and possibly exhibit growth retardation, anemia, or osteomalacia. There is also the risk of developing malignant lymphoma of the small intestine, esophageal cancer, and other gastrointestinal malignancies.

Several resources are available to assist parents in all aspects of coping with celiac disease. The American Celiac Society* has cookbooks with gluten-free recipes and a booklet, "Pointers for parents: coping with celiac sprue", is available† that provides information on shopping, cooking, and otherwise living with an affected child.

SHORT GUT (BOWEL) SYNDROME

The short gut syndrome is a condition in which there is a loss of intestine resulting in a diminished ability to digest and absorb a regular diet normally. The major causes in children are: (1) congenital, such as small intestine atresias or gastroschisis, (2) volvulus involving a large segment of bowel, and (3) inflammation, such as that of necrotizing enterocolitis or Crohn's disease.

Both the amount and location of gut lost are important in determining the severity of the condition. Up to 50% of the intestine can be lost without affecting the health of the child, unless it includes the distal ileum. A loss of greater than 75% of the small bowel results in malabsorption. However, the remaining intestine and stomach can adapt to the loss through compensatory growth provided the child is kept alive with special nutritional support.

Therapeutic management

The goals of treatment are (1) to preserve as much length of bowel as possible during surgery and (2) to maintain the child's nutritional status until adaptation to the altered bowel takes place. For the severely affected child total parenteral nutrition is the treatment of choice.

Nursing considerations

Nursing care is directed toward maintaining the child's nutritional state. Every effort is made to preserve the intravenous line in parenteral alimentation and to prevent complications such as infection. When long-term parenteral nutrition is required, preparing the family for home care of the child is a major nursing responsibility. Since hospitalization may be prolonged, the child's developmental and emotional needs must be met as well.

*Dept. N83, 45 Gifford Ave., Jersey City, NJ 07304.
†Clinical Dietetics Department, Children's Memorial Hospital, 2300 Children's Plaza, Chicago, IL 60614

OBSTRUCTIVE DISORDERS

Obstruction of the bowel occurs when the passage of intestinal contents is mechanically impeded by a constricted or an occluded lumen or when there is interference with normal muscular contraction. Intestinal obstruction from any cause is characterized by similar signs and symptoms, although the progression may vary greatly. For example, in acute conditions, such as intussusception, the clinical manifestations are apparent within a few hours of the onset of the disorder. In other conditions, such as pyloric stenosis, the signs and symptoms usually develop more gradually and can be missed in the early stages.

Clinical manifestations

Classically acute mechanical intestinal obstruction is characterized by colicky abdominal pain, nausea and vomiting, abdominal distention, and constipation. *Abdominal distention* is the result of accumulation of gas and fluid above the level of the obstruction. As these secretions continue to accumulate, the gut becomes excessively irritated and stimulates the vomiting center in the medulla to rid itself of the irritants with or without nausea. *Vomiting* is often the earliest sign of a high obstruction and a later sign in lower obstructions. Conversely *constipation* and *obstipation* are early signs of low obstructions and later signs of higher obstructions.

If the obstruction is below the stomach, reflux from the small intestine causes intestinal secretions to flow back into the stomach, where they are vomited along with stomach contents. As this progresses, large quantities of fluid and electrolytes are lost, resulting in *dehydration*.

As distention progresses, the abdomen may be rigid and boardlike, with moderate to severe *tenderness. Bowel sounds* gradually diminish and cease. *Respiratory distress* occurs as the diaphragm is pushed up into the pleural cavity. As proteins are lost from the bloodstream into the intestinal lumen, the plasma volume diminishes and *shock* may occur.

HYPERTROPHIC PYLORIC STENOSIS (HPS)

Obstruction at the pyloric sphincter by hypertrophy of the circular muscle of the pylorus is one of the most common surgical disorders of early infancy. This functional anomaly is seen soon after birth with vomiting that becomes progressively more severe and projectile. It is five times more common in male than female infants, affecting approximately five of every 1000 males and only one of every 1000 females. It is seen less frequently in black and

Oriental than in white infants. It is more likely to affect a full-term than a premature infant.

Etiology

The cause of the increased size of the pyloric musculature is unknown. A higher incidence in first-degree relatives and in monozygotic as opposed to dizygotic twins implicates heredity in the etiology, although the nature of the hereditary factors is only speculative.

Pathophysiology

The circular muscle of the pylorus is grossly enlarged as a result of both hypertrophy and hyperplasia. This produces severe narrowing of the pyloric canal between the stomach and duodenum. Consequently the lumen at this point is partially obstructed. Over a period of time inflammation and edema further reduce the size of the opening until the partial obstruction may progress to complete obstruction. The muscle is thickened to as much as twice its usual size—2 to 3 cm long—and is almost cartilaginous in consistency. The distal portion ends abruptly and is externally distinct and easily palpated, but the proximal end merges into the gastric antrum. The stomach is usually dilated (Fig. 21-9, *A*).

Clinical manifestations

Typically infants with pyloric hypertrophy are well during the first weeks of life. Initially there is only regurgitation or occasional nonprojectile vomiting that begins about the second to the fourth week after birth, although in a few infants symptoms begin at birth. Others do well for the first few weeks and then suddenly develop vomiting that becomes projectile in nature, usually within a week, and may lead to complete obstruction by 4 to 6 weeks. The vomiting is forceful, and vomitus may be ejected 3 to 4 feet from the child in a side-lying position and 1 foot or more when the infant is lying on the back. Vomiting most often occurs shortly after a feeding, although it may not occur for several hours. In some instances the vomiting may follow each feeding; in others it appears intermittently. The infant is hungry and an avid nurser who eagerly accepts a second feeding after a vomiting episode. The vomitus is nonbilious, containing only gastric contents, but may be blood-tinged. The infant does not appear to be in pain other than the discomfort of chronic hunger.

The infant may show weight loss and signs of dehydration. The upper abdomen is distended, and diagnosis can be established on the basis of (1) a readily palpable olive-shaped tumor in the epigastrium just to the right of the umbilicus and (2) visible gastric peristaltic waves that move from left to right across the epigastrium. The pyloric tumor is most easily felt when the abdominal muscles are relaxed during a feeding or immediately after vomiting.

Diagnostic evaluation

If diagnosis is inconclusive from the history and physical signs, upper gastrointestinal x-ray studies will reveal de-

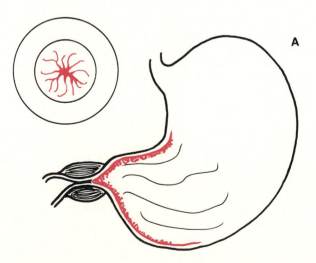
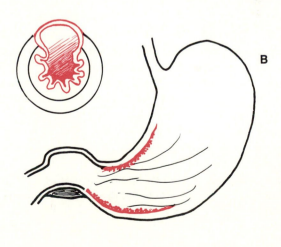

FIG. 21-9

Hypertrophic pyloric stenosis. **A,** *Enlarged muscular tumor nearly obliterates pyloric channel.* **B,** *Longitudinal surgical division of muscle down to submucosa establishes adequate passageway.*

layed gastric emptying and an elongated, threadlike pyloric channel. Many are finding that ultrasound is as accurate and less traumatic for diagnosis of pyloric stenosis. Laboratory findings reflect the metabolic alterations created by severe depletion of both water and electrolytes from extensive and prolonged vomiting. There are decreased serum levels of both sodium and potassium, although these may be masked by the hemoconcentration from extracellular fluid depletion. Of greater diagnostic value are a decrease in serum chloride levels and increases in pH and bicarbonate (carbon dioxide content) characteristic of metabolic alkalosis.

Therapeutic management

Surgical relief of the pyloric obstruction by pyloromyotomy is simple, safe, and effective and is, with very few exceptions, the standard treatment for this disorder. The surgical procedure is performed through a right upper quadrant muscle-splitting incision and consists of a longitudinal incision through the circular muscle fibers of the pylorus down to, but not including, the submucosa (Fredet-Ramstedt operation, Fig. 21-9, *B*). The procedure has a very high success rate when infants receive careful preoperative preparation to correct fluid and electrolyte imbalances.

Feedings are usually begun 4 to 6 hours postoperatively, beginning with small, frequent feedings of glucose in water or electrolyte solutions. If clear fluids are retained, about 24 hours after surgery formula is started in the same stepwise increments, gradually increasing the amount and the interval between feedings until a full feeding schedule is reinstated, which usually takes about 48 hours. The infant is ready to be discharged from the hospital by about the fourth postoperative day. The prognosis is excellent, and the mortality rate is low.

Medical treatment of pyloric stenosis is not widely used, since there is such a high success rate with surgical management. It consists of a long-term regimen of small, frequent feedings of formula thickened with cereal, maintaining an upright position after feedings, refeeding, sedation, and administration of a cholinergic blocking agent. Parenteral fluids are administered as needed, and stomach lavage for epigastric distention reduces the likelihood of vomiting.

Nursing considerations

Nursing care of the infant with hypertrophic pyloric stenosis involves primarily observation for physical signs and behaviors that help establish the diagnosis, careful regulation of fluid therapy, and reestablishment of normal feeding behaviors. Hypertrophic pyloric stenosis should be considered as a possibility in the very young infant who

appears alert but fails to gain weight and has a history of vomiting after meals.

Preoperative care. Preoperatively the emphasis is placed on restoring hydration and electrolyte balance and beginning replacement of depleted body fat and protein stores. These infants are usually given no oral feedings and placed on intravenous fluids with glucose and electrolyte replacement based on laboratory serum electrolyte values. Careful monitoring of the intravenous infusion and diligent attention to intake, output, and urine-specific gravity measurements are important to the success of fluid replacement. Any vomiting, as well as the number and character of stools, is observed and recorded accurately.

No matter what the infant is fed, special techniques are needed to minimize the likelihood of vomiting. Feedings are given slowly with the infant held in a semiupright position. Because these infants tend to suck their fingers and hands, they swallow a good deal of air; therefore, bubbling before and frequently during feedings will lessen gastric distention. After a feeding the infant is turned slightly on the right side in high-Fowler's position in an infant seat or propped in the crib to facilitate gastric emptying. Minimum handling, especially after a feeding, helps prevent vomiting. If vomiting occurs, the type, amount, character, and its relationship to the feeding are observed and recorded. Refeeding of formula is usually ordered in an amount equivalent to the volume lost.

Observations include assessment of vital signs, particularly those that might indicate fluid or electrolyte imbalances. These infants are especially prone to metabolic alkalosis from loss of hydrogen ions and to potassium, sodium, and chloride depletion. The skin and mucous membranes are assessed for alterations in hydration status, and daily weight provides added clues to water gain or loss.

When stomach decompression and gastric lavage are part of preoperative management, it is the responsibility of the nurse to ensure that the tube is patent and functioning properly and to measure and record the type and amount of drainage. The infant is usually positioned flat or with the head slightly elevated. The infant who is receiving intravenous fluids and/or has a nasogastric tube to continuous drainage must be adequately restrained to prevent the needle and/or tube from becoming dislodged.

General hygienic care, with particular attention to skin and mouth in dehydrated infants, is an important part of care. Protection from infection is also important, since infants with impaired nutritional status are even more susceptible than normal newborn infants. Sensory stimulation is incorporated into nursing care, and parental involvement is encouraged and promoted.

Postoperative care. Postoperative vomiting is not uncommon, and most infants, even with successful surgery, exhibit some vomiting during the first 24 to 48

SUMMARY OF NURSING CARE OF THE CHILD WITH PYLORIC STENOSIS

GOALS	RESPONSIBILITIES

Help establish diagnosis	Recognize signs of pyloric stenosis and refer for medical evaluation
	Obtain specimens and assist with diagnostic tests and procedures
	Observe and record
	  Physical signs of upper gastrointestinal obstruction, hyperperistalsis
	  Amount, type, and character of vomiting
	  Amount, type, and character of stools
	Observe oral behaviors, including eating, hand-sucking, and so on

Prevent vomiting	Give small, frequent feedings; feed slowly Bubble before and frequently during feedings Position in high-Fowler's position and slightly on right side after feeding Handle minimally and gently after feeding
Promote gastric decompression	Give nothing by mouth Carry out lavage as ordered Maintain patency of nasogastric tube Measure and record amount and type of drainage
Recognize signs of complications	Observe, report, and record any signs of upper gastrointestinal fluid loss, such as alkalosis, hypokalemia, hypochloremia, dehydration, altered neurologic signs, shock Postoperatively, check incision site
Prevent removal of intravenous or nasogastric tube	Apply and maintain adequate restraining devices

Prevent infection	Continue general protective measures, including
	  Avoidance of contact with infected persons
	  Good hand washing before handling infant
	  Only clean or sterile supplies in contact with infant

Provide nutrition	Administer feedings as ordered Feed frequently in small amounts to avoid overdistending the stomach Administer and monitor parenteral fluids as ordered at desired rate of flow
Maintain warmth	Place infant in Isolette or warmer or provide adequate covering

Assess adequacy of intake	Weigh daily or as ordered
	Assess status of skin and mucous membranes
	Measure carefully
	  Intake—oral and/or parenteral
	  Output—vomitus, nasogastric tube drainage, stools, and urine
	  Urine specific gravity

Maintain general hygiene	Administer good skin care Change diapers immediately when wet or soiled Administer special care to reddened or excoriated areas Administer mouth care
Provide comfort	Provide pacifier to meet oral needs Provide sensory stimulation Encourage the parents' visitation and involvement in care Whenever possible, arrange to hold, or have others hold, the infant

Continued.

SUMMARY OF NURSING CARE OF THE CHILD WITH PYLORIC STENOSIS—cont'd

GOALS	RESPONSIBILITIES
Support parents	Keep parents informed regarding the infant's progress Assure the mother or other caregiver that the problem is organic and is in no way a reflection of inadequate mothering skills Allow the parents to express concerns and anxieties
Teach parents	Instruct the parent in feeding and positioning techniques Instruct in care of incision Instruct regarding signs of 　Expected behavior 　Behaviors and signs that should be reported
Administer follow-up care	Instruct the parents regarding posthospitalization evaluation Refer to public health agency if needed

hours. Intravenous fluids are administered until the infant is taking and retaining adequate amounts by mouth. Therefore, much of the same care that was instituted prior to surgery is continued postoperatively, that is, observation of physical signs, monitoring intravenous fluids, and careful observation and recording of intake and output. In addition the infant is observed for responses to the stress of surgery. The nasogastric tube may be maintained after surgery for a variable length of time.

Feedings are usually instituted relatively soon, beginning with clear liquids containing glucose and electrolytes. They are offered slowly, in small amounts, and at frequent intervals as ordered by the physician. If the infant has been breast-fed, breast milk, expressed by the mother, is given by bottle when the infant is able to tolerate feedings, and breast-feeding is resumed as soon as feasible. Observation and recording of feedings and the infant's responses to feedings and feeding techniques are a vital part of postoperative care. Positioning with the head elevated is usually continued postoperatively. Care of the operative site consists of observation for any drainage or signs of inflammation and care of the incision as directed by the surgeon.

As with any child in the hospital, parents are encouraged to visit and become involved in the child's care. Vomiting of a projectile nature is frightening to parents, and they often believe that they may have done something wrong. Most mothers need support and reassurance that the condition is caused by a structural problem and is in no way a reflection on their mothering skills and capacities.

INTUSSUSCEPTION

Intussusception, the invagination or telescoping of one portion of the intestine into another, is one of the most frequent causes of intestinal obstruction during later infancy and early toddlerhood. Half of the cases occur in children younger than age 1 year, more commonly between 3 and 12 months of age, and most of the others occur in children during the second year. Intussusception is three times more common in males than females. Although specific intestinal lesions can be found in a small percentage of the children, generally the cause is not known.

Pathophysiology

The most common site of intussusception is the ileocecal valve, where the ileum invaginates into the cecum and colon (Fig. 21-10) producing an obstruction to the passage of intestinal contents beyond the defect. In addition the two walls of the intestine press against each other, causing inflammation, edema, and eventually decreased blood flow. Continued incarceration results in necrosis with hemorrhage, perforation, and peritonitis. If left untreated this condition is incompatible with life.

Clinical manifestations

The classic presentation of intussusception is a healthy, thriving child, usually between 3 and 12 months of age, who suddenly develops an episode of acute abdominal pain, vomiting, and passing of one normal brown stool. Typically there are episodes of severe pain during which the child screams and draws the knees onto the chest. Characteristically, the child appears normal and comfortable during the intervals between these episodes of pain. As the condition becomes worse, the vomiting increases, the child becomes apathetic, and subsequent stools are red currant jelly-like from the passage of stool mixed with blood and mucus.

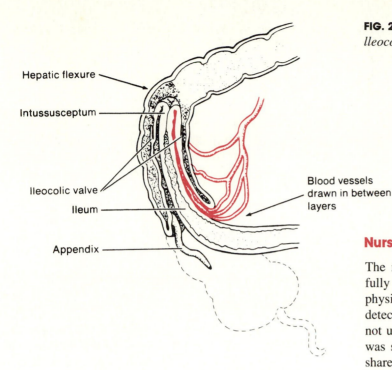

Hepatic flexure

Intussusceptum

Ileocolic valve

Ileum

Appendix

Blood vessels
drawn in between
layers

FIG. 21-10
Ileocolic intussusception.

The abdomen becomes tender and distended and a sausage-shaped mass may be felt in the upper right quadrant. In contrast the lower right quadrant usually feels empty (Dance's sign) as the bowel distal to the obstruction is less involved and free of contents. If the condition is allowed to progress, the child becomes acutely ill with fever, prostration, and other signs of peritonitis.

Diagnostic evaluation

Frequently the diagnosis can be made on subjective findings alone. However, definitive diagnosis is based on a barium enema, which clearly demonstrates the obstruction to the flow of barium. A rectal examination reveals mucus, blood, and, occasionally, a low intussusception itself.

Therapeutic management

In most cases the initial treatment of choice is nonsurgical hydrostatic reduction by barium enema at the time of diagnostic testing. The force exerted by the flowing barium is usually sufficient enough to push the invaginated portion of the bowel into its original position, similar to pushing an inverted "finger" out of a glove. Successful reduction is accomplished in about 75% to 85% of uncomplicated cases. This procedure is not recommended if there are clinical signs of shock or perforation.

Since this procedure is not always successful, the child is prepared for surgery before the barium enema. Surgical intervention consists of reducing the invagination manually and, where indicated, resecting any nonviable intestine.

Nursing considerations

The nurse can assist in establishing a diagnosis by carefully listening to the parent's description of the child's physical and behavioral symptoms. Parents are astute in detecting that something is wrong with their child and it is not unusual for parents to express that they felt something was seriously wrong with their child before the physician shared their concerns. The description of the child's severe colicky abdominal pain combined with vomiting is a significant clue to intussusception.

Physical care of the child with intussusception differs little from the preparation of any child for abdominal surgery. Even though nonsurgical intervention may be successful, usual preoperative procedures, such as withholding fluids, routine laboratory testing (complete blood count and urinalysis), signed parental consent, and preanesthetic sedation, are carried out. The parents are also prepared for the child's undergoing the nonsurgical technique of barium enema as well as the possibility of surgery.

For the child with signs of electrolyte imbalance, hemorrhage, or peritonitis, additional medical preparation such as replacement fluids, whole blood or plasma, and nasogastric suctioning may be performed. Prior to surgery the nurse monitors all stools. Passage of a normal brown stool usually indicates that the intussusception has reduced spontaneously. This is reported immediately to the physician who may choose to alter the diagnostic/therapeutic plan of care.

Postprocedural care is the same as for any child with abdominal surgery including vital signs, blood pressure, intact sutures and dressing, and the return of bowel sounds. In the case of hydrostatic or autoreduction, the nurse observes for passage of barium and the stool patterns, since recurrences of the intussusception are most likely to occur within the first 36 hours after reduction; therefore, the child is kept in the hospital for 2 to 3 days.

Since this hospitalization may be the child's first separation from his parents, it is especially important to preserve the parent-child relationship by encouraging rooming-in or extended visiting. Also, it may be the parents' first experience with hospital care for their child; therefore, it is important that they are prepared for procedures such as intravenous therapy, frequent vital signs and blood pressure, dressings, and special orders, such as nothing by mouth. Because of the rapidity of the onset, diagnosis, and treatment, parents may be left with the feeling of stunned numbness. They may either ask few questions or constantly make inquiries, sometimes the same ones repeatedly. If the nurse realizes the circumstances surrounding this condition, the parents' reactions are more likely to be understood and supported.

IMPERFORATE ANUS

Malformations in the anorectal region of the gastrointestinal tract are among the more common congenital malformations caused by abnormal development (approximately one in 5000).

The most widely used classification describing anorectal malformations is illustrated and described in Fig. 21-11. The rectal defect may consist of a stenosis, a membrane obliterating the anal opening, a blind rectal pouch,

or a fistulous connection to the perineum, urethra, bladder, or, in females, vagina.

Clinical manifestations

Inspection of the perineal area reveals absence of an anal opening or the thin translucent membrane of anal membrane atresia. Failure to pass meconium is cause for investigation. Fistulas associated with types B and C anomalies are not usually apparent at birth, but as peristalsis gradually forces the meconium through the fistula they can be identified by careful examination. With a rectourinary fistula meconium appears in the urine. Stenosis may not become apparent until 1 year of age or older when the child has a history of difficult defecation, abdominal distention, and ribbonlike stools.

Diagnostic evaluation

Checking for patency of the anus and rectum is a routine part of the newborn assessment, including observation or inquiries regarding the passage of meconium. Digital and

FIG. 21-11

Anorectal stenosis and imperforate anus. **A,** *Congenital anal stenosis.* **B,** *Anal membrane atresia.* **C,** *Anal agenesis.* **D,** *Rectal atresia.* **E,** *Rectoperoneal fistula.* **F,** *Rectovaginal fistula.*

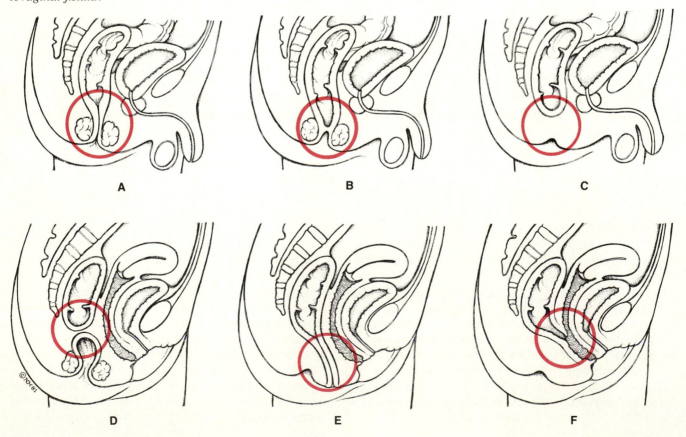

endoscopic examinations identify constriction or the blind pouch of rectal atresia.

Definitive diagnosis of the extent and location of the rectal pouch is made by radiographic examination. With the infant inverted and an opaque marker at the anal dimple, air ascending into the rectum and lower bowel will outline the location of the pouch in relation to the anal depression.

Therapeutic management

Successful treatment for anal stenosis is generally accomplished by manual dilations. The procedure, begun by the physician, is repeated on a regular basis by the nurses in the hospital and continued at home by the parents, after they are carefully instructed in the technique. An imperforate anal membrane is excised and followed by daily anal dilations.

Reconstruction of an anus in the proper position is the goal of surgical treatment of other anorectal malformations. Malformations of the lower rectum often can be corrected in the neonatal period by way of an abdominal-perineal pull-through procedure and/or anoplasty. Infants with higher anomalies require a divided sigmoid colostomy in the newborn period. Final correction of higher defects is usually postponed for a year.

Nursing considerations

The first nursing responsibility is identification of undetected anorectal malformations. A newborn who does not pass a stool within 24 hours of birth requires further assessment, and meconium that appears at an inappropriate orifice should be reported.

Postoperative nursing care ordinarily presents few problems and is primarily directed toward healing of the anoplasty without infection or other complications. Where the infant has undergone a pull-through procedure with anoplasty, special nursing care involves maintaining the anal area as clean as possible with scrupulous perineal care. There may or may not be a temporary dressing and drain, but, when the infant is passing stool, dressings are of little value. The preferred position is a side-lying prone position with the hips elevated or a supine position with the legs suspended at a 90-degree angle to the trunk to prevent pressure on perineal sutures. Periodic application of a heat lamp facilitates healing.

The infant is administered regular infant formula as soon as peristalsis returns. In the meantime there may be a nasogastric tube for abdominal decompression and intravenous feedings. Care of the infant with a colostomy involves frequent dressing changes, meticulous skin care, and correct application of a collection device (p. 584).

INFLAMMATORY CONDITIONS

Inflammatory conditions involving large or small segments of the gastrointestinal tract are not uncommon in childhood. They may be acute or chronic and some are more likely to affect one age-group more than another; for example, necrotizing enterocolitis is seen in the newborn, ulcerative colitis occurs most frequently in the prepubescent and adolescent child, whereas acute appendicitis presents at any age.

ACUTE APPENDICITIS

Appendicitis, inflammation of the vermiform appendix or blind sac at the end of the cecum, is the most common condition requiring abdominal surgery during childhood. Although rare in children younger than 2 years of age, it is associated with increased complications and mortality in this age-group. Primarily an acute condition, appendicitis rapidly progresses to perforation and peritonitis if it remains undiagnosed. It is a significant pediatric problem, because early diagnosis is frequently delayed as a result of the child's inability to verbalize his symptoms and professionals' failure to interpret behavioral clues correctly.

Etiology

The exact cause of appendicitis is poorly understood but it is almost always a result of obstruction of the lumen, usually by a fecalith (a hard fecal concretion). Sometimes a fold of peritoneum causes the appendix to adhere to the cecum causing an obstructive kink. Other causes include lymphoid hyperplasia, fibrous stenosis from an earlier inflammation, and tumors. Although worms are frequently found in the appendix, there is no substantiated evidence that they are a cause of appendicitis.

Pathophysiology

With acute obstruction the outflow of mucous secretions is blocked, pressure builds within the lumen, resulting in compression of blood vessels. The resulting ischemia is followed by ulceration of the epithelial lining and bacterial invasion. Subsequent necrosis causes perforation or rupture with fecal and bacterial contamination of the peritoneal cavity. The resulting inflammation spreads rapidly throughout the abdomen (*peritonitis*)—especially in young children who are unable to localize infection. Progressive peritoneal inflammation results in functional intestinal obstruction of the small bowel, since intense gastrointestinal reflexes severely inhibit bowel motility.

Clinical manifestations

The most common signs and symptoms of appendicitis are colicky abdominal pain, tenderness, and fever. Initially the pain is generalized or periumbilical; however, it usually descends to the lower right quadrant. The most intense site of pain may be at McBurney point, which is located at a point midway between the anterior superior iliac crest and the umbilicus. Other important signs are a rigid abdomen, decreased or absent bowel sounds, and rebound tenderness (the sudden pain at the point of tenderness elicited by pressing firmly over a part of the abdomen distal to the area of tenderness). Jumping or riding over bumps in an automobile or gurney aggravates the pain.

Vomiting commonly follows the onset of pain, especially in younger children, and constipation or diarrhea may be present. Anorexia is a constant feature. The child also displays tachycardia, rapid shallow breathing, pallor, irritability, and restlessness. Probably the most significant clinical manifestation is a change in the child's behavior. The nonverbal child will assume a rigid, motionless, side-lying posture with the knees flexed on the abdomen. The older child may exhibit all of these behaviors, while complaining of abdominal pain.

Diagnostic evaluation

Diagnosis is based primarily on history and examination. The white blood cell count is usually elevated but is seldom higher than 15,000 to 20,000/mm³, and radiographic studies of the abdomen may reveal possible contributing causes of appendicitis, such as fecaliths or a foreign body.

Diagnosis is not always straightforward. Numerous infectious processes have features in common. Fever, vomiting, abdominal pain, and elevated blood count are associated with inflammatory bowel disease, gastroenteritis, urinary tract infection, pneumonia and numerous hematologic disorders, for example.

Therapeutic management

Treatment of appendicitis before perforation is surgical removal of the appendix (appendectomy). Recovery is rapid.

Ruptured appendix. Management of the child diagnosed with peritonitis caused by a ruptured appendix often begins preoperatively with intravenous administration of fluid and electrolytes, systemic antibiotics, and nasogastric suction. Postoperative management includes fluid and electrolyte balance maintenance, continued administration of antibiotics, and nasogastric suction for abdominal decompression until intestinal activity returns.

Most surgeons provide for external drainage when abscess formation has occurred, there is necrotic or severely damaged tissue, or where there are purulent collections within the peritoneum. This is accomplished by sump drainage or a Penrose drain and wound irrigations. The child is maintained in semi-Fowler position to reduce spread of the infection to other parts of the peritoneum, one of the most common of which is the subdiaphragmatic area.

Nursing considerations

Because successful treatment of appendicitis is based on prompt recognition of the disorder, a primary nursing objective is assisting in establishing a diagnosis. Since abdominal pain is the most common childhood complaint, the nurse needs to make some preliminary evaluation of the severity of pain (see p. 512 for assessment of pain). One of the most reliable estimates is the degree of change in behavior. For example, a child who stays home from school and voluntarily lies down or refuses to play is much more likely to have considerable pain than the child who is absent from school but plays contentedly at home.

Preoperative care. Physical preparation of the child with appendicitis is the same as that for any child with abdominal surgery (see p. 653). In any instance when severe abdominal pain is expected, the nurse must be aware of the danger of administering laxatives, enemas, or applying heat to the area. Such measures stimulate bowel motility and increase the risk of perforation.

Postoperative care. Postoperative care for the nonperforated appendix is the same as for most abdominal operations. Care of the child with a ruptured appendix and peritonitis involves more complex care. The course of recovery is considerably longer and may require 2 weeks or more of hospitalization, in contrast to a week or less for an uncomplicated appendectomy.

The child is maintained on intravenous fluids, allowed nothing by mouth, and remains on low intermittent gastric decompression until there is evidence of intestinal activity. The nurse listens for bowel sounds as part of the routine assessment and observes for other signs of bowel activity such as passage of stool. Management of intravenous therapy is the same as for any child and parenteral antibiotics are usually infused for 7 to 10 days, after which oral preparations may be continued even longer.

Positioning the child in semi-Fowler's position or lying on the right side after surgery for a ruptured appendix facilitates drainage from the peritoneal cavity as well as prevents the formation of a subdiaphragmatic abscess. A Penrose drain is placed in the wound, and frequent dressing changes with meticulous skin care are essential to prevent excoriation of the surgical area. Sometimes the abdominal wound is irrigated with antibacterial solution.

Psychologic care of the child and parents is similar to that employed in other emergency situations. Parents and older children need an opportunity to express their feelings postoperatively. It is especially important for the nurse to

SUMMARY OF NURSING CARE OF THE CHILD WITH APPENDICITIS

GOALS	RESPONSIBILITIES
Preoperative	
Assist with diagnosis	Obtain history, if appropriate Observe for symptoms of appendicitis
Anticipate possible surgery	Initiate nothing by mouth Prepare for surgery (p. 533) Collect and order needed specimens
Prevent aggravating the condition	Maintain complete bed rest Avoid heat to abdomen Apply cold applications to abdomen (ice pack) Caution against administering laxative or enemas

Relieve discomfort	Position for comfort
	   Semi-Fowler's position
	   Side-lying position
	Avoid palpating the abdomen unless necessary
	Apply cold applications to abdomen

Relieve anxiety in the child and parents	Maintain calm, reassuring manner Explain procedures and other activities before initiating them Answer questions and explain purposes of activities Keep informed of progress
Postoperative Simple appendectomy	See postoperative care of the child with abdominal surgery (p. 653)

Postoperative
Ruptured appendix
  Prevent abdominal distention
	See postoperative care of the child with abdominal surger (p. 653)
	Allow nothing by mouth
	Maintain abdominal decompression as ordered
	   Assess and assure patency of nasogastric tube
	   Irrigate with normal saline as indicated
	   Maintain intermittent suction at appropriate negative pressure
	Insert rectal tube if indicated

Assess status of bowel activity	Gently palpate abdomen to determine degree of distention (if present) Auscultate abdomen for sounds of peristaltic activity Observe and record type and amount of any bowel movement
Prevent spread of infection	Position in semi-Fowler's position to localize infection and prevent upward spread of infection Administer antibiotics as prescribed Implement appropriate isolation precautions Careful wound care and disposal of wound dressings

Detect presence of infection	Take vital signs every 2-4 hours
	Collect or request needed specimens
	   Wound culture
	   White blood count
	   Blood culture (if indicated)
	Inspect wound for signs of infection: redness, swelling, heat, pain, purulent drainage

Facilitate wound healing	When on oral feedings, provide nutritious diet
	Perform careful wound care
	   Keep wound clean and dry
	   Cleanse with prescribed preparation
	   Advance Penrose drain as ordered (if present)
	   Apply antibacterial solutions and/or ointments as ordered
	   Administer vitamins A and/or C if prescribed

Continued.

SUMMARY OF NURSING CARE OF THE CHILD WITH APPENDICITIS—cont'd

GOALS	RESPONSIBILITIES
Postoperative—cont'd	
Maintain adequate nutrition and hydration	Monitor intravenous infusion (p. 569)
	Provide fluids and food by mouth as ordered when bowel activity evident
	Give progressive diet
Relieve discomfort	Position for comfort
	Fowler's position
	Avoid strain on abdomen
	Administer analgesic as prescribed
	Insert rectal tube if indicated
	Encourage to void if appropriate
Prevent other complications	Turn, cough, deep breathe every 2 hours
	Ambulate as prescribed
	Assess for bladder distention
	Encourage to void
Provide reassurance	Remain with the child as much as possible
	Explain activities and procedures
	Give encouragement and positive feedback for cooperation in care
Support and reassure parents	See postoperative care of the child with abdominal surgery

---

encourage the child to relate all the events he remembers concerning admission and treatment in order to clarify misconceptions.

MECKEL DIVERTICULUM

Meckel diverticulum is a vestigial remnant of a fetal structure that connects the yolk sac with the intestinal cavity during fetal life. The diverticulum is located at the distal ileum and varies in size from a small appendiceal process to a pouch several inches long and almost as wide. At times it may be connected to the umbilicus by a cord.

Meckel diverticulum is the most common congenital malformation of the gastrointestinal tract and is present in 1% to 2% of the population. It is twice as common in males as in females, and complications are several times more frequent in males. Most symptomatic cases are seen in the first 2 years of life, but it frequently exists without causing symptoms.

Pathophysiology

Meckel diverticulum is a sac subject to inflammation (diverticulitis) in the same manner as appendicitis. In over half the cases the diverticulum contains gastric mucosa, which produces hydrochloric acid and pepsin. The acid continually irritates the bowel and erodes the surface resulting in bleeding and, in some instances, may lead to perforation. Mechanical obstruction can occur as a result of volvulus, or twisting of the bowel around the fibrotic Meckel cord.

Clinical manifestations

Over half of the individuals with Meckel diverticulum are symptomatic, and the signs and symptoms reflect the pathologic process as, for example, intestinal obstruction. Acute diverticulitis presents the same clinical picture as acute appendicitis, although the pain may be vague and recurrent. In the majority of children the presenting sign is painless bright or dark red rectal bleeding representing acute (sometimes massive) hemorrhage. In infants, however, the bleeding may be accompanied by pain. Severe anemia and shock occur as consequences of the hemorrhage.

Diagnostic evaluation

Diagnosis is ordinarily based on the history. Rectosigmoidoscopy and barium enema are usually performed to eliminate other possible diagnoses, such as anal fissure, polyps, and intussusception. Radiologic studies are not helpful in confirming the diagnosis, because the diverticulum may be too small to be visualized or may fail to fill with barium. Blood studies are usually part of the general laboratory workup to rule out any bleeding disorders and to evaluate the severity of the anemia.

Therapeutic management

Treatment is surgical removal of the diverticulum. In instances in which severe hemorrhage increases the surgical risk, medical intervention to correct hypovolemic shock, such as blood replacement, intravenous fluids, and oxygen, may be necessary. In diverticulitis antibiotics may be used preoperatively to control infection. If intestinal obstruction has occurred, appropriate preoperative measures are used to reverse electrolyte imbalances and prevent abdominal distention.

Nursing considerations

Nursing objectives are similar to those for the child with appendicitis. Since the onset is usually rapid, psychologic support parallels that for other conditions, such as appendicitis. It is important to remember that the the massive rectal bleeding is most often traumatic to both the child and the parent and may significantly affect their emotional reaction to hospitalization and surgery.

Specific preoperative considerations when rectal bleeding is present include (1) frequent monitoring of vital signs and blood pressure for shock, (2) keeping the child on bed rest, and (3) recording the approximate amount of blood lost in stools. In the absence of frank rectal hemorrhage, the nurse tests the stools for occult blood.

ULCERATIVE COLITIS

Ulcerative colitis is a disease characterized by a chronic inflammatory reaction involving the mucosa and submucosa of the large intestine. It occurs in both sexes and in all age-groups. It is basically a disease of young adults, although close to 15% of the cases begin in children younger than 16 years of age. The peak onset in children is between ages 10 and 19 years. This disorder and Crohn disease are together referred to as *inflammatory bowel disease (IBD)*.

Etiology

The cause of ulcerative colitis is unknown, although infectious, nutritional, immunologic, and psychogenic etiologies have been proposed but not substantiated. Several genetic and environmental factors influence the incidence of ulcerative colitis: (1) there is a familial tendency in about 5% to 15% of the cases, (2) individuals from higher socioeconomic levels and more whites than nonwhites are affected, (3) the incidence is four times greater in Jewish populations than in the general population; and (4) there is a higher occurrence of allergic disease in relatives of these patients.

At present the feeling is that ulcerative colitis is an organic disease caused by a combination of physical and emotional factors. Psychologic influences, such as stress, significantly affect the exacerbation and chronicity of the illness.

Pathophysiology

The mucous membranes of the bowel become hyperemic and edematous with the formation of patchy granulations over the intestinal surface that bleed easily and eventually develop irregular areas of superficial ulcerations. In longstanding disease, the bowel becomes narrowed, smooth, and inflexible with thin or absent mucosa heavily infiltrated by scar tissue.

Clinical manifestations

The most common feature of ulcerative colitis is persistent or recurring diarrhea. In the acute, fulminating disease there is bloody diarrhea preceded by cramping abdominal pain and followed by abdominal distention. Diarrhea may be very severe with marked urgency and frequency (20 to 30 stools per day). It is usually associated with fever, marked weight loss, anorexia, and sometimes nausea and vomiting. Pallor and anemia may result from bleeding and reduced dietary intake, and the numerous watery bowel movements often cause depletion of water and electrolytes (Fig. 21-12).

The course of the disease is marked by exacerbations and remissions that occur at unpredictable intervals. Rarely is an affected child completely free of symptoms. Exacerbations can be frequent but, in most cases, the disease pattern tends to stabilize and the affected children arrive at a state of control that is compatible with their individual way of life, the illness varying in intensity from child to child and from time to time in any individual child. The most critical episode is usually the initial attack but frequently recurring exacerbations can be severe.

Diagnostic evaluation

Diagnosis is suspected on the basis of history and physical examination and is confirmed by rectosigmoidoscopy. Barium enema is often helpful and mucosal biopsy is useful in differentiating the disease from other forms of colitis, but the procedure carries the risk of perforation. Stool ex-

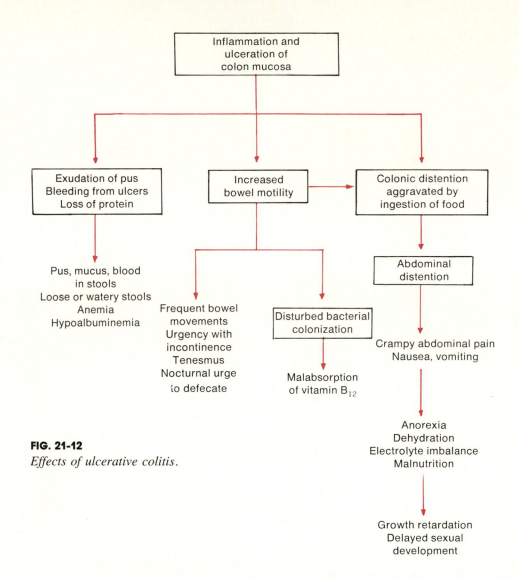

FIG. 21-12
Effects of ulcerative colitis.

amination is carried out to rule out infections and malabsorptive defects, and blood studies determine the state of anemia, electrolytes, and immunoglobulin levels.

Therapeutic management

Medical treatment is based on a combination of therapies: (1) dietary management to allow the colon a rest and improve the child's nutritional status, (2) medication to reduce the abdominal pain and rectal spasm, (3) steroids to reduce bowel inflammation and (4) antibacterial agents (sulfasalazine) to prevent infection. The child is usually hospitalized both to ensure proper medical management and to reduce the familial/environmental factors that may be contributing to the disease. Other medical therapies that may be warranted include intravenous fluids to correct dehydration and associated electrolyte imbalances, parenteral alimentation when malnutrition is severe and the colitis is further aggravated by oral diet, and antibiotics to combat

secondary colonic infection. Emergency surgical intervention is required for complications such as perforation, massive hemorrhage, or toxic megacolon (fulminating distention of the colon with progressive inflammation).

In some instances a poor response to medical treatment necessitates elective surgery either to allow the bowel a period of rest, in which a temporary colostomy is performed, or to arrest the disease process by removing the entire section of ulcerated bowel, in which case a total colectomy and ileostomy are usually required.

Nursing considerations

Many of the nursing considerations relate directly to the therapeutic management in treating colitis. However, the scope of nursing responsibilities extends beyond the immediate period of hospitalization and involves (1) continued guidance of families in terms of dietary management, (2) coping with those factors that increase stress and emotional lability, (3) adjusting to a disease of remission and exacerbations or one of chronic ill health, and (4) when indicated, preparing the child and parents for the possibility of diversionary bowel surgery.

Dietary management. During the acute stage the diet has the following characteristics: high protein, to replace lost protein from the ulcerated bowel, plasma lost through bleeding, and decreased intake resulting from anorexia; high calorie, to restore daily losses in the stool, to combat weight loss, and to promote positive nitrogen balance; normal fat; and low residue or residue-free, to decrease bowel irritation. Vitamin and mineral supplements are usually provided.

Encouraging the anorexic child to consume sufficient quantities of this diet while avoiding emotional conflict at mealtime is a nursing challenge. Including the child in meal planning; encouraging small, frequent meals or snacks rather than three large meals a day; serving meals around medication schedules when diarrhea, mouth pain, and intestinal spasm are controlled; and preparing high-protein, high-calorie foods (such as eggnog, milk shakes, cream soups, puddings, or custard) are approaches that are more likely to meet with success. Good mouth care prior to eating and the selection of bland foods help relieve the discomfort of mouth sores that sometimes complicate the disease.

Reducing stress and facilitating adjustment to chronic illness. Attending to the emotional components of the disease requires a thorough assessment of those stress factors that are disease related or circumstantial. Frequently the nurse can be instrumental in helping these children adjust to the problems of growth retardation, delayed sexual maturation, dietary restrictions, feelings of being ''different'' or ''sickly,'' inability to compete with peers, and necessary absence from school during exacerbations of the illness.

In the event that a permanent colectomy/ileostomy is required, the nurse can assist the child and family in accepting and adjusting to the change by teaching them how to care for the ileostomy, by emphasizing the positive aspects of surgery, particularly accelerated growth and sexual development, permanent recovery, and eliminated risk of colonic cancer, and by stressing a normal life despite bowel diversion. Introducing the child and parents to other ostomy patients, especially those of the child's age, can be the greatest therapeutic measure in fostering eventual acceptance.

The nurse must also recognize a dysfunctional relationship between the child and parents such as the dependent child–overprotective mother dyad. The nurse's own feelings toward what is viewed as a ''negative relationship'' may actually increase stress for the child. For example, if the nurse intervenes to encourage the child's independence and consequently discourages the mother's attempts to care for her child, the nurse may be forcing alterations in the parent-child relationship that are more stressful. Beneficial changes in a relationship are a gradual process. The child needs to be helped to find independence from his parent more rewarding then dependence, and the parent needs assistance in finding a substitute object for his or her attention.

The National Foundation for Ileitis and Colitis, Inc.* has branches in many of the major communities in the country to provide education and other services for families and health professionals involved in the management of persons with inflammatory bowel diseases. The United Ostomy Association† is also available to assist with ileostomy care and management.

REGIONAL ENTERITIS (CROHN DISEASE)

Crohn disease is an inflammatory disease of the bowel that is being recognized in both children and adolescents with increasing frequency. It occurs in both sexes and, like ulcerative colitis, is more prevalent in the adolescent and young adult. It is rare in children less than 6. The incidence is equal to that of ulcerative colitis in children.

Etiology

The cause of Crohn disease is unknown but infectious, genetic, psychologic, and immunologic factors have been implicated. The disease occurs with greater frequency in Jews than in non-Jews and in blacks more than in white populations.

Pathophysiology

Crohn disease may involve any part of the gastrointestinal tract but most commonly affects the terminal ileum. The disease characteristically involves all layers of the bowel wall (transmural). Acute edema and inflammation eventually progress to deep, transverse, or longitudinal ulcerations often associated with fissure formation. The thickened bowel wall may lead to obstruction. The asymmetric and patchy distribution of the lesions helps to differentiate Crohn disease from the contiguous and symmetric lesions of ulcerative colitis. Local lymph nodes are enlarged.

Clinical manifestations

The onset of Crohn disease is usually insidious with nonspecific symptoms including anorexia, lethargy, fever, and

---

*295 Madison Avenue, New York, NY 10017
†Dept. N80, 2001 Beverly Blvd., Los Angeles, CA 90052

SUMMARY OF NURSING CARE OF THE CHILD WITH INFLAMMATORY BOWEL DISEASE

GOALS	RESPONSIBILITIES
Assist with diagnosis	Take careful history of illness Order diagnostic tests Collect needed specimens—stool, blood Assist with diagnostic tests—barium enema, rectosigmoidoscopy, mucosal biopsy
Rest bowel	Withhold oral intake as indicated
Provide nutrition	Monitor total parenteral nutrition infusion in acute illness Offer nutritious diet in recovery phase High protein, high calorie, low fat, low residue diet Administer supplementary vitamins and minerals
Maintain hydration	Monitor intravenous infusion Provide oral fluids as indicated
Relieve discomfort	Administer antispasmodics as ordered Administer analgesics if ordered
Relieve nausea	Administer antiemetics as needed
Prevent infection	Carry out conscientious medical asepsis Administer antibacterial agents as prescribed Avoid contact with infected persons and items
Reduce bowel inflammation	Administer corticosteroids as prescribed
Reduce distress of diarrhea	Provide meticulous perianal care Apply soothing preparations to perianal area as ordered Provide ready access to bedpan Keep hand-cleansing materials readily available Empty and clean bedpan as soon as possible after use Provide room deodorizer
Prevent skin breakdown	Provide sheepskin or egg-crate mattress Keep the child clean and dry
Provide nonstressful environment	Provide for privacy Plan to spend segments of uninterrupted time with the child Discuss nonstressful everyday topics Provide relaxing games and reading materials suited to the child's age and interests
Promote rest	Provide quiet environment Administer sedatives as ordered Schedule treatments and activities around rest periods Keep visiting periods with friends and family short Schedule visiting to allow for sufficient rest
Prepare for tests and therapies	Explain procedures and their relationship to disease process
Prepare the child for surgery (if prescribed)	Carry out preoperative teaching (pp. 533-537) Consult with enterostomal therapist for joint teaching sessions Explore the child's feelings regarding outcome of surgery
Assess parent-child relationships	Explore the child's attitudes and feelings Explore the parent's attitudes and feelings Elicit clues to possible parent-child disharmony Secure psychologic counseling if indicated

Prepare for discharge	Teach the child and parent about
	   Hygiene
	   Diet
	   Need for rest and reduced stress
	   Ileostomy care (if performed)
	   Maintaining normal activities and interests

fatigue. There is diarrhea and intermittent, cramping pain that often resembles that of acute appendicitis. As the disease progresses, however, the abdominal pain becomes a constant aching or soreness. The diarrhea may contain blood but this is a less frequent finding in children. Weight loss, pallor, anemia, and finger clubbing are not uncommon and may precede the abdominal symptoms.

Diagnostic evaluation

The diagnosis is established by sigmoidoscopic examination and biopsy. Barium enema and small bowel series demonstrate characteristic bowel changes. The stools are examined for occult blood, white blood cells, fat, and ova and parasites to help rule out infectious processes. An elevated erythrocyte sedimentation rate is usually found and a red cell count and hemoglobin analysis reveal the extent of anemia.

Therapeutic management

The general principles of care outlined for ulcerative colitis are applied to children with Crohn disease. This includes primarily nutritional management with a high-protein diet, corticosteroids, antibiotics, and general supportive therapy. Sometimes total parenteral nutrition is needed for short periods to alleviate severe malnutrition. Sedatives and analgesics are administered as indicated according to the individual case. Surgical removal of affected areas has not proved satisfactory; the disease tends to recur in approximately 2 years in a large number of patients.

Nursing considerations

The nursing care for Crohn disease is the same as nursing care of the child with ulcerative colitis.

PEPTIC ULCER

A *peptic ulcer*, or peptic ulcer disease (PUD), is an erosion of the mucosal wall of the stomach, pylorus, or duodenum. *Gastric ulcers* affect the lining of the stomach, whereas *duodenal ulcers* involve the pylorus or duodenum. Although peptic ulcers are more common in adults, they are also a significant pediatric problem, occurring at any age but most frequently between the ages of 12 and 18 years. Males are affected more than three times as often as females.

Etiology

The exact cause of peptic ulcer is not known, although both genetic and environmental factors appear to be important in the etiology of peptic ulcers. There is an increased frequency among relatives and a positive relationship to blood group O. However, emotional stress has been implicated as an important contributing factor toward the development, severity, and prognosis of peptic ulcers.

Pathophysiology

The precise mechanism is not understood, but one of two mechanisms probably reflects the basic defect: (1) an increase in the rate of production of gastric juice or (2) interference with the normal protective mechanisms of the mucosal lining. As a result of either of these two conditions, the gastric mucosa is highly vulnerable to the digestive effects of gastric juice. Prolonged contact with the highly acidic contents of the stomach and duodenum causes an erosion of the mucosal wall, especially in those areas least protected, such as the cardia and lesser curve of the stomach and the area immediately beyond the pylorus.

Secondary or *stress ulcers* are also known to occur as a complication of a number of acute disorders (such as encephalitis, meningitis, or sepsis) and several chronic conditions (for example, burns, rheumatoid arthritis, cirrhosis of the liver, or chronic obstructive lung disease). Also, certain drugs, particularly aspirin and corticoseroids, are ulcerogenic.

Clinical manifestations

Signs and symptoms of peptic ulcers vary according to the age of the child and the location of the ulcer (Table 21-5). Symptoms that suggest peptic ulcer show the adult pattern in children over 9 to 12 years of age, including chronic abdominal pain, especially when the stomach is empty, such as during the night or early morning, recurrent vomiting after meals, chronic anemia with occult blood in the stools, and vague gastrointestinal complaints with a positive family history for peptic ulcer.

The classic pain-food-relief syndrome seen in adults with peptic ulcer is usually absent in young children. The pain can be anywhere in the mid or upper abdomen, shows no definite pattern, is unrelated to meals, and is not always relieved by antacids. Children with chronic illness and especially those on aspirin or corticosteroid therapy are especially prone to develop peptic ulcers.

Diagnostic evaluation

Diagnosis is based on the history (pattern of pain), physical examination (pain in the epigastric area), and diagnostic testing such as radiologic studies, barium swallow, and panendoscopy (visualization of the gastric wall with a fiberoptic instrument). Other tests include blood studies

TABLE 21-5. CLINICAL MANIFESTATIONS OF PEPTIC ULCER

AGE-GROUP	TYPE OF ULCER	MANIFESTATIONS	COMMENTS
Neonates	Usually gastric	Usually perforation Often massive hemorrhage Almost the same as seen in stress ulcers	Usually catastrophic More likely in infants with hypoxia, sepsis, difficult labor/delivery, or nasogastric feeding Prognosis often poor
Infants to 2-year-old children	Gastric or duodenal, primary or secondary	Poor eating, vomiting, crying spells after feeding, abdominal distention, tarry stools, melena Vague discomfort Irritability	Primary ulcers more likely to be gastric with slow onset Usually bleed rather than perforate
2- to 6-year-old children	Gastric or duodenal	No really positive physical findings May have vomiting related to eating, generalized or periumbilical pain, melena, hematemesis Wake at night crying with pain	Diagnosis often made on basis of social history Duodenal ulcers 5:1 over gastric Perforation more likely in secondary ulcers
6- to 9-year-old children	Usually duodenal and primary Often with obstruction	Pain—burning or gnawing sensation in epigastrium related to fasting state, melena, hematemesis, vomiting	Often related to school achievement, change, relationship with peers and/or teachers
Over 9 years	Usually duodenal	Same as above	More typical of adult type Chances of recurrence greater than 50%

(anemia), stool samples (occult blood), and, occasionally, gastric acid measurements (to isolate hypersecretors).

Therapeutic management

The objectives of therapy for children with peptic ulcers is to relieve discomfort, promote healing, prevent complications, and prevent recurrence. The management of ulcers is primarily medical and consists of administration of medications that reduce or neutralize gastric acid secretion and, when possible, implement measures to eliminate or reduce stresses. Nonrecurrence and healing of a primary ulcer is more favorable in young children than in the older age-groups.

Antacids are the principal agent employed in the treatment of peptic ulcers. The antacid of choice, usually a magnesium preparation, is administered every 1 to 2 hours during the acute phase, the dosage determined by the size of the child. As healing progresses, the frequency is gradually reduced to 1 hour after meals and at bedtime. This schedule is maintained for approximately 3 months, after which the drug is discontinued.

In some children the anticholinergic drug propantheline (Pro-Banthine) may be useful in decreasing gastric motility and acid secretion. It is usually administered at bedtime to reduce acid secretion during the night. The newer histamine$_2$ blocking agent cimetidine (Tagamet) is proving effective in the management of acute episodes in children over 12 years of age, and carbenoxolone is sometimes administered to promote ulcer healing.

The child is provided with a nutritious diet but advised to avoid foods that are associated with aggravation of symptoms. Sedatives are seldom helpful and are not generally prescribed. Since aspirin is known to have a damaging effect on gastric mucosa, acetaminophen is recommended as a substitute.

A child with an acute ulcer who has developed complications, such as massive hemorrhage, requires emergency care. A nasogastric tube is inserted to remove the blood, prevent abdominal distention, and provide a means of calculating blood loss. Blood replacement, intravenous fluids, and oxygen are usually necessary. Surgical closure of the perforation or bleeding point may be required to stop the hemorrhage.

Surgical management is *very* uncommon, except for the catastrophic ulcerations of the newborn. For intractable ulcers (those that do not respond to medical therapy) vagotomy and pyloroplasty are the preferred procedures. A gastric resection is seldom done unless absolutely necessary and usually for stress ulcers.

Nursing considerations

The main nursing objective is to promote healing of the ulcer through dietary management and reduction of stress.

Dietary management. At present there is considerable controversy concerning the benefits of strict, rigid, and slowly advanced dietary control and more liberalized diet therapy. Since children are less likely to comply with a rigid bland diet and power struggles over food restriction are likely to increase emotional tension, a liberal regimen is usually recommended. This includes: (1) avoiding secretagogues (substances that enhance gastric secretion), such as tea, coffee, spices, carbonated beverages (especially cola), meat extractives (beef broth), fried foods, citrus fruit juices, and alcohol where indicated and (2) eliminating any food that causes the child pain.

The nurse also stresses feeding practices that help neutralize gastric acid, such as (1) eating small frequent meals evenly spaced throughout the day and evening—a typical meal plan may be breakfast at 8:00 AM, a snack of milk and cereal at 10:00 AM, lunch at 12:30 PM, a bowl of soup with crackers at 3:30 PM, dinner at 5:30 PM, and a snack of fruit, ice cream, or pudding and a glass of milk before bedtime; (2) maintaining this regular schedule and especially avoiding prolonged fasting; whenever adhering to a regular meal plan is difficult, such as when traveling, attending school, or working, modifications may be necessary such as carrying packaged foods (instant soups, cheese and crackers, a sandwich, nutritious milk drinks, or fruit) or discussing the importance of in-between meals with the teacher or employer; (3) avoiding overeating, which distends the stomach, thus stimulating the production of increased gastric juice; and (4) drinking small amounts of liquid with meals to avoid diluting stomach contents, thus decreasing emptying time.

Reducing stress and facilitating adjustment to chronic illness. Another nursing responsibility is helping the child and parent reduce stress and adjust to the condition. Many of the suggestions discussed under ulcerative colitis apply here. Sometimes psychotherapy is necessary to prevent recurrence of peptic ulcer as a lifelong problem. When hospitalization is required, manipulating the environment to reduce stress factors, such as separation from parents and home, absence from school, frightening procedures, and possible surgery, can enhance healing of the ulcer.

Surgical care. When surgical intervention is required for intractable ulcers, the nurse can help the child adjust to a gastrectomy. Although the psychologic trauma of losing part of one's stomach is significantly less than that of adjusting to bowel diversion, still there are necessary dietary controls to promote optimum nutrition and prevent a complication called the "dumping syndrome," a physiologic reaction to a high-carbohydrate solution passing directly into the jejunum. To prevent this reaction, carbohydrates, especially simple sugars, are reduced to a minimum, small frequent meals are served, proteins and fats are increased to provide sufficient calories and retard bowel emptying, and fluid with meals is kept to a minimum to decrease bowel distention and motility. Ideally the child should eat slowly and regularly, avoid any emotional upset at mealtime, and rest after meals. These instructions can be particularly difficult for adolescents to adhere to, with "fast foods" high in carbohydrates considered a symbol of teenage living. The nurse needs to stress the importance of following dietary instructions for the child to maintain an optimum weight and prevent nutritional deficiencies.

HEPATIC DISORDERS

The liver is a vital organ that performs multiple important functions: (1) secretion of bile, (2) enzyme secretion, (3) storage depot, (4) detoxification, (5) synthesis of blood proteins, and (6) heat production. Inflammatory, obstructive, or degenerative disorders that affect the liver will also interfere with all or some of these functions with greater or lesser consequences for the affected child.

ACUTE HEPATITIS

Hepatitis, or inflammation of the liver, is rapidly emerging as one of the major causes of morbidity and a significant cause of mortality in children. The discussion that follows is focused primarily on acute hepatitis, although the chronic disease may involve many of the same mechanisms.

SUMMARY OF NURSING CARE FOR THE CHILD WITH PEPTIC ULCER

GOALS	RESPONSIBILITIES

Assist with diagnosis	Take careful history
	Assist with diagnostic procedures
	    Radiographs
	    Panendoscopy
	    Gastric acid measurements
	Collect specimens as needed
	    Stool for occult blood
	    Blood analysis

Relieve discomfort	Administer antacids as prescribed Administer anticholinergic agents as ordered Offer soothing foods such as milk, custard, etc.
Reduce gastric acidity	Administer antacids every 1 to 2 hours as ordered to absorb or neutralize acids Administer anticholinergic drugs to decrease gastric motility and acid secretion Administer histamine$_2$ (H$_2$) receptor antagonist if ordered

Reduce stress	Place in quiet environment
	Employ measures to reduce anxiety
	    Spend as much time as possible with the child
	    Schedule activities around rest periods
	    Explain procedures and therapies
	Explore feelings and attitudes for clues to stress-provoking situations
	Secure psychologic counseling if indicated

Detect complications	Be alert for signs of hemorrhage
	    Overt bleeding
	    Shock

Regulate eating practices	Provide and encourage well-balanced nutritious diet Avoid foods that increase gastric secretions Avoid foods found to produce discomfort Maintain regular meal schedule Encourage small frequent meals evenly spaced throughout the day Avoid overeating Discourage drinking large amounts of fluids with meals

Prepare for discharge	Teach the child and family regarding
	    Meal planning and scheduling
	    Administration of medications
	    Adequate rest and appropriate exercise schedules
	Encourage normal activities
	Help the child and family to recognize and avoid stress-producing situations
	Refer to public health agency

Etiology

Hepatitis of viral etiology is caused by at least two types of virus, which produce the same pathologic changes in the liver and very similar clinical manifestations but which are distinct in their epidemiologic and immunologic characteristics. These are hepatitis virus A (HAV, formerly "infectious hepatitis") and hepatitis virus B (HBV, formerly "serum hepatitis"). A third type of hepatitis virus (non-A, non-B or NANBV) is an important cause of disease in the adult population and is responsible for most posttransfusion hepatitis. Although persons in any age-group are susceptible to hepatitis, HAV is most common

TABLE 21-6. COMPARISON OF TYPES A AND B HEPATITIS

CHARACTERISTICS	TYPE A	TYPE B
Incubation period	15-40 days, average 25 days	6 weeks to 6 months
Period of communicability	Unknown Virus in blood and feces 2 to 3 weeks before onset of jaundice and for at least 1 week after onset of jaundice	Variable Virus in blood (probably in stool but no direct proof) during late incubation period and acute stage of disease; may persist in carrier state for years
Mode of transmission	Principal route—oral-fecal Less frequent route—parenteral Fetal transfer—from transplacental blood during last trimester, but more commonly at time of delivery	Principal route—parenteral Less frequent route—oral, venereal (semen, menstrual secretions, saliva) Fetal transfer—from transplacental blood during last trimester, but more commonly at time of delivery
Clinical features		
Onset	Usually rapid, acute	More insidious
Fever	Common and early	Less frequent
Anorexia	Extreme	Mild to moderate
Nausea and vomiting	Common	Less common
Rash	Rare	Common
Arthralgia	Rare	Common
Pruritus	Rare	Sometimes present
Jaundice	Present	Present
Immunity	Present after one attack, but no crossover to type B	Present after one attack, but no crossover to type A
Prophylaxis		
Immune serum globulin (ISG)	Passive immunity Successful, especially during early incubation period	Passive immunity Inconsistent benefits; probably of no use
Hepatitis B immune globulin (HBIG)	No benefit	Postexposure protection possible if given immediately after definite exposure Recommended for newborn or affected mother
Hepatitis B vaccine (Heptavax-B)	Not indicated	Provides active immunity Recommended for those persons at high risk of exposure

in children under 15 years of age, especially in low socioeconomic groups, where housing conditions are crowded. See Table 21-6 for a comparison of hepatitis A and hepatitis B.

Hepatitis A. HAV is highly contagious and is transmitted from one person to another primarily by the oral route, usually from ingestion of contaminated food or water. This includes eating shellfish caught in contaminated water and from swimming in such water. Persons at highest risk of acquiring HAV are persons sharing a household and sexual contacts. Additional sources for children are day care centers (especially those that have children in diapers) and in custodial care facilities. School contacts are considered a relatively low risk.

Hepatitis B. HBV is most commonly transmitted by direct (needles) or indirect (cuts, burns, abrasions) parenteral means although it can be spread to mucous surfaces (intimate contact, contaminated secretions splashed into mouth or eyes during irrigations) and certain fomites (contaminated equipment, gloves). The virus can be found in almost all body fluids and secretions (except perhaps feces)—saliva, tears, sweat, urine, genital secretions, nasopharyngeal secretions, and possibly mother's milk. Persons at risk include close family contacts, clients and staff of custodial institutions for retarded children, those requiring frequent blood transfusions, hemodialysis, and health workers—especially those in operating rooms, emergency rooms, dialysis units, intensive care units, laboratories, personnel of and those providing dental care. With the abuse of parenteral drugs, the incidence of HBV is significant in adolescent drug users and their contacts. Most HBV in children is acquired by the nonparenteral route. Newborn infants are also at risk for neonatal hepatitis, especially if the mother is infected with HBV or was a carrier of HBV during pregnancy.

Pathophysiology

The pathologic changes occur primarily in the parenchymal cells of the liver and result in variable degrees of swelling, infiltration of liver cells by mononuclear cells, subsequent degeneration, necrosis, and autolysis. Structural changes within the hepatocyte are thought to account for altered liver functions.

The pathology is usually self-limited and complete regeneration of liver cells without scarring occurs within 2 to 3 months. However, some forms of hepatitis do not result in complete return of liver function. These include *fulminant hepatitis,* which is characterized by a severe, acute course with death frequently occurring within 1 to 2 weeks, and *subacute* or *chronic active hepatitis,* characterized by progressive liver destruction and uncertain regeneration with the possibility of scarring.

Clinical manifestations

The clinical manifestations for both types of viral hepatitis are similar except for a more rapid, acute onset in type A and a slower, more insidious onset in type B. Both types may present with the flu-like symptoms. Some may never be recognized as actual cases of hepatitis.

However, the classic picture is predictable and begins with nausea and vomiting, extreme anorexia, malaise, easy fatigability, and slight to moderate fever. The child may have abdominal pain, especially in the epigastrium or upper right quadrant. He usually acts ill, preferring to rest in bed, and is fretful or irritable. The most significant finding on physical examination is liver tenderness with or without enlargement. This initial *anicteric* (absence of jaundice) *phase* usually lasts 5 to 7 days.

Following this period, evidence of jaundice (the *icteric phase*) is present, beginning with darkening of the urine and the presence of light-colored stools and followed by yellowing of the sclera and skin, which commonly lasts less than 4 weeks. Complete recovery with return of normal liver function and a feeling of well-being with absence of fatigue or malaise may take 1 to 3 months. Generally children recover promptly.

Not all affected children exhibit signs of disease. Because the manifestations of hepatitis are the body's response to the viral antigen, individuals who are unable to muster an adequate defense will develop few if any symptoms. However, they will still harbor the virus as carriers. Newborn infants of mothers with HBV who have been exposed to the virus during prenatal life do not recognize the virus as a foreign protein and, thus, become chronic carriers. The American Academy of Pediatrics also recommends that carrier mothers should not breast-feed their infants if an acceptable milk substitute is available.

Diagnostic evaluation

Diagnosis is based on history, physical examination, laboratory evidence of the virus, and liver function tests. Blood and stool cultures can prove the existence of virus A; however, diagnosis of virus B is usually based on the presence of hepatitis-associated antigen. No liver function test is specific for hepatitis. Serum glutamic-oxaloacetic transaminase (SGOT) and serum glutamic-pyruvic transaminase (SGPT) levels are markedly elevated. Serum bilirubin levels peak 5 to 10 days after clinical jaundice appears.

Therapeutic management

There is no specific treatment for either type of viral hepatitis. Management is primarily treatment of symptoms. For example, antiemetics may be helpful to reduce the nausea or vomiting. The value of bed rest in promoting overall recovery is controversial. Since the child feels ill and tired in the anicteric phase, he usually chooses to stay in bed. However, once improvement of physical complaints begins, the child prefers to resume normal activity gradually. The best approach is probably to allow the child to regulate his own pace. Hospitalization is rarely necessary, although proper isolation practices at home are imperative.

The child is allowed to choose foods he prefers, especially during the initial stage when anorexia is severe. Generally low-fat foods cause less stomach distention and are better tolerated than foods high in fat content. Carbohydrates should be encouraged to ensure an adequate caloric intake to spare proteins for cell growth. Vitamin K is administered if prothrombin time is prolonged.

Prevention. Isolation or quarantine of the infected child is not necessary as long as measures are employed to prevent spread of the virus. An attack of either virus confers long-lasting immunity to that virus, however, there is no crossover protection to the other virus. Prophylactic use of immune serum globulin (ISG) is effective in preventing hepatitis virus A during the early part of the incubation period and, to a lesser extent, before the onset of the disease. It is of inconsistent benefit in preventing type B virus.

Passive immunity to HBV can be achieved with hyperimmune gamma globulin (hepatitis B immune serum globulin, HBIG) but it is very expensive. However, it is used in special situations, for example it has been found that the carrier state can be avoided in newborn infants of infected mothers if given within 24 hours of birth and repeated at 3 and 6 months of age. The new hepatitis B vaccine, the first to be manufactured from human blood, is proving to be highly effective in providing protection against HBV. At present the vaccine is recommended for those persons with frequent exposure to blood.

Nursing considerations

Nursing objectives depend largely on the severity of the hepatitis, the rigidity of medical treatment, and factors influencing the control and transmission of the disease. Since children with benign viral hepatitis are frequently cared for at home, the responsibility of explaining any medical therapies and control measures is frequently left to the clinic or office nurse. In instances in which further assistance is needed for parents to comply with such instructions, a public health nursing referral may be necessary.

The emphasis is on encouraging a well-balanced diet and a realistic schedule of rest and activity adjusted to the child's condition. Since hepatitis type A is not infectious within a week or so after onset of jaundice, the child may feel well enough to resume school shortly thereafter. The parents are also cautioned about administering any medication to the child without the physician's knowledge, since normal doses of many drugs may become dangerous because of the liver's inability to detoxify and excrete them. Common drugs that are affected by hepatic failure include acetaminophen (Tylenol), ferrous sulfate (oral iron), and propoxyphene hydrochloride (Darvon).

Hand washing is the single most critical measure in prevention and control of hepatitis in any setting. The nurse explains to parents and children the usual ways in which hepatitis virus A (oral-fecal route) and hepatitis virus B (parenteral route) are spread. However, regardless of which type of virus is present, the same general precautions are followed, since each virus is spread by both modes of transmission.

Hospitalized children are not usually isolated in a separate room unless they are fecally unreliable or incontinent or if their toys and other items might become contaminated with feces. They are discouraged from sharing their toys. All personnel should wear gowns and gloves when caring for the child directly in addition to following other enteric precautions. Contaminated items (such as a stethoscope) are cleaned with a detergent solution and appropriate disinfectant. Special attention must be given to handling and disposing of all blood products and invasive equipment. Only disposable needles and syringes are used. Any contaminated equipment and blood samples are labeled "possibly infectious." The nurse explains to parents and older children the reason for isolation and specific precautions to help them adjust to hospitalization and to reinforce practice of control measures before and after discharge.

In those children with type B virus who have a known or suspected history of illicit drug use, the nurse has the additional responsibility of helping them realize the associated dangers of drug abuse, stressing the parenteral mode of transmission, and encouraging them to seek counseling from a drug program.

CIRRHOSIS

Cirrhosis, which means "yellow" and refers to the typical orange-colored nodules of a fibrotic liver, is a result, not a primary cause, of liver dysfunction. It represents the end stage of chronic disease in which there is generalized destruction of hepatic cells. Cirrhosis is not a common cause of morbidity in children; therefore, the diagnosis may be easily missed.

Pathophysiology

Cirrhosis is believed to be the result of some type of injury or insult to the liver including prior hepatitis, metabolic disease, drug toxicity, hepatobiliary obstruction, and cystic fibrosis. Following injury fibrous connective tissue forms throughout the liver, which interferes with normal hepatic function and impedes the blood supply causing further destruction and fibrosis.

The consequences of liver malfunction are evident in the various processes that depend on the products of liver function. For example, diminished formation of blood proteins results in hypoproteinemia and impaired coagulation, inability to conjugate bilirubin produces jaundice, reduced bile causes malabsorption of fats, and depressed detoxification and destruction result in accumulation of toxic substances. Interference with liver circulation causes hypertension in the portal circulation. This together with the decreased protein in the blood leads to fluid accumulation in the abdomen (ascites).

Clinical manifestations

Clinical manifestations depend on the etiology. In cirrhosis from congenital biliary atresia, jaundice is usually the first sign, although all the pathologic effects eventually become evident, especially since most cases are not amenable to surgical correction. In cirrhosis from other causes, the symptoms are usually vague and the onset insidious.

The three major complications of chronic liver disease are (1) bleeding from esophageal varices, (2) ascites, and (3) hepatic encepalopathy (hepatic coma). Not infrequently the first evidence of severe liver decompensation is failure to thrive, ascites, or bleeding esophageal varices.

Diagnostic evaluation

Diagnosis rests on (1) the history, especially evidence of prior liver disease, such as hepatitis, (2) physical examination, particularly hepatosplenomegaly, and the cutaneous changes, and (3) laboratory evaluation, especially liver function tests. Definitive diagnosis is a liver biopsy for evidence of histologic changes.

Therapeutic management

There is no specific treatment for cirrhosis, except in those cases in which a treatable cause, such as an infection, exists. Therapy is directed primarily toward (1) frequent assessment of liver status with physical examination and liver function tests and (2) management of pathologic changes based on these findings.

For cirrhosis uncomplicated by ascites or encephalopathy the diet is one that provides sufficient calories and essential nutrients to maintain growth and prevent specific deficiencies. A high-calorie diet with low or moderate fats, moderate high-quality protein, and high carbohydrates is recommended. In addition supplements of water-soluble preparations of vitamins A, D, E, and K are given. In children with vitamin B_{12} deficiency, injectable supplements are necessary.

The child and his parents are advised against strenuous physical exercise and cautioned regarding the role of trauma, infection, and hepatotoxic drugs as factors that can aggravate his condition.

Complications.   The complications of cirrhosis require special treatment:

Hemorrhage from esophageal varices is managed, as in adults, with blood transfusions, fluid and electrolyte replacement, administration of vitamin B complex and vitamin K, and, in life-threatening bleeding, with a Sengstaken-Blakemore balloon tube and oxygen.

Ascites is managed with diuretics and restriction of dietary sodium, limitation of protein, and sometimes intravenous administration of albumin. Fluid restriction may be necessary but drainage by paracentesis is rarely needed unless abdominal pain or respiratory distress is present.

Hepatic encephalopathy is related to the harmful effects of ammonia; therefore, much of the management is aimed at reducing ammonia formation. Treatment attempts to (1) reduce dietary protein, (2) inhibit the growth of organisms active in the formation of ammonia by administration of lactulose, (3) administer antibiotics to reduce the

bacterial flora, and (4) correct any other causes that might precipitate coma, such as infections or fluid and electrolyte imbalances.

Nursing considerations

Nursing objectives in caring for the child with cirrhosis depend on several factors, including the precipitating cause of the cirrhosis, the severity of complications, and the prognosis. Overall the last factor has the greatest impact because the prognosis for life is poor. Since treatment of cirrhosis ideally is treatment of the cause, in many instances a fatal outcome is determined by the inability to surgically correct biliary atresia (see next section), reverse hepatic necrosis, or stop the progressive damage as a result of cystic fibrosis. Therefore, nursing care of this child is the same as that for a potentially terminally ill child (see Chapter 16). Hospitalization is usually required when complications occur.

BILIARY ATRESIA

Biliary atresia is the congenital obstruction or absence of a portion of the bile ducts. Blockage may be either *intrahepatic,* the absence of bile ducts within the liver, or *extrahepatic,* in which there is absence or obstruction of the main bile passages outside the liver. Numerous variations are encountered but the most common abnormality is complete atresia of the extrahepatic structures. The cause is unknown but recent evidence favors a viral infection before or shortly after birth. The predictable course of the disease terminates in complete and irreversible obliteration of the extrahepatic bile ducts.

Clinical manifestations

Jaundice is usually the earliest evidence of biliary atresia and is the most striking feature of the disorder. It is first observed in the sclera. It may be present at birth but is not usually apparent until the child is 2 to 3 weeks of age. The urine becomes dark and stains the diaper and the stools are lighter than expected. Hepatomegaly and abdominal distention are common and splenomegaly occurs later. Poor fat metabolism results in poor weight gain and general failure to thrive. Pruritis is a distressing feature of the jaundice of unconjugated bilirubin. As the disease progresses the child becomes irritable and difficult to comfort.

Diagnostic evaluation

No single test or combination of tests is diagnostic. The disease is suspected on the basis of clinical signs but surgical exploration is needed for confirmation.

Therapeutic management

The major hope in care of these children is that the condition will benefit from surgery. Although surgical correction is possible in only a few cases of extrahepatic atresia, surgery is most successful when performed early; therefore, diagnosis is urgent. Occasionally a duct obstruction can be relieved. More often the Kasai procedure is employed in which a substitute duct is formed from a segment of jejunum if there are any hepatic duct remnants. Liver transplantation offers hope for some, but the success rate has not been impressive.

Medical management is primarily supportive. It is the method of choice for intrahepatic atresia and supplemental to surgical therapy in extrahepatic atresia. Medical management consists of a high-calorie formula containing fats that can be digested without bile (Pregestimil, Portagen) and water-miscible vitamins. The bile acid-binding drug cholestyramine (Questran, Cuemid) is sometimes useful in reducing pruritis and improving liver function. Phenobarbital helps reduce irritability. A low-salt diet and diuretics may reduce ascites formation. Phototherapy is not effective in reducing the jaundice of unconjugated bilirubin.

Nursing considerations

Nursing care of the infant with biliary atresia is primarily supportive. Initially the infant is not uncomfortable and requires care suited to any infant of the same age. As the disease progresses the accumulation of toxic products causes the child to become irritable, restless, and difficult to comfort. Efforts are extended to allow as much sleep and rest as possible. The child is cared for when he awakens and provided with sedatives and comforting measures that he is able to tolerate.

During the diagnostic phase of the illness the nurse assists with tests and procedures as ordered. The child who has undergone exploratory or corrective surgery is given the same care as any infant following abdominal surgery. Infants with the Kasai operation require care of the double stoma and collection, measurement, and replacement of bile via the stomal openings. Parental teaching includes this practice, administration of antibiotics, and observation for signs of cholangitis.

BIBLIOGRAPHY
Gastroesophageal reflux

Boyd, C.W.: Postural therapy at home for infants with gastroesophageal reflux, Pediatr. Nurs. **8**:395-398, 1982.
Kurfiss-Daniels, D.: Positioning as treatment for infant gastroesophageal reflux, Am. J. Nurs. **82**:1535-1537, 1982.

Diarrhea

Castle, M.: Isolation. Precise procedures for better protection, Nursing 75 **5**:50-57, May 1975.

Copeland, L.: Chronic diarrhea in infancy, Am. J. Nurs. **77**:461-463, 1977.
Diarrhea as caused by *Salmonella* and *Shigella,* Nursing 75 **5**:59-60, Nov. 1975.
Hamm, P., and Jemison-Smith, P.: Salmonella, Crit. Care Update **9**(1):41-44, 1982.
Ling, L., and McCamman, S.P.: Dietary treatment of diarrhea and constipation in infants and children, Issues Compr. Pediatr. Nurs. **3**(4):17-28, 1978.

Hirschsprung disease

Bishop, W.S., and Head, J.J.: Care of the infant with a stoma, Am. J. Maternal Child Nurs. **1**:315-319, 1976.
Cooney, D.E., and Grosfeld, J.L.: Care of the child with a colostomy, Pediatrics **59**(3):469-472, 1977.
Sugar, E.C.: Hirschsprung's disease, Am. J. Nurs. **81**:2065-2067, 1981.

Helminthic infections

Abadie, S.H., Blumenthal, D.S., and Wang, C.C.: When the name of the game is worms, Patient Care **9**(10):96-101, May 15, 1975.
Kuntz, R.E.: Parasites of children in the United States, Pediatr. Nurs. **5**(6):12-17, 1979.
Malarkey, L.M.: Ridding school children of parasites—a community approach, Am. J. Maternal Child Nurs. **4**(6):363-366, 1979.

Structural defects

Ashcraft, K.W., and Holder, T.M.: Esophageal atresia and tracheoesophageal fistula malformations, Surg. Clin. North Am. **56**:299, 1976.
Brueggemeyer, A.: Omphalocele: coping with a surgical emergency, Pediatr. Nurs. **5**(4):54-56, 1979.
Darling, D.B., and others: Hiatal hernia and gastroesophageal reflux in infants and children, Pediatrics **54**:450-455, 1974.
Hazle, N.: An infant who survived gastroschisis, Am. J. Maternal Child Nurs. **6**(1):35-40, 1981.
Huddart, A.G.: The care and management of the newborn cleft palate infant, Nurs. Mirror **140**:61, 1975.
Kim, S.: Omphalocele, Surg. Clin. North Am. **56**:361, 1976.
Martin, L.W.: A new "gravity-flow" nipple for feeding infants with congenital cleft palate, Pediatrics **72**:244, 1983.
Ravitch, M.: The non-operative treatment of surgical conditions in children, Pediatrics **51**:435, 1973.

Malabsorption syndromes

Hartwig, M.S.: Sticking to a gluten free diet, Am. J. Nurs. **83**:1308-1310, 1983.
Feigenberg, M., and Sotman, J.W.: A toddler with a malabsorption syndrome, Am. J. Nurs. **75**:978-979, 1975.
Robinson, L.A.: Nontropical sprue (gluten intolerance and vitamins), Pediatr. Nurs. **7**(5):61, 1981.
Rosenberg, F.H.: Lactose intolerance, Am. J. Nurs. **77**:823-824, 1977.

Obstructive disorders

Durham, N.: Looking out for complications of abdominal surgery, Nursing 75 **5**(2):24-31, 1975.
Grosfeld, J.L.: Alimentary tract obstruction in the newborn, Curr. Probl. Pediatr. **5**(3):3-47, 1975.
Literte, J.W.: Nursing care of patients with intestinal obstruction, Am. J. Nurs. **72**(6):1003-1006, 1977.
McConnell, E.A.: All about gastrointestinal intubation, Nursing 75 **5**(9):31-37, 1975.

Inflammatory conditions

Brunner, L.S.: What to do and what to teach your patient about peptic ulcer, Nursing 76 **6**(11):27-34, 1976.

Gryboski, J.D.: Crohn's disease in children, Pediatr. Rev. **2**(8):239-244, 1981.

Kneut, C.: Acute stress ulcers in childhood, Issues Compr. Pediatr. Nurs. **3**(4):42-50, 1978.

Kroner, K.: Are you prepared for your ulcerative colitis patient? Nursing 80, **10**(4):43-49, 1980.

Meyers, S.A.: Crohn's disease, Crit. Care Update **7**(1):12-22, 1980.

Nursing grand rounds: Supporting the patient with Crohn's disease, Nursing 83 **13**(11):46-51, 1983.

Rosenberg, J.M., and Kirschenbaum, H.L.: Antacids, Am. J. Nurs. **82:**54-56, 1982.

Hepatic disorders

Altman, R.P., Lilly, J.R., and Smith, E.I.: When an infant needs bile duct surgery, Patient Care **13**(6):156-163, 1979.

Baranowski, K., Greene, H.L., and Lamont, J.T.: Viral hepatitis: how to reduce its threat to the patient and others (including you), Nursing 76 **6**(5):31-39, 1976.

Barkin, R.M., and Lilly, J.R.: Biliary atresia and the Kasai operation: continuing care, J. Pediatr. **96:**1015-1019, 1980.

Dolan, P.O., and Greene, H.L.: Conquering cirrhosis of the liver and a dangerous complication, Nursing 76 **6**(11):44-53, 1976.

Fredette, S.L.: When the liver fails, Am. J. Nurs. **84:**64-67, 1984.

Guenter, P.: Hepatic disease: nutritional implications, Nurs. Clin. North Am. **18:**71-80, 1983.

Gurevich, I.: Hepatitis in critical care: area of concern, Crit. Care Update **10**(4):14-17, 1983.

Gurevich, I.: Viral hepatitis, Am. J. Nurs. **83:**572-586, 1983.

Hamm, P., and Jemison-Smith, P.: Viral hepatitis, Crit. Care Update **10**(2):37-44, 1983.

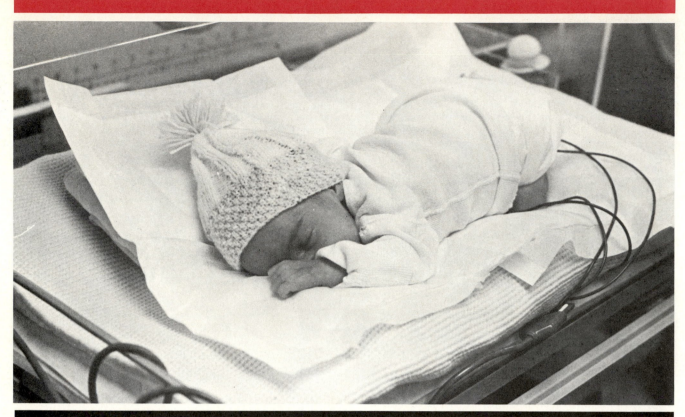

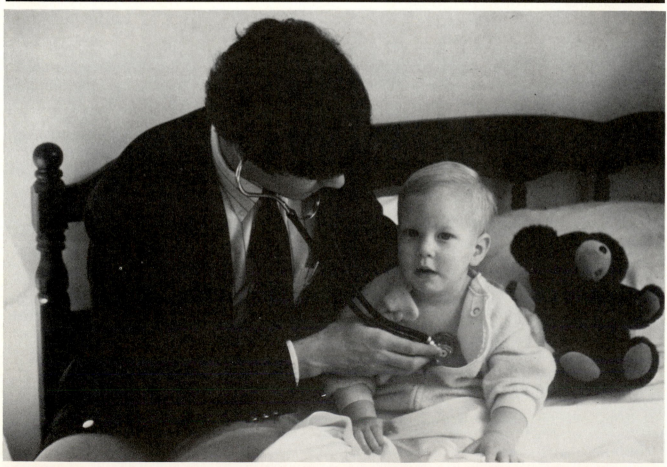

UNIT 10

THE CHILD WITH PROBLEMS RELATED TO PRODUCTION AND CIRCULATION OF BLOOD

Some of the most common and serious childhood conditions are related to the heart and the formed elements of the blood. Many of these disorders are inherited and present at birth, whereas others are acquired. Most of them necessitate medical/surgical intervention to prevent complications and permit normal growth. Nursing care at the time of diagnosis, prior to and during corrective or palliative procedures, and after treatment is essential to promote physical and emotional recovery.

Chapter 22, *The Child with Cardiovascular Dysfunction,* discusses the types of congenital and acquired cardiac disorders and the physical consequences of impaired functioning. It focuses on caring for the child with heart disease, preparation of the family for surgery, diagnostic procedures, and postoperative nursing interventions. It also discusses problems of short- and long-term circulatory impairment in children. Chapter 23, *The Child with Dysfunction of the Blood or the Blood-forming Organs,* deals with several disorders related to the formed elements of the blood. Since most of these conditions are inherited and chronic, nursing interventions stress helping the family adjust to the disorder and cope with and prevent its complications.

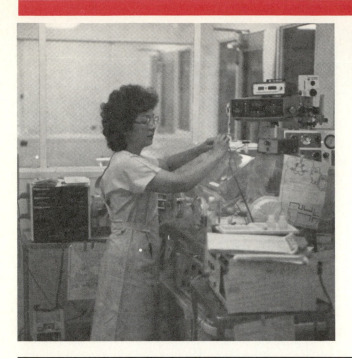

THE CHILD WITH CARDIO-VASCULAR DYSFUNCTION

OBJECTIVES

On completion of this chapter the reader will be able to:

- Design a plan for assisting a child during a cardiac diagnostic procedure

- Demonstrate an understanding of the hemodynamics, distinctive manifestations, and therapeutic management of congenital heart disease

- Describe the care for an infant or a child with a congenital heart defect

- Outline a plan of care for an infant or child with congestive heart failure

- Discuss the role of the nurse in assisting the child and family to cope with congenital heart disease

- Discuss the assessment and management of hypertension in children and adolescents

- Contrast the causes and mechanisms of shock in children

- Outline a plan of care for the child with Kawasaki disease

NURSING DIAGNOSES

Nursing diagnoses identified for the child with cardiovascular dysfunction include, but are not restricted to, the following:

Health perception-health management pattern

- Injury, potential for, related to disease process

- Noncompliance related to (1) concept of disorder; (2) knowledge deficit

Nutritional-metabolic pattern

- Fluid volume deficit, actual, related to (1) inadequate intake; (2) fluid loss

- Nutrition alteration in, less than body requirements related to inadequate intake

Activity-exercise pattern

- Activity intolerance, related to fatigue

- Airway clearance, ineffective, related to decreased energy/fatigue

- Breathing pattern, ineffective, related to (1) insufficient environmental oxygen; (2) decreased energy/fatigue

- Diversional activity, deficit related to (1) decreased activity tolerance; (2) prolonged illness

- Self-care deficit, feeding, bathing/hygiene, dressing/grooming, toileting related to (1) developmental level; (2) decreased energy

Sleep-rest pattern

- Sleep pattern disturbance related to (1) discomfort; (2) schedule of therapies

Cognitive-perceptual pattern

- Sensory perceptual alterations, visual, auditory, related to therapeutic environment

Self-perception—self-concept pattern

- Anxiety related to (1) strange environment; (2) perception of impending events; (3) separation; (4) anticipated discomfort; (5) knowledge deficit; (6) discomfort

- Self-concept, disturbance in body image, self-esteem, personal identity, related to (1) nonintegration of body changes; (2) perceived body imperfection; (3) unrealistic self-expectations

Role-relationship pattern

- Family process, alteration in, related to situational crisis

- Parenting, alteration in: potential related to (1) anxiety; (2) hospitalization

- Social isolation related to physical restrictions

Coping-stress tolerance pattern

- Coping, family: potential for growth

- Coping, ineffective family, compromised related to (1) situational crisis; (2) temporary family disorganization

Disorders involving the heart and blood vessels include those that are present at birth and those that are acquired as the result of some disease process that directly or indirectly affects cardiovascular function. Some conditions are asymptomatic and detected only on examination. Many conditions place minimal limitations on a child's activities, while others are serious enough to impose severe restrictions. A few are incompatible with life.

The most common form of heart disease in children is congenital heart disease, predominantly structural defects that result from developmental arrest or deviation. The acquired heart lesion most frequently encountered in pediatrics is carditis and subsequent valvular stenosis related to childhood rheumatic fever. Congestive heart failure is a serious consequence of congenital or acquired heart disease, and it is also a complication of other diseases, including chronic lung disease, muscular dystrophy, advanced kidney disease, and a variety of acute disorders and infections that place undue demands on the heart.

Rhythm disturbances are relatively uncommon in children. Occasionally, bradycardia is recognized during the prenatal period and the infant is closely monitored before and after birth for any untoward effects. Paroxysmal atrial tachycardia, a potentially serious disorder, is amenable to therapy when it is recognized early.

Any disorder that affects the heart provokes anxiety in the family, the nurse, and, subsequently, the child. In many instances this anxiety is not unfounded, but in some cases it is greater than that called for by the seriousness of the condition. To help the child and his family to adjust to a heart condition and to live a life without overprotection and excessive restriction requires guidance and support from many health professionals, particularly nurses.

DIAGNOSTIC PROCEDURES

Diagnosis of congenital or acquired heart disease is based on a comprehensive history and physical examination and on a variety of specific and related diagnostic procedures. The most frequently conducted diagnostic tests are outlined in Table 22-1. Cardiac catheterization, which generates more anxiety than any other test, is discussed in detail. Specific findings are included in the discussions of the various heart defects presented in this chapter.

CARDIAC CATHETERIZATION

The most valuable diagnostic procedure is cardiac catheterization, in which a radiopaque catheter is inserted through a peripheral blood vessel into the heart. The catheter is usually introduced by way of the femoral vein— either through a cutdown procedure, in which a small incision is made to expose the vessel, or through a percutaneous technique, in which the catheter is threaded through a large-bore needle that is inserted into the vein. The catheter is guided through the heart with the aid of fluoroscopy. Once the tip of the catheter is within a heart chamber, dye is injected and films are taken of the dilution and circulation of the material. At various times blood samples are taken and oxygen concentrations and blood pressures within the chambers are measured and recorded.

There are two main types of cardiac catheterization: (1) right-sided catheterization, in which the catheter is introduced from a vein into the right atrium, and (2) left-sided catheterization, in which the catheter is threaded by way of a systemic artery retrograde into the aorta and left ventricle or, from a right-sided approach, into the left atrium by means of a septal puncture. In children the most common method is right-sided catheterization, since septal defects permit entry into the left side of the heart from the right side.

Nursing considerations

Although cardiac catheterization has become a routine diagnostic procedure, it is not without risks, especially in neonates, infants, and seriously ill children. Therefore, nursing judgment prior to and after the procedure is essential. Since cardiac catheterization is performed more frequently than cardiac surgery, consideration of this necessary but potentially frightening procedure is of utmost importance for nurses.

Preprocedural care. Preparing the child and his family for the procedure is the joint responsibility of physician, nurse, and parents. The cardiologist usually explains the procedure to the parents, but nurses can reinforce and clarify the information they have received. Many parents of children who undergo both cardiac catheterization and cardiac surgery say, in retrospect, that they were more anxious about the catheterization than about the surgery.

Little psychologic preparation can be made for infants and toddlers, who comprise the bulk of pediatric cardiac catheterization candidates. However, the older child's preparation must be individualized to his level of development (especially his cognitive skills), his past experiences, and his understanding and perception of the situation. He should be neither underprepared nor overprepared for the experience.

As a general guideline, it is best to inform the child about what he will see, feel, and hear during the procedure and about what he will be expected to do to cooperate. He needs to know what preparations will begin before he goes to the cardiac catheterization laboratory and something

TABLE 22-1. PROCEDURES USED IN THE DIAGNOSIS OF HEART CONDITIONS

PROCEDURE	DESCRIPTION	SIGNIFICANCE
History		
Family	Elicit information regarding heart disease in other family members	Identifies probable hereditary factors, such as a sibling with congenital heart disease or a disease known to be associated with a high incidence of heart conditions
Pregnancy	Elicit information regarding contact with known teratogenic agents	Infections such as rubella can cause heart defects in the unborn child
Patient	Identify evidence of prior murmurs, poor weight gain, poor feeding behavior; frequent respiratory infection; recent streptococcal infection	Presence of deviations may indicate heart disease; failure to thrive is a constant feature of congenital heart disease; streptococcal infection is associated with rheumatic fever
Physical examination	Perform complete assessment of physical status	
Inspection	Assess nutritional state	Poor weight gain associated with heart disease
	Observe for	Cyanosis a common feature of congenital heart disease
	Cyanosis at rest or after exertion	
	Pallor	Pallor often associated with anemia
	Chest deformities	Visible pulsations seen in some patients
	Unusual cardiac pulsations	Dyspnea and expiratory grunt consistent with congestive heart disease
	Respiratory rate and character	
	Observe behavior	Squatting typical of some types of heart disease
Palpation and percussion	Percuss chest	Helpful in discerning heart size and other characteristics associated with heart disease
	Palpate for thrills	
	Palpate liver and spleen	Hepatomegaly and splenomegaly evident in congestive heart failure
	Palpate peripheral pulses for rate, regularity, and amplitude (strength)	Discrepancies apparent in some heart diseases
Auscultation	Assess	Detects presence of heart murmurs
	Cardiac rate, rhythm	Deviations in heart sounds, intensity help localize heart defects
	Character of sounds—intensity, timing	
	Determine peripheral blood pressure	Deviations present in some cardiac conditions
Electrocardiography	Measures electrical potential generated from heart muscle	Detect arrhythmias, muscular damage, hypertrophy, and some electrolyte imbalances
Echocardiography	Short pulses of ultrasound transmitted through the heart bounce off heart structures; reflected on a screen	Aids in diagnosis of structural defects
Ultrasonography	Similar to echocardiography; it is synchronized with ECG to provide a three-dimensional recording of heart structures	Provides information about heart structure and function
Roentgenography		
Fluoroscopy	Provides direct observation of heart size, position, contour, and relationships	Size and contour of heart altered in some types of heart disease
Radiography	Provides permanent record of heart size and configuration	Provides baseline for comparison, record for review
Angiocardiography	Opaque media injected into circulatory system outlines blood flow through the heart and vessels performed in conjunction with cardiac catheterization	Course of blood flow through abnormal openings is visible; allows defects to be localized

Continued.

TABLE 22-1. PROCEDURES USED IN THE DIAGNOSIS OF HEART CONDITIONS—cont'd

PROCEDURE	DESCRIPTION	SIGNIFICANCE
Cardiac catheterization	Opaque catheter introduced into the heart chambers via large peripheral vessels is observed by fluoroscopy or image intensification; pressure measurements and blood samples provide additional source of information.	Yields information about pressures within structures, oxygen saturation of chambers, and presence and location of abnormal openings (see discussion)
Digital subtraction angiography (DSA)	Opaque media injected into circulatory system Provides computerized images of vessels and tissues containing dye—''subtracts'' all tissues not containing dye	Yields information regarding venous and arterial structures May eventually replace cardiac catheterization

about what he will experience during the time he is there. Familiar and strange aspects of the procedure are explained and, whenever possible, related to past experiences, for example, electrocardiograph leads on the chest, a thermometer to monitor body temperature, and restraints to ''help him remember to lie very still.'' It is helpful to include parents and to enlist their aid as participants, since they are often aware of the child's fears and concerns.

The child who is old enough to understand should be told that he will receive medication that will make him ''very, very sleepy'' and that he will ride on a special bed (if he has not had experience with a gurney) to a special room (some institutions routinely take a child on a brief tour of the area the day before the test.) It is important to describe some of the things he will see, feel, or hear that may be anxiety-provoking, such as what the ''cath'' room looks like, because the x-ray machinery can have a frightening appearance. Since the test is done under sterile conditions, all health personnel wear surgical garb. If the child is unfamiliar with this, he may become frightened by their masked appearance unless he has been prepared beforehand.

Although the child is very heavily sedated he can be told about some of the sensations that he will experience during the procedure such as people working and talking close around him. He should be told that a special medicine will make him feel warm for a few seconds and then the lights will go out and a machine that is taking his picture will make a ''funny noise.''

The last point is important to stress, because younger children may associate the lights going off with ''causing'' the warm feeling from the dye. As a result they may become fearful of the dark and the noise from the machines. It is also advisable to avoid using the word ''dye'' for the radiopaque solution, since children may interpret the word as ''die.'' Older children may appreciate a more detailed explanation of how the dye aids in the diagnostic procedure, since this point can be elaborated on during the test to prevent boredom. An adequate explanation is helpful in ensuring the older child's cooperation during the long procedure, which may last from 2 to 5 hours. With a younger child, reading him stories during the test or allowing him to hold a favorite toy is helpful in maintaining cooperation.

Overpreparing the child, especially a preschooler, can add to the level of anxiety rather than decrease it. The best course of action is to explain what is going on and what he can expect as the procedure progresses rather than to explain the entire process ahead of time.

Physical preparation of the child is the same as the preparation for any surgical procedure. He is allowed nothing by mouth for 4 to 6 hours before the catheterization, and he is given sedation, usually a combination of an analgesic such as injectable meperidine (Demerol) in combination with a tranquilizing agent. Usually, the morning dose of oral digoxin is withheld (for those children who are receiving the drug), although this is clarified beforehand with the physician.

Infants are not premedicated and it is not advisable to withhold fluids for more than 2 to 3 hours prior to the scheduled time of the procedure because any state of dehydration will cause difficulty in entering the veins. It is a good idea to send along extra diapers and a pacifier and/or a bottle of water if these items are not part of the laboratory's inventory.

Postprocedural care. Essentially, the care following cardiac catheterization is the same as postoperative care. However, since the child is not anesthetized during the procedure, he usually returns directly to his room.

Cardiac catheterization involves several potential complications, including arrhythmias, cardiac perforation, hemorrhage, arterial obstruction, reactions to contrast media, infection, phlebitis, and hypoxia. The most important

SUMMARY OF NURSING CARE OF THE CHILD WHO UNDERGOES CARDIAC CATHETERIZATION

GOALS	RESPONSIBILITIES

Preprocedural care	Obtain parental consent for procedure
	Arrange for preoperative diagnostic procedures as ordered:
	    electrocardiogram, complete blood count, chest radiograph, vectorcardiogram,
	      phonocardiogram, echocardiogram

Provide physical preparation	Assure nothing by mouth for a stated period of time prior to the procedure Take and record vital signs Administer preoperative medication to older infants and children Prepare requests to accompany child, such as x-rays, cardiopulmonary, according to routine of hospital
Anticipate needs	Provide extra diapers for infants Provide pacifier and/or sugar nipple for smaller infants, if irritable Provide K-pad or other device for warming small infant

Provide psychologic preparation
   Explain procedure to parents and older
   children
	Reinforce and clarify explanations provided by the cardiologist
	Give nonthreatening information at their level of understanding

Prepare for experience	Describe what the child will experience
	   Honestly
	   In simple terms
	   Appropriate to the child's level of development and past experiences
	Stress the familiar and relate the unfamiliar to known objects or experiences
	Avoid overpreparing the child with
	   Too much information
	   Unneeded information
	   Information beyond the child's ability to comprehend
	Allow the child to experience unfamiliar pieces of equipment in the safe environment of play
	   Ride a gurney in the hallway
	   Wear gown and mask
	   Play with real hospital equipment and/or miniature replicas or models
	Describe sensations the child will feel, in simple terms, at the appropriate time (not far in advance of the experience)

Provide comfort	Allow the child the comfort of a familiar toy or object, such as a favorite blanket Permit parents to be with the child as long as possible Be available and accessible to the child Answer questions Maintain a calm, reassuring manner Arrange to remain with the child if possible
Take to cardiac catheterization laboratory	Transport infants in bassinet, crib, or Isolette Transport older children by gurney

Continued.

SUMMARY OF NURSING CARE OF THE CHILD WHO UNDERGOES CARDIAC CATHETERIZATION—cont'd

GOALS	RESPONSIBILITIES
Support and reassure parents	Reinforce and clarify information given by the physician
	Explain associated diagnostic tests and procedures, such as x-ray examinations, ECG
	Explain the child's schedule
	When the child will receive premedication
	Time the child will leave for the cardiac catheterization laboratory
	Where the parents can wait for the child to return
	Room to which the child will return
	Explore the parents' feelings regarding the procedure and its implications
	Include the parents in the preparation of the child
Postprocedural care	
Assess physiologic status	Check vital signs until stable, as ordered: pulse (apical), respiration, temperature, blood pressure (if prescribed)
	Assess general color
	Assess circulation in involved extremity and compare with opposite extremity: pedal or radial pulses, color, temperature
	Assess operative site for bleeding and/or swelling
	Administer withheld digitalis, if ordered
Provide nutrition and hydration	Give sips of water first
	Advance intake to include other fluids and foods as tolerated
Prevent complications	Keep leg or arm on operative side as straight as possible
	Keep incision and dressing clean and dry
	Carry out routine physical assessments
	Keep the child relatively quiet
	Avoid undue excitement
Maintain optimum body temperature	Provide warmth if the infant or child is chilled from exposure during procedure
	Avoid either overheating or chilling

nursing responsibility is observation of the following: (1) temperature, respirations, and apical pulse; (2) blood pressure; (3) pulses, especially below the catheterization site, which are checked for equality and symmetry (pulse distal to the site may be weaker for the first few hours after catheterization but should gradually increase in strength); (4) temperature and color of the affected extremity, since coolness, cyanosis, or blanching may indicate vessel obstruction; and (5) dressing, which are checked for evidence of bleeding or hematoma formation in the femoral or antecubital area.

Usually, the child is kept in bed for up to 24 hours after the procedure. Infants and small children can be held, especially if restless. He is allowed his usual diet as soon as it is tolerated. It is best to begin with sips of water and advance as his condition indicates.

Generally, there is only slight discomfort at the cutdown or percutaneous site. The area is protected from possible contamination, such as that resulting from soiling if the child wears diapers. If keeping the dressing dry is a problem, it can be covered with a piece of plastic film and the edges sealed to the skin with tape. The nurse must be careful, however, to continue to observe the site for any evidence of bleeding.

It is important at this time to evaluate the child's conception of what occurred during the procedure, in order to clarify any misconceptions and allow him a feeling of triumph and satisfaction in having gone through the experience.

CONGENITAL HEART DISEASE (CHD)

The incidence of congenital heart disease in children is approximately 8 to 10 per 1000 live births; it is the major cause of death in the first year (other than prematurity).

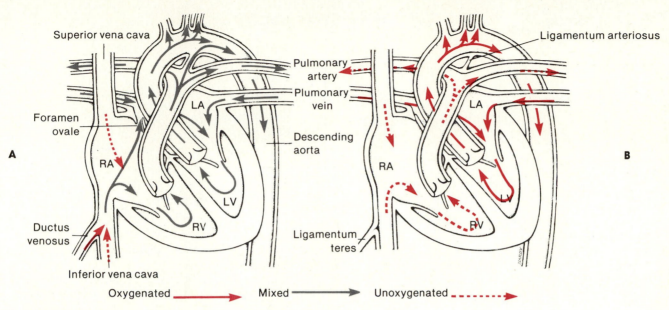

FIG. 22-1

Changes in circulation at birth. **A,** *Prenatal circulation.* **B** *Postnatal circulation. Arrows indicate direction of blood flow.* RA, *Right atrium.* LA, *Left atrium.* RV, *Right ventricle.* LV, *Left ventricle. Note: Although four pulmonary veins enter the left atrium, for simplicity this diagram shows only two.*

The sexes are affected differently, depending on the defect, and defects are found in a much higher percentage of stillbirths and spontaneous abortions.

GENERAL CONCEPTS

The etiology of most congenital heart defects is not known. However, several factors are associated with a higher than normal incidence of the disease. These include *prenatal factors* such as maternal rubella, poor nutrition, diabetes, and maternal age over 40 years. Several genetic factors are also implicated. For example, there is an increased risk of congenital heart disease in the child who (1) has a sibling with a heart defect, (2) has a parent with congenital heart disease, (3) has a chromosomal aberration, such as Down syndrome, or (4) is born with other, noncardiac congenital anomalies.

Circulatory changes at birth

During fetal life, blood carrying oxygen and nutritive materials from the placenta enters the fetal system through the umbilicus via the large umbilical vein. Oxygenated blood enters the heart by way of the inferior vena cava. Because of the higher pressure of blood entering the right atrium, it is directed posteriorly in a straight pathway across the right atrium and through the *foramen ovale* to the left atrium. In this way the better-oxygenated blood enters the left atrium and ventricle, to be pumped through the aorta to the head and upper extremities. Blood from the head and upper extremities entering the right atrium from the superior vena cava is directed downward through the tricuspid valve into the right ventricle. From here it is pumped through the pulmonary artery, where the major portion is shunted to the descending aorta via the *ductus arteriosus*. Only a small amount flows to and from the nonfunctioning fetal lungs (Fig. 22-1).

Before birth the high pulmonary vascular resistance created by the collapsed fetal lung causes greater pressures in the right side of the heart and the pulmonary arteries. At the same time the free-flowing placental circulation and the ductus arteriosus produce a low vascular resistance in the remainder of the fetal vascular system. With the cessation of placental blood flow from clamping of the umbilical cord and the expansion of the lungs at birth, the hemodynamics of the fetal vascular system undergo pronounced and abrupt changes.

Types of defects

Congenital heart defects are usually divided into two types, which reflect the alteration in circulation: (1) *acyanotic,* in which there is no mixing of unoxygenated blood in the systemic circulation, and (2) *cyanotic,* in which unoxygenated blood enters the systemic circulation, re-

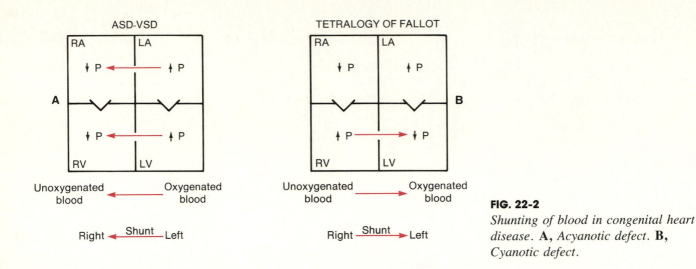

FIG. 22-2
Shunting of blood in congenital heart disease. **A,** *Acyanotic defect.* **B,** *Cyanotic defect.*

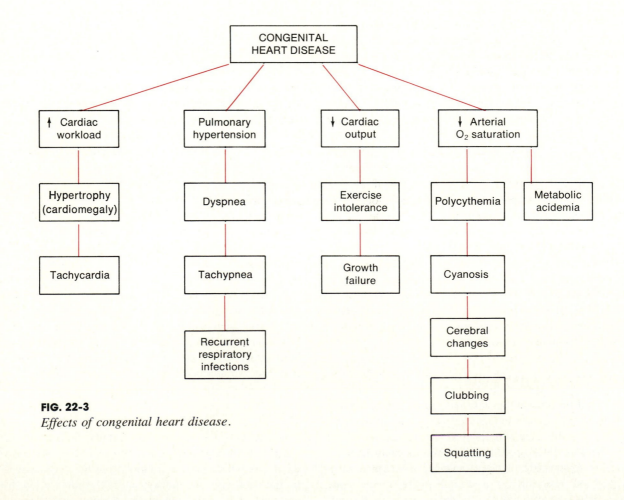

FIG. 22-3
Effects of congenital heart disease.

gardless of whether cyanosis is clinically evident. Clinical manifestations depend on the severity of the defect and the degree of cyanosis more than on the specific type of abnormality.

Altered hemodynamics. A knowledge of pressure and resistance is necessary to an understanding of physiology of heart defects. Normally the pressure on the right side of the heart is lower than that on the left side. Likewise, vessels entering or exiting these chambers have corresponding pressures. Therefore, if there is an abnormal connection between the heart chambers, such as a septal defect, blood will necessarily flow from an area of higher pressure (left side) to one of lower pressure (right side). Such a flow of blood is termed a left-to-right shunt. No unoxygenated blood flows directly into the left side of the heart; hence the term "acyanotic defect" (Fig. 22-2, *A*). If the hole is small and high on the septum, the amount of blood shunted to the atrium or ventricle may be easily compensated for by a moderately increased cardiac effort.

Primary obstruction of the outflow of blood from the right side of the heart or pulmonary hypertension causes the blood flow to shift from the area of high pressure on the right to one of lower pressure on the left, with mixing of unoxygenated and oxygenated blood and, consequently, cyanosis (Fig. 22-2, *B*). Severe acyanotic defects are potentially cyanotic, either as a result of pulmonary vascular changes or as a result of associated or secondary defects.

Physical consequences. The general effects of heart malformation may be summarized as (1) increased workload in terms of systolic or diastolic overloading of the chambers, (2) pulmonary hypertension (increased vascular resistance), (3) inadequate systemic cardiac output, and possibly (4) arterial unsaturation as a result of the shunting of unoxygenated blood directly into the systemic circulation. The principal physical consequences of these changes, which may vary in severity, are growth retardation, decreased exercise tolerance, recurrent respiratory infections, dyspnea, tachypnea, tachycardia, cyanosis, and tissue hypoxia (Fig. 22-3).

The body attempts to compensate for the decreased arterial oxygen saturation by increasing the pumping action of the heart, through *increased force* (which causes *cardiomegaly*) and *tachycardia*, the heart's attempt to increase cardiac output by increasing the number of beats per minute.

Dyspnea is also caused by increased pulmonary resistance as the lungs are unable to oxygenate adequate supplies of blood, resulting in "air hunger." It may be associated with *tachypnea* as the lungs try to compensate through an increased respiratory effort.

Cyanosis results from deoxygenated hemoglobin in the skin blood vessels, especially in the capillaries. Any event that increases metabolism and thus causes a demand for additional oxygen will result in a more severe degree of cyanosis. (See p. 95 for a discussion of evaluation of skin color.)

Growth retardation and *decreased exercise tolerance* are direct consequences of inadequate nutrient intake and oxygen supply for cellular metabolism. Failure to gain weight and poor muscular development, both from decreased metabolism and disuse, are consistent findings. Exercise intolerance is usually first noted by the parent during feedings, when the infant is too fatigued to consume the entire formula.

Recurrent respiratory infection occurs as a result of pulmonary vascular congestion as large amounts of blood pool in the lungs, making it readily susceptible to bacterial or viral invasion and growth.

Murmurs, abnormal sounds produced by vibrations within the heart chambers or vessels, are characteristic of many heart defects. Individual heart defects produce distinctive murmurs that aid in the diagnosis of the anomaly.

ACYANOTIC DEFECTS

Most acyanotic defects involve primarily left-to-right shunting through an abnormal opening. Others result from obstructive lesions that reduce the flow of blood to various areas of the body. The more common acyanotic defects, with the distinctive manifestations associated with them and the surgical correction available, are outlined on pp. 710-712.

The majority of acyanotic defects are amenable to surgical correction, and the tendency is toward early diagnosis and surgical repair. Patent ductus arteriosus is repaired as soon as the defect is discovered, sometimes in the newborn period in severe conditions. Defects of the septum are corrected surgically sometime prior to school entry. The child is placed on a regimen of oral digitalis to strengthen heart action and reduce the incidence of congestive heart failure, and some form of iron preparation is prescribed to enhance the iron carrying capacity of hemoglobin. Since children with congenital heart disease are more susceptible to upper respiratory infections than other children are, every effort is exerted to prevent unnecessary exposure to infections.

Palliative surgical procedures may be performed on symptomatic infants until permanent repair can be safely carried out. The usual procedure is banding of the pulmonary artery to decrease the blood flow to the pulmonary circulation.

MAJOR ACYANOTIC DEFECTS

Defect: Patent ductus arteriosus (PDA)

Description: failure of the fetal ductus arteriosus to completely close after birth. Complete anatomic closure may take several weeks.

Altered hemodynamics: blood from the aorta (a vessel of high pressure) flows into the pulmonary artery (a vessel of lower pressure) to be reoxygenated in the lungs and returned to the left atrium and left ventricle. The effects of this altered circulation are increased workload on the left side of the heart and increased pulmonary vascular congestion.

Distinctive manifestations: characteristic, machinery-like murmur, which is heard best at the mid to upper left sternal border; widened pulse pressure; cardiomegaly; bounding pulses; tachycardia.

Complications: congestive heart failure, bacterial endocarditis (potential).

Medical management: administration of indomethacin has proved successful in closing a patent ductus in low-birth-weight infants.

Surgical correction: surgical division or ligation of the patent vessel.

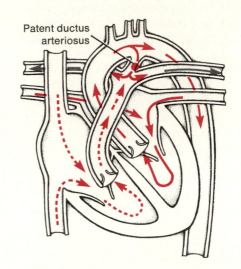

Patent ductus arteriosus

Defect: Coarctation of the aorta

Description: localized narrowing of the aorta.
Preductal, proximal to the insertion of the ductus arteriosus; *postductal,* distal to the ductus arteriosus.

Altered hemodynamics: increased pressure proximal to the defect and decreased pressure distal to it.

Distinctive manifestations (postductal): high blood pressure and bounding pulses in areas of the body that receive blood from vessels proximal to the defect. Femoral pulses are weak or absent, the lower extremities may be cooler than the upper ones, and muscle cramps may result during increased exercise from tissue anoxia. Child may experience dizziness, headaches, fainting, and epistaxis due to hypertension. A murmur may or may not be present.

Complications: intracranial hemorrhage and stroke, hypertension, ruptured aorta, hypertensive heart disease, congestive heart failure, possibility of a ruptured dissecting aortic aneurysm, and infective endocarditis.

Surgical correction: resection of the coarcted portion with an end-to-end anastomosis or graft replacement of the constricted section.

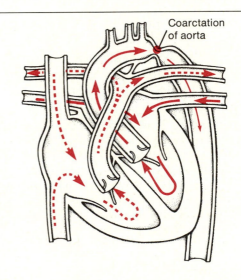

Coarctation of aorta

Defect: Atrial septal defect (ASD)

Description: abnormal opening between the two atria.

Altered hemodynamics: pressure in the left atrium exceeds that in the right atrium, causing blood to flow from left to right. Thus, there is an increased flow of oxygenated blood into the right side of the heart.

Distinctive manifestations: characteristic, crescendo-decrescendo type of systolic ejection murmur over the second to third interspace along the left sternal border; dyspnea and fatigue on exertion.

Complications: congestive heart failure, pulmonary vascular disease, bacterial endocarditis, and atrial arrhythmias (probably from atrial enlargement and effect on conduction system).

Surgical correction: surgical closure of moderate to large defects similar to closure of ventricular septal defects. Open repair with cardiopulmonary bypass.

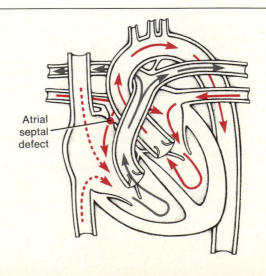

Atrial septal defect

Defect: Ventricular septal defect (VSD)

Description: abnormal opening between the right and left ventricles. May vary in size from a small pinhole to absence of the septum, resulting in a common ventricle. Frequently associated with other defects.

Altered hemodynamics: pressure within the left ventricle causes blood to flow through the defect to the right ventricle, resulting in increased pulmonary vascular resistance.

Distinctive manifestations: loud, harsh, pansystolic murmur heard best at the left lower sternal border and radiating throughout the precordium. A systolic thrill is associated with loud murmurs.

Complications: congestive heart failure, infective endocarditis, aortic insufficiency, pulmonary stenosis, and progressive pulmonary vascular disease.

Surgical correction

Palliative: pulmonary banding in symptomatic infants. *Complete repair:* small defects are repaired with a purse-string approach. Large defects usually require a knitted Dacron patch sewn over the opening. Both procedures are performed via cardiopulmonary bypass.

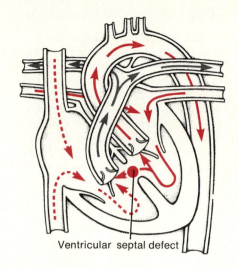

Ventricular septal defect

Defect: Pulmonary stenosis (PS)

Description: narrowing at the entrance to the pulmonary artery.

Altered hemodynamics: resistance to blood flow causes right ventricular hypertrophy and decreased pulmonary blood flow.

Distinctive manifestations: can range from only the presence of a murmur to cyanosis and congestive heart failure. Systolic ejection murmur is heard best over the second left intercostal space lateral to the sternum. Systolic thrill. Cardiomegaly.

Complications: with severe defects cyanosis, congestive heart failure, decreased systemic output, and increased venous resistance.

Surgical correction: in infants, transventricular (closed) valvotomy (Brock) procedure. In children, pulmonary valvotomy with cardiopulmonary bypass.

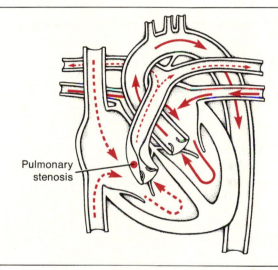

Pulmonary stenosis

Defect: Aortic stenosis (AS)

Description: narrowing or stricture of the aortic valve.

Altered hemodynamics: stricture causes resistance to blood flow in the left ventricle, decreased cardiac output, left ventricular hypertrophy, and pulmonary vascular congestion.

Distinctive manifestations: systolic ejection murmur. Infants with severe defects demonstrate evidence of decreased cardiac output, such as faint peripheral pulses, severe physical limitations. Children show exercise intolerance, epigastric or anginal pain, and dizziness after prolonged standing.

Complications: coronary insufficiency, ventricular failure.

Surgical correction: opening the valve orifice (commissurotomy).

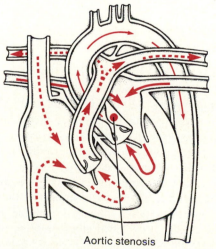

Aortic stenosis

MAJOR ACYANOTIC DEFECTS—cont'd

Defect: Endocardial cushion defect (ECD)

Description: incomplete fusion of endocardial cushions. Consists of a low atrial septal defect that is continuous with a high ventricular septal defect and clefts of the mitral and tricuspid valves creating a large central atrioventricular valve that allows blood to flow between all four chambers of the heart. May be complete or partial.

Altered hemodynamics: the openings between chambers allow blood to flow freely from one chamber to another. The directions and pathways of flow are determined by pulmonary and systemic resistance, left and right ventricular pressures, and the compliance of each chamber.

Distinctive manifestations: in the complete form dyspnea, fatigability, pulmonary infections, and a harsh pansystolic murmur. Cyanosis is generally mild or absent. Gross cardiomegaly is evident. Symptoms occur later and with less severity in the incomplete types.

Complications: congestive heart failure is common; pulmonary vascular obstruction.

Surgical correction

Palliative: pulmonary artery banding for infants with severe symptoms due to increased pulmonary blood flow.
Complete repair: open repair with cardiopulmonary bypass. Consists of mitral and tricuspid valve repair and patch closure of septal defects.

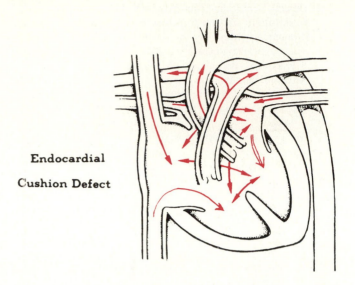

Endocardial Cushion Defect

CYANOTIC DEFECTS

Cyanotic defects are those in which unoxygenated blood is mixed with oxygenated blood in the systemic circulation. Diminished circulatory oxygenation is usually caused by right-to-left shunting of blood through an abnormal opening and/or vessel configuration. Improvements in surgical techniques have significantly increased the outlook for children with these defects. Some of the most frequently encountered cyanotic disorders are outlined on pp. 713-714.

Compensatory mechanisms observed in cyanotic heart disease

In addition to the physical consequences of congenital heart defects children with cyanotic lesions often develop other compensatory mechanisms. The body responds to decreased oxygen supply by increased production of erythrocytes (*polycythemia*) in an attempt to carry more available oxygen to tissues. However, the additional number of red blood cells increases the viscosity of the blood. As a result circulation becomes sluggish and is often impeded, especially in the capillaries. Consequently, the blood that is able to carry additional oxygen is not able to reach the peripheral circulation. Dehydration presents further hazards to the child because of the increased hemoconcentration.

Posturing is a compensatory mechanism automatically learned by the child. Infants assume either a flaccid posture with the extremities extended or a side-lying or prone position with the knees bent toward the chest (knee-chest position). The former position, in contrast to the normal flexed posturing of infants, is a response to tissue hypoxia. Continual muscle contraction demands additional oxygen supply. Flaccidity is usually a sign of progressive heart failure.

The knee-chest position and, later in childhood, the squatting position serve to decrease venous return by occluding the femoral vein through hip flexion, to lessen the workload on the right side of the heart, and to increase arterial oxygen saturation, especially to vital organs in the body (Fig. 22-4).

A characteristic finding in cyanotic cardiac lesions is *clubbing* of the fingers, a thickening and flattening of the distal phalanges (Fig. 22-5). Although the exact cause is unknown, some theories are soft tissue fibrosis and hypertrophy from anoxia and formation of increased numbers of capillaries to enhance blood supply.

Decreased oxygen to the brain is often manifested in cerebral changes, such as fainting (*syncope*), mental confusion, seizures, and sometimes mental slowness.

FIG. 22-4

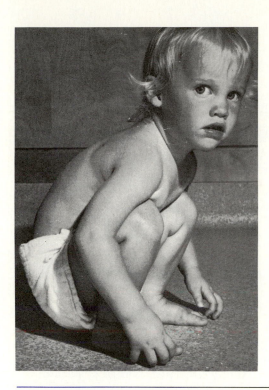

The characteristic squatting position assumed by the child with tetralogy of Fallot. (From Ingalls, A.J., and Salerno, M.C.: Maternal and child health nursing, ed. 5, St. Louis, 1983, The C.V. Mosby Co.)

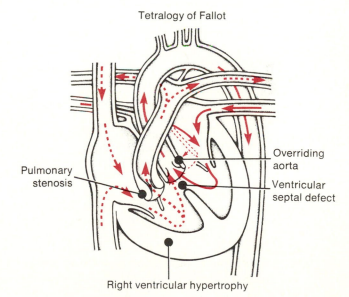

FIG. 22-5
Clubbing of the fingers.

MAJOR CYANOTIC DEFECTS

Defect: Tetralogy of Fallot (TOF)

Description: the classic form includes four defects: (1) ventricular septal defect, (2) pulmonic stenosis, (3) overriding aorta, and (4) right ventricular hypertrophy.

Altered hemodynamics: the pulmonic stenosis impedes the flow of blood to the lungs, and thus causes increased pressure in the right ventricle, forcing unoxygenated blood through the septal defect to the left ventricle. The increased workload on the right ventricle causes hypertrophy. The overriding aorta receives blood directly from both the right and left ventricles.

Distinctive manifestations

Infants: acute severe episodes of cyanosis and hypoxia, often called "blue spells." Anoxic spells occur when the infant's oxygen requirements exceed the blood supply, usually during crying or after feeding. The infant may assume a knee-chest position rather than an extended position.

Children: physical evidence of cyanosis, markedly delayed physical growth and development, clubbing of the fingers, squatting to relieve the chronic hypoxia. Fainting and/or mental slowness may occur from chronic hypoxia to the brain. Seizures may occur after exertion. A pansystolic murmur is usually heard at the mid to lower left sternal border; it is usually associated with a thrill. Radiographic studies reveal a "boot-shaped" configuration of heart and great vessels.

Complications: polycythemia, thrombophlebitis, emboli, cerebrovascular disease, brain abscess. Hyperpnea with severe cyanosis may lead to unconsciousness and death.

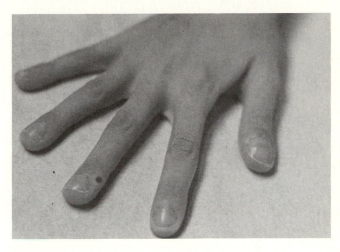

Tetralogy of Fallot

Overriding aorta

Ventricular septal defect

Pulmonary stenosis

Right ventricular hypertrophy

Surgical correction

Palliative: artificial opening created between aorta and pulmonary artery to increase pulmonary blood flow (Waterston shunt, a side-to-side anastomosis of the ascending aorta to the right pulmonary artery in neonates; Blalock-Taussig operation, a subclavian artery–pulmonary artery anastomosis in older infants and children).

Corrective: repair of the defects—that is, closure of the ventricular septal defect, pulmonic valvotomy, as well as (when indicated) correction of the overriding aorta.

MAJOR CYANOTIC DEFECTS—cont'd

Defect: Transposition of the great arteries (TGA), or vessels (TGV)

Description: pulmonary artery leaves the left ventricle and the aorta exits from the right ventricle, with no communication between systemic and pulmonary circulations.

Associated defects and hemodynamics: associated defects such as septal defects or patent ductus arteriosus permit blood to enter the systemic circulation and/or the pulmonary circulation for mixing of unoxygenated and oxygenated blood. However, presence of these defects can increase the problems of congestive heart failure, which results from large amounts of blood flowing through the heart to the lungs.

Distinctive manifestations: depend on the type and size of the associated defects. Children with minimum communication are severely cyanotic and depressed at birth. Those with large septal defects or a patent ductus arteriosus may be less severely cyanotic but have symptoms of congestive heart failure. Heart sounds vary according to the type of defect present. Cardiomegaly is usually evident a few weeks after birth.

Complications: congestive heart failure is the main complication; hypoxia is the major cause of death.

Surgical correction

Palliative: to prevent pulmonary vascular resistance and congestive heart disease until the child is able to tolerate complete cardiac repair: (1) surgical creation of an atrial septal defect (Blalock-Hanlon operation), (2) enlargement of an existing atrial septal defect by pulling a balloon through the defect (balloon septotomy) during a cardiac catheterization (Rashkind procedure), (3) pulmonary artery banding to decrease blood flow to the lungs, and (4) creation of a ductus arteriosus if pulmonic stenosis is present.

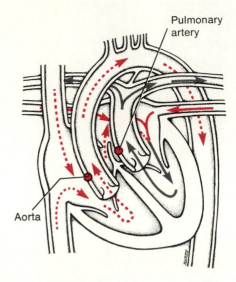

Transposition of the great vessels

Complete repair: atrioseptopexy. Involves removing the entire atrial septum and creating a new atrial septum from existing pericardium (Senning's operation) or a prosthesis (Mustard operation) that tunnels or baffles blood for more effective oxygenation.

Defect: Truncus arteriosus (TA)

Description: failure of normal septation and division of the embryonic bulbar trunk into the pulmonary artery and aorta, resulting in a single vessel that overrides both ventricles.

Altered hemodynamics: blood ejected from the left and right ventricles enters the common artery and flows either to the lungs or to the aortic arch and body. Pressure in both ventricles is high, and blood flow to the lungs is markedly increased.

Distinctive manifestations: marked cyanosis, left ventricular hypertrophy, dyspnea, marked activity intolerance, and retarded growth.

Complications: congestive heart failure, hypoxia, infective endocarditis, brain abscess.

Surgical correction:

Palliative: banding both pulmonary arteries as they arise from the truncus arteriosus, to decrease the amount of blood flow to the lungs.

Corrective: closing the ventricular septal defect and inserting a prosthetic valved conduit (Rastelli's operation).

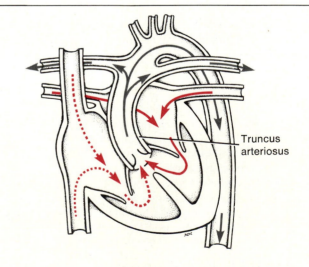

NURSING CARE OF THE CHILD WITH CONGENITAL HEART DISEASE

When a child is born with a severe cardiac anomaly, the parents are faced with the immense psychologic and physical tasks of adjusting to the birth of a defective child and raising a child with physical limitations. Many of the concepts and interventions related to the management of the child with a physical handicap or a chronic, and potentially life-threatening, illness have been discussed in Chapter 16.

The present discussion is concerned with the family whose child has a serious heart defect that requires an indefinite period of home care prior to corrective surgery. The goal for this child is to live as normal a life as possible within the limitations of his condition. Since the prognosis is often variable, such a goal allows him time to live as a child first and as a patient second. Since many defects are correctable, it also prepares the child to abandon the sick role following surgery and adjust to the privileges and responsibilities of a well child.

Observation

Nursing care of the child with a congenital heart defect begins as soon as the diagnosis is suspected. However, in many instances symptoms suggestive of a cardiac anomaly are not present at birth or, if manifest, are so subtle they are easily overlooked. (See consequences of congenital heart disease p. 709.)

Many heart defects are not evident until the child's growth and/or energy expenditure exceeds the heart's ability to supply oxygenated blood. Since the onset is gradual, the child may curtail his activity so that the signs of exercise intolerance are less obvious. However, a careful history yields important clues to this change. For example, toddlers are normally extremely mobile and their energies are directed toward learning gross motor skills. It is very unusual to hear of a toddler who prefers to sit rather than crawl or walk. Such histories should alert the nurse to assess cardiac function. Likewise, a child who needs frequent rests after limited play periods may also be exhibiting exercise intolerance.

Other clues, which have already been discussed, are a history of retarded weight gain, poor feeding habits, especially the need to pause during feeding, frequent respiratory infections, particularly when the child is well cared for and isolated from known sources of infection, and any unusual posturing, such as squatting. Since parents may not view any of these findings as abnormal, the nurse must ask about them specifically during a physical assessment. Children with suspected heart murmurs are referred for evaluation.

Help parents and child adjust to the disorder

When parents and older children learn of the heart defect, they are in a period of shock initially followed by high anxiety. They are especially fearful that the child may die. The diagnosis may be made soon after the child's birth or at a later period in life. Whatever its timing, the family needs a period of grief before assimilating the meaning of the defect. Unfortunately, the demands for medical treatment may not allow this, which requires that the parents be informed of the condition in order to consent to various procedures. However, the nurse can support parents in their loss, assess their level of understanding, supply information as needed, and help other members of the health team to understand the parents' reactions.

Parental adjustment. Once parents are ready to hear about the heart condition, it is essential that they be given a clear explanation, based on their level of understanding. One tool for illustrating heart defects simplistically is to depict the heart as a four-room structure (house) with normal exits and entrances (representing the valves and vessels). A septal defect can then be illustrated as an abnormal entrance to one side of the structure that allows mixing of blood that should remain only in one room. Although this explanation may not suffice for all parents, it does allow for clarification of basic information. Parents also appreciate receiving written information about the specific defect.*

Parents are primarily interested in two kinds of information—prognosis and whether surgery will be required—and are upset about indefinite answers to their questions. In addition, all members of the health team may not use the same terms to present identical information. If this is identified as a problem, the nurse should encourage parents to write down the term or ask the informant to clarify it.

Parents also need an explanation regarding the symptoms of the disease. Watching a child become cyanotic and dyspneic is frightening. However, offering parents suggestions of what to do during and after an episode decreases their anxiety by providing them some control. After a cyanotic and/or dyspneic episode, the child needs to rest and attain a position of comfort, which usually consists of lying on his side or on his stomach with knees flexed and the head and chest elevated. An infant is cuddled against an adult's shoulder with his knees and hips flexed. This serves to decrease the return of deoxygenated blood to the heart and to provide comfort. He is kept warm to prevent increased metabolism and vasoconstriction. Most important, he should remain calm. The cyanotic spell is treated

---

*One booklet that can be given to parents is ''If your child has a congenital heart defect,'' New York, 1970, American Heart Association.

casually to prevent parental emotions from being transferred to the child.

An essential intervention is prevention of cyanosis and dyspnea by tailoring energy expenditure to cardiac output and arterial oxygenation. For older children this involves little difficulty, because activity restrictions are self-imposed. Even in infants there is little need to prevent crying because it usually ceases when hypoxia increases. Deliberate attempts to prevent crying should be avoided because it can establish a maladaptive parental pattern of relating to the infant. Strenuous spontaneous activity and competitive sports may be restricted in selected children and adolescents.

An important area of intervention for distressed infants is decreasing energy requirements needed for feeding. The infant may need to be fed small amounts of formula every couple of hours to insure an adequate intake. If several nighttime feedings are required, the nurse should discuss with parents the need to share the responsibility and to enlist the help of others whenever possible. Parents do not feel confident leaving the child in the care of someone else. They believe that the child will be upset by a change in routine and that the individual will be unable to cope with the child's symptoms.

Since growth retardation is believed to be a result of inadequate caloric intake, the nurse assists parents in finding ways to provide highly nutritious foods. The physician may order protein-calorie supplements. Less energy is required for sucking if the nipple hole is enlarged by cutting a cross in the center to facilitate flow of the formula.

Self-feeding techniques such as the use of a spoon or cup may be delayed in order to conserve energy. However, the benefit of this practice must be weighted against the consequent lag in development, especially in learning to chew. Parents may wish to encourage finger foods and self-feeding as a method of play rather than at mealtime, when ingesting sufficient nutrients is the priority.

Children with severe cardiac defects are often anorexic and tempting them to eat can be a tremendous challenge. Because of the parents' concern over eating, children learn at an early age to manipulate them through eating behavior, such as making unrealistic demands for foods that are not available. The nurse advises parents of this potential problem, since prevention yields greater success than intervention.

Child adjustment. Children of various ages form different ideas about the heart. Children between 4 and 6 years of age have heard about the heart, know its approximate anatomic location in the chest or back, illustrate it as valentine shaped, and characterize it by its sounds—tick-tock, thump, and so on. Children 7 to 10 years of age have a clearer concept of the heart, realizing that it is not shaped like a valentine and that it has vital functions—for example, "It makes you live." However, their knowledge of its integrated functions in pumping blood through a system of vessels to all parts of the body is still vague. By the age of 10 or 11 years, children have a much more involved concept of the heart, with knowledge of veins, valves, pumping action, and circulation. They are beginning to appreciate its mechanisms and the reason that death occurs when the heart stops.

Information about his condition must be tailored to the child's developmental level. Preschoolers need basic information about what they may experience and what they are allowed to do more than they need information about what is actually occurring physiologically. School-age children benefit from a concrete explanation of the defect. Using the "house" model can be very effective. Preadolescents and adolescents often appreciate a more detailed description of how the defect affects the heart. Children of all ages need an opportunity to express their feelings concerning the diagnosis and its particular meaning to them.

Foster growth-promoting family relationships. The effect of a child with a serious heart defect on the family is complex. No member, regardless of the degree of positive adjustment, is unaffected. The mother frequently feels inadequate in her mothering ability because she is unable to continually satisfy the child. She may view the child's failure to feed well as evidence of her failure, not as a direct consequence of the disease. The usual joys of watching a child grow and thrive are limited. Frequently, attainment of gross motor milestones is delayed because of physical inability to practice crawling or sitting unsupported. Mothers often feel constantly exhausted from the pressures of caring for these children and the other members of the family.

The need to maintain discipline and to set limits cannot be overemphasized. Behavior modification techniques, either in the form of concrete awards, such as a favorite food, or social reinforcement, such as approval, can be effective. However, such techniques are most beneficial if they are employed *before* the child learns to control the family. Therefore, guiding parents toward the need for discipline while the child is in infancy is necessary to prevent problems later on. These children must be taught how to tolerate frustration and delayed gratification, an ability that is difficult to attain because of the early need for immediate satisfaction of all their needs.

Although the child may not be able to participate in physical activity, he is encouraged in acceptable pursuits, such as reading, quiet hobbies, and less demanding physical activities. Allowing the child to watch television as his total means of recreation is not fostering his development. If the child enters school prior to corrective surgery, the parents should discuss appropriate activity levels with the teacher, the school nurse, and the principal.

Another problem that frequently develops within family relationships is the child's overdependency, especially

SUMMARY OF NURSING CARE OF THE CHILD WITH CONGENITAL HEART DISEASE

GOALS	RESPONSIBILITIES
Prevent congenital heart disease	Encourage immunization against rubella in all females Detect rubella infection early in pregnant women; discuss possibility of elective abortion Encourage genetic counseling of parents of child with congenital heart disease regarding risk to subsequent offspring Discuss risks of congenital heart disease in diabetic or alcoholic women or in women of advanced age Encourage prevention through general measures of optimum nutrition, prenatal supervision, and avoidance of any drugs unless medically indicated
Observe for signs or symptoms of congenital heart disease	Be alert for physical and behavioral characteristics that indicate congenital heart disease Report suspected heart murmurs
Assist with diagnosis	Take careful history with special attention to poor weight gain, poor feeding habits, exercise intolerance, unusual posturing, or frequent respiratory tract infections Perform general physical assessment with special emphasis on color, pulse (apical and peripheral), respiration, blood pressure, and examination and auscultation of chest Order or draw blood for CBC Perform or assist with electrocardiography Order and/or assist with x-ray examinations, echocardiography, angiography, fluoroscopy, ultrasonography Prepare the child and family for and assist with cardiac catheterization (p. 702)
Help the parents and child adjust to diagnosis	Allow period of grief Accept initial shock and disbelief Repeat information as often as necessary Foster parent-child attachment, especially in the case of newborn Introduce the parents to other families who have similarly affected children
Improve efficiency of the heart	Administer digoxin (Lanoxin) as ordered, using established precautions to prevent toxicity (see p. 723)
Reduce cardiac demands	Adjust physical activity to child's condition and capabilities Avoid extremes of environmental temperature
Maintain nutrition	Assure well-balanced diet Discourage food with high salt content; no added salt
Prevent infection	Avoid contact with infected persons Provide for adequate rest
Prevent potassium depletion	Encourage potassium-rich foods to prevent depletion Mix potassium supplements (if prescribed) with fruit juice to camouflage bitter taste and prevent intestinal irritation
Improve iron-carrying capacity of blood	Administer iron preparations as prescribed Encourage iron-rich foods in the diet

Continued.

SUMMARY OF NURSING CARE OF THE CHILD WITH CONGENITAL HEART DISEASE—cont'd

GOALS	RESPONSIBILITIES

Recognize signs of complicating factors	Be alert for signs of complications such as
	    Congestive heart failure (CHF) (p. 721)
	    Digitalis toxicity
	    Pneumonia
	    Hypoxemia
	    Cerebral thrombosis
	    Cardiovascular collapse
	    Cerebral vascular accident

Prepare the parents for home care of the infant or child	Instruct the parents in
	    Administration of medications
	    Feeding techniques
	    Interventions for conserving energy and relieving frightening symptoms
	    Signs that indicate complications
	    Where to go and whom to contact for help and guidance

Increase the parents' understanding of the child's condition	Assess their understanding of the diagnosis Reinforce and clarify physician's description of the child's condition and the prognosis Explore their feelings regarding prescribed therapies Reinforce and clarify physician's explanation of suggested diagnostic procedures and palliative or corrective surgery

Reduce the parents' fears and anxieties	Explore the parents' concerns and feelings of irritation, guilt, anger, disappointment, or adequacy
	Help the parents distinguish between realistic fears and unfounded fears
	Discuss with the parents their fears regarding
	    The child's symptoms, such as pounding heart, cyanotic spells, irritability
	    Dealing with the child's anxiety about his condition
	    Fear of dreadful developments
	    Fear of death
	    Fear of tests and procedures

Help the parents cope with symptoms of disease	During dyspneic cyanotic spell, place the child in side-lying, knee-chest position, with head and chest elevated Minimize crying by anticipating needs Keep the child warm; encourage rest and sleep Decrease the child's anxiety by remaining calm Encourage the parents to include others in the child's care, to prevent own exhaustion
Facilitate feeding	Feed the child slowly Administer small, frequent meals Enlarge hole in nipple to facilitate sucking Delay self-feeding to minimize exertion Encourage the anorexic child to eat

SUMMARY OF NURSING CARE OF THE CHILD WITH CONGENITAL HEART DISEASE—cont'd

GOALS	RESPONSIBILITIES
Help the child understand his defect	Assess level of understanding
	Use visual aids to describe heart defect
	Provide written information
	Keep technical information simple
	Convey same information as other health team members convey
	Stress that prognosis and plans for surgery may change
	Base explanation of heart on the child's developmental level of understanding
	Allow the child to express feelings about heart condition
	Explore the child's feelings regarding his disorder
	Clarify misconceptions the child may have acquired
	Help the child select activities appropriate to his age and condition
	Support positive coping mechanisms and extinguish negative ones
Palliate or correct defects	Assist with parental decision regarding surgery
	Explore feelings regarding palliative or corrective surgery
	Explain or clarify information presented to the parents by the physician and surgeon
	Prepare the child and parents for the procedure
	Administer nursing care to the child who has undergone cardiac surgery (p. 720)
Foster growth-promoting family relationships	Assess the family's support systems
	Reinforce positive coping mechanisms
	Encourage family members to discuss their feelings about each other
	Maintain as equal expectations from all the siblings as possible
	Impress upon the parents the importance of providing as normal a life as possible for the affected child
	Assist the parents in determining apropriate physical activity and disciplining methods for the child
	Provide consistent discipline, especially from infancy, to prevent behavioral problems
	Encourage acceptable pursuits for the child
	Discuss school entry with teacher and school nurse
	Counsel parents about the eventual hazards of fostering overdependency
	Help the parents feel adequate in their maternal or paternal roles by emphasizing growth and developmental progress of their child
	Help the parents foster the child's development by stimulating the child to age-appropriate goals consistent with his activity tolerance
	Provide social experiences for the child
Assist in providing financial support	Investigate state and local agencies that may be able to provide financial assistance, such as state crippled children's services
	Collaborate with social service agencies to ensure optimum utilization of community services

on his mother. Mothers, in turn, frequently respond to the dependency with overprotectiveness, resulting in a cycle that is mutually satisfying although destructive in terms of developing maturity and responsibility. The nurse should encourage parents to begin early to stimulate the infant toward feasible developmental goals, such as holding his own bottle, learning to amuse himself for short periods rather than always being held, and picking up finger foods. Unless parents are helped to see what the child can do, they often will focus only on his physical limitations.

The child also needs opportunities for social development. Often these children are isolated from known sources of infection and not allowed to play with other children because of overexertion. Such limitations only add to the dangers of increased dependency on the home environment. Parents need to be encouraged to seek appropriate social activity, especially prior to kindergarten. One approach is to introduce the family to other families with similarly affected children who can help them adjust to the daily stresses of coping with a child with a heart defect. Sometimes several parents who have children with heart disease are willing to form a cooperative group to share such responsibilities, form a play group for their children, and provide respite care for one another.* (See Chapter 16 for further approaches to care of the chronically ill child).

Nursing care of the child undergoing heart surgery

The child is usually admitted to the hospital for diagnostic tests 1 or 2 days prior to surgery. Few surgical procedures demand as much planning for preoperative and postoperative care; therefore, this interval allows additional time to prepare the child and parents for surgery. Since a great deal of information is conveyed, it is important to schedule teaching to prevent information overload and to be alert to signs of overload (see p. 585 for suggestion on preparing children and parents for surgical procedures).

The preparation is divided into three major categories: environment, equipment, and procedures. Ideally, when the child is admitted he should be assigned to one nurse for each shift—preferably the nurses who will be responsible for his care postoperatively. A visit to the recovery room and/or intensive care unit is desirable and should take place when there is least activity in the unit, when the parents can accompany the child, and when the child is well rested. Usually the day before surgery is ample time to allow the child to ask questions but prevent undue fantasizing about the experience. All positive, nonfrightening aspects of the environment are emphasized, such as the

play area, visitors' section, pictures or mobiles in the room, or television.

Pieces of equipment that are new and unfamiliar are shown to the child and the family, and demonstrated either on him or on a doll. This might include such items as the oxygen mask, the oxygen tent, suction, chest tubes, the endotracheal tube, incentive spirometer, and intravenous tubing. With a younger child, displaying miniature equipment that is suitable for use with a doll or puppet is often less anxiety producing than showing the actual objects. If other children in the unit are receiving intravenous infusions or are in oxygen tents, an older child may benefit from seeing them. The more sensations he experiences beforehand, the less likely it is that he will be frightened by them later.

The type and size of dressing the child will have after surgery are discussed and demonstrated on a doll. Usually, one of two types of incision is made: a median sternotomy (which splits the sternum) or a lateral thoracotomy (which extends from the midaxillary line to the scapula). In either instance the suture line and dressing are extensive. Frequently no sutures are visible because subcuticular, absorbable sutures may be used. If this is done, it should be pointed out to the child and parents, who may fear that the incision might open.

The older child is told about chest tubes, their purpose, and that he will be expected to move while they are in place. He is also told about the presence of a postsurgery endotracheal tube, which will be removed as soon as possible, but he should be assured that, although he will be unable to talk, he will be able to communicate his desires by other means.

Several postoperative procedures are imperative to prevent postsurgical complications—especially coughing, turning, deep breathing, and postural drainage and percussion. Each of these is practiced several times before surgery. Although they can be presented as a game, the child is told that each procedure will not be as easy after surgery and may cause discomfort.

Deep breathing is demonstrated by having the child watch the nurse's chest rise and fall. The child is told to imitate the nurse's actions, emphasizing that the higher the chest rises, the more air enters the lung. For a young child the nurse can explain that the lungs are like balloons that expand when air is inspired. The use of incentive spirometers is also demonstrated to encourage breathing. If these are not available, the child can blow bubbles through a straw placed in water. Coughing is demonstrated by taking a deep breath and forcibly attempting to bring up secretions. It is emphasized that coughing is not the same as clearing the throat. The nurse also performs percussion and vibration on the child to demonstrate the procedure and clarify that the clapping is not hitting.

---

*Some local chapters of the American Heart Association have organized parent groups.

The child also practices turning in bed while in a semi-Fowler's position and using the bedpan or urinal. He is told that following surgery he will have a special tube (Foley catheter) so that he will not have to urinate for a day or two but after that he will be expected to use the other equipment.

The child is also prepared for preoperative procedures, such as taking nothing by mouth for 12 hours prior to surgery, skin preparation, which includes shaving or the use of a topical depilatory in adolescent males and females, and preoperative sedation. Physical preoperative care differs little from that for any type of surgery. Skin preparation may involve a tub bath with special bacteriocidal cleanser the day before surgery. The nurse clarifies with the physician exactly what preoperative procedures are to be done, to avoid the hazard of overpreparing or underpreparing the child. (See also the discussion of preparing the child for surgery, p. 585.)

Postoperative care. Immediate postoperative care is usually provided by specially trained nurses in intensive care units. Many of the procedures, such as intra-arterial and central venous pressure monitoring and the observations related to vital functions, require advanced education and technical training. These procedures will not be elaborated here.

The child will be returned to the pediatric unit as soon as his condition warrants. Physical care is the same as for any child recovering from major surgery. He is encouraged to be as active and as involved in his own care as his age and condition indicate. This seldom creates difficulty, since most children are naturally active, although children with cardiac lesions tend to prefer more quiet activities as a result of their preoperative behavior patterns.

Planning for discharge. Ideally, planning for discharge begins on admission, when the nurse assesses the readiness and ability of the parents and child to give up the sick role and adjust to the responsibilities and privileges of a healthy child. If parents have been guided in caring for the child as they would for a normal child, the transition to full recovery is facilitated. Unfortunately, this is not always the case, necessitating that the nurse discuss this phase of recovery with the parents.

Emotional adjustment involves a gradual resumption of physical ability as well as responsibility. For an older child who has never had the opportunity to develop athletic competence, a sense of competition, or fine muscle coordination, it may be unrealistic to pursue a goal in this direction, despite physical ability to do so. In such an instance it is more beneficial to encourage interests that have already been developed. This may be very difficult for fathers who may anticipate that after corrective heart surgery their sons will be able to join them in competitive sports.

Fostering a sense of responsibility is equally difficult.

Parents may have a great need to continue a dependent relationship for themselves. Likewise, the child may be unwilling to accept new limits or to give up privileges of the sick role. The nurse investigates the family relationships to identify those roles or needs that may prevent parents or children from establishing a new set of expectations.

The nurse can facilitate adjustment by gradually expecting more from the child in the recovery period and stressing to parents the importance of gradual achievement of new skills and responsibilities. Since the postoperative period is quite short—only 7 to 10 days for an uncomplicated recovery—the nurse should make a referral to a public health nursing agency for follow-up care in the home.

ACQUIRED HEART DISEASE

Acquired heart disease, as opposed to congenital heart disease, occurs as a result of a previously existing disease or defect or as a complication of an acute disease. The most common condition classified as acquired heart disease is congestive heart failure—usually as a complication of congenital heart disease. *Cor pulmonale* is the term applied to congestive failure that results from pulmonary hypertension associated with chronic lung disease, principally cystic fibrosis.

CONGESTIVE HEART FAILURE (CHF)

Congestive heart failure is inability of the heart to pump an adequate amount of blood to the systemic circulation to meet the body's metabolic demands. In children congestive heart failure most frequently occurs secondary to structural abnormalities that result in increased blood volume and pressure. Congestive heart failure is a symptom caused by an underlying cardiac defect, not a disease in itself, since it is usually the result of an excessive workload imposed on a normal myocardium. Most children who experience congestive heart failure are infants.

Pathophysiology

Heart failure is often separated into two categories, right-sided and left-sided failure. In *right-sided failure* the right ventricle is unable to pump blood into the pulmonary artery, resulting in less blood being oxygenated by the lungs and increased pressure in the right atrium and systemic venous circulation. Systemic venous hypertension causes edema in the extremities and viscera. In *left-sided failure* the left ventricle is unable to pump blood into the systemic circulation, resulting in increased pressure in the left atrium and pulmonary veins. The lungs become congested with blood, causing elevated pulmonary pressures and pulmonary edema.

Although each type produces different systemic and pulmonary alterations, clinically it is unusual to observe solely right- or left-sided failure. Since each side of the heart depends on adequate function of the other side, failure of one chamber causes a reciprocal change in the opposite chamber. For example, in left-sided failure an increase in pulmonary vascular congestion will cause back pressure in the right ventricle, resulting in right ventricular hypertrophy, decrease myocardial efficiency, and eventu-

ally cause pooling of blood in the systemic venous circulation.

Clinical manifestations

If the abnormalities precipitating heart failure are not corrected, the heart muscle becomes damaged. Despite compensatory mechanisms, the heart is unable to maintain an adequate cardiac output. Decreased blood flow to the kidneys continues to stimulate sodium and water reabsorption, leading to hypervolemia, increased workload on the heart, and congestion in the pulmonary and systemic circulations (Fig. 22-6).

Cardiac manifestations include tachycardia (heart rate

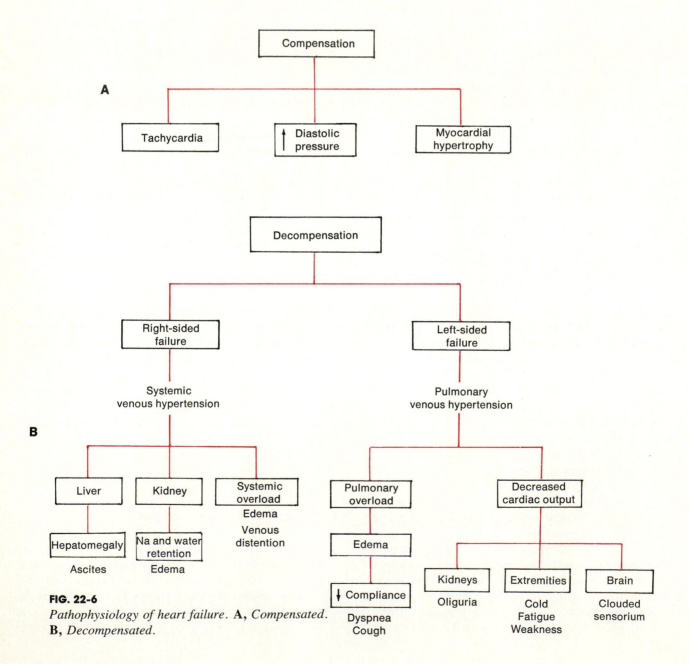

FIG. 22-6
Pathophysiology of heart failure. **A**, *Compensated.*
B, *Decompensated.*

above 160 beats/minute in infants), pulsus alternans (alternating of one strong beat and one weak one), and cardiomegaly. Pulmonary congestion is evidenced by dyspnea and tachypnea (respiratory rate above 60 breaths/minute), costal and substernal retractions, orthopnea, coughing, and grunting on expiration. Rales, moist respirations, rhonchi, and wheezing can be heard on auscultation. Cheyne-Stokes respirations (rapid, deep breathing alternating with slow, shallow breathing) are a late sign.

Systemic congestion is evidenced by distended neck and peripheral veins, edema (reflected in weight gain), and hepatomegaly. Inappropriate sweating, especially on the head, is a sympathetic response characteristic of infants in congestive failure.

Therapeutic management

The goals of treatment are to (1) improve cardiac function, (2) remove accumulated fluid and sodium, (3) decrease cardiac demands, and (4) improve tissue oxygenation.

Improve cardiac function. Myocardial efficiency is improved through the use of digitalis glycosides. The beneficial effects are increased cardiac output, decreased heart size, decreased venous pressure, and relief of edema. In pediatrics digoxin (Lanoxin) is used almost exclusively, because of its more rapid onset and the decreased risk of toxicity as a result of a much shorter half-life. It is available as an elixir (0.05 mg/ml) for oral administration. For infants the dose is often calculated in micrograms (1000 $\mu g = 1$ mg).

Treatment consists of a digitalizing dose, given orally, intramuscularly, or intravenously as one large dose or in divided doses over a short time span to produce optimum cardiac effects, and a maintenance dose, usually one fourth to one third the digitalizing dose, given orally twice a day to maintain blood levels. During digitalization the child is monitored by means of an electrocardiograph, to observe for the desired effects (prolonged P-R interval and reduced ventricular rate) and detect side effects, especially arrhythmias.

Remove accumulated fluid and sodium. Treatment consists of diuretics, fluid restriction, and possible sodium restriction. Diuretics are the mainstay of therapy to eliminate excess water and salt to prevent reaccumulation. The most commonly used agents are furosemide (Lasix), the thiazides (chlorothiazide suspension or hydrochlorothiazide tablets), and spironolactone. Since furosemide and the thiazides are potassium-losing diuretics, potassium supplements may be prescribed and rich sources of the electrolyte are encouraged in the diet. A fall in serum potassium enhances the effects of digitalis, increasing the risk of digitalis toxicity; therefore, serum potassium levels are carefully monitored.

Fluid restriction may be required in the acute states of CHF or if fluid retention is accompanied by loss of sodium. For example, diuretics cause additional sodium loss whereas limited oral fluids preserve the serum sodium levels. Fluids must be carefully calculated to avoid dehydrating the child, especially if significant polycythemia is present.

Sodium-restricted diets are used less often in children than in adults to control congestive heart failure, because of their potential negative effects on appetite. For example, low-sodium milk is unpalatable and poorly tolerated by infants. If salt intake is restricted, the diet usually consists of avoiding additional table salt and highly salted foods.

Decrease cardiac demands. The workload on the heart is reduced when metabolic needs are kept to a minimum. This is accomplished by limiting physical activity (bed rest), preserving body temperature, treating any existing infections, reducing the effort of breathing (semi-Fowler's position), and using medication to sedate an irritable child (usually morphine sulfate, 0.1 mg/kg). Since meeting these objectives effectively depends on nursing intervention, they are discussed in more detail in the next section.

Improve tissue oxygenation. All of the preceding measures serve to increase tissue oxygenation, either by improving myocardial function or by lessening tissue oxygen demands. Iron supplements are administered to enhance the oxygen carrying capacity of red blood cells. Supplemental cool humidified oxygen is usually provided to increase the amount of available oxygen during inspiration. The amount of cool humidity is carefully regulated to prevent overhydration and chilling.

Nursing considerations

The objectives of nursing care include (1) assisting in measures to improve cardiac function, (2) decreasing cardiac demands, (3) reducing respiratory distress, (4) maintaining nutritional status, (5) assisting in measures to promote fluid loss, and (6) providing emotional support. Although the objectives are the same, the interventions differ depending on the child's age; interventions for infants are quite different from those for older children.

Improve cardiac function. The responsibility of the nurse in administering digitalis includes calculating and administering the correct dose, observing for signs of toxicity, and instituting parental teaching regarding drug administration in the home.

Digitalis is a potentially dangerous drug because the differences between therapeutic, toxic, and lethal doses are very small and there is no known antidote. Many toxic responses are extensions of the drug's therapeutic effects. Therefore, when administering digitalis, the nurse must observe carefully for the following signs of toxicity.

The earliest indication of toxicity is vomiting although

one episode does not warrant cessation of the drug since it is such a common occurrence in infants. The principal manifestations of cardiac toxicity are abnormalities in heart rate, rhythm, and conduction. An early sign is bradycardia; therefore, the *apical* pulse (counted for one full minute) is always checked before administering digitalis. As a general rule the drug is not given if the pulse is below 90 to 110 beats/minute in infants and young children or below 70 beats/minute in older children. Since the pulse rate varies in children within different age-groups, the physician should specify at what heart rate the drug is to be withheld as part of the written order. The nurse should also use judgment in evaluating the pulse rate. If it is significantly lower than the previous recording, the dose should be withheld until the physician is notified.

In no other drug is it more important to employ the safe practice of checking for correct drug preparation, dose, patient, time, and route. An accidental overdose can be fatal. As an added safety precaution, the nurse administering the drug always checks the dose with another nurse before giving the drug to the child.

A problem arises when the child vomits or spits out the medication, since regiving it may result in overdose. In general, the physician is notified prior to administering another dose, especially since vomiting may be an early sign of toxicity. To minimize this problem, it is important to administer the drug carefully, by slowly squirting it on the side and back of the mouth. It should not be mixed with foods or fluids, since refusal to consume these substances results in inaccurate dosage of the drug.

Decrease cardiac demands.   The infant or child with CHF is placed at complete rest although the manner of attainment varies with the age of the child. The infant requires rest and conservation of energy for the task of feeding; therefore, every effort is made to organize nursing activities to allow for periods of uninterrupted sleep. Whenever possible, the parents are encouraged to stay with their infant to provide the holding, rocking, and cuddling that help children sleep more soundly and to preserve the parent-child relationship.

To minimize disturbing the infant, changing bedclothes and complete bathing are done only when necessary. Feeding is planned to accommodate the infant's sleep and wake patterns. He is fed as soon as he appears hungry, for example, when he is sucking on his fists. He should be fed before he begins to cry for a bottle, since the stress of crying exhausts his limited energy supply. If he is sleeping, he is fed after he awakens.

Usually, the older child is placed on a regimen of complete bed rest to minimize any unnecessary physical activity. This usually means dependence on others for feeding, bathing, and elimination (use of bedpan for older child). Encouraging parents to stay with the child and participate in his care is most beneficial to ensuring bed rest, since the child's physical and emotional needs are anticipated and quickly met. They need an explanation of what is happening to them, to decrease anxiety about their physical status, for example, an explanation of equipment and procedures. Sometimes the sense of urgency associated with admission of a child in severe congestive heart failure overshadows the need for psychologic preparation. However, the few minutes it takes to reassure a child that electrocardiograph leads do not hurt or to familiarize him with the way the world appears through a plastic tent reduce the physiologic responses to stress.

Temperature is carefully monitored because hyperthermia or hypothermia increases the need for oxygen. Febrile states are reported to the physician, since infection must be promptly treated. Maintaining body temperature is of special importance in children who are receiving cool, humidified oxygen and in infants, who tend to be diaphoretic and lose heat by way of evaporation.

Reduce respiratory distress.   To facilitate respiratory effort, the child is placed in semi- to high Fowler's position; infants are placed in an infant or cardiac seat. Infants and children with cyanotic heart disease often breathe better in the knee-chest position, which decreases venous return and reduces the workload of the right side of the heart. An infant can be maintained in this position by placing him on his side (maintaining Fowler's position), with the knees bent toward the chest and pillows propped behind the back and buttocks. If he must be transported, either position is maintained. Shirts and diapers are pinned loosely to allow maximum chest expansion. Safety restraints, such as those used with the infant seats, are applied low on the abdomen; they should be secure enough to provide safety but loose enough to allow maximum expansion.

Respiration is carefully monitored, the rate counted for 1 full minute during a resting state, and any unusual breathing patterns or other evidence of respiratory distress are reported to the physician. If morphine sulfate is given, the nurse observes for respiratory depression from the drug.

The child is usually placed in a high humidified oxygen environment—the infant in an incubator or under an oxygen hood; a child in a Croupette. However, supplemental oxygen may or may not be helpful in relieving the respiratory distress or cyanosis. If a trial period is ordered to determine its effectiveness, the nurse evaluates the child's response by noting respiratory rate, ease of respiration, degree of cyanosis, and interval of sleep. (See p. 572 for care of the child receiving oxygen therapy).

Since children with congestive heart failure are susceptible to recurrent respiratory infection, they are placed in rooms with patients who have noninfectious conditions.

With an older child, it is advantageous to choose a roommate who is also confined to bed and relatively quiet, in order to promote a restful environment. Visitors and hospital personnel with active respiratory infection are isolated from the child. Good hand-washing technique is practiced before and after caring for either an infant or an older child. Antibiotics are given to combat respiratory infection. The nurse ensures that the drug is given at equally divided times over a 24-hour schedule, to maintain high blood levels of the antibiotic.

Maintain nutritional status. Many infants with severe cardiac defects are poorly nourished and physically retarded. Because of the dyspnea on exertion, sucking becomes an exhausting activity and the infant is unable to consume his needed nutrients. To minimize the effort of eating, small frequent feedings are scheduled, allowing for needed rest periods. The nipple should be soft, with a hole that is large enough to permit entry of milk without the danger of aspiration. To reduce the respiratory effort, the infant is fed in an upright position and burped frequently. If these measures are still exhausting to the infant, he may require gavage for all or part of the feedings. For the infant who is unable to tolerate extended periods without supplemental oxygen, the source can be held near his face during feeding or comforting.

Food selections for older children need to be highly nutritious, easy to ingest, and palatable. They should also provide sufficient fluid to maintain hydration. Blenderized preparations, such as shakes and malted milks, or commercially available food supplements are usually well tolerated by children, especially if prepared with their favorite flavors, such as chocolate or strawberry. The use of a straw, a special cup, or rewards for drinking or eating, such as reading a story or playing a quiet game, can be incentives. To minimize the fatigue of eating, mealtimes should be carefully planned around rest periods and spaced at frequent intervals.

Promote fluid loss. When diuretics are given, the nurse continues to record fluid intake and output and to monitor body weight at the same time each day, to evaluate the effectiveness of the drug. Since profound diuresis may cause dehydration and electrolyte imbalance (loss of sodium, potassium, chloride, and bicarbonate), the nurse observes for signs that indicate either complication. Diuretics are given early in the day to children who are toilet trained, to avoid the need to urinate at night. If potassium-losing diuretics are given, the nurse observes for signs of hypokalemia and encourages foods high in potassium, such as bananas, oranges, whole grains, legumes, and leafy vegetables. A potassium supplement, if given, is mixed with fruit juice (red punch or grape juice works well) to disguise the bitter taste and to prevent intestinal irritation from a concentrated solution.

Fluid restriction is rarely necessary in infants because of their difficulty in feeding. When fluids are restricted, the nurse plans fluid-intake schedules. With toddlers and preschoolers it is psychologically advantageous to give small amounts of liquid in vessels of appropriate size, since young children associate volume with size of the container. Suitable utensils are decorated medicine cups, paper Dixie cups, doll-sized teacups, or measuring cups. It is also important to avoid leaving extra fluids at the bedside, since older children may help themselves to additional servings. The cooperation of older children can be gained by placing them in charge of recording fluid intake.

If salt intake is limited, the nurse discusses food sources of sodium with the parents and discourages their bringing salt-containing treats to the child. At mealtime the nurse checks the child's tray to make sure that salt was not mistakenly given.

Provide emotional support. CHF is a serious, potentially fatal complication of heart disease and parents and older children are usually acutely aware of the critical nature of the condition. Since stress places additional demands on cardiac function, nurses focus on reducing anxiety through anticipatory preparation, frequent communication with the parents regarding the child's progress, and constant reassurance that everything possible is being done.

The imposed bed rest and placement of the child in an oxygen tent severely limit physical contact between the child and the parents. This separation can be minimized by encouraging parents to participate in care, such as feeding, bathing, positioning, and stimulating the child. As was mentioned earlier, active parent participation also optimally meets the infant's physical and emotional needs, with minimum exertion. However, parents must feel comfortable and well accepted by the staff. For example, positioning the child may be cumbersome with the interfering electrocardiogram leads, but, with practice, parents become expert in functioning despite such equipment.

If congestive heart failure is the final stage of a severe heart defect, the nurse cares for the child as for any terminally ill child, using principles discussed in Chapter 16.

INFECTIVE ENDOCARDITIS (IE)

Infective endocarditis, an infection of the valves, inner lining, or a septal defect of the heart, is one of the most serious of the cardiac complications and a significant cause of morbidity in the pediatric age-group. It develops most often as a complication of congenital or rheumatic heart disease but can occur without an underlying heart disorder. The most common causative agents are bacteria (streptococci, especially *Streptococcus viridans,* staphylococci,

SUMMARY OF NURSING CARE OF THE CHILD WITH CONGESTIVE HEART FAILURE

GOALS	RESPONSIBILITIES

Reduce cardiac demands and oxygen consumption	Maintain neutral thermal environment for minimal oxidative metabolism
	    Place infant in Isolette with servocontrol or under warmer
	Maintain in resting state at 10 to 30 degrees
	Feed small volumes at frequent intervals (every 2-3 hours) using soft nipple with moderately large opening
	Implement gavage feeding if infant becomes fatigued before taking an adequate amount
	Time nursing activities to disturb infant as little as possible
	Implement measures to reduce anxiety
	Minimize crying by anticipating child's needs
	    Respond promptly to crying or other expressions of distress

Reduce respiratory distress	Administer oxygen via Isolette or Croupette
	Place in inclined posture of 10 to 30 degrees
	    Tilt mattress support of Isolette
	    Place older infant in cardiac chair or infant seat
	Avoid any constricting clothing or tight restraints around abdomen and chest
	Provide humid atmosphere
	Perform percussion, vibration, and suction as ordered
	Place in knee-chest position (some infants with cyanotic heart disease)

Improve tissue oxygenation	Administer oxygen as above Reduce tissue demands for oxygen as above
Improve contractility of heart	Administer digoxin as prescribed, employing appropriate precautions (pp. 723-724)
Assess cardiac status	Attach cardiac monitor Carry out frequent assessments of vital signs Take ECG as prescribed and/or indicated by infant's condition
Maintain hydration	Provide or restrict fluids, depending on amount of fluid retention Plan schedule for restricted fluid intake on child's usual drinking habits Administer fluids child prefers; use small container Do not leave additional fluid at bedside (if restricted) Gain older child's cooperation in monitoring his fluid intake
Maintain nutrition	Provide feedings appropriate to age and capabilities relative to feeding techniques Replace electrolytes as indicated

enterococci, and pneumococci), fungi such as *Candida albicans,* and *Rickettsia.*

Pathophysiology

Organisms usually gain entrance to the bloodstream by: (1)lymphatic spread from a wound site, (2) infected thrombi, which attain direct access into the general circulation, and (3) infected materials inserted into the peripheral circulation during surgical or traumatic procedures. The most common portals of entry are oral, particularly with dental procedures (*S. viridans*); urinary tract infections following catheterization (gram-negative bacilli); and the bloodstream, as a result of long-term infusions.

Following an infection, vegetations (*verrucae*) consisting of deposits of platelets, fibrin, and fibrinoid material, form at a weakened spot on the endocardium. Infective endocarditis results when these vegetations become contaminated with microorganisms from the bloodstsream. Infected emboli may travel through the bloodstream to other areas of the heart and to other organ systems producing extensive damage.

SUMMARY OF NURSING CARE OF THE CHILD WITH CONGESTIVE HEART FAILURE—cont'd

GOALS	RESPONSIBILITIES

Remove accumulated tissue fluid	Administer diuretics as prescribed
	    Observe for side effects of electrolyte depletion, especially potassium
	    Administer early in day to avoid need for frequent voiding at night

Prevent increased accumulation of fluids	Feed low-salt formula, such as Lonalac (Mead-Johnson) or Similac PM 60/40 (Ross) Reduce salt intake
Assess fluid gain or loss	Weigh daily at same time and on same scale Maintain strict record of intake and output Assess for evidence of increased or decreased edema
Prevent infection	Avoid exposure to persons with infections Administer antibiotics if prescribed Employ thorough hand-washing techniques and meticulous cleansing procedures for any equipment coming in contact with the infant
Provide adequate systemic oxygen transport	Administer supplemental iron preparation as prescribed
Reduce anxiety	Employ flexible feeding schedule that reduces fretfulness associated with hunger Handle the child gently Hold and comfort the infant Employ comfort measures found to be effective in individual cases Encourage parents to provide comfort and solace Administer morphine sulfate judiciously, if ordered
Support parents	Employ active listening techniques Explain and clarify the child's behavior and the therapies prescribed Keep parents informed of the child's condition Reassure family that everything is being done for the child Encourage parents to remain with the child Demonstrate acceptance of the parents' willingness to participate in the child's care If CHF is terminal stage for the child, support the parents' grief, make the child as comfortable as possible, and remain with the family

Clinical manifestations

The onset is usually insidious, with unexplained fever, anorexia, malaise, and weight loss. The most characteristic findings result from emboli formation elsewhere in the body, especially splinter hemorrhages (thin black lines) under the nails, Osler's nodes (red, painful intradermal nodes with white centers found on the pads of the phalanges), Janeway lesions (painless hemorrhagic areas on the palms and soles), and petechiae on the oral mucous membranes. Congestive heart failure and cardiac arrhythmias may be present, and a new murmur or a change in a previously existing one may be found as a result of damage to valves or perforation of the myocardium.

Diagnostic evaluation

Several laboratory findings may suggest infective endocarditis, for example, electrocardiographic changes (prolonged P-R interval), x-ray evidence of cardiomegaly, anemia, elevated erythrocyte sedimentation rate, leukocytosis, and microscopic hematuria. Definitive diagnosis rests on growth and identification of the causative agent in the blood.

Therapeutic management

Treatment should be instituted immediately and consists of administration of high doses of appropriate antibiotics intravenously and/or intramuscularly for at least 4 weeks. Blood cultures are taken periodically to evaluate response to antibiotic therapy.

Prevention of infective endocarditis in susceptible children is achieved by administering prophylactic antibiotic therapy both prior to and for a short period after procedures known to increase the risk of entry of organisms, including dental work and any manipulation of the respiratory, genitourinary, or gastrointestinal tract. In female adolescents this includes childbirth.

Nursing considerations

Ideally, the objective of nursing care is prevention through counseling parents of high-risk children about the need for prophylactic antibiotic therapy prior to procedures such as dental work. Unless parents are aware of the risk inherent in exposing their child to these procedures, they may not be inclined to seek medical treatment beforehand. The family's regular dentist should be advised of existing cardiac problems in the child, as an added precaution and to ensure that preventive treatment is carried out.

Treatment requires hospitalization for the duration of parenteral drug therapy. Nursing goals during this period are (1) preparation of the child for continuous intravenous infusion, possibly for multiple intramuscular injections, and for several venipunctures for blood cultures; (2) prevention of boredom, resulting especially from restricted mobility caused by intravenous infusion and the need for partial bed rest, if required; (3) observation for side effects of antibiotics; and (4) observation for complications, especially from embolism, and the possibility of heart failure. For specific interventions see the nursing care summary for the child with congestive heart failure.

RHEUMATIC FEVER (RF)

Rheumatic fever is an inflammatory disease affecting the heart, joints, central nervous system, and subcutaneous tissue. It derives its name from involvement of joints and the presence of fever in the acute stage. The most significant sequela of rheumatic fever is *rheumatic heart disease*, especially damage to and scarring of the mitral valve. Because the disease has declined so rapidly in North America and Western Europe during recent years it is rarely encountered in children today, although valvular damage is still observed in the adult population.

The disease was known to be a sequelae of streptococcal pharyngitis; therefore, prophylactic administration of penicillin following such infections has become standard practice. At present the rare cases of rheumatic fever are observed primarily in socioeconomically deprived black school children.

CARDIAC TAMPONADE

Cardiac tamponade is compression of the heart by blood and other fluids in the pericardial sac, which severely restricts the normal heart movement. A characteristic sign is *paradoxical pulse pressure,* in which the systolic pressure drops during inspiration because inhaling causes the accumulated blood to compress the heart, resulting in a drop in cardiac output. Other signs include rising venous pressure, falling arterial pressure, narrowing pulse pressure, dyspnea, cyanosis, apprehension, and compensatory posturing that consists of sitting and leaning forward. Any evidence of this potentially fatal complication is immediately reported to the physician. Treatment consists of pericardiocentesis to remove the blood. If active hemorrhage is present, steps are taken to enhance blood clotting.

CIRCULATORY DYSFUNCTION

Disorders of the circulatory system in children involve primarily the shock states and hypertension. The vascular degenerative disorders seen in adults are almost nonexistent in children; however, vascular anomalies and cerebrovascular accidents are an uncommon cause of cerebral dysfunction in children.

SYSTEMIC HYPERTENSION

Hypertension occurs in a variety of acute and chronic illnesses of childhood and adolescence. Secondary hypertension of a sustained nature accompanies renal, cardiovascular, adrenal, and some neurologic disorders. In recent years there has been increasing interest in primary hypertension as it occurs in adolescents and children. Routine blood pressure measurements of children in the pediatric age-group have detected hypertension similar to essential hypertension in adults with surprising frequency in asymptomatic children, especially teenagers. Evidence is accumulating to indicate that the essential hypertension of adulthood may have its origin in childhood; therefore, its early detection has significance for prevention and treatment.

Pathophysiology

The causes of primary hypertension are undetermined, but there is evidence to indicate that both genetic and environmental factors play a role. Hypertension has been shown to be increased in children whose parents are considered to be hypertensive. American blacks have a higher incidence of hypertension than whites, and in these persons it develops earlier, is frequently more severe, and results in mortality at an earlier age.

Clinical manifestations

Most of the confusion regarding hypertension is related to a cutoff point to differentiate normal from abnormal blood pressure in children, especially in borderline cases. It is generally agreed, however, that any child or adolescent who has a diastolic blood pressure repeatedly in the range of 90 to 95 mm Hg in the supine position should be considered hypertensive. Recent studies suggest that children or teenagers whose systolic and/or diastolic pressures are repeatedly in the 90th percentile for age or occasionally above the 90th percentile constitute a borderline group who are probably at high risk to develop hypertension at a later age.

Diagnostic evaluation

Although clinical manifestations associated with hypertension depend largely on the underlying cause, there are some observations that can provide clues to the examiner that an elevated blood pressure may be a factor. Adolescents and older children with hypertension complain of frequent headaches, dizziness, and/or changes in vision. In infants or young children who cannot communicate symptoms, observation of behavior provides clues, although gross behavioral changes may not be apparent until complications are present. Parents of infants and small children who have been treated for hypertension report that their child had previously been irritable, often indulged in an abnormal degree of head banging or rubbing, and may have wakened screaming in the night (when blood pressure tends to be highest).

Therapeutic management

Therapy for secondary hypertension involves diagnosis and treatment of the underlying cause. Children or adolescents who have consistently elevated blood pressure readings with no known etiology or those in whom secondary hypertension is not amenable to surgical correction are placed on hypotensive drug therapy. The type of drug and the dosage are tailored to meet the needs of individual children and are determined by the hypotensive effect produced and the appearance of any side effects. The aim is to achieve a normotensive state throughout the day without any accompanying side effects. The drug regimen is kept simple, preferably with a single antihypertensive agent in combination with a suitable diuretic.

Nursing considerations

The nurse is a valuable link in the health-care delivery system in relation to hypertension in the pediatric age-group. Blood pressure measurement should always be part of the routine assessment of infants and children. In carrying out the procedure it is most important to make certain that the cuff used is suited to the individual child and that any questionable reading is repeated, using different instruments if necessary. When an elevated pressure is detected the procedure is carried out in the standing, sitting, and supine positions and comparison readings made between both upper extremities to ascertain if they are equal.

To obtain an accurate reading, care is taken to quiet the child or relax the adolescent while the measurement is recorded to avoid false readings caused by excitement. The chief cause of falsely elevated blood pressure readings is the use of improperly fitting, narrow cuffs. Sphygmomanometer cuffs must be selected according to the weight and build of the child. (See p. 92 for techniques and selection of cuff and inside front cover for expected readings at various ages.)

Following a medical regimen is seldom a problem in the younger child. Parents and child are instructed in the administration of the medications and observation for side effects. They are taught the technique of blood pressure measurement and instructed regarding what to do when findings exceed the desired levels. The major problem in hypertensive adolescents is compliance in relation to maintaining contact with the physician or clinic for follow-up care, taking antihypertensive drugs as prescribed, and allowing home blood pressures to be taken. An important aspect of nursing care is to convince these youngsters that their disorder is probably a lifelong concern and that management must include drug therapy, perhaps some modification in diet and activity, and regular follow-up care.

SHOCK

Shock, or circulatory failure, is a clinical syndrome characterized by prostration and tissue perfusion that is inadequate to meet the metabolic demands of the body. The physiologic consequences of shock are: hypotension, tissue hypoxia, and metabolic acidosis.

The most common type of circulatory failure in children is hypovolemia, or *hypovolemic shock*, in which there is a loss of blood or plasma from the vascular compartment with a falling blood pressure, poor capillary filling, and a low central venous pressure. *Septic shock (bacteremic shock, endotoxic shock)*, caused by overwhelming sepsis and circulating bacterial toxins, is not uncommon in children.

Less common causes are *dysrhythmias* such as paroxysmal atrial tachycardia, atrioventricular block, and ventricular arrhythmias, and shock secondary to myocarditis or biochemical abnormalities.

Pathophysiology

In the healthy child the circulation is able to transport oxygen and metabolic substrates to body tissues, which require a constant source for these essential needs. The cardiac output and distribution to the various body tissues can change very rapidly in response to intrinsic (myocardial and intravascular) or extrinsic (neuronal) control mechanisms. In shock states these mechanisms are altered or challenged.

Reduced blood flow, as in hypovolemic shock, causes diminished venous return to the heart, low central venous pressure, low cardiac output, and hypotension. Vasomotor centers in the medulla are signaled, causing a compensatory increase in the force and rate of cardiac contraction and constriction of arterioles and veins, thereby increasing peripheral vascular resistance. At the same time the mechanisms are activated in an effort to conserve body fluids. This causes reduced blood flow to the skin, kidneys, muscles, and viscera in order to shunt the available blood to the brain and heart. Consequently the skin feels cold and clammy, there is poor capillary filling, and glomerular filtration and urine output are significantly reduced.

Oxygen depletion in tissue cells as a result of impaired perfusion causes the cells to revert to anaerobic metabolism, thus producing lactic acidosis. The acidosis places an extra burden on the lungs as they attempt to compensate for the metabolic acidosis by increased rate. Prolonged vasoconstriction results in fatigue and atony of the peripheral arterioles, which leads to vessel dilation. Venules, less sensitive to vasodilator substances, remain constricted for a time, causing massive pooling in the capillary and venular beds to further deplete blood volume.

Clinical manifestations

The outcomes of circulatory failure are tissue hypoxia, metabolic acidosis, and eventually organ dysfunction. Initially, early clinical signs of shock are subtle and include apprehension, irritability, unexplained tachycardia, normal blood pressure, narrowing pulse pressure, thirst, pallor, and diminished urinary output. As the shock state advances, signs are more obvious, including confusion and somnolence, tachypnea, moderate metabolic acidosis, oliguria, and cool, pale extremities with decreased skin turgor and poor capillary filling. Thready, weak pulse, hypotension, periodic breathing or apnea, anuria, and stupor or coma are signs of impending cardiopulmonary arrest.

Additional signs may be present depending on the type and etiology of the shock. In early septic shock there are chills, fever, and vasodilation with increased cardiac output that results in warm, flushed skin (hyperdynamic or "hot" shock). A later and ominous development is disseminated intravascular coagulation (p. 753), the major hematologic complication of septic shock. Anaphylactic shock (caused by an extreme allergy or hypersensitivity to a foreign substance) is frequently accompanied by urticaria and angioneurotic edema, which is life-threatening when it involves the respiratory passages.

Diagnostic evaluation

The etiology of shock can be discerned from the history and the physical examination. The extent of the shock is determined by measurements of vital signs, including central venous pressure and capillary filling. Laboratory tests that assist in assessment are blood gas measurements, pH, and sometimes liver function tests. Coagulation tests are evaluated when there is evidence of bleeding, such as oozing from a venipuncture site, bleeding from any orifice, or petechiae. Cultures of blood and other sites are indicated when there is a high suspicion of sepsis. Renal function tests are performed when impaired renal function is evident.

Therapeutic management

Treatment of the child in shock begins with establishment of an airway and administration of oxygen. Once the airway is assured, circulatory stabilization is the major concern. Placement of an intravenous catheter for rapid volume replacement is the most important action for reestablishment of circulation. In the majority of cases rapid restoration of blood volume is all that is needed for resuscitation of the child in shock. Successful resuscitation will be reflected by an increase in blood pressure and a reduction in heart rate; increased cardiac output will result in improved capillary circulation and skin color. Central venous pressure measurements of right atrial pressure help guide fluid therapy, and urinary output measurement is an important indicator of adequacy of circulation. Correction of acidosis, hypoxemia, and any metabolic derangements is mandatory.

Temporary pharmacologic support may be required to enhance myocardial contractility, to reverse metabolic or respiratory acidosis, and/or to maintain arterial pressure. The principal agents used to improve cardiac output and circulation are the sympathetic amines administered by constant infusion pump. Those given most often to pediatric patients are the catecholamines dopamine (Intropin), epinephrine (Adrenalin), and isoproterenol (Isuprel). Vasodilators that are sometimes employed include nitroprusside (Nipride) and hydralazine (Apresoline).

Acidosis is corrected with adequate ventilatory support, including oxygen, and the administration of sodium bicarbonate. Calcium chloride may be administered to improve cardiac function. Appropriate antibiotics are administered to patients with septic shock. In cases of septic shock caused by gram-negative organisms, corticosteroids are of value. Other complicating disorders are treated appropriately.

Nursing considerations

When shock is a likely complication, the child is observed carefully for any early signs such as irritability, unexplained increase in heart rate, thirst, pallor, or diminished urinary output. Appearance of any of these signs requires further evaluation and initiation of therapy.

The child who is in shock requires intensive observation and care. The initial action is assuring adequate tissue oxygenation. The nurse should be prepared to administer oxygen by the appropriate route and to assist with any intubation and ventilatory procedures indicated. Other procedures and activities that require immediate attention are establishing an intravenous line, weighing the child, obtaining baseline vital signs, placing an indwelling catheter, obtaining blood gas and other measurements, and administering medications as indicated.

The nurse's responsibilities are to monitor the intravenous infusion, intake and output, vital signs (including central venous pressure), and general systems assessments on a routine basis. Intravenous medications are titrated according to patient responses, and vital signs are taken every 15 minutes during the critical periods and thereafter as needed. Urine output is measured hourly, and blood gases, hematocrit, pH, and electrolytes are monitored frequently to assess the status of the child and the efficacy of therapy. An apnea and cardiac monitor is attached and monitored continuously. In the initial stages of acute shock the care of the child often requires the attendance of more than one nurse in order to manage all the necessary activities that must be carried out simultaneously.

Throughout the intense activity the parents must not be overlooked. Someone should contact them at frequent intervals to inform them about what is being done and if there is any progress. Ideally someone should remain with the parents to serve as liaison between them and the intensive care team. However, this is not always feasible in such a critical situation. As soon as possible they are allowed to see the child. A clergyman may be called to help provide comfort and support.

TOXIC SHOCK SYNDROME (TSS)

A recently recognized disease entity, toxic shock syndrome, is a relatively rare disease that occurs predominantly (but not exclusively) in previously healthy young women during their menstrual periods. Studies have shown a striking relationship between the disease and the use of tampons (Centers for Disease Control, 1980). In its acute form the disease is characterized by sudden onset of high fever, vomiting, and diarrhea, with a rapid progression to hypotension and shock.

Pathophysiology

Evidence from several sources suggests that the toxic shock syndrome is generated by infection with phage group-1 *Staphylococcus aureus*, which is believed to produce an epidermal toxin. The disease has been observed primarily in women who use tampons during a menstrual period. The tampons may carry the organism from the fingers or the vulva into the vagina during insertion, the tampon might traumatize the vaginal wall and provide a focus of infection, or the tampon itself may provide a favorable environment for growth of the organism or elaboration of its toxin.

Clinical manifestations

The sudden development of high fever, vomiting and diarrhea, profound hypotension, shock, oliguria, and an erythematous macular rash with subsequent desquamation are characteristic manifestations of toxic shock syndrome. Other manifestations might include headache, blurred vision, purulent conjunctivitis, abdominal guarding, and purulent vaginal discharge.

Complications of the shock state are respiratory distress, cardiac dysfunction, hematologic changes (particularly disseminated intravascular coagulation), and abnormal liver function. Impaired perfusion to extremities may become severe with eventual necrosis and loss of extremities.

Diagnostic evaluation

Diagnosis is established on the basis of the criteria established by the Centers for Disease Control's toxic case definition. A history of tampon use contributes to the diagnosis. Additional laboratory tests include cultures from blood, vagina, cervix, and any discharge. Other laboratory tests are those that facilitate the management of shock.

Therapeutic management

The management of toxic shock syndrome is the same as management of shock of any etiology. Since the disease is highly varied in intensity, therapy is directed toward supportive care in mild cases to hospitalization and intensive care in severe cases. Appropriate parenteral antibiotics are usually administered after cultures are obtained. The drugs do not appear to alter the course of the disease but seem to be effective in preventing recurrences. Preventing complications of impaired circulation demands constant observation and immediate therapeutic intervention for hypotension, pulmonary dysfunction, acidosis, hematologic changes, and renal impairment.

Nursing considerations

Nursing care and observation of the acutely ill patient are the same as those described for shock of any etiology. Since the disease is relatively rare, the major efforts of nursing are directed toward prevention. The association between the disease and the use of tampons provides some direction for education. Avoiding the use of tampons offers the most certain preventive measure, although this approach is probably unacceptable to most adolescent girls. Most young women prefer the freedom, comfort, and inconspicuousness that tampons afford and are unlikely to comply with this advice.

Adolescent girls who use tampons can be advised to modify their use. For example, tampons may be used intermittently during the menstrual cycle, alternating with sanitary napkins—perhaps using the napkins during the night and tampons during the day. It is probably advisable to encourage young girls not to use superabsorbent tampons and not to leave any tampon in the body for more than 12 hours. Instruction in general hygienic measures, such as hand washing before insertion of the tampon, is an important part of patient teaching.

It is also advisable to teach patients how to recognize the early symptoms of toxic shock syndrome. They should understand that they should remove the tampon and consult their physician if they develop a sudden high fever, vomiting and diarrhea, and muscle pain, dizziness, or rash.

HENOCH-SCHÖNLEIN PURPURA (HSP)

Henoch-Schönlein purpura (Schönlein-Henoch vasculitis, allergic purpura, anaphylactoid purpura) is a relatively common acquired disorder in children characterized by a nonthrombocytopenic purpura and variable joint and visceral abnormalities. The etiology is unknown but the disease often follows an upper respiratory infection, and allergy or drug sensitivity play a role in some instances. The disease occurs in children aged 6 months to 16 years but more frequently between ages 2 to 8 years. It is observed more often in white children and in boys three times more often than in girls.

Pathophysiology

The disease is characterized by inflammation of small blood vessels and the manifestations observed are influenced by the size and distribution of the affected vessels. A generalized vasculitis of dermal capillaries (and to a lesser extent small arterioles and veins) causing extravasation of red blood cells produce the petechial skin lesions. Inflammation and hemorrhage may also occur in the gastrointestinal tract, synovium, glomeruli, and central nervous system.

Clinical manifestations

The onset of the disease may be abrupt with simultaneous appearance of several manifestations or gradual with sequential appearance of different manifestations. The primary feature, however, is a symmetrical purpura involving the buttocks and lower extremities but may extend to include the extensor surfaces of the upper extremities and, less commonly, the upper trunk and face. The rash may be associated with maculopapular lesions and variable elements of urticaria and erythema. There is often marked edema of scalp, eyelids, lips, ears, and dorsal surfaces of hands and feet—especially in infants and younger children.

Arthritic effects are evident in two thirds of affected children and range from asymptomatic swelling around a single joint to painful tender swelling of several joints, most often the knees and ankles. The involvement is periarticular and resolves in a few days without permanent damage or deformity.

Two thirds of the children have gastrointestinal involvement manifested by recurrent colicky midabdominal pain often associated with nausea and vomiting. The stools contain gross or occult blood and mucus.

Renal involvement occurs in up to 50% of affected children and is potentially the most serious long-term complication. Initially the nephritis is manifest as hematuria, casts, and proteinuria. Although the majority of children with renal involvement recover completely, some develop chronic renal disease with eventual renal failure.

Diagnostic evaluation

Diagnosis is usually established on the basis of clinical manifestations. Laboratory tests are employed to assess gastrointestinal and renal involvement and to determine adequacy of hematostatic function.

Therapeutic management

Management is primarily supportive with close observation for signs of renal or gastrointestinal manifestations. Edema, rash, malaise, and arthralgia are usually managed with appropriate analgesics, such as acetaminophen, and mild sedation if necessary. Corticosteroids may be prescribed for relief of more severe edema, arthralgia, and colicky abdominal pain but are not warranted in all cases.

The majority of children recover without the need for hospitalization and, in most instances, a single acute episode clears spontaneously within a month. Others may have periodic recurrences for as long as 2 to 3 years before permanent remission from symptoms. Rarely death occurs from severe gastrointestinal complications, acute renal failure, or central nervous system involvement.

Nursing considerations

Nursing care of the child hospitalized with Henoch-Schönlein purpura is primarily supportive with vigilant observation for signs of complications. Vital signs are taken and recorded at regular intervals, specimens obtained for laboratory examination, and medication administered as prescribed. Urine and stools are carefully observed for fresh and occult blood.

If the child suffers from joint pain positioning, careful movement and administration of analgesics help reduce discomfort. Anaglesics also relieve the discomfort of fever and malaise. More severe involvement such as gastrointestinal symptoms and nephritis are managed as for any such disorder (see appropriate nursing care).

The child may be concerned about the unsightly appearance of the rash. He and his parents can be reassured that it is only a temporary phenomenon and encourage wearing of clothing that helps to hide the rash, such as long sleeves, pants, and robe. Emphasizing good grooming and attractive apparel help promote a more positive self-image.

MUCOCUTANEOUS LYMPH NODE SYNDROME (MCLS) (KAWASAKI DISEASE [KD])

Mucocutaneous lymph node syndrome, or Kawasaki disease, is an acute febrile illness of unknown etiology that occurs primarily in infants and young children. In the United States the peak incidence is 3 years of age, with a slightly higher incidence in males. In Japan, where it was first described, the peak incidence is 9 to 12 months of age. There appears to be no regional, seasonal, or socioeconomic prevalence associated with the disease, and no organism or environmental toxins have been implicated. There is some evidence to indicate that susceptibility is associated with histocompatibility antigens, however.

Pathophysiology

The principal area of involvement is the cardiovascular system. During the initial stage of the illness there is extensive inflammation of the arterioles, the venules, and the capillaries, which later progresses to include the main coronary arteries, the heart, and the larger veins. When death occurs, it is usually the result of coronary thrombosis or severe scar formation and stenosis of the main coronary artery.

Clinical manifestations

The child appears ill with a prolonged high fever that is unresponsive to antibiotics, and within 5 days of onset develops inflamed mucous membranes of the eye and oropharynx and diffuse and tender indurative swelling and erythema of the extremities, followed by characteristic desquamation. The cervical lymph nodes are often enlarged. In addition, the child may display other signs, including diarrhea, photophobia, tympanitis, and arthralgia and arthritis, especially involving the larger joints such as elbows, wrists, knees, and ankles.

Diagnostic evaluation

Diagnosis is established on the basis of the clinical findings. The child must exhibit five of the following six criteria, including fever:

1. Fever for 5 or more days
2. Bilateral congestion of the ocular conjunctiva without exudation
3. Changes of the mucous membranes of the oral cavity, such as erythema, dryness, and fissuring of the lips, oropharyngeal reddening, or ''strawberry tongue''
4. Changes in the extremities, such as peripheral edema, peripheral erythema, and desquamation of palms and soles—particularly periungual peeling
5. Polymorphous rash, primarily of the trunk
6. Cervical lymphadenopathy

No laboratory tests are of significant value in the diagnosis of the disease.

Therapeutic management

There is no definitive treatment for the disease; therefore, the management is primarily supportive and aimed at controlling fever, preventing dehydration, and minimizing possible cardiac complications. Large doses of aspirin are administered in the acute stage to control fever and symptoms of inflammation and during the recovery period to prevent platelet aggregation. Corticosteroids may be administered. Monitoring the cardiac status for possible complications is essential in follow-up care.

Nursing considerations

The nursing care of children with Kawasaki disease is primarily concerned with assisting in the diagnosis and case finding, supportive treatment as outlined by the physician, and supportive care to the child and family during both the acute and the chronic phases of the illness. Nurses should be aware that children with prolonged fever may be victims of this disorder and should encourage early medical evaluation. Administration of aspirin involves an understanding of the reasons for administration and teaching the family how it can best be administered, the importance of compliance, and the early signs of toxicity. The child requires careful monitoring during the acute phase and conscientious follow-up in the chronic phase. It is during the long-term stage of the disease that the nurse can be especially valuable in monitoring progress and preparing the child for health visits and diagnostic tests that may be ordered to assess cardiac status, such as echocardiography and electrocardiography. The importance of nutrition, hygiene, and normal activities is emphasized.

REFERENCES

Centers for Disease Control: Follow-up on toxic shock syndrome, Morbid. Mort. Weekly Rep. **29**:441-445, 1980.

BIBLIOGRAPHY
General cardiac

Coats, K.: Non-invasive cardiac diagnostic procedures, Am. J. Nurs. **75**:1980-1984, 1975.
Cortez, A., Mendoza, M., and Muniz, G.: The utilization of nurses in expanded roles to deliver pediatric cardiology health care, Pediatr. Nurs. **1**(3):22-29, 1975.
Freis, P.C.: Sounds of a healthy heart, Issues Compr. Pediatr. Nurs. **3**(7):1-4, 1979.
Friedberg, D.Z., and Caldart, L.: A center for pediatric cardiovascular patients, Am. J. Nurs. **75**(9):1480-1482, 1975.
Hedenkamp, E.A.: Humanizing the intensive care unit for children, Crit. Care Q. **3**(1):63-73, 1980.
Reif, K.: A heart makes you live, Am. J. Nurs. **72**(6):1085, 1972.
Shor, V.Z.: Long-term implications of cardiovascular disease. Issues Compr. Pediatr. Nurs. **2**(5):36-50, 1978.

Werner, B.L.: Cardiovascular crises. In Vestal, K.W.: Pediatric critical care nursing, New York, 1981, John Wiley & Sons.
Westfall, U.E.: Electrical and mechanical events in the cardiac cycle, Am. J. Nurs. **76**:231-235, 1976.

Cardiac catheterization

Armstrong, F., and Finesilver, C.: Cardiac catheterization, Crit. Care Update **10**(7):39-46, 1983.
Cogen, R.: Preventing complications during cardiac catheterizations, Am. J. Nurs. **76**(3):401-405, 1976.
Hinz, E.: Coping strategies of a two year old girl hospitalized for cardiac catheterization, Maternal Child Nurs. J. **9**(1):1-6, 1980.
Tesler, M., and Hardgrove, C.: Cardiac catheterization: preparing the child, Am. J. Nurs. **73**:80-82, 1983.
Uzark, K.: A child's cardiac catheterization—avoiding potential risks, Am. J. Maternal Child Nurs. **3**(3):158-161, 1978.
Youssef, M.M.: Self control behaviors of school-age children who are hospitalized for cardiac diagnostic procedures, Maternal Child Nurs. J. **10**:219-284, 1981.

Congenital heart disease

Bindler, R.M.: Home care for a child with a cardiac defect, Issues Compr. Pediatr. Nurs. **3**(7):48-60, 1979.
Cloutier, J., and Measel, C.P.: Home care for the infant with congenital heart disease, Am. J. Nurs. **82**:100-103, 1982.
D'Antonio, I.G.: Cardiac infant's feeding difficulties, West. J. Nurs. Res. **1**:53-55, 1979.
Gottesfeld, I.B.: The family of the child with congenital heart disease, Am. J. Maternal Child Nurs. **4**:101-104, 1979.
Meyer, R.A., and Lindower, B.: Management of the symptomatic neonate with congenital heart disease, Heart Lung **3**:392-395, 1974.
Sacksteder, S., Congenital heart defects. Embryology and fetal circulation, Am. J. Nurs. **78**:262-264, 1978.
Sacksteder, S., Gildea, J.H., and Dassy, C.: Common congenital cardiac defects, Am. J. Nurs. **78**(2):266-272, 1978.
Sasso, S.C.: Prostaglandin 1 for infants with congenital heart disease, Am. J. Maternal Child Nurs. **8**:29, 1983.
Shor, V.Z.: Congenital cardiac defects: assessment and case finding, Am. J. Nurs. **78**(2):256-261, 1978.
Weinberg, A.D., Christiansen, C.H., and Wise, D.J.: Respiratory rate: forgotten clue in the early detection of congenital heart disease, Pediatr. Nurs. **3**(3):38-41, 1977.

Cardiac surgery

Filipek, J.E.: Post-operative care of the pediatric cardiac patient, Crit. Care Q. **3**(1):45-52, 1980.
Gildea, J.H., and others: Congenital heart defects; pre- and postoperative nursing care, Am. J. Nurs. **78**:273-278, 1978.
Hazinski, M.F.: Critical care of the pediatric cardiovascular patient, Nurs. Clin. North Am. **16**:671-679, 1981.
Kaplan, S., Achtel, R.A., and Callison, C.B.: Psychiatric complications following open-heart surgery, Heart Lung **3**:423-428, 1974.
Lewandowski, L.A.: Stresses and coping styles of parents of children undergoing open-heart surgery, Crit. Care Q. **3**:75-84, 1980.
Miles, M.S.: Impact of the intensive care unit on parents, Issues Compr. Pediatr. Nurs. **3**(7):72-90, 1979.
Peterson, M.C.: Preparation of the cardiac child and the family for surgery, Issues Compr. Pediatr. Nurs. **3**(7):61-71, 1979.

Congestive heart failure

Agarevala, B., and Boffes, T.: Congestive heart failure in the infant, Heart Lung **5:**63-68, 1976.

Albeit, S., and others: Recognizing digitalis toxicity, Am. J. Nurs. **77**(12):1935-1945, 1977.

Cohen, S.: New concepts in understanding congestive heart failure. I. How the clinical features arise, Am. J. Nurs. **81**(1):119-142, 1981.

Cohen, S.: New concepts in understanding congestive heart failure. II. How the therapeutic approaches work, Am. J. Nurs. **81**(2):357-380, 1981.

Jackson, P.L.: Digoxin therapy at home: keeping the child safe, Am. J. Maternal Child Nurs. **4**(2):105-109, 1979.

McCauley, K.: Probing the ins and outs of congestive heart failure, Nursing '82 **12**(11):60-65, 1982.

Modrcin, M.A., and Schott, J.: An update on congestive heart failure in infants, Issues Compr. Pediatr. Nurs. **3**(7):6-22, 1979.

Smith, K.M.: Recognizing cardiac failure in neonates, Am. J. Maternal Child Nurs. **4**(2):98-100, 1979.

Infective endocarditis

Jenkins, J.: Infective endocarditis: a clinical overview, Crit. Care Update **10**(5):42-47, 1983.

Updated antibiotic labeling for prevention of bacterial endocarditis, FDA Drug Bull. **10**(2):12-13, 1980.

Hypertension

Botwin, E.D.: Should children be screened for hypertension? Am. J. Maternal Child Nurs. **1**(3):152-158, 1976.

Britton, C.V.: Blood pressure measurement and hypertension in children, Pediatr. Nurs. **7**(4):13-17, 1981.

Buckley, K.M.: Pediatric and adolescent hypertension, Crit. Care Update **6**(2):14-26, 1979.

Greenfield, D., Grant, R., and Lieberman, E.: Children can have high blood pressure, too, Am. J. Nurs. **76:**770-772, 1976.

Grim, C.M., and Grim, C.E.: The nurse's role in hypertension control, Fam. Comm. Health **4:**29-40, 1981.

Hill, M.N., and Foster, S.B.: Seeking and finding all those patients with high blood pressure, Nursing 82 **12**(2):72-75, 1982.

Hutchins, L.N.: Drug treatment of high blood pressure, Nurs. Clinics North Am. **16:**365-376, 1981.

Long, M.L., and others: Hypertension: what patients need to know, Am. J. Nurs. **75:**765-770, 1976.

Loustau, A., and Blair, B.J.: A key to compliance: systematic teaching to help hypertensive patients follow through on treatment, Nursing 81 **11:**84-87, 1981.

Maloney, R.J.: Hypertension update! Crit. Care Update **9**(10):7-18, 1982.

Marcinek, M.A.: Hypertension, Crit. Care Update **9**(3):22-32, 1982.

Marsh B., Dubes, M., and Boosinger, J.K.: Adolescent hypertension and significant variables: weight, height, and skinfold thickness, Pediatr. Nurs. **9:**287-289, 1983.

Mitchell, E.S.: Protocol for teaching hypertensive patients, Am. J. Nurs. **77:**808-809, 1977.

Moser, M.: Hypertension: how therapy works, Am. J. Nurs. **80:**937-941, 1980.

Nauright, L.P., and others: Identifying hypertensive adolescents, Pediatr. Nurs. **5**(2):34-37, 1979.

Pasternack, S.B.: Hypertension in children and adolescents, Issues Compr. Pediatr. Nurs. **3**(7):23-47, 1979.

Vogel, M.A.: Hypertension in children, Pediatr. Nurs. **3**(6):37-39, 1977.

Shock

Barrows, J.J.: Shock demands drugs, Nursing 82 **12**(2):34-41, 1982.

Lamb, L.S.: You think you know septic shock, Nursing 82 **12**(1):34-43, 1982.

Molyneux-Luick, M., and Knecht, J.: Hypovolemic shock, Nursing 77 **7**(11):32-37, 1977.

Purcell, J.A.: Shock drugs. Standardized guidelines, Am. J. Nurs. **82:**965-975, 1982.

Taylor, M.: When to anticipate septic shock, Nursing 75 **5**(4):34-38, 1975.

Thompson, M.A.: Shock syndrome: mechanisms and manifestations, nursing intervention, and evaluation, Reading, Mass., 1978, Addison-Wesley Publishing Co., Inc.

Thorp, G.D.: Shock: the overall mechanisms, Am. J. Nurs. **74:**1108-1122, 1974.

Toxic shock syndrome

Brown, B.S.: Tampons, teen-agers, and toxic shock syndrome (editorial), Pediatr. Nurs. **7**(3):7, 1981.

Brown, L.K.: Toxic shock syndrome, Am. J. Maternal Child Nurs. **6:**57-60, 1981.

Cestaro-Seifer, D.J.: Developing an instructional unit on toxic shock syndrome for adolescent girls, Issues Compr. Pediatr. Nurs. **6:**107-126, 1983.

Stein, A.P., and Baughman, D.C.: Nursing implications of toxic shock syndrome, Crit. Care Update **8**(6):17-19, 1981.

Toxic shock syndrome: an update, Crit. Care Update **8**(2):33-35, 1981.

Kawasaki disease

Hall, C.B.: Exploring clues to Kawasaki disease, Patient Care, Aug. 15, 1980, pp. 64-81.

L'Orange, C.: Kawasaki disease: a new threat to children, Am. J. Nurs. **83:**558-562, 1983.

Lynch, M.H., and Gray, J.L.: Kawasaki disease, Pediatr. Nurs. **8:**96-101, 1982.

Sealy, S.: Kawaski disease: a worldwide problem, Am. J. Maternal Child Nurs. **5:**331-334, 1980.

Yanagihara, R., and Todd, J.K.: Acute febrile mucocutaneous lymph node syndrome, Am. J. Dis. Child. **134:**603-614, 1980.

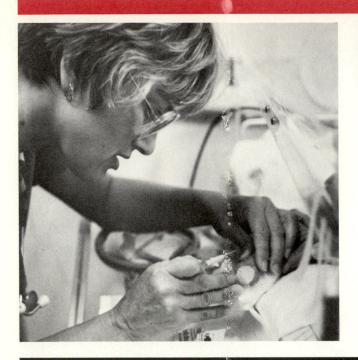

THE CHILD WITH DYSFUNCTION OF THE BLOOD OR THE BLOOD–FORMING ORGANS

OBJECTIVES

On completion of this chapter the reader will be able to:

- Distinguish between the various categories of anemia

- Describe the prevention of and care of the child with iron-deficiency anemia

- Compare the pathophysiology and care of children with sickle cell anemia and thalassemia major

- Describe the mechanisms of inheritance and nursing care of the child with hemophilia

- Relate the pathophysiology and clinical manifestations of leukemia

- Demonstrate an understanding of the rationale of therapies for neoplastic disease

- Outline a plan of care for the child with neoplastic disease and his family

- Contrast the pathophysiology and management of the immune-deficiency disorders

NURSING DIAGNOSES

Nursing diagnoses identified for the child with a disorder of the blood or blood forming organs include, but are not restricted to, the following:

Health perception-health management pattern

- Injury, potential for, related to (1) increased tendency to bleed; (2) presence of infective organisms; (3) damaged tissues

Nutritional-metabolic pattern

- Nutrition, alterations in: less than body requirements related to (1) anorexia; (2) increased metabolism

- Nutrition, alteration in: potential for more than body requirements related to inactivity

- Skin integrity, impairment of: related to effects of disease process

Activity-exercise pattern

■ Activity intolerance related to weakness

■ Diversional activity deficit related to hospitalization

■ Mobility, impaired physical, related to physical weakness

■ Self-care deficit: feeding, bathing/hygiene, dressing/grooming, toileting, related to (1) developmental level; (2) discomfort; (3) immobility

Sleep-rest pattern

■ Sleep pattern disturbance related to (1) discomfort; (2) schedule of therapies

Cognitive-perceptual pattern

■ Comfort, alteration in, pain related to physical injury

■ Sensory-perceptual alteration: visual, auditory, related to protective isolation

Self-perception—self-concept pattern

■ Anxiety related to (1) strange environment; (2) perception of impending events; (3) separation; (4) anticipated discomfort; (5) knowledge deficit; (6) pain

■ Fear related to perception of disease process

■ Powerlessness related to perceived lack of control

■ Self-concept disturbance in: body image, self-esteem related to perception of (1) effects of disease; (2) unrealistic self-expectations

Role-relationship pattern

■ Family process, alteration in, related to situational crisis

■ Parenting, alterations in: potential related to (1) skill deficit; (2) family stress

■ Social isolation related to (1) impaired mobility; (2) perception of body (3) physical isolation

Coping-stress tolerance pattern

■ Coping, family: potential for growth

■ Coping, ineffective family: compromised related to (1) situational crisis; (2) knowledge deficit; (3) temporary family disorganization

Disorders involving the blood and/or blood-forming organs in childhood encompass a wide range of diseases and pathologic states. Since the blood is a multipurpose fluid concerned with the functions of so many tissues and organs, either primary or secondary changes in the blood are reflected in the essential functions of these structures. Disorders of blood and blood-forming organs in childhood include the anemias, defects in hemostasis, neoplastic disorders, and the immunologic-deficiency disorders.

THE ANEMIAS

Anemia is defined as a condition in which the number of red blood cells and/or the hemoglobin concentration is reduced below the range of values found in healthy persons. As a result of this decrease the oxygen-carrying capacity of the blood is diminished, causing a reduction in the oxygen available to the tissues.

GENERAL CONCEPTS

The anemias constitute the most common hematologic disorders of infancy and childhood. Anemia is an indication or manifestation of a nutritional deficiency or of an underlying pathologic process or disease. Therefore, it is important that the cause be determined by appropriate laboratory examination before extensive therapeutic measures are instituted.

Classification of anemia

Anemias are classified in several ways under the broad categories of etiology and morphology.

Etiology. Etiologic factors are those in which the anemia results from (1) excessive blood loss or destruction (hemolysis), or (2) a decrease or impairment in the rate of production of red blood cells (erythrogenesis). Excessive loss occurs in acute or chronic hemorrhage (either internal or external). Excessive hemolysis is caused by either an intracorpuscular defect (usually a hereditary defect such as sickle cell disease) or an extracorpuscular factor (such as infectious agents, chemicals, or immune mechanisms).

Impaired production occurs when there is (1) a deficiency in products required for synthesis of red cells or hemoglobin (such as nutritional deficiencies), (2) diseases or chemicals that depress the bone marrow, (3) mechanical interference and replacement by abnormal cells (such as occurs in neoplastic disease), and (4) defective erythropoiesis (such as takes place in a number of diseases).

Morphology. Morphologic changes in red blood cells are described as *normocytic* in which cell size and shape are normal, *microcytic* in which cell size is smaller than normal, or *macrocytic* in which cell size is larger than normal. In any of these three types the hemoglobin may be sufficient *(normochromic)* or reduced *(hypochromic)*.

Clinical manifestations

Most of the clinical manifestations of anemia are attributed directly to tissue hypoxia. Muscle weakness and easy fatigability are common, although children seem to have a remarkable ability to function quite well despite low levels of hemoglobin. The skin is usually pale; a waxy pallor is seen with severe anemia. Cyanosis (the result of the quantity of deoxygenated hemoglobin in arterial blood) is typically not evident. Central nervous system manifestations include headache, dizziness, light-headedness, irritability, slowed thought processes, decreased attention span, apathy, and depression. Growth retardation resulting from decreased cellular metabolism and coexisting anorexia is a common finding in chronic severe anemia. It is frequently accompanied by delayed sexual maturation in the older child.

The effects of anemia on the circulatory system can be profound. Because the viscosity of blood depends almost entirely on the concentration of red blood cells, the resulting hemodilution of severe anemia decreases peripheral resistance, causing greater quantities of blood to return to the heart. As a result, the cardiac workload is markedly increased (especially during exercise, infection, or emotional stress), and cardiac failure may ensue.

Diagnostic evaluation of erythrocytes

Several tests are used to evaluate the morphologic and quantitative changes that result from anemia. These include red blood cell (RBC) count, hemoglobin (Hb), hematocrit (Hct) or packed cell volume (PCV), mean corpuscular volume (MCV), mean corpuscular hemoglobin (MCH), mean corpuscular hemoglobin concentration (MCHC), reticulocyte count, and a stained peripheral blood smear. In general, few physiologic disturbances take place because of decreased oxygen-carrying capacity of the blood until the Hb falls below 7 to 8 g/100 ml. Therefore, a hemoglobin below this level is considered diagnostic of anemia. In all anemias the measurement of the packed cell volume, which reflects the total mass of cells in a unit volume of blood, serves as an essential guide for diagnosis and therapy. (See Appendix A for normal values.) Other tests used to diagnose the underlying cause of anemia are included in the discussion of the particular disorder.

Therapeutic management

The objective of medical management is to reverse the anemia by treating the underlying cause and to make up for any deficiency of blood, blood component, or substance the blood needs for normal functioning. For example, blood or blood cells are replaced after hemorrhage; in nutritional anemias the specific deficiency is replaced. In cases of severe anemia supportive medical care may include oxygen therapy, bed rest, and replacement of intravascular volume with intravenous fluids.

Nursing considerations

Since anemia is not a disorder but a symptom of some underlying problem, nursing care is directed toward determining the cause, fostering appropriate supportive and therapeutic treatments, and decreasing tissue oxygen requirements.

IRON DEFICIENCY ANEMIA

Anemia that is caused by an inadequate supply of dietary iron is the most prevalent nutritional disorder in the United States. It occurs most frequently in children between 6 and 24 months of age and during adolescence. The prevalence of iron deficiency anemia in these age-groups is a result of the rapid growth rate of each and because of the poor eating habits of adolescents.

Etiology and pathophysiology

Iron is stored in the fetal erythrocytes, liver, spleen, and bone marrow during the final weeks of gestation. These iron stores are adequate for the first 4 to 5 months of life in the full-term infant but are reduced considerably in premature infants or infants of multiple births. When exogenous sources of iron are not supplied to meet the infant's growth demands following depletion of fetal iron stores, iron deficiency anemia results. The primary cause is an inadequate supply of iron in the diet, usually the result of excessive milk intake and delayed addition of solid foods. Other factors include inadequate iron stores at birth, impaired absorption, blood loss, lactose intolerance, or excessive demands for iron required for growth. Less commonly it may be caused by deficiency diseases such as pernicious anemia.

Clinical manifestations

The clinical manifestations of iron deficiency anemia are directly attributed to the reduction in the amount of oxygen available to tissues and do not differ from those in other types of anemia. The signs are usually insidious and obscure and the severity is directly related to the duration of the dietary deficiency.

Frequently infants with iron deficiency anemia are overweight because of excessive milk ingestion (so-called milk babies). These children become anemic when milk, a poor source of iron, is given almost to the exclusion of solid foods. Although chubby, these infants are pale, usually demonstrate poor muscle development, and are prone to infection. The skin color is sometimes described as porcelain-like.

Diagnostic evaluation

Since iron deficiency primarily affects hemoglobin synthesis, laboratory tests are usually performed that measure or describe hemoglobin, the morphologic changes in the red blood cell, and iron concentration. For the purpose of differential diagnosis, a stool analysis for occult blood (guaiac test) is frequently performed to confirm or rule out the possibility of chronic fecal blood loss, especially from milk (lactose) intolerance or structural anomalies, such as diverticulitis.

Therapeutic management

Nutritional anemia is usually treated with oral iron supplements. Ferrous iron, more readily absorbed than ferric iron, results in higher hemoglobin levels. Dietary addition of iron-rich foods is usually inadequate as a sole treatment for iron deficiency anemia because the iron is poorly absorbed and provides insufficient supplemental quantities of iron. Therefore, oral iron supplements are prescribed for approximately 3 months to replace body stores. Ascorbic acid appears to facilitate absorption of iron and may be prescribed in addition to the iron preparation.

If the hemoglobin is very low or if levels fail to rise after 1 month of oral therapy, intramuscular injections of iron dextran (Imferon) are administered. Transfusions are indicated for the most severe anemia and, in cases of serious infection, cardiac dysfunction, or surgical emergency where anesthesia is required. Packed red cells, not whole blood, should be used to minimize the chance of circulatory overload. Supplemental oxygen is administered when tissue hypoxia is severe.

Nursing considerations

There are several considerations in the administration of iron preparations and in the instruction of parents for administration. When iron dextran is ordered, it must be injected deeply into a large muscle mass using the Z-tract method, and the injection site should not be massaged after injection to minimize skin staining and irritation. Since no more than 1 ml should be given in one site, multiple injections are sometimes required.

An essential nursing responsibility is instructing parents in the administration of iron. It should be given as prescribed in three divided doses between meals when the presence of free hydrochloric acid is greatest, because more iron is absorbed in the acid environment of the upper gastrointestinal tract. A citrus fruit or juice taken with the medication aids in absorption. An adequate dosage of iron turns the stools a tarry green color. The nurse advises parents of this normally expected change and inquires about its occurrence on follow-up visits. Absence of the greenish black stool may be a clue to poor administration of iron, either in schedule or in dosage. Vomiting and/or diarrhea are not uncommon complications of iron therapy. If the parents report these symptoms, the iron can be given with meals and the dosage reduced and gradually increased until tolerated.

Liquid preparations of iron may temporarily stain the teeth. If possible the medication should be taken through a straw or given through a syringe or medicine dropper placed toward the back of the mouth. Brushing the teeth after administration of the drug lessens the discoloration.

The primary nursing objective is prevention of nutritional anemia through parent education. The nurse discusses with parents the importance of using iron-fortified formula and the introduction of solid foods by 5 to 6 months of age. The best solid food source of iron is the commercial infant cereals.

One of the difficulties in discouraging the parents from feeding milk to the exclusion of other foods is dispelling the popular myth that milk is a ''perfect food.'' Many parents believe that milk is best for the infant and equate the resultant weight gain with a ''healthy child.'' The nurse can also stress that overweight is not synonymous with good health.

SICKLE CELL ANEMIA

Sickle cell anemia is one of a group of diseases collectively termed *hemoglobinopathies,* in which normal adult hemoglobin (hemoglobin A or HbA) is partly or completely replaced by an abnormal hemoglobin. Sickle cell disease includes all those hereditary disorders, the clinical, hematologic, and pathologic features of which are related to the presence of sickle hemoglobin (HbS). The degree of dysfunction is directly related to the amount of HbS contained in the red blood cells. The gene that determines the production of HbS is situated on an autosome; therefore, the inheritance is essentially that of any autosomal recessive disorder (see p. 49). Heterozygous persons who have hemoglobin containing both normal HbA and abnormal

HbS are said to have *sickle cell trait*. Persons who are homozygous have predominantly HbS and suffer from *sickle cell anemia*.

Sickle cell anemia is observed primarily in blacks, although infrequently it affects caucasians, especially those of Mediterranean descent. The incidence of the disease varies in different geographic locations. Among American blacks, the incidence of sickle cell trait ranges between 7% and 13.4%. In East Africa the incidence is reported to be as high as 45% among native blacks. The high incidence of sickle cell trait in these individuals is believed by some to be the result of selective protection afforded trait carriers against malaria caused by one specific parasite.

Sickle cell–hemoglobin C (HbC) disease is the second most frequent form of sickle cell anemia in black Americans. Persons can have various combinations of the abnormal hemoglobins, including the thalassemias, but this discussion is restricted to HbS.

Pathophysiology

Hemoglobin S is structurally different from hemoglobin A. Under conditions of decreased oxygen tension and lowered pH, the relatively insoluble HbS changes its molecular structure to form long slender crystals. The rapid growth of these crystals causes the formation of crescent or sickle-shaped red blood cells. These rigid cells, unable to flow through a narrow diameter, accumulate and obstruct the flow of blood through small vessels (Fig. 23-1). The thickened blood slows the circulation, causing capillary stasis, obstruction by elongated and pointed erythrocytes, and thrombosis. Eventually tissue ischemia and necrosis result with pathologic changes in tissues and organs that constitute the sickle cell crisis.

This decreased blood flow causes further oxygen depletion and more sickling. The body responds by rapidly destroying these fragile sickled cells before the process can be reversed, producing a severe anemia.

Clinical manifestations

In addition to the effects of sickling on various organ structures, the child with sickle cell anemia may have a variety of complaints, such as weakness, anorexia, joint, back, and abdominal pain, fever, and vomiting. Although sickle cell anemia has been reported during the neonatal period and early part of infancy, it most commonly is recognized after 4 months of age when fetal hemoglobin (HgF) levels are diminished. It is particularly apparent during the toddler and preschool period, and is frequently first diagnosed during a crisis that follows acute upper respiratory or gastrointestinal infection.

Other generalized effects include growth retardation in

SUMMARY OF NURSING CARE OF THE CHILD WITH ANEMIA

GOALS	RESPONSIBILITIES
Assist in establishing diagnosis	Take careful history regarding common causes of anemia in childhood Assist with diagnostic tests Be aware of significance of various blood tests
Prepare the child for laboratory tests	Explain to older children the need for repeated venipunctures or fingersticks for blood analysis, particularly why a sequence of tests is required Allow children to play with laboratory equipment and/or participate with test Older children may enjoy looking at blood smears under a microscope or at pictures of blood cells Explain to the parents the reason for replacing withdrawn blood and the need for forming tests
Decrease tissue oxygen needs Minimize physical exertion	Assess the child's level of physical tolerance Anticipate and assist the child in those activities of daily living that may be beyond his tolerance Provide diversional play activities that promote rest and quiet but prevent boredom and withdrawal Choose an appropriate roommate of similar age and interests and one who requires restricted activity
Minimize emotional stress	Anticipate the child's irritability, short attention span, and fretfulness by offering to assist him in activities rather than waiting for him to ask Assess the parents' awareness of the child's need for dependency to conserve strength Explain to older children and their parents the reason for behavioral changes caused by anemia Encourage the parents to remain with the child
Prevent and observe for infection	Place the child in room with noninfectious children; restrict visitors with active illnesses Advise visitors (and hospital personnel) to practice good handwashing Report any temperature elevation to the physician Observe for leukocytosis Maintain adequate nutrition
Promote safety	Alert ancillary hospital personnel regarding the child's physical tolerance and need for assistance during activity Keep the side rail raised and use safety restraints when applicable
Improve tissue oxygenation	Administer oxygen as indicated Monitor for benefit of oxygen but avoid prolonged use
Observe for complications Cardiac decompensation	Be alert to signs of heart failure from excessive cardiac demands or from cardiac overload during blood transfusion

Transfusion reaction	Practice all precautions
	  Check blood with another nurse and physician to ensure correct blood group/type with that of the child
	  Run blood slowly and remain with the child for infusion of initial 50 ml
	  Stop blood immediately if any untoward reaction occurs
	  Attach blood to piggyback setup with normal saline or other intravenous solution to maintain open venous line
	Observe for signs and symptoms of reaction

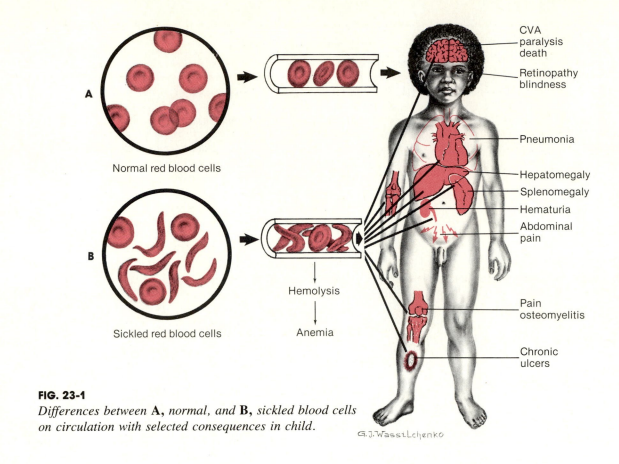

FIG. 23-1

*Differences between **A,** normal, and **B,** sickled blood cells on circulation with selected consequences in child.*

G.J.Wassilchenko

both height and weight, delayed sexual maturation, decreased fertility, and priapism (constant penile erection). If the child reaches adulthood, sexual development and adult height are usually achieved.

Diagnostic evaluation

The simplest of the various methods to detect sickling is to produce deoxygenation by placing a drop of blood on a slide and covering it with a sealed cover slip. Eventually sickling of the red blood cell occurs. The hemoglobin electrophoresis ("fingerprinting") test is accurate, rapid, and specific for detecting the homozygous and heterozygous forms of the disease, as well as the percentage of the various hemoglobins.

For screening purposes either the sickling test or the sickle-turbidity test (Sickledex) is commonly used. The Sickledex is a reliable screening method because it can be performed on blood from a fingerstick and because it yields accurate results in 3 minutes. However, it does not differentiate between the trait and the disease, and it yields false negatives in anemic children (hemoglobin less than 10 g/100 ml) or in infants less than 4 to 6 months of age who have not completely converted to adult hemoglobin. If the test is positive, hemoglobin electrophoresis is nec-

essary to distinguish between those children with the trait and those with the disease.

Therapeutic management

There is no cure for sickle cell anemia. The aims of therapy are (1) to prevent the sickling phenomenon, which is responsible for the pathologic sequelae, and (2) to treat sickle cell crisis, which constitutes a medical emergency. Prevention consists of promoting adequate oxygenation and maintaining hemodilution. The successful implementation of these two goals depends more often on nursing interventions than on medical therapies.

Medical management of a crisis is usually directed at supportive and symptomatic treatment. The main objectives are to provide (1) bed rest to minimize energy expenditure and oxygen use, (2) hydration through oral and intravenous therapy, (3) electrolyte replacement, (4) analgesics for the severe abdominal and joint pain, (5) blood replacement to treat anemia, and (6) antibiotics to treat any existing infection. Administration of the newly developed pneumococcal and meningococcal vaccine is recommended for these children who are over 2 and 5 years of age, respectively, because of their susceptibility to infection as a result of functional asplenia.

Short-term oxygen therapy may be helpful in severe anoxia, especially in children with cardiac failure. Although oxygen may prevent more sickling, it usually is not effective in reversing sickling, because the oxygen is unable to reach the enmeshed sickled erythrocytes in clogged vessels.

Exchange transfusion, which reduces the number of circulating sickle cells and slows down the vicious cycle of hypoxia, thrombosis, tissue ischemia, and injury, has been successful. The procedure is sometimes advocated as a possible preventive technique. However, multiple transfusions carry the risk of hepatitis, hemosiderosis, and transfusion reactions.

The spleen is the major site of sickling, sequestration (pooling of blood), and destruction of red blood cells in children with recurrent splenic sequestration. Therefore, splenectomy may be a life-saving measure. However, since the spleen usually atrophies on its own through progressive fibrotic changes, routine splenectomy is not recommended, especially since any procedure that requires anesthesia has increased risk for these children.

Nursing considerations

The primary nursing objectives are (1) preventing sickling and (2) helping the child and parents adjust to a lifelong, potentially fatal, hereditary disease. Many of the measures that prevent sickling are also appropriate when a crisis occurs. In addition, special cautions are mandatory when the child undergoes surgery of any kind. Nurses may also be faced with the dilemmas of sickle cell screening and their role in genetic counseling. Taking time to establish a sound basis of understanding why certain measures are beneficial to the child encourages parents to practice them.

To prevent tissue hypoxia the child should avoid situations that cause increased cellular metabolism. This includes (1) strenuous physical activity (especially contact sports if the spleen is enlarged, since rupture will cause massive internal hemorrhage), (2) emotional stress, (3) environments of low-oxygen concentration, such as high altitudes or nonpressurized airplane flights, and (4) known sources of infection. If the child has even a mild infection, the parents must seek medical attention at once.

The nurse emphasizes the importance of adequate hydration to prevent sickling and to delay the stasis-thrombosis-ischemia cycle in a crisis. It is seldom sufficient to advise parents to ''force fluids'' or ''encourage drinking.'' They need specific instructions on how many glasses or bottles of fluid are required. Many foods are also a source of fluid, particularly soups, gelatin, and puddings; these can be included as liquid sources. Parents are advised to be particularly alert during situations where dehydration may be a possibility, such as hot weather, and to recognize early signs of reduced intake, such as decreased urine output.

Forced fluids combined with renal diuresis result in the problem of enuresis. Parents who are unaware of this fact frequently employ the usual measures to discourage bedwetting, such as limiting fluids at night, and many revert to punishment and shame to force bladder control. It is advisable to treat the enuresis as a complication of the disease, such as joint pain or some other symptom, in order to alleviate parental pressure on the child.

Since infection is often a predisposing factor toward a crisis and since the body's natural ability to resist infection is compromised, the nurse stresses to parents the importance of adequate nutrition, frequent medical supervision, and isolation from known sources of infection. The last measure must be tempered with an awareness of the child's need for living a normal life.

The need for a surgical procedure poses an additional risk for the child with sickle cell anemia. The main surgical risk is hypoxia from anesthesia. However, emotional stress, the demands of wound healing, and the possibility of infection potentially increase the sickling phenomenon, both in children with the disease and in those with the trait. The primary nursing objectives are aimed at minimizing each of these threats preoperatively and postoperatively.

Promote supportive therapies during crises. The success of many of the medical therapies relies heavily on nursing implementation. Management of pain is an especially difficult problem and often involves experimentation with various analgesics and schedules before relief is achieved. Heat to the affected area is often soothing, as well as passive exercises to promote circulation. Applying cold compresses to the area is avoided, because this enhances sickling and vasoconstriction.

Bed rest is usually well tolerated during a crisis, although actual rest depends a great deal on pain alleviation and organized schedules of nursing care. Although the object of bed rest is to minimize oxygen consumption, some activity, particularly passive range of motion exercises, is beneficial to promote circulation. Usually the best course of action is to let the child dictate his activity tolerance.

Intake, especially intravenous fluids, and output are recorded. The child's admission weight serves as a baseline for evaluating hydration. Vital signs and blood pressure are also closely monitored for impending shock. If blood transfusions or exchange transfusions are administered, the nurse has the responsibility of observing for signs of transfusion reaction. Since hypervolemia from too rapid transfusion can increase the workload of the heart, the nurse also is alert to signs of cardiac failure.

If oxygen is administered, the nurse notes the child's response in terms of decreased pain and improved physical

SUMMARY OF NURSING CARE OF THE CHILD WITH SICKLE CELL ANEMIA

GOALS	RESPONSIBILITIES
Recognize sickle cell disease	Be alert for signs and symptoms in infants and children of black or Mediterranean descent
	Assist with diagnostic procedures
	Prepare the child and family for procedures
Explain the disease	Inform the parents and older children of basic defect and measures that promote sickling
	Stress importance of informing significant health personnel of the child's condition and benefit of Medic Alert tag
	Explain signs of developing crisis, especially fever, pallor, and pain
Prevent sickling	
Promote tissue oxygenation	Explain prevention measures
	Avoid strenuous physical exertion
	Avoid emotional stress
	Prevent infection
	Avoid low oxygen environment
Promote hydration	Calculate recommended daily fluid intake and base the child's fluid requirements on this *minimum* amount
	Give parents written instructions regarding specific quantity of fluid required
	Encourage the child to drink
	Teach parents signs of dehydration
	Stress importance of avoiding overheating as source of fluid loss
Prevent infection	Stress importance of adequate nutrition, protection from known sources of infection and frequent medical supervision
	Report any sign of infection to the physician immediately
Promote supportive therapies during crisis	
Control pain	Administer analgesics
	Position for comfort
	Apply warmth to painful areas
Promote rest	Maintain bed rest
	Schedule caregiving activities to allow for optimum rest
Assure adequate hydration	Record intake and output
	Monitor intravenous fluids carefully
	Observe for signs of hydration; diuresis is not a valid indication
	Observe for electrolyte imbalance

status and reports signs of diminished therapeutic benefit, such as restlessness, increased pallor, and continued pain.

Screening and genetic counseling. Although screening children for sickle cell anemia is generally accepted since it allows earlier, more prevention-oriented treatment, there is much controversy concerning the proposed benefits and potential hazards of screening for the trait. One of the basic issues behind this controversy involves genetic counseling. Since the carrier is generally asymptomatic, there is little direct benefit in informing him of his genetic makeup. The advantages of trait identification lie in selective reproduction of offspring not afflicted with hemoglobin S.

Long-term care. Besides genetic counseling, parents need the opportunity to discuss their feelings regarding transmitting a potentially fatal, chronic illness to their child. Because of the widely publicized prognosis for children with sickle cell anemia, many parents express their prevalent fear of the child's death. Prognosis varies; the greatest risk is usually in children under 5 years of age;

SUMMARY OF NURSING CARE OF THE CHILD WITH SICKLE CELL ANEMIA—cont'd

GOALS	RESPONSIBILITIES
Replace blood	Administer blood Observe for signs of transfusion reactions and cardiac overload
Increase tissue oxygenation	Administer oxygen Promote circulation through passive range of motion exercises Monitor for evidence of benefit from oxygen
Observe for complications of crises	Monitor for evidence of increasing anemia; use appropriate nursing interventions Measure size of spleen, if ordered Monitor for signs of shock Assess neurologic status for evidence of cerebrovascular accident
Decrease surgical risks	Keep the child well hydrated Decrease fear through appropriate preparation Avoid unnecessary exertion Promote pulmonary hygiene postoperatively Use passive range of motion exercises to promote circulation Observe for signs of infection
Prevent psychologic problems	Encourage normal activities and relationships within the child's capabilities Implement measures to reduce the unpleasant side effects of the disease, such as enuresis Explore feelings and attitudes toward disease, its side effects, and its complications
Promote long-term care	Allow the parents to express their feelings regarding transmitting disease to offspring Refer to public health nurse for follow-up in home Refer the child for medical care through comprehensive sickle cell clinic Refer the parents to agencies that provide assistance and education Discuss prognosis, especially increased chances of survival when sickling is prevented Care for the child as one with life-threatening illness
Prevent sickle cell anemia Screening	Participate in screening programs Be aware of controversial aspects of screening and genetic control
Genetic counseling	Refer all heterozygous (HbSA) parents for genetic counseling Reinforce basics of trait transmission, especially concerning subsequent pregnancies Discuss with parents their feelings regarding selective birth methods
Public education	Participate in education projects, dissemination of literature, and political decisions

the majority of deaths in these children are caused by overwhelming infection. However, as the child grows older, the crises usually become less severe and less frequent. Since there is no way to predict which child will follow a favorable course, nursing care for the family should be the same as for any family with a child with a life-threatening illness. Particular emphasis is placed on the siblings' reactions, the stress on the marital relationship, and the child-rearing attitudes displayed toward the child (see Chapter 16).

The nurse advises parents to inform all treating personnel of the child's condition. The use of a Medic Alert bracelet is another way of ensuring awareness of the disease. Some people view such identification as "negative labeling." The nurse can stress the positive benefits of displaying this information, especially in emergencies when the use of anesthesia may be required.

THALASSEMIA MAJOR (COOLEY ANEMIA)

The term "thalassemia," which is derived from the Greek word "thalassa" meaning sea, is applied to a variety of inherited blood disorders characterized by deficiencies in the rate of production of specific globin chains in hemoglobin. The name appropriately refers to descendents of or those people living near the Mediterranean sea who have the highest incidence of the disease, namely, Italians, Greeks, and Syrians. There is evidence to suggest that the high incidence of the disorders among these groups is a result of selective advantage of the trait to malaria, as is postulated in sicklemia.

β-Thalassemia is the most common of the thalassemias and occurs in a heterozygous (minor) form which produces a mild microcytic anemia, and in a homozygous (major) form (also known as Cooley anemia), which results in an anemia of variable severity.

Pathophysiology

Normal postnatal hemoglobin is composed of equal amounts of α- and β-polypeptide chains. In β-thalassemia there is a partial or complete deficiency in the synthesis of the β-chain of the hemoglobin molecule. Consequently, there is a compensatory increase in the synthesis of α-chains, and γ-chain production remains activated, resulting in defective hemoglobin formation. This unbalanced polypeptide unit is very unstable; when it disintegrates it damages the red blood cells, causing severe anemia.

To compensate for the hemolytic process an overabundance of red blood cells is formed. This excessive and largely ineffective erythropoietic activity causes a hyperexpansion of the bone marrow volume that is reflected in skeletal abnormalities of the involved bone. Especially noticeable are those of the frontal, malar, and maxillary bones. Extramedullary hematopoiesis causes enlargement of the liver, spleen, and kidneys. Excess iron from hemolysis of supplemental erythrocytes in transfusions and from the rapid destruction of defective red blood cells is stored in various organs (hemosiderosis).

Clinical manifestations

The onset of thalassemia major is usually insidious and is usually not recognized until the latter half of infancy. Signs of anemia, unexplained fever, poor feeding, and a markedly enlarged spleen, particularly in a child of Mediterranean extraction, are descriptive of β-thalassemia. The bone changes from accelerated medullary hematopoiesis produce characteristic facies in older children: (1) an enlarged head, (2) prominent frontal and parietal bosses, (3) prominent malar (cheek bone) eminences, (4) a flat or depressed bridge of the nose, (5) enlargement of the maxilla, with protrusion of the lip and upper central incisors and eventual malocclusion, and (6) a mongoloid appearance to the eyes. Other features that are common to these children are small stature, infantile genitalia, a bronzed freckled complexion, and protrusion of the abdomen from hepatosplenomegaly.

With progressive anemia one can also expect to see signs of chronic hypoxia, including headache, precordial and bone pain, decreased exercise tolerance, listlessness, and anorexia. Another common symptom in these children is frequent epistaxis, although the exact reason for this is unknown. Hyperuricemia and gout from rapid cellular catabolism are also seen. In those children who require multiple transfusions for several years, the eventual effects of hemochromatosis (iron storage with cellular damage) in various organs are evident.

Diagnostic evaluation

Hematologic studies reveal the characteristic changes in the red blood cells and immature erythrocytes. Low hemoglobin and hematocrit levels are seen in severe anemia, although they are typically lower than the reduction in red blood cell count because of the proliferation of immature erythrocytes. Hemoglobin electrophoresis confirms the diagnosis, and radiographs of involved bones reveal characteristic findings.

Therapeutic management

There is no specific treatment and no known cure for children with thalassemia major. The objective of supportive therapy is to maintain sufficient hemoglobin levels to prevent tissue hypoxia. Transfusions are the foundation of medical management, although they greatly increase the risk of siderosis (excess iron in blood and tissues). At the present time there is no completely successful method of preventing excessive iron storage, although the use of the iron-chelating agent deferoxamine (Desferal or DFO), which increases iron excretion, is the current treatment of choice.

In some children with severe splenomegaly who require repeated transfusions, a splenectomy may be necessary to decrease the disabling effects of abdominal pressure and to increase the life span of supplemental red blood cells. A major postsplenectomy complication is severe and overwhelming infection. Therefore, these children are usually kept on prophylactic antibiotics with close medical supervision for many years and are considered candidates for the pneumococcal and meningococcal vaccines.

Nursing considerations

The objectives of nursing care involve (1) observing for complications of multiple blood transfusions, (2) assisting the child in coping with the effects of the illness, and (3)

SUMMARY OF NURSING CARE OF THE CHILD WITH β-THALASSEMIA (Cooley anemia)

GOALS	RESPONSIBILITIES
Recognize thalassemia early	Be alert for signs and symptoms in older infants or young children of Mediterranean descent (Italian, Greek, Syrian)
Assist with diagnosis	Order or collect blood for analysis Order and assist with radiographs
Prevent infection	Avoid contact with persons with infections Administer prophylactic antibiotics
Increase circulating hemoglobin and prevent tissue hypoxia	Assist with administration of whole blood or packaged red cells
Prepare for surgical care	Prepare the child and family for surgery (if applicable) Provide postoperative care
Prevent complications Transfusion reaction	Carry out careful observation during transfusion
Hemosiderosis	Administer chelating agents as ordered
Folic acid deficiency	Administer folic acid
Fractures	Instruct the child to avoid activities that increase the risk of fractures
Cholelithiasis	Observe for signs of cholecystitis in adolescents
Support the child during tests and procedures	Prepare the child for procedures according to age and level of understanding Remain with the child
Assist the child to cope with disorder and its effects	Explore the child's feelings about being different from other children Emphasize the child's abilities and focus on realistic endeavors Encourage quiet activities, creative efforts, and ''thinking'' games Emphasize good hygiene and grooming Encourage interactions with peers Help plan therapies and medical care so they do not interfere with the child's regular activities and social interaction Assist the child with vocational planning Introduce the child to other children who have adjusted well to this or a similar disorder
Support the parents	Explore feelings of guilt regarding the hereditary nature of the disease Institute appropriate teaching Refer to appropriate agencies for additional assistance: financial, social, and supportive Emphasize the need for the child to lead as normal a life as possible Help the family deal with the potentially fatal nature of the disease
Prevent occurrence of thalassemia	Refer for genetic counseling Reinforce and clarify counseling information

fostering the parents' and child's adjustment to a life-threatening illness. Basic to each of these goals is explaining to parents and older children the defect responsible for the disorder and its effect on red blood cells. Since the prevalence of this condition is high among families of Mediterranean descent, the nurse also inquires regarding the family's previous knowledge about thalassemia. All families with a child with thalassemia should be tested for the trait and referred for genetic counseling.

The prognosis of thalassemia major is variable and relies heavily on the severity of the anemia. The chief cause of death is heart failure, and, once signs of this complication become evident, death may occur within a year. Unfortunately it is not possible to predict which severely afflicted child will follow a more favorable course. Since many children with the severe form die before puberty and since few survive beyond the third decade, thalassemia is considered a potentially fatal disease. The nurse must care for families of these children in light of this knowledge. (See also Chapter 16.)

APLASTIC ANEMIA

Aplastic anemia refers to a condition in which all formed elements of the blood are simultaneously depressed. The peripheral blood smear demonstrates pancytopenia or the triad of profound anemia, leukopenia, and thombocytopenia. *Hypoplastic anemia* is characterized by a profound depression of erythrocytes but normal or slightly decreased white blood cells and platelets. Aplastic anemia can be primary (congenital) or secondary (acquired).

Etiology

The best known congenital disorder of which aplastic anemia is an outstanding feature is *Fanconi syndrome*. The syndrome appears to be inherited as an autosomal-recessive trait with varying penetrance; therefore, affected siblings may demonstrate several different combinations of defects. Prognosis is variable but is better than for acquired types. The treatment is the same as for other causes of aplastic anemia.

Several factors contribute to the development of acquired hypoplastic anemia, including suppressed erythropoiesis from multiple transfusion therapy, hemolytic syndromes, such as sickle cell anemia, infections, toxic substances, drugs, and autoimmune or allergic states. The following discussion, however, focuses on acquired aplastic anemia, which carries a poorer prognosis and follows a more rapidly fatal course than the primary types.

The most common causes of acquired aplastic anemia are (1) irradiation; (2) drugs, such as the chemotherapeutic agents and several antibiotics, most notable of which is chloramphenicol; (3) industrial and household chemicals, including benzene and its derivatives, which are found in petroleum products, dyes, paint remover, shellac, and lacquers; (4) infections, especially hepatitis or overwhelming infection; (5) infiltration and replacement of myeloid elements, such as in leukemia or the lymphomas; and (6) idiopathic causes, in which no identifiable precipitating cause can be found. Prognosis is the worst for children in the idiopathic group. There is a generalized depletion of hematopoietic elements in the bone marrow caused by insufficient stem cells or some factor that limits their ability to proliferate.

Clinical manifestations and diagnosis

The onset of clinical manifestations, which include anemia, leukopenia, and decreased platelet count, is usually insidious, not unlike that seen in leukemia. Definitive diagnosis is determined from bone marrow aspiration, which demonstrates the conversion of red bone marrow to yellow, fatty bone marrow.

Therapeutic management

The objectives of treatment are to eliminate the causative agent whenever possible and to provide therapeutic approaches, including (1) supportive care, such as transfusions to maintain hemoglobin levels and prevent tissue hypoxia and antibiotic therapy for intercurrent infections, (2) androgens to stimulate erythropoiesis and glucocorticoids to offset the bone-maturing effects of the androgens, (3) immunosupressives, and (4) bone marrow transplantation, the current treatment of choice for severe aplastic anemia.

Response to drug therapy is usually gradual. Elevations in hemoglobin and red blood cells may take as long as 3 to 6 months. During this period the child must be protected from infection and hemorrhage and treated for the anemia with transfusions. Unfortunately the prognosis is poor. The mortality rate is about 70% for acquired aplastic anemia. Almost 50% of these children die within 4 to 6 months after diagnosis. Prospects for improved survival lie in preventing the condition and in researching better approaches to treatment.

Nursing considerations

The care of the child with aplastic anemia is similar to that of the leukemic child (p. 758)—specifically, preparing the family for the diagnostic and therapeutic procedures, preventing complications from the severe pancytopenia, and emotionally supporting them in terms of a potentially fatal outcome. Since each of these nursing considerations is discussed in the section on leukemia, only the exceptions are presented here.

Testosterone produces several undesirable effects that, when combined with the effects of steroid therapy, such as moon face, result in dramatic body image alterations. The virilizing effects of testosterone include deepening of the voice, hirsutism, growth of pubic hair, enlargement of the penis in males, flushing of the skin, and acne. Potentially testosterone can cause muscular and skeletal maturation, resulting in severely retarded height in a young child. Not only are these changes difficult to accept, they are especially difficult to explain to children not approaching puberty. Parents may feel embarrassed because they are unprepared for the sexual changes.

The nurse can help by deemphasizing the sexual nature of the effects and by matter-of-factly explaining each in the same tone as moon face, truncal obesity, and so on. Expressing embarrassment or surprise to the child at observing mature sexual characteristics must be avoided. New members of the staff who may be assigned to care for the child need to be prepared for the experience of seeing a sexually mature ''6-year-old male with a slight beard and a deep masculine voice.''

Since chemotherapeutic agents are not used, many of the reactions, such as nausea and vomiting, alopecia, mucosal ulceration, and so on, are not encountered. However, extensive ecchymotic areas of the oral mucosa that result from thrombocytopenia require meticulous mouth care to prevent breakdown, bleeding, and infection. Fortunately these lesions are not painful, although their appearance may lead one to expect discomfort. Local anesthetics are not necessary, but anorexia is still a consequence because of the edematous nature of the lesions. Liquid, bland, and soft diets are usually tolerated best.

DEFECTS IN HEMOSTASIS

The body controls excessive bleeding through three processes: (1) vascular spasm, (2) platelet aggregation, and (3) coagulation and clot formation. Defects in platelets and clotting factors are the most common causes of bleeding during childhood. The following discussion focuses on the major conditions that require nursing intervention. The reader is urged to apply these principles to other medical conditions that involve similar nursing considerations.

HEMOPHILIA

The term *hemophilia* refers to a group of bleeding disorders in which there is a deficiency of one of the factors necessary for coagulation of the blood. Although the symptomatology is similar despite the missing factor, the identification of specific factor deficiencies has allowed definitive treatment with replacement agents.

In about 80% of all cases of hemophilia, the inheritance is demonstrated as X-linked recessive. The two most common forms of the disorder are classic hemophilia (hemophilia A or factor VIII deficiency) and Christmas disease (hemophilia B or factor IX deficiency). The following discussion is primarily concerned with the classic form, which accounts for about 75% of all cases.

Pathophysiology

The basic defect of hemophilia A is a deficiency of factor VIII—antihemophilic factor (AHF) or antihemophilic globulin (AHG). This factor is necessary for the formation of thromboplastin in phase I of blood coagulation. The degree of severity of the disease is inversely correlated with the amount of antihemophilic globulin found in the blood. The source of the factor in the body is unknown.

Clinical manifestations

The effect of hemophilia is prolonged bleeding anywhere from or in the body. With severe factor deficiencies hemorrhage can occur as a result of minor trauma, such as after circumcision, during loss of deciduous teeth, or as a result of a slight fall or bruise.

Subcutaneous and intramuscular hemorrhages are common. *Hemarthrosis,* bleeding into the joint cavities, especially the knees, ankles, and elbows, is the most frequent type of internal bleeding and often results in bone changes and, consequently, crippling, disabling deformities. Spontaneous hematuria is not uncommon. Epistaxis may occur but is not as frequent as other kinds of hemorrhage. Children are very reliable in telling the examiner where a bleed is.

Bleeding into the tissue can occur anywhere, but it is serious if it occurs in the neck, mouth, or thorax, since the airway can become obstructed. Intracranial hemorrhage can result in fatal consequences, although this occurs less frequently than expected because the brain tissue has a high concentration of thromboplastin. Hemorrhage anywhere along the gastrointestinal tract can lead to obstruction, and hematomas in the spinal cord can cause paralysis.

Petechiae are uncommon in persons with hemophilia because repair of small hemorrhages depends on platelet function, not on blood-clotting mechanisms.

Diagnostic evaluation

The diagnosis is usually made on a history of bleeding episodes, evidence of X-linked inheritance (only one third are new mutations), and laboratory findings. The tests specific for hemophilia are those that depend on specific factors for a reaction to occur, such as the partial thromboplastin time test, thromboplastin generation test, and prothrombin consumption test. Specific determination of factor deficiencies requires assay procedures normally performed in specialized laboratories.

Therapeutic management

The primary therapy for hemophilia is to prevent spontaneous bleeding by replacement of the missing factor VIII. The products currently used, either alone or in conjunction, are (1) *cryoprecipitated AHF,* a concentrated form of AHF that also contains fibrinogen and immunoglobulins and that has less risk of hepatitis, and (2) *lyophilized AHF*, an easily stored AHF concentrate to be reconstituted with sterile water immediately before use.

Vigorous therapy is instituted to prevent chronic crippling effects from joint bleeding. If replacement therapy is begun immediately, local measures such as ice applications and splinting are seldom needed. Local application of ε-aminocaproic acid (Amicar) prevents clot destruction; however, its use is limited to mouth surgery or trauma. Assistive devices, such as splints or traction, may be recommended and surgical decompressive procedures are sometimes needed for muscle bleeds.

A regular program of exercise and physical therapy is an important aspect of management. Physical activity, within reasonable limits, strengthens muscles around joints, which will help retard or confine bleeding in the area.

Treatment without delay results in more rapid recovery and a decreased likelihood of complications; therefore, most hemophiliac children are treated at home. The family is taught the technique of venipuncture and to administer the AHF to children over 3 years of age. The child himself learns the procedure for self-administration at 9 to 12 years of age. Home treatment is highly successful and the rewards, in addition to the immediacy, are less disruption of family life, fewer school or work days missed, and enhancement of the child's self-esteem.

Nursing considerations

The objectives for nursing care can be divided into immediate needs and long-term goals. The most immediate consideration is control of bleeding episodes. However, the ultimate adjustment and prognosis for the hemophiliac person rely heavily on the family's ability to cope with the disorder, to learn effective methods of control and prevention, and to temper child-rearing practices with judicious protection from injury while fostering independence and development.

Decrease risk of injury. Prevention of bleeding through control of behavior is not an easy task. During infancy and toddlerhood the normal acquisition of motor skills creates innumerable opportunities for falls, bruises, and minor wounds. Restraining the child from mastering motor development can herald more serious long-term problems than allowing the behavior. However, the child and his environment can be made as safe as possible to minimize the incidental injuries (for example, padding the clothing of a toddler, especially the knees). Close supervision should be maintained during playtime.

One of the objectives for older children and for the family is preparation of the child for school. The nurse can help the family and school personnel plan jointly for an appropriate schedule of activity. Since almost all hemophiliacs are boys, the physical limitations in regard to active sports are a difficult adjustment. Encouraging the pursuit of intellectual and/or creative endeavors from early childhood helps foster a life-style that is fulfilling and less conflicting than one focused on unrealistic goals. Often within a group of children with the same health problem they can find acceptance, healthy competition, and a sense of camaraderie. In fact, such a setting may be the first time that these children have felt a sense of belonging, because, even with their sibling relationships, they commonly see themselves as outsiders. However, it may serve to emphasize their differentness.

Since the mucous membranes bleed easily, the young child is given food that is easily masticated. For the older child food choices need not be limited as long as he understands the need for chewing thoroughly and eating slowly. Dental care is very important and may require some readjustment in terms of daily hygiene. For example, the nurse can recommend using a Water Pik,* softening the toothbrush in warm water before brushing, or using a sponge-tipped disposable toothbrush, which is available in many drugstores. A regular toothbrush should be soft bristled and small in size. Adolescents also need to be advised of the dangers of shaving with a safety razor.

Diet is also an important consideration. Excessive body weight can increase the strain on affected joints, especially the knees, and predispose the child to hemarthrosis. Since limited activity is frequently the result of a more sedentary life-style and of occasional periods of bed rest after tissue bleeding, calories need to be supplied in accordance with energy requirements.

Since any trauma can lead to a bleeding episode, all persons caring for these children must be aware of their disorder. Children with hemophilia should wear Medic Alert identification, and older children are encouraged to recognize situations in which disclosing their condition is important. During procedures such as dental extraction or injections, health personnel need to take special precautions to stop the bleeding. Unnecessary venipunctures are avoided. A peripheral fingerstick is better for blood samples and the subcutaneous route is substituted for intramuscular injections whenever possible. Hemophiliac children need to avoid salicylates and any aspirin-containing compound. Aspirin inhibits platelet aggregation, prolongs bleeding time, and weakly inhibits prothrombin synthesis. Acetaminophen (Tylenol) is a suitable aspirin substitute, especially for use during control of pain at home.

Recognize and treat bleeding. Bleeding that occurs from a wound or that occurs close to the skin can be

---

*Teledyne Water Pik, 1730 E. Prospect St., Ft. Collins, CO 80525.

controlled by (1) applying pressure to the area for at least 10 to 15 minutes to allow clot formation, (2) immobilizing and elevating the area above the level of the heart to decrease blood flow, and (3) applying cold to promote vasoconstriction. By teaching parents and older children such measures beforehand, they can be prepared to initiate immediate treatment before blood loss is excessive. Plastic bags of ice should be kept in the freezer for such emergencies. If the bleeding does not stop within 15 minutes, the factor may need to be replaced. In a home-care program this would be done by the child or parent. In other situations the child would require emergency medical treatment.

The nurse, who is skilled in venipuncture techniques, is often the person who teaches families to administer AHF concentrates. The nurse must be familiar with the properties of the concentrates, for example factor VIII and to a lesser extent factor IX are very labile at room temperature. They must be stored at cool temperatures (slightly above freezing) and administered immediately after their preparation. To hasten the mixing process of reconstituting dried antihemophilic factor with diluent, the solution may be warmed or the vial gently rotated. Excessive heating or shaking of the container will cause loss of active antihemophilic factor. A filtered intravenous setup is usually supplied with the drug to filter any particles in the solution, and if the solution is not thoroughly mixed before administration, the filter will also remove the active factor.

Transfusion reactions and viral hepatitis are potential complications from replacement products. Transfusion reactions to cryoprecipitate and, to a lesser degree, the concentrates are possible because anti-A and anti-B isohemagglutinins are present in the solution. Hepatitis virus may have been transferred in the plasma from an infected donor. When cryoprecipitate is given, the plasma should be cross-matched to the recipient's blood type. The nurse teaches the parents and/or child the signs of transfusion reactions and stresses the need to notify a physician if they occur.

Currently there is widespread concern regarding the risk for contracting acquired immune deficiency syndrome (AIDS) from blood products. There have been a few reported cases in hemophiliacs, and this has generated high anxiety in parents to the extent that they are delaying treatment. This delay is reflected in an increase in the incidence of joint complications. Although the risk is relatively low, many families now prefer to solicit their own blood donors.

Foster independence. The discovery of factor concentrates has greatly changed the outlook for these children. With scheduled infusions of the missing factor, bleeding can be prevented and the child can live a much more normal, unrestricted life.

Constructive teaching about the disease and measures to control or prevent bleeding must follow a period of parental adjustment to the diagnosis (see Chapter 16 for suggestions for dealing with the parents of a chronically ill child). Genetic counseling is essential as soon as possible after diagnosis. Unlike many other disorders in which both parents carry the trait, the feeling of responsibility for this condition usually rests with the mother. Without an opportunity to discuss her feelings, the marital relationship can suffer. Technology is now available to identify carriers in approximately 80% of cases and may reduce the anxiety regarding childbearing in females who may be at risk of carrying the defective gene, such as sisters or maternal aunts of an affected male.

The needs of families with hemophiliac children are best met through a comprehensive team approach of physicians (pediatrician, hematologist, orthopedist), nurse, social worker, and physical therapist. Parent-group discussions are beneficial in meeting those needs often best met by similarly affected families. For example, with the improved prognosis for these children, parents and adolescent hemophiliacs are faced with vocational and financial problems in addition to concern over future childbearing. Once children reach 21 years of age, many insurance companies no longer wish to carry them. This can be disastrous in terms of the cost of treatment. A person with severe hemophilia may require factor replacement therapy and other medical treatments in excess of $20,000 a year. The National Hemophilia Foundation* provides numerous services and publications for both health providers and families.

THROMBOCYTOPENIC PURPURA

Idiopathic thrombocytopenic purpura (ITP) is an acquired hemorrhagic disorder that is characterized by (1) excessive destruction of platelets (thrombocytopenia) and (2) purpura (a discoloration caused by petechia beneath the skin). Although the cause is unknown, it is believed to be an autoimmune response to disease-related antigens. It is the most frequently occurring thrombocytopenia of childhood.

Clinical manifestations

Idiopathic thrombocytopenic purpura occurs in one of two forms: an acute, self-limiting course or a chronic condition interspersed with remissions. The acute form is most commonly seen after upper respiratory infections or after the childhood diseases measles, rubella, mumps, and chickenpox. The most common clinical manifestations of either

---

*25 W. 39th Street, New York, NY 10018.

SUMMARY OF THE NURSING CARE OF THE CHILD WITH HEMOPHILIA

GOALS	RESPONSIBILITIES
Prevent bleeding	Prepare and administer intravenous cryoprecipitate or concentrates as needed
Decrease risk of injury	Make environment as safe as possible Encourage pursuit of intellectual/creative activities Encourage the older child to choose activity but accept responsibility for own safety Plan with the schoolteacher appropriate activity schedule Confer with the school nurse regarding severity of bleeding episodes Discuss with the parents appropriate limit-setting patterns Stress need for oral hygiene using soft toothbrush or available substitute Discuss diet, especially effect of overweight on hemarthrosis Advise use of Medic Alert identification in case of emergency During nursing procedures, especially injections, use local measures to control bleeding

Control bleeding	Administer replacement factor immediately
	Apply local measures
	    Apply pressure to area for 10 to 15 minutes
	    Immobilize area
	    Elevate site to above level of heart
	    Apply cold compresses; encourage the family to have frozen plastic bags of water prepared in advance

Prevent crippling effects of joint degeneration	Administer replacement factor to control bleeding Institute passive range of motion exercises after acute phase Exercise unaffected joints and muscles Administer analgesics before physical therapy Avoid use of aspirin or its compounds; substitute acetaminophen for pain relief at home Consult with the physical therapist concerning exercise program Refer to the public health nurse and/or physical therapist for supervision at home Stress to the family serious long-range consequences of hemarthrosis Support any orthopedic measures in joint rehabilitation
Assist in coping with disorder	Provide opportunity for the parents and older child to adjust to discovery of diagnosis Assess factors that promote or retard the family's adjustment to crisis
Prevent the disorder	Refer the parents for genetic counseling, including identification of carrier offspring Assess the parents' understanding of X-linked inheritance Provide opportunity for the parents, especially the mother, to discuss feelings regarding genetic transmission
Support the parents	Refer to local chapter of National Hemophilia Foundation for parent groups Whenever possible provide care through comprehensive hemophilia program
Foster independence	Assess the family for potential strength in home-care program Institute appropriate teaching Encourage independence and self-help during hospitalizations Introduce the child to other hemophiliac children who have adjusted well Encourage the parents to promote sense of independence and responsibility in the older child Have the adolescent investigate job opportunities in appropriate vocation Discuss financial costs, especially insurance coverage at age 21 years Discuss future plans regarding marriage and childbearing; include daughters who carry the trait in discussion

type include (1) easy bruising with petechiae and/or ecchymoses, particularly over bony prominences, (2) bleeding from mucous membranes, such as epistaxis, bleeding gums, and internal hemorrhage with evidence of hematuria, hematemesis, melena, hemarthrosis, and hypermenorrhea, and (3) hematomas over the lower extremities that may result in chronic leg ulcers.

Therapeutic management

Management is primarily supportive since the course of the disease is self-limited in the majority of cases. Activity is restricted at the onset while the platelet count is low and while active bleeding or progression of lesions is occurring. This restriction is most easily accomplished in the hospital. Corticosteroids are employed for children with the highest risk for serious bleeding, for chronic cases with increased bleeding tendencies, as an adjunct to life-threatening hemorrhage, or before splenectomy to decrease the risk of surgical bleeding. Administration of intravenous gammaglobulin has proved successful in increasing the platelet count of children with chronic disease. Splenectomy is reserved for symptomatic children with chronic disease or as an emergency measure in the event of life-threatening hemorrhage. Packed red blood cells may be given to replace blood lost in symptomatic children. Platelets are seldom administered.

Nursing considerations

Nursing care is largely supportive and is directed toward restricting the activity of an otherwise normal child. Children and parents need careful explanations of the rationale behind the therapies employed and support in their efforts to comply.

The nursing considerations of controlling bleeding, preventing bruising, and preventing crippling effects of hemarthrosis are similar to those discussed in the section on hemophilia. The deleterious effects of using aspirin to control joint pain are critical for these children; therefore, salicylate substitutes should always be used.

DISSEMINATED INTRAVASCULAR COAGULATION (DIC)

Disseminated intravascular coagulation, also known as *consumption coagulopathy,* is not a primary disease. It is a secondary disorder of coagulation that complicates a number of pathologic processes (such as hypoxia, acidosis, shock, and endothelial damage) and many severe systemic disease states (such as congenital heart disease, necrotizing enterocolitis, gram-negative bacterial sepsis, rickettsial in-

fections, and some severe viral infections). The disease is characterized by inappropriate systemic activation and acceleration of the normal clotting mechanism.

Pathophysiology

Disseminated intravascular coagulation occurs when the first stage of the coagulation process is abnormally stimulated. Although there is no well-defined sequence of events, two distinct phases can be identified. First, when the clotting mechanism is triggered in the circulation, thrombin is generated in greater amounts than can be neutralized by the body. Consequently, there is rapid conversion of fibrinogen to fibrin with aggregation and destruction of platelets. If local and widespread fibrin deposition in blood vessels takes place, obstruction and eventual necrosis of tissues occur. Second, the fibrinolytic mechanism is activated, causing extensive destruction of clotting factors. With a deficiency of clotting factors the child is vulnerable to uncontrollable hemorrhage into vital organs. An additional complication is damage and hemolysis of red blood cells (Fig. 23-2).

Clinical manifestations

Signs of DIC are the same as those of many other diseases; this often confuses the diagnosis. There is evidence of bleeding: petechiae, purpura, bleeding from openings in the skin, such as a venipuncture site or surgical incision, hypotension, and dysfunction of organs from infarction and ischemia.

Diagnostic evaluation

DIC is suspected when there is an increased tendency to bleed, such as from venipuncture or blood taken from the heel and bleeding from umbilicus, trachea, or gastrointestinal tract. Hematologic findings include prolonged prothrombin (PT), partial thromboplastin (PTT), and thrombin times. There is a profoundly depressed platelet count, fragmented red blood cells, and depleted fibrinogen.

Therapeutic management

Treatment of DIC is directed toward control of the underlying or initiating cause, which, in most instances, stops the coagulation problem spontaneously. Platelets and fresh-frozen plasma may be needed to replace lost plasma components, especially in the child whose underlying disease remains uncontrolled. The extremely ill newborn infant may require exchange transfusion with fresh blood. The administration of heparin to inhibit thrombin formation is most often restricted to severe cases.

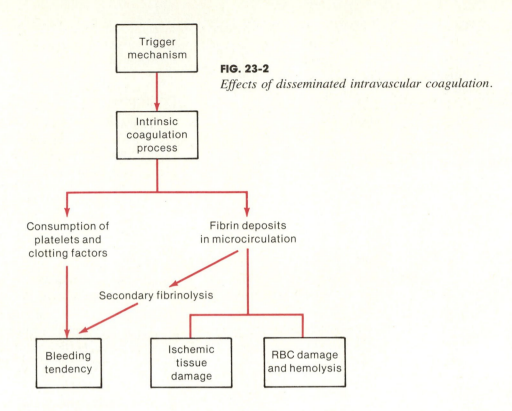

FIG. 23-2
Effects of disseminated intravascular coagulation.

Nursing considerations

The goals of nursing care are to be aware of the possibility of DIC in the severely ill child and to recognize signs that might indicate its presence. The skills needed to monitor intravenous infusion and blood transfusions and to administer heparin are the same as for any child receiving these therapies.

EPISTAXIS (NOSEBLEEDING)

Isolated and transient episodes of epistaxis, or nosebleeding, are common in childhood. The nose, especially the septum, is a highly vascular structure and bleeding usually results from direct trauma, including blows to the nose, foreign bodies, and nose picking, or from mucosal inflammation associated with allergic rhinitis and upper respiratory infections. The bleeding ordinarily stops spontaneously or with minimum pressure and requires no medical evaluation or therapy.

Recurrent epistaxis and severe bleeding may indicate an underlying disease, particularly vascular abnormalities, leukemia, thrombocytopenia, and clotting factor deficiency diseases, such as hemophilia and von Willebrand disease. Nosebleeds are sometimes associated with administration of aspirin, even in normal amounts. Persistent episodes of epistaxis require medical evaluation.

Nursing considerations

In the event of a nosebleed, the foremost intervention is to remain calm. If not, the child becomes more agitated, his blood pressure will increase, and he will not cooperate. To control the bleeding the child is instructed to sit up and lean forward (not to lie down) to avoid aspiration of blood. Most of the nosebleeding originates in the anterior part of the nasal septum and can be controlled by applying pressure to the soft lower portion of the nose with the thumb and forefinger. Pressure is maintained for at least 10 minutes to allow clotting to occur. During this time the child breathes through his mouth.

If bleeding has not stopped, a piece of cotton or tissue (on which some petroleum jelly has been placed) is inserted into each nostril and compressed for another 10 minutes. If the hemorrhaging continues, the child should be evaluated by a physician, who may pack the nose with epinephrine-soaked gauze.

After a nosebleed, petroleum jelly can be inserted into each nostril to prevent crusting of old blood and to lessen the likelihood of the child's picking at his nose and restarting the hemorrhage.

NEOPLASTIC DISORDERS

Neoplastic disorders are the leading cause of death from disease in children past infancy, and almost half of all childhood cancer involves the blood or blood-forming organs. Problems related to the various solid tumors of childhood are discussed elsewhere in relation to the tissues or organs involved.

The leukemias are neoplastic diseases of the blood-forming tissues; the lymphomas are a group of neoplastic diseases that arise from the lymphoid and reticuloendothelial system. Lymphomas are more common in males than in females and are usually divided into the Hodgkin and non-Hodgkin lymphomas. This discussion is concerned with the leukemias and the lymphomas.

LEUKEMIAS

Leukemia is the most common form of childhood cancer. It occurs more frequently in males than females after age 1 year, and the peak onset is between 2 and 5 years of age. It is one of the forms of cancer that has demonstrated dramatic improvements in survival rates. Before the use of antileukemic agents in 1948, a child with acute lymphocytic leukemia (ALL) lived only a few weeks or months. Today 5-year survival rates for children with ALL exceed 50% in major research centers, and a proportion of these children may be cured. However, even for the child with the most favorable prognosis, leukemia presents innumerable physical, emotional, financial, and familial stresses.

Classification

"Leukemia" is the broad term applied to a complex and heterogenous group of malignant diseases of the bone marrow and lymphatic system. Classification of the leukemias is necessary for therapeutic and prognostic purposes and is based on the morphologic (structural), cytochemical, and immunologic characteristics of the cells.

Morphology. Leukemia is classified according to its predominant cell type and level of maturity as follows:

Lympho—indicates leukemias involving the lymphoid or lymphatic system

Myelo—indicates those leukemias of myeloid (bone marrow) origin

Blastic and acute—indicate those leukemias involving immature cells

Cytic and chronic—indicate those leukemias involving mature cells

In children two forms of leukemia are generally recognized: (1) *acute lymphoid leukemia (ALL)* and *(2) acute nonlymphoid leukemia (ANLL)*. Synonyms for ALL include acute lymphatic, lymphocytic, lymphoblastic, and lymphoblastoid leukemia. The term "stem cell" or "blast cell" usually refers to the lymphoid type of leukemia. Synonyms for ANLL include myelogenous (AML), myelocytic, monocytic, monoblastic, monomyeloblastic, and acute granulocytic.

Because of the confusion and inconsistency in classifying the leukemias, ALL and ANLL are further subdivided after thorough study of the cell morphology. They are also classified according to whether or not they contain cell elements. These more definitive classifications are significant for purposes of prognosis but will not be discussed here.

Immunology. A number of cell-surface antigens allow for differentiation of ALL into three broad categories: T-lymphocytes (T cells), B-lymphocytes (B cells), or "null" cells (those cells that lack T or B cell characteristics). This further classification of lymphocytic leukemia appears to have prognostic importance in that persons with leukemias of the "null" category (about 85% of ALL) demonstrate better survival rates. Unfortunately, immunologic markers are not available for ANLL at the present time.

Prognostic factors

The three most important factors for determining long-term survival for childen with acute leukemia, in addition to treatment, are the type of cell involved, the initial white blood cell count (WBC), and the child's age at the time of diagnosis. The most optimistic outlook is for the child with ALL who has greater than a 90% chance to attain an initial remission; more than 50% are expected to survive for 5 years or more. With ANLL the chances of attaining an initial remission are about 75%, but with considerably shorter duration of remissions and higher mortality than for ALL.

Children with normal or low white blood count appear to have a much better prognosis than those with a high count. Children diagnosed between 2 and 10 years of age have consistently demonstrated a better outlook than those diagnosed before 2 or after 10 years of age, and females appear to have a more favorable prognosis than males. In addition, it appears that the more rapid is the induction of a remission in ANLL, the better is the chance for an ultimate long-term continuous remission.

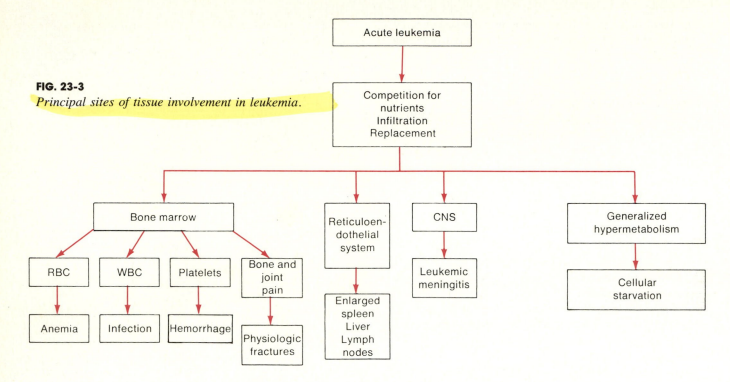

FIG. 23-3

Principal sites of tissue involvement in leukemia.

Onset

The precise time of onset of leukemia is unknown. Its clinical appearance varies markedly from acute to insidious. In most instances the child displays remarkably few symptoms. For example, it is quite typical for leukemia to be diagnosed when a minor infection, such as a cold, fails to completely disappear. The child continues to be pale, listless, irritable, febrile, and anorexic. Parents often suspect some underlying problem when they observe the weight loss, petechiae, bruising without cause, and continued complaints of bone and joint pain.

At other times leukemia is diagnosed after an extended history of signs and symptoms that mimic such conditions as rheumatoid arthritis or mononucleosis. There are also occasions when the diagnosis of leukemia accompanies some totally unrelated event, such as a routine physical examination or accidental injury.

The history not only yields valuable medical information regarding the subsequent course of the illness but also bears heavily on the parents' emotional reaction to the discovery of the diagnosis. In most instances the diagnosis is an unexpected revelation of catastrophic proportion.

Pathophysiology and clinical manifestations

Leukemia is an unrestricted proliferation of immature white blood cells in the blood-forming tissues of the body. Although not a "tumor" as such, the leukemic cells demonstrate the same neoplastic properties of solid cancers.

Therefore, the resulting pathology and clinical manifestations are caused by infiltration and replacement of any tissue of the body with nonfunctional leukemic cells. Highly vascular organs of the reticuloendothelial system are most severely affected.

In order to understand the pathophysiology of the leukemic process, it is important to clarify two common misconceptions. First, although leukemia is an overproduction of white blood cells, most often in the acute form the leukocyte count is low (hence, the term "leukemia"). Second, these immature cells do not deliberately attack and destroy the normal blood cells or vascular tissues. Cellular destruction takes place by infiltration and subsequent competition for metabolic elements (Fig. 23-3).

Bone marrow dysfunction. In all types of leukemia the proliferating cells depress the production of formed elements of the blood in bone marrow by competing for and depriving the normal cells of the essential nutrients for metabolism. The three main consequences are (1) *anemia* from decreased erythrocytes; (2) *infection* from neutropenia; and (3) *bleeding tendencies* from decreased platelet production.

The invasion of the bone marrow with leukemic cells gradually causes a weakening of the bone and a tendency toward physiologic fractures. As leukemic cells invade the periosteum, increasing pressure causes severe pain.

The most frequent presenting signs and symptoms of leukemia are a result of infiltration of the bone marrow. These include fever, pallor, fatigue, anorexia, hemorrhage (usually petechiae), and bone and joint pain. In the presence of neutropenia the body's normal bacterial flora can become aggressive pathogens. Any break in the skin is a potential site of infection. Frequently, vague abdominal pain is caused by areas of inflammation from normal flora within the intestinal tract.

Disturbance of involved organs.   The organs of the reticuloendothelial system—the spleen, liver, and lymph glands—demonstrate marked infiltration, enlargement, and eventually fibrosis. Hepatosplenomegaly is typically more severe than lymphadenopathy. Toxic chemotherapeutic agents seem to account for more liver and spleen damage than the disease process.

The next most important site of involvement is the central nervous system. Initially leukemic cells do not tend to invade this area, probably as a result of the protective blood-brain barrier. However, this normal protective mechanism also prevents the antileukemic drugs, with the exception of steroids, from entering the brain in sufficient therapeutic doses to be effective. The usual effect of leukemic infiltration is increased intracranial pressure, which causes the signs and symptoms normally associated with this condition, such as severe headache, vomiting, papilledema, irritability, lethargy, and eventually coma. Irritation of the meninges also causes pain and stiffness in the neck and back. Cranial nerves may be involved also and the signs and symptoms observed reflect the area affected.

Other sites of involvement in long-term disease include the kidneys, testes, prostate, ovaries, gastrointestinal tract, and lungs. With the increased length of survival becoming more common, it is likely that such sites of leukemic invasion will become more important clinically.

Hypermetabolism.   The immense metabolic needs of proliferating leukemic cells eventually deprive all body cells of nutrients necessary for survival. Muscle wasting, weight loss, anorexia, and fatigue are natural consequences. Obviously, in addition to the risk of death from infection and hemorrhage, uncontrolled growth of leukemic cells can also terminate in metabolic starvation.

Diagnostic evaluation

Leukemia is usually suspected by the history, physical manifestations, and a peripheral blood smear that contains immature forms of leukocytes, frequently combined with low blood counts. Definitive diagnosis is based on bone marrow aspiration or biopsy.

Once the diagnosis is confirmed, a lumbar puncture is performed to determine if there is any central nervous system involvement. Only about 10% of children demonstrate the presence of leukemic cells in the spinal fluid at the time of diagnosis.

Therapeutic management

Treatment of leukemia involves the use of chemotherapeutic agents and irradiation in three phases: (1) *induction therapy,* which achieves a complete remission or disappearance of all leukemic cells; (2) *sanctuary therapy,* which prevents leukemic cells from invading or destroying leukemic cells in those areas of the body normally protected from cytotoxic drug levels; and (3) *maintenance therapy,* which serves to maintain the remission phase. Although the combination of drugs and radiation may vary according to institutions and the type of leukemia being treated, the following general principles for each phase are quite consistently employed.

Remission induction.   Almost immediately after confirmation of the diagnosis, induction therapy is begun and lasts 4 to 6 weeks. The two main drugs used for induction in ALL are oral corticosteroids (especially prednisone) and intravenous vincristine, with the possible addition of doxorubicin or asparaginase (L-asparaginase). Since the use of combination-drug therapy has been more successful in inducing remissions than single-agent schedules, the two drugs are used simultaneously.

The chemotherapeutic agents used to treat leukemia cause massive cell destruction resulting in the formation of uric acid, which can eventually accumulate and precipitate in the renal tubules. Therefore, allopurinol is administered in conjuncion with these drugs to inhibit the formation of uric acid. Diuresis is also helpful in assuring an adequate excretion of the harmful metabolites.

A complete remission is determined by the absence of leukemic cells in the bone marrow and disappearance of all signs and symptoms of the disease. Since many of the drugs also cause suppression of some blood elements, the period immediately following a remission can be critical when the child is highly susceptible to invading organisms and spontaneous hemorrhage.

Sanctuary therapy.   The second phase of therapy consists of prophylactic treatment of the central nervous system with cranial irradiation and/or intrathecal administration of methotrexate. Therapy is usually begun during the first 6 to 8 weeks after diagnosis and consists of daily high-dose radiation treatments for about 2 weeks and weekly or twice weekly doses of methotrexate for a total of five to six injections. An alternative therapy involves combination chemotherapy without irradiation.

The testes have been found resistant to chemotherapy and a site of relapse; therefore, a routine bilateral testicular biopsy is often recommended to identify any evidence of disease and to implement aggressive therapy in that area.

Maintenance therapy.   Maintenance or continuation therapy is begun after completion of successful induction and sanctuary therapy to preserve the remission and further lessen the number of leukemic cells. It most often begins after the child is discharged from the hospital and when blood values begin to approach normal levels. As with induction therapy, combined drug regimens have been more successful in maintaining remissions and preventing drug resistance. Also, during maintenance therapy weekly or monthly complete blood counts are taken to evaluate the marrow's response to the drugs.

Reinduction therapy. For many children a fourth phase of therapy becomes necessary when a relapse occurs, as evidenced by the presence of leukemic cells within the bone marrow. Usually reinduction includes the use of prednisone and vincristine with a combination of other drugs not previously used. Sanctuary and maintenance therapy follow as outlined before if a remission is induced.

Bone marrow transplant. Bone marrow transplants have been used successfully for treating children who have ANLL or poor-prognosis ALL. The most promising results have occurred when transplantation is performed during a remission rather than a relapse.

Nursing considerations

Nursing care of the child with leukemia is directly related to the regimen of therapy. Secondary complications that necessitate supportive physical care are caused by myelosuppression, drug toxicity, and leukemic infiltration. Although this discussion is primarily concerned with the physical problems requiring nursing care, it also focuses on the specific emotional needs during diagnosis, treatment, and relapse. The general psychologic interventions during each phase of therapy are discussed in Chapter 16.

Prepare family for diagnostic and therapeutic procedures. From the time before diagnosis to cessation of therapy, children must undergo several tests, the most traumatic of which are bone marrow aspiration or biopsy and lumbar punctures. Multiple fingersticks and venipunctures for blood analysis and drug infusion are common occurrences for several years after the diagnosis. Therefore, the child needs an explanation of why each procedure is done and what can be expected.

Prevent complications of myelosuppression. The leukemic process and most of the chemotherapeutic agents cause myelosuppression. The reduced numbers of blood cells result in secondary problems of infection, bleeding tendencies, and anemia. Supportive care involves both medical and nursing management. Because they are so closely linked, they are discussed together rather than separately.

Infection. The most frequent cause of death from leukemia is overwhelming infection. The leukemic child is most susceptible to overwhelming infection during three phases of his disease: (1) at the time of diagnosis and relapse when the leukemic process has replaced normal leukocytes, (2) during immunosuppressive therapy, and (3)

after prolonged antibiotic therapy that predisposes to the growth of resistant organisms.

Because the usual viral infecions of childhood are particularly dangerous, the child is not immunized against these diseases until his immune system is capable of responding appropriately to the vaccine. If given when the immune system is depressed, the attenuated virus can result in an overwhelming infection. (Salk vaccine for poliomyelitis is recommended in lieu of Sabin's oral vaccine.)

The first defense against infection is prevention. When the child is hospitalized, the nurse employs all measures to control transfer of infection. This may include strict protective isolation or, more frequently, the use of a private room, restriction of all visitors and health personnel with active infection, and strict handwashing technique with an antiseptic solution. In some research centers special germ-free environments are available during complete myelosuppression from intensive chemotherapy or for bone marrow transplant.

If an infection does not respond to antibiotics, transfusions of concentrated granulocytes obtained by leukapheresis (removal of white blood cells only from the donor) can be administered.

Febrile reactions from leukocyte antigens are common, especially from repeated transfusions. Although the patient may experience moderate to severe chills and an elevated temperature, this is not an indication to stop the transfusion. The nurse records and reports these reactions and explains their significance to the child and family. Also, if the child's blood type is rare, parents are encouraged to locate suitable donors in case leukocytes or platelets are needed.

At home, parents should encourage quiet periods during the day, such as before dinner and bedtime, to avoid exhaustion. A well-rested child is more likely to resist infection than one who is continually fatigued.

Nutrition is another important component of infection prevention. An adequate protein-calorie intake provides the child with better host defenses against infection and increased tolerance to chemotherapy and irradiation. However, providing optimum nutrition during periods of anorexia is a tremendous challenge.

Hemorrhage. Epistaxis and gingival bleeding are the most common bleeding complications of myelosuppression; therefore, the nurse teaches parents and older children measures to control bleeding. Pressure at the site without disturbing clot formation is the general rule.

Since infection increases the tendency toward hemorrhage, and since bleeding sites become more easily infected, a combined effort at controlling and preventing infection and hemorrhage has cumulative beneficial effects. Skin care is important, and special care is taken in cleaning all puncture sites, such as fingersticks, venipunctures, and intramuscular injections. Meticulous mouth care is essential since gingival bleeding is a frequent problem. Because of various drugs the rectal area is prone to ulceration; therefore, feces and urine are removed immediately and the perineal area washed. Frequent turning, the use of a flotation or alternating-pressure mattress, and sheepskin placed under bony prominences prevent pressure areas and decubitus ulcers.

Before the use of transfused platelets, hemorrhage was a leading cause of death in leukemia. Now most bleeding episodes can be prevented or controlled with judicious administration of platelet concentrates or platelet-rich plasma. These therapies are generally reserved for active bleeding episodes that do not respond to local treatment.

During bleeding episodes the parents and child need a good deal of emotional support. The sight of oozing blood is very upsetting. Often parents will request a platelet transfusion, unaware of the need to try local measures first. The nurse can be instrumental in allaying anxiety by explaining the reason for delaying a platelet transfusion until absolutely necessary.

Anemia. Initially anemia from complete replacement of the bone marrow by leukemic cells may be profound. During induction therapy, blood transfusions with whole blood or packed red cells may be necessary to raise hemoglobin to levels approaching 10 g. The nurse institutes usual precautions in caring for the anemic child (p. 741).

Manage problems of irradiation and drug toxicity. The toxic effects of the drugs and irradiation used in the treatment of leukemia often create as much distress as the disease itself. This poses numerous problems for the nurse who must use judgment in recognizing which side effects are normal reactions and which indicate toxicity.

Nausea and vomiting. The nausea and vomiting that occur shortly after administration of several of the drugs and as a result of cranial irradiation can be profound. They can be controlled with antiemetics such as prochlorperazine (Compazine), metoclopramide (Reglan), or trimethobenzamide (Tigan), which are available in oral, injectable, or suppository form. For children, the oral or suppository form is recommended. However, if rectal ulcers are a problem, the suppository is not advisable because of increased tissue trauma. The antiemetics are most beneficial when given before nausea and vomiting begin.

Loss of appetite. This is a direct consequence of the chemotherapy, irradiation, and nausea and vomiting. It is a major problem for parents because it is the one area for which they feel responsible, particularly when so many other facets of care are outside their control. There are no panaceas for encouraging a sick child to eat.

The most important measure is to encourage parents to relax. Forcing a child to eat only meets with rebellion and negativism. In turn, refusing to eat becomes a controlling mechanism for the child. Second, it is impressed on parents that during the period of intense therapy the child legitimately does not feel like eating. This is a time for the parents to concentrate on giving the child anything he wants to eat. Sometimes it is helpful to encourage the child to participate in noneating activities, such as grocery shopping, menu planning, and food preparation (see p. 541 for feeding the sick child).

Mucosal ulceration. One of the most distressing side effects of several drugs is gastrointestinal mucosal cell damage, which can produce ulcers anywhere along the alimentary tract. Oral ulcers greatly compound anorexia because eating is extremely uncomfortable, but the following interventions may be helpful: (1) provide a bland, moist, soft diet, (2) use of a soft sponge toothbrush (Toothettes)* or cotton-tipped applicator, (3) administer frequent mouthwashes with diluted hydrogen peroxide (1 part hydrogen peroxide and 4 parts normal saline), and (4) apply local anesthetics such as Chloroseptic spray or viscous lidocaine.

Rectal ulcers are managed by meticulous toilet hygiene, warm sitz baths after each bowel movement, and periodic exposure of the ulcerated area to warm heat to promote healing. Parents should be advised to record bowel movements since the child may voluntarily avoid defecation to prevent discomfort. Taking temperatures rectally is contraindicated since it may cause further trauma to the area.

Peripheral neuropathy. Vincristine and, to a lesser extent, vinblastine can cause various neurotoxic effects. Nursing interventions for management of these effects include: administer stool softeners or laxatives for severe constipation caused by decreased bowel innervation; maintain good body alignment and a footboard to minimize or prevent footdrop; carry out safety measures during ambulation because of weakness and numbing of the extremities, that may cause difficulty in walking or fine hand movement; and, provide a soft or liquid diet for severe jaw pain.

Hemorrhagic cystitis. Sterile hemorrhagic cystitis, a side effect of chemical irritation to the bladder from cyclophosphamide, can be prevented by a liberal fluid intake (at least one and a half times the recommended daily fluid requirement) and frequent voiding (including nighttime voiding). If signs of cystitis occur (such as burning on urination), fluids are increased, and the physician is notified of these symptoms immediately. Hemorrhagic cystitis warrants cessation of the drug.

Alopecia. Hair loss is a side effect of several chemotherapeutic drugs and cranial irradiation. Although nothing can prevent alopecia from cranial irradiation, the use of a scalp tourniquet may prevent hair loss from drug administration. A scalp tourniquet is a wide rubber band that is

---

*Manufactured by Halbrand, Inc., Willoughby, OH.

placed around the head near the hairline during drug infusion and kept in place for 5 minutes after administration of the drug. It is not recommended for induction therapy, since leukemic cells may be missed. However, it is used by some physicians when the child is in remission.

Not all children lose their hair during drug therapy; however, this is the exception rather than the rule. It is better to warn children and parents of this side effect than to allow them to think that it is only a remote possibility. Encouraging a child to choose a wig similar to his own hairstyle and color before the hair falls out is helpful in fostering later adjustment to hair loss. The nurse should also inform the family that hair regrows in 3 to 6 months and may be of a different color and texture. Frequently, the hair is darker, thicker, and curlier than before.

If the child chooses not to wear a wig, attention to some type of head covering, especially in cold climates, and scalp hygiene are important. The scalp should be washed like any other body part.

Moon face. Short-term steroid therapy produces no acute toxicities and produces two beneficial reactions—increased appetite and a sense of well-being. However, it does produce alterations in body image, which, although not clinically significant, can be extremely distressing to older children. One of these is moon face in which the child's face becomes rounded and puffy, and it is not unusual for other children to make fun of the child with such remarks as "porky-pig" or "fat face." For the child who experiences such name-calling, it is helpful to reassure him that after cessation of the drug the facial changes will return to normal. Unlike hair loss, little can be done to camouflage this obvious change. If the child resumes activity early in the course of treatment, the change may be less noticeable to peers than after a long absence.

Mood changes. Shortly after beginning steroid therapy, children experience a feeling of well-being that may be a striking change in behavior after a period of depression following hospitalization, impact of the diagnosis, and induction therapy. When the drug is discontinued, the loss of the euphoric effect may also be noticeable. If parents are unaware of these drug-induced changes, they may interpret the mood swings erroneously. Therefore, the nurse warns them of the reactions and encourages them to discuss the behavioral changes with each other and the child.

Relieve pain. Toward the terminal stages of the disease there are two complications—central nervous system meningitis and bone pain—that may require nursing intervention. The main objective in each is relief of discomfort with environmental manipulation, positioning, and analgesics.

Environmental manipulation. Depending on the type of pain, manipulating the environment to avoid unnecessary exertion or altering sensory input may be bene-

ficial. For example, dimming the lights and diminishing ambient noise may be helpful for headaches caused by central nervous system involvement.

Positioning. Good body alignment is important when bone pain is present. However, pressure against these tender sites produces more pain. Some devices that may be helpful are reclining chairs, a water bed, or a beanbag chair. The last is relatively inexpensive and may be worth the investment if the child remains at home.

Once the child assumes a position of comfort, he is usually reluctant to move. However, frequent turning and repositioning are necessary to prevent pressure sores. To facilitate movement, it is advisable to coordinate position changes with pain medication schedules. Also, moving the television to the opposite side of the bed may be sufficient incentive to encourage the child to assume a new position.

Analgesics. Because aspirin enhances the effects of methotrexate and promotes bleeding tendencies, nonsalicylate analgesics are used for pain. Acetaminophen (Tylenol) is recommended for home use; however, it is only effective for mild to moderate pain. Management of more severe pain requires experimentation with various analgesics, such as oxycodone hydrochloride (Percocet), levorphanol tartrate (Levo-Dromoran), or methadone. The oral form of the drug is least addicting and used whenever possible. The physician must prescribe these drugs, but the nurse should be familiar with each. Guidelines for managing pain are discussed on p. 513.

Provide continued emotional support. The preceding discussion of nursing care of the leukemic child is based on typical problems that confront the family during the treatment phases. It is not unlikely for a child who discontinues therapy after 2 or 3 years and maintains a permanent remission to experience many of these side effects. Therefore, the nurse's role is continually one of support, guidance, clarification, and judgment. Parents need to know how to recognize symptoms that demand medical attention. Although some of the reactions discussed are expected, parents should still report them to their physician. Warning parents of their possible occurrence beforehand, however, allows parents the opportunity to prepare for them. At the same time it reassures them that these reactions are not caused by a return of leukemic cells.

HODGKIN DISEASE

Hodgkin disease is a neoplastic disease that originates in the lymphoid system and primarily involves the lymph nodes. Although Hodgkin disease is extremely rare before 5 years of age, there is a striking increase during adolescence and until 30 years of age. In children in the 15- to 19-year-old age-group, Hodgkin disease occurs with almost equal frequency as leukemia. It predictably metastasizes to nonnodal or extralymphatic sites, especially the

SUMMARY OF NURSING CARE OF THE CHILD WITH LEUKEMIA

GOALS	RESPONSIBILITIES
Assist in establishing diagnosis	Recognize signs that indicate leukemia and encourage the family to seek medical care Assist with diagnostic procedures and tests Prepare the family and child for procedures Collect specimens as indicated
Help the family cope with impact of diagnosis	Allow expression of feelings Provide explanations and reinforce information given by medical staff Be available to the family for support
Prepare the family for diagnostic/therapeutic procedures	Explain reason for each test (fingersticks, venipunctures, bone marrow aspirations, lumbar punctures, x-ray treatments) Explain basic elements of blood to provide foundational information for tests and therapies Encourage older children and parents to learn the meaning of various blood values Explain bone marrow aspiration and lumbar puncture with a step-by-step approach and point out those few procedures that are painful Use the recall of each step as a method of distraction Whenever possible, make use of newer procedures that minimize discomfort, such as the anesthetic patch, heparin lock, or Ommaya reservoir
Support the child during treatment for myelosuppression	Explain reason for antibiotics and/or transfusions Anticipate need for crossmatched platelets and white blood cell count; encourage parents to locate potential donors Observe for signs of transfusion reaction; a febrile reaction is common with leukocyte transfusion and is *not* a contraindication for its use Record approximate time for hemostasis to occur after administration of platelets Minimize limited activity and boredom imposed by continuous intravenous infusion Encourage appropriate quiet activities Choose site for intravenous infusion that allows maximum mobility
Prevent complications of myelosuppression	Be aware of which drugs cause bone marrow depression Interpret current peripheral blood counts to guide implementation of specific infection/bleeding precautions
Infection	Institute protective isolation Evaluate the child for any potentital sites of infection (needle punctures, mucosal ulceration, minor abrasions, and dental problems) Monitor temperature elevations closely, although steroids may depress this symptom Administer meticulous skin care, especially in the mouth and perianal regions Prevent skin breakdown with frequent change of position Encourage adequate calorie-protein intake Avoid exertion or fatigue Teach preventive measures at discharge (handwashing and isolation from crowds) Stress importance of isolating the child from any known cases of chickenpox or other childhood communicable diseases Work with the school nurse and physician to determine optimum time for school reattendance

Continued.

SUMMARY OF NURSING CARE OF THE CHILD WITH LEUKEMIA—cont'd

GOALS	RESPONSIBILITIES
Hemorrhage	Use all measures to prevent infection, especially in ecchymotic areas Use local measures to stop bleeding Restrict strenuous activity that could result in accidental injury Involve the child in responsibility for limiting activity when platelet count drops
Anemia	Allow the child to monitor his activity tolerance Encourage rest periods throughout the day and at least 8 to 10 hours of sleep at night For severe anemia, see the box on p. 741 for nursing interventions
Manage problems of radiotherapy and drug toxicity Nausea and vomiting	Be aware of treatment protocols and expected reactions/toxicities resulting from each Give antiemetic prior to onset of nausea and vomiting Calculate optimum time by establishing when nausea and vomiting occur after the first dose Administer about 20 minutes before the expected reaction during subsequent doses Whenever possible, give drug before bedtime and/or on an empty stomach Stress that this side effect is usually only temporary If dehydration occurs, notify the physician
Loss of appetite	Encourage the parents to relax; stress legitimate nature of loss of appetite Allow the child *any* food he tolerates; plan to improve quality of food selections when appetite increases Stress expected increase in appetite from steroids Take advantage of any hungry period; serve small "snacks" Fortify foods with nutritious supplements, such as powdered milk in foods and nutritious beverages Allow the child to be involved in food preparation and selection (grocery shopping, trying new recipes, eating "picnic" lunch) Make food appealing (for example, "face" on hamburger) Remember usual food practices of children in each age-group, such as food jags of toddlers or normal occurrence of physiologic anorexia If anorexia persists despite improved physical status, assess the family for additional problems (for example, use of food by the child as a control mechanism)
Oral ulcers	Inspect mouth daily for oral ulcers Institute meticulous oral hygiene as soon as a drug is used that causes oral ulcers Use a soft-sponge toothbrush, cotton-tipped applicator, or gauze-wrapped finger Administer mouthwashes frequently (at least every 4 hours and after meals) Report evidence of ulcers to the physician Apply local anesthetics to ulcerated areas before meals and as needed Serve bland, moist, soft diet Encourage fluids, drinking through a straw may help bypass painful areas
Rectal ulcers	Wash perineal area after each bowel movement Use warm sitz baths or tub baths as frequently as necessary for comfort Expose ulcerated area to warm heat to hasten healing Apply A and D Ointment or other nonporous lubricant, especially before a bowel movement Observe for constipation resulting from the child's voluntary refusal to defecate Avoid rectal temperatures or suppositories

SUMMARY OF NURSING CARE OF THE CHILD WITH LEUKEMIA—cont'd

GOALS	RESPONSIBILITIES

Peripheral neuropathy	Advise the parents of possible reactions
	Record bowel movements
	  May use stool softener to prevent constipation
	  May need stimulants for evacuation
	Encourage ambulation when the child is able
	If weakness occurs alter activity to prevent accidents (including school attendance)
	Use footboard to prevent footdrop
	Administer analgesics (not aspirin) for jaw pain
	Provide fluids and soft foods to lessen chewing movements
	Allow the child to rest
	Advise the parents of neurologic syndrome from central nervous system irradiation (5 to 8 weeks after treatment)

Hemorrhagic cystitis	Observe for signs (burning and pain on urination) Give liberal (3000 ml/m^2/day) fluid intake Encourage frequent voiding, including during nighttime
Alopecia	May be lessened with use of scalp tourniquet; discuss this procedure with the physician Introduce idea of a wig prior to hair loss Administer good scalp hygiene Provide adequate covering during sunlight, wind, or cold Keep hair clean, short, and fluffy to camouflage partial baldness Stress that hair begins to regrow in 3 to 6 months and may be a slightly different color or texture Stress that alopecia during a second treatment with the same drug may be much less severe
Moon face	Understand often conflicting reactions of the child (negative) and parents (positive) to moon face Encourage rapid reintegration with peers to lessen contrast of changed facial appearance Stress that this reaction is temporary Evaluate weight gain carefully (in weight gain resulting from administration of steroids, extremities remain thin)
Mood changes	Prepare the family for expected euphoric effect from steroids Interpret mood changes based on drugs or reactions to disease/treatment
Relieve pain	Carefully assess pain to determine its true cause—may be a manifestation of fear, loneliness, or depression During terminal stage, appreciate that pain control is necessary component of physical and emotional care
Environmental manipulation	Avoid excess noise or light Place all commodities within easy reach Use gentle, minimal physical manipulation Avoid pressure (bedclothes, sheets) on painful areas Experiment with heat or cold applications on painful areas (use cautiously because of easy skin breakdown)

Continued.

SUMMARY OF NURSING CARE OF THE CHILD WITH LEUKEMIA—cont'd

GOALS	RESPONSIBILITIES
Positioning	Change position frequently; if difficult for the child, coordinate with pain relief from analgesics Avoid pressure on bony prominences or painful sites (water bed, bean bag chair, flotation mattress) Ensure good body alignment
Analgesics	Administer analgesics as needed; never use aspirin or any of its compounds Select narcotic drugs carefully to use them when most needed Administer drugs before the pain becomes severe (administration as needed for severe pain is inadequate to provide optimum relief) Evaluate effectiveness of pain relief with degree of alertness vs sedation

Provide continued emotional support	Advise the parents of expected therapy side effects vs toxicities
	   Clarify which demand medical evaluation
	   Reassure the parents that such reactions are not caused by return of leukemic cells
	Interpret prognostic statistics carefully, realizing the parents' temporary need to interpret them as they see necessary
	(For additional interventions, refer to Chapter 16)

spleen, liver, bone marrow, and lungs, although no tissue is exempt from involvement (Fig. 23-4).

It is usually classified according to four histologic types: (1) lymphocytic predominance, (2) nodular sclerosis, (3) mixed cellularity, and (4) lymphocytic depletion. Histologic pattern and staging of the extent of disease have significant prognostic implication. The first two types and stages are most likely to result in a 90% chance of cure.

Accurate staging of the extent of disease is the basis for treatment protocols and expected prognoses. The specific classification for each patient is derived from the history, physical examination, roentgenographic studies, laboratory tests, and biopsy findings. The staging system proceeds from stages I to IV, or from most to least favorable prognosis, respectively.

Clinical manifestations

Hodgkin disease is characterized by painless enlargement of the lymph nodes. The most common finding is enlarged, firm, nontender, movable nodes in the cervical area. In children the "sentinel" node located near the left clavicle may be the first enlarged node. Enlargement of axillary and inguinal lymph nodes is less frequent.

Other signs and symptoms depend on the extent and location of involvement. Mediastinal lymphadenopathy may cause a persistent nonproductive cough. Enlarged retroperitoneal nodes may produce unexplained abdominal pain. Systemic symptoms include low-grade and/or inter-

FIG. 23-4

Main areas of lymphadenopathy and organ involvement in Hodgkin's disease.

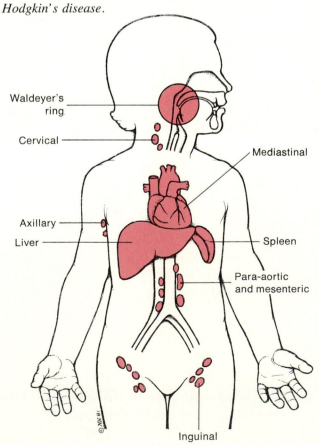

Waldeyer's ring

Cervical

Mediastinal

Axillary

Liver

Spleen

Para-aortic and mesenteric

Inguinal

mittent fever (Pel-Ebstein disease), anorexia, nausea, weight loss, night sweats, or pruritus. Generally such symptoms indicate advanced lymph node and extralymphatic involvement.

Diagnostic evaluation

Because of the multiple organs that can become involved, diagnosis consists of several tests to confirm the presence of Hodgkin disease and to assess the extent of involvement for accurate staging. Routine laboratory tests include complete blood count, uric acid levels, liver function tests, urinalysis, and erythrocyte sedimentation rate. Radiographic examinations of the chest and/or tomograms and liver, spleen, and bone scans are done to detect metastasis. An intravenous pyelogram may be done if renal involvement is suspected.

The most definitive diagnostic procedure is the lymphangiogram, in which a dye is injected intradermally in the first interdigital space of each foot allowing the lymphatic vessels to be visualized within seconds. Radiographs are taken during the procedure, 24 hours later, and sometimes after therapy to chart the progression of treatment or disease. The contrast material remains in the vessels for up to 1 year.

Approximately 24 to 48 hours after the lymphangiogram an inferior venacavogram may be performed. In this procedure a radiopaque dye is infused through a catheter in the right femoral vein, and radiograms are taken to visualize the larger veins of the abdomen.

Biopsy, which is essential to diagnosis and staging, is usually carried out in two stages. First the enlarged lymph node is excised and histologically analyzed for evidence of the *Sternberg-Reed cell*. Second, in some centers laparotomy with splenectomy is performed for definitive staging purposes.

Therapeutic management

The primary modalities of therapy are radiation and chemotherapy. Each may be used alone or in combination based on the clinical staging. The most widely used chemotherapeutic agent is MOPP, which consists of mechlorethamine (Mustargen), vincristine (Oncovin), prednisone, and procarbazine. The length of chemotherapy depends on the individual's response to the drugs. Chemotherapy usually lasts at least 6 months, but it is more likely to last 12 to 18 months.

Prognosis

The prognosis for patients with Hodgkin disease has improved dramatically in the past few years, largely as a result of the systematic staging procedure and treatment pro-

tocols. The overall 5-year survival rate for any type or stage of disease is 90%; 10-year survival rates decrease to 80%. The prognosis is excellent in children with localized disease, and even in those with disseminated disease, long-term remissions are possible in about half of the patients. However, late recurrences are not uncommon and 5-year survival rates should not be equated with a cure.

Nursing considerations

Nursing care for patients with Hodgkin disease involves the same objectives as for patients with other types of cancer—specifically, (1) preparation for diagnostic and operative procedures and (2) explanation of treatment side effects. Since this is most often a disease of adolescents and young adults, the nurse must have an appreciation of their psychologic needs and reactions during the diagnostic and treatment phases.

Once the child is hospitalized for suspected Hodgkin disease, a battery of diagnostic tests is ordered. The family needs an explanation of why each test is performed, since many of them, such as a bone marrow aspiration, are not routine. The one test that deserves special explanation is lymphography. If a laparotomy is performed, preparation is similar to that for any other surgery.

The most common side effect of irradiation is malaise, which may last for a year after treatment. This is particularly difficult for active, outgoing adolescents, because it prevents them from keeping up with their peers. Sometimes the adolescent will push himself to the point of physical exhaustion rather than admit and succumb to the decreased activity tolerance. The nurse cautions parents to observe for such behavior, such as extreme fatigue at the end of the day, falling asleep at the dinner table, inability to concentrate on homework, or an increased susceptibility to infection. A regular bedtime and scheduled rest periods are important for these children, especially during chemotherapy when myelosuppression increases the risk of infection and debilitation. Prior to discharge the nurse should discuss a feasible school schedule with the parents and child.

An area of concern for adolescents is the high risk of sterility from irradiation and chemotherapy. Both irradiation to the gonads and drugs, particularly procarbazine and alkylating agents, can lead to infertility. Sexual function is not altered, although the appearance of secondary sexual characteristics and menstruation may be delayed in the pubescent child. Adolescents should be informed of these side effects early in the course of the diagnosis and treatment. Delayed sexual maturation may be an extremely sensitive and painful area for children (see Chapter 15). It is important for the nurse to respect their concern and refrain from casually placating them with expressions, such as, ''You'll catch up someday.''

Families require the same emotional care as that discussed for any family with a potentially fatally ill child (see Chapter 16).

NON-HODGKIN LYMPHOMA (NHL)

Non-Hodgkin lymphoma in children is strikingly different from Hodgkin disease and adult types of non-Hodgkin lymphoma in several aspects:

1. The disease is usually diffuse rather than nodular.
2. The cell type is either undifferentiated or poorly differentiated.
3. Dissemination occurs early, more often, and rapidly.
4. Control of the primary tumor, especially mediastinal presentation, is difficult.
5. Current methods of treatment are less effective.
6. Prognosis is much poorer.

Non-Hodgkin lymphoma exhibits a variety of morphologic, cytochemical, and immunologic features, not unlike the diversity seen in leukemia. Their classification is based on the histologic pattern, either nodular (circumscribed) or diffuse (spread out), and immunologically as T-cells, B-cells, or null cells (lacking immunologic properties).

The clinical staging system used in Hodgkin disease is of little value in non-Hodgkin lymphoma, although other systems have been developed. Basically, children present with two types of disease: (1) involvement of *supradiaphragmatic* lymph nodes, often in association with an anterior mediastinal mass; or (2) *infradiaphragmatic* tumors, often involving the ileocecal region, mesentary, ovaries, and/or retroperitoneum.

Clinical manifestations

Clinical manifestations depend on the anatomic site and extent of involvement. Many of the manifestations seen in Hodgkin disease may be present in non-Hodgkin lymphoma, although rarely does a single symptom give rise to the diagnosis. Rather metastasis to the bone marrow or central nervous system may produce signs and symptoms typical of leukemia. Lymphoid tumors compressing various organs may cause intestinal or airway obstruction, cranial nerve palsies, or spinal paralysis.

Diagnostic evaluation

Because most children with non-Hodgkin lymphoma present with widespread disseminated disease, thorough pathologic staging is unnecessary. Current recommendations include a surgical biopsy, histopathologic confirmation of disease with cytochemical and immunologic evaluation, bone marrow examination, radiographic studies (especially tomograms of lungs and gastrointestinal organs), and lumbar puncture.

Therapeutic management

The present treatment protocols for non-Hodgkin lymphoma include combination irradiation and chemotherapy. The drug regimens vary and include cyclophosphamide, vincristine, methotrexate, and prednisone (COMP) or the substitution of hydroxydaunorubicin (Doxorubicin) for methotrexate (CHOP) and other combinations of 6-thioguanine, cytarabine (Cytosine arabinoside), and asparaginase (L-asparaginase). Generally 6 to 9 weeks of chemotherapy are required to induce a remission. If relapse does not occur, treatment is usually continued for 18 to 24 months.

Prognosis

The prognosis for children with non-Hodgkin lymphoma has improved greatly in the past few years as a result of intensive multimodal therapy. Important prognostic factors include the amount of bulky, widespread disease at initial presentation, early and aggressive therapy, and the achievement of a complete remission within 1 to 2 months from onset of therapy. Since relapse after 12 months is rare, a 24-month survival rate essentially equals the cure rate.

Nursing considerations

Nursing care of the child with non-Hodgkin lymphoma is very similar to that for Hodgkin disease; therefore, the principles of care are appropriate for the child with non-Hodgkin lymphoma.

IMMUNOLOGIC-DEFICIENCY DISORDERS

The immune system consists of the *primary lymphoid organs* (thymus, bone marrow, and probably liver) and the *secondary lymphoid organs* (lymph nodes, spleen, and gut-associated lymphoid tissue). The defense functions of the immune system are basically of two types: nonspecific and specific. *Nonspecific immune defenses* are activated on exposure to any foreign substance but react similarly regardless of the type of antigen; they are unable to identify the antigen. *Phagocytosis*, the ingestion and digestion of foreign substances, is the principle process of this system.

Specific (adaptive) defenses are those that have the

ability to recognize the antigen and respond selectively. Adaptive immunity consists of (1) *humoral immunity,* which includes antibodies in the form of the immunoglobulins and which is concerned primarily with response to foreign antigens; and, (2) *cell-mediated immunity,* which provides protection against most invading organisms. Conditions that cause interference with any or all of these protective mechanisms leaves the body vulnerable to disease.

SEVERE COMBINED IMMUNODEFICIENCY DISORDER (SCID)

Severe combined immunodeficiency disorders are congenital (usually hereditary) deficiencies that involve both humoral and cell-mediated immunity. They are distinguished by their apparent absence of all adaptive immune function. The inheritance patterns are either X-linked recessive or autosomal-recessive, and males outnumber females 3 to 1. SCID is characterized by an early onset of severe infections that can progress rapidly to early death.

Pathophysiology

The exact cause of SCID is unknown. All patients with SCID have nearly total lack of cellular immune function, absent or extremely low responses of lymphocytes to substances that stimulate their proliferation, more rapid skin responses to antigens, and an inability to reject transplants. Serum concentrations of immunoglobulins are extremely low and no antibodies are formed following immunization. The consequence of the immunodeficiency is an overwhelming susceptibility to infections and to the *graft-vs-host reaction*.

Clinical manifestations

Susceptibility to infection is evident early in life, often in the first month of life when the infant develops oral thrush that disseminates to the gastrointestinal tract and skin. Following the initial limited passive protection provided by maternal antibodies, children with the disorder are subject to chronic infections, failure to completely recover from an infection, frequent reinfection, and infection with unusual agents. Frequently, the history reveals no logical source of infection. Failure to thrive is a consequence of the persistent illnesses.

If the child should receive a foreign tissue, such as blood supplements, signs of graft-vs-host reaction are expected, including fever, skin rash, alopecia, hepatosplenomegaly, and diarrhea. Since the reaction requires 7 to 20 days for tissue damage to become evident, the symptoms may be mistaken for an infection. However, the presence of a graft-vs-host reaction increases the child's susceptibility to overwhelming infection and is, therefore, a grave complication.

Diagnostic evaluation

Diagnosis is usually based on a history of recurrent, severe infections from early infancy, a familial history of the disorder, and specific laboratory findings, which include lymphopenia, lack of lymphocyte response to antigens, and absence of plasma cells in the bone marrow. Documentation of immunoglobulin deficiency is difficult during infancy because of the normally delayed response of the infant to produce his own immunoglobulins and maternal transfer of immunoglobulin G.

Therapeutic management

The only definitive treatment is a histocompatible bone marrow transplant. The perfect donor is an identical twin because the histocompatibility (HL-A) antigens and blood type are exactly the same. The second best choice is a sibling. Bone marrow transplants are usually performed at medical centers where measures to control postrantsplantation infection, such as a sterile environment, and other specialized facilities are available. Since the host's immunologic system is incompetent, graft rejection is not a problem. However, a graft-vs-host reaction is always a possibility in a nonidentical twin graft, and, once it occurs, little can be done to reverse the process.

Other approaches to SCID are to provide passive immunity with gamma globulin injections and maintain the child in a sterile environment. The latter is effective only if instituted prior to the existence of any infectious process in the infant. Other investigational transplant procedures include nonidentical HLA bone marrow grafts and fetal liver or thymus transplants.

Nursing considerations

Since the prognosis for SCID is very poor if a compatible bone marrow donor is not available, nursing care is directed at supporting the family in caring for a fatally ill child. Genetic counseling is essential because of the modes of transmission in either form of the disorder. Nursing goals are directed at (1) helping parents prevent sources of infection in the child, such as cautious isolation from crowded facilities and individuals with active infection, (2) meticulous skin and mouth care, (3) good general nutrition, and (4) careful supervision during periods of activity to prevent skin trauma.

Even with exacting environmental control, these children are prone to opportunistic infection. Chronic fungal infections of the mouth and nails with *Candida albicans* are frequent problems despite vigorous efforts at prevention or treatment.

Children who receive frequent injections of immune serum globulin (ISG) need support during the procedure because the injections are painful. To prevent tissue damage and provide maximum absorption, the total amount may be divided between two injection sites. A modified preparation of ISG (MISG) is reported to be more effective and less painful.

Care of the child undergoing bone marrow transplantation is mainly directed at preventing infection. Because it takes 7 to 20 days before evidence of bone marrow functioning becomes evident, hospitalization is long. It is not the purpose of this discussion to detail the care of the child with a bone marrow transplant, except to emphasize that the psychologic needs of the parents and child are tremendous. For the parents, it represents the last hope for successful therapy and survival. For the child, it means sensory deprivation because of isolation, numerous blood tests, and the possibility of more pain and suffering if a graft-vs-host reaction occurs.

ACQUIRED IMMUNE DEFICIENCY SYNDROME (AIDS)

Acquired immune deficiency syndrome is a disease characterized by (1) any of a variety of opportunistic infections, (2) unusual malignant neoplasms, such as Kaposi sarcoma, (3) autoimmune phenomena, such as thrombocytopenia, and (4) defective cell-mediated immunity. Although it is most prevalent in adult populations (especially homosexual males, intravenous drug users, and persons with hemophilia A), it may also affect children. What appears to be AIDS has been reported in a number of children. The reported cases in children have been those who have received transfused blood products or those who have lived in households with recognized risks for AIDS, especially infants born to mothers with the disease. The mode of transmission remains unknown but it appears that, in children, (1) an infectious agent is responsible, (2) sexual contact or drug abuse is not required for transmission, and, (3) the disease can be transmitted to an otherwise normal host (Oleske and Minnefor, 1983).

Children with the disease develop recurrent infections and/or chronic infections and, although they may have severe disease, they do not show a characteristic inflammatory reaction because of the diminished or absent immune response. Their symptoms are nonspecific including fever, weight loss, anemia, hepatosplenomegaly, an eczema-like rash, and generalized, persistent lymphadenopathy.

There is no known cure for the disease, but animicrobial therapy and supportive measures are implemented and intravenous gamma globulin has been of benefit in some cases. The condition is not reversible with present knowledge and treatment at present is disappointing.

Nursing considerations

Nursing care of children suspected of AIDS is essentially the same as for children with other diseases with depressed immune response. The Centers for Disease Control* has published guidelines for hospitalized patients with suspected AIDS. Essentially, there appears to be little risk in casual exposure to affected persons. Handwashing is practiced and gloves are worn when in direct contact with patient's body fluids, secretions, or excretions; gowns are worn when there are copious secretions or excretions; and, a mask is recommended when secretions or excretions may splatter inadvertently.

Patients and families are extremely anxious regarding the prognosis and communicability of this relatively recent health problem. It is important for health personnel to maintain an attitude of acceptance and not to convey the impression that caring for the patient is distasteful. With reasonable caution there should be no danger to health workers.

WISKOTT-ALDRICH SYNDROME

The Wiskott-Aldrich syndrome is a sex-linked recessive disorder characterized by several abnormalities: (1) thrombocytopenia, (2) eczema, (3) recurrent infection, (4) an inability to form specific antibodies to polysaccharide antigens, and (5) acquired thymic system deficiency. At birth the major effect of the disorder is bleeding as a result of the thrombocytopenia. As the child grows older, recurrent infection and eczema become more severe and the bleeding becomes less frequent.

Eczema is typical of the allergic type and easily becomes superinfected. Chronic infection with herpes simplex is a frequent problem and may lead to chronic keratitis of the eye with loss of vision. Chronic pulmonary disease, sinusitis, and otitis media result from repeated infections. In those children who survive the bleeding episodes and overwhelming infections, malignancy presents an additional risk to survival.

Medical treatment involves (1) counteracting the bleeding tendencies with platelet transfusions, (2) providing gamma globulin to provide passive immunity, and (3) administering prophylactic antibiotics to prevent and con-

---

*1600 Clifton Rd., NE, Atlanta, GA 30333

trol infection. Bone marrow transplants have been attempted but, even if successful, do not reverse all the defects of this disorder.

Nursing considerations

Because of the grave prognosis for these children, the main nursing consideration is supporting the family in the care of a fatally ill child. Physical care is directed at controlling the problems imposed by the disorder. The measures used to control bleeding are similar to those for hemophilia. Another major goal is prevention or control of infection. Since eczema is a troublesome problem, nursing measures specific to this condition are especially important.

The genetic implications of this sex-linked recessive disorder differ little from those of any other X-linked disorder. However, because of the multiplicity of defects, the emotional adjustment and physical care required for these children are greater than those of many other conditions. The nurse can be especially supportive by providing short-term goals during periods of hospitalization and by focusing on long-range needs through coordinated efforts with a public health nurse.

REFERENCES

Oleske, J.M., and Minnefor, A.B.: Acquired immune deficiency syndrome in children, Pediatr. Infect. Dis. **2**:85-65, 1983.

BIBLIOGRAPHY
Iron deficiency anemia

Calbreath, D.: Serum iron and iron-building capacity, J. Nurs. Care **12**(9):30, 1979.
Gever, L.N.: New thinking about parenteral iron supplements, Nursing 80 **10**(8):60, 1980.
Habersang, R., and Marsh, A.: Iron and infant nutrition, Issues Compr. Pediatr. Nurs. **2**(1):43-49, 1978.
Pipes, P.L.: Nutrition in infancy and childhood, ed. 2, St. Louis, 1981, The C.V. Mosby Co.
Robinson, L.A., Brown, A.L., and Underwood, T.: Iron therapy: helps and hazards, Pediatr. Nurs. **4**(6):9-13, 1978.
Weeks, H.F.: Iron supplements, Am. J. Maternal Child Nurs. **5**:354, 1980.

Sickle cell anemia

Bonner, S.E.: Nursing care of a child with sickle cell disease. In Brandt, P., Chinn, P.L., and Smith, M.E., editors: Current practice in pediatric nursing, vol. 1, St. Louis, 1976, The C.V. Mosby Co.
Doswell, W.M.: Sickle cell anemia, Nursing 78 **8**(4):65-70, 1978.
Flanagan, C.: Home management of sickle cell anemia, Pediatr. Nurs. **6**(2):B-D, 1980.
Gibbons, P.T.: Transfusion therapy in sickle cell disease, Nurs. Clin. North Am. **18**:201-205, 1983.

Godwin, M., and Baysinger, M.: Understanding antisickling agents and the sickling process, Nurs. Clin. North Am. **18**:207-214, 1983.
Greene, P.: Teaching aid for children with sickle cell disease, Am. J. Nurs. **77**(12):1953, 1977.
McFarlane, J.M.: Sickle cell disorders, Am. J. Nurs. **77**(2):1948-1954, 1977.
Richardson, E.A.W., and Milne, L.S.: Sickle-cell disease and the childbearing family: an update, Am. J. Maternal Child Nurs. **8**:417-422, 1983.
Rooks, Y., and Pack, B.: A profile of sickle cell disease, Nurs. Clin. North Am. **18**:131-138, 1983.
Rozzell, M.S., Hijazi, M., and Pack, B.: The painful episode, Nurs. Clin. North Am. **18**:185-199, 1983.
Walters, I., and others: Complications of sickle cell disease, Nurs. Clin. North Am. **18**:139-184, 1983.
Williams, I., Earles, A.N., and Pack, B.: Psychological considerations in sickle cell disease, Nurs. Clin. North Am. **19**:215-229, 1983.

Thalassemia

Cohen, A., Markenson, A.L., and Schwartz, E.: Transfusion requirements and splenectomy in thalassemia major, J. Pediatr. **79**:100-102, 1980.
Ohene-Frempong, K., and Schwartz, E.: Clinical features of thalassemia, Pediatr. Clin. North Am. **27**:403-420, 1980.

Aplastic anemia

Alter, B.P.: Bone-marrow failure in children, Pediatr. Ann. **8**(7):53-70, 1979.
Hutchison, M.M.: Aplastic anemia. Care of the bone-marrow-failure patient, Nurs. Clin. North Am. **18**:543-551, 1983.

Hemophilia

Boutaugh, M., and Patterson, P.C.: Summer camps for hemophiliacs, Am. J. Nurs. **77**(8):1288-1289, 1977.
Dressler, D.: Understanding and treating hemophilia, Nursing 80 **10**(8):72-73, 1980.
Sergis-Davenport, E., and Varni, J.W.: Behavioral techniques in teaching hemophilia factor replacement to families, Pediatr. Nurs. **8**:416-419, 1982.
Tetrick, A.P.: Ambulatory care of the hemophiliac, J. Assoc. Care Child. Hosp. **7**(2):19-27, 1978.

Miscellaneous coagulation problems

Ingram, N.M.: Stanching nosebleeds: your guide to all the measures available, RN **45**(9):51-53, 115, 1982.
Klosky, L.: Nose picking in children, Pediatr. Nurs. **4**(6):47-48, 1978.
Lightsey, A.L., Jr.: Thrombocytopenia in children, Pediatr. Clin. North Am. **27**:293-308, 1980.
McClure, P.D.: Idiopathic thrombocytopenic purpura in children, Am. J. Dis. Child. **131**:357, 1977.
McGillick, K.: DIC: the deadly paradox, RN **45**(8):41-43, 1982.
O'Brian, B.S., and Woods, S.: The paradox of DIC, Am. J. Nurs. **78**:1878-1880, 1978.

Leukemias/Lymphomas

Baker, L.S.: You and leukemia: a day at a time, Philadelphia, 1978, W.B. Saunders Co.
Cameron, C.O., and Wallace, N.: Having a bone marrow test: a child's perspective, Child Health Care, **12**(1):41-42, 1983.

Campbell, J.B., Preston, R., and Smith, K.Y.: The leukemias. Definition, treatment, and nursing care, Nurs. Clin. North Am. **18:**523-541, 1983.

Collins, M.M.: The leukemic child, Issues Compr. Pediatr. Nurs. **4**(1)49-59, 1980.

Craft, M., and others: Nursing care in childhood cancer: coping, Am. J. Nurs. **82:**440-442, 1982.

Desotell, S.: A brighter future for leukemia patients, Nursing 77 **7**(1):19-24, 1977.

Fochtman, D., and Foley, G.V.: Nursing care of the child with cancer, Boston, 1982, Little, Brown and Co.

Gaddy, D.S.: Nursing care in childhood cancer: update, Am. J. Nurs. **82:**416-421, 1982.

Greene, P.E., and Fergusson, J.H.: Nursing care in childhood cancer: late effects of therapy, Am. J. Nurs. **82:**443-446, 1982.

Griffiths, S.S.: Changes in body image caused by antineoplastic drugs, Issues Compr. Pediatr. Nurs. **4**(1):17-27, 1980.

Hagan, S.J.: Bring help and hope to the patient with Hodgkin's disease, Nursing 83 **13**(8):58-63, 1983.

Houlihan, N.G.: Leukemia: nursing management, Cancer Nurs. **4:**397-405, 1981.

Klopovich, P.: Immunosuppression in the child who has cancer, Am. J. Maternal Child. Nurs. **4:**288-292, 1979.

Mattia, M.A., and Blake, S.L.: Hospital hazards: cancer drugs, Am. J. Nurs. **83:**759-762, 1983.

McCaffery, M.A.: Pain relief for the child: problem areas and selected nonpharmacological methods, Pediatr. Nurs. **3**(4):11-16, 1977.

Ostchega, Y.: Preventing and treating cancer chemotherapy's oral complications, Nursing 80 **10**(8):47-52, 1980.

Sontesgard, L., and others: A way to minimize side effects from radiation therapy, Am. J. Maternal Child Nurs. **1**(1):27-31, 1976.

Stagner, S.A., and Wood, A.: The child with cancer on immunosuppressive therapy, Nurs. Clin. North Am. **11**(1):21-34, 1976.

Sutow, W.W., Fernbach, D.J., and Vietti, T.J.: Clinical pediatric oncology, ed. 3, St. Louis, 1983, The C.V. Mosby Co.

Walker, P.: Bone marrow transplant: a second chance for life, Nursing 77 **7**(1):24-25, 1977.

Wiley, F.M., and Rhein, M.: Challenges of pain management: one terminally ill adolescent, Pediatr. Nurs. **3**(4):26-27, 1977.

Wolf, W.J., and Bancroft, B.: Early detection of childhood malignancies, Pediatr. Nurs. **5**(1):43-46, 1980.

Zimmerman, S., and others: Bone marrow transplantation, Am. J. Nurs. **77**(8):1311-1315, 1977.

Immunologic-deficiency disorders

Brandt, E.N.: The public health service's number one priority, Public Health Reports **98**:306-307, 1983.

Dharan, M.: Immunoglobulin abnormalities, Am. J. Nurs. **76**(10):1626-1628, 1976.

Donley, D.L.: Nursing the patient who is immunosuppressed, Am. J. Nurs. **76**(10):1619-1625, 1976.

Jemison-Smith, P., and Hamm, P.: Immune responses, Crit. Care Update **10**(8):45-46, 1983.

Nursing Grand Rounds: Caring for the AIDS patient—fearlessly, Nursing 83 **13**(9):50-55, 1983.

Nysather, J.O., Katz, A.C., and Lenth, J.L.: The immune system: its development and functions, Am. J. Nurs. **76**(10):1614-1616, 1976.

Phillips, J.L: As a nurse, I want to find out what the facts are about AIDS, Crit. Care Update **10**(9):37-38, 1983.

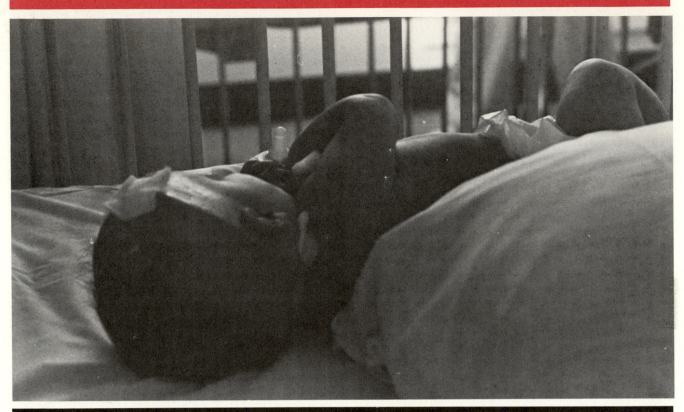

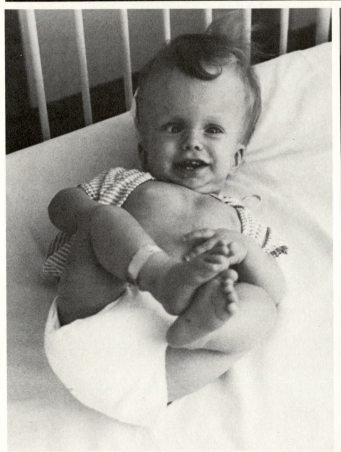

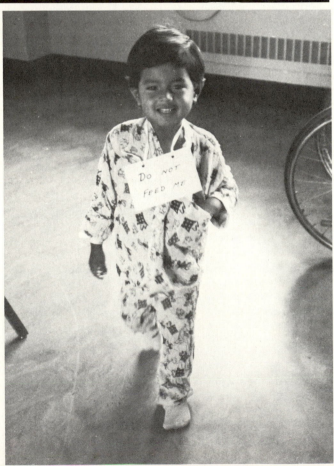

UNIT 11

THE CHILD WITH A DISTURBANCE OF REGULATORY MECHANISMS

In an organism such as a human being, the maintenance of dynamic equilibrium involves a complex interaction of many systems and subsystems. All the activities within the individual cells, tissues, and organs that comprise these systems depend on the function of other systems, and, like all systems, each component part has one or more factors that act on it or affect it. A change in a component part can affect all other component parts. Basic to this interaction are (1) the processes whereby messages are communicated from one area or subsystem to the other and (2) feedback mechanisms, which enable the system to counteract any disturbance that causes a deviation from the normal.

Regulation is the function of automatically maintaining an important biologic variable within a narrow range regardless of disturbances that may act on the system and prevent excessive deviations that are incompatible with life. Regulation enables the organism to maintain the function of cells, tissues, organs, and systems within the parameters described as normal for that system despite changes in the internal or external environment. Communication between the various systems and subsystems is carried by chemical or neural mechanisms. Disturbances in the regulatory processes can create disturbances in one or more of the interrelated component parts of the system with consequences that affect other systems and the organism as a whole.

Genetic and numerous chemical regulatory mecha-

nisms, for example, acid-base equilibrium and oxygen–carbon dioxide disturbances, have been discussed in previous segments. The major regulatory mechanisms of the body are the endocrine and neural systems. The portion of the endocrine regulation that involves the pituitary gland is so closely associated with the neurologic system that it is frequently referred to as the neuroendocrine system. It is sometimes difficult to determine whether dysfunctions in this interrelated system are caused by impaired function in the target glands that secrete hormones, the tropic substances that stimulate the target glands to secrete hormones, or the portions of the midbrain that produce releasing factors that stimulate the pituitary gland.

The kidneys are important regulatory organs and principally concerned with regulation of fluid and acid-base equilibrium. Although the function of the skin is primarily protective, its integrity and metabolism markedly affect the structures encased within this protective shelter.

Renal impairment is discussed in Chapter 24, *The Child with Genitourinary Dysfunction.* Dysfunction of the central nervous system is discussed in Chapter 25, *The Child with Cerebral Dysfunction.* Chapter 26, *The Child with Endocrine Dysfunction,* describes the problems related to impairment of the complex endocrine system and the pancreatic hormones. Chapter 27, *The Child with Integumentary Dysfunction,* is concerned with the multiple disorders of the skin.

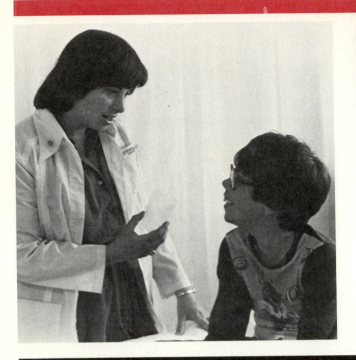

THE CHILD WITH GENITOURINARY DYSFUNCTION

OBJECTIVES

On completion of this chapter the reader will be able to:

- Describe the various factors that contribute to urinary tract infections in infants and children

- Demonstrate an understanding of the causes and mechanisms of edema formation in nephrotic syndrome

- Outline a nursing care plan for a child with nephrotic syndrome

- Compare the manifestations and nursing care of the child with minimal change nephrotic syndrome and a child with acute glomerulonephritis

- Contrast the causes, complications, and management of acute and chronic renal failure

- Discuss the preoperative preparation of the child and parents when the child has a structural defect of the genitourinary tract

- Discuss the role of the nurse in assisting the parents to cope with the problems of a newborn with ambiguous genitalia

NURSING DIAGNOSES

Nursing diagnoses identified for the child with renal dysfunction include, but are not restricted to, the following:

Health perception–health management pattern

- Injury, potential for, related to (1) the presence of infectious organisms; (2) residual urine

Nutritional-metabolic pattern

- Fluid volume, alteration in: excess related to intake greater than output

- Skin integrity, impairment of: potential, related to (1) presence of incontinent urine; (2) irritation to edematous tissues; (3) presence of artificial drainage system and/or appliance

Elimination pattern

- Urinary elimination, alterations in, patterns related to (1) urinary retention; (2) artificial drainage system

Activity-exercise pattern

- Activity intolerance, related to fatigue

- Diversional activity deficit related to (1) environmental restrictions; (2) fatigue

- Self-care deficit: feeding, bathing/hygiene, dressing/grooming, toileting related to (1) developmental level; (2) activity intolerance

Sleep-rest pattern

- Sleep pattern disturbance related to (1) anxiety; (2) schedule of therapies.

Cognitive-perceptual pattern

- Comfort, alteration in: pain, related to (1) response to disease; (2) postoperative response

Self-perception—self-concept pattern

- Anxiety related to (1) a strange environment; (2) perception of impending events; (3) separation; (4) anticipated discomfort; (5) knowledge deficit; (6) discomfort

- Self-concept, disturbance in: body image, self-esteem, personal identity related to (1) perception of physical defect; (2) perception of surgical outcome

Role-relationship pattern

- Family process, alteration in, related to situational crisis

- Parenting, alterations in: potential related to (1) skill deficit; (2) family stress

- Social isolation related to (1) frequent illness and/or hospitalization; (2) body image disturbance

Coping—stress tolerance pattern

- Coping, family: potential for growth

- Coping, ineffective family: compromised, related to (1) situational crisis; (2) temporary family disorganization

The primary responsibility of the kidney is to maintain the composition and volume of the body fluids in equilibrium. To maintain this constant internal environment, the kidney must respond appropriately to alterations in the internal environment caused by variations in dietary intake and extrarenal losses of water and solutes. A secondary function of the kidney is the production of certain humoral substances important in stimulating erythropoiesis in the bone marrow and the regulation of blood pressure.

When pathologic processes interfere with these functions the consequences are manifest in a variety of systems and processes. Diseases involving the kidneys are relatively common in childhood and are caused by a variety of etiologic factors, including infectious processes and structural abnormalities.

INFLAMMATORY DISEASES OF THE GENITOURINARY TRACT

Kidneys react to tissue injury in the same manner as all other body tissues. Acute inflammation evokes a pattern of exudation, white blood cell accumulation, and tissue damage; chronic long-standing inflammation results in scarring and permanent destruction of tissue elements. This discussion focuses on inflammations of the renal system, including bacterial infections and those nonsuppurative disorders collectively described as *nephritis*.

URINARY TRACT INFECTION (UTI)

Urinary tract infection is a significant childhood problem, probably second only to infection of the respiratory tract. Although its exact incidence is not known, studies suggest that from 1% to 2% of school-age children have urinary tract infections as demonstrated by significant bacteriuria; it accounts for unexplained fever in the majority of children under 3 years of age. The peak incidence for urinary tract infection is between 2 and 6 years of age, and females have a 10 to 30 times greater risk for developing urinary tract infections than males, except during infancy, when males outnumber females.

Infection of the urinary tract may be present with or without clinical symptoms. As a result, the site of infection is often difficult to pinpoint with any degree of certainty. Therefore, the term ''urinary tract infection'' has been used to designate instances of bacteriuria with or without signs or symptoms of inflammation in the bladder, kidneys, or both. Various other terms used to delineate specific areas of inflammation are:

bacteriuria growth of bacteria in uncontaminated urine
urethritis inflammation of the urethra
cystitis inflammation of the bladder
ureteritis inflammation of the ureters
pyelonephritis inflammation of the kidney and upper tract (may be acute or chronic)

Predisposing factors

Several factors influence the development of urinary tract infection in childhood. These include anatomic, physical, and chemical factors that may operate individually or collectively.

Anatomic factors. Anatomic or structural factors appear to account for the increased incidence of asymptomatic bacteriuria and clinical urinary tract infection in females. Unlike the longer male urethra, the short, straight urethra in young females provides a ready channel for invading organisms especially during certain activities such as a squatting position while at play and bathing in a tub. Soap or water softeners, which decrease the surface tension of the water, increase the possibility of fluid entry into the short urethra. Tight clothing or diapers, poor hygiene, and local inflammation, such as vaginitis or pinworm infestation, may also increase the risk of ascending infection.

Physical factors. Physical factors associated with bladder function are of major importance in the incidence and spread of infection. Ordinarily urine is sterile, but at 37° C (98.6° F) it serves as an excellent culture medium. Under normal conditions the act of completely and repeatedly emptying the bladder flushes away any organisms before they have an opportunity to multiply and invade surrounding tissue. However, urine that remains in the bladder allows bacteria from the urethra to rapidly become established in the rich medium.

Incomplete bladder emptying may result from reflux, anatomic abnormalities, or dysfunction of the voiding mechanism. *Vesicoureteral reflux* refers to the backward flow of bladder urine into the ureters that occurs when urine is swept into the ureters during voiding. The urine then flows into the bladder after voiding, where it remains as a reservoir for bacterial growth until the next void (Fig. 24-1). Primary reflux results from the congenitally abnormal insertion of the ureters into the bladder; secondary reflux occurs as a result of infection.

Chemical factors. Several chemical characteristics of the urine and bladder mucosa help maintain urinary sterility. An increased fluid intake promotes flushing of the normal bladder and lowers the concentration of organisms in the infected bladder. Water diuresis also seems to enhance the antibacterial properties of the renal medulla.

Most pathogens favor an alkaline medium. Although

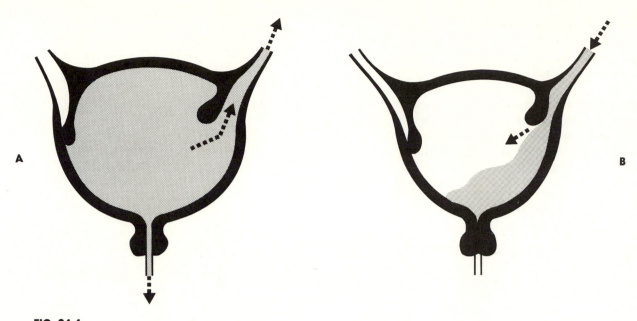

FIG. 24-1

Mechanisms of vesicoureteral reflux. **A,** *During voiding, urine refluxes into the ureter.*
B, *After voiding, residual urine from the ureter remains in the bladder.*

urine is normally slightly acidic, the pH can be lowered by acid-forming drugs, such as ascorbic acid, or by certain foods, such as apple or cranberry juices and animal protein. A urine pH of about 5 inhibits bacterial growth, although the acidification rarely eliminates the bacteriuria. However, it may enhance the therapeutic effectiveness of drugs and of the natural defense mechanisms, as well as help relieve some of the symptoms.

Clinical manifestations

Symptoms of bacteriuria of the lower urinary tract are frequently vague and not unlike the symptoms observed in a number of other disorders. Many infants and children are essentially asymptomatic, with symptoms that appear unrelated to the urinary tract.

Signs in infants are especially nonspecific and resemble sepsis from any source and, therefore, can be easily overlooked or misinterpreted. These signs include low-grade fever, irritability, poor feeding, increased voiding, and failure to gain weight. Fever and systemic symptoms are often absent; colic or jaundice may be seen. Parents should be alerted to observe for specific clues of urinary tract infection in cases with no evidence of respiratory tract infection, such as frequent or infrequent voiding, constant squirming and irritability, foul-smelling urine, and abnormal stream. Checking the diaper every half hour increases the opportunity for observing the stream for such findings as straining or fretting before voiding begins, signs of dis-

comfort before and when urinating, starting and stopping the stream intermittently, and frequent dripping of small amounts of urine. A persistent diaper rash may also be a helpful clue.

Signs and symptoms in children may include urgency, frequency, dysuria, dribbling, nocturnal enuresis, daytime wetting in a previously dry child, and foul-smelling urine. Fever, irritability, abdominal pain, anorexia, vomiting, inflammation of the external genitalia, and observed hematuria are not uncommon. Symptoms often subside in untreated cases, but recurrences are very common.

Acute upper urinary tract infection is usually evidenced by more severe symptoms, such as fever, chills, flank pain, and vomiting. Neonates and young infants may become acutely ill with high temperature, convulsions, and gastrointestinal disturbances. Except for flank pain and tenderness, there may be no other indication on physical examination that suggests pyelonephritis.

Diagnostic evaluation

Bacteriuria is diagnosed by the presence of organisms in the urine. Clean-voided specimens may grow bacteria from contamination of the normal urethral flora but may represent a contaminated specimen and should alert the nurse to the need for more careful urine collecting technique. Low bacteria counts in cases of suspected infection may be a result of diuresis before the test. Therefore, children are not encouraged to drink large volumes of water in an attempt to obtain a specimen quickly. Urine obtained by suprapubic aspiration or from catheterization is normally sterile. Therefore, any growth of bacteria in these cases represents infection.

Other tests, such as intravenous pyelogram (IVP), voiding cystourethrogram (VCUG), and cystoscopy, are sometimes indicated (after the infection subsides) to identify anatomic abnormalities that might contribute to the development of infection and existing kidney changes in cases of recurrent infection.

Therapeutic management

Treatment is directed at clearing the primary infection and preventing recurrence. Antibiotic therapy should be initiated after identification of the pathogen. Antibacterial compounds used in the management of urinary tract infection include (1) systemic penicillins and sulfonamides, which are used for a short, intensive course of therapy, and (2) antiseptic preparations, such as nitrofurantoin, methenamine mandelate, and nalidixic acid, which are often continued over longer periods of time to maintain urinary sterility. If anatomic defects such as primary reflux or bladder neck obstruction are present, surgical correction of these abnormalities may be necessary to prevent recurrent infection. Medical management of constipation may be required if "functional" bladder obstruction is present.

Follow-up study is an important component of medical management, since recurrence (often asymptomatic) is high. Urine cultures are recommended every 1 to 4 months for 1 to 2 years in order to prevent morbidity rather than to reduce the chance of renal failure. Some children are placed on prophylactic antimicrobials. The hazard of progressive renal injury is greatest when infection occurs in young children (especially under 2 years of age) and is associated with congenital renal malformations and reflux. Therefore, early diagnosis of children at risk is particularly important during infancy and toddlerhood. There is as yet no definitive therapy for vesicoureteral reflux.

Nursing considerations

Nursing objectives include identification of children with urinary tract infection and education of parents and children regarding prevention and treatment of infection. This involves identifying those children at risk for developing urinary tract infection and helping to confirm the diagnosis of existing infection. Mass screening is difficult; however, children who are receiving annual health examinations should have routine urinalysis performed. In addition, nurses should instruct parents to observe routinely for clues that suggest urinary tract infection. Many cases go undetected because of vague symptoms, and many parents fail to investigate this very common problem. Because in-

fants and young children are unable to communicate their distress verbally, there is no way to know if they suffer from dysuria. A careful history regarding voiding habits and episodes of unexplained irritability may well "diagnose" less obvious cases of urinary tract infection.

When infection is suspected, a midstream clean-catch voided specimen is essential (see p. 553 for procedure). Although older children can be instructed in the proper collection, the nurse performs the procedure on infants and young children. It is the nurse's responsibility to take every precaution to obtain acceptable clean-voided specimens in order to avoid the use of other collecting procedures. Suprapubic aspiration may be the method of choice for collecting specimens in infants. If so, the nurse assists the physician with the procedure.

Frequently other tests are performed to detect anatomic defects and assess renal status. Children are prepared for these tests as appropriate for their age. Except for intravenous pyelography, voiding cystography and cystoscopy are usually performed under general anesthesia.

TABLE 24-1. PREVENTION OF URINARY TRACT INFECTION

FACTORS PREDISPOSING TO DEVELOPMENT	MEASURES OF PREVENTION
Short female urethra close to vagina and anus	Perineal hygiene—wipe from front to back Avoid tub baths, especially with bubble-bath or water softener; use showers Avoid tight clothing or diapers; wear cotton panties rather than nylon Check for vaginitis or pinworms, especially if child scratches between legs
Incomplete emptying (reflux) and overdistention of bladder	Avoid "holding" urine; encourage child to void frequently, especially before a long trip or other circumstances where toilet facilities are not available Empty bladder completely with each void Avoid straining at stool
Concentrated and alkaline urine	Encourage generous fluid intake Acidify urine with juices such as apple or cranberry and a diet high in animal protein

SUMMARY OF NURSING CARE OF THE CHILD WITH URINARY TRACT INFECTION

GOALS	RESPONSIBILITIES
Recognize urinary tract infection	Be alert for symptoms that indicate infection
Assist with diagnosis	Collect specimens as needed Assist the child with collecting specimens, if needed Teach the child clean-catch technique Explain purpose of specimen
Eradicate infectious organisms	Administer antibiotics as prescribed
Prevent bacterial growth	Encourage acidifying beverages Administer urinary antiseptics as prescribed
Assure sufficient fluid intake	Encourage fluid intake Employ play techniques to encourage fluid intake
Prevent urinary tract infection	Teach appropriate hygienic practices Encourage adequate fluid intake Encourage tests to detect possible anatomic defects that predispose to urinary tract infections Emphasize importance of continued antibiotic therapy and regular urine examinations following an infection Provide needed follow-up care or refer to appropriate health agency

However, children still need an explanation of the procedure, its purpose, and a simple description of what they will experience. When explaining to children about the urinary tract, especially to preschool children, the nurse must clarify that the urinary tract is separate from any sexual function and that the test is for a problem that they did not cause. It is not uncommon for children to associate blame for activities (such as masturbation), wrongdoing, or unacceptable thoughts with the reason for the illness or the tests.

Since antibacterial drugs are always indicated in urinary tract infection, the nurse advises parents of proper dosage and administration. It is important for parents to be aware that the drug should be administered as prescribed and for the length of time indicated. When prophylactic medications are ordered for prolonged therapy, the nurse must emphasize to parents and older children the need for continued administration even when no signs of infection are present.

Prevention is certainly the most important goal in both primary and secondary infection. The suggestions listed in Table 24-1 are very simple, commonplace habits that should be practiced by all females. The other measures, with the exception of avoiding tub baths, are applicable to

males as well. Urinary tract infections have also been traced to hot tubs and whirlpool baths. For sexually active adolescent females, it is also advisable for them to urinate as soon as possible after intercourse to flush out bacteria introduced during sex play.

MINIMAL CHANGE NEPHROTIC SYNDROME (MCNS)

The *nephrotic syndrome* is a clinical state that may develop during the course of several different renal disorders in which increased glomerular permeability to plasma protein results in massive urinary protein loss. Approximately 80% of cases of nephrotic syndrome in children occur in the absence of recognizable systemic disease and are categorized as idiopathic. The following discussion is limited to the disorder now known as minimal change nephrotic syndrome (also called "minimal lesion" nephrosis, idiopathic nephrotic syndrome, childhood nephrosis, lipoid nephrosis, or uncomplicated nephrosis).

The cause of minimal change nephrotic syndrome remains obscure. Often a nonspecific illness, usually a viral upper respiratory infection, precedes the manifestations by

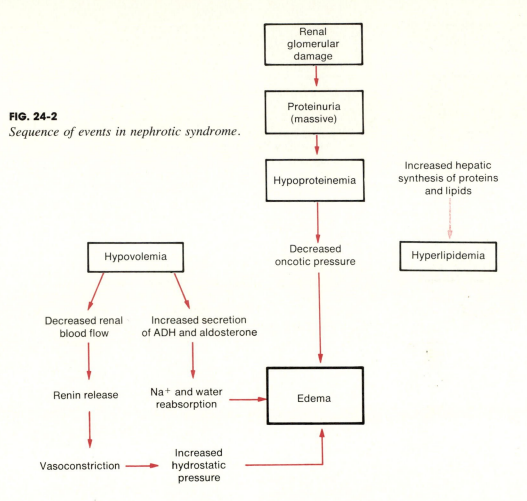

FIG. 24-2

Sequence of events in nephrotic syndrome.

4 to 8 days but is considered a precipitating factor rather than a cause. It is doubtful that this syndrome has a single cause; the disease probably represents several different pathologic processes affecting the glomerular membranes.

Pathophysiology

The pathogenesis of this disorder is not understood. There may be a metabolic, biochemical, or physiochemical disturbance that causes the basement membrane of the glomeruli to become increasingly permeable to protein, but the cause and mechanisms are only speculative.

The glomerular membrane, normally impermeable to albumin and other proteins, becomes permeable to proteins, especially albumin, which leak through the membrane and are lost in urine (hyperalbuminuria). This reduces the serum albumin level (hypoalbuminemia), decreasing the colloidal osmotic pressure in the capillaries. As a result, the vascular hydrostatic pressure exceeds the pull of the colloidal osmotic pressure causing fluid to accumulate in the interstitial spaces (edema) and body cavities, particularly in the abdominal cavity (ascites). The shift of fluid from the plasma to the interstitial spaces re-

duces the vascular fluid volume (hypovolemia), which in turn stimulates the renin-angiotensin system and the secretion of antidiuretic hormone and aldosterone. Tubular reabsorption of sodium and water is increased in an attempt to increase intravascular volume. The elevation of serum lipids is unexplained. The sequence of events in nephrotic syndrome is diagrammed in Fig. 24-2.

Clinical manifestations

A previously healthy child begins to gain weight; this weight gain progresses insidiously over a period of days or weeks. Puffiness of the face, especially around the eyes, is apparent on arising in the morning but subsides during the day, when swelling of the abdomen and lower extremities is more prominent. The generalized edema develops so slowly that parents may consider it a sign of healthy growth. Although an acute infection may precipitate severe generalized edema (anasarca), the usual course is one of progressive weight gain until either rapid or gradual increase in edema prompts the family to seek medical evaluation. Usually present are abdominal swelling from ascites, respiratory difficulty from pleural effusion, and

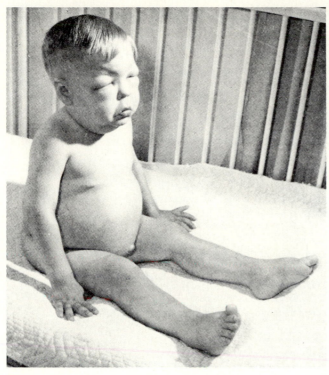

FIG. 24-3

Child with nephrosis. Note edema of face, eyelids, abdomen, and lower extremities. (From Benz, G.S.: Pediatric nursing, ed. 5, St. Louis, 1964, The C.V. Mosby Co. Courtesy University of Minnesota Photographic Laboratory.)

labial or scrotal swelling (Fig. 24-3). Edema of the intestinal mucosa may cause diarrhea, anorexia, and poor intestinal absorption. The volume of urine is decreased, and the urine appears darkly opalescent and frothy. Neurologic examinations are negative, and the sensorium is clear.

Extreme skin pallor is often present, and the child has a tendency toward skin breakdown during periods of edema. The child is irritable and may be easily fatigued or lethargic but does not appear seriously ill. Malnutrition from poor appetite and loss of protein is not uncommon, although it is frequently obscured by edema. However, changes in the quality of the hair give evidence of the malnourished state. The blood pressure is usually normal or slightly decreased. The child is more susceptible to infection, especially cellulitis, pneumonia, peritonitis, or septicemia.

Diagnostic evaluation

Massive proteinuria is reflected in urine excretion of large amounts of protein with high specific gravity proportionate to the concentration of protein. Hyaline casts, fat bodies, and a few red blood cells, can be found in the urine of most affected children, although there is seldom gross hematuria. If hypovolemia is not significant and if the child is well hydrated, the glomerular filtration rate is usually normal.

Total serum protein concentrations are lowered, with the albumin fractions significantly reduced and globulins and plasma lipids elevated. Hemoglobin and hematocrit are usually normal or even elevated as a result of hemoconcentration. Serum sodium concentration is usually low.

Renal biopsy and the appearance of renal tissue under the light and electron microscope provide information regarding the glomerular status and type of nephrotic syndrome, response to drugs, and probable course of the disease. Under the microscope the foot processes of the basement membrane appear fused.

Therapeutic management

Children with severe symptoms or those whose disease is newly recognized are hospitalized for assessment and observation for evidence of infection and response to therapy. During the edema phase the child is often placed on bed rest, but activity is not restricted during remission. Acute and intercurrent infections are treated with appropriate antibiotics, and efforts are made to eliminate possible infection.

The child who is in remission is allowed a regular diet; however, during periods of massive edema, salt is restricted. This restriction is usually tolerated by the child for a time. Although edema cannot be removed by a low-sodium diet, its rate of increase may be reduced. Water is seldom restricted.

Oral corticosteroid (prednisone) therapy is begun as soon as the diagnosis has been established and is continued until the urine is free from protein and remains normal for 10 days to 2 weeks. In most patients diuresis occurs, urine protein excretion disappears within 7 to 21 days, and other clinical manifestations stabilize or return to normal. In 90% of patients urine returns to normal within 4 weeks; in many patients this occurs as early as 3 or 4 days. When the child is free of proteinuria and edema, the medication is given as a single dose every 48 hours for a time, then gradually tapered to discontinuance over a variable period of time.

It is estimated that approximately 80% of nephrotic children have this favorable prognosis. However, children who require frequent courses of steroid therapy are highly susceptible to complications of steroids, such as growth retardation, hypertension, gastrointestinal bleeding, Cushing's syndrome, bone demineralization, infections, and diabetes mellitus. Children who do not respond to steroid therapy, children who have frequent relapses, and those in

SUMMARY OF NURSING CARE OF THE CHILD WITH MINIMAL CHANGE NEPHROTIC SYNDROME

GOALS	RESPONSIBILITIES
Assist with diagnosis	Recognize signs and symptoms that indicate nephrosis Collect specimens as needed Assist with diagnostic procedures
Prevent and control acute infection	Avoid contact with infected persons Do not place the child in room with infectious children Observe medical asepsis Administer antibiotics if ordered Keep the child dry and warm Monitor vital signs for early signs of infectious processes Collect specimens, such as urine for culture, blood
Prevent skin breakdown	Provide meticulous skin care Clean and powder opposing skin surfaces several times daily Separate skin surfaces with soft cotton Support edematous organs, such as scrotum Clean edematous eyelids with warm saline wipes Change position frequently; maintain good body alignment
Prevent further edema formation	Provide salt-restricted diet Administer steroids and diuretics, if ordered Administer salt-poor albumin intravenous infusion, if ordered
Prevent hypovolemia	Monitor vital signs to detect physical signs Assess pulse quality and rate Take blood pressure Report deviations
Conserve energy	Maintain bed rest initially Balance rest and activity when ambulatory Plan and provide quiet activities Instruct the child to rest when he begins to feel tired
Control edema	Administer corticosteroids as ordered Administer diuretics, if ordered Limit intake, if ordered

whom the side effects threaten their growth and general health are considered for a course of immunosuppressant drug therapy with an oral alkylating agent, usually cyclophosphamide (Cytoxan), alternating with prednisone. Both drugs are administered for up to 2 months, after which cyclophosphamide is discontinued abruptly and the prednisone is decreased gradually.

Nursing considerations

Children hospitalized with nephrotic syndrome are placed on bed rest during the edema phase of the disease. They seldom offer resistance, since they are usually lethargic and easily fatigued, and their cumbersome edematous bulk is not conducive to movement. Most are content to lie in the prone position and must be encouraged and helped to turn regularly to prevent tissue breakdown. Areas that are particularly edematous, such as the scrotum, abdomen, and legs, may require support, and skin surfaces should be cleaned and separated with clothing, cotton, or antiseptic powder to prevent intertrigo.

Infection is a constant source of danger to edematous children and those on corticosteroid therapy. These children are particularly vulnerable to upper respiratory infection; therefore, they must be kept warm and dry, turned frequently, and protected from contact with infected roommates, visitors, and personnel. Vital signs are monitored to detect any early signs of an infective process.

Strict intake and output records are essential but may be difficult in very young children. Application of collection bags is highly irritating to sensitive skin that is readily subject to breakdown. Application of diapers or weighing wet pads may be necessary. Other methods of monitoring progress include urine examination for specific gravity and

SUMMARY OF NURSING CARE OF THE CHILD WITH MINIMAL CHANGE NEPHROTIC SYNDROME—cont'd

GOALS	RESPONSIBILITIES
Assess changes in edema	Weigh daily (or more often if ordered) Measure abdominal girth at umbilicus Measure accurately intake and output Test urine for specific gravity, albumin Collect specimens for laboratory examination
Establish good nutrition	Administer high-protein, high-carbohydrate diet (restrict sodium during edema) Administer supplementary vitamins and iron as ordered
Stimulate appetite	Enlist aid of the child, parents, and dietitian in formulation of diet Provide cheerful, clean, relaxed atmosphere during meals Serve small quantities initially to stimulate appetite; encourage seconds Provide special and preferred foods Serve foods in an attractive manner
Establish good mental hygiene	Encourage activity within limits of tolerance Encourage socialization with persons without active infection Provide positive feedback Explore areas of interest and encourage their pursuit

Prepare for home care	Instruct the parents
	  Testing urine for albumin daily
	  Administration of medications
	  Initial signs of relapse
	  Side effects of drugs
	  Prevention of infection
	Impress on the parents importance of following prescribed regimen

Support the parents	Listen to the parents Assist the parents with problem solving Provide education when indicated Provide positive feedback Refer to parent groups
Continue follow-up care	Maintain contact with the family Refer to appropriate persons or agencies for assistance

albumin and measurement of daily weight and abdominal girth. Assessment of edema, such as increased or decreased swelling around the eyes and dependent areas, degree of pitting (if noted), and color and texture of skin are part of nursing care.

Loss of appetite accompanying active nephrosis creates a perplexing problem for nurses. During this time the combined efforts of nurse, dietitian, parents, and the child himself are needed to formulate a nutritionally adequate and attractive diet. Salt is usually restricted, but not eliminated, during the edema phase, and fluid restriction is limited to short-term use during massive edema. A generous protein intake is highly desirable to minimize negative nitrogen balance but is poorly accepted by most children. Every effort should be made to serve attractive meals with preferred foods and a minimum of fuss, but it usually requires a considerable amount of ingenuity and enticement

to get the child to eat (see the discussion on feeding the sick child on p. 541).

As the edema subsides, children are allowed increased activity, which is desirable in order to prevent bone demineralization from immobilization and corticosteroid administration. Although easily fatigued, they usually adjust activities according to their tolerance level. However, they may require guidance in selecting play activities. Suitable recreational and diversional activities are an important part of their care. Once edema fluid has been lost, children are allowed to resume their usual activities with discretion. Irritability and mood swings that accompany the inactivity, disease process, and steroid therapy are not unusual manifestations in these children, and they create an additional challenge to the nurse and the family.

The prolonged up-and-down course of remissions and exacerbations with periodic disruption of family life by hospitalization places a severe strain on the child and family, both psychologically and financially. Children over 5 or 6 years of age and parents need reassurance regarding the characteristic course of the disease so that they will not become discouraged with the frequent relapses. At the same time, to gain cooperation, it is important to impress on them the importance of long-term care and compliance. A satisfactory response is more likely when relapses are detected and therapy instituted early, and remissions are prolonged when instructions are carried out faithfully. For example, one child had a relapse when his mother reduced the dosage of his drug because it was so expensive.

ACUTE GLOMERULONEPHRITIS (AGN, POSTSTREPTOCOCCAL)

Acute glomerulonephritis is the most common of the noninfectious renal diseases in childhood and is the one for which cause can be established in the majority of cases. Acute nephritis occurs most frequently in children 2 to 12 years of age, with a peak incidence at about age 6 years. It is uncommon in children younger than 2 years of age, and males outnumber females two to one in most series studied.

Etiology

It is now generally accepted that acute glomerulonephritis is caused by a reaction to streptococcal infection with certain strains of the group A β-hemolytic *Streptococcus* with a period of 10 to 14 days between the streptococcal infection and the onset of clinical manifestations. The peak incidence of disease is in the school-age years and corresponds to the incidence of streptococcal infections. Disease secondary to streptococcal pharyngitis is more common in the winter or spring, but, when associated with pyoderma (principally impetigo), it may be more prevalent in later summer or early fall, especially in warmer climates.

Pathophysiology

In the inflammatory process that follows a streptococcal infection, the glomeruli become edematous and infiltrated with polymorphonuclear leukocytes, which occlude the capillary lumen. The resulting decrease in plasma filtration results in an excessive accumulation of water and retention of sodium that expands plasma and interstitial fluid volumes, leading to circulatory congestion and edema. It is unclear whether the decreased glomerular filtration rate, increased capillary permeability, or vascular spasm is responsible for these various manifestations. The cause of the hypertension associated with acute glomerulonephritis is also unexplained.

Clinical manifestations

Typically, affected children are in good health until they experience the streptococcal infection. In some instances there is no history of an infection, or it is only described as a mild cold. The onset of nephritis appears after an average latent period of about 10 days. Since the child appears well during this time, the association is not recognized by parents.

Initial signs of renal response include puffiness of the face, especially around the eyes (periorbital edema), anorexia, and passage of dark urine. The edema is more prominent in the face in the morning but spreads during the day to involve the extremities and abdomen. The edema is relatively moderate and may not be appreciated by someone unfamiliar with the child's normal appearance. The urine is cloudy, smoky brown, or what parents describe as resembling tea or cola, and severely reduced in volume.

The child is pale, irritable, and lethargic. He appears ill but seldom expresses specific complaints. Older children may complain of headaches, abdominal discomfort, and dysuria. Vomiting is not uncommon. On examination there is usually a mild to moderate elevation in blood pressure (diastolic, 80 to 120 mm Hg; systolic, 120 to 180 mm Hg).

Diagnostic evaluation

Urinalysis during the acute phase characteristically shows hematuria, proteinuria, and increased specific gravity. The specific gravity is moderately elevated and seldom exceeds 1.020. Proteinuria generally parallels the hematuria, and the content usually shows 3+ or 4+ but is not the massive proteinuria seen in nephrotic syndrome. Gross discoloration of urine reflects its red blood cell and hemoglobin content. Microscopic examination of the sediment shows many red blood cells, leukocytes, epithelial cells, and casts, primarily composed of epithelial and red blood cells. Bacteria are not seen, and urine cultures are negative.

Azotemia that results from impaired glomerular filtration is reflected in elevated blood urea nitrogen and creatinine levels in at least 50% of cases. When proteinuria is heavy, there may be changes associated with nephrotic syndrome, that is, transient hypoproteinemia and hyperlipidemia.

Cultures of the pharynx are positive for streptococci in only a few cases, and the numbers are not significantly greater than the normal carrier incidence in many communities. Positive cultures help to establish a diagnosis. Cultures should be obtained from other household members, and persons positive for group A streptococci should receive a course of antistreptococcal therapy.

Some serologic tests may help in the diagnosis of acute glomerulonephritis. The antistreptolysin O (ASO) titer is the most familiar and readily available test for streptococcal infection. It is used to detect the presence of antibodies, which documents a recent infection, especially a rising titer in two samples taken a week apart. More consistent and reliable antibody tests following streptococcal skin infections are elevated antihyaluronidase and antideoxyribonuclease B titers.

Nonspecific acute-phase reactants that reflect acute inflammatory processes, such as the erythrocyte sedimentation rate (ESR), C-reactive protein (CRP), and serum mucoprotein tests, are elevated during the early stages of acute disease and then gradually return to normal as healing takes place. The erythrocyte sedimentation rate is sometimes used as a guide to the progress of the nephritis.

Therapeutic management

There is no specific treatment for acute glomerulonephritis, and recovery is spontaneous and uneventful in most cases. Bed rest is recommended during the acute phase, but ambulation does not seem to have an adverse effect on the course of the disease once the gross hematuria, edema, hypertension, and azotemia have abated. Since they are generally listless and experience fatigue and malaise, most children voluntarily restrict their activities during the most active phase of the disease. After diuresis has occurred, ambulation is allowed for those children without hypertension and gross urine abnormalities.

Regular measurement of vital signs, body weight, and intake and output is essential in order to monitor the progress of the disease and to detect complications that may appear at any time during the course of the disease. A record of daily weight is the most useful means to assess fluid balance and is kept for children treated at home as well as for those who are hospitalized. Water restriction is seldom necessary unless the output is significantly reduced. Children on restricted fluids, especially those who are not severely edematous or those who have lost weight, are observed for signs of dehydration.

Dietary restrictions depend on the severity of the edema. A regular diet is permitted in uncomplicated cases, but the intake of sodium is usually limited (no salt is added to foods). Moderate sodium restriction is usually instituted for children with hypertension or edema. Severe sodium restriction is not well tolerated by children and may interfere with caloric intake in these already anorexic youngsters. Foods with substantial amounts of potassium are generally restricted during the period of oliguria. Protein restriction is reserved only for patients with severe azotemia resulting from prolonged oliguria. The anorexia as-

sociated with the disease usually limits the protein intake sufficiently.

Antibiotic therapy is indicated only for those children with evidence of persistent streptococcal infections. Hypertension is controlled with hydralazine (Apresoline), usually in conjunction with reserpine. Some authorities recommend hydralazine with furosemide (Lasix). The diuretic furosemide has been used with some success in severe cases. A mild sedative may help to control mild hypertension.

Almost all children correctly diagnosed as having acute poststreptococcal glomerulonephritis recover completely, and specific immunity is conferred so that subsequent recurrences are uncommon. Deaths from complications still occur but are, fortunately, rare. A few of these children may develop chronic disease, but many of these cases are believed to be different glomerular diseases misdiagnosed as poststreptococcal disease.

Nursing considerations

Nursing care of the child with glomerulonephritis involves careful assessment of the disease status, with regular monitoring of vital signs (including blood pressure), fluid balance, and behavior. Vital signs provide clues to the severity of the disease and early signs of complications. They are carefully measured, and any abnormalities are reported and recorded. The volume and character of urine are noted, and the child is weighed daily.

Assessment of the child's appearance for signs of cerebral complications is an important nursing function, since the severity of the acute phase is variable and unpredictable. The child with edema, hypertension, and gross hematuria may be subject to complications, and anticipatory preparations such as seizure precautions and intravenous equipment are included in the nursing care plan.

For most children a regular diet is allowed, but it should contain no added salt. Foods high in sodium and salted treats are eliminated, and parents and friends are advised not to bring items such as potato chips or pretzels. However, the total amount of salt ingested is usually less than prescribed because of the child's poor appetite. Fluid restriction, if included in care, is more difficult, and the amount permitted is evenly divided throughout the waking hours and served in small cups to give the illusion of larger servings. Meal preparation and service require special attention, since the child is indifferent to meals during the acute phase. Again, collaboration with parents and the dietitian and special consideration for food preferences facilitate meal planning.

During the acute phase children are generally quite content to lie in bed. Activities should be those that require little expenditure of energy. As they begin to feel better and as their symptoms subside, activities are planned to allow for frequent rest periods and avoidance of fatigue.

Children who have mild edema and no hypertension and convalescent children who are being treated at home need follow-up care. Parents are instructed regarding general measures, including activity, diet, and prevention of infection. The children are permitted to be ambulatory but should not attend school or participate in outside games and sports until the risk of complications has passed. Strenuous activity is usually restricted until there is no microscopic evidence of proteinuria or hematuria, which may persist for months.

Health supervision is continued with weekly, followed by monthly, visits for evaluation and urinalysis. Parent education and support in preparation for discharge and home care include education in home management and the need for follow-up care and health supervision.

CHRONIC OR PROGRESSIVE GLOMERULONEPHRITIS

The majority of cases of renal glomerular disease are acute glomerulonephritis, minimal change nephrotic syndrome, and glomerulonephritis associated with systemic diseases, such as systemic lupus erythematosis. *Persistent glomerulonephritis* is a term used to describe those cases of glomerulonephritis that have no specific histologic picture but that fail to show the rapid recovery expected in acute nephritis. *Chronic glomerulonephritis* (CGN) describes advanced glomerular disease caused by a variety of different disease processes. *Rapidly progressive glomerulonephritis* is a term used to describe an acute illness with severe, acute onset resembling acute poststreptococcal glomerulonephritis but that causes rapidly progressive deterioration of renal function in 6 to 12 months.

Etiology

Chronic glomerulonephritis is a progressive disorder that can be caused by a variety of diseases. It may begin abruptly; more often there is no history of an attack of acute glomerular disease, or it may represent one of a succession of exacerbations of a preexisting disease. Chronic glomerulonephritis that is not associated with other diseases may go undetected for years and be relatively asymptomatic until kidney destruction produces marked reduction in renal function. Consequently the disease is more common in adolescents than in younger children. Renal insufficiency with all its manifestations occurs as the ultimate event.

Clinical manifestations

The varied clinical manifestations and laboratory findings generally reflect deteriorating renal function. Nephrotic syndrome, with its usual clinical picture develops frequently. Hypertension, edema, proteinuria, cardiac failure, dyspnea, osteodystrophy, and anemia are common manifestations of progressive disease.

Diagnostic evaluation

Laboratory findings may include proteinuria with casts and red and white blood cells. Failing renal function is evident from elevated blood urea nitrogen, creatinine, and uric acid levels. Electrolyte alterations include metabolic acidosis, decreased sodium from the chronic salt-losing state, elevated potassium, elevated phosphorus, and decreased calcium levels. As the disease progresses, urine specific gravity eventually stabilizes at an isotonic state (about 1.012) as a result of the inability of the kidney to reabsorb solutes or respond to antidiuretic hormone. The renal insufficiency may extend from 5 to 15 years and even longer, or rapid deterioration may cause death in 1 to 2 years.

Therapeutic management

Early in the course of the disease, treatment is appropriate to the underlying disease and is largely symptomatic in most cases. Efforts are directed toward providing optimum conditions for the child's physical, psychologic, and social development. As few restrictions as feasible are imposed, and the child is allowed to live as normal a life as possible for as long as possible. Drug treatment offers little lasting benefit, although diuretic therapy may be helpful occasionally for edema or hypertension. Marked hypertension is controlled with antihypertensive agents, and anemia may require periodic transfusion with fresh packed cells. Salt is only moderately restricted. Ultimately dialysis and transplantation may restore relatively good health; however, these are usually not available alternatives until renal failure is far advanced. (See the discussion of chronic renal failure on pp. 793 to 798 for more detailed management of specific problems.) Children with rapidly progressive glomerulonephritis are usually referred to a center specializing in renal disease.

Nursing considerations

The problems of chronic glomerulonephritis and those encountered in chronic renal insufficiency from any cause will be discussed in association with chronic renal failure on p. 793.

SUMMARY OF NURSING CARE OF THE CHILD WITH ACUTE GLOMERULONEPHRITIS

GOALS	RESPONSIBILITIES
Prevent glomerulonephritis	Refer children with sore throats or impetigo for throat culture Ensure compliance with antibiotic therapy for diagnosed streptococcal infections
Assist with diagnosis	Recognize signs and symptoms that suggest kidney dysfunction Assist with diagnostic procedures Collect specimens as needed
Prevent infection	Avoid contact with infected persons Administer antibiotics if ordered Keep the child warm and dry
Prevent or control progress of edema	Help plan and serve restricted or low-sodium diet Limit fluids if ordered
Prevent hyperkalemia	Restrict foods high in potassium during oliguria Monitor laboratory findings Observe for incipient signs of hyperkalemia
Assess progress of edema	Assess general appearance and behavior Weigh daily Measure intake and output
Reduce blood pressure	Institute bed rest Administer antihypertensive agents Administer diuretics if ordered

Observe for signs of complications	Report significant deviations of
	    Vital signs—blood pressure, pulse, respiration, temperature
	    Appearance and volume of urine
	    Weight gain relative to size of the child
	Report any dyspnea
	Report unusual symptoms
	    Vomiting
	    Visual disturbances
	    Motor disturbances
	    Seizure activity
	    Severe headache
	    Abdominal pain
	    Changes in behavior and/or activity level, for example, lethargy, restlessness

Provide nourishment	Administer high-carbohydrate diet Allow sodium and protein as prescribed
Stimulate appetite	Serve attractive meals in small portions Serve preferred foods Arrange meals with other children or family
Provide comfort	Encourage the parents to visit Spend time with the child Provide opportunity to socialize with noninfectious children Provide appropriate play activities
Educate the parents for home care	Teach urine testing for blood and protein Teach early signs of complications
Continue follow-up care	Arrange for regular checkups Provide for public health nurse if needed Refer to proper agency for home tutoring if needed
Promote growth and development	Encourage normal activity within limitations imposed by state of disease process Allow for regression when appropriate

MISCELLANEOUS RENAL DISORDERS

Renal damage occurs as a major or minor complication in many systemic diseases and with varying degrees of severity. In some the renal complications may be the principal cause of death or one of several complications with fatal consequences. In others it may be only a source of discomfort but no direct threat to life.

HEMOLYTIC-UREMIC SYNDROME (HUS)

Hemolytic-uremic syndrome is an uncommon, acute renal disease that occurs primarily in infants and small children between the ages of 6 months and 3 years. It appears worldwide but is seen more often in white children than in black children. Although uncommon, hemolytic-uremic syndrome represents one of the most frequent causes of acute renal failure in children.

In the majority of cases no causative agents have been identified; however, many possible agents or precipitating events have been suggested. The appearance of the disease has been associated with rickettsial, viral, pneumococcal, and gastrointestinal disorders. The disease usually follows an acute gastrointestinal or upper respiratory infection and tends to occur in scattered outbreaks in small geographic areas. There is a familial tendency in some cases.

Pathophysiology

The primary site of injury appears to be the endothelial lining of the small glomerular arterioles, which become swollen and occluded with deposits of platelets and fibrin clots. Red cells are damaged as they attempt to move through the partially occluded blood vessels. These damaged cells are removed by the spleen, causing acute hemolytic anemia. The platelet aggregation within the damaged blood vessels or the damage and removal of platelets produce the characteristic thromboyctopenia.

Clinical manifestations

The hemolytic process persists from several days to 2 weeks. During this time the child is anorectic, irritable, and lethargic. There is marked and rapid onset of pallor, accompanied by hemorrhagic manifestations such as bruising, purpura, or rectal bleeding. Usually there is oliguria or anuria, although nonoliguric acute renal failure may be manifested. Convulsions and stupor suggest central nervous system involvement, and there may be signs of acute heart failure.

Diagnostic evaluation

The presence of anemia, thrombocytopenia, and renal failure is sufficient for diagnosis. Renal involvement is evidenced by proteinuria, hematuria, and the presence of urinary casts; blood urea nitrogen and serum creatinine levels are elevated. A high reticulocyte count confirms the hemolytic nature of the anemia.

Therapeutic management

The most consistently effective treatment of hemolytic-uremic syndrome is peritoneal dialysis, which is instituted in any child who has been anuric for 24 hours or who demonstrates oliguria with hypertension and seizures. Blood transfusions with fresh, washed packed cells are administered for severe anemia but are used with caution to prevent circulatory overload from added volume.

There is no substantial evidence that heparin, corticosteroids, or fibrinolytic agents are beneficial. With prompt treatment the recovery rate is about 95%, but there may be residual renal impairment. Renal impairment or central nervous system injury are the usual causes of death.

Nursing considerations

Nursing care is the same as that provided in acute renal failure and, for children with continued impairment, includes management of chronic disease.

FAMILIAL GLOMERULOPATHY (ALPORT SYNDROME)

The syndrome of familial glomerulopathy (a chronic hereditary nephritis) consists of hematuria, nerve deafness, ocular disorders, and chronic renal failure. The disease appears to be inherited as an autosomal-dominant trait. Although uncommon, the disease is not rare and accounts for a significant percentage of persistent glomerular disease in childhood.

The clinical manifestations are indistinguishable from mild acute nephritis. Initial symptoms include hematuria, proteinuria, malaise, and mild edema. The symptoms are often associated with an acute respiratory infection. The condition begins in infancy and slowly progresses until uncontrollable renal failure develops in adolescence or early adulthood. Most untreated boys develop severe symptoms, whereas affected girls generally have a milder disease and a normal life expectancy.

Treatment is symptomatic and supportive, and every effort should be made to restrict the activities of affected children as little as possible. Dialysis and renal transplantation are ultimate therapeutic measures for renal involvement. Hearing loss and ocular disorders should receive appropriate attention, and families should be counseled regarding the genetic implications of the disease.

WILMS TUMOR

Wilms tumor, nephroma, or nephroblastoma is the most frequent intraabdominal tumor of childhood and the most common type of renal cancer. Its frequency is estimated to be 1 in 10,000 live births; there is a slightly higher incidence in males. The peak incidence is 3 years of age.

Etiology

Wilms tumor probably arises from a malignant, undifferentiated cluster of primordial cells capable of initiating the regeneration of an abnormal structure. Its occurrence slightly favors the left kidney, which is advantageous because surgically this kidney is easier to manipulate and remove. In about 10% of the cases both kidneys are involved. Although the tumor may become quite large, it remains encapsulated for an extended period of time.

Clinical manifestations

The most common presenting sign is a swelling or mass within the abdomen. The mass is characteristically firm, nontender, confined to the midline, and deep within the flank. If the tumor is on the right side, it may be difficult to distinguish from the liver, although, unlike that organ, it does not move with respiration. Parents usually first discover the mass while bathing or dressing the child.

Other clinical manifestations are the result of compression from the tumor mass, metabolic alterations secondary to the tumor, or metastasis. Hematuria occurs in less than one fourth of children with Wilms tumor. Anemia, usually secondary to hemorrhage within the tumor, results in pallor, anorexia, and lethargy. Hypertension occurs occasionally, probably because of secretion of excess amounts of renin by the tumor. Other effects of malignancy include weight loss and fever. If metastasis has occurred, symptoms of lung involvement, such as dyspnea, cough, shortness of breath, and pain in the chest, may be evident.

Diagnostic evaluation

The usual tests include abdominal and radiographic chest examinations, an intravenous pyelogram, and organ and skeletal surveys. In difficult cases, ultrasonography, tomography, and angiography may be employed to help as-

sess an abdominal mass. A complete blood count and peripheral smear are done preoperatively to evaluate the degree of anemia, especially in terms of increasing surgical risks. Liver function tests are performed to assess liver dysfunction from metastasis or any preexisting abnormality that may alter antineoplastic drug metabolism and excretion. Renal function tests determine function of the unaffected kidney.

Therapeutic management

The principal modes of treatment are surgery, irradiation, and chemotherapy. Although in some institutions the exact sequence of treatment varies, with some institutions preferring the administration of chemotherapy before surgery, the following is the usual approach.

Surgery. Surgery is scheduled as soon as possible after confirmation of a renal mass, usually within 24 to 48 hours after admission, and the tumor, affected kidney, and adjacent adrenal gland are removed. Great care is taken to keep the encapsulated tumor intact, since rupture can seed cancer cells throughout the abdomen, lymph channel, and bloodstream. The contralateral kidney and regional lymph nodes are carefully inspected for evidence of disease or dysfunction. Lymph nodes are biopsied when indicated and any involved structures, such as part of the colon, diaphragm, or vena cava, are removed. Metal clips are placed around the tumor site for exact marking during radiotherapy.

Radiotherapy. Postoperative radiotherapy is usually indicated for all children with Wilms tumor except those under 18 months of age with stage I disease. The normal tissues of infants are extremely radiosensitive and are, therefore, at risk for developing skeletal and soft-tissue deformities. Irradiation of the tumor site and metastasized areas may be started within 1 to 3 days postoperatively if the child's condition is stable.

Chemotherapy. The most effective agents for treating Wilms tumor following surgery are the antineoplastic drugs actinomycin D and vincristine. For stage I tumors these medications alone are usually sufficient. For stage II tumors and for those that have advanced past stage II the drug regimen is accompanied by irradiation. If the neoplasia is bilateral, the surgeon often attempts to save the less involved kidney with a wedge resection and careful irradiation to prevent nephritis.

Prognosis

The survival rate for Wilms tumor is one of the highest among all childhood cancers. Children with localized tumor (stages I and II) have a 90% chance of cure with multimodal therapy (surgical extirpation, irradiation, and chemotherapy). In children with metastasis, survival rates are approximately 50%. Metastasis is most commonly to the lungs, followed by the liver, bone, and brain.

Nursing considerations

Nursing care of the child with Wilms tumor is similar to that of other cancers treated with surgery, irradiation, and chemotherapy. However, there are some significant differences; these are discussed for each phase of nursing intervention.

Preoperative care.   The preoperative period is one of swift diagnosis. Typically surgery is scheduled within 24 to 48 hours of admission. The nurse is faced with the challenge of preparing the child and parents for all laboratory and operative procedures. Because of the little time available, explanations are kept simple and they are repeated often.

There are several special preoperative concerns, the most important of which is that the tumor is not palpated unless absolutely necessary because manipulation of the mass may cause dissemination of cancer cells to adjacent and distant sites. In teaching hospitals in which many medical and nursing students are assigned to one patient, it may be necessary to post a sign on the bed, such as, *Do not palpate abdomen*. This same precaution is extended to parents as soon as Wilms tumor is suspected. Careful bathing and handling are also important in preventing trauma to the tumor site.

Children and parents need preparation for the size of the incision and dressing. An extensive abdominal incision is required to adequately view the internal organs. Postoperatively a large dressing and retention sutures are in place. If the child is unprepared, he may become upset and angry when he sees the surgical area.

In addition to the usual preoperative observations, the nurse carefully monitors blood pressure, since hypertension from excess renin production is a possibility. This is particularly important in young children in whom improperly sized blood pressure cuffs can yield inaccurate readings.

Postoperative care.   Despite the extensive surgical intervention necessary in many children with Wilms tumor, the recovery is usually rapid. The major nursing responsibilities are the same as those following any abdominal surgery (see the boxed material on p. 653). Since these children are at risk for intestinal obstruction from vincristine-induced adynamic ileus, radiation-induced edema, and postsurgical adhesion formation, gastrointestinal activity, such as bowel movements, bowel sounds, distention, vomiting, and pain are carefully monitored.

The nurse also monitors blood pressure for a possible drop after removal of the tumor, urinary output to assess functioning of the remaining kidney, and signs of infec-tion, especially during chemotherapy. Because of the myelosuppression from the drugs, pulmonary hygiene measures are instituted in the immediate postoperative period to prevent lung involvement.

The postoperative period is frequently difficult for parents. The shock of seeing their child immediately after surgery may be the first realization of the seriousness of the diagnosis. It also marks the confirmation of the stage of the tumor. Again, during this period, the nurse should be with the parents to assure them of the child's recovery after surgery and to assess the parents' understanding of the operative report. They need an opportunity to express their feelings and to realize that they are normal and realistic. The same emotional care discussed in Chapter 16 for families who have a child with a life-threatening disorder is applied to these individuals.

Older children need an opportunity to deal with their feelings concerning the many procedures to which they have been subjected in rapid succession. Play therapy with dolls or puppets or through drawing can be extremely beneficial in helping them adjust to the surgery and hair loss. It is not unusual for children to feel betrayed because they were not adequately prepared for the extent of surgery, the need for additional therapy, or the seriousness of the disorder.

Discharge planning.   The overall objective in discharge planning is returning the child to his normal preoperative life-style. The nurse emphasizes the usual needs for discipline and moderate protection from infection. Treatment schedules are planned to allow uninterrupted school attendance.

RENAL FAILURE

Renal failure is the inability of the kidneys to excrete wastes, concentrate urine, and conserve electrolytes. It can occur suddenly (acute renal failure) in response to inadequate perfusion, kidney disease, or urinary tract obstruction, or it can develop slowly (chronic renal failure) as the result of long-standing kidney disease.

ACUTE RENAL FAILURE (ARF)

Acute renal failure exists when the kidneys suddenly are unable to regulate the volume and composition of urine appropriately in response to food and fluid intake and the needs of the organism. The principal feature is oliguria* associated with azotemia, acidosis, and diverse electrolyte

---

*The definition of oliguria varies extensively in the literature, from 100 to 400 ml/m^2/24 hours.

SUMMARY OF NURSING CARE FOR THE CHILD WITH WILMS TUMOR

GOALS	RESPONSIBILITIES
Recognize presence of tumor	Suspect tumor with presence of an asymptomatic swelling or mass within the abdomen

Assist with diagnosis	Take detailed history
	Observe for signs of associated congenital anomalies
	Assist with collection of specimens
	  Complete blood count
	  Liver function tests
	  Renal function tests
	  Urinalysis
	Assist with bone marrow aspiration
	Assist with radiographic examination

Prevent rupture of tumor capsule	Avoid palpating abdomen Post signs at head of bed stating the above
Provide preoperative care	Take routine vital signs Take blood pressure using proper size cuff Prepare the child and family for surgery (p. 585), including anticipation of large incision and dressing Prepare the family for anticipated postoperative therapies and their probable effects
Provide postoperative care Assess function of remaining kidney	Provide postoperative care for the child with abdominal surgery (p. 653) Monitor blood pressure Monitor intake and output
Prevent infection	Avoid contact with infected persons Employ meticulous medical and surgical asepsis Institute pulmonary hygiene measures
Observe for signs of intestinal obstruction	Monitor gastrointestinal activity Assess bowel sounds Assess abdomen for distention and pain Evaluate any vomiting
Eradicate any remaining tumor cells	Administer antimetabolites as prescribed Assist with radiation therapy
Support and reassure the child	Prepare the child for therapies and their expected side effects Assist the child in coping with distressing side effects of therapy such as hair loss, nausea and vomiting, peripheral neuropathy Allow the child the opportunity to express and play out his feelings and fears
Support the parents	Clarify misconceptions and reinforce information given by the physician and surgeon Provide anticipatory guidance regarding expected outcomes and side effects Prepare the parents to identify untoward reactions Prepare the parents for discharge of the child Help the parents acquire needed auxiliary services Maintain continuity of care

disturbances. Acute renal failure is not common in childhood, but the outcome depends on the cause, associated findings, and prompt recognition and treatment.

The terms *azotemia* and *uremia* are often used in relation to renal failure. Azotemia is the accumulation of nitrogenous waste within the blood. Uremia is a more advanced condition in which retention of nitrogenous products produces toxic symptoms. Azotemia is not life threatening, whereas uremia is a serious condition that often involves other body systems.

Pathophysiology

The pathology that produces acute renal failure caused by glomerulonephritis, hemolytic-uremic syndrome, and other renal disorders has been discussed in relation to those disease processes. Acute renal failure can also develop as a result of a large number of related or unrelated clinical conditions—poor renal perfusion, acute renal injury, or the final expression of chronic, irreversible renal disease. The most common cause in children is transient renal failure resulting from dehydration or other causes of poor perfusion that responds to restoration of fluid volume.

Acute renal failure is usually reversible, but the deviations of physiologic function can be extreme and the mortality rate in the pediatric age-group is still high. There is severe reduction in the glomerular filtration rate, an elevated blood urea nitrogen level, and a significant reduction in renal blood flow.

Clinical manifestations

The prime manifestation of acute renal failure is oliguria, generally a urine output less than 50 ml in 24 hours. Anuria is uncommon except in obstructive disorders. No other symptoms are specific to acute renal failure, although nausea, vomiting, and drowsiness may develop. Some nonspecific physical findings, such as edema or hypertension, may serve to identify the underlying cause. With continued oliguria, biochemical abnormalities can develop rapidly and circulatory and central nervous system manifestations appear. Laboratory data reflect the kidney dysfunction—hyperkalemia, hyponatremia, metabolic acidosis, hypocalcemia, anemia, or azotemia.

In many instances of acute renal failure the infant or child is already critically ill with the precipitating disorder and the explanation for development of oliguria is readily apparent.

The clinical course is variable and depends on the cause. In reversible acute renal failure there is a period of severe oliguria, or a low-output phase, followed by an abrupt onset of diuresis, or a high-output phase, followed by a gradual return to, or toward, normal urine volumes.

Diagnostic evaluation

When a previously healthy child develops acute renal failure without obvious cause, a careful history is taken to reveal symptoms that may be related to disorders of the urinary tract or regarding exposure to nephrotoxic chemicals, such as ingestion of heavy metals, inhalation of carbon tetrachloride or other organic solvents, or drugs known to be toxic to kidneys. Significant laboratory measurements that are elevated during renal shutdown and that serve as a guide for therapy are blood urea nitrogen and serum creatinine, pH, sodium, potassium, and calcium.

Therapeutic management

Treatment of acute renal failure is directed toward (1) treatment of the underlying cause, (2) management of the complications of renal failure, and (3) provision of supportive therapy within the constraints imposed by the renal failure.

Treatment of poor perfusion resulting from dehydration consists of volume restoration as described previously in treatment of dehydration. If oliguria persists after restoration of fluid volume or if the renal failure is caused by intrinsic renal damage, the physiologic and biochemical abnormalities that have resulted from kidney dysfunction must be corrected or controlled.

Initially a Foley catheter is inserted to rule out urine retention, to collect available urine for analysis, and to monitor results of mannitol or furosemide administration. The catheter may or may not be removed. Many authorities who believe that it serves little purpose during the oliguric phase and that it predisposes the bladder to infection prefer collection bags for measuring urine output. Others maintain a catheter for hourly urine measurements.

The amount of exogenous water provided should not exceed the amount needed to maintain zero water balance. It is calculated on the basis of estimated endogenous water formation and losses from sensible (primarily gastrointestinal) and insensible sources. No allotment is calculated for urine as long as oliguria persists.

The child with acute renal failure has a tendency to develop water intoxication and hyponatremia, which make it difficult to provide calories in sufficient amounts to meet the needs of the child and reduce the tissue catabolism, metabolic acidosis, hyperkalemia, and uremia. If the child is able to tolerate oral foods, concentrated food sources high in carbohydrate and fat but low in protein, potassium, and sodium may be provided. However, many children have functional disturbances of the gastrointestinal tract, such as nausea and vomiting; therefore, the intravenous route is generally preferred and usually consists of highly concentrated carbohydrate solutions in small volumes of water administered by the central venous route.

Control of water balance in these patients requires careful monitoring of feedback information, such as accurate intake and output, body weight, and electrolyte measurements. In general, during the oliguric phase, no sodium, chloride, or potassium is given unless there are other large ongoing losses. Regular measurement of plasma electrolyte, pH, blood urea nitrogen, and creatinine levels is required to assess the adequacy of fluid therapy and to anticipate complications that require specific treatment.

Elevated serum potassium is the most immediate threat to the life of the child with acute renal failure. Hyperkalemia can be minimized and sometimes avoided by eliminating potassium from all food and fluid, by reducing tissue catabolism, and by correcting acidosis. Measures employed for the reduction of serum potassium levels are rectal administration of an ion-exchange resin such as sodium polystyrene sulfonate (Kayexalate) and peritoneal dialysis or hemodialysis. The resin produces its effect by exchange of its sodium for the potassium, thus binding potassium for removal from the body. Dialysis removes potassium and other waste products from the serum by diffusion through a semipermeable membrane.

Complications.   Other complications that may occur with acute renal failure are hypertension, anemia, convulsions, coma, cardiac failure, and pulmonary edema. The most common cause of hypertension in acute renal failure is hypervolemia, or overexpansion of the extracellular fluid and plasma volume, together with hypersecretion of renin. Hypertension is controlled by limiting water and sodium; antihypertensive drugs are often used with caution.

Anemia is frequently associated with acute renal failure, but transfusion is not recommended unless the hemoglobin drops below 6 g/100 ml. Transfusions, if used, consist of fresh, packed red blood cells given slowly to reduce the likelihood of increasing blood volume, hypertension, and hyperkalemia.

Seizures occur rather often when renal failure progresses to uremia and are also related to hypertension, hyponatremia, and hypocalcemia. Treatment is directed to the specific cause, when it is known. More obscure causes are managed with anticonvulsant drugs.

Cardiac failure with pulmonary edema is almost always associated with hypervolemia. Treatment is directed toward reduction of fluid volume, with water and sodium restriction and administration of diuretics.

Nursing considerations

Nursing care of the infant or child with acute renal failure supports medical care and management. The major goal is reestablishment of renal function, with emphasis on pro-

viding an adequate caloric intake to minimize reduction of protein stores, preventing complications, and monitoring fluid balance, laboratory data, and physical manifestations. The probability of dialysis must be considered and the necessary equipment made available in anticipation of such an eventuality. Because the child requires intensive observation and, often, specialized equipment, he is usually admitted to an intensive care unit in which needed equipment and trained personnel are available.

Meticulous attention to fluid intake and output is mandatory, including all the physical measurements discussed previously in relation to problems of fluid balance. Monitoring fluid balance is a continuous process, and nursing measures, such as maintaining an optimum thermal environment, reducing any elevation of body temperature, and reducing restlessness and anxiety, are employed to decrease the rate of tissue catabolism. Although these children are usually quite ill and voluntarily diminish their activity, infants may become restless and irritable and children are often anxious and frightened. There are frequent, painful, and stress-producing treatments and tests that must be performed. The presence of a supportive, empathetic nurse can provide comfort and stability in a threatening and unnatural environment.

The nurse must be continually alert for changes in behavior that indicate the onset of complications. Infection from reduced resistance, anemia, and general morbidity is a constant threat. Fluid overload and electrolyte disturbances can precipitate cardiovascular complications such as hypertension and cardiac failure. Fluid and electrolyte imbalances, acidosis, and accumulation of nitrogenous waste products can produce neurologic involvement manifest by coma, convulsions, or alterations in sensorium.

Parental support and reassurance are among the major nursing responsibilities. The seriousness and emergency nature of acute renal failure are stressful to parents, and most parents feel some degree of guilt regarding the child's condition, especially when the illness is the result of ingestion of a toxic substance, dehydration, or genetic disease. They need reassurance and a sympathetic listener. They also need to be kept informed of the child's progress and provided explanations regarding the therapeutic regimen. The equipment and the child's behavior are sometimes frightening and anxiety provoking. Nurses can do much to help them comprehend and deal with the stresses of the situation.

CHRONIC RENAL FAILURE (CRF)

The kidneys are able to maintain the chemical composition of fluids within normal limits until more than 50% of functional renal capacity is destroyed by disease or injury.

SUMMARY OF NURSING CARE OF THE CHILD WITH ACUTE RENAL FAILURE

GOALS	RESPONSIBILITIES
Distinguish between urine retention and diminished urine formation	Insert Foley catheter Measure output Send urine obtained (if any) for laboratory analysis
Help establish diagnosis and extent of renal function	Assist with diagnostic procedures Collect specimens for laboratory examinations Perform tests as ordered Observe, record, and report clinical manifestations

Monitor fluid balance	Weigh the child daily or as ordered
	Measure intake and output accurately
	Measure urine specific gravity
	Monitor vital signs
	   Blood pressure
	   Heart rate
	   Respiratory status
	   Central venous pressure, if indicated
	Replace fluid losses as ordered (gastrointestinal, perspiration, and so on)
	Observe for signs of dehydration or fluid overload

Prevent complications Infection	Observe medical asepsis Avoid contact with infected persons Keep skin clean and dry Change position at least every 2 hours Administer aseptic care of intravenous, hyperalimentation, or dialysis sites Administer antibiotics if ordered
Hypertension	Administer antihypertensives if ordered Carefully regulate fluid administration Observe for signs of fluid overload Monitor blood pressure and central venous pressure Administer diuretics as ordered
Minimize catabolism	Provide nutrition as ordered Reduce energy expenditure

Reduce elevated levels of electrolyte and nitrogenous waste	Oral
	   Become well acquainted with protein, potassium, and sodium content of common foods and beverages
	   Provide low-protein, low-sodium, and low-potassium diet
	Parenteral
	   Administer hyperalimentation formula as ordered
	Prevent catabolism
	Assist with peritoneal dialysis
	   Gather necessary equipment
	   Warm dialysate solution
	   Assist with catheter insertion
	   Carry out procedure as ordered
	   Observe response to treatment
	   Monitor vital signs frequently
	   Collect specimens as ordered
	Hemodialysis
	   Transport to specialized unit as ordered

SUMMARY OF NURSING CARE OF THE CHILD WITH ACUTE RENAL FAILURE—cont'd

GOALS	RESPONSIBILITIES
Support the child	Remain with the child during treatment Provide as much comfort as possible within limitations imposed by treatment regimen Provide means for the child to express his feelings
Support the parents	Allow the parents to visit the child Explain or reinforce explanations of treatments Keep the parents informed of the child's progress Allow the parents to express their feelings and concerns Provide reassurance where possible Refer to agencies for social service and financial aid

Chronic renal insufficiency or failure begins when the diseased kidneys can no longer maintain normal chemical structure of body fluids under normal conditions. Progressive deterioration over a period of months or years produces a variety of clinical and biochemical disturbances that eventually culminate in the clinical syndrome known as *uremia*.

A variety of diseases and disorders can result in chronic renal failure. The most frequent causes of chronic renal failure before age 5 years are congenital renal and urinary tract malformations (particularly renal hypoplasia and dysplasia) and vesicoureteral reflux. Glomerular and hereditary renal disease predominate in children 5 to 15 years of age. Glomerular diseases that most frequently lead to chronic renal failure are chronic pyelonephritis, chronic glomerulonephritis, and glomerulonephropathy associated with systemic diseases such as anaphylactoid purpura and lupus erythematosus. Hereditary nephritis, congenital nephrotic syndrome, Alport syndrome, polycystic kidney, and several other hereditary disorders result in renal failure in childhood. Renal vascular disorders such as hemolytic-uremic syndrome, vascular thrombosis, or cortical necrosis are less frequent causes.

Pathophysiology

Early in the course of progressive nephron destruction the child remains asymptomatic with only minimum biochemical abnormalities. Unless its presence is detected in the process of routine assessment, signs and symptoms that indicate advanced renal damage frequently emerge only late in the course of the disease. Midway in the disease process, as increasing numbers of nephrons are totally destroyed and as most others are damaged in varying degree, the few that remain intact are hypertrophied but functional.

These few normal nephrons are able to make sufficient adjustments to stresses to maintain reasonable degrees of fluid and electrolyte balance. Definitive biochemical examination at this time will reveal restricted tolerance to excesses or restrictions. As the disease progresses to the terminal stage, because of severe reduction in the number of functioning nephrons, the kidneys are no longer able to maintain fluid and electrolyte balance, and the features of the uremic syndrome appear.

The accumulation of various biochemical substances in the blood, those that result from diminished renal function, produces complications such as:

1. Retention of waste products, especially the blood urea nitrogen and creatinine
2. Inability to maintain water and sodium balance, which contributes to edema and vascular congestion
3. Dangerous hyperkalemia
4. A sustained metabolic acidosis
5. A complex disturbance of calcium and phosphorus hemostasis resulting in altered bone metabolism, which in turn causes growth arrest or retardation, bone pain, and deformities known as *renal osteodystrophy* (sometimes called *renal rickets,* since the disorganization of bone growth and demineralization is similar to that caused by vitamin D–resistant rickets)
6. Hematologic disturbances such as shortened life span of red blood cells, impaired red blood cell production, prolonged bleeding time, and nutritional anemia
7. Disturbed growth, probably caused by such factors as poor nutrition, anorexia, and bone demineralization

Children with chronic renal failure seem to be more than usually susceptible to infection, especially pneumonia, urinary tract infection, and septicemia, although the reason for this is unclear.

Clinical manifestations

The first evidence of difficulty is loss of normal energy and increased fatigue on exertion. The child may be somewhat pale, but it is often so inconspicuous that the change may not be evident to parents or others. Sometimes the blood pressure is elevated. As the disease progresses, other manifestations may appear. The child eats less well (especially breakfast), shows less interest in normal activities, such as schoolwork or play, and has an increased urinary output with a compensatory intake of fluid. Pallor becomes more evident and skin develops a characteristic sallow, muddy appearance as the result of anemia and deposition of urochrome pigment in the skin. The child may complain of headache, muscle cramps, and nausea. Other signs and symptoms include weight loss, facial puffiness, malaise, bone or joint pain, growth retardation, dryness or itching of the skin, bruised skin, and sometimes sensory or motor loss. Amenorrhea is common in adolescent girls.

Therapy is generally instigated before the appearance of the *uremic syndrome*. Manifestations of untreated uremia reflect the progressive nature of the homeostatic disturbances and general toxicity. Gastrointestinal symptoms include anorexia, nausea, and vomiting. Bleeding tendencies are apparent in bruises, bloody diarrheal stools, stomatitis, and bleeding from the lips and mouth. There is intractable itching and deposits of urea crystals appear on the skin as "uremic frost." There may be an unpleasant "uremic" odor to the breath. Respirations become deep as a result of metabolic acidosis, and circulatory overload is evident in hypertension, congestive heart failure, and pulmonary edema. Neurologic involvement is manifest by progressive confusion, dulling of sensorium, and, ultimately, coma. Other signs may include tremors, muscular twitching, and seizures.

Diagnostic evaluation

Laboratory and other diagnostic tools and tests are of value in assessing the extent of renal damage, biochemical disturbances, and related physical dysfunction. Often they can help establish the nature of the underlying disease and differentiate between other disease processes and the pathologic consequences of renal dysfunction.

Therapeutic management

In irreversible renal failure the goals of medical management are (1) to promote effective renal function, (2) to maintain body fluid and electrolyte balance within acceptable limits, (3) to treat systemic complications, and (4) to promote as active and normal a life as possible for the child for as long as possible. The child is allowed unrestricted activity, and he is allowed to set his own limits regarding rest and extent of exertion. He is encouraged to attend school as long as he is able. When the effort is too great, home tutoring is arranged.

Diet.   Regulation of diet is the most effective means, short of dialysis, for reducing the quantity of materials that require renal excretion. The goal of the diet in renal failure is to provide sufficient calories and protein for growth while limiting the excretory demands made on the kidney, to minimize metabolic bone disease (osteodystrophy), and to minimize fluid and electrolyte disturbances. Dietary phosphorus is restricted, principally the intake of cow's milk. Protein is limited and the proteins allowed should be those high in essential amino acids. Bottle-fed infants are placed on a low-protein, low-electrolyte formula with additional caloric supplements. Sodium and water are not usually limited, unless there is evidence of edema or hypertension, and potassium is not restricted. However, restrictions of any or all three may be imposed in later stages or at any time at which factors cause abnormal serum concentrations.

Dietary phosphorus is controlled to prevent or correct the calcium phosphorus imbalance by the reduction of protein and milk. Phosphorus levels can be further reduced by the oral administration of aluminum hydroxide gel (Amphojel) or tablets that combine with the phosphorus to decrease gastrointestinal absorption and, thus, the serum levels of phosphate. At the same time, serum calcium levels are increased with supplementary calcium preparations, calcium gluconate, calcium carbonate, or calcium lactate.

Metabolic acidosis is alleviated through administration of alkalizing agents such as sodium bicarbonate or a combination of sodium and potassium citrate (Shohl's solution*). Sufficient sources of folic acid and iron should be provided in the diet, and iron losses that may occur should be replaced.

Osseous deformities that result from renal osteodystrophy, especially those related to ambulation, are troublesome and require correction as soon as feasible. However, until the osteodystrophy is under control, the deformities will recur. Blood transfusions carry the risk of aggravating or precipitating cardiovascular disturbances and also tend to inhibit erythropoiesis. If needed for symptomatic anemia, packed red blood cells are given slowly over several hours.

Hypertension of advanced renal disease may be managed initially by cautious use of a low-sodium diet, fluid restriction, and perhaps diuretics, such as hydrochlorothiazide or furosemide. Severe hypertension requires the use of antihypertensive agents, usually reserpine, hydralazine, and methyldopa, singly or in combinations.

---

*Each milliliter of Shohl's solution contains 1 mEq of citrate ion, which metabolizes to yield 1 mEq of bicarbonate. Citric acid exerts no effect on acid-base balance but enhances the palatability of the mixture.

Intercurrent infections are treated with appropriate antimicrobials at the first sign of infection; however, any drug eliminated through the kidneys is administered with caution. Other complications are treated symptomatically, for example, chlorpromazine (Thorazine) or prochlorperazine (Compazine) for nausea, anticonvulsants for seizures, and diphenhydramine (Benadryl) for pruritus.

Once symptoms of uremia appear in a child, the disease runs its relentless course and terminates in death in a few weeks, unless waste products and toxins are removed from body fluids by dialysis and/or kidney transplantation. Since these techniques have been adapted for infants and small children, these alternatives are implemented in most cases of renal failure once palliative management is no longer effective.

Dialysis. Dialysis is the process of separating substances in solution by the difference in their rate of diffusion through a semipermeable membrane. Two methods of dialysis are currently available for clinical management of renal failure:

1. **Peritoneal dialysis** the abdominal cavity acts as a semipermeable membrane through which water and solutes of small molecular size move by osmosis and diffusion according to their respective concentrations on either side of the membrane
2. **Hemodialysis** blood is circulated outside the body through artificial cellophane membranes that permit a similar passage of water and solutes

As a rule, hemodialysis is reserved for children who have end-stage renal disease (ESRD), since it requires creation of a vascular access and special equipment. Peritoneal dialysis is preferred for children in acute renal failure, because it is usually a temporary therapy, it is generally an emergency procedure, and, therefore, it is more readily available, requires less expertise, and does not require specialized facilities.

Most children show rapid clinical improvement with the implementation of dialysis, although it is directly related to the duration of uremia before dialysis and the extent to which dietary regulations are followed. Growth rate and skeletal maturation usually improve, but recovery of normal growth is infrequent. In many cases sexual development, although delayed, progresses to completion.

Home dialysis. With appropriate implantation or cannulization and proper training and education of both the child and the parents, either peritoneal dialysis or hemodialysis can be performed at home. Time spent in transportation is eliminated, the environment is more pleasant and secure, and the child is able to assume a more active role in the treatment program.

Home dialysis units are available to some children, and the preparation and management for its use are similar to that required for hemodialysis in the hospital. The child is equipped with a dialysis unit that is used with the vascular access established for outpatient dialysis.

The recent development of a satisfactory method for continuous ambulatory peritoneal dialysis (CAPD) has provided an additional means for managing end-stage renal disease at home. It provides more mobility and eliminates the need for intermittent hemodialysis. A special soft catheter is surgically implanted in the abdomen and permanently sutured in place. Through this catheter the warmed dialysate enters the peritoneal cavity by gravity, the line is clamped off, and the empty bag is rolled up and worn attached to the abdomen or thigh or placed in a pocket. The solution is allowed to remain in the peritoneum for 4 to 6 hours. The bag is then unrolled and placed on the floor, the line is unclamped, and the fluid is drained into the bag by gravity. Another heated bag is hung and the process repeated.

Transplantation. Renal transplantation is now an acceptable and effective means of therapy in the pediatric age-group. The criteria for selection are quite liberal, and uniform criteria have not been established among the various centers that specialize in the procedure. Many children with systemic disease and tumors have had successful transplants. On the other hand, there is a high incidence of recurrent disease in the donor kidney in children who receive a transplant for rapidly progressive glomerulonephritis with irreversible renal failure.

Nursing considerations

The child with chronic renal failure is a prime example of an individual whose life is maintained by drugs and artificial means, and the multiple stresses placed on these children and their families are often overwhelming. The unrelenting course of the disease process is one of progressive deterioration. The affected child progresses from renal insufficiency to uremia and then to hemodialysis and transplantation. As the need for therapy intensifies, the need for supportive nursing care is also intensified. Team effort is more important than ever and involves coordination of personnel from medicine, nursing, social services, dietetics, and psychologic or psychiatric specialties.

End-stage renal disease places the same nonspecific stresses on the child and family as any other potentially fatal illness (see Chapter 16). There is a continuing need for repeated examinations that often entail painful procedures, side effects, and frequent hospitalizations. Diet therapy becomes progressively more restricted and intense, and the child is required to take a variety of medications. Ever present in all aspects of the treatment regimen is the agonizing realization that without treatment death is the inevitable outcome.

Some specific stresses related to end-stage renal disease and its treatment are predictable. When it first becomes apparent that kidney failure is inevitable, both parents and child experience great depression and anxiety. Acceptance is particularly difficult if renal failure progresses rapidly after diagnosis. Denial and disbelief are usually pronounced, especially among the parents. Once the kidney failure is established and once symptoms become progressively more distressing, the initiation of hemodialysis is usually perceived as a positive experience, and, after the initial concerns of implementing the treatment, the child begins to feel better and parental anxiety is relieved for a time.

Initiating a hemodialysis regimen is a traumatic and anxiety-provoking experience for most children, since it involves surgery for implantation of the shunt or fistula. The initial experience with the hemodialysis machine and its implication is frightening to most children. They need reassurance about the nature of the preparations for dialysis and conduct of the treatment.

Adolescents, with their increased need for independence and their urge for rebellion, usually adapt less well. They resent the control and enforced dependence imposed by the rigorous and unrelenting therapy program. They resent being dependent on a machine, their parents, and the professional staff. Depression and/or hostility are common in adolescents undergoing hemodialysis.

The availability of home dialysis has offered a greater degree of freedom for persons undergoing long-term dialysis. The family must learn the technique and the nurse is responsible for teaching this technique to the family. The family must learn how to take vital signs before and after the dialysis, and they must learn the significance of blood pressure and temperature variations. They need to know how to manage the various aspects of the procedure, how to maintain accurate records, and how to observe for signs of complications that need to be reported to the proper persons.

Body changes related to the disease process, such as skin color, growth retardation, and lack of sexual maturation, are stress provoking. Dietary restrictions are particularly burdensome for both children and parents. Children feel deprived when unable to eat foods previously enjoyed and unrestricted for other family members. Consequently failure to cooperate is not uncommon. Diet restrictions are interpreted as punishment and, since they may not be able to fully understand the purpose of restrictions, some will sneak forbidden food items at every opportunity. Allowing children, especially adolescents, maximum participation in and responsibility for their own treatment program is helpful.

After weeks or months of hemodialysis, the parents and child feel anxiety associated with the prognosis and continued pressures of the treatment. The relentless need for treatment interferes with family plans. Transportation to and from the dialysis unit and the time spent on the machine cut into time for outside activites, including school. Shunt and fistula problems are not uncommon and present a common source of aggravation. Eventually most severely affected children face nephrectomy, which predictably causes depression in both the child and family.

The possibility of renal transplantation often comes as a hope for relief from the rigors of hemodialysis and the hated diet restrictions. Except for children with preexisting personality problems or residual physical disabilities, most children and families respond well to kidney transplant and the majority return to normal life within a year after surgery.

The National Kidney Foundation* and numerous other agencies provide services and information for families, including pamphlets and descriptive literature. Particularly useful are easily understandable booklets for children with renal disease.†

DEFECTS OF THE GENITOURINARY TRACT

External defects of the genitourinary tract are usually obvious at birth. Several, such as hypospadias, epispadias, and undescended testes (cryptorchism), do not necessitate immediate repair but may require one or more staged repairs during early childhood. Others, such as exstrophy of the bladder, require initial intervention at birth with repeated medical and surgical treatment for several years. The anatomic location of these defects frequently causes more psychologic concern to children and parents than does the actual condition or treatment.

HYPOSPADIAS

Hypospadias refers to a condition in which the urethral opening is located behind the glans penis or anywhere along the ventral surface of the penile shaft (Fig. 24-4). In very mild cases the meatus is just off center from the tip of the penis. In the most severe malformations the meatus is located on the perineum between the two halves of the scrotum. Chordee, or ventral curvature of the penis,

---

*116 E. 27th Street, New York, NY 10016.
†Recommended is Pamplin, H.H., Light, J.A., and Hyman, L.R.: Sidney Kidney, Washington, DC, 1974, Walter Reed Army Medical Center.

SUMMARY OF NURSING CARE FOR THE CHILD WITH CHRONIC RENAL FAILURE

GOALS	RESPONSIBILITIES

Recognize impending renal failure	Be suspicious of symptoms of chronic renal failure such as
	    History of renal dysfunction
	    Loss of energy
	    Increased fatigue on exertion
	    Pale (often muddy appearance) and listless
	    Loss of appetite, especially at breakfast
	    Polyuria, polydipsia, and bed wetting in previously continent child
	    Amenorrhea in adolescent girls

Assess extent of renal dysfunction	Collect specimens for analysis—urine; blood Prepare the child for and assist with renal biopsy Prepare to assist with radiographic examinations
Do ongoing evaluation	Take history for new or increasing symptoms Carry out frequent physical assessments with particular attention to blood pressure, signs of edema, or neurologic dysfunction Assess psychologic responses to the disease and its therapies

Prevent retention of waste products	Provide diet that reduces excretory demands on kidney
	    Limit protein to essential amino acids and no more than required for growth
	    Allow no added salt
	    Discourage foods high in potassium

Prevent osteodystrophy	Restrict protein and phosphorus-containing foods in the diet, especially milk Administer aluminum hydroxide Provide supplementary calcium Administer alkalizing agents Administer supplementary vitamin D
Prevent or treat hypertension	Monitor fluid intake Provide low-sodium diet Administer diuretics as prescribed Administer antihypertensive agents as ordered
Treat anemia	Provide foods rich in folic acid and iron Administer supplementary iron Administer packed red blood cells periodically as prescribed
Prevent infection	Avoid contact with infected persons Employ careful medical asepsis Administer appropriate antibiotics, as prescribed, at first sign of infection
Remove waste products and toxins from body fluids	Prepare the child and family for hemodialysis and/or kidney transplantation Assist with dialysis procedure
Maintain as normal a life as possible	Avoid limiting activities Allow the child to set his own pace for activity and rest Encourage the child to attend school as much as possible; when unable to attend arrange for home tutoring Help the child to adjust to therapies and diet regulations Encourage interaction with peers

Continued.

SUMMARY OF NURSING CARE FOR THE CHILD WITH CHRONIC RENAL FAILURE—cont'd

GOALS	RESPONSIBILITIES
Assist the child to cope with stresses of disease	Explore fears and clarify misconceptions
	Support positive coping mechanisms
	Encourage activities that promote self-image
	Reassure the child that necessary therapies are not punishment
	Assist the child to plan acceptable alternatives for restricted foods
	Provide anticipatory guidance regarding probable and expected events such as symptoms, diet, and effects of medications
	Prepare the child for hemodialysis and surgeries
Provide parental support	Explore parental feelings of guilt, helplessness, and threat of the child's death
	Explain and clarify information about the disease and its therapy
	Refer the parents to specialized service agencies, such as the National Kidney Foundation, Special Child Health Services, etc.
	Introduce to other parents who have a similarly affected child
	Assist the parents in diet planning and support their efforts to adjust their diet to meet needs of all members of the family
	Assist the parents in decision regarding dialysis and transplantation
	Maintain periodic contact with the family

FIG. 24-4

Hypospadias. (Courtesy M.C. Gleason, M.D., San Diego, Calif. From Ingalls, A.J., and Salerno, M.C.: Maternal and child health nursing, ed. 5, St. Louis, 1983, The C.V. Mosby Co.)

FIG. 24-5

Hypospadias with significant chordee. (From Shirkey, H.C.: Pediatric therapy, ed. 6, St. Louis, 1980, The C.V. Mosby Co.)

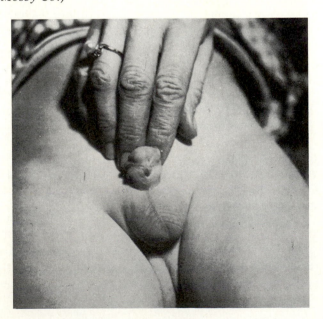

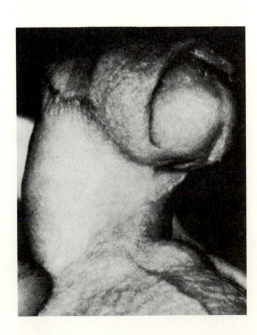

results from the replacement of normal skin with a fibrous band of tissue, causing constriction of the penis. In addition, the foreskin is usually absent ventrally and, when combined with chordee, gives the organ a hooded and crooked appearance (Fig. 24-5). The altered appearance may leave the sex of the child in doubt at birth. The perineal position of the meatus may be mistaken for a female urethra and, with the presence of undescended testes, the small penis may appear to be an enlarged clitoris.

Surgical correction

The prinicipal objectives in surgical correction are (1) to enable the child to void in the standing position by voluntarily directing the stream in the usual manner, (2) to improve the physical appearance of the genitalia for psychologic reasons, and (3) to produce a sexually adequate organ. The procedure involves releasing the chordee, extending the length of the urethra, and constructing a new meatal opening. Since the prepuce is valuable skin for use in reconstructive surgery, circumcision should not be performed on these infants. A minimum defect without chordee usually requires no treatment except perhaps for cosmetic reasons; when the meatus is located on the glans penis, no intervention may be required except to release the chordee. Repair of more severe hypospadias often requires more than one surgical procedure to progressively extend the length of the urethra. The surgery is usually performed at about 3 years of age when the phallus is of sufficient size, when the child has not yet developed mutilation anxiety, and before entrance into school in order to prevent criticism and embarrassment from peers and to foster a more positive body image.

Psychologic problems

The location of the defect and the need for repeated surgery cause these children more emotional concern than does the actual defect. Voiding usually presents no problem when diapers are used, and the infant and young child are not unduly affected by an altered body image. When surgery is performed at an early age (such as release of chordee) the problems are those related to hospitalization and possible separation from parents. Delayed repair until the preschool years increases the fear of castration and mutilation anxiety typical of that age-group. In addition, parental concerns for acceptable physical appearance and adequate future sexual competency may be transmitted to the child.

Nursing considerations

Preparation of the parents and child for the type of procedure to be done and for the expected cosmetic result helps to avert later problems. Surgical correction is explained to parents but, often, they are not advised of what to expect as a reasonable consequence. As a result, they may be greatly disappointed to see a physically imperfect penis. If the child is old enough to understand, he is also prepared for the operation and the expected outcome. It is particularly important to emphasize that the operation is needed because of a problem with which he was born and that it is in no way a punishment for misdeeds or thoughts. Considering the sexual curiosity of preschoolers, the operation can be mistakenly viewed as retribution for masturbation, sex play, or erotic feelings.

Urethroplasty usually requires some type of urinary diversion to promote optimum healing and to maintain the position and patency of the newly formed urethra. The nurse employs all measures to avoid infection of the urinary tract and operative site.

EPISPADIAS

In this congenital anomaly the urethra is located on the dorsal surface of the penis. As in hypospadias the defect can occur in differing degrees of severity. In the mildest cases the meatus is located in front of the glans penis. In the most severe instance epispadias extends to exstrophy of the bladder. The treatment is surgical and usually requires more than one procedure. The psychologic problems and nursing considerations are similar to those discussed under hypospadias.

PHIMOSIS

Phimosis is an abnormal narrowing or stenosis of the preputial opening in the uncircumcised male so that the foreskin cannot be retracted over the glans penis. In most normal males there is some degree of adherence of the foreskin that does not become completely retractable until the child is approximately 3 years of age. In rare cases the narrowing obstructs the flow of urine, resulting in straining at urination and a dribbling stream rather than a steady flow of urine during voiding.

Phimosis can occur as a congenital anomaly, or, more commonly, as a result of poor hygiene. In the latter case smegma accumulates between the prepuce and the glans, infections occur, and adhesions form, preventing the easy retraction of the foreskin.

Therapeutic management

Mild phimosis that does not interfere with urination is treated by instructing the parents to carefully cleanse and then gently retract the foreskin during the bath to gradually release the adhesions and widen the opening. More severe phimosis is managed by an incision to widen the opening or a circumcision is performed.

Nursing considerations

True cases of congenital phimosis are rare, and proper hygiene prevents most instances of acquired phimosis. Circumcision for older children may be done to relieve the phimosis, but psychosexual factors are important to consider.

When manual retraction is prescribed, parents are taught the technique. However, parents are cautioned that care must be exercised when replacing the foreskin back over the glans penis. If left retracted, the tight band of skin constricts the blood vessels, causing edema, bluish discoloration, pain, dysuria, and eventually necrosis. The resulting edema and pain further complicate attempts to replace the foreskin in its normal position.

CRYPTORCHISM

Cryptorchism, or undescended testicle, is failure of one or both testes to descend in the scrotal sac. There are two types of cryptorchism. In *true, undescended testes* the organ has never been in the scrotal sac but lies somewhere along the path of descent above the inguinal ring. In *ectopic testes* the organ has passed down the inguinal canal through the external rings but is fixed in an upward direction, such as in the perineum or proximal scrotum. Because the testes normally descend during the seventh to ninth month of gestation, it is common in infants born prematurely. Congenital hydrocele or inguinal hernias frequently accompany the defect. The cause of cryptorchism is not known.

Diagnostic evaluation

Diagnosis of undescended testes is complicated by the normal retraction of testes by the cremasteric reflex, which is particularly sensitive to touch and cold. However, it can be obviated by placing the child in a squatting or tailor-like position or by applying firm finger pressure on the external ring before palpating the abdomen or genitalia (see p. 117). Retracted testes can be "milked" or pushed back into the scrotum, but truly undescended ones cannot. Ectopic testes may be felt along the inguinal canal; those in the abdominal cavity usually cannot.

Therapeutic management

In some cases hormonal therapy with human chorionic gonadotropin may be attempted in the child 1 to 4 years of age to help enlarge the scrotum or testes. Testes below the external ring may descend by hormonal treatment, but those lodged inside the inguinal canal or fixed in an abnormal position usually require surgical intervention (orchiopexy). In the routine procedure, the testes are brought down into the scrotum, then secured in that position by one end of a rubber band attached to a retraction suture in the scrotum and the other end to the inner thigh with adhesive tape and left in place for about 5 to 7 days.

The optimum age for treatment of cryptorchism is influenced by several factors. Many testes descend spontaneously during the first year, especially in premature infants. During the second year surgery is complicated by tissue that is still very fragile and easily traumatized. It should be performed before the child is 5 years of age. If left in the abdomen longer, there is risk that the testes will be damaged by the higher body temperature, resulting in sterility. Also, having both testes in the scrotum by school age prevents psychologic problems related to body image and peer group embarrassment, since the empty scrotum is smaller in size and altered in shape.

Adequate treatment usually results in functional testes, although infertility from impaired sperm production may be a problem. Undescended testes are regarded as worth saving because of their unimpaired secretion of testosterone, which is necessary for pubertal changes. Also, cancers in undescended testes are more frequent than in descended ones, although testicular cancer is rare and is not prevented by orchiopexy. Because of their increased propensity toward neoplastic changes, cryptorchid testes are better observed in the scrotal position.

Nursing considerations

Preparation for surgery is managed as that for any child undergoing a surgical procedure, taking into consideration the probable trauma to any preschool child and the psychologic effects of surgery associated with the genitals. Care must be exercised to preserve the necessary tension on the rubber band or else the testes may reascend to an abnormal location. Infection of the operative site is prevented by careful cleansing of stool and urine. If surgery is done after the child is toilet trained, prevention of contamination is simplified.

INGUINAL HERNIA

Inguinal hernia is derived from persistence of all or part of the processus vaginalis, the tube of peritoneum that precedes the testicle through the inguinal canal into the scrotum during the eighth month of gestation (Fig. 24-6). The hernial sac is present at birth but does not usually become apparent until the infant is able to build up sufficient in-

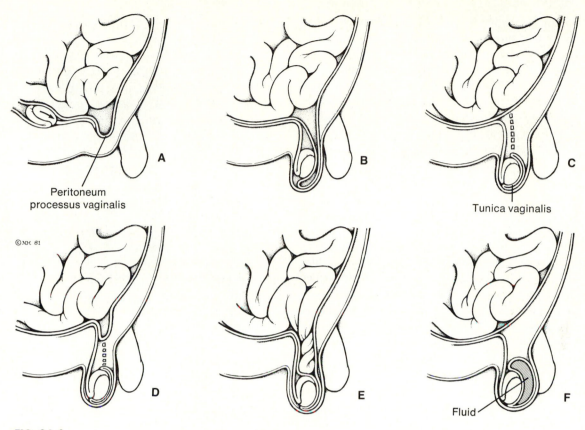

FIG. 24-6
Development of inguinal hernias. **A,** *and* **B,** *Prenatal migration of processus vaginalis.*
C, *Normal.* **D,** *Partially obliterated processus vaginalis.* **E,** *Hernia.* **F,** *Hydrocele.*

traabdominal pressure to open the sac, usually 2 to 3 months of age. Since the inguinal canal is short, hernias occur relatively early. Inguinal hernia occurs much more frequently in boys (90%), but it is also seen in girls.

Clinical manifestations

This very common defect is asymptomatic unless the abdominal contents are forced into the patent sac. Most often it appears as a painless inguinal swelling that varies in size. It disappears during periods of rest or is reducible by gentle compression; it appears when the infant cries or strains or when the older child strains, coughs, or stands for a long period. The defect can be palpated as a thickening of the cord in the groin, and the "silk glove" sign can be elicited by rubbing together the sides of the empty hernial sac.

Sometimes the herniated loop of intestine becomes partially obstructed, producing variable symptoms that may include fretfulness and irritability, tenderness, anorexia, abdominal distention, and difficulty in defecating. Occasionally the loop of bowel becomes incarcerated (ir-

reducible), with symptoms of complete intestinal obstruction that, if left untreated, will progress to strangulation and gangrene. Incarceration occurs more often in infants under 10 months of age and is more common in girls.

Therapeutic management

In healthy infants and children the treatment for hernias is prompt, elective surgical repair as soon as the defect is diagnosed. Many physicians advocate exploration of both sides since there is a high incidence of recurrence on the contralateral side. This remains controversial, however. It is preferable to attempt reduction of a recently incarcerated hernia in order that surgery can be delayed to allow the injured tissues to recover somewhat, but irreducible or strangulated hernias are treated as emergencies.

Nursing considerations

Both infants and children tolerate surgery very well. There is usually no restriction placed on their activities, and it is not uncommon for the child to be discharged from the hospital on the day of surgery. Every attempt is made to keep the wound clean and reasonably dry. With infants and small children who are still in diapers, the wound is left without a dressing. Changing diapers as soon as they become damp helps reduce the chance of irritation or infection of the incision, or the child may be left undiapered. It is seldom necessary to apply a urine-collecting device, and in doing so it is often difficult or impossible to avoid the incision.

HYDROCELE

Hydrocele is the presence of fluid in the persistent processus vaginalis and is the result of the same developmental process as inguinal hernia (see Fig. 24-6). When the upper segment of the processus vaginalis has been obliterated but the tunica vaginalis still contains peritoneal fluid, this is called a *noncommunicating hydrocele*. This type of hydrocele is common in newborns and often subsides spontaneously as fluid is gradually absorbed.

A *communicating hydrocele* is one in which the processus vaginalis remains open and into which peritoneal fluid may be forced by intraabdominal pressure and gravity. The length of the hydrocele depends on the length of the processus vaginalis and may extend into the tunica vaginalis within the scrotum. The hydrocele is asymptomatic except for a palpable bulge in the inguinal or scrotal areas. Unlike a hernia, the hydrocele cannot be reduced and it cannot be produced by a sudden increase in intraabdominal pressure (such as straining). The scrotum appears larger after an active day and smaller in the mornings. Since a hydrocele represents a patent processus vaginalis, it can predispose to herniation; therefore, surgical repair is indicated.

EXSTROPHY OF BLADDER

Exstrophy of the bladder is an obvious and serious congenital defect that occurs three times more frequently in males than in females (Fig. 24-7). There is no familial tendency, and it rarely occurs in siblings.

In males the defect may be associated with other problems, such as undescended testes, a short penis, epispadias, or inguinal hernia. The sexual handicap in males may be severe because the penis protrudes inadequately. In females the genitalia may be affected, with a cleft clitoris, completely separated labia, and absent vagina. In either sex, separation of the pubic bones causes difficulty in walking, such as a waddling gait.

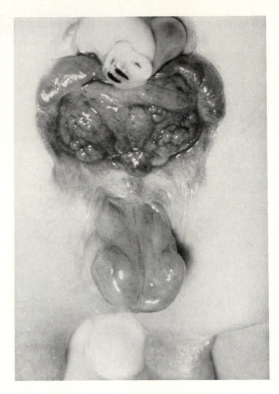

FIG. 24-7
Exstrophy of bladder. (Courtesy E.S. Tank, M.D., Division of Urology, University of Oregon Health Sciences Center, Portland, Ore.)

Therapeutic management

The objectives of treatment include (1) preservation of renal function, (2) attainment of urinary control, (3) adequate reconstructive repair for psychologic benefit, and (4) improvement of sexual function, particularly in males. The success of each of these goals depends on the severity of the exstrophy. The exact surgical intervention is frequently a matter of preference. However, in those cases where continence is not possible, some type of urinary diversion is generally necessary, such as ureteral sigmoid implant, bilateral ureterostomy, or ileal conduit.

A satisfactory procedure, and the one that is usually performed, is an *ileal conduit*, also called a ureteroileal cutaneous ureterostomy. A small section of the ileum or colon is resected and the distal ends of the ureters are severed from the bladder and attached to the ileum, which then acts as a bladder, but without voluntary control of voiding. The infant is diapered as a normal infant, although the surrounding skin must be kept clean and relatively dry of urine to prevent excoriation. The older child is fitted with an ileostomy appliance over the stoma, to collect the continuously flowing urine.

In a cutaneous *ureterostomy* the ureters are attached directly to the abdominal wall, usually at a site proximal to the level of the kidneys. A collecting appliance may also be worn, although in exstrophy of the bladder two appliances are necessary to accommodate the bilateral openings. Infection is more common because of the short length of the ureters, and general care is more cumbersome. Usually ureterostomy is a method of choice for temporary urinary diversion to prevent renal function deterioration.

Nursing considerations

One of the most devastating aspects of exstrophy of the bladder is its gross appearance. Frequently surgical intervention is delayed until the infant has attained more physiologic maturity to withstand the operation and increased body growth to allow for improved abdominal closure. As a result the newborn may be discharged from the nursery before the parents have had sufficient opportunity to adjust to the defect and learn the procedures for home care. It is advisable to prolong the hospital stay of mother and child until at least one parent feels somewhat comfortable in caring for the child and until there is ample opportunity to evaluate that parent's capabilities. Although the actual procedures are not difficult, it is not easy for parents to assume responsibility for what to them seems an enormous task because of the emotional impact of the defect.

Surgical correction may require more than one procedure. Depending on the age of the child, preparation for hospitalization includes an adequate description of what can be expected postoperatively. As difficult as it was for parents to adjust to the defect at the time of the child's birth, it may be equally disturbing for them to accept the fact that surgical closure does not ensure normal urination and that urinary diversion is necessary. The prospect of a permanent ileal conduit or other similar procedure provokes powerful emotional responses. Parents often worry about the child's sexual adjustment, even though they may not voice such thoughts.

Preoperative care is similar to that for any major abdominal surgery. Since a routine urinalysis is part of most admission procedures, a urine specimen can be obtained by allowing urine to drip into a container by holding the child prone over a basin or by aspirating some urine directly from the bladder area into a medicine dropper or syringe. If a sterile specimen is needed for evaluation of existing infection, the former procedure is preferable, but a sterile container must be used.

Postoperative care differs little from that given to any surgical patient. An abdominal dressing is placed over the closure site, kept clean, and checked for any presence of urine. If an ileal conduit or ureterostomy was performed, a separate absorbent dressing is placed over the stoma to collect the urine and prevent contamination of the other dressing. An appliance is usually fitted as soon as possible to allow the child and parents adequate time to learn its proper use and to adjust to the change in body image.

Even with improved reconstructive surgery for these patients, substantial psychologic support and guidance are needed to help them adjust to their fears of inadequate penile size, unsightly genitalia, potential inability to procreate, and rejection by peers, especially the opposite sex. Ongoing discussion groups for parents and children are particularly useful in promoting resolution of these fears and in allowing for optimum emotional adjustment, particularly during adolescence.

OBSTRUCTIVE UROPATHY

Structural or functional abnormalities of the urinary system that interfere with the normal flow of urine can produce renal pathology. When urine flow is obstructed, the collecting system above the obstruction causes hydronephrosis (the collection of urine in the renal pelvis to the extent of cyst formation from the distention) with eventual pressure destruction to renal parenchyma. Glomerular filtration ceases when intrapelvic pressure equals the filtration pressure in glomerular capillaries. However, the dilating ureters form a reservoir that reduces the effect on the kidneys for a long time.

Obstruction may be unilateral or bilateral, complete or incomplete, and can occur at any level of the upper or lower urinary tract (Fig. 24-8). Partial obstruction may not be symptomatic unless there is a water or solute diuresis, but it will result in progressive loss of renal function as a result of irreversible damage to the nephrons.

Pooled urine serves as a medium for bacterial growth; therefore, urinary tract infection further increases the extent of renal damage. Early diagnosis and surgical correction or amelioration are essential in order to prevent progressive renal damage.

AMBIGUOUS GENITALIA

The birth of a child with ambiguous genitalia is a situation that constitutes a crisis situation quite different from that of many other congenital anomalies. Uncertain sex is no threat to life in a physical sense but is a potential lifelong social tragedy for the child and family. The problem of appropriate sex must be solved quickly and accurately; it

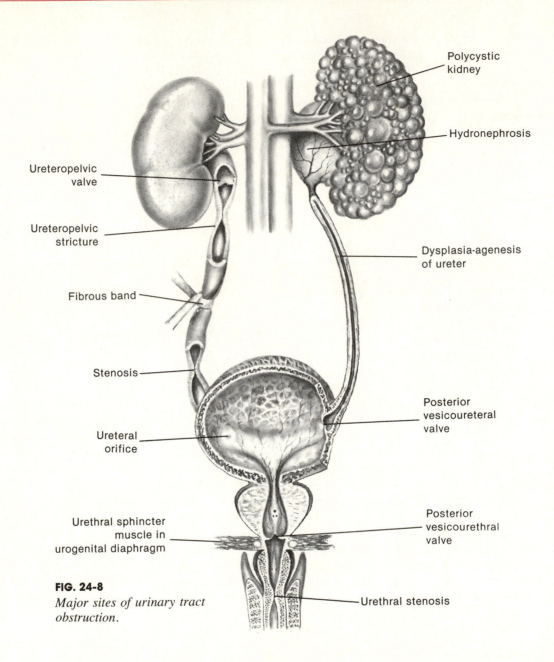

Ureteropelvic valve

Ureteropelvic stricture

Fibrous band

Stenosis

Ureteral orifice

Urethral sphincter muscle in urogenital diaphragm

Polycystic kidney

Hydronephrosis

Dysplasia-agenesis of ureter

Posterior vesicoureteral valve

Posterior vesicourethral valve

Urethral stenosis

FIG. 24-8
Major sites of urinary tract obstruction.

requires no less speed and skill than life-threatening anomalies.

Disturbances in the normal order of events in sex determination will produce abnormal sexual development, with the presence of ambiguous or inappropriate external genitalia at birth. The degree of ambiguity varies from case to case and the physical appearance often closely conforms to one sex or the other. In some instances, however, the external sexual structures represent those of a perfectly normal male or female, whereas the genetic sex is the direct opposite. A situation in which the phenotypic sex differs from the chromosomal sex is often termed *intersex*.

Types of abnormalities

Some disorders with abnormal sexual development are not characterized by ambiguous genitalia in the newborn period. For example, the most common sex chromosomal disorders do not become apparent until later childhood, adolescence, or even young adulthood when the individual seeks medical attention because of problems of delayed development or infertility. The four conditions producing ambiguous genitalia in the newborn that require prompt and accurate evaluation are (1) the masculinized female (female pseudohermaphrodite), (2) the incompletely masculinized male (male pseudohermaphrodite), (3) the true hermaphrodite, and (4) mixed gonadal dysgenesis.

The most common condition that produces ambiguous genitalia in the newborn is the masculinized female, resulting from virilization by adrenal androgens after the time of early differentiation of gonadal tissues. The second most frequently seen disorder is mixed gonadal dysgenesis, in which affected infants are sex chromosome mosaics (see Table 3-2). Genitalia vary greatly, but, in affected infants who appear predominantly female, the dysplastic testis may cause masculinzation at puberty.

In the incompletely masculinated male, the external genitalia may be incompletely masculinized, ambiguous, or completely female. The complex nature of virilization offers numerous opportunities for disturbance in the process. In some disorders there is deficient production of fetal androgen, and in others there is deficiency of any of the enzymes needed in the numerous steps of testosterone biosynthesis. More commonly there is unresponsiveness or subresponsiveness of genital structures to testosterone.

True hermaphrodites are rare and may be either genetic males or females with *both* ovarian and testicular tissues (an ovary on one side and a testis on the other), or they may have a combination of ovary and testis, known as an ovotestis. The external genitalia may be male, usually cryptorchid, or normal female, but in the majority of cases the genitalia are ambiguous.

Diagnostic evaluation

Diagnostic tools, with their corresponding significant findings that help determine gender assignment, include:

History previous abortions may help identify chromosomal aberrations; ingestion of steroids; relatives with ambiguous genitalia or death in the first weeks of life

Physical examination seldom of significant value

Buccal smear detects presence or absence of sex chromatin

Chromosomal analysis detects chromosomal abnormalities and precise genetic sex

Endoscopy and radiographic contrast studies reveal presence, absence, or nature of internal genital structures

Biochemical tests urinary steroid excretion patterns help detect several of the adrenal cortical syndromes; tests include 17-ketosteroids, 17-hydroxycorticoids, and urinary pregnanediol

Laparotomy or **gonad biopsy** in some instances this is the only way to arrive at a definitive diagnosis

Therapeutic management

The assignment of a gender sex to the infant whose sex is doubtful constitutes a social emergency. The long-term implications are such that a hasty decision based on appearance alone may be disastrous, and the optimum sex of rearing may not be the same as the genetic or gonadal sex. The infant's anatomy rather than genetic sex is the primary criterion on which the choice of gender should be based. An incomplete female is better able to adjust than is an inadequate male. A functional vagina can be constructed surgically, and with appropriate administration of hormones the anatomically incomplete female can lead a relatively normal life. It is as yet impossible to construct a satisfactory penis from an inadequate phallus to make possible an equally satisfactory adjustment of the incomplete male.

In most instances of ambiguous genitalia it is recommended that the infant be reared as a female. Genetic males with a phallus of adequate size that will respond to testosterone at the time of puberty can be considered for male rearing. Thorough studies should be carried out early to assist in gender selection, even though they may delay final sex assignment for several days or even weeks. Supportive measures such as appropriate surgical reconstruction techniques that provide normal-appearing external structures are carried out. Removal of inappropriate internal structures and dysgenic gonads is recommended.

Nursing considerations

Families need a great deal of support and encouragement from nurses and other members of the health team to cope with this emotionally charged situation. Parents are confused, anxious, and overwhelmed by feelings of guilt and shame. They may pressure for immediate sex assignment because not only are they concerned about the child and the child's future, but they must also face questioning relatives and friends. There are some things a nurse can suggest to parents in order to help them cope with this problem while awaiting the diagnosis. The parents might give the child a unisex name such as Frances(is), Leslie, or Pat, or they may announce the birth of twins, a boy and a girl. When a gender sex is assigned to the child, the parents can inform friends and relatives that only one twin survived—the one with the appropriate sex. It requires sympathy and understanding to deal with parental anxiety during this trying period and to guide them throughout the long-term management.

BIBLIOGRAPHY
General

Bielski, M.: Preventing infection in the catheterized patient, Nurs. Clin. North Am. **15:**703-713, 1980.

Brundage, D.J.: Nursing management of renal problems, ed. 2, St. Louis, 1980, The C.V. Mosby Co.

Hetrick, A., Frauman, A.C., and Gilman, C.M.: Nutrition in renal disease: when the patient is a child, Am. J. Nurs. **79:**2152-2154, 1979.

Juliani, L.M.: Assessing renal function, Nursing 78 **8**(1):34-35, 1978.

Leonard, M.: Health issues and primary nursing in nephrology care, Nurs. Clin. North Am. **10:**413-420, 1975.

Murphy, L.M., and Cole, M.J.: Renal disease: nutritional implications, Nurs. Clin. North Am. **18:**57-70, 1983.

Pickering, L., and Robbins, D.: Fluid, electrolyte, and acid-base balance in the renal patient, Nurs. Clin. North Am. **15**:577-592, 1980.

Winter, C.C., and Morel, A.: Nursing care of patients with urologic diseases, ed. 4, St. Louis, 1977, The C.V. Mosby Co.

Urinary tract infection

American Academy of Pediatrics, Section of Urology: Screening school children for urologic disease, Pediatrics **60**(2):239-240, 1977.

Stann, J.H.: Urinary tract infections in children, Pediatr. Nurs. **5**(4):49-52, 1979.

Thomas, C.K.: Childhood urinary tract infection, Pediatr. Nurs. **8**:114-119, 1982.

Renal diseases

Gorrell, J.F.: Hemolytic-uremic syndrome: an overview and a pediatric case report, J. Maternal Child Nurs. **3**(4):235-241, 1978.

Hekelman, F.P., and Ostendarp, C.A.: Nursing approaches to conservative management of renal disease, Nurs. Clin. North Am. **10**:431-434, 1975.

Juliani, L.M.: When infection leads to acute glomerulonephritis: here's what to do, Nursing 79 **9**(9):40-45, 1979.

Oestreich, S.J.K.: Rational nursing care in chronic renal disease, Am. J. Nurs. **79**:1096-1099, 1979.

Renal failure

Fearing, M.O.: Osteodystrophy in patients with chronic renal failure, Nurs. Clin. North Am. **10**:461-468, 1975.

Frauman, A.C., and Lansing, L.: The child with chronic renal failure: I. Change and challenge, Issues Compr. Pediatr. Nurs. **6**:127-133, 1983.

Frauman, A.C., and Lansing, L.: The child with chronic renal failure: II. Developmental habilitation, Issues Compr. Pediatr. Nurs. **6**:135-146, 1983.

Lewis, S.M.: Pathophysiology of chronic renal failure, Nurs. Clin. North Am. **16**:501-513, 1981.

Lopes, G.S.: A dietary approach to chronic renal failure, Issues Compr. Pediatr. Nurs. **6**:23-62, 1983.

Rodriguez, D.J., and Hunter, V.M.: Nutritional intervention in the treatment of chronic renal failure, Nurs. Clin. North Am. **16**:573-585, 1981.

Stark, J.L.: How to succeed against acute real failure, Nursing 82 **12**(7):26-33, 1982.

Stark, J.L., and Hunt, V.: Helping your patient with chronic renal failure, Nursing 83 **13**(9):56-61, 1983.

Tichy, A.M.: Renal failure, Crit. Care Update **9**(8):7-19, 1982.

Topor, M.: Chronic renal failure in children, Nurs. Clin. North Am. **16**:587-597, 1981.

Tyndall, M.G.: Chronic renal failure: past and future trends, Nurs. Clin. North Am. **16**:489-499, 1981.

Dialysis

Ceccarelli, C.M.: Hemodialytic therapy for the patient with chronic renal failure, Nurs. Clin. North Am. **16**:531-550, 1981.

Chambers, J.K.: Assessing the dialysis patient at home, Am. J. Nurs. **81**:750-754, 1981.

Chambers, J.K.: Bowel management in dialysis patients, Am. J. Nurs. **83**:1051-1052, 1983.

Davis, V., and Lavandero, R.: Caring for the catheter carefully . . . before, during, and after peritoneal dialysis, Nursing 80 **10**(12):67-71, 1980.

Denniston, D.J., and Burns, K.T.: Home peritoneal dialysis, Am. J. Nurs. **80:**2022-2026, 1980.

Duffy, M.M.: Peritoneal dialysis, Crit. Care Update **10**(8):7-19, 1983.

Gross, S.: Teaching young patients—and their families—about home peritoneal dialysis, Nursing 80 **10**(10):72-73, 1980.

Irwin, B.C.: Hemodialysis means vascular access and the right kind of nursing care, Nursing 79 **9**(10):49-53, 1979.

McDaid, T.K.: Chronic hemodialysis in children, Issues Compr. Pediatr. Nurs. **2**(6):53-68, 1978.

McNamara, R.M.: The bioinstrumentation of hemodialysis, Nurs. Clin. North Am. **13:**611-624, 1978.

Melber, S., Leonard, M., and Primack, W.: Hemodialysis at camp, Am. J. Nurs. **76:**935-938, 1976.

Reed, S.B.: Giving more than dialysis, Nursing 82 **12**(4):58-62, 1982.

Sorrels, P.A.J.: Peritoneal dialysis: a rediscovery, Nurs. Clin. North Am. **16:**515-529, 1981.

Wheeler, D.: Teaching home-dialysis for an eight-year-old boy, Am. J. Nurs. **77:**273-274, 1977.

Williams, J.A.: Hypotension during hemodialysis, Crit. Care Update **10**(6):44-49, 1983.

Kidney transplantation

Cianci, J., Lamb, J., and Ryan, R.K.: Renal transplantation, Am. J. Nurs. **81:**354-355, 1981.

Irwin, B.C.: Renal transplantation, Crit. Care Update **10**(2):28-35, 1983.

Juliani, L., and Reamer, B.: Kidney transplant: your role in aftercare, Nursing 77 **7**(10):46-53, 1977.

Kobrzycki, P.: Renal transplant complications, Am. J. Nurs. **77:**641-643, 1977.

Korsch, R.M., and others: Kidney transplantation in children: psychosocial follow-up study on child and family, J. Pediatr. **83:**399, 1973.

Powers, A.M.: Renal transplantation: the patient's choice, Nurs. Clin. North Am. **16:**551-564, 1981.

Reckling, J.B.: Safeguarding the renal transplant patient, Nursing 82 **12**(2):47-49, 1982.

Topor, M.A.: Kidney transplantation especially in pediatric patients, Nurs. Clin. North Am. **10:**503-516, 1975.

Wolf, Z.R.: What patients awaiting kidney transplant want to know, Am. J. Nurs. **76:**92-94, 1976.

Wilms tumor

Fochtman, D.: Malignant solid tumors in children, Pediatr. Nurs. **2**(6):11-17, 1976.

Schwartz, A.D.: Neuroblastoma and Wilms' tumor, Med. Clin. North Am. **61**(5):1053-1071, 1977.

Structural defects of genitourinary tract

Cross, P.S.: Ureteral reimplantation: nursing care of the child, Am. J. Nurs. **76**(11):1800-1803, 1976.

Hill, S.: The child with ambiguous genitalia, Am. J. Nurs. **77:**810-814, 1977.

Mazur, T.: Ambiguous genitalia: detection and counseling, Pediatr. Nurs. **9:**417-422, 431, 1983.

McCoy, N.L.: Innate factors in sex differences, Nurs. Forum **15:**277-293, 1976.

Stevens, M.S., and Reinitz, M.: Nursing a child through exstrophic bladder reconstruction surgery, J. Maternal Child Nurs. **5:**265-270, 1980.

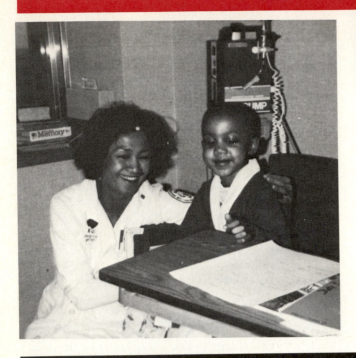

THE CHILD WITH
CEREBRAL DYSFUNCTION

OBJECTIVES

On completion of this chapter the reader will be able to:

- Describe the various modalities for assessment of cerebral function

- Differentiate between the stages of consciousness

- Formulate a plan of care for the unconscious child

- Distinguish between the types and serious complications of head injuries

- Describe the nursing care of a child with a tumor of the central nervous system

- Outline a plan of care for the child with bacterial meningitis

- Differentiate between the various types of seizure disorders

- Demonstrate an understanding of the manifestations and management of a child with a convulsive disorder

- Describe the preoperative and postoperative care of a child with hydrocephalus

NURSING DIAGNOSES

Nursing diagnoses identified for the child with cerebral dysfunction include, but are not restricted to, the following:

Health perception-health management pattern

- Injury, potential for, related to (1) environmental hazards; (2) immobility

Nutritional-metabolic pattern

- Fluid volume deficit, potential, related to inability to manage own intake

- Nutrition, alteration in: less than body requirements related to inability to manage own intake

- Oral mucous membranes, alteration in, related to mouth breathing

- Skin integrity, impairment of: actual or potential, related to immobility

Coping-stress tolerance pattern

■ Coping, family: potential for growth

■ Coping, ineffective family: compromised related to (1) situational crisis; (2) temporary family disorganization

Elimination pattern

■ Bowel elimination, alteration in, constipation related to immobility

■ Urinary elimination, alteration in patterns, related to inability to communicate

Activity-exercise pattern

■ Airway clearance, ineffective, related to inability to handle secretions

■ Diversional activity deficit related to immobility

■ Mobility, impaired physical, related to neuromuscular impairment

■ Self-care deficit: feeding, bathing/hygiene, dressing/grooming, toileting, related to (1) developmental level; (2) neuromuscular impairment; (3) immobility

Sleep-rest pattern

■ Sleep pattern disturbance related to schedule of therapies

Cognitive-perceptual pattern

■ Comfort, alterations in: pain, related to (1) positioning; (2) post-injury response

■ Sensory-perceptual alterations: visual, auditory, kinesthetic related to environmental factors

Self-perception—self-concept pattern

■ Anxiety related to (1) strange environment; (2) perception of impending events; (3) separation; (4) knowledge deficit; (5) discomfort

■ Powerlessness related to immobility

■ Self-concept, disturbance in: self-esteem, body image related to perception of disability

Role-relationship pattern

■ Communication, impaired verbal, related to effects of disability

■ Family process, alteration in, related to situational crisis

■ Parenting, alterations in, related to (1) skill deficit; (2) family stress; (3) long-term implications of disability

■ Social isolation related to (1) impaired mobility; (2) perception of disability

The brain is the center for multiple vital body functions. Any disturbance in this regulating, controlling, and communicating mechanism can produce alterations in the way in which the system receives, integrates, and/or responds to stimuli entering the system. These disturbances are reflected in a variety of clinical manifestations, depending on the focus of the disturbance and the integrity of the conducting mechanism.

This chapter is concerned with some of the major sources of insult to the brain and the way in which a skilled observer can assess the clinical evidence of neurologic dysfunction and intervene appropriately. The feature common to most cerebral disturbances is alterations in consciousness and is, therefore, presented as a concept to be applied in the subsequent discussions of problems with specific etiologies and manifestations. Diagnostic methods used to assess cerebral dysfunction and the neurologic assessment universally employed in nursing care of cerebral dysfunction are outlined early and applied throughout the remainder of the discussion.

THE UNCONSCIOUS CHILD

Consciousness implies the awareness of self and the environment. An altered state of consciousness usually refers to varying states of unconsciousness that may be momentary or may extend for hours, days, or indefinitely; it can be partial or complete. The causes of unconsciousness are numerous but, in a large number of instances, it is the result of increased intracranial pressure (ICP). Because increased intracranial pressure is common to so many of the cerebral disorders the concept is discussed briefly and followed by methods for assessment of cerebral function.

INCREASED INTRACRANIAL PRESSURE

The brain, tightly enclosed in the solid, bony cranium, is well protected but highly vulnerable to pressure that may accumulate within the enclosure. Its total volume, including brain, cerebrospinal fluid, and blood, must remain approximately the same at all times. A change in the proportional volume of one of these components produces an increase in intracranial pressure (ICP). This results in compensatory changes in the other components, which are manifest in neurologic signs and symptoms. An increase in intracranial pressure may be caused by tumors or other space-occupying lesions, accumulation of fluid within the ventricular system, bleeding, or edema of cerebral tissues.

Early signs and symptoms of increased ICP are often subtle and assume many patterns, such as personality changes, irritability, and fatigue. In older children subjective symptoms are headache, especially when lying flat (such as on awakening in the morning) or when coughing, sneezing, or bending over, and nausea and vomiting. The child may complain of double vision or of blurred vision on movement of the head. Funduscopic examination often reveals papilledema, the most reliable sign of increased ICP in older children. Seizures are not uncommon. In children prior to closure of the cranial sutures there is an increase in the head circumference and bulging fontanels. As pressure increases, pupils may be dilated and accompanied by an altered level of consciousness that progresses from drowsiness to eventual coma.

ASSESSMENT OF CEREBRAL DYSFUNCTION

Since the brain is impossible to assess by direct observation and measurement, most of the information about its status is obtained by indirect measurements. Some of these measurements are discussed in relation to numerous aspects of child care. The neurologic examination is an integral part of the health assessment (p. 124), assessment of gestational age (p. 182), and the newborn assessment (p. 149). Children younger than 2 years of age are more difficult to evaluate neurologically. Therefore, most information regarding infants and small children is gained through observation of their spontaneous and elicited reflex responses, by their development of increasingly complex locomotor and fine motor skills, and by eliciting more sophisticated communicative and adaptive behaviors.

General observations

In evaluating the infant or young child, physical evaluation includes observation of the size and shape of the head, spontaneous activity and postural reflex activity, and sensory responses. The attitude is observed. It is noted whether the infant assumes a normal flexed posture or one of extreme extension, opisthotonos, or hypotonia. Extremities are observed for symmetry of movement. Excessive tremulousness or frequent twitching movements may be significant signs indicating the onset of a seizure disorder. Seizure activity is suspected if holding the extremity snugly does not stop the activity. An abnormal respiratory cycle such as prolonged apnea, ataxic breathing, paradoxical chest movement, and unilateral expansion of the chest wall may be the result of a neurologic problem. Skin and hair texture may be important in detecting certain neurologic diseases. Facial features may suggest a specific syndrome, and a high-pitched, piercing cry is associated with central nervous system disorders. Abnormal eye movements, inability to suck or swallow, lip smacking, asymmetric contraction of facial muscles, and yawning may indicate cranial nerve involvement.

Older children can be evaluated by the usual methods employed in a neurologic examination. In addition, an estimation of the level of development provides essential information about neurologic function. The Denver Developmental Screening Test (Appendix C) serves as an excellent screening tool for assessing developmental progress in the young child.

Altered states of consciousness

Consciousness consists of (1) *cognitive power*—the sum of the mental processes including mood, behavior, memory, vision, speech, language, and so on; and (2) *alertness*—the state of wakefulness including the ability to respond to stimuli. Alteration of consciousness occurs as a continuum and reflects the awareness of self and surroundings.

Consciousness implies awareness, the ability to respond to sensory stimuli and have subjective experiences. *Unconsciousness* is depressed cerebral function, the inability to respond to sensory stimuli and have subjective experiences. *Coma* is a state of unconsciousness from which the patient cannot be aroused even with powerful stimuli.

Levels of consciousness (LOC). Various terms are used to describe alterations in level of consciousness that are determined by observations of the patient's responses to his environment. The most consistently used terms are:

  Sleep (normal unconsciouness) is a regular, recurring physiologic state in which there is absence of alertness, cognition, and voluntary movement that is readily reversed by auditory, visual, or tactile stimulation.
  Confusion is failure to comprehend one's surroundings—disorientation relative to time, inability to follow even simple directions, misidentification of persons, short attention span, loss of proper bearings, inability to estimate direction or location, ability to give relevant answers to simple questions, such as their age and location of pain, but inability to give relevant and accurate answers to more complex questions. Alert with intact arousal responses.
  Delirium is a state characterized by confusion, agitation, and hyperactivity, and marked by illusions (false interpretation of sensory perceptions), hallucinations (false sensory perceptions), and delusions (false ideas).
  Pseudowakeful states are demonstrated by wakefulness but inability to follow objects or lights, turn eyes toward noise, or speak. In less developed states the patient may follow objects or persons with eyes, turn slowly, but remain silent.
  Comatose states are characterized by diminished alertness that extends from somnolence or semistupor to deep coma.

Comatose states. Several scales have been devised in an attempt to standardize the description and interpretation of the comatose state. The most popular of these scales is the Glasgow Coma Scale (GCS) (see the box on p. 814), which consists of a three-part assessment: eye opening, verbal response, and motor response. Numerical values are assigned to the levels of response in each category and the sum of these numerical values provides an objective measure of the patient's level of consciousness. The lower the score, the deeper the comatose state. A normal person would score the highest, 15; a score of 7 or below is generally accepted as a definition of coma; the lowest score, 3, indicates deep coma.

Vital signs

Pulse, respiration, and blood pressure provide information regarding the adequacy of circulation and the possible underlying cause of altered consciousness. Autonomic activity is most intensively disturbed in deep coma and in brainstem lesions. Body temperature is often elevated, and sometimes the elevation may be extreme. Coma of a toxic origin may produce hypothermia.

A fever is most frequently a sign of an acute infectious process or heat stroke but may be caused by ingestion of some intoxicant drugs (especially alcohol and barbiturates) or intracranial bleeding. A fever sometimes follows a cerebral seizure.

The pulse is variable and may be rapid, slow and bounding, or feeble. Blood pressure may be normal, elevated, or at shock levels. With increased intracranial pressure, the pressor response causes a slowing of the pulse and an increase in blood pressure. This is an extremely serious sign that requires immediate action. This rise in blood pressure is greater in the systolic than the diastolic pressure, producing an increased, or widened, pulse pressure. This response is not so common in children; in children, a *change* in heart rate is considered more significant than the direction of the change.

Respirations are more often slow, deep, and irregular. The respiratory rate and rhythm are believed to be the most sensitive indicators of increased intracranial pressure. Hyperventilation is usually the result of metabolic acidosis or of abnormal stimulation of the respiratory center in the medulla as a result of salicylate poisoning, hepatic coma, or Reye syndrome. A description of the pattern of the respirations is useful in determining the level of injury. The odor of the breath may provide additional clues, for example, the fruity, acetone odor of ketosis, foul odor of uremia, fetid odor of hepatic failure, or odor of alcohol.

The skin may offer clues to the etiology of unconsciousness. The body surface should be examined for the presence of injury, needle marks, petechiae, bites, and ticks. Evidence of toxic substances may be found on the hands, face, mouth, and clothing—especially in small children.

PEDIATRIC COMA SCALE*

	Score	Over 1 year	Less than 1 year	
Eyes opening	4	Spontaneously	Spontaneously	
	3	To verbal command	To shout	
	2	To pain	To pain	
	1	No response	No response	
		Over 1 year	**Less than 1 year**	
Best motor	6	Obeys		
response	5	Localizes pain	Localizes pain	
	4	Flexion withdrawal	Flexion withdrawal	
	3	Flexion—abnormal (decorticate rigidity)	Flexion—abnormal (decorticate rigidity)	
	2	Extension (decerebrate rigidity)	Extension (decerebrate rigidity)	
	1	No response	No response	
		Over 5 years	**2-5 years**	**0-23 months**
Best verbal	5	Oriented and converses	Appropriate words and phrases	Smiles, coos, cries appropriately
	4	Disoriented and converses	Inappropriate words	Cries
	3	Inappropriate words	Cries and/or screams	Inappropriate crying and/or screaming
	2	Incomprehensible sounds	Grunts	Grunts
	1	No response	No response	No response
Total	3-15			

*Modification of Glasgow Coma Scale

Eyes

Pupil size and reactivity are assessed. Pinpoint pupils are commonly observed in poisoning, such as opiate or barbiturate poisoning, or in brainstem dysfunction. Widely dilated and reactive pupils are often seen after seizures and may involve only one side. Dilated pupils may also be caused by eye trauma. Widely dilated and fixed pupils suggest paralysis of cranial nerve III secondary to pressure from herniation of the brain through the tentorium. A unilateral fixed pupil usually suggests a lesion on the same side. Bilateral fixed pupils usually imply brainstem damage if present for more than 5 minutes. Dilated and unreactive pupils are also seen in hypothermia, poisoning with atropine-like substances, or prior instillation of mydriatic drugs.

Eye movements are assessed by the doll's-head maneuver, in which the child's head is rotated quickly to one side and then to the other. When brainstem centers for eye movement are intact, there is conjugate (paired or working together) movement of the eyes in the direction opposite to the head rotation. Absence of this response suggests dysfunction of the brainstem or oculomotor nerve (cranial nerve III). Downward or lateral deviation is frequently observed in association with pupillary dilation in dysfunction of cranial nerve III because of tentorial herniation.

The caloric test, or oculovestibular response, is elicited by irrigating the external auditory canal with ice water. This normally causes conjugate movement of the eyes toward the side of stimulation. This is lost when the pontine centers are impaired and, therefore, the caloric test provides important information in assessment of the comatose patient.

Funduscopic examination reveals additional clues. Papilledema indicates increased intracranial pressure. However, this may not be evident early in the course of unconsciousness since papilledema takes 24 to 48 hours to develop. The presence of preretinal (subhyaloid) hemorrhages in children is almost invariably the result of acute trauma with intracranial bleeding, usually subarachnoid or subdural hemorrhage.

Motor function

Observation of spontaneous activity, posture, and response to painful stimuli provides clues to the location and extent of cerebral dysfunction. Asymmetric movements of the limbs or absence of movement suggest paralysis. In hemiplegia the affected limb lies in external rotation and will fall uncontrollably when lifted and allowed to drop.

In the deeper comatose states there is little or no spon-

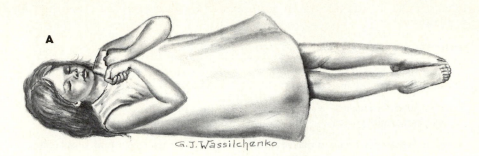

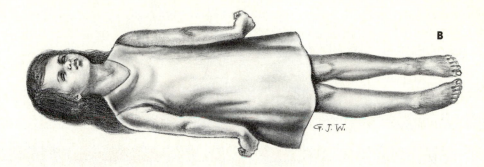

Fig. 25-1
A, *Decorticate posturing.*
B, *Decerebrate posturing.*

taneous movement and the musculature tends to be flaccid. There is considerable variability in the motor behavior in lesser degrees of coma. For example, the child may be relatively immobile or restless and hyperkinetic; muscle tone may be increased or decreased. Tremors, twitching, and spasms of muscles are common observations. The patient may display purposeless plucking or tossing movements. Combative or negativistic behavior is not uncommon. Hyperactivity is more common in acute febrile and toxic states than in cases of increased intracranial pressure. Convulsions are common in children and may be present in coma as a result of any cause.

Posturing.   As cortical control over motor function is lost in brain dysfunction, primitive postural reflexes emerge. These are evident in posturing and motor movement that are directly related to the area of the brain involved. *Decorticate posturing* is seen when there is severe dysfunction of the cerebral cortex. Typical decorticate posturing includes adduction of arms at the shoulders, the arms are flexed on the chest with the wrists flexed and the hands fisted, and the lower extremities extended and adducted (Fig. 25-1, *A*). *Decerebrate posturing*, a sign of dysfunction at the level of the midbrain, is characterized by rigid extension and pronation of the arms and legs (Fig. 25-1, *B*). The posturing may not be evident when the child is quiet but can usually be elicited by applying painful stimuli, such as knuckle pressure to the sternum.

Reflexes.   Testing of some reflexes may be of limited value. In general the corneal, pupillary, muscle-stretch, superficial, and plantar reflexes tend to be absent in deep coma. The state of reflexes is variable in lighter grades of unconsciousness and depends on the underlying pathologic process and the location of the lesion. Absence

of corneal reflexes and the presence of a tonic neck reflex are associated with severe brain damage. The Babinski reflex (p. 124) may be of value if it is found to be present consistently in children who are older than 1 year of age. A positive Babinski reflex is significant in assessment of pyramidal tract lesions when it is unilateral and associated with other pyramidal signs.

In the presence of symptoms that suggest meningeal irritation, the Kernig or Brudzinski signs may be elicited:

Kernig sign inability to extend the leg (or pain on extension) from a supine position with the hips flexed.
Brudzinski sign pain and involuntary flexion of knees and hips on flexion of the head while the child is lying supine.

Diagnostic procedures

Numerous diagnostic procedures are employed to determine the cause of unconsciousness and cerebral function. Some are common laboratory tests, which help to rule out metabolic or toxic etiologies; tests used to detect structural abnormalities and mechanical interference are highly technical and carried out with specialized equipment by skilled personnel. Table 25-1 outlines the major characteristics of tests used in neurologic diagnosis.

Laboratory tests.   Tests that may help to determine the cause of unconsciousness include blood glucose, urea nitrogen, electrolytes (pH, sodium, potassium, chloride, calcium, and bicarbonate) tests; clotting studies, hematocrit, and a complete blood count; liver function tests; blood cultures if there is fever; and sometimes studies to detect lead or other toxic substances, such as drugs.

Special procedures.   A variety of technical procedures is used in the diagnosis of cerebral dysfunction,

TABLE 25-1. DIAGNOSTIC PROCEDURES

TEST	PURPOSE	COMMENTS
Lumbar puncture (LP)	Measure spinal fluid pressure Obtain spinal fluid for analysis	Contraindicated in patients with increased intracranial pressure
Subdural tap	Rule out subdural effusion Relieve intracranial pressure	Infants only Requires scalp shaving
Ventricular puncture	Remove cerebrospinal fluid to relieve pressure	Used if lumbar puncture unsuccessful or contraindicated
Transillumination	Screening device to detect absence of vital structures	Simple to perform
Electroencephalography (EEG)	Measure electric activity of cerebral cortex	Patient should rest quietly during procedure—may require sedation
Brain scan	Identify focal brain lesions	Requires sedation in young or uncooperative children
Echoencephalography	Identifies shifts in midline structures	Simple, safe, rapid procedure
Radiography	Identify fractures, dislocations, spreading sutures	Simple procedure
Imaging techniques		
Computerized tomography (CT) or (CAT)	Yields precise cross-sectional views of desired area	Requires complete immobilization of head
Real-time ultrasound (RTUS)	Similar to CT but uses ultrasound	Subjects not exposed to ionizing radiation
Digital subtraction angiography (DSA)	Outline vascular system	Able to visualize arterial as well as venous vessels
Nuclear magnetic resonance (NMR)	Similar to CT but uses radio frequency	Subjects not exposed to ionizing radiation

which can be very frightening to children. Children who are old enough to understand require careful explanation of the procedure, why it is being done, what they will experience, and how they can help.

It is helpful for nurses to become acquainted with the equipment and the general environment in which the test will take place so that they can better explain the procedure to the child at his level of understanding. Equipment is often strange and ominous to a child and may even appear as a frightening monster. It is especially frightening to young children to experience a large mechanical device coming toward them as if to crush or devour a small, helpless child. They need constant reassurance from a trusted companion (Fig. 25-2).

Physical preparation may involve administration of a sedative. If so, the child should be helped through the preparation and administration and assured that someone will remain with him (if this is possible). The child will need continual support and reinforcement during the procedures in which he remains conscious. The child's vital signs and physiologic response to the procedure are moni-

tored throughout. Care after the test depends on the nature of the procedure.

Children who have undergone a procedure with general anesthesia require postanesthesia care, including positioning to prevent aspiration of secretions and frequent assessment of vital signs and level of consciousness. Also, other neurologic functions, such as pupillary responses, motor strength, and movement, are tested at regular intervals. After some procedures, for example, ventriculogram and pneumoencephalogram, the child should be kept flat and at bed rest. Any surgical wound is checked for bleeding, oozing, and other complications.

THERAPEUTIC MANAGEMENT OF THE UNCONSCIOUS CHILD

Emergency measures are directed toward assuming a patent airway, treatment of shock, and reduction of intracranial pressure (if present). Delayed treatment often leads to increased damage. A history is very important since it pro-

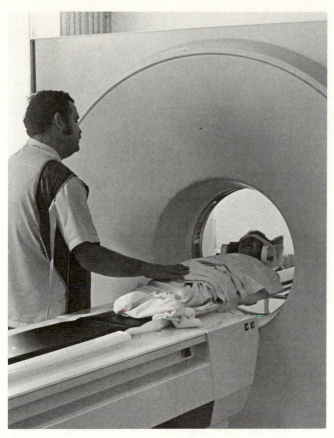

FIG. 25-2

A child reflects stress and a feeling of powerlessness during tomography, even when he is accompanied by a kind and supportive person.

vides valuable cues regarding the etiology of unconsciousness. There may have been an injury or short febrile illness, or the child may be a known diabetic. As soon as emergency measures have been implemented—in many cases concurrently—specific therapies for specific causes are initiated.

Respiratory status

Respiratory effectiveness is the primary concern in the unconscious child and demands immediate evaluation and intervention. Cerebral hypoxia that extends longer than 4 minutes causes irreversible brain damage. The child is positioned to prevent aspiration of secretions, and the stomach is emptied to reduce the likelihood of vomiting. An endotracheal tube or tracheostomy is frequently needed to assure an adequate airway and to facilitate removal of secretions. Also, upper airway obstruction, that is, laryngospasm, is a frequent complication in comatose children. When the respiratory center is involved, mechanical ventilation is usually indicated.

Blood gas analysis is performed regularly, and oxygen is administered when indicated. Moderately severe hypoxia and respiratory acidosis are often present and are not always evident from clinical manifestations. Hyperventilation frequently accompanies unconsciousness and can lead to respiratory alkalosis, or it may represent the body's attempt to compensate for metabolic acidosis. Therefore, blood gas and pH determinations are essential guides for electrolyte therapy.

Neurologic assessment

Continual observation of vital signs, pupillary reaction, and level of consciousness is essential to management of central nervous system disorders. Diagnostic tests are performed as indicated for diagnosis and observation of progress.

Sedatives are usually avoided but may be indicated when marked agitation or restlessness may result in further damage. If so, chloral hydrate or diphenhydramine (Benadryl) and, occasionally, paraldehyde are preferred. These drugs are less likely to produce respiratory depression. However, favorable results are achieved with the administration of codeine. Sometimes a large initial dose of phenobarbital is administered, even to the extent that short-term respiratory support is required. Anticonvulsants, primarily phenytoin (Dilantin), are ordered for control of seizure activity.

Increased intracranial pressure

Prompt intervention is lifesaving in the comatose patient who has evidence of marked increase in ICP. When increased ICP is the result of accumulation of cerebrospinal fluid from obstruction of cerebrospinal fluid flow, a ventricular tap will provide relief quickly and effectively. Evacuation of a hematoma reduces pressure from this source.

The child is positioned to facilitate venous return and ease respiratory efforts. The body is maintained in good alignment with the head elevated 10 to 30 degrees. The position is changed from side to back at least every 2 hours.

ICP is monitored directly by one of three methods. The most accurate means of measuring ICP is the intraventricular catheter. Sometimes a catheter is threaded between the skull and the dura to measure pressure, but the method most frequently used for children is the subarachnoid screw, or bolt.

For increased intracranial pressure resulting from cerebral edema, several medical measures are available. Osmotic diuretics may provide rapid relief in emergency situations. Although their effect is transient, lasting only about 6 hours, they can be lifesaving in emergencies. Mannitol or urea administered intravenously is most frequently employed for rapid reduction. The infusion is given slowly and, because of the profound diuretic effect of the drug, an indwelling catheter is inserted to ensure bladder emptying. Digitalis may be given to improve cerebral circulation. Adrenal corticosteroids are also used to reduce cerebral edema. The effect is less rapid than that of the osmotic diuretics, but high doses can be used over an extended period of time for prolonged control. A tube or other device is sometimes placed into the subarachnoid space or ventricle to monitor intracranial pressure directly. The simplest device is a subdural catheter attached to a standard manometer.

Nutrition

Fluids and calories are supplied initially by the intravenous route. Later, if the child remains unresponsive, fluids and nutrition are supplied by nasogastric tube or gastrostomy.

An intravenous infusion is started early, and the type of fluid administered is determined by the general condition of the patient. Fluid therapy requires careful monitoring and adjustment based on neurologic signs and electrolyte determinations. Often the comatose child is unable to cope with the same amounts of fluid that he could handle at other times and overhydration must be avoided to prevent fatal cerebral edema.

Hyperthermia

Fever often accompanies cerebral dysfunction, and, if present, measures are implemented to reduce the temperature to prevent brain damage from hyperthermia. Hypothermia by way of a cooling blanket is frequently prescribed for several days. The body temperature is reduced to 30.5° to 32.2° C (87° to 90° F) to decrease the oxygen demand by the brain.

Specific therapies

The foregoing treatments are nonspecific for comatose children in general. In addition, specific therapies for specific disorders are initiated as soon as the diagnosis is determined. For example, if diabetic ketoacidosis is diagnosed or suspected, insulin is administered intravenously, antibiotics are administered for cerebral infections, and tumors or cysts are removed.

Nursing considerations

The unconscious child requires continuous nursing attendance with observation, recording, and evaluation of changes in objective signs. These observations provide valuable information regarding the patient's progress. Often they serve as a guide to diagnosis and treatment. In addition, vital functions must be maintained and compli-

cations prevented through conscientious and meticulous nursing care. The outcome of unconsciousness may be early and complete recovery, death within a few hours or days, persistent and permanent unconsciousness, or recovery with varying degrees of residual mental and/or physical disability.

Respiratory status. Maintaining a patent airway is a primary consideration. Children in lighter stages of coma may be able to cough and swallow, but those in deeper states of coma are unable to handle secretions, which tend to pool in the throat and pharynx. A temporary airway can be used for the child who is suffering a temporary loss of consciousness, such as after a seizure or anesthesia. For children who remain unconscious for a period of time, a nasotracheal or orotracheal tube is inserted to maintain the open airway. A tracheostomy is performed in cases in which laryngoscopy for introduction of an endotracheal tube would be difficult or dangerous. Suctioning is used as often as needed to clear the airway.

Respiratory status is observed and evaluated regularly. When making an assessment of respirations it is usually best to describe what is observed rather than attempt to place a label to the respirations because terms are frequently used incorrectly. Signs of respiratory embarrassment may be an indication for ventilatory assistance. Particular care should be taken in positioning these patients to avoid neck vein compression, which may further increase intracranial pressure by interfering with venous return.

Neurologic assessment. Regular assessment of neurologic signs is a vital part of nursing comatose children. Vital signs are taken and recorded regularly. The frequency depends on the cause of coma, the status, and the progression of the cerebral involvement. The intervals may be as frequent as every 15 minutes or as long as every 2 hours. Significant alterations are reported immediately. Temperature is taken every 2 to 4 hours, depending on the patient's condition.

An elevated temperature is not uncommon in children with central nervous system dysfunction; therefore, a light covering is sufficient. Vigorous efforts are needed, such as tepid sponge baths or application of a hypothermia blanket, to prevent brain damage.

The level of consciousness is assessed periodically, including size, equality, and reaction to light of pupils; signs of meningeal irritation, such as nuchal rigidity; and level of consciousness. This includes response to vocal commands, spontaneous behavior, resistance to care, and response to painful stimuli, such as sternal or supraorbital pressure. It is important to record the type of stimulus needed to elicit any movement. Voluntary motions of any kind, changes in muscle tone or strength, and body position are noted. Seizure activity is described according to type and length of seizure and body areas involved (p. 845).

Hygienic care. Routine measures for cleansing and maintaining skin integrity are an integral part of nursing care of the unconscious child. Skin folds require special attention to prevent excoriation. Children who are unable to move are prone to develop tissue breakdown and pressure necrosis; therefore, the child is placed on a sheepskin, egg-carton pad, or other resilient appliance (alternating pressure mattresses and water-filled mattresses are also used) to prevent pressure on prominent areas of the body. The goal is prevention by regular change of position and inspection of vulnerable areas, such as the ankle, trochanter, and shoulder. Since supine positioning is seldom employed, the occiput and sacrum are less likely to be involved. Bed linen and any clothing are kept dry and free of wrinkles. Rubbing the back and extremities with lotion or other lubricating preparation stimulates circulation and helps prevent drying of the skin.

Mouth care is performed at least twice daily, since the mouth tends to become dry or coated with mucus. The teeth are carefully brushed with a soft toothbrush or cleaned with gauze saturated with mouthwash. Commercially prepared cleansing devices, such as Toothettes, are convenient for cleansing the mouth and teeth. Saline or other solutions, such as dilute hydrogen peroxide, can be used to cleanse and moisten mucous surfaces. Lips are coated with ointment, petrolatum, or other preparations to protect them from drying, cracking, or blistering.

The deeply comatose child is also prone to eye irritation. The corneal reflexes are absent; therefore, the eyes are easily irritated or damaged by linen, dust, or other substances that may come in contact with them. There is excessive dryness as a result of decreased secretions, especially if the child is undergoing osmotherapy to reduce or prevent brain edema, and incomplete closure of the eyes. The eyes are examined regularly and carefully for early signs of irritation or inflammation. Artificial tears (methylcellulose) are placed in the eyes at frequent intervals. Sometimes eye dressings may be needed to protect the eyes from possible damage.

The hair is combed and styled neatly. Long hair is usually braided and secured with rubber bands. The scalp is kept clean with dry or wet shampoos as needed. The child's head may be shaved for tests or surgical procedures. If so, the hair is saved if possible.

Nutrition and hydration. Initially, unconscious children are fed by intravenous infusion or hyperalimentation. Later, nutrition is provided in a balanced formula given by nasogastric or gastrostomy tube. The nasogastric tube is usually taped in place with care to prevent pressure on the nares. The tube is rinsed carefully after each feeding and is replaced frequently (usually every 24 hours) to prevent bacterial growth and to alternate nostrils to prevent nasal irritation and pressure. Overfeeding is avoided to prevent vomiting with the danger of aspiration. The stomach contents are aspirated and measured prior to feeding to ascertain the amount remaining in the stomach. If the residual volume is excessive (depending on the size of the child), the dietitian and physician should be consulted regarding alteration of the formula composition to provide the needed calories and nutrients in a smaller volume. The aspirated contents should always be refed.

Hydration is maintained in the same manner. When cerebral edema is a threat, the fluids may be restricted to reduce the chance of fluid overload. Skin and mucous membranes are examined for signs of dehydration.

Elimination. A retention catheter is usually inserted in the older child, and a plastic collection bag is placed on the infant or small child. The child who formerly had bowel and bladder control is generally incontinent. The collecting devices help keep the skin clean and provide a means for obtaining an accurate intake and output measurement. If the child remains comatose for a long period of time, the indwelling catheter may be removed and periodic bladder emptying accomplished by pressure applied over the suprapubic area (Credé). Stool softeners are usually sufficient to maintain bowel function, but suppositories or enemas may be needed occasionally for adequate elimination.

Positioning and exercise. The unconscious child is positioned to prevent aspiration of saliva, nasogastric secretions, and vomitus and to minimize intracranial pressure. The head of the bed is slightly elevated, and the child is placed on the side or in a semiprone position. A small, firm pillow is placed under the head, and the uppermost limbs are flexed and supported with pillows. The weight of the body should not rest on the dependent arm. In the semiprone position the child lies with the dependent arm at the side behind the body and the opposite side supported on pillows with the uppermost arm and leg flexed and resting on the pillows. This position prevents undue pressure on the dependent extremities. The dependent position of the face encourages drainage of secretions and prevents the flaccid tongue from obstructing the airway.

Normal range of motion exercises are carried out to maintain function and prevent contractures of joints. Exercises are performed gently and with full range of motion. A small rolled pad can be placed in the palms to help maintain proper position of fingers; footboards or boots can be used to help prevent foot-drop, and sometimes splinting may be needed to prevent severe contractures of the wrist, knee, or ankle in decerebrate children.

Medications. The cause of unconsciousness determines specific drug therapies. Children with infectious processes are given antibiotics appropriate to the disease and the infecting organism, and corticosteroids are prescribed for inflammatory conditions and edema. Cerebral edema is an indication for osmotherapy with osmotic diuretics and/or hypertonic glucose solution. Sedatives are often indicated for extreme restlessness, agitation, and hyperresponsiveness to stimuli. Sedatives or anticonvulsants are prescribed for seizure activity. The unconscious child requires stool softeners to maintain bowel function.

Medications such as antibiotics and corticosteroids may be ordered intravenously during the early days of unconsciousness. When nasogastric or gastrostomy feedings are implemented, most medications are given by this route. It is particularly important to be alert to signs of adverse drug reactions, since many of the side effects or toxic effects of drugs involve observation of changes in behavior or responsiveness, which are rendered invalid by the child's unconscious state.

Stimulation. Sensory stimulation is important in the care of the unconscious child, just as it is in the care of the alert child. For the temporarily unconscious or semiconscious child, sensory stimulation helps to arouse him to the conscious state and orient him in terms of time and place. Unconscious children need sensory stimulation as much as conscious children. Auditory and tactile stimulation are especially valuable. Tactile stimulation is not appropriate for the child in whom it may elicit an undesirable response. However, for other children, tactile contact often has a relaxing and calming effect. When the child's condition permits, holding or rocking the child has a soothing effect on him and provides the body contact needed by young children.

The auditory sense is often present in a state of coma. Hearing is the last sense to be lost and the first sense to be regained; therefore, the child is spoken to as any other child. Conversation around the child should not include thoughtless or derogatory remarks. A radio playing soft music, a music box, or a record player is frequently employed to provide auditory stimulation. Singing the child's favorite songs or reading a favorite story within his hearing is a tactic used to maintain his contact with a familiar world. Above all, it is important to remember that this is a child who has all the needs of any ill child.

Parents. Dealing with the parents of an unconscious child is especially difficult. They may demonstrate all the guilt, fear, and anxiety of any parent of a seriously ill child. In addition they are faced with the uncertain outcome of the cerebral dysfunction. The fear of death, mental retardation, or other permanent disability is present. Nursing intervention with parents depends on the nature of the pathology, the personality of the parents, and the parent-child relationship prior to injury or illness.

The child may regain consciousness within a short period of time. If there is little or no residual effect, the child will be dismissed to home care fairly soon. The parents need the most intensive nursing intervention during the period of crisis and uncertainty. During the recovery phase they are given information, information is clarified, and they are encouraged to become involved in the child's care. Often the child's hospitalization is brief; however, some children require extended hospitalization for intensive therapy and rehabilitation.

The parents of children who die within hours or days require the support and guidance that the parents of any dying child would (see Chapter 16) in coping with the reality and resolving their grief.

Probably the most difficult situations are those that involve children who are unconscious permanently or for an indefinite period. Unlike parents who lose a child through death, the finality is lacking for these parents, often leaving them in a state of suspended grief. The presence of the child renders the parents unable to resolve the loss. Superimposed on the process of grieving for the "lost" child, parents may be faced with difficult decisions. First there is the child whose brain is so severely damaged that his vital functions must be maintained by artificial means. When brain death has been determined according to established criteria, the parents must make the final decision to remove the life-support systems.

Second there is the child who has survived the illness or injury that produced the brain damage but who is left unconscious permanently. These parents must decide whether to place the child in a rest home or other institution for comatose children or make arrangements to care for the child at home. The parents who choose to care for their child at home will need education and support in learning to care for the child, regular follow-up observation and assessment of the home management, and planning for some respite care of the child. Parents need to understand that it is important to plan for periodic relief from the continual care of the child.

CRANIOCEREBRAL TRAUMA

Accidental injury is the major single cause of death in the pediatric age-group, and, although it cannot be stated with certainty, most of these injuries are probably the result of central nervous system trauma. Whereas serious injury contributes significantly to childhood mortality and morbidity, the majority of accidental head traumas do not leave the injured child with permanent neurologic impairment.

Head injury can be defined as any pathologic process involving the scalp, skull, meninges, or brain as the result of mechanical force. The exposed nature of the head renders it particularly vulnerable to external violence, and many of the physical characteristics of children predispose to craniocerebral trauma. Incomplete motor development contributes to falls at all ages, and the natural curiosity, exuberance, and exploring nature of children frequently place them in situations in which they are more likely to incur an accidental injury. The highest incidence occurs during the ages of 8 to 9 years, with a secondary peak incidence in boys at around 12 to 13 years of age. Because of the relative frequency of craniocerebral injuries in the pediatric age-groups and the potential for damaging se-

SUMMARY OF NURSING CARE OF THE UNCONSCIOUS CHILD

GOALS	RESPONSIBILITIES

Maintain patent airway	Position to prevent aspiration
	    Semiprone position
	    Side-lying position
	Aspirate airway as needed
	Insert oral airway if indicated
	Administer care of endotracheal tube or tracheostomy if appropriate; have equipment available for emergency insertion if indicated for respiratory distress
	Avoid neck hyperextension

Minimize intracranial pressure	Elevate head of the bed 10 to 30 degrees Avoid pressure on neck veins

Prevent cerebral hypoxia	Maintain patent airway
	Provide oxygen as indicated by objective signs or as ordered
	If on mechanical ventilation
	    Monitor for
	        Correct settings
	        Proper functioning
	Prepare to provide artificial ventilation in case of ventilatory failure; have AMBU bag at hand
	Administer medications as ordered to prevent cerebral edema and improve cerebral circulation

Detect early signs of cerebral hypoxemia	Monitor vital signs Observe changes in color of face, lips, extremities Observe for changes in responsiveness Observe for seizure activity

Assess neurologic status	Monitor vital signs as ordered
	    Temperature
	    Pulse quality, rate, rhythm
	    Respirations—rate, rhythm, depth
	    Blood pressure
	    Pulse pressure
	Monitor central venous pressure (if attached)
	Monitor intracranial pressure (if device is in place)
	Check pupillary reaction for size, reaction to light and accommodation, and equality of responses
	Note and describe
	    Voluntary movements of extremities, for example, purposeful, random
	    Changes in muscular tone
	    Changes in position of body and/or head
	    Tremor, twitching
	    Seizure activity, for example, generalized or focal
	    Signs of meningeal irritation, for example, nuchal rigidity, opisthotonos
	In infants measure occipital-frontal circumference
	    Assess status of fontanel—full or sunken, tense or soft

Assess level of consciousness	Observe and record
	    Changes in spontaneous behavior
	    Resistance to care
	    Response to verbal commands
	    Response to noxious stimuli
	    Type of verbalization or crying

Continued.

SUMMARY OF NURSING CARE OF THE UNCONSCIOUS CHILD—cont'd

GOALS	RESPONSIBILITIES
Prevent cerebral edema	Monitor fluid intake and output Observe for signs of impending overhydration and take appropriate action Elevate head of bed to 15 to 30 degrees Administer osmotic diuretics and/or hypertonic glucose as ordered Administer corticosteroids as ordered Weigh daily or as ordered to detect fluid accumulation or reduction
Prevent or control hyperthermia	Assess temperature regularly to detect elevation Remove excess coverings Administer antipyretics, if prescribed Administer tepid sponge bath for elevated temperature Apply and monitor hypothermia blanket if indicated or ordered
Assist with diagnostic tests	Collect specimens as ordered Carry out examinations as indicated or ordered, such as urine specific gravity, blood samples Prepare for and assist with diagnostic procedures, such as lumbar puncture, radiographic examination Interpret and report results of tests
Prevent respiratory complications	Position for optimum ventilation Turn frequently—at least every 2 hours Avoid contact with persons with upper respiratory infection Maintain patent airway Perform percussion, vibration, and suctioning every 3 to 4 hours Remove accumulated secretions promptly Provide good oral hygiene

Maintain skin integrity	Place child on sheepskin, egg-carton pad, or other resilient surface
	Change position frequently
	Protect pressure points, for example, trochanter, sacrum, ankle, shoulder, occiput
	Inspect skin surfaces regularly for signs of irritation, redness, evidence of pressure
	Cleanse skin regularly, at least once daily
	Protect skin folds and surfaces that rub together
	Keep clothing and linen clean and dry
	Apply urine collecting device or insert indwelling catheter (if ordered) to prevent irritation from urine
	   Carry out proper care of catheter
	   Carry out good perineal care under collection device
	Stimulate circulation by gentle rubbing with lotion, ointment, or other lubricating substance
	Protect lips with cream, glycerine, or ointment

Protect from injury	Keep side rails up Pad hard surfaces that may injure extremities during spontaneous or involuntary movements Place protective device between teeth if biting movements have occurred during a previous seizure Administer sedatives or anticonvulsants as prescribed
Maintain limb flexibility and function	Perform gentle, passive range of motion exercises Position to reduce contractures—splint contracting joints if needed
Provide nutrition and hydration	Monitor intravenous feedings when ordered Feed prescribed formula by means of nasogastric or gastrostomy tube

SUMMARY OF NURSING CARE OF THE UNCONSCIOUS CHILD—cont'd

GOALS	RESPONSIBILITIES
Assure adequate elimination	Provide sufficient liquid intake, unless contraindicated by cerebral edema or if overhydration is threat Administer stool softener Administer suppositories or enema as indicated
Prevent overstimulation	Avoid stimulation that precipitates undesirable responses Time nursing activities for minimum disturbance
Provide sensory stimulation	Provide tactile stimulation (if it does not cause undesirable muscle response, for example, seizures) Provide auditory stimulation by voice, radio, music box, and so on Provide visual stimuli appropriate for age Provide proprioceptive stimulation by rocking, cuddling, and so on
Support the parents	Explain therapies; clarify and reinforce information given to family by physician Interpret the child's behaviors and responses Allow expression of feelings and concerns Accept aggressive behavior
Assist in child placement	Provide needed information Answer the parents' questions Refer to persons or agencies for further information and clarification Support the parents' decision
Arrange for discharge and follow-up care	Teach the parents techniques and procedures needed in care of the child (if appropriate) Arrange for follow-up visit by appropriate persons, for example, public health nurse

quelae, they present a common and serious clinical entity. There is also a high incidence of head injury associated with other manifestations of battering.

Pathophysiology

Blows to the head involving a small area, such as when the head is struck by an object such as a rock or bat, produce a depressed area corresponding to the object. Blows involving larger areas, such as those sustained when the head strikes a hard surface, are more likely to produce more extensive damage.

Injury to the brain occurs by way of compression, tearing, or shearing, either singly, in combination, or in succession. When the stationary head receives a blow, the sudden movement causes deformation of the skull and mass movement of the brain. Continued movement of the intracranial contents allows the brain to strike parts of the skull (such as the sharp edges of the sphenoid or the irregular surface of the anterior fossa) or the edges of the tentorium. Although the brain volume remains unchanged, significant distortion takes place as it changes shape in response to the force of the impact to the skull. This movement can cause bruising at the point of impact *(coup)* and/

or at a distance as the brain collides with the unyielding surfaces far removed from the point of impact *(contrecoup)* (Fig. 25-3). Thus a blow to the occipital region can cause severe injury to the frontal and temporal areas of the brain. Sudden deceleration, such as takes place during a fall, causes the greatest cerebral injury at the point of impact.

Another effect of brain movement is shearing stresses, which tear small arteries and cause subdural hemorrhages. Another source of damage occurs when severe compression of the skull causes the brain to be forced through the tentorial opening. This can produce irreparable damage to the brainstem (see Figs. 25-4 and 25-5).

Types of injury

As a whole, head injuries can be regarded as localized or generalized. In localized injuries the force is concentrated on a local area of both skull and underlying tissues; in generalized injuries the force is transmitted to the entire skull.

Concussion.   The most common head injury is concussion, a transient and reversible neuronal dysfunction with instantaneous loss of awareness and responsiveness

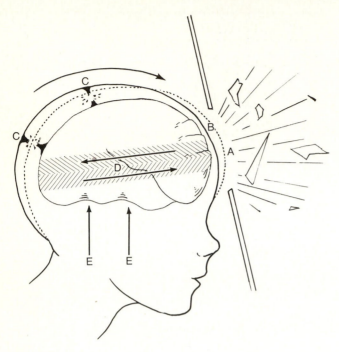

FIG. 25-3

Mechanical distortions of cranium during closed head injury. **A,** *Preinjury contour of skull.* **B,** *Immediate postinjury contour of skull.* **C,** *Torn subdural vessels.* **D,** *Shearing forces.* **E,** *Trauma from contact with floor of cranium.* *(Redrawn from Grubb, R.L., and Coxe, W.S.: Central nervous system trauma: cranial. In Eliasson, S.G., Prensky, A.L., and Hardin, W.B., Jr., editors: Neurological pathophysiology, New York, 1974, Oxford University Press.)*

from trauma to the head that persists for a relatively short time, usually minutes or hours. It is generally followed by amnesia for the moment of the injury and a variable period prior to the injury.

Contusion and laceration. The terms "contusion" and "laceration" are used to describe visible bruising and tearing of cerebral tissue. Contusions represent petechial hemorrhages at the site of impact (coup injury) and/or a lesion remote from the site of direct trauma (contrecoup injury). In serious accidents there may be multiple sites of injury. Contusions may cause focal disturbances in strength, sensation, or visual awareness. The degree of brain damage in the contused areas varies according to the extent of vascular injury. Cerebral lacerations are generally associated with penetrating wounds or depressed skull fractures.

Fractures. The immature skull, because of its flexibility, is able to sustain a greater degree of deformation than the adult skull before it incurs a fracture. It requires a great deal of force to produce a fracture in the skull of an infant. A fracture may occur with little or no brain

damage, or severe and fatal brain injury can take place without fracture. The undersurface of the skull contains grooves in which the meningeal arteries lie. A fracture that runs through one of these grooves may tear the artery and produce severe and damaging hemorrhage.

The majority of skull fractures (about 70%) are linear. Depressed fractures are those in which the bone is locally broken usually into several irregular fragments that are pushed inward, causing pressure on the brain. The inner portion of the bone is more extensively fragmented than the outer portion, which almost invariably produces tears in the dura. Both linear and comminuted depressed fractures are uncommon before 2 to 3 years of age. In infants and very young children, the soft, malleable bone may become dented in a peculiar rounded or "Ping-Pong ball" depression without laceration of either skin or dura.

Complications of head injuries

The major complications of trauma to the head are hemorrhage, infection, edema, and tentorial herniation. Infection is always a hazard in open injuries, and edema is related to tissue trauma. Vascular rupture may occur even in minor head injuries, causing hemorrhage between the skull and cerebral surfaces. Compression of the underlying brain produces effects that can be rapidly fatal or insidiously progressive.

Increased intracranial pressure. Increase in the volume of the intracranial contents from any cause is the greatest threat to the head-injured child. The increased volume can be the result of hemorrhage or edema, but the damage is caused by the pressure. The description and management have been discussed elsewhere and will not be elaborated here, but nurses should be alert to this ever-present and serious complication of head injury.

Epidural hemorrhage. In epidural hemorrhage the blood accumulates between the dura and the skull to form a hematoma, which, because of the difficulty with which dura is stripped from bone, forces the underlying brain contents downward and inward as they expand (Fig. 25-4). Since bleeding is generally arterial, brain compression occurs rapidly. Most often the expanding hematoma is located in the parietotemporal region, forcing the medial portion of the temporal lobe under the edge of the tentorium, where it causes pressure on nerves and blood vessels.

The classic clinical picture of epidural hemorrhage is one in which the individual loses consciousness momentarily or is merely stunned by the injury and is then free of symptoms (the lucid period). Within a few minutes or hours (occasionally days), he develops signs and symptoms of intracranial compression. Sometimes signs of increased pressure develop without evidence of a lucid period, however. Clinical signs include headache, vomiting,

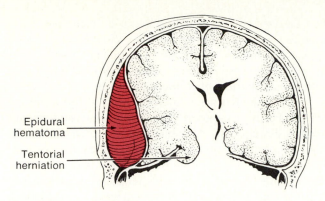

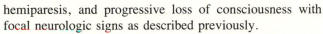

FIG. 25-4
Epidural (extradural) hematoma and compression of portion of temporal lobe through tentorial hiatus.

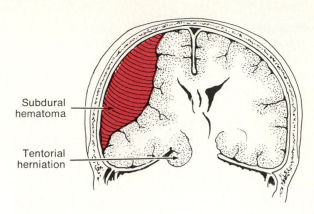

FIG. 25-5
Subdural hematoma.

hemiparesis, and progressive loss of consciousness with focal neurologic signs as described previously.

In children this classic picture is seldom evident. The period of impaired consciousness is frequently lacking, and the symptom-free period is atypical because of nonspecific complaints such as irritability, headache, and vomiting. It frequently lasts longer than 48 hours. Clinically significant epidural hematomas are uncommon in children younger than 4 years of age.

Subdural hemorrhage. A subdural hemorrhage is bleeding between the dura and the cerebrum, usually as a result of rupture of cortical veins that bridge the subdural space (Fig. 25-5). Unlike epidural hemorrhage, which develops inwardly, subdural hemorrhage tends to develop more slowly and spreads thinly and widely until it is limited by the dural barriers—the falx and tentorium. Subdural hematoma is fairly common in infants, frequently as the result of birth trauma.

The clinical course and manifestations are variable and depend on the damage sustained by the brain substance and the age of the child. Delayed symptoms are common in children with open fontanels and sutures. The most common presenting manifestations in children are seizures, vomiting, and irritability, drowsiness, or other personality changes. Older children may complain of headache. Less common signs are developmental retardation and failure to thrive. Presenting signs include evidence of increased intracranial pressure such as increased head size and bulging fontanels (in the infant), retinal hemorrhages, extraocular palsies (especially cranial nerve VI), hemiparesis, quadriplegia, and sometimes fever. Older children may display an unsteady gait, and papilledema is usually present.

Cerebral edema. Some degree of brain swelling is expected after craniocerebral trauma and often accompanies any of the previous disorders. Cerebral edema caused by direct cellular injury or vascular injury induces

vascular stasis, anoxia, and further vasodilation. If the progression continues unchecked, intracranial pressure exceeds arterial pressure and fatal anoxia ensues and/or the pressure causes herniation of a portion of the brain over the edge of the tentorium.

Diagnostic evaluation

After a thorough clinical examination, a variety of diagnostic tests are helpful in providing a more definitive diagnosis of the type and extent of the trauma. Skull x-ray films and other radiographic tests are indicated, especially when the patient has lost consciousness after injury. Electroencephalography is not particularly helpful for early diagnosis but is useful for defining seizure activity or focal destructive lesions after the acute phase of illness. Lumbar puncture is rarely employed in craniocerebral trauma and is contraindicated in the presence of increased intracranial pressure.

Where available, imaging techniques such as computerized tomography (CT) are especially valuable in diagnosis of neurologic trauma and usually make other diagnostic procedures unnecessary. CT is easily carried out, is noninvasive, and can be repeated periodically for reassessment in the patient who remains unconscious or shows progressive neurologic deterioration.

In the infant or small child a subdural tap through a fontanel or coronal suture may establish the diagnosis of subdural or epidural hemorrhage.

Therapeutic management

The majority of children with mild to moderate concussion who have not lost consciousness can be cared for and observed at home after careful examination reveals no serious intracranial injury. The parents are instructed to check the child every 2 hours to determine any changes in responsiveness. The sleeping child is wakened to see if he can be roused normally. Parents are advised to maintain contact with the attending physician, who usually wishes to examine the child again in 1 or 2 days. The manifestations of epidural hematoma in children do not generally appear until 24 hours or more after injury.

Children with severe injuries, those who have lost consciousness for more than a few minutes, and those with prolonged and continued seizures or other focal or diffuse neurologic signs must be hospitalized until their condition is stable and their neurologic signs have diminished. As a rule the outlook of a head injury in children is more optimistic than a similar injury in the adult. Children have a greater ability to recover from major intracranial trauma, especially those less than 24 months of age.

The child is maintained on clear liquids, if he is able to take fluids by mouth, until it is determined that vomiting will not occur. Intravenous fluids are indicated in the child who is comatose or displays dulled sensorium and/or in the child with persistent vomiting. Fluid balance is closely monitored by daily weight, accurate intake and output measurement, and serum osmolality to detect early signs of water retention, excessive dehydration, and states of hypertonicity or hypotonicity.

Restlessness can be satisfactorily managed, if necessary, with diphenhydramine (Benadryl) or chloral hydrate, and headache is usually controlled with aspirin in age-appropriate dosages. Anticonvulsants are employed for seizure control and, frequently, in cases of suspected contusion or laceration. Antibiotics are administered if there are lacerations, cerebrospinal fluid leakage, or excessive cerebral tissue damage. Prophylactic tetanus toxoid is given for open scalp wounds according to the policy of the institution.

Cerebral edema is managed as described for the unconscious child, including administration of corticosteroids and hypertonic solutions. Hyperthermia is controlled with tepid sponges.

Surgical therapy.   Scalp lacerations are sutured after careful examination of underlying bone. Depressed fractures require surgical reduction and removal of bone fragments. Torn dura is sutured. Ping-pong ball skull fractures in very young infants ordinarily correct themselves within a few weeks and do not require specific treatment.

Nursing considerations

Since all but the most minor head injuries are managed in the hospital, close observation of the child is essential. Careful neurologic assessment and evaluation, including vital signs, repeated at frequent intervals provide information needed to establish a correct diagnosis, determine clinical management, and prevent many complications.

Bed rest is prescribed, usually with the head of the bed elevated slightly, and appropriate safety measures, such as side rails kept up for older children and seizure precautions for children of all ages, are implemented. The extremely restless child may require that hard surfaces be padded and the use of restraint to prevent the possibility of further injury. Care is individualized according to the specific needs of the child. The unconscious child is managed as described in the previous section, but most childhood head injuries are those causing momentary stunning or temporary unconsciousness. The child may be restless and irritable, but more often his reaction is to fall asleep when left undisturbed. A quiet environment helps reduce the restlessness and irritability. Bright lights shining directly into the child's face are irritating. This often makes checking the ocular responses more difficult to perform and more aggravating to the child.

Frequent examinations of vital signs, neurologic signs, and level of consciousness are extremely important nursing observations. When possible they are performed by a single observer in order to better detect subtle changes that may indicate worsening of neurologic status. Pupils are checked for size, equality, and reaction to light and accommodation. After the initial elevations usually seen after injury, the vital signs generally return to normal unless there is brainstem involvement. A rectal or axillary temperature is the safest method of measuring temperature, since seizures are not uncommon and vomiting is a frequent response in children, especially when the child is disturbed. Hand grasps and motor function, both spontaneous and elicited, are observed, evaluated relative to strength, and compared bilaterally.

Probably the most important nursing observation is assessment of the child's level of consciousness. Alterations in consciousness appear earlier in the progression of an injury than alterations of vital signs or focal neurologic signs (see p. 812 for evaluation of responsiveness). Some expected responses may be interpreted as deviations from the normal. Frequent examinations of alertness are fatiguing to the child; therefore, he often desires to fall asleep, which may be confused with depressed consciousness. When left alone the child promptly dozes.

Observations of position and movement provide additional information. Any abnormal posturing is noted as well as whether or not it occurs continuously or intermittently.

The child may complain of headache or other discomfort. The child who is too young to describe a headache will be fussy and resist being handled. The child who suffers from vertigo will often assume a position and vigorously resist efforts to move him. Seizures, relatively common in children with craniocerebral trauma, may be of any type but are more often generalized regardless of the type of injury. Any seizure activity is carefully observed and described in detail (p. 846).

Drainage from any orifice is noted. Bleeding from the ear suggests the possibility of a basal skull fracture. The amount and characteristics of the drainage are observed, and, since the auditory canal may be a source of infection, dry, sterile cotton can be placed loosely at the orifice and changed when soiled. Continued drainage of clear fluid from the nose is tested with Dextrostix and the amount and reaction recorded. The presence of glucose is evidence of cerebrospinal fluid drainage, and suctioning through the nares is contraindicted, since there is a high risk of secondary infection and the probability of the catheter entering the brain substance through the fracture.

Head trauma is frequently accompanied by other undetected injuries; therefore, any bruises, lacerations, or evidence of internal injuries or fractures of the extremities is noted and reported. Associated injuries are evaluated and treated appropriately.

The child is usually allowed clear liquids unless fluid is restricted. If the child has an intravenous infusion, it is maintained as prescribed. The diet is advanced to that appropriate for the child's age as soon as his condition permits. Intake and output are measured and recorded, and any incontinence of bowel or bladder is noted in the child who has been toilet trained.

The child is observed for any unusual behavior, but interpretation of behavior is made in relation to the child's normal behavior. Information obtained from parents at or shortly after admission is helpful in evaluating the child's behavior, for example, the ease with which the child is roused normally, his usual sleeping position, how much he sleeps during the day, motor activity of which he is capable (rolling over, sitting up, climbing), hearing and visual acuity, appetite, and manner of eating (spoon, bottle, cup). There would be less concern about a child who falls asleep several times during the day if this particular type of behavior is consistent with his usual behavior.

Children may require sedation for severe restlessness, acetaminophen (Tylenol) or Tylenol with codeine for headache, and anticonvulsants to control seizure activity. They are rarely given central nervous system depressants.

When the child is discharged the parents are advised of probable posttraumatic symptoms that may be expected. They need to understand observations that should be made and how to contact the physician, nurse, or health facility in case the child develops any unusual signs or symptoms.

NEOPLASMS OF THE CENTRAL NERVOUS SYSTEM

Tumors of the central nervous system are second only to leukemia as a cause of death from cancer in children. Brain tumors, although less common in children than in older age-groups, constitute a significant nursing concern. Neuroblastoma, a tumor that usually arises in the autonomic nervous system or adrenal medulla, is not a cerebral tumor but is the most common solid tumor in children and is included here for convenience.

BRAIN TUMORS

The majority of tumors in children (about 60%) are *infratentorial,* which means that they occur in the lower posterior third of the brain beneath the tentorium (the tent-shaped portion of the dura mater that lies between the cerebrum and the cerebellum), primarily in the cerebellum or brainstem. This anatomic distribution accounts for the frequency of symptoms caused by increased intracranial pressure and the high incidence of fatalities. A smaller number are *supratentorial,* or within the superior two thirds of the brain, mainly the cerebrum. In adults the majority of tumors are of the latter type.

Classification

Neoplasms can arise from any cell within the cranium, and the tumor reflects the type of cell in which the tumor has its origin. Some major intracranial tumors of childhood are in the box on p. 830. Gliomas, which arise from glial cells, the supporting structures of the brain, are the most common brain tumors in children. Except where indicated all the tumors described are gliomas.

Clinical manifestations

Except for a general ''failure to thrive,'' the signs and symptoms of brain tumors are directly related to their anatomic location, their size, and to some extent the age of the child. In infants, in whom sutures remain open, virtually no early detectable signs develop. It is not until intracranial pressure from spinal fluid obstruction causes a marked increase in head size that a lesion may be suspected.

Headache. Recurrent and progressive headaches in the frontal or occipital areas may indicate a brain tumor. They are characteristically worse on arising, lessen during the day, are affected by position (intensified by lowering the head), and increase during straining, such as during a bowel movement, coughing, or sneezing. In infants persistent irritability, crying, and head rolling are often a sign of headache.

Vomiting. Vomiting with or without nausea or feeding and which progressively becomes projectile is an early clue to increased intracranial pressure or direct tumor compression of the emetic control center. Like headaches,

SUMMARY OF NURSING CARE OF THE CHILD WITH CRANIOCEREBRAL TRAUMA

GOALS	RESPONSIBILITIES
Protect from bodily injury	Maintain bed rest—head flat or slightly elevated Keep side rails up on beds Apply padding around bed if the child is extremely agitated Place net over crib if indicated Apply restraints if needed in extremely restless children

Determine neurologic status
  Vital signs
	Take frequently and report changes immediately—serious signs are
	  Rectal or axillary temperature—hypothermia or hyperthermia
	  Pulse—rapid or slow for age; irregularities
	  Respirations—rapid and shallow; slow and deep; intermittent
	  Blood pressure—decreased (shock) or widening pulse pressure

Ocular signs	Pupil size—dilated; pinpoint; unequal Pupil reaction—sluggish; absent; different Position of globes—divergence; conjugate deviation; skewed Movement of globes—extraocular palsy; nystagmus; fixed gaze
Motor function	Spontaneous—normal but reduced; involuntary Evoked—purposeful; reflex withdrawal Paresis—mild or severe; flaccid, tonic, continuous, or transient Posturing—decerebrate states; any lateralized difference in function
Level of consciousness	Depressed—easily roused Stupor—difficulty in rousing Comatose—unable to rouse; roused only with painful stimuli Speech—present or absent; conversant or confused; monosyllabic; jargon Type of cry—piercing, difficult to hear

Detect additional neurologic data
  Seizure activity
	Observe and record
	  Nature, onset, characteristic
	  Precipitating factors
	  Postictal behavior

Nuchal rigidity	Presence or absence

Drainage from orifice (nose, ear)	Note and record amount and characteristics of drainage
	  Bloody
	  Serosanguinous
	  Clear

Enlarged head (infants)	Measure occipital-frontal circumference Check size and tension of fontanels
Headache	Note presence or absence Note type and location (if this information can be elicited) Determine if continuous or intermittent
Wounds	Describe location, extent, type
Vomiting	Note amount, kind, frequency Determine precipitating factors (such as movement)
Unusual behavior	Note nature and frequency Note circumstances related to behavior
Elimination	Note bowel or bladder incontinence (in toilet-trained child) Spontaneous or associated with other phenomena (such as seizure activity)

SUMMARY OF NURSING CARE OF THE CHILD WITH CRANIOCEREBRAL TRAUMA—cont'd

GOALS	RESPONSIBILITIES

Cranial nerve dysfunction	Note disturbance of taste, smell, sight, hearing, facial sensation
	Note inability voluntarily to
	  Roll eyes up, down, or to side
	  Wrinkle forehead

Provide adequate nutrition and hydration	Provide clear liquids as ordered—that is, ad lib or restricted Progress to regular diet as tolerated and condition indicates
Prevent overhydration or dehydration	Measure accurately intake and output Provide fluids as prescribed Weigh daily if ordered If child has intravenous infusion, monitor to maintain as prescribed Use minidropper to prevent too rapid infusion rate
Promote venous return from brain	Elevate head of bed 15 to 30 degrees Maintain head in straight position
Prevent hypoventilation	Turn and position for maximum diaphragm excursion and to reduce dependent edema in lungs Hyperventilate, if prescribed
Reduce cerebral edema	Position to increase venous drainage Administer corticosteroids as prescribed Administer osmotic diuretic as prescribed Hyperventilate and/or administer oxygen to reduce blood P_{CO_2} and cerebral blood flow Perform arterial blood gas assessments
Assist in definitive diagnosis	Collect specimens as needed Prepare the child for diagnostic procedures Assist with procedures as needed Provide supportive care after procedure
Reduce restlessness and anxiety	Provide comfort and reassurance Administer sedatives as ordered

Prevent complications	Observe for early signs of complications, such as
	  Shock—decreasing blood pressure; rapid, weak pulse; reduced sensorium
	  Increased intracranial pressure—increased blood pressure, widening pulse pressure
	  Infection—elevated temperature; nuchal rigidity, redness and swelling at wound site(s)
	  Gastrointestinal bleeding—guaiac all stools and/or nasogastric aspirant
	  Emotional disturbances

Support family	Explain therapies Clarify and reinforce information given to family Interpret child's behaviors Allow expression of feelings and concerns

Prepare for discharge	Teach parents about observations to be made and what to report
	Make certain parents know how to contact appropriate persons if needed
	Instruct in administration of medication if ordered
	Arrange for follow-up care
	  Appointment with clinic or physician's office
	  Public health nurse referral if needed
	Refer to appropriate agencies, such as social service, for assistance if indicated

MAJOR INTRACRANIAL NEOPLASMS OF CHILDHOOD

INFRATENTORIAL		SUPRATENTORIAL	
Cerebellar astro-cytoma	Most common type of brain tumor Benign, usually cystic, and slow growing Surgical excision associated with high rate of cure	Craniopharyngiomas	Most common nongliomatous neo-plasm of childhood Located near sella turcica Causes cerebrospinal fluid obstruc-tion, disturbed pituitary function, visual problems, and depressed hypothalamic function Total surgical extirpation may not be possible Radiation therapy and repeated sur-gery reduce tumor size Hormone replacement needed
Medulloblastomas	Fast-growing, highly malignant Cerebellum most common site Surgical excision difficult Radiation and chemotherapy produce longer survival rates		
Brainstem gliomas	Usually astrocytomas or glioblasto-mas Location within vital centers makes surgical excision impossible Few children survive beyond 12 months of age Palliative therapy by radiation shrinks tumor to prolong survival	Cerebral tumors	Astrocytomas and ependymomas most common Astrocytomas grow rapidly, invade adjacent structures Ependymomas most frequently in lat-eral ventricles Surgical excision often difficult
Ependymomas	Varying speed of growth Frequently occur in fourth ventricle, producing cerebrospinal fluid ob-struction Close to vital centers; therefore, only partial surgical removal possible Postoperative radiation of entire cranio-spinal axis	Optic nerve gliomas	Invade optic nerves and chiasm Most often astrocytomas Variable ocular symptoms Increased intracranial pressure from obstruction of foramen of Monro Optic nerves atrophy from tumor compression

vomiting is usually more severe in the morning but re-lieved when the child moves about and changes position.

Ataxia. Ataxia is the most frequent sign of cerebel-lar involvement. Early signs may be missed because par-ents or teachers regard the incoordination as clumsiness. Loss of balance may only be evident when the child is asked to turn quickly and must resort to a wide-based stance in order to maintain an upright position. Later on, falling, tripping, banging into objects, and poor fine motor control become more obvious signs of a cerebellar insult. (See Chapter 5 for tests of muscular coordination.)

Weakness. Hypotonia and hyporeflexia are fre-quent signs of cerebellar involvement. Neoplasms of the cerebrum, brainstem, or spinal cord may also produce lower-extremity weakness with hyperreflexia, positive Ba-binski sign, spasticity, and paralysis. Early signs that may be missed include subtle changes of handedness, posture, dexterity, and recently acquired motor skills.

Head tilt. Abnormal posturing of the head is an im-portant sign of a possible brain tumor, particularly of the posterior fossa. Head tilt may be the result of extraocular

muscle paresis, particularly with cranial nerve IV involve-ment, and is frequently the first sign of decreased visual acuity. *Nuchal rigidity* caused by traction on the dura by the tumor may also be present.

Visual defects. Several visual defects may be pres-ent with infratentorial neoplasms, the most common of which are nystagmus, diplopia, strabismus, decreased vi-sual acuity, and visual field defects.

Behavioral changes. Behavioral changes such as decreased appetite, irritability, lethargy, and coma may re-sult from the tumor but more likely are caused by in-creased pressure. Obvious personality changes are more related to cerebral tumors than the types of tumors most commonly seen in children.

Cranial neuropathy. Any of the cranial nerves can be involved and the manifestations observed depend on the tumor location and intensity of pressure on the nerve. Brainstem gliomas characteristically cause cranial nerve damage by infiltration and compression. In general cranial neuropathy is bilateral, mixed, and incomplete. (See p. 127 for assessment of cranial nerves.)

Seizures. Seizures are most often a sign of cerebral neoplasms and generally cause electroencephalographic changes. When accompanied by changes in vital signs, the seizures may indicate a herniation of a cerebellar tumor through the foramen magnum into the brainstem.

Vital sign disturbance. Tumors invading the brainstem most commonly cause regulatory disturbance in the cardiorespiratory center. This is usually manifest by decreased pulse and respiration, increased blood pressure, and decreased pulse pressure (difference between systolic and diastolic blood pressure). Hypothermia or hyperthermia is also related to involvement of the hypothalamus from craniopharyngiomas.

Cranial enlargement. Widening of the sutures may appear before complete closure has occurred, usually by age 18 months. However, it is not noticeable once the skull has no flexible openings. Exophthalmos may be present, especially with optic nerve tumors, but is regarded as a late sign of tumor involvement.

Papilledema. Papilledema is visible under ophthalmoscopy as a swelling of the optic disc, blurring of the disc margins, and dilation of disc capillaries and veins. It is ordinarily a late sign of increased intracranial pressure but may be the only sign of a posterior fossa neoplasm.

Diagnostic evaluation

Diagnosis of a brain tumor is based subjectively on presenting clinical signs and objectively on a battery of neurologic tests. The more recently developed imaging techniques offer major advantages over previous procedures because they are noninvasive tests that provide an exact estimation of the tumor's location and extent (Fig. 25-6). They also provide valuable information about the tumor's properties, such as whether it is solid, semisolid, or cystic.

Therapeutic management

The treatment of choice is total extirpation of the tumor without residual neurologic damage. With the exception of brainstem gliomas, surgery is usually attempted in order to determine the type of tumor, the extent of invasiveness, and potential for removal. In those cases in which surgical resection is limited, radiation and/or chemotherapy are begun. The drugs most commonly used are nitrosoureas, vincristine, methotrexate, procarbazine, cis-platinum, prednisone, and nitrogen mustard in various combinations.

One major postoperative medical problem that may require intervention is brain edema and postoperative seizures may be a concern, especially if they were present preoperatively.

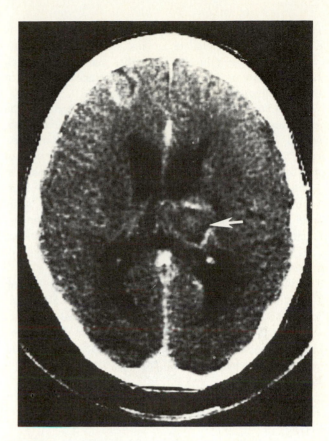

FIG. 25-6
Computed tomography (CT) scan showing brain tumor. Arrow indicates location of tumor.

Nursing considerations

Nursing care of the child with a brain tumor consists of (1) observing for signs and symptoms related to the tumor, (2) preparing the child and parents for the diagnostic tests and operative procedure, (3) preventing postoperative complications, and (4) planning for discharge. The principles of care are similar regardless of the type of intracranial lesion. Since a brain tumor is a potentially fatal diagnosis, the reader is urged to incorporate psychologic interventions with those that follow (see Chapter 16).

Assessment. A child admitted to the hospital with neurologic dysfunction is often suspected of having a brain tumor, although the actual diagnosis is as yet unconfirmed. Establishing a baseline of data on which to compare preoperative and postoperative changes is essential toward planning physical care and preventing complications. It also allows the nurse to assess the degree of physical incapacity and the family's emotional reaction to the diagnosis.

Vital signs, including blood pressure, are taken routinely and more often when any change is noted. The nurse should also chart pulse pressure. Any sudden variations in vital signs are reported immediately to the physician. It is essential to note a change in vital signs after diagnostic procedures, especially after a lumbar puncture, in which sudden release of spinal fluid may precipitate herniation of the brainstem and cardiorespiratory arrest.

A routine neurologic assessment is performed at the same time as the vital signs. In addition, the child is observed for evidence of headache, vomiting, and any seizure activity. The location, severity, and duration of the headache are noted and, if the child is unable to verbalize these characteristics, the nurse relies on observations of behavior such as lying flat and facing away from light or refusing to engage in play. Although acetaminophen may be given for pain or fever, depressant analgesics are avoided because they obscure state of consciousness.

Vomiting is charted for time, amount, and relationship to feeding and nausea. If the child vomits soon after waking in the morning, breakfast should be delayed until after vomiting has occurred. Head circumference is measured daily and any seizure activity is recorded. Seizure precautions are implemented on all children suspected to have a brain tumor.

The nurse observes the child's gait at least once daily. Head tilt and any other change in posturing is always recorded.

Preparation of child and family for procedures. The suspected diagnosis of a brain tumor is always a crisis event. Despite the fact that some tumors are removed with excellent results, the physician can rarely give definitive answers regarding prognosis until after surgery. Therefore, parents and older children require a great deal of emotional support to face the diagnostic procedures and a craniotomy.

The preparation given a child before a procedure depends on his age and previous experience. The child may have been exposed to tests with large pieces of equipment; many have had radiographs. School-age children usually appreciate a more detailed description. The importance of lying still for tests, particularly tomography and lumbar puncture, is stressed.

Once surgery is scheduled, the child needs preparation for what will take place. By the time most children are late preschoolers, they know that the head and brain are important parts of their body and this knowledge can be a source of anxiety. It may be helpful to have a child draw his concept of the brain in order to clarify misconceptions and base the explanation on his level of understanding. As in preparing for any surgical procedure, the temptation to explain too much should be recognized. The child needs to know what he will experience and what will be expected of him.

Two aspects of preoperative preparation need empha-

sis. Usually the night before surgery the child's head is shaved. This can be traumatic to the child and parents. However, it can be approached in a sensitive, positive way. If the child's hair is long, it is braided so that the long swatch is easily saved. Showing the child how he looks at different stages of the process helps him prepare for the final appearance. A scarf or cap can be in readiness for the child to wear in order to camouflage the baldness after the hair is removed. The nurse takes every precaution to protect the child from teasing or ridicule by other children prior to surgery. It is also emphasized that the hair will regrow shortly after the operation. Depending on the child's immediate adjustment to the hair loss, the nurse may introduce the idea of wearing a wig until the hair is grown in, particularly if additional irradiation or chemotherapy is anticipated.

The child is told about the size of the dressing. Usually the entire scalp is covered to maintain a tight wound closure, even when a small incision is made. Infratentorial head dressings may be attached to the upper back and around toward the neck in order to maintain slight extension and alignment as a precaution against wound rupture. Applying a similar dressing or "special hat" to a doll is a useful technique and a less traumatic way to demonstrate the physical appearance.

The child also needs a brief explanation of how he will feel after surgery and where he will be. Ordinarily he will return to a special intensive care unit, which he may visit beforehand. Unlike other postsurgical instructions, which include frequent moving and coughing, the nurse stresses that he will sleep for awhile, sometimes even a couple of days, and that when he wakens it will be important for him to lie still. He should be forewarned to expect a headache, but it is stressed that the discomfort will go away after a few days.

Parents need similar explanations prior to surgery, especially in relation to special equipment used in the intensive care unit, dressings, and their child's general appearance and behavior. For example, they should know that it is not unusual for the child to be comatose or lethargic for a few days after surgery. The nurse may wish to encourage less frequent visiting during this period so that parents can rest and recoup their resources to support their child when he awakens.

Although the temptation is to justify the need for surgery by stating that removing the tumor will take away various symptoms, the nurse should refrain from emphasizing this point too strenuously. Postsurgery headaches and cerebellar symptoms, such as ataxia, may be aggravated rather than improved. Surgery may not improve vision. With optic gliomas the child will be blind in one eye. Finally surgical removal of the mass may be impossible, and, if so, there may be temporary deterioration of functioning following surgery. Honesty before surgery most often makes honesty after the operation easier because no false hopes were created.

Postoperative care. Neurologic signs are part of the routine postoperative assessment following surgery and rectal or axillary temperatures are particularly important because surgical intervention in the area of the temperature control and some types of general anesthesia predispose to hyperthermia. A cooling blanket is placed on the bed *before* the child returns to the unit to be ready for use when needed. Body temperature is monitored carefully when any cooling measures are employed, because hypothermia can occur suddenly.

Observations for signs of complications include increased intracranial pressure, meningitis, and respiratory tract infection. There is an especially high risk of respiratory infections because of the imposed immobility, danger of aspiration, and possible depression from the brainstem.

Observations for function are not instituted until the child regains consciousness. However, testing reflexes, handgrip, and functioning of the cranial nerves begins as soon as possible. Muscle strength is usually less after surgery from general weakness but should improve daily. Ataxia may be significantly worse with cerebellar intervention but usually improves slowly. Edema near the cranial nerves may depress important functions such as the gag, blink, or swallowing reflex.

Behavior is recorded at regular intervals, including sleep patterns, response to stimuli, and level of consciousness. Although a child may be comatose for a few days, once he regains consciousness there should be a steady increase in alertness. Regression to a lethargic, irritable state indicates increasing pressure, possibly caused by meningitis. Seizure precautions are maintained.

Dressings are observed for evidence of drainage. If a drain is in place the physician specifies this, since drainage frequently soaks through the dressing. If soiled, the dressing is not removed but reinforced with dry sterile gauze. This approximate amount of drainage is estimated and recorded.

Once the child is alert, his arms may need to be restrained to prevent him from removing the dressing. Even a child who has been cooperative before surgery must be closely supervised during the initial stages of regaining consciousness, when disorientation and restlessness are common. Elbow restraints are satisfactory to prevent the hands from reaching the head, although additional restraint may be necessary to preserve an infusion line and maintain a side-lying position.

The child with an infratentorial operation is usually positioned flat and on either side. He is kept off his back to prevent pressure against the operative site and to avoid the danger of aspiration. He should be positioned with pillows placed against his back, not his head, to maintain the desired position. The surgeon will specify the degree of neck flexibility allowed. Ordinarily the head and neck are kept in midline with the body and slightly extended. When the child is turned this alignment must be preserved to prevent undue strain on the sutures. Two nurses are needed, one to support the head and the other the body. The use of turning sheet will facilitate moving a heavy child.

In a supratentorial craniotomy the head is usually elevated above the heart to facilitate cerebrospinal fluid drainage and decrease excessive blood flow to the brain to prevent hemorrhage. The Trendelenburg position is contraindicated in both types of surgeries because it increases intracranial pressure and the risk of hemorrhage.

With an infratentorial craniotomy, the alert child is allowed nothing by mouth for at least 24 hours and longer if the gag and swallowing reflexes are depressed. Following a supratentorial operation, feeding may be resumed soon after the child is alert, sometimes within 24 hours. Clear water is always started first, because of the possible danger of aspiration. If the child vomits, oral liquids are discontinued. Vomiting not only predisposes to aspiration but also increases intracranial pressure and incisional rupture.

When the child is able to take fluids, he should be fed to conserve strength and minimize movement. If there is any sign of facial paralysis, the child is fed slowly to prevent choking or aspiration. Scrupulous mouth care is essential to prevent oral infection.

Unlike most other types of surgery, postoperative analgesics are not routinely prescribed since they can mask signs of altered consciousness or neurologic functioning. Narcotics, especially morphine, are contraindicated because of their depressant effect on the respiratory center. The one exception is the use of antipyretics, usually acetaminophen, to control hyperthermia. Also their moderate analgesic benefits help relieve the discomfort of headache pain. When oral intake is limited, the suppository forms are used.

Severe headache as a result of cerebral edema is expected following a craniotomy. Measures to relieve some of the discomfort include providing a quiet, dimly lit environment, restricting visitors to a minimum, avoiding any sudden jarring movement (such as banging into the bed), and preventing an increase in intracranial pressure. The last is most effectively achieved by proper positioning and prevention of straining, such as during coughing, vomiting, or defecating. Bowel movements are monitored to prevent constipation.

Planning for discharge. Discharge planning depends on many variables including any neurologic deficits, expected prognosis, and additional therapy. It begins in the

SUMMARY OF NURSING CARE OF THE CHILD WITH A BRAIN TUMOR

GOALS	RESPONSIBILITIES
Observe for signs and symptoms	Keep daily records of signs and symptoms to help locate site and extent of tumor, to assess child's physical capabilities, and to assist parents in adjusting to insidious or acute deterioration
Vital signs and blood pressure	Record more frequently whenever a change occurs Monitor vital signs for 1 full minute to note subtle difference in rate or rhythm Record values with child's activity Report changes immediately (signs of increasing intracranial pressure are decreased pulse and respiratory rates and rising blood pressure) Institute measures to lower temperature
Ocular signs	Check pupils for size, equality, reaction to light and accommodation (PERRLA) Evaluate nystagmus, strabismus, diplopia, visual acuity, and peripheral vision Perform funduscopic examination for papilledema Chart sequentially with vital signs
Level of consciousness	Record intervals of sleep and wakefulness; observe level of activity when awake Assess mental functioning by asking simple questions (name, age, residence, and so on) Assess ease of arousal if child sleeps for a long interval
Function	Test cranial nerves, especially cranial nerves V through X Assess muscle strength (extremities) Assess coordination Observe gait and changes in posture, especially head tilt Keep side rails up and assist child during ambulation if weakness is present
Headache	Assess location, severity, duration, and relationship to time of day and position
Vomiting	Chart time, amount, and relationship to feeding and nausea Delay breakfast until after emesis if child characteristically vomits in morning Refeed after vomiting whenever possible Observe for signs of dehydration (*sunken* fontanel is not a sign, since it usually remains bulging because of increased intracranial pressure)
Cranial enlargement	In child with open sutures, measure head circumference daily In older child, note evidence of setting-sun sign
Seizures	Have seizure precautions at bedside Record seizures accurately Record vital signs and blood pressure; depressed pulse and respiratory rates may indicate brainstem involvement

Prepare family for diagnostic/operative procedures	Explain reason for each test and radiotherapy
	Explain responsibility of the child, e.g., need to remain motionless during test and/or radiotherapy
	Explain operative procedure honestly
	  Avoid overpreparation
	  Avoid overemphasis on positive benefits, which may not be evident for several days postoperatively
	Arrange for child and parents to visit special intensive care unit where he will be postoperatively
	Prepare child and parents for head shaving
	  Provide absolute privacy
	  Save long hair by braiding it first
	  Allow child to look into mirror at different stages to lessen shock of total baldness
	  Provide an attractive scalp covering (lacy nightcap or baseball cap)

Prepare child's head for surgery	Prepare child and parents for the large dressing; may help to show a picture or wrap gauze around a doll's head

GOALS	RESPONSIBILITIES
	Explain to child what he will experience following surgery, for example, he may be very sleepy, have a headache, and must remain quiet
	Advise parents, if appropriate, to visit less frequently during immediate postoperative period because of child's decreased state of consciousness
	Shave the head with care to avoid skin cuts, which can become infected
	Cleanse scalp as prescribed
Prevent postoperative complications	Take vital signs, blood pressure, and ocular signs every 15 to 30 minutes until stable
	Place hypothermia blanket on bed prior to child's return to room
	View any temperature elevation as potential sign of infection
	Auscultate respiratory status, especially for evidence of decreased breath sounds
	Institute breathing exercises (use of blow bottle) when child is awake
	Institute tests for function after child is alert
	Observe level of consciousness, noting sleep pattern and response to stimuli
	Observe dressings for drainage; reinforce with sterile gauze pads but do not remove bandage; circle area of drainage to note further seepage; report evidence of clear fluid (cerobrospinal fluid) immediately; restrain child's hands as necessary to preserve intact dressing
Positioning	Consult with surgeon regarding specific orders, which may differ from the following positioning
	Infratentorial—position child flat and on either side, not on back; neck is usually slightly extended to prevent strain on sutures
	Supratentorial—elevate head, usually above level of heart; do not lower head unless ordered by physician
	Post sign above bed noting exact position of head
	Turn child cautiously to maintain proper position
Eye care	Apply ice compresses to eyes for short intervals to relieve edema
	Keep eyes closed or apply eye dressings
	Instill normal saline eye drops to prevent corneal ulceration if blink reflex is depressed
Fluid regulation	Check gag and swallowing reflexes before beginning clear water
	Stop fluids if vomiting occurs
	Calculate all fluids very carefully to prevent overload
	Measure urinary output, especially if hypertonic solutions for brain edema are given
	Feed child to conserve energy
Pain relief	Most analgesics/sedatives are contraindicated because they mask level of consciousness and/or depress respiratory center
	Provide pain relief with environmental manipulation (dimly lit room, no noise, no sudden movement)
	Prevent increasing intracranial pressure (no straining at stool, coughing, or sneezing)
Plan for discharge	Help parents plan for future, especially toward helping child live a normal life
	Encourage parents to discuss their feelings regarding child's course prior to diagnosis and his prospects for survival
	Discuss with parents how they will tell the child about the outcome of surgery and need for additional treatment
	Help parents plan a realistic activity schedule, including resumption of school; child may need limited physical activity (for example, may have to wear a helmet to protect the skull until it is completely healed) but should be encouraged to pursue academic goals
	Help child prepare for questions from peers regarding "brain surgery," hair loss, or any residual neurologic deficit
	Provide continuing support for family through comprehensive oncology clinic and/or community nursing service

immediate postoperative period and involves a great deal of emotional support for parents. Few definitive answers can be given prior to surgery; therefore, much of the planning depends on the surgical findings, which can vary from a completely benign, resected neoplasm to a highly malignant, invasive, and only partially removed tumor.

Until surgery there is always hope and, although parents try to prepare themselves, the impact of a potentially fatal diagnosis is a shock. In some ways it is fortunate that the child is unconscious for a brief period of time to allow parents the opportunity to deal with their acute grief before they must cope with the child's postoperative distress. This is an opportune time for the nurse and physician to discuss with parents the expected prognosis and plan of therapy. Parents may hear only a fraction of what they are told, but they can begin to put the future into perspective. For example, with most brain tumors, except those of the brainstem and a metastasized medulloblastoma, survival time may be years or indefinitely. Although the parents are in acute grief, their thinking must be directed toward helping the child recover and regain a normal life to his fullest potential, not toward preparing for imminent death.

During this period the nurse should also discuss with parents what they plan to tell the child when he regains consciousness. If he was prepared honestly the diagnosis can be expressed in a similar manner. As the child improves he will need additional explanation about the treatment (similar to that discussed for leukemia) as well as the reason for residual neurologic effects, such as ataxia or blindness.

At the time of discharge the nurse discusses with parents the child's activity schedule, especially the need for resumption of normal activity such as returning to school. Until the skull is completely healed, the child may need to wear a helmet if he engages in any physical activity. The Association for Brain Tumor Research* provides information for patients and health professionals, including several easy-to-understand publications designed to assist patients and families in coping with chronic or terminal disease.

NEUROBLASTOMA

Neuroblastoma is probably the most common malignant solid tumor in children. It occurs in about one per 10,000 live births, with a slightly higher incidence in males. About half the cases occur in children under 2 years of age, and another fourth occur in children under age 4 years. Because these tumors develop from embryonic

---

*Suite 200, 6232 North Pulaski Road, Chicago, IL 60646.

neural crest tissue, they may arise anywhere along the craniospinal axis. The primary site for the majority of tumors is the abdomen and they most often arise from the adrenal gland or from the retroperitoneal sympathetic chain. Other sites are the head, neck, chest, or pelvis.

Clinical manifestations

The signs and symptoms of neuroblastoma depend on the location and stage of the disease. Most presenting signs are caused by compression of adjacent structures. With abdominal tumors the most common presenting sign is a firm, nontender, irregular mass in the abdomen that crosses the midline (in contrast to Wilms tumor, which is usually confined to one side). Compression of the kidney, ureter, or bladder may cause urinary frequency or retention.

Distant metastasis frequently causes supraorbital ecchymosis, periorbital edema, and proptosis (exophthalmos) from invasion of retrobulbar soft tissue (Fig. 25-7). Lymphadenopathy, especially in the cervical and supraclavicular areas, may also be an early presenting sign. Bone pain may or may not be present with skeletal involvement. Vague symptoms of widespread metastasis include pallor, weakness, irritability, anorexia, and weight loss.

Other primary tumors may cause significant clinical effects, such as neurologic impairment from an intracranial lesion, respiratory obstruction from a thoracic mass, or varying degrees of paralysis from compression of the spinal cord. Infrequently a child may have symptoms of increased catecholamine excretion, such as flushing, hypertension, tachycardia, and diaphoresis.

Diagnostic evaluation

The primary object of diagnosis is to locate the primary site and areas of metastasis. Skull, neck, chest, and abdominal radiographic examinations are used to locate a tumor mass and an intravenous pyelograph shows a kidney that is displaced by an adrenal tumor. Bone marrow aspiration may be performed to rule out metastases, and peripheral smears that reveal anemia and thrombocytopenia are indications of generalized malignancy.

Urinary excretion of catecholamines is increased in children with adrenal or sympathetic involvement. A 24-hour urine collection for vanillylmandelic acid (VMA) is the most accurate measurement.

Therapeutic management

The ideal treatment is complete extirpation of the tumor. However, because of the high frequency of metastasis at

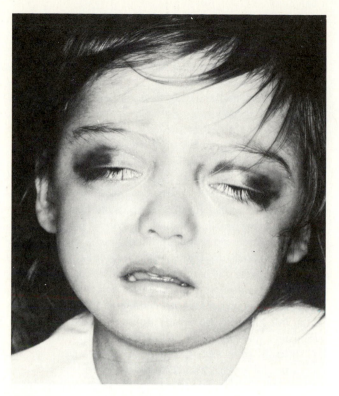

FIG. 25-7

Supraorbital ecchymoses associated with periorbital metastases. (Courtesy Howard A. Britton.) (From Sutow, W.W., Vietti, T.J., and Fernbach, D.J., editors: Clinical pediatric oncology, ed. 2, St. Louis, 1977, The C.V. Mosby Co.)

the time of diagnosis, total removal is often impossible. Both radiotherapy and chemotherapy are used in the treatment of neuroblastoma. The methods and the combinations depend on the stage of the tumor. Neuroblastoma is one of the few tumors that demonstrates spontaneous regression.

Nursing considerations

Nursing considerations are similar to those discussed previously for brain tumors, such as psychologic and physical preparation for diagnostic and operative procedures, prevention of postoperative complications for abdominal, thoracic, or cranial surgery, and explanation of radiotherapy and drug actions and side effects.

Since this tumor carries a poor prognosis for many children, every consideration must be given the family in terms of coping with a fatal illness. Because of the high percentage of metastasis at the time of diagnosis, many parents suffer much guilt for not having recognized signs earlier. Often the guilt is expressed as anger toward the physician for not diagnosing it sooner. Parents need much support in dealing with these feelings and expressing them to the appropriate people, particularly the physician.

INTRACRANIAL INFECTIONS

The nervous system and its coverings are subject to infection by the same organisms that affect other organs of the body. However, the nervous system is limited in the ways in which it responds to injury. The inflammatory process can affect the meninges (meningitis), brain (encephalitis), or spinal cord (myelitis). Infectious processes share virtually the same clinical and pathologic features. They differ primarily in the growth and virulence of the specific organism. It is generally difficult to distinguish between the various etiologic agents from clinical manifestations. Laboratory studies are needed to identify the causative agent.

The most common infection of the central nervous system is meningitis. Meningitis can be caused by a variety of organisms, but the three main types are (1) *bacterial,* or pyogenic, caused by pus-forming bacteria, especially meningococci, pneumococci, and the influenza bacilli; (2) *tuberculous,* caused by tubercle bacilli; and (3) *viral,* or aseptic, caused by a wide variety of viral agents. Encephalitis is usually caused by a virus.

BACTERIAL MENINGITIS

Bacterial meningitis is a potentially fatal disease, and, although the advent of antimicrobial therapy has had a marked effect on the course and prognosis, it remains a significant cause of illness in the pediatric age-groups. Its importance lies primarily in the frequency with which it occurs in infancy and childhood and the unnecessarily high death rates and residual damage caused by undiagnosed and untreated or inadequately treated cases.

Bacterial meningitis can be caused by any of a variety of bacterial agents. *Hemophilus influenzae* (type B), *Streptococcus pneumoniae,* and *Neisseria meningitidis* (meningococcal) organisms are responsible for bacterial meningitis in 95% of children older than 2 months of age. *H. influenzae* is the predominant organism in children 3 months to 3 years of age but is rare in the infant younger than 3 months of age, who is apparently protected by passively acquired bactericidal substances, and in children older than 5 years of age. The leading causes of neonatal meningitis are the group B streptococci and *Escherichia coli* organisms. *E. coli* infection is seldom seen beyond infancy. Meningococcic (epidemic cerebrospinal) meningitis occurs in epidemic form and is the only form readily transmitted to others. It is transmitted by droplet infection from nasopharyngeal secretions. Although it may develop at any age, the risk of meningococcal infection increases with the number of contacts; therefore, it occurs predominantly in school-age children and adolescents. The highest incidence of meningitis occurs between ages 6 and 12 months.

Pathophysiology

Meningitis appears to occur as an extension of a variety of bacterial infections, probably as a result of the lack of acquired resistance to the various causative organisms. The presence of preexisting central nervous system anomalies, neurosurgical procedures or injuries, sickle cell anemia, or primary infections elsewhere in the body are factors related to an increased susceptibility.

The most common route of infection is by vascular dissemination from a focus of infection elsewhere. Organisms also gain entry by direct implantation after penetrating wounds, skull fractures that provide an opening into the skin or sinuses, lumbar puncture or surgical procedures, and anatomic abnormalities such as spina bifida or foreign bodies such as a ventricular shunt. Once implanted, the organisms spread into the cerebrospinal fluid by which the infection spreads throughout the subarachnoid space.

The infective process is that seen in any bacterial infection—inflammation, exudation, white blood cell accumulation, and varying degrees of tissue damage. The brain becomes hyperemic and edematous, and the entire surface of the brain is covered with a layer of purulent exudate. As infection extends to the ventricles, thick pus, fibrin, or adhesions may occlude the narrow passages, thereby obstructing the flow of cerebrospinal fluid to cause obstructive hydrocephalus. Subdural effusions occur frequently, and thrombosis may occur in meningeal veins or venous sinuses. Destructive changes may take place in the cerebral cortex, and brain abscesses may form by direct extension of the infection or by vascular dissemination.

Clinical manifestations

The clinical manifestations of acute bacterial meningitis depend to a large extent on the age of the child. The picture is also influenced to some degree by the type of organism, the effectiveness of therapy for antecedent illness, and whether it occurs as an isolated entity or as a complication of another illness or injury.

Children and adolescents. The illness is likely to be abrupt, with fever, chills, headache, and vomiting that are associated with or quickly followed by alterations in sensorium. Often the initial sign is a seizure, which may recur as the disease progresses. The child is extremely irritable and agitated and may develop delirium, aggressive or maniacal behavior, or drowsiness, stupor, and coma. Sometimes the onset is slower, frequently preceded by several days of respiratory or gastrointestinal symptoms.

The child resists flexion of the neck, and, as the disease progresses, the neck stiffness becomes marked until the head is drawn into extreme overextension (opisthotonos). The Kernig and Brudzinski signs are positive. Reflex responses are variable, although they show hyperactivity.

Other signs and symptoms may appear that are peculiar to individual organisms. Petechial or purpuric rashes usually indicate a meningococcal infection, especially when the eruption is associated with a shocklike state. Joint involvement is seen in meningococcic and *H. influenzae* infection. A chronically draining ear commonly accompanies pneumococcal meningitis.

Infants and young children. The classic picture of meningitis is rarely seen in children between 3 months and 2 years of age. The illness is characterized by fever, vomiting, marked irritability, and frequent seizures, which are often accompanied by a high-pitched cry. A bulging fontanel is the most significant finding, and nuchal rigidity may or may not be present. The Brudzinski and Kernig signs are not usually helpful in diagnosis, since they are difficult to elicit and evaluate in children in this age-group.

Neonatal. Meningitis in newborn and premature infants is extremely difficult to diagnose. The vague and nonspecific manifestations, characteristic of all neonatal sepsis, bear little resemblance to the findings in older children. These infants are usually well at birth but within a few days begin to look and behave poorly. They refuse feedings, have poor sucking ability, and may vomit or have diarrhea. They display poor tone, lack of movement, and a poor cry. Other nonspecific signs that may be present include hypothermia or fever (depending on the maturity of the infant), jaundice, irritability, drowsiness, seizures, respiratory irregularities or apnea, cyanosis, and weight loss. The full, tense, and bulging fontanel may or may not be present until late in the course of illness, and the neck is usually supple.

Diagnostic evaluation

A definitive diagnosis of acute bacterial meningitis is made only by examination of the cerebrospinal fluid by means of a lumbar puncture. The fluid pressure is measured and samples are obtained for culture, Gram stain, blood cell count, and determination of glucose and protein content. The findings are usually diagnostic. There is generally an elevated white blood cell count, predominantly polymorphonuclear leukocytes, but it may be extremely variable. The glucose level is reduced, generally in proportion to the duration and severity of the infection.

A blood culture is advisable for all children suspected of meningitis and occasionally proves positive when cerebrospinal fluid culture is negative. Nose and throat cultures may provide helpful information in some cases.

Therapeutic management

Acute bacterial meningitis is a medical emergency that requires early recognition and immediate institution of therapy to prevent death and avoid residual disabilities. The initial therapeutic management includes (Committee on Infectious Diseases, 1982):

    Isolation
    Initiation of antimicrobial therapy
    Maintenance of optimum hydration
    Maintenance of ventilation
    Reduction of increased intracranial pressure
    Management of bacterial shock
    Control of seizures
    Control of extremes of temperature
    Correction of anemia

The child is isolated from other children. An intravenous infusion is started as soon as the lumbar puncture has been completed in order to facilitate the administration of antimicrobial agents, fluids, anticonvulsive drugs, and blood if needed.

Until the causative organism is identified, the choice of antibiotic is based on the known sensitivity of the organism most likely to be the infective agent in any given situation and the probable interactions with the specific patient. Except under special circumstances, the drugs are administered intravenously throughout the course of treatment. The drugs are given in large doses, and the period of therapy is determined by cerebrospinal fluid findings (normal glucose level and negative culture) and the child's clinical condition.

Maintaining hydration is a prime concern, and intravenous fluids and the type and amount of fluid are determined by the patient's condition. The optimum hydration involves correction of any fluid deficits followed by low maintenance levels to prevent cerebral edema. If indicated, measures are employed to reduce intracranial pressure as described previously (p. 817).

Complications are treated appropriately. Subdural effusions in infants are managed by aspirations to relieve symptoms, and heparin therapy may be required for children who develop disseminated intravascular coagulation syndrome. Shock, if it occurs, requires restoration of blood volume and maintenance of electrolyte balance.

Lumbar puncture is carried out as needed to determine the effectiveness of therapy. The patient is evaluated neurologically during the convalescent period and at regular intervals during the succeeding year. Prognosis is related to a variety of factors: the age of the child, the type of organisms, the severity of the infection, the duration of the illness prior to the onset of therapy, and the sensitivity of the organism to antimicrobial drugs. The younger the patient, the higher the mortality.

Prevention. Two vaccines are now available for types A and C meningococci (a third is currently being developed for type B). At the present time type A is the only one recommended for use in children over 5 years of age who are close contacts of a primary case or who are considered high risk because of asplenia.

Nursing considerations

The primary nursing responsibilities immediately following admission of the child suspected of bacterial meningitis are to prevent transmission of the disease to others and to begin intravenous antibiotic therapy if it has not been initiated before admission (for example, in the emergency room or outpatient department).

The child remains in respiratory isolation for at least 24 hours after implementation of antimicrobial therapy. Nurses should take necessary precautions to protect themselves and others from possible infection. Parents are taught the proper protective procedures and supervised in their application.

The room is kept as quiet as possible and environmental stimuli kept at a minimum, since most affected children are sensitive to noise, bright lights, and other external stimuli. Most children are more comfortable without a pillow and with the head of the bed slightly elevated. A side-lying position is more often assumed because of nuchal rigidity. The nurse should avoid actions, such as lifting the child's head, that cause pain or increase his discomfort. Measures are employed to assure safety, since the child is often restless and subject to seizures.

The nursing care of the child with meningitis is determined by the child's symptoms and treatment. Observation of vital signs, neurologic signs, level of consciousness, urine output, and other pertinent data is carried out at frequent intervals. The child who is unconscious is managed as described previously (p. 818), and all children are observed carefully for signs of complications just described, especially signs of increased intracranial pressure, shock, or respiratory distress.

Fluids and nourishment are determined by the child's status. The child with dulled sensorium is usually given nothing by mouth. Other children are allowed clear liquids initially and progressed to a diet suitable for their age. Careful monitoring and recording of intake and output are needed to determine deviations that might indicate impending shock or increasing fluid accumulation, such as cerebral edema or subdural effusion.

One of the most difficult problems in nursing care of children with meningitis is maintaining the intravenous infusion for the length of time needed to provide adequate antimicrobial therapy. Older infants and small children require restraining devices to maintain the integrity of the infusion site, but they are released from the restraints as often as possible to reduce the ill effects of long-term immobilization. These children are particularly in need of attendance and opportunities for play.

Children are allowed ambulation and other normal activities as soon as the condition allows and as often as feasible. In some children, especially older ones, a heparin-lock device can be employed to allow for more freedom of movement. The infusion site is monitored for signs of inflammation as well as for patency. Some medications are highly irritating to veins and may tend to produce phlebitis if continued in the same site over a prolonged period of time.

Emotional support. The sudden nature of the illness makes emotional support of the child and parents extremely important. Parents are very upset and concerned about their child's condition and frequently feel guilty for not having suspected the seriousness of the illness sooner. They need much reassurance that the natural onset of meningitis is sudden and that they acted responsibly in seeking medical assistance when they did. The nurse encourages them to openly discuss their feelings to minimize blame and guilt. They also are kept informed of the child's progress and of all procedures and treatments. In the event that the child's condition worsens, they need the same psychologic care as parents facing the possible death of their child (see Chapter 16).

NONBACTERIAL (ASEPTIC) MENINGITIS

Aseptic meningitis is a benign syndrome caused by a number of agents, principally viruses, and is frequently associated with other diseases, such as measles, mumps, herpes, and leukemia. Enteroviruses and mumps viruses account for a large number of cases.

The onset may be abrupt or gradual. The initial manifestations are headache, fever, malaise, gastrointestinal symptoms, and signs of meningeal irritation that develop a day or two after the onset of illness. Abdominal pain and nausea and vomiting are common; sore throat, chest pain, and generalized muscular aches or pains are found occasionally. There may be a maculopapular rash. These symptoms usually subside spontaneously and rapidly, and the child is well in 3 to 10 days with no residual effects.

Diagnosis is based on clinical features and cerebrospinal fluid findings, which include increased lymphocytes, predominantly mononuclear cells. It is important to differentiate this benign disorder from the more serious form of meningitis and to diagnose and treat any disease of which it is a manifestation.

Treatment is primarily symptomatic, such as acetaminophen for headache, moist heat for muscle aches and pains, and positioning for comfort. Antimicrobial agents may be administered and isolation enforced until a definitive diagnosis is made as a precaution against the possibility that the disease might be of bacterial origin.

Nursing care is similar to nursing care of the child with bacterial meningitis.

ENCEPHALITIS

Encephalitis is an inflammatory process of the central nervous system producing altered function of various portions of the brain and spinal cord. Encephalitis can be caused by a variety of organisms, including bacteria, spirochetes, fungi, protozoa, helminths, and viruses. Most infections are associated with viruses, and this discussion will be limited to these etiologic agents.

Etiology

The disease can occur as the result of (1) direct invasion of the central nervous system by a virus or (2) postinfectious involvement of the central nervous system after a viral disease. Encephalitis as a result of direct invasion is most often caused by the arboviruses (arthropod-borne viruses) accidentally acquired through an arthropod vector. The vector reservoir for these arboviruses is the mosquito; therefore, most cases of encephalitis appear during the hot summer months and subside during the autumn.

Diagnostic evaluation

The clinical features are similar regardless of the agent involved. Manifestations can range from a mild benign form that resembles aseptic meningitis, lasting a few days and being followed by rapid and complete recovery, to a fulminating encephalitis with severe central nervous system involvement. The onset may be sudden or gradual with malaise, fever, headache, dizziness, apathy, stiffness of

SUMMARY OF NURSING CARE OF THE CHILD WITH ACUTE BACTERIAL MENINGITIS

GOALS	RESPONSIBILITIES
Eradicate causative organism	Administer antibiotics as prescribed and as soon as possible after admission
Prevent spread of infection	Place the child in isolation for at least 24 hours after initiation of antibiotic therapy Protect self by observing proper precautions Identify close contacts and high-risk children who might benefit from meningococci vaccinations
Help to establish diagnosis	Assist with diagnostic procedures Order laboratory tests Send obtained specimens, for example, spinal fluid, to laboratory for analysis Obtain specimens, for example, nasopharyngeal smears, as needed
Provide and maintain route for rapid administration of medication	Assist with establishment of intravenous infusion Monitor intravenous infusion—type of fluid, rate of flow, amount of fluid Maintain integrity of infusion Immobilize intravenous site Apply restraint as needed Change tubing and so on as dictated by hospital policy Observe for signs of inflammation at infusion site and along course of vein
Assess neurologic status	Monitor Vital signs Neurologic signs Level of consciousness Behavior Posturing
Detect early signs of complications	Observe for signs of impending Vasomotor collapse or shock Increased intracranial pressure Respiratory distress Altered state of consciousness Intravascular coagulation
Maintain optimum hydration	Regulate intake as prescribed; restrict or encourage fluids as determined by the child's status Measure intake and output Weigh daily (if ordered)
Maintain nutrition	Provide diet as ordered; give nothing by mouth or clear liquids initially but appropriate for age as tolerated
Decrease effects of long-term intravenous therapy and immobilization	Remove restraining devices frequently Allow as much freedom of movement as possible and encourage normal activities Provide diversional activities Encourage play
Provide emotional support to parents	Keep the parents informed regarding the child's progress Interpret the child's behavior and neurologic signs Explain diagnostic procedures and therapeutic management Encourage expression of feelings regarding the child's illness

the neck, nausea and vomiting, ataxia, tremors, hyperactivity, and speech difficulties. In severe cases there is high fever, stupor, seizures, disorientation, spasticity, and coma that may proceed to death. Ocular palsies and paralysis may be seen, also.

Therapeutic management

Patients suspected of having encephalitis are hospitalized promptly for skilled nursing care and observation. Treatment is primarily supportive, including conscientious nursing care, control of cerebral manifestations, and adequate nutrition and hydration, with observations and management as for other disorders involving cerebral injury. Follow-up care with periodic reevaluation and rehabilitation are important aspects of survivors with residual effects of the disease.

Nursing considerations

Nursing care of the child with encephalitis is the same as for any unconscious child and the child with meningitis. Neurologic monitoring, administration of medications, and support to the child and parents are the major aspects of care.

REYE SYNDROME

Acute encephalopathy with fatty degeneration of the liver is a disorder identified with increasing frequency and characterized by fever, profoundly impaired consciousness, and disordered hepatic function. The disease affects white children primarily and the ages of affected children range from 2 months to adolescence, with peak incidences at 6 and 11 years of age.

Etiology

The etiology of the disorder is obscure and a number of theories have been advanced, but it is usually associated with an antecedent viral illness. It has also been consistently observed that children who develop Reye syndrome have been administered aspirin. Although no causal relationship can be identified, the Committee on Infectious Diseases (1982) has cautioned against the use of aspirin for children with viral illnesses.

Pathophysiology

The pathologic changes of Reye syndrome are marked cerebral edema and enlargement of the liver with marked fatty infiltration.

Clinical manifestations

The disease has essentially two phases, a prodromal illness and an encephalopathic stage. The prodromal stage is similar in all age-groups and consists of a viral infection, which may be quite mild, usually gastroenteritis or a respiratory tract infection. There is a high incidence of varicella and influenza. The manifestations of the encephalopathic stage differ according to the age of the child.

Children over 1 year of age. The child appears to be recovering from the infection but develops recurrent, intractable vomiting. In 24 to 48 hours central nervous system dysfunction becomes apparent with behavioral changes including delirium, irrational behavior, disorientation, hallucinations, and combativeness, which may alternate with lethargy and stupor. Clinically liver involvement is limited to mild hepatomegaly.

To help evaluate the child's progress and predict a probable outcome a set of staging criteria have been developed as follows:

Stage I vomiting, lethargy, and drowsiness
Stage II disorientation, delirium, aggressiveness and combativeness, central neurologic hyperventilation (or sometimes shallow breathing), hyperactive reflexes, stupor, appropriate response to noxious stimuli
Stage III obtundent, comatose, hyperventilation, and decorticate posturing, preserved pupillary reflexes
Stage IV deepening coma, decerebrate posturing, loss of ocular reflexes, large fixed pupils, and divergent eye movements
Stage V absent deep tendon reflexes, seizures, flaccidity, respiratory arrest

The clinical course of the disease is rapid, and the mortality rate is high (40% to 80% in various studies), particularly in children younger than 2 years of age and in those in whom convulsions are part of the clinical picture. Fortunately recovery is rapid and complete in those who survive, and residual disability is uncommon.

Infants under 1 year of age. Clinical features in infants less than 1 year of age are somewhat different. In infants the prodromal infection is followed by mild vomiting but marked seizure activity (often the initial manifestation) and respiratory disturbances, especially hyperventilation. Most have hepatomegaly.

Diagnostic evaluation

Evidence of liver dysfunction is reflected by elevated serum glutamic-oxaloacetic transaminase (SGOT), serum glutamic-pyruvic transaminase (SGPT), and lactic dehydrogenase (LDH) levels. Liver-dependent clotting factors, such as prothrombin time, are diminished. Serum bilirubin and alkaline phosphatase levels are usually unaffected. Blood urea nitrogen and ammonia levels are often elevated, indicating mild renal dysfunction. In the majority of children blood sugar levels fall to below 50 mg/100 ml, with reduced insulin levels and diminished glucagon response.

Therapeutic management

Treatment is primarily supportive and directed toward restoring blood sugar levels, controlling cerebral edema, and correcting acid-base imbalances. Intravenous administration of hypertonic (10%) glucose solution with added insulin help to replace glycogen stores, but it is controlled to avoid overhydration. The pH and electrolytes are monitored and replaced according to regular assessments. Anticonvulsant medication is given for seizure activity. Sometimes corticosteroids are useful, and mannitol may be administered to reduce cerebral edema if the kidneys are not compromised. Endotracheal intubation with respiratory assistance is implemented for respiratory distress, and interventions are initiated to reduce an elevated temperature. Exchange transfusions or peritoneal dialysis has been used in some cases to reduce elevated blood ammonia levels. A craniectomy, temporarily creating bilateral bone flaps, has been performed to reduce pressure from an edematous brain.

A radical approach now used extensively is curarization and sedation. Skeletal muscles are paralyzed with administration of *d*-tubocurarine or pancuronium (Pavulon) to prevent any activity, especially coughing, that might increase intracranial pressure. Curarization does not affect sensory input; therefore, the child's anxiety may be sufficient to cause cerebral hypertension. Placing the child in a drug-induced coma with barbiturates arrests almost all neurologic functions.

Nursing considerations

The child who is acutely ill with Reye syndrome requires continuous and intensive nursing care. On admission to the hospital numerous procedures and observations must be carried out as quickly as possible. In addition to an appraisal of vital functions and neurologic status, the nurse assists with a lumbar puncture, obtaining blood for laboratory examination, and insertion of various intravenous lines such as peripheral, arterial, and central venous pressure. A retention catheter and a nasogastric tube are inserted, and, when respirations are compromised, an endotracheal tube is inserted and attached to a respirator for controlled respirations. If equipment is available, a line is inserted for continuous monitoring of intracranial pressure.

Care and observations are implemented as for any child with an altered state of consciousness (p. 818) and increasing intracranial pressure (p. 817). Accurate and frequent monitoring of intake and output is essential for adjusting fluid volumes to prevent both dehydration and cerebral edema. Since hypovolemic shock is a constant danger in children with Reye syndrome, vital signs, including central venous pressure, are monitored frequently. Laboratory analysis of serum electrolytes, pH, blood urea nitrogen, glucose, osmolality, and blood gases serves as a guide for therapy, and arranging for their collection is a nursing responsibility. Because of related liver dysfunction, the nurse must observe for signs of impaired coagulation such as prolonged bleeding, petechiae, and so on.

Recovery from Reye syndrome is rapid, usually without sequelae. However, a trend in the behaviors has been observed when children waken from the unconscious state. The stress and anxiety they appear to feel in a strange and unfamiliar environment are consistently expressed in silent and withdrawn behavior. They respond to basic questioning but do not display their prehospitalization personality and social behavior until they are transferred from the critical care area.

The children awaken disoriented with no recollection of events that took place during the critical phase of their illness. Strange equipment being used in their care that was started while they were unconscious requires explanation. The appearance of other ill children is puzzling and frightening, increasing their anxiety and stress concerning their own situation. They are powerless to control what is happening to them. Nurses can help these children deal with their stress by orienting them to where they are and the circumstances of their being there, describing what is expected of them, and giving them a sense of control whenever possible. Even if they are heavily sedated or comatose, they may hear some of what is going on around them. Therefore, they are treated as if they see and hear. Encouraging parents to visit and providing other items associated with home, such as a favorite toy, a photograph, or other item, help them maintain a link with their lives outside the confines of the critical care environment. Understanding and individualized care help children to weather the stresses and tension of this period of crisis.

Emotional support. Because of the rapidity of the illness parents need much of the same emotional support as that discussed for meningitis. Their distress is increased if they believe that their actions may have contributed to a delay in diagnosis. Parents are encouraged to verbalize their guilt feeling and are provided with reassurance that they did not contribute to the child's condition, that the development of the disease cannot be anticipated, and that their care was proper under the circumstances. They need to be kept informed regarding the child's progress, to have diagnostic procedures and therapeutic management explained, and to be given concerned and sympthetic support.

Some of these children recover with residual disability and require assistance in accepting and adjusting to the handicap (see Chapter 16). A helpful resource for both parents and health professionals is the National Reye's Syndrome Foundation* which has been established for the purpose of research and education regarding this frightening disease.

RABIES

Rabies is an acute infection of the nervous system caused by a virus that is almost invariably fatal. It is transmitted to humans by the saliva of an infected mammal introduced through a bite or skin abrasion. The domestic dog is the principal source of infection, although any animal, including raccoons, bats, cats, foxes, skunks, squirrels, and coyotes, may be responsible for human infection.

The disease is uncommon in humans, but the highest incidence occurs in children under 15 years of age. The incubation period usually ranges from 1 to 3 months but may be as short as 10 days or as long as 8 months. Only 10% to 15% of persons bitten develop the disease, but, once symptoms are present, rabies progresses inexorably to a fatal outcome. The disease is characterized by period of general malaise, fever, and sore throat followed by a phase of excitement featured by hypersensitivity and increased reaction to external stimuli, convulsions, maniacal behavior, and choking. Attempts at swallowing may cause such severe spasm of respiratory muscles that apnea, cyanosis, and anoxia are produced—the characteristics from which the term "hydrophobia" was derived.

Diagnosis is made on the basis of history and clinical features. Once symptoms appear, treatment is of little avail, but the long incubation period allows time for induction of active as well as passive immunity before the onset of illness. The current therapy for a rabid animal bite consists of thorough cleansing of the wound and inoculation with human rabies immune globulin (RIG) or hyperimmune antirabies serum (ARS) as soon as possible after exposure to provide rapid, short-term passive immunity. Active immunity is conferred by administration of the recently developed human diploid cell rabies vaccine (HDCV). The first dose of the vaccine is given at the same time as the immune globulin and followed by injections at 3, 7, 14, and 21 days. An additional dose in 90 days is recommended by the World Health Organization.

Nursing considerations

Nursing care of the child who has been bitten involves reducing the child's and his family's anxiety, caring for the wound, and preparing the child for the required injections. The proper authorities are notified, if this has not

*P.O. Box R.S., Benzonia, MI 49616.

been done, in order that the animal in question can be dealt with correctly.

Although the care of the bitten child is critical, prevention should be the major thrust in rabies infection. Ordinances in most areas require vaccination of dogs and, often, other household pets. Children are taught proper treatment of pets and to avoid unknown animals and seemingly friendly or tame wild animals. Although the vaccine is available and well tolerated by children, mass immunization is not warranted except when a child is being taken to an area of the world where rabies in stray dogs is still a problem.

CONVULSIVE DISORDERS

Convulsive phenomena are among the most frequently observed neurologic dysfunctions in children and can occur with a wide variety of conditions involving the central nervous system. A *convulsion* is defined as involuntary muscular contractions and relaxation; a *seizure* is a sudden attack. The two words are often used synonymously. In general the term "seizure," "convulsion," or "spell" is used to designate a single episode, whereas "convulsive disorder" is the preferred term for a chronic and recurring disorder. These chronic forms are also known as the *epilepsies*.

GENERAL CONCEPTS

Seizures are more common during the first 2 years of life than during any other period of childhood. In very young infants the most frequent causes are birth injuries, that is, intracranial trauma, hemorrhage, or anoxia, and congenital defects of the brain. Acute infections are a frequent cause of seizures in late infancy and early childhood but become an infrequent cause in middle childhood. In children older than 3 years of age the most common factor is idiopathic epilepsy.

A seizure disorder can also be acquired as a result of brain injury during prenatal, perinatal, or postnatal periods. This injury may be caused by trauma, hypoxia, infections, exogenous or endogenous toxins, and a variety of other causes.

Pathophysiology

Regardless of the etiologic factor or the type of seizure, the basic mechanism is the same. There are electric discharges that (1) may arise from central areas in the brain that affect consciousness immediately, (2) may be restricted to one area of the cerebral cortex, producing manifestations characteristic of that particular anatomic focus, or (3) may begin in a localized area of the cortex and spread to other portions of the brain, which, if sufficiently extensive, produce generalized neurologic manifestations.

Seizure activity is believed to be caused by spontaneous electric discharge initiated by a group of hyperexcitable cells referred to as the *epileptogenic focus.* These cells display increased electric excitability but may remain quiescent over a period of time while discharging intermittently as evidenced on electroencephalographic tracings. Normally these discharges are restrained from spreading beyond the focal area by normal inhibitory mechanisms.

Clinical manifestations

Convulsive seizures are described according to several types within the categories of generalized or focal seizures and varied clinical features (see the discussion following diagnostic evaluation). The onset of a seizure is abrupt, paroxysmal, and transitory, and signs may vary from behavioral abnormalities to continuous and prolonged motor convulsions.

Diagnostic evaluation

The process of diagnosis in a child with a convulsive disorder has two major foci: (1) to ascertain the type of seizure the child has experienced, and (2) to attempt to understand the cause of the attacks. The assessment and diagnosis rely heavily on a thorough history, skilled observation, and employment of several diagnostic tests.

A complete, accurate, and detailed history should be obtained from a reliable and knowledgeable informant. History of the seizure(s) should be equally detailed, and a complete physical and neurologic examination often provides clues to neurologic disturbances.

Laboratory studies that may prove to be of value include a complete blood cell count (for evidence of lead poisoning) and white blood cell count for signs of infection. Blood and cerebrospinal fluid glucose may give evidence of hypoglycemic episodes, and serum electrolytes, blood urea nitrogen, calcium, and other blood studies may indicate metabolic disturbances. Lumbar puncture may confirm a suspected diagnosis of cerebrospinal infection or trauma.

Skull radiographs, computerized tomography, echoencephalograms, brain scans, and other studies help to identify skull abnormalities, separation of sutures, and intracranial calcifications. Other imaging studies may be used to visualize blood vessel configuration.

The electroencephalogram is obtained for all children with convulsive manifestations and is the most useful tool for evaluating seizure disorders. The electroencephalogram is carried out under varying conditions—with the child asleep, awake, awake with provocative stimulation (flashing lights, noise), and hyperventilating. Stimulation elicits abnormal electric activity, which is recorded on the electroencephalogram. Various seizure types produce characteristic electroencephalographic patterns.

PARTIAL OR FOCAL SEIZURES

Focal or partial seizures are caused by abnormal electric discharges from epileptogenic foci limited to a more or less circumscribed region of the cerebral cortex. Focal seizures may arise from any area of the cerbral cortex, but the frontal, temporal, and parietal lobes are the ones most often affected. The area of cerebral involvement is reflected by clinical manifestations. Partial or focal seizures may spread to other areas and become generalized convulsions. This is known as secondary generalization.

Psychomotor seizures

Psychomotor seizures are observed more often in children from 3 years of age through adolescence and are more common in adults than in children. The seizures are most characteristically associated with focal lesions of the temporal lobe and are sometimes referred to as temporal lobe seizures. The attack is characterized by a period of altered behavior for which the individual is amnesic and during which he is unable to respond to his environment. Though the child does not lose consciousness during an attack, he has no recollection of his behavior during the seizure. Drowsiness or sleep usually follows the seizure. Confusion and amnesia may be prolonged.

Complex sensory phenomena associated with the beginning of a seizure reflect the complicated connections and integrative functions of that area of the brain. The most frequent sensation is a strange feeling in the pit of the stomach that rises toward the throat. This feeling is often accompanied by odd or unpleasant odors or tastes, complex auditory or visual hallucinations, or ill-defined feelings of elation or strangeness (such as *déjà vu,* a feeling of familiarity in a strange environment). Small children may emit a cry or attempt to run for help as a manifestation of an aura. The child may suddenly cease his activity, appear dazed, stare into space, become confused and apathetic, and become limp, stiff, or display some form of posturing. The primary feature may be confusion, and the child may perform purposeless, complicated activities in a repetitive manner (automatisms), such as walking, running, kicking, laughing, or speaking incoherently, most often followed by postictal confusion or sleep. The predominant observations may be oropharyngeal activities, such as smacking, chewing, drooling, swallowing, and nausea or abdominal pain followed by stiffness, a fall, and postictal sleep.

Other seizures

Focal seizures are characterized by localized motor symptoms. The most common focal motor seizure in children is the *adversive seizure,* in which the eye or eyes and head turn away from the side of the focus. *Focal sensory seizures* are characterized by various sensations, including numbness, tingling, prickling, paresthesia, or pain that originates in one area (such as the face or extremities) and spreads to other parts of the body. Visual sensations or formed images may be manifestations.

NONEPILEPTIC SEIZURES

Nonepileptic seizures are those that do not manifest as convulsions (with the exception of febrile convulsions). They include such varied manifestations as breath-holding spells, migraine, and recurrent abdominal pain (p. 430).

Febrile convulsions

Febrile convulsions are a transient disorder of children that occur in association with a fever. They are one of the most common neurologic disorders of childhood, affecting 3% to 5% of children. Most febrile convulsions occur after 6 months of age and usually before age 3 years, with increased frequency in children younger than 18 months of age. They are unusual after 5 years of age. Boys are affected about twice as often as girls, and there appears to be an increased susceptibility in families, indicating a possible genetic predisposition.

The cause of febrile convulsions is still uncertain. In most children the height and rapidity of the temperature elevation seem to be factors. The fever usually exceeds 38.8° C (101.8° F) and occurs during the temperature rise rather than after a prolonged elevation. Sometimes it constitutes the dramatic beginning of an illness. Febrile convulsions usually accompany an upper respiratory or gastrointestinal infection, and 25% of children with simple febrile convulsions have a recurrence of the seizure with subsequent infections. Since fevers are almost impossible to prevent in children, efforts are directed toward preventing an increase in the temperature.

Treatment consists of controlling the seizure with phenobarbital or diazepam (Valium) in appropriate dosage, reducing the temperature by administration of antipyretics and conductive and evaporative cooling of the child, and treatment of the intercurrent infection. Antipyretics and cooling sponge baths are administered early as a preventive measure in the event of subsequent infections (see p.

542 for management of the child with a fever). Whether or not to implement continuous prophylactic anticonvulsant therapy in children who have experienced their initial febrile convulsion is still controversial. Anticonvulsant therapy is usually reserved for children who have prolonged convulsions or who have experienced a second seizure.

Breath-holding spells

Breath-holding spells (reflex hypoxic crisis) are a benign entity, characterized by violent crying and cessation of breathing that is precipitated by fright, frustration, or anger, in infants between the ages of 6 and 18 months of age. Many children appear to use an attack or the threat of an attack to assert themselves and to express anger, particularly during a "temper tantrum." Parents need reassurance that the attacks do not represent a danger to the child, and this knowledge may even help to decrease or eliminate the incidence of attacks.

Migraine

Migraine is the most common paroxysmal disorder that affects the brain. It is characterized by chronic recurrent headache, often preceded by visual disturbances and accompanied by nausea and vomiting. The cause is unknown. The diagnosis is seldom made until the child is old enough to relate his symptoms, although one in five children has his first attack before age 5 years. Early in life the symptoms are nonspecific, such as recurrent abdominal pain, car sickness, and restlessness, and the child may display head banging or sudden alterations in personality. Sleep ordinarily terminates an attack. Treatment is symptomatic.

GENERALIZED SEIZURES (EPILEPSY)

Generalized seizures may occur at any age. Children, as opposed to adults, seldom report a warning or aura, the peculiar sensation experienced by some persons just prior to the onset of a seizure. Seizures occur at any time, day or night, and the interval between attacks may be minutes, hours, weeks, or even years.

Grand mal (major motor) seizures

The generalized seizure occurring alone or in combination with other forms and either with or without focal onset is the most common and most dramatic of all seizure manifestations of childhood. The seizure usually occurs without warning. There is a rolling of the eyes upward and immediate loss of consciousness. If the child is standing, he falls to the floor or ground. The child stiffens in a generalized and symmetric tonic contraction of the entire body musculature. The arms usually flex, whereas the legs, head, and neck extend. The child may utter a peculiar piercing cry produced as the jaws clamp shut and the thoracic and abdominal muscles contract, forcing air through tightly closed vocal cords. This tonic phase lasts approximately 10 to 20 seconds, during which the child is apneic and may become cyanotic. Autonomic stimulation causes increased salivation.

The tonic rigidity is replaced by the violent jerking movements as the trunk and extremities undergo rhythmic contraction and relaxation of the clonic phase. During this time the child may foam at the mouth and be incontinent of urine and feces. As the attack ends the movements become less intense and occur at longer intervals, until they cease entirely. The clonic phase generally lasts about 30 seconds but can vary from only a few seconds to a half hour or longer. A series of seizures at intervals too brief to allow the child to regain consciousness between the time one attack ends and the next begins is known as *status epilepticus*. This requires emergency intervention. A succession of interrupted seizures can lead to exhaustion, respiratory failure, and death.

In the postictal state (the period following a seizure), the child appears to relax but may remain semiconscious and difficult to rouse. He may waken in a few minutes but remains confused for several hours. He is poorly coordinated with mild impairment of fine motor movements. He may have visual and speech difficulties, and he may vomit or complain of severe headache. When left alone, he usually sleeps for several hours. On awakening he is fully conscious but usually feels tired and complains of sore muscles and headache and has no recollection of the entire event.

Petit mal (absences)

Petit mal seizures, also called absences or lapses, are characterized by a brief loss of consciousness with minimum or no alteration in muscle tone and may go unrecognized since the child's behavior is altered very little. Attacks almost always first appear during childhood. In most instances the onset occurs between 5 and 9 years of age. Attacks are rarely detected before 5 years of age and usually cease at puberty, although they may be seen in adults. They are more common in girls than in boys.

The onset of petit mal seizures is abrupt, and the child suddenly develops 20 or more attacks daily. Characteristically the brief loss of consciousness appears without warning or aura and usually lasts about 5 to 10 seconds. Slight loss of muscle tone may cause the child to drop objects, but he is able to maintain postural control and seldom falls. There are frequently minor movements such as lip

smacking, twitching of eyelids or face, or slight hand movements. The sudden arrest of activity and consciousness is not accompanied by incontinence, and the child is amnesic for the episode but may need to reorient himself to the previous activity. An attack is often mistaken for inattentiveness or daydreaming. Frequent attacks can result in slowed intellectual processes and deterioration in schoolwork and behavior, which is sometimes the first indication of the problem. Attacks can be precipitated by hyperventilation, hypoglycemia, stresses (emotional and physiologic), fatigue, or sleeplessness.

Other seizures

Less frequently occurring seizures are *akinetic seizures,* manifested as a sudden, momentary loss of muscle tone and postural control; *myoclonic seizures,* characterized by sudden, brief contractures of a muscle or group of muscles, occurring singly or repetitively without loss of consciousness or postictal state; and *infantile myoclonic spasms,* which most commonly occur between 3 and 12 months and which consist of a series of sudden, brief, symmetric, muscular contractions in which the head is flexed, the arms are extended, and the legs are drawn up. Infantile spasms are almost always associated with cerebral abnormalities, such as structural malformations, chronic edema, and degenerative changes.

Therapeutic management

The objective of treatment of convulsive disorders is to control the seizures or to reduce their frequency, discover and correct the cause when possible, and help the child who has recurrent seizures to live as normal a life as possible. Seizures of a recurrent nature are treated as soon as the diagnosis is established. If the seizure activity is a manifestation of an infectious, traumatic, or metabolic process, the seizure therapy is instituted as a part of the general therapeutic regimen.

The primary therapy for convulsive disorders is the administration of the appropriate anticonvulsant drug or combination of drugs in a dosage that provides the desired effect without causing undesirable side effects or toxic reactions. Therapy is begun with a single drug known to be effective for the child's particular type of seizure, and the dosage is gradually increased until the seizures are controlled or the child develops signs of toxicity. If the drug is effective but does not sufficiently control the seizures, a second drug is added in gradually increasing doses. Once seizures are controlled, the drug or drugs are continued for a prolonged period of time.

Phenobarbital is effective for all types of seizures. For control of grand mal seizures phenytoin (Dilantin) is most often prescribed but has the undesirable side effect of gingival hyperplasia in many children. Petit mal seizures are managed with ethosuximide (Zarontin), valproic acid (Depakene), or trimethadione (Tridione).

Status epilepticus is managed by supportive measures, including maintenance of an adequate airway, administration of oxygen, and hydration, and by the intravenous administration of either diazepam or phenobarbital. Most physicians prefer diazepam for its dramatic effect on persistent seizures. The child must be closely monitored during administration to detect early alterations in vital signs that may indicate impending cardiac arrest or respiratory depression.

The beneficial effects of fasting have been known to be effective in reducing seizures for decades. A ketogenic diet that simulates the ketosis and acidosis of starvation has been advocated as therapy for epilepsy. The diet restricts protein and carbohydrate intake and supplies 80% of the caloric requirements in fats. It appears that the ketones have a tranquilizing effect. This diet has proved most effective in controlling myoclonic seizures and is of value in grand mal seizures, particularly in younger children. The practical difficulties of maintaining the diet limit is usefulness in most instances, especially for older children.

Nursing considerations

Nursing care of the child with a convulsive disorder involves both acute care during a seizure and long-term management, including support to the child and his family and education of the child, family, and community regarding the disorder.

Acute care. Nurses, when they first witness a child in a generalized cerebral seizure, are often frightened, puzzled, and immobilized. These reactions are normal but can reduce the effectiveness of care for the child and of significant observations of the event. The child must be protected from injury during the seizure, and nursing observations that are made during the attack provide valuable information for diagnosis and management of the disorder.

It is impossible to halt a seizure once it has begun, and no attempt should be made to do so. The nurse must remain calm, stay with the child, and prevent him from sustaining any harm during the attack. If possible the child is isolated from the view of others by closing a door or pulling screens around him. A seizure can be very upsetting to visitors and to other children and their families. If other persons are present they are assured that the affected child is in no danger, and, after the attack, they can be provided with a simple explanation to meet their needs.

The convulsing child is not moved or forcefully restrained, and force is not exerted in an attempt to place a solid object between his teeth. If it is possible at the beginning of an attack, a rubber wedge, padded tongue depressor, or the corner of a collar, blanket, wallet, or similar item can be used if it can be placed without difficulty. Nurses should never place their own fingers in the child's mouth during a seizure since the forceful muscular contractions can produce a serious bite. If the child is standing and the nurse is able to reach him in time or if he is seated in a chair (including a wheelchair), he is eased to the floor immediately. The nurse can protect the child from injury by supporting his head and gently restraining his hands to decrease the likelihood of injury from violent movements against the floor. After the attack the child is placed on his side in his bed or a similar place to allow him to sleep until he awakens. If he is at school or away from his home, the parents are contacted so that he can be taken home to rest.

A child who is known to have convulsive attacks or one who is under observation for seizures will require special precautions. The extent of these measures will depend on the type and frequency of the seizure. The child who is subject to daily seizures should not be permitted to engage in activities in which he might be injured, such as climbing, swimming, or handling sharp implements, and most of these children are advised to wear lightweight protective helmets. They should have side rails on beds with the hard surfaces padded if there is danger that they could hurt themselves. A padded tongue depressor or rubber wedge is usually placed in a convenient spot so that it can be quickly inserted between the child's teeth, if possible.

A child who has infrequent seizures or who is relatively free of seizures will have few restrictions on his activities. When he is hospitalized appropriate precautions should be implemented, such as side rails kept up when he is sleeping or resting, especially if his seizures are of the grand mal variety, since many of these children are subject to nocturnal attacks. The bed should be protected with a waterproof mattress or sheeting.

An important nursing function during a convulsion is to observe the seizure and describe its pertinent features. This includes the child's behavior before, during, and after the attack. Grand mal seizures and other seizures with dramatic manifestations are easily detected, but petit mal episodes may be more difficult to detect. They are easily misinterpreted as inattention. Any unusual behavior, even seemingly inconsequential behavior such as a momentary interruption of activity, staring, or mental blankness, are described. The more detailed these descriptions, the more valuable they are for purposes of assessment.

Records include the time that the seizure began and the length of the seizure. This is especially important if the child becomes cyanotic.

SUMMARY OF NURSING CARE OF THE CHILD DURING A GENERALIZED CONVULSIVE SEIZURE

GOALS	RESPONSIBILITIES

Protect child during seizure	If child is standing or sitting in wheel-chair at beginning of attack, ease child down so that he will not fall; when possible place cushion or blanket under child
	Remain with child
	Loosen restrictive clothing
	Prevent child from hitting hard or sharp objects that might cause injury
	    Remove object(s)
	    Pad object(s)
	    Gently support child
	Do not force hard object between the teeth when jaw is tightly closed

Observe seizure	Describe and record
	    Only what is actually observed
	    Order of events
	    Duration of seizure

Onset	Describe and record
	    Significant preseizure events—bright lights, noise, excitement, emotional outbursts
	    Behavior
	        Change in facial expression such as of fear
	        Cry or other sound
	        Stereotyped or automatous movements
	        Random activity
	    Position of head, body, extremities
	        Head turned to side or straight
	        Unilateral or bilateral posturing of one or more extremities
	        Body deviation to side
	    Time of onset

Movement	Describe and record
	    Change of position, if any
	    Site of commencement—hand, thumb, mouth, generalized
	    Tonic phase, if present—length, parts of body involved
	    Clonic phase—twitching or jerking movements, parts of body involved, sequence of parts involved, generalized, change in character of movements
	    Lack of movement of any extremity

Face	Describe and record
	    Color change—pallor, cyanosis, flushing
	    Perspiration
	    Mouth—position, deviating to one side, teeth clenched, tongue bitten, frothing at mouth, flecks of blood or bleeding

Eyes	Describe and record
	    Position—straight ahead, deviation upward, deviation outward, conjugate or divergent
	    Pupils (if able to assess)—change in size, equality, reaction to light and accommodation

Respiratory effort	Describe and record
	    Presence and length of apnea
	    Presence of stertor

Other	Describe and record
	    Involuntary urination
	    Involuntary defecation

Continued.

SUMMARY OF NURSING CARE OF THE CHILD DURING A GENERALIZED CONVULSIVE SEIZURE—cont'd

GOALS	RESPONSIBILITIES
Observe postictally	Describe and record 　Method of termination 　State of consciousness—unresponsiveness, drowsiness, confusion 　Orientation to time, place, persons, and so on 　Sleeping but able to be roused Motor ability 　Any change in motor power 　Ability to move all extremities 　Any paresis or weakness 　Ability to whistle (if appropriate to age) Speech—changes, pecularities, type and extent of any difficulties Sensations 　Complaint of discomfort or pain 　Any sensory impairment of hearing, vision 　Recollection of preseizure sensations, warning of attack 　Awareness that attack was beginning
Promote rest	Make child comfortable Allow child to rest after seizure Reduce sensory stimuli Record length of postictal sleep Notify physician if seizure is followed by other seizures in rapid succession or if duration of seizure is excessive
Reduce parental anxiety	Provide calm, relaxed atmosphere Explain purposes of nursing activities Provide emotional support

Long-term care.   Care of the child with a recurrent convulsive disorder involves the physical care and instruction regarding the importance of the drug therapy and, probably more importantly, the problems related to the emotional aspects of the disorder. There are few diseases that generate as much anxiety among relatives as epilepsy. Fears and misconceptions about the disease and its treatment abound in the lay person's mind. For many it represents the archetype of severe hereditary affliction. Therefore, the foci of nursing care are directed toward helping the child and his family to deal with the psychologic and sociologic problems related to the disorder and to educate the child, his family, his peers, and the public in general toward a more realistic and liberal view of the disease.

Parental attitudes and management of a child with a convulsive disorder are as varied as those of other parents of children with a chronic disorder, and they are subject to the same long-term problems (see Chapter 16). The parents want to know if it will affect the child's mental capacities. To many persons epilepsy is erroneously associated with mental deficiency. Seizures do frequently accompany other manifestations of severe brain damage from disease or injury, but the majority of children with seizures, like any population of healthy children, display a wide range of intelligence.

It is important to impress on the family the necessity of continuing the medication regularly without interruption for as long as required. This is usually 2 to 3 years after the last seizure, after which the drug is discontinued slowly over a period of time to avoid the possibility of precipitating a seizure. Planning ahead to replace a nearly empty bottle will prevent the risk of running out of the medication. It is sometimes easy to skip doses or omit them for any of a variety of reasons, especially when the child is free of seizures most of the time. This is particularly so when the child is older and assumes the responsibility for his medication. Omitting medication is the most frequent cause of status epilepticus.

The degree to which activities are restricted is individualized for each child and depends on the type, frequency, and severity of the seizures, the child's response to therapy, and the length of time the seizures have been controlled. Normal healthy activities are encouraged for children, and participation in competitive sports is determined on an individual basis. With encouragement most older children can accept the restrictions placed on activities.

Contact sports such as football, karate, or wrestling are avoided, but basketball, baseball, and tennis are allowed. Climbing trees or an apparatus from which the child might fall and be seriously injured is not usually permitted. The well-controlled epileptic child can ride a bicycle or swim if accompanied by a companion. The child who is subject to seizures induced by bright flashing lights should be cautioned against playing many of the video games so attractive to youngsters.

It is important to encourage a healthy attitude toward the child and his disease and to help the parents feel competent in their ability to meet their responsibilities to the child. The child should be reared as any normal child with natural concern tempered by the understanding of his need not to be overprotected. Many parents refrain from correcting or punishing the child, especially if they have had the experience of such an emotional stress precipitating an attack. The child should not be made to feel that he is different. Behavioral problems are common in children with epilepsy and can become a more serious problem than the seizures. Much of the behavioral difficulties, especially aggressive or delinquent behaviors, has been attributed to the child's reaction to parental rejection.

The suddenness and unpredictability of the attacks and the reactions of others further influence his feelings. The child needs to learn about his disease and the role that the medication plays in contributing to his prolonged well-being. As soon as he is old enough, the child should assume responsibility for taking his own medication. He should be advised to carry a card or a Medic Alert bracelet with pertinent information about his condition. Planning activities with the child and emphasizing those in which he can engage rather than those in which he cannot participate help the child to succeed and to gain satisfaction in his achievements. The Epilepsy Foundation of America* is a national organization that works toward and for the welfare of epileptic persons and their families, helps with employment and legal problems, and provides education to patients, families, and communities.

MALFORMATIONS OF THE CENTRAL NERVOUS SYSTEM

Defects of the central nervous system are usually the result of embryologic developmental failures. Some can be attributed to prenatal insults (caused by factors such as maternal infections or radiation), anoxia, or genetic factors; others may be a result of postnatal infections; however, in most cases the etiology is obscure. The defects that will be discussed are (1) cranial deformities caused by failure

*4351 Garden City Drive, Landover, MD 20785

of cranial sutures to remain open during the period of brain growth, (2) defects of neural tube closure, and (3) those characterized by an increase of free fluid in the cranial cavity, such as hydrocephalus.

CRANIAL DEFORMITIES

Various types of cranial deformities are encountered in early infancy. These include the enlarged head with frontal protrusion or bossing characteristic of hydrocephalus, the parietal bossing that is seen in chronic subdural hematoma, the small head, and a variety of skull deformities caused by premature closure of the cranial sutures. The principal sutures in the infant's skull are the sagittal, coronal, and lambdoid sutures, and the major soft areas at the juncture of these sutures are the anterior and posterior fontanels. Following birth, growth occurs in a direction perpendicular to the line of the suture and normal closure occurs in a regular and predictable order. Although there are wide variations in the age at which closure takes place in individual children, normally all sutures and fontanels should be ossified by the following ages:

2 months—posterior fontanel closed
6 months—fibrous union of suture lines and interlocking of serrated edges
18 months—anterior fontanel closed
12 years—sutures unable to be separated by increased intracranial pressure

Solid union of all sutures is not completed until very late childhood. Closure of a suture before the expected time inhibits growth of the skull *perpendicular* to the line of fusion. Since normal increase in brain volume requires expansion, the skull is forced to grow in a direction *parallel* to the fused suture. This alteration in the growth pattern of the skull always produces a distortion of the head shape when the underlying brain growth is normal. The small head with closed and normal shape is the result of deficient brain growth; the suture closure is secondary to this brain growth failure. Failure of brain growth is not secondary to suture closure.

Microcephaly

Primary microcephaly reflects a small brain and may be caused by a single gene, a chromosomal abnormality, or the result of application of a toxic stimulus during a critical period in prenatal development. These stimuli may be irradiation (especially between 4 and 20 weeks of gestation), maternal infection (notably toxoplasmosis, rubella, or cytomegalovirus), or chemical agents. *Secondary microcephaly* can result from a variety of insults that occur during the third trimester of pregnancy, the perinatal period, or early infancy. Infection, trauma, metabolic disorders, and anoxia are all capable of causing decreased brain growth and early closure of cranial sutures.

In both types the neurologic manifestations range from decerebration, complete unresponsiveness, and/or autistic behavior to mild motor impairment, educable mental retardation, and/or mild hyperkinesis. There appears to be a decided relationship between microcephaly and mental retardation of varying degrees; however, children with microcephaly may have normal intelligence. There is no treatment. Nursing care is directed toward helping parents adjust to rearing a brain-damaged child (see Chapter 17), if this is the case.

Craniostenosis (craniosynostosis)

Premature closure of the sutures of the skull produces deformities of the head, frequently with damage to the brain and eyes. In contrast to microcephaly, suture closure is the primary defect and is not the result of impaired brain growth. Consequently brain growth continues and the clinical picture depends on which sutures close, the duration of the closure process, and the success or failure of the other sutures to compensate by expansion. Usually the skull growth is inhibited in a direction at right angles to the closed sutures. The most common form is premature closure of the sagittal suture with consequent elongation of the skull in the anteroposterior direction. (A similar head shape is seen as a result of postnatal position maintenance in some premature infants.)

Treatment, if any, involves surgical excision of long bars of bone along or parallel to the fused suture and placement of a polyethylene- or silicone-coated film over the bony margins to delay closure. Surgery is performed for cosmetic reasons or, when multiple sutures are fused, to relieve cerebral pressure symptoms and complications.

Nursing considerations

Since craniosynostosis is present at birth, one of the first nursing implications is identification. Early diagnosis leads to improved prognosis. Premature closure of the sutures is characterized by absent fontanels and a suture line that feels prominent and bony. Obvious cephalic and facial deformity may be present at birth.

As with all birth defects, parents must be allowed to grieve for the loss of a perfect child. Since this is a very visible deformity, body image is a long-range problem. Demonstrating acceptance of the child assists parents in their progress toward acceptance. Since dysfunction of the brain can occur, particularly in coronal synostosis, continued care and developmental assessment are essential. Vision testing should be done periodically, and if exophthalmos is severe, preventive measures, such as the use of artificial tears or a patch, may be necessary to prevent corneal damage.

HYDROCEPHALUS

Hydrocephalus is a pathologic entity characterized by an excessive accumulation of cerebrospinal fluid (CSF), usually under increased pressure, as a consequence of obstructed drainage that produces passive dilation of the ventricles. The variations in manifestations depend primarily on the site of obstruction and the age at which obstruction develops.

Pathophysiology

The causes of hydrocephalus can be classified into three general categories:

1. **Excess secretion:** caused by a choroid plexus papilloma, a tumor composed of a large aggregate of choroidal fronds structurally similar to the choroid plexus that produces large quantities of cerebrospinal fluid.
2. **Noncommunicating (intraventicular):** the circulation of cerebrospinal fluid is blocked somewhere within the ventricular system, preventing its flow to the subarachnoid spaces. This is sometimes referred to as obstructive hydrocephalus (Fig 25-8).
3. **Communicating (extraventricular):** no interference to the flow of cerebrospinal fluid within the ventricular system. Fluid pathways are open so that fluid moves freely into the spinal subarachnoid space but is not absorbed from the cerebral subarachnoid space.

Most cases of noncommunicating hydrocephalus are a result of developmental malformations and, although the defect usually becomes apparent in early infancy, it may become evident at any time from the prenatal period to late childhood or early adulthood. Other causes include neoplasms, infections, and trauma. An obstruction to the normal flow can occur at any point in the cerebrospinal fluid pathway to produce increased pressure and dilation of the pathways proximal to the site of obstruction.

During infancy hydrocephalus is usually a major developmental defect. From birth to 2 years of age most cases are the result of the *Arnold-Chiari malformation* (a congenital anomaly in which the cerebellum and medulla oblongata extend down through the foramen magnum), aqueduct stenosis, and a glial tumor of the aqueduct. Hydrocephalus is so often associated with meningomyelocele that all such infants should be observed for its development. In the remainder of cases there is a history of intrauterine infection, perinatal hemorrhage (anoxic or traumatic), and neonatal meningoencephalitis (bacterial or viral). In older children hydrocephalus is most often the result of space-occupying lesions, preexisting developmental defects (aqueduct stenosis, Arnold-Chiari malformations), intracranial infections, or hemorrhage.

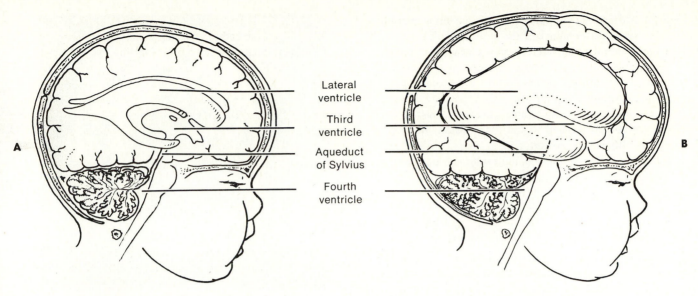

	Lateral ventricle
	Third ventricle
	Aqueduct of Sylvius
	Fourth ventricle

Fig. 25-8

Hydrocephalus: a block in the flow of cerebrospinal fluid. **A,** *Patent cerebrospinal fluid circulation.* **B,** *Enlarged lateral and third ventricles caused by obstruction of circulation—stenosis of the aqueduct of Sylvius.*

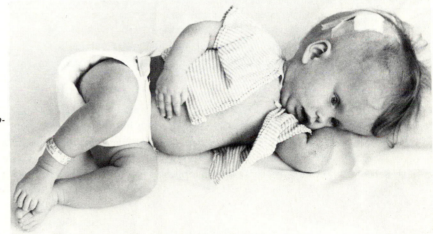

Fig. 25-9

Child with enlarged head caused by hydrocephalus.

Clinical manifestations

The two factors that influence the clinical picture in hydrocephalus are the time of onset and preexisting structural lesions. In infancy prior to closure of the cranial sutures, head enlargement is the predominant sign of hydrocephalus, whereas in older infants and children the lesions responsible for hydrocephalus produce other neurologic signs through pressure on adjacent structures before causing cerebrospinal fluid obstruction.

In infants the head grows at an abnormal rate, although the first signs may be bulging fontanels without head enlargement (Fig. 25-9). With the increase in intracranial volume the bones of the skull become thin and the sutures become palpably separated to produce the "cracked-pot" sound (Macewen sign) on percussion of the skull. The anterior fontanel is tense, often bulging, and nonpulsatile. Scalp veins are dilated and markedly so when the infant cries. There may be frontal enlargement or "bossing" with depressed eyes and a "setting-sun" sign in which the sclera is visible above the iris. Typical behaviors include irritability, opisthotonos (often extreme), and lower extremity spasticity. Early infantile reflex acts may persist, and normally expected responses fail to appear, indicating failure in the development of normal cortical inhibition.

If hydrocephalus is allowed to progress, development of lower brainstem functions is disrupted as manifested by difficulty in sucking and feeding and a shrill, brief, and high-pitched cry. Eventually the skull becomes enormous and the cortex is destroyed. If the hydrocephalus is rapidly progressive, the infant may display emesis, somnolence, seizures, and cardiopulmonary embarrassment. Severely affected infants usually do not survive the neonatal period.

The signs and symptoms in early to late childhood are caused by increased intracranial pressure, and specific manifestations are related to the focal lesion. Most commonly resulting from posterior fossa neoplasms and aqueduct stenosis, the clinical manifestations are primarily those associated with space-occupying lesions, that is, headache on awakening with improvement following emesis or upright posture, papilledema, strabismus, and extrapyramidal tract signs such as ataxia. In one of the congenital defects with later onset, the Dandy-Walker syndrome (congenital obstruction of the foramina of Luschka and Magendie), characteristic manifestations are bulging occiput, nystagmus, ataxia, and cranial nerve deficits.

Diagnostic evaluation

In infancy the diagnosis of hydrocephalus is based on head circumference that crosses one or more grid lines on the measurement chart within a period of 2 to 4 weeks and on associated neurologic signs that are present and progressive. However, other diagnostic studies are needed to localize the site of cerebrospinal fluid obstruction. Routine daily head circumference measurements are carried out in infants with meningomyelocele and intracranial infections.

The diagnostic tool of choice is computerized axial tomography (Fig. 25-10). The child is sedated prior to the test since he must remain absolutely still for an accurate picture. Diagnostic evaluation of children who have symptoms of hydrocephalus after infancy is similar to that employed in those with suspected intracranial tumor.

Therapeutic management

The treatment of hydrocephalus is almost exclusively surgical. Medical therapy directed toward reduction of the production of cerebrospinal fluid has proved to be ineffective in all but a few selected cases that involve overproduction. The surgical procedures employed most frequently are direct removal of the obstruction (tumor, cyst, or hematoma), ventricular bypass into a normal intracranial channel (for example, shunting of cerebrospinal fluid from the lateral ventricle into the cisterna magna—the Torkildsen procedure), or ventricular bypass into an extracranial compartment.

At present the most widely used procedure and the treatment of choice for communicating hydrocephalus and infantile noncommunicating hydrocephalus is drainage of the fluid from a lateral ventricle into an extracranial compartment (the most common being the right atrium or peri-

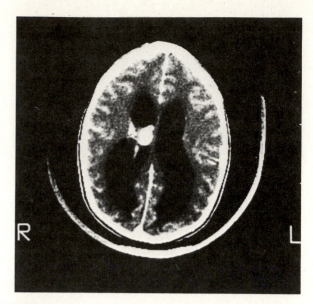

FIG. 25-10
Computed tomography scan reveals enlarged ventricles of child with hydrocephalus.

toneum) by way of an artificial passage, or shunt (Fig. 25-11). Shunts from the lateral ventricle are accomplished with plastic tubing and one-way valves. Slit one-way valves are designed to open at a predetermined intraventicular pressure and close when the pressure falls below that level. Thus backflow of blood or other secretions is prevented.

The initial success rate with shunting procedures is relatively high; however, they are associated with complications that interfere with continued shunt function or that threaten the life of the child. All are subject to mechanical difficulties, such as kinking, plugging, or separation of the tubing, and to bacterial infection, the most common serious complication. In case of infection, massive doses of antibiotics are administered by the intravenous route or directly into the ventricles. A persistent infection necessitates removal of the shunt until the infection is controlled.

Children with surgically treated hydrocephalus and continued neurosurgical and medical management have a survival rate of about 80% with the highest incidence of mortality occurring within the first year of treatment. Of the surviving children approximately one third are both intellectually and neurologically normal and one half have neurologic disabilities.

Nursing considerations

Preoperatively the infant with diagnosed or suspected hydrocephalus is observed carefully for signs of increasing intracranial pressure. In infants the head is measured daily at the point of largest measurement—the occipitofrontal

FIG. 25-11
A, *Ventriculoarterial shunt.*
B, *Ventriculoperitoneal shunt.*

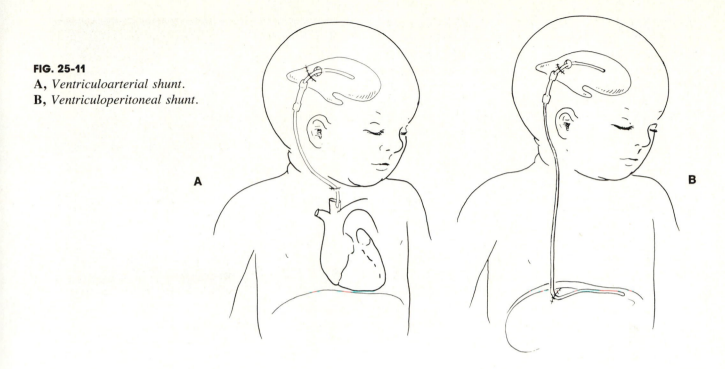

circumference (OFC). Fontanels and suture lines are gently palpated for size, signs of bulging, tenseness, and separation. However, an infant with normal intracranial pressure will display bulging under certain circumstances such as straining or crying; therefore, such accompanying behavior is noted. Irritability, lethargy, or seizure activity as well as altered vital signs and feeding behavior may indicate advancing pathology.

General nursing care of the infant with hydrocephalus may present special problems. Maintaining adequate nutrition often requires flexible feeding schedules to accommodate diagnostic procedures since feeding before or after handling can precipitate an episode of vomiting. Small feedings at more frequent intervals are frequently better tolerated than are larger ones spaced farther apart. These infants are often difficult to feed and require extra time and innovation. Care must be exercised to see that the large head is well supported when the infant is fed or moved to prevent extra strain on the infant's neck, and measures must be taken to prevent development of pressure areas. As the hydrocephaly progresses, untreated children become increasingly helpless and prone to the multiple problems of immobility, for example, pressure sores, contracture deformities, and so on. Not infrequently infants with irreversible brain damage or with severe developmental defects such as hydranencephaly, in which both cerebral hemispheres fail to develop and are replaced with a membranous sac filled with cerebrospinal fluid, are placed in long-term institutions designed for these infants.

Postoperative care. In addition to routine postoperative care and observation, the infant or child is posi-
tioned on the unoperated side to prevent pressure on the shunt valve with care to avoid pressure areas and is kept flat to help avert complications resulting from too rapid reduction of intracranial fluid. When the ventricular size is reduced too rapidly, the cerebral cortex may pull away from the dura and tear the small interlacing veins, producing a subdural hematoma. Sedation is avoided since the level of consciousness is an important observation.

Observation for signs of increased intracranial pressure, which indicate obstruction of the shunt, is continued. Sometimes the valve can be pumped several times to relieve the pressure and the procedure is repeated routinely a prescribed number of times every hour or two as ordered. If these measures are unsuccessful, the shunt may require replacement.

Since infection is the greatest hazard of the postoperative period, nurses are continually on the alert for the usual manifestations of cerebrospinal fluid infection, which may include elevated vital signs, poor feeding, vomiting, decreased responsiveness, and seizure activity. There may be signs of local inflammation at the operative sites and along the shunt tract. Antibiotics are administered by the intravenous route as ordered, and the nurse may also need to assist the physician with intraventricular instillation.

Emotional support. Helping parents cope with the hydrocephalic child or the child with a functioning shunt is an important nursing responsibility. Specific needs and concerns of parents during periods of hospitalization are related to the reason for the child's hospitalization (that is, shunt revision, infection, diagnosis) and the diagnostic and/or surgical procedures to which the child must be sub-

SUMMARY OF NURSING CARE OF THE CHILD WITH HYDROCEPHALUS

GOALS	RESPONSIBILITIES
Assess hydrocephalus	Assist with diagnostic evaluation Measure head circumference daily Observe for signs of increased intracranial pressure Prepare for procedures Assist with diagnostic procedures when appropriate, for example, ventricular tap, transillumination
Prevent pressure sore on head	Administer skin care and general hygiene measures Change position every 2 hours
Prevent postoperative complications	Position flat to prevent subdural hematoma Turn every 2 hours to prevent hypostatic pneumonia Position on unoperated side Observe for signs of infection or increased intracranial pressure Maintain care of and observe shunt and operative sites Observe and evaluate state of consciousness
Maintain nutrition and hydration	Institute flexible feeding schedule Give small, frequent feedings
Administer comfort measures	Administer general hygiene Provide tactile stimulation Encourage parental involvement in care
Reduce parental anxiety	Support parents Explain procedures and medical plan Answer questions Give anticipatory guidance
Guide posthospital care	Refer to appropriate agencies (public health, Special Child Health Services, social service) If parents are unable or unwilling to care for child, arrange placement in long-term care facility or refer to social service for foster home care

mitted. They are especially frightened of any procedure that involves the brain, and the fear of retardation or brain damage is very real and pervasive. Nurses can do much to allay their anxiety with explanations of the rationale underlying the various nursing and medical activities such as positioning or testing and by simply being available and willing to listen to their concerns.

REFERENCES

Committee on Infectious Diseases of the Academy of Pediatrics: Aspirin and Reye's syndrome, Pediatrics **69**:810, 1982.

BIBLIOGRAPHY
General

Bracke, M., Taylor, A.G., and Kinney, A.B.: External drainage of cerebrospinal fluid, Am. J. Nurs. **78**:1355-1358, 1978.
Conway, B.L.: Pediatric neurologic nursing, St. Louis, 1977, The C.V. Mosby Co.
Conway-Rudtkowski, B.L.: Carini and Owens' neurological and neurosurgical nursing, ed. 8, St. Louis, 1982, The C.V. Mosby Co.
Johnson, L.K.: If your patient has increased intracranial pressure, your goal should be: no surprises, Nursing 83 **13**(6):58-63, 1983.
Mitchell, P.H., and Mauss, N.: Intracranial pressure: fact and fancy, Nursing 76 **6**(6):53-57, 1976.
Ransohoff, J.: Death, dying and the neurosurgical patient, J. Neurosurg. Nurs. **10**(4):198-201, 1978.

The unconscious child

Adams, N.R.: Prolonged coma: your care makes the difference, Nursing 77 **7**(8):21-27, 1977.
Mauss-Clum, N: Bringing the unconscious patient back safely: nursing makes the critical difference, Nursing 82 **12**:34-42, 1982.
Surveyer, J.A.: Coma in children: how it affects parents, Am. J. Maternal Child Nurs. **1**(1):17-21, 1976.
Surveyer, J.A.: The emotional toll on nurses who care for comatose children, Am. J. Maternal Child Nurs. **1**:243-247, 1976.

Assessment and diagnosis

Bachman, D.S., Hodges, F.J., and Freeman, J.M.: Computerized axial tomography in neurologic disorders of children, Pediatrics **59**:352-363, 1977.

Bell, M., and Rekate, H.L.: Cerebrospinal fluid dynamics, J. Neurosurg. Nurs. **10**:46-48, 1978.

Blount, M., Kinney, A.B., and Donohoe, K.M.: Obtaining and analyzing cerebrospinal fluid, Nurs. Clin. North Am. **9**:593-610, 1974.

Bolin, K.L.: Assessing the status of neurological patients, Am. J. Nurs. **77**:1478-1479, 1977.

Jackson, P.L.: Assessing increased intracranial pressure in infants and young children, Crit. Care Update **10**(9):8-15, 1983.

Jones, C.: Glasgow coma scale, Am. J. Nurs. **79**:1551-1553, 1979.

King, R.C.: Checking the patient's neurological status, RN **44**(12):57-62, 1982.

Mills, G.: Preparing children and parents for cerebral computerized tomography, Am. J. Maternal Child Nurs. **5**(6):403-407, 1980.

Rudy, E.: Early omens of cerebral disaster, Nursing 77 **7**(2):59-62, 1977.

Stone, B.H.: Computerized transaxial brain scan, Am. J. Nurs. **77**:1601-1605, 1977.

Vernberg, K., Jagger, J., and Jane, J.A.: The Glasgow Coma Scale: how do you rate? Nurs. Educator, Autumn 1983, pp. 33-37.

Walleck, C.A.: A neurologic assessment procedure that won't make you nervous, Nursing 82 **12**(12):50-58, 1982.

Craniocerebral trauma

Bailey, J.: Head trauma, RN **41**(3):44-51, 1979.

Benjamin, R., and McKay, R.: Working with a brain-injured child, J. Assoc. Care Child Hosp. **8**(4):99-104, 1980.

Kunkel, J., and Wiley, J.K.: Acute head injury: what to do when and why, Nursing 79 **9**(3):23-33, 1979.

Meier, E.M.: Evaluating head trauma in infants and children, Am. J. Maternal Child Nurs. **8**:54-57, 1983.

Meyd, C.J.: Acute brain trauma, Am. J. Nurs. **78**:40-44, 1978.

Miller, M.E.: Cycle trauma: nursing's three key roles, Nursing 80 **10**(7):26-31, 1980.

Nezamis, F.K.: The child with a head, nurse, Issues Compr. Pediatr. Nurs. **2**(2):29-37, 1977.

Neoplasms of the central nervous system

Cleaveland, M.J.: Nursing care in childhood cancer: brain tumor, Am. J. Nurs. **82**:422-425, 1982.

Fochtman, D.: Malignant solid tumors in children, Pediatr. Nurs. **2**(6):11-17, 1976.

Hardin, K.: Solid tumors in children, Issues Compr. Pediatr. Nurs. **4**(1):29-47, 1980.

Hausman, K.A.: Brain tumors in children, J. Neurosurg. Nurs. **10**(1):8-21, 1978.

Petito, C.K., De Girolami, U., and Earle, K.M.: Craniopharyngiomas, Cancer **37**:1944-1952, 1976.

Pochedly, C.: Neuroblastoma, Nurse Pract. **4**(1)12-14, 1979.

Schwartz, A.D.: Neuroblastoma and Wilms' tumor, Med. Clin. North Am. **61**(5):1053-1071, 1977.

Walker, M.D.: Treatment of brain tumors, Med. Clin. North Am. **61**(5):1045-1051, 1977.

Wheeler, P.: Care of patient with a cerebellar tumor, Am. J. Nurs. **77**(2):263-266, 1977.

Intracranial infections

Jacob, J., and Kaplan, R.A.: Bacterial meningitis, Am. J. Dis. Child. **131**:46-56, 1977.

Krugman, S., and Katz, S.L.: Infectious diseases of children, ed. 7, St. Louis, 1981, The C.V. Mosby Co.

Langner, B.E., and Schott, J.R.: Nursing implications of central nervous system infections in children, Issues Compr. Pediatr. Nurs. **2**(2):38-53, 1977.

Smith, D.H.: The challenge of bacterial meningitis, Hosp. Pract. **11**:71, 1976.

Reye syndrome

Belkengren, R.P., and Sapala, S.: Reye syndrome: clinical guidelines for practitioners in ambulatory care, Pediatr. Nurs. **7**(2):26-28, 1981.

Budd, R.A., and Rothwell, R.: Spotting Reye's syndrome while there's still time, RN **45**(12):39-42, 1983.

Dalgas, P.: Reye's syndrome update, Am. J. Maternal Child Nurs. **8**:345-349, 1983.

Dunne, R.S., and Perez, R.C.: Reye's syndrome: a challenge not limited to critical care nurses, Issues Compr. Pediatr. Nurs. **5**:253-263, 1981.

Flammang, M., and Hohm, J.: The child with Reye's syndrome, Nursing 76 **6**:80C-80E, 1976.

Jemison-Smith, P., and Hamm, P.: Reye's syndrome, Crit. Care Update **10**(7):54-55, 1983.

Miller, J., and Arsenault, L.: Reye's syndrome, Neurosurg. Nurs. **15**:154-164, 1983.

Page-Goertz, S.S., and Lansky, L.L.: Reye's syndrome: an overview of nursing and medical management, Issues Compr. Pediatr. Nurs. **1**(6):41-56, 1977.

Shaywitz, B.A., and others: Prolonged continuous monitoring of intracranial pressure in severe Reye's syndrome, Pediatrics **59**:595-605, 1977.

Sinatra, F., Yoshida, T., and Sunshine, R.: Reye syndrome, Am. J. Dis. Child. **130**:781-782, 1976.

Weeks, H.L.: What every ICU nurse should know about Reye's syndrome, Am. J. Maternal Child Nurs. **1**:231-238, 1976.

Wright, E.: Reye's syndrome: epidemiology and treatment. In Chinn, P., and Leonard, K., editors: Current practice in pediatric nursing, St. Louis, 1980, The C.V. Mosby Co.

Rabies

Ferguson, C.K: Rabies in humans, Crit. Care Update **10**(7):11-16, 1983.

Ferguson, C.K., and Roll, L.J.: Human rabies, Am. J. Nurs. **81**:1175-1179, 1981.

Immunization Practices Advisory Committee: Rabies prevention, Morbid. Mortal. Weekly Rep. **29**:278, 1980.

Nichols, A.O.: Taking the fear out of rabies treatment, Nursing 83 **13**(6):42-43, 1983.

Convulsive disorders

Berkowitz, C.D., and Jones, C.R.: The PNP's role in evaluation and management of febrile seizures, Pediatr. Nurs. **9**:432-434, 1983.

Bindler, R.M., and Howry, L.B.: Nursing care of children with febrile seizures, Am. J. Maternal Child. Nurs. **3**:270-273, 1978.

Bruya, M.A., and Bolin, R.H.: Epilepsy: a controllable disease. Part I. Classification and diagnosis of seizures, Am. J. Nurs. **76**:389-392, 1976.

Bruya, M.A., and Bolin, R.H.: Epilepsy: a controllable disease. Part II. Drug therapy and nursing care, Am. J. Nurs. **76**:393-397, 1976.

Cooper, C.R.: Anticonvulsant drugs and the epileptic's dilemma, Nursing 76 **6**(1):45-50, 1976.

Coughlin, M.K.: Teaching children about their seizures and medications, Am. J. Maternal Child. Nurs. **4:**161-162, 1979.

Coulter, D.L.: The psychosocial impact of epilepsy in childhood, Child Health Care, **11**(2):48-53, 1983.

Farley, J.N.: Valproic acid for children with uncontrolled epilepsy, Am. J. Maternal Child Nurs. **15:**22, 1982.

Livingston, S., Pauli, L.L., and Pruce, I.M.: Epilepsy! Diagnosis and treatment, Pediatr. Nurs. **2**(3):23-27, 1976.

McGrath, D.M.: Nursing management of the child in status epilepticus, Issues Compr. Pediatr. Nurs. **5:**2173-2177, 1981.

McGrath, D.M.: Video recording seizure activity in children, Am. J. Maternal Child Nurs. **8:**218-220, 1983.

Mills, M.: When a child has surgery for focal epilepsy, Am. J. Maternal Child Nurs. **7:**304-308, 1982.

Muehl, J.N.: Seizure disorders in children: prevention and care, Am. J. Maternal Child. Nurs. **4:**154-160, 1979.

Norman, S.E.: Surgical treatment of epilepsy, Am. J. Nurs. **81:**994-996, 1981.

Norman, S.E., and Browne, T.R.: Seizure disorders, Am. J. Nurs. **81:**985-994, 1981.

Parish, M.A.: A comparison of behavioral side effects related to commonly used anticonvulsants, Pediatr. Nurs. **10:**149-152, 1984.

Robinson, L.A.: Phenytoin in anticonvulsant therapy, Pediatr. Nurs. **5**(3):57-58, 1979.

Santilli, N., and Tonelson, D.: Screening for seizures, Pediatr. Nurs. **7**(2):11-15, 1981.

Trekas, J.: Managing epilepsy: don't forget the patient, Nursing 82 **12**(10):63-65, 1982.

Williams, A., Swisher, C., and Bremer, H.L.: Critical care of seizures, Crit. Care Update **8**(7):22-25, 1981.

Wills, J.K., and Oppenheimer, E.Y.: Children's seizures and their management, Issues Compr. Pediatr. Nurs. **2**(2):55-67, 1977.

Zenk, K.E.: Drugs used for neurological disorders, Crit. Care Update **6**(9):19-24, 1979.

Zwang, H.J.: Epilepsy, Crit. Care Update **4**(7):5-15, 1977.

Hydrocephalus

Bernardo, M.L: When your caseload includes a hydrocephalic child, Pediatr. Nurs. **5**(3):27-29, 1979.

Bracke, M., and others: External drainage of cerebrospinal fluid, Am. J. Nurs. **78**:1355-1358, 1978.

Jackson, P.L.: Peritoneal shunting for hydrocephalus, Crit. Care Update **10**(4):33-39, 1983.

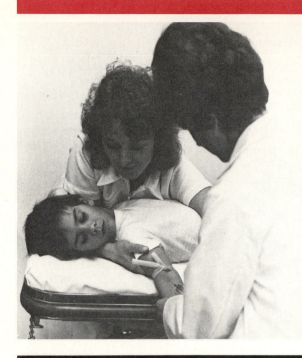

THE CHILD WITH ENDOCRINE DYSFUNCTION

OBJECTIVES

On completion of this chapter the reader will be able to:

■ Differentiate between the disorders caused by hypo- and hyperpituitary dysfunction

■ Describe the manifestations and management of the child with thyroid hypo- and hyperfunction

■ Distinguish between the manifestations of adrenal hypo- and hyperfunction

■ Differentiate between the various categories of diabetes mellitus

■ Describe the characteristics of the three major types of insulin

■ Discuss the management and nursing care of the child with diabetes mellitus in the acute care setting

■ Distinguish between a hypo- and hyperglycemic reaction

■ Design a teaching plan for a child with diabetes mellitus

■ Formulate a teaching plan for the parents of a child with diabetes mellitus

NURSING DIAGNOSES

Nursing diagnoses identified for the child with endocrine dysfunction include, but are not restricted to, the following:

Health perception-health management pattern

■ Injury: potential for, related to impaired circulation

■ Noncompliance, related to (1) knowledge deficit; (2) denial of disease

Nutritional-metabolic pattern

■ Fluid volume deficit related to osmotic diuresis

■ Nutrition, alteration in: more than body requirements, related to decreased activity

■ Skin integrity, impairment of: potential related to impaired circulation

Activity-exercise pattern

■ Diversional activity deficit related to inactivity

■ Self-care deficit: feeding, bathing/hygiene, dressing/grooming, toileting related to (1) developmental level; (2) knowledge deficit; (3) denial of illness

■ Tissue perfusion, alteration in: peripheral, related to disease process

Sleep-rest pattern

■ Sleep pattern disturbance related to diuresis

Self-perception—self-concept pattern

■ Anxiety related to (1) knowledge deficit; (2) previous experiences; (3) perception of impending events

■ Self-concept, disturbance in: body image, self-esteem, personal identity, related to perception of disease

Role-relationship pattern

■ Family process, alteration in, related to situational crisis

■ Parenting, alterations in: potential, related to (1) skill or knowledge deficit; (2) family stress

Coping-stress tolerance pattern

■ Coping, family: potential for growth

■ Coping, ineffective family: compromised, related to (1) situational crisis; (2) temporary family disorganization

■ Coping, ineffective individual, related to perception of disease

The major chemical regulators of the body are substances produced and secreted by a diverse group of tissues collectively known as the endocrine system. These substances, the hormones, are synthesized intracellularly and secreted into the circulation where they are transported to other tissues to stimulate, catalyze, or serve as pacemaker substances for metabolic processes. Together with the closely related but more rapidly reacting nervous system, they serve to integrate the various physiologic functions of the body in its adjustment to external and internal environmental demands. Endocrine substances even in extremely small concentrations are effective in modifying metabolism, behavior, and development (Table 26-1).

This chapter is primarily concerned with problems associated with oversecretion or undersecretion of the major hormones or defective responses in those organs and tissues that are sensitive to these hormones. It is the endocrine system that affects all aspects of body function including growth, feelings of physical and emotional well-being, appearance, and body function. It is largely responsible for the size, shape, texture, and sexual characteristics of the body and, therefore, has a profound influence on body image. Most endocrine disorders are relatively uncommon; however, the most common endocrine disturbance in childhood, diabetes mellitus, is a health problem with lifelong health implications and will be discussed at length.

PITUITARY DYSFUNCTION

The pituitary gland, or hypophysis, is often referred to as the *master gland* because of its role in regulating other endocrine glands. Under the influence of secretions from the hypothalamus, the anterior lobe of the pituitary (adenohypophysis) releases or withholds seven hormones. These hormones control the secretion of hormones from other endocrine glands and influence somatic and sexual development. Because of this relationship a dysfunction observed in target tissues can be either the result of malfunction of the target gland, the hypothalamus, or the pituitary gland.

Most often excesses or deficiencies of pituitary hormones are idiopathic and occur as a single hormonal problem or in combination with other hormonal dysfunction. The clinical manifestations depend on the hormones involved and the age of onset. If the tropic hormones are involved, the resulting disorder is related to the target gland and will be discussed in relation to those glands. This discussion is limited to dysfunction related primarily to the secretion of growth hormone.

HYPOPITUITARISM

Hypopituitarism is primarily a disorder associated with deficient secretion of growth hormone (somatotropin). It may be caused by a variety of conditions: developmental defects; destructive lesions such as tumors, trauma, vascular abnormalities, and surgery; a manifestation of certain hereditary disorders; or, it may be the result of functional disorders such as anorexia nervosa and psychosocial dwarfism. In more than half of children with hypopituitarism no lesion is evident and the cause is unknown—*idiopathic hypopituitarism* or idiopathic pituitary growth failure.

The primary site of dysfunction in the syndrome of idiopathic hypopituitarism appears to be in the hypothalamus. In half the affected children there is deficiency of somatotropin only; in the other half there is also impaired secretion of other pituitary hormones. The disorder is seen more frequently in boys than in girls and in children who experienced some type of birth trauma such as, breech birth, hypoxia, or intrapartal maternal bleeding.

Clinical manifestations

The child with idiopathic hypopituitarism is usually of normal height and weight at birth but approximately half will demonstrate retarded growth by 1 year of age. Others will appear to grow normally but are always below their age-mates in height, or will alternate periods of lack of growth with short growth spurts. Their body proportions are normal but remain immature. Consequently they appear younger than their chronologic age. Sexual development is usually delayed but is otherwise normal.

The facial structure may be normal or short and broad with prominent frontal bone and the bridge of the nose depressed. Primary teeth usually appear at the expected age, but the eruption of the permanent teeth is delayed. An underdeveloped jaw causes the teeth to become overcrowded and malpositioned. The neck is short and a small larynx produces a high-pitched voice that remains past puberty.

Most of these children have normal intelligence and, in early childhood, often appear precocious in their learning because their ability seems to exceed their small size. However, emotional problems are not uncommon, especially as they near puberty and their diminished size becomes increasingly apparent when compared to their peers.

Eventual height is difficult to predict. Because the period of growth is prolonged beyond adolescence and into the third or fourth decade, many of them reach a permanent height of 4 to 5 feet.

Diagnostic evaluation

Definitive diagnosis is based on radioimmunoassay of plasma growth hormone levels. Radiographic examination

TABLE 26-1. ENDOCRINE GLANDS AND THEIR FUNCTION

GLAND/HORMONE	PRIMARY EFFECT
Adenohypophysis (Anterior pituitary)	
Growth hormone (GH)	Promotes growth of bone and soft tissues
Thyroid-stimulating hormone (TSH)	Stimulates thyroid hormone secretion
Adrenocorticotropic hormone (ACTH)	Stimulates adrenal cortex to secrete glucocorticoids and androgens
Gonadotropins:	
Follicle-stimulating hormone (FSH)	Stimulates gonads to mature and produce sex hormones and germ cells
Luteinizing hormone (LH)	Same as above
Prolactin or luteotropic hormone (LTH)	Stimulates milk secretion
Melanocyte-stimulating hormone (MSH)	Promotes pigmentation of skin
Neurohypophysis (Posterior pituitary)	
Antidiuretic hormone (ADH)	Acts on kidney tubules to reabsorb water
Oxytocin	Stimulates uterine contractions
	Causes milk-ejection reflex
Thyroid gland	
Thyroid hormones	Regulate metabolic rate
	Control rate of body cell growth
Thyrocalcitonin	Influences ossification and development of bone
Parathyroid glands	
Parathyroid hormone (PTH)	Regulates calcium metabolism
Adrenal cortex	
Aldosterone	Regulates sodium retention and excretion
Sex hormones	Same as hormones from gonads
Glucocorticoids	Promote metabolism
	Mobilize body defenses during stress
	Suppress inflammatory reaction
Adrenal medulla	
Catecholamines	Produce a sympathetic response
Islands of Langerhans of pancreas	
Insulin	Promotes utilization of glucose by cells; reduces blood sugar
Glucagon	Increases blood sugar
Somatostatin	Inhibits secretion of insulin and glucagon
Ovaries	
Estrogen	Stimulates ripening of ova
	Produces female secondary sex characteristics
Progesterone	Prepares uterus for fertilization
Testes	
Testosterone	Stimulates spermatogenesis
	Produces male secondary sex characteristics

of the wrist for centers of ossification is an important procedure in evaluating growth. Endocrine studies to detect tropic hormone deficiencies are also performed if there is evidence of hypothyroidism or hypoadrenalism.

Therapeutic management

Treatment involves replacement of growth hormone. The only natural source of the substance is human cadaver pituitary glands; however, the development of synthetic growth hormone now offers hope to children with growth retardation. Not all children benefit from hormone replacement. A small number demonstrate circulating antibodies to growth hormone that inhibit its activity. Children who respond to the therapy eventually achieve a normal adult height.

Nursing considerations

Nursing care is primarily directed toward assisting in establishing the diagnosis and providing emotional support to the child and family (see Chapter 15). Since these children appear younger than their chronologic age, others frequently relate to them in infantile or childish ways. Parents and teachers benefit from guidance directed toward realistic expectations of the child, based on his age and abilities. Children require additional support because even when hormone replacement is successful, their eventual adult height is attained at a slower rate than that of their peers. They need assistance in setting realistic expectations regarding improvement.

PITUITARY GIGANTISM

Excess growth hormone prior to closure of the epiphyseal shafts results in proportional overgrowth of long bones, until the individual reaches a height of 8 feet or more. Vertical growth is accompanied by rapid and increased development of muscles and viscera. Weight is increased but is usually in proportion to height. Proportional enlargement of head circumference also occurs and may result in delayed closure of the fontanels. Children with a pituitary secreting tumor may also demonstrate signs of increasing intracranial pressure, especially headache.

If hypersecretion of growth hormone occurs after epiphyseal closure, growth is in the transverse direction, producing a condition known as *acromegaly*. Typical facial features include overgrowth of head, lips, nose, tongue, jaw, and paranasal and mastoid sinuses, separation and malocclusion of the teeth in the enlarged jaw, disproportion of the face to the cerebral division of the skull, increased facial hair, and thickened, deeply creased skin.

Diagnostic evaluation

Diagnosis is based on a history of excessive growth during childhood and evidence of increased levels of growth hormone. Radiologic studies may reveal a tumor in an enlarged sella turcica, normal bone age, enlargement of bones, such as the paranasal sinuses, and evidence of joint changes. Endocrine studies to confirm excess of other hormones, such as cortisol and sex hormones, are also included in the differential diagnosis.

Therapeutic management

If a lesion is present, surgical treatment, including cryosurgery or hypophysectomy, may be warranted to remove the tumor whenever feasible. Other therapies that destroy pituitary tissue include external irradiation and radioactive implants. Depending on the extent of surgical extirpation and the degree of pituitary insufficiency, hormone replacement with thyroid extract, cortisone, and sex hormones may be necessary.

Nursing considerations

The primary nursing consideration is early identification of children with excessive growth rates. Although medical management does not diminish the height already attained, it can retard height. The earlier the treatment is begun, the better the chance to attain a normal adult height.

These children require the same emotional support as those with short stature. However, girls may suffer from the effects of excessive height much more than boys who may find the tallness an asset when pursuing sports such as basketball. A compassionate nurse can be very supportive to these children, especially prior to adolescence when they are larger than their peers. The nurse can emphasize to a tall girl that as boys grow older they become taller and that she will not always be looking down at them. Since early adolescence is a time of idol worship, the nurse can point out marriages of celebrities in which the woman is taller than the man to help the girl gain a perspective that not all heterosexual relationships must follow stereotypic models.

PRECOCIOUS PUBERTY

Precocious puberty is the manifestation of pubertal development that appears before the expected age of onset. Although puberty is gradually appearing earlier in most societies, manifestations of sexual development before age 10 in boys or age 8½ in girls are considered precocious and should be investigated. Early sexual development can be a result of a number of causes, for example, a disorder of the gonad, the adrenal gland, or the hypothalamic-pituitary mechanism.

Precocious sexual development can be divided into two types: (1) true, or complete, precocious puberty in which there is premature development of the gonads with secretion of sex hormones, development of secondary sex characteristics, and sometimes production of mature sperm or ova; and, (2) precocious pseudopuberty (incomplete puberty) in which there is no maturation of the gonads, but there is appearance of secondary sex characteristics. The latter may be caused by a tumor on the adrenals or an organic brain lesion.

Psychologic management and guidance of children with true precocious puberty and their families constitute the most important aspects of treatment. Parents need a detailed explanation and reassurance of the benign nature of the condition. Dress and activities for the physically precocious child should be appropriate to the age. Heterosexual interest is not usually advanced beyond the child's chronologic age, and parents need to understand that the child's normal, overt manifestations of affection are age-appropriate and do not represent sexual advances.

DIABETES INSIPIDUS

The principal disorder of the posterior pituitary is hyposecretion of antidiuretic hormone that produces a condition known as diabetes insipidus. Primary diabetes insipidus may be the result of a hereditary vasopressin deficiency or an idiopathic etiology. Secondary diabetes insipidus is caused by damage to the posterior pituitary, usually as a result of head trauma or neoplasms (craniopharyngioma). *Nephrogenic diabetes insipidus* (vasopressin-insensitive diabetes insipidus) is a rare hereditary disorder caused by unresponsiveness of the renal tubules to the hormone, not to pituitary hyposecretion of antidiuretic hormone.

Clinical manifestations

The cardinal signs of diabetes insipidus are polyuria and polydipsia. In the older child excessive urination accompanied by a compensatory insatiable thirst may be so intense that the child does little else other than go to the toilet and drink fluids. Frequently enuresis is the first sign of the disorder. In the infant the initial symptom is irritability that is relieved with feedings of water but not milk. The infant is especially prone to dehydration, electrolyte imbalance, hyperthermia, azotemia, and potential circulatory collapse.

Diagnostic evaluation

The most simple test used to diagnose this condition is restriction of oral fluids and observations of consequent changes in urine volume and concentration. In diabetes insipidus fluid restriction has little or no effect on urine formation but causes weight loss from dehydration. If this test is positive the child is given a test dose of injected aqueous vasopressin (Pitressin), which should alleviate the polyuria and polydipsia. The child with nephrogenic diabetes insipidus is unresponsive to exogenous vasopressin administration.

Other tests employed in the diagnostic evaluation include a skull x-ray film to detect a tumor, kidney function tests and blood electrolyte levels to rule out renal failure, and specific endocrine studies to isolate associated problems.

Therapeutic management

The usual treatment of diabetes insipidus is hormone replacement with vasopressin by intramuscular or subcutaneous injection in peanut oil or by nasal sprays of aqueous vasopressin (lypressin).

Children with the nephrogenic type do not benefit from antidiuretic hormone replacement. The polyuria can be controlled by reducing the solute load on the kidney, both with dietary restriction of salt and protein and with the use of diuretics, such as chlorothiazide, which diminish reabsorption of sodium and chloride ions. These children still require a sufficient intake of fluids to prevent dehydration.

Nursing considerations

The initial objective of care is identification of the disorder. After confirmation of the diagnosis, parents need a thorough explanation of the condition with special emphasis on distinguishing the difference between diabetes insipidus and diabetes mellitus. They must realize that treatment is lifelong. If the child is to receive the injectable vasopressin (Pitressin), ideally both parents should be taught the correct procedure for preparation and administration of the drug. Once the child is old enough he should be encouraged to assume full responsibility for his care.

For emergency purposes these children should wear Medic Alert tags. Older children are advised to carry the nasal vasopressin spray with them for temporary relief of symptoms. School personnel should be made aware of the problem in order that the child is granted unrestricted use of the lavatory and drinking water. Failure to permit this may result in embarrassing accidents that often result in the child's unwillingness to attend school.

SYNDROME OF INAPPROPRIATE ANTIDIURETIC HORMONE SECRETION (SIADH)

Hypersecretion of the posterior pituitary antidiuretic hormone (ADH, vasopressin) produces the disorder known as the syndrome of inappropriate ADH secretion. SIADH is observed with increased frequency in a variety of conditions, especially those involving infections, tumors, and trauma of the central nervous system.

The manifestations observed are directly related to fluid retention and hypotonicity. Increased secretion of ADH causes the kidneys to reabsorb water, which increases the fluid volume and decreases serum osmolality. When serum sodium levels are diminished to 120 mEq/L, the child displays anorexia, nausea (and sometimes vomiting), irritability, and personality changes. With progressive reduction in sodium other neurologic signs, stupor, and convulsions may be evident. The symptoms disappear when the underlying disorder is corrected. Immediate management consists of restricting fluids.

THYROID DYSFUNCTION

The thyroid gland secretes two types of hormones: the thyroid hormones, thyroxine (T_4) and triiodothyronine (T_3), and thyrocalcitonin. The main physiologic actions of thyroid hormones are regulation of metabolic activities essential to all tissues, mobilization of fats and gluconeogenesis for energy production, and thereby control of the processes of growth. The secretion of thyroid hormone is controlled by thyroid-stimulating hormone of the anterior pituitary. Consequently hypothyroidism or hyperthyroidism can be caused by a defect in the thyroid gland or from a disturbance in the secretion of thyroid-stimulating hormone from the pituitary or its releasing factor in the hypothalamus.

Thyrocalcitonin is essential for calcium and phosphorus metabolism. It reduces the serum calcium concentration by inhibiting bone demineralization and promoting calcium deposition in the bone.

Hypothyroidism is one of the most common endocrine problems of childhood and may be either congenital or acquired. Hypothyroidism from dietary insufficiency of iodine is now rare in the United States because the use of iodized salt has permitted a readily available source of the nutrient.

Hyperthyroidism is much less common in children than hypothyroidism. In most instances it is the result of Graves disease; less often it is caused by adenoma of the thyroid. A benign, self-limiting hyperplasia of the thyroid is also observed in some children during adolescence.

CONGENITAL HYPOTHYROIDISM

Congenital hypothyroidism (sometimes called by the undesirable term cretinism) may be caused by aplasia or hypoplasia of the thyroid gland, radioiodine administered to the mother prenatally, pituitary dysfunction, defective synthesis of thyroid hormones, or tissue unresponsiveness to thyroid hormones. No matter what the etiology the manifestations and management are similar. In some of these conditions the thyroid deficiency is severe and manifestations develop early; in others the symptoms may be delayed for months or years. It is twice as common in girls as in boys.

Clinical manifestations

Symptoms of hypothyroidism are seldom recognized in the newborn period but close observation may reveal initial signs such as prolonged physiologic jaundice, feeding difficulties, excessive sleeping, and choking spells during feeding. There may be respiratory difficulties. The affected infant continues to sleep a great deal and cry very little, has a poor appetite, and is generally sluggish. The behavioral characteristics often lead parents to describe the infant as exceptionally "quiet and good."

As the disease progresses impaired physical and mental development become obvious; by 3 to 6 months the manifestations are fully evident. Anemia is often present and the infant may develop problems resulting from hypotonic abdominal musculature, such as constipation, diastasis recti, protruding abdomen, and umbilical hernia. The temperature is subnormal and the pulse is slow; the skin becomes mottled and cold.

The symptoms may be less severe in partial thyroid deficiency and in breast-fed infants and hypothyroidism may be delayed until the child is weaned, at which time the characteristic features become evident. Because breast milk contains suboptimal amounts of thyroid hormone, intellectual functioning remains near normal. However, bone age is greatly retarded, usually comparable to that of a newborn.

Because skeletal growth is severely stunted, the child is short. Unlike pituitary dwarfism, infantile proportions persist in that the length of the trunk remains long in relation to the legs. The decreased metabolic rate results in weight gain and often leads to obesity. Characteristic infantile facial features of myxedema include a short forehead, wide, puffy eyes, wrinkled eyelids, broad short upturned nose, and a large protruding tongue. The hair is often dry, brittle, or lusterless and extends far down onto the forehead. Dentition is delayed and usually defective. Such facial features give the child a characteristic dull expression.

The severity of the intellectual deficit is related to the degree of hypothyroidism and the duration of the condition

SUMMARY OF NURSING CARE OF THE CHILD WITH HYPOTHYROIDISM

GOALS	RESPONSIBILITIES
Recognize hypothyroidism	Be suspicious of disorder in infants less than 3 months of age with characteristic signs Be alert to signs of delayed physical and mental growth in child over 3 months
Assist with diagnosis	Take careful history Perform physical assessment Order or draw blood for analysis Assist with thyroid function tests Assist with radiographic examination
Replace deficient thryoid hormone	Administer desiccated thyroid or synthetic thyroid as prescribed
Provide parent education	Reinforce physician's explanation of disorder and clarify misconceptions Emphasize importance of compliance regarding thyroid administration Instruct parents in administration of medication Alert parents to signs of overdosage, such as rapid pulse, dyspnea, irritability, weight loss, insomnia, fever, sweating
Support parents	Support and reassure parents in their care of infant and child Provide for follow-up care as appropriate If diagnosis is delayed, assist parents in adjusting to sequelae such as mental retardation

prior to treatment. Other nervous system manifestations include slow, awkward movements, somnolence, lethargy, and abnormal deep tendon reflexes (often referred to as "hung-up" because the relaxation phase is slow following the contraction).

Diagnostic evaluation

Several tests are available to assess thyroid activity. The more common ones are measurement of protein-bound iodine (PBI), free thyroxine, thyroid-stimulating hormone, and thyrotropin-releasing factor and radioimmunoassay of thyroxine and triiodothyronine. Tests of thyroid gland function usually involve oral administration of a radioactive isotope of iodine (^{131}I) and measurement of the iodine uptake by the thyroid, usually within 24 hours. In congenital hypothyroidism protein-bound iodine, thyroxine, triiodothyronine, and free thyroxine levels are low and thyroid uptake of ^{131}I is decreased. Neonatal screening is now possible with a highly sensitive and specific radioimmunoassay for thyroxine or thyroid-stimulating factor and is mandatory in most states. Diagnosis rests on the detection of a high serum level of thyroid-stimulating factor and a low level of thyroxine during the early days of life.

Therapeutic management

Treatment involves replacement therapy with desiccated thyroid to abolish all signs of hypothyroidism and reestab-

lish normal physical and mental development. If started before 3 months of age the chance for completely normal growth is possible and the chance for normal intelligence is increased.

To avoid the risk of overdosage of thyroid hormones, thyroxine and triiodothyronine levels should be measured regularly. Bone age surveys are also performed to assess the progress of growth.

Nursing considerations

The most important nursing objective in hypothyroidism is early identification of the disorder. Nurses caring for neonates and those in ambulatory settings for well-infant care need to be alert to the earliest signs of hypothyroidism such as parental remarks about an unusually "good" baby and observation of any early physical manifestations. Unfortunately many parents harbor guilt about their impressions of the infant prior to the diagnosis because the child's inactivity may not have alerted them to a problem, resulting in delayed treatment.

Once the diagnosis is confirmed, parents need an explanation about the disorder and the necessity of lifelong treatment. They should be aware of signs indicating overdose, namely, rapid pulse, dyspnea, irritability, insomnia, fever, sweating, and weight loss. Ideally they should know how to count the pulse and be instructed to withhold a dose and consult the physician if the pulse rate is above a certain value.

If the diagnosis was delayed past early infancy, the chance of permanent mental retardation is great. Parents need the same guidance in caring for their child as others who have a retarded offspring (Chapter 17), including an opportunity to discuss their feelings regarding late recognition of the disorder. Although treatment will not reverse the intellectual deficit, it will prevent further damage. Helping the parents deal with future prospects for the child, encouraging them to stimulate him to his potential, and directing their focus to his strengths rather than disabilities can promote an earlier and more positive adjustment to the diagnosis of mental retardation.

JUVENILE HYPOTHYROIDISM

Hypothyroidism in a previously euthyroid (normal functioning) child can result from a variety of defects in addition to an undetected thyroid deficiency that becomes manifest as rapid growth increases body demands for the hormone. Some of these conditions include partial or complete thyroidectomy, irradiation to the neck area, and, sometimes, infections or prolonged ingestion of iodine or cobalt. The usual cause of juvenile hypothyroidism is lymphocytic thyroiditis.

Clinical manifestations depend on the age of the child at onset and the extent of dysfunction. The later the detection, the less will be the physical and mental impairment. Diagnostic studies and treatment are the same as for congenital hypothyroidism.

GOITERS

A goiter is an enlargement or hypertrophy of the thyroid gland and may occur in hypothyroid, hyperthyroid, or euthyroid (normal) states. When thyroid hormone production is impaired, such as in congenital hypothyroidism resulting from enzymatic defects or from lymphocytic thyroiditis, thyroid-stimulating hormone stimulation results in hypertrophy and hyperplasia of the gland. A large gland, if untreated, can cause severe respiratory distress.

If an infant is born with a goiter, immediate precautions are instituted for emergency ventilation, such as supplemental oxygen and a tracheostomy set at the bedside. Positioning the child with the neck hyperextended often facilitates breathing. Immediate surgery to remove part of the gland may be life-saving.

Thyroid hormone replacement reverses the thyroid-stimulating hormone effect on the gland.

LYMPHOCYTIC THYROIDITIS

Lymphocytic thyroiditis (autoimmune thyroiditis, or Hashimoto's thyroiditis) is the most common cause of goiters and acquired hypothyroidism in children. There is a genetic predisposition to development of the disease and the incidence is much higher in girls than in boys. Although it is more common after the age of 6 years, the disease may be manifest during the first year of life. However, the peak age of appearance is during the early pubertal changes of adolescence. Because of the marked increase at that time, thyroiditis during adolescence was thought to be a separate disorder and given the term *thyroid hyperplasia of adolescence*.

Clinical manifestations

The presence of the enlarged thyroid gland is usually detected by the physician or pediatric nurse practitioner during a routine examination, although it may be noted by parents when the youngster swallows. The entire gland is enlarged symmetrically with one side usually more dominant than the other, but it is extremely rare for nontoxic diffuse goiter to enlarge to the extent that its size causes mechanical symptoms. Most often the goiter is transient, asymptomatic, and regresses spontaneously within a year or two.

Laboratory studies of thyroid function are usually sufficient to establish the diagnosis or to determine whether further tests should be carried out for more complex thyroid pathology. High serum titers of antibodies suggest an autoimmune process.

Therapeutic management

Therapy of nontoxic diffuse goiter is usually simple, uncomplicated, and effective. Oral administration of thyroid hormone will decrease the size of the gland significantly. Supplemental oral thyroid extract provides the feedback needed to suppress thyroid-stimulating hormone stimulation, and the hyperplastic thyroid gland regresses in size. Surgery is contraindicated in this disorder.

Nursing considerations

Nursing care consists of identifying the youngster with thyroid enlargement, reassuring him that the condition is probably only temporary, and reinforcing the instructions for thyroid therapy.

GRAVES DISEASE

Graves disease is the most common cause of thyrotoxicosis in childhood and is believed to be an autoimmune process that has a stimulatory effect on the thyroid gland. It occurs about 5 times more frequently in females and has a significant increase in incidence prior to and during puberty.

Clinical manifestations

Symptoms of Graves disease develop gradually and consist of three types of manifestations: goiter (enlarged thyroid gland), exophthalmos (protruding eyeballs), and hypermetabolism. The signs of hypermetabolism are those of excessive motion, such as irritability, hyperactivity, short attention span, tremors, insomnia, and emotional lability. Gradual weight loss is common despite a voracious appetite. Linear growth and bone age are usually accelerated. Muscle weakness often occurs. Hyperactivity of the gastrointestinal tract may cause vomiting and frequent stooling. The skin is warm, flushed, and moist. Heat intolerance may be severe and is accompanied by diaphoresis. The hair is unusually fine and unable to hold a curl. Cardiac manifestations include a rapid pounding pulse even during sleep, widened pulse pressure, systolic murmurs, and cardiomegaly. Dyspnea occurs during slight exertion, such as climbing stairs.

Exophthalmos is accompanied by a wide-eyed staring expression, increased blinking, lid lag, lack of convergence, and absence of wrinkling of the forehead when looking upward. As protrusion of the eyeball increases, the child may not be able to completely cover the cornea with the lid. Visual disturbances may include blurred vision and loss of visual acuity.

Thyroid crises may occur from sudden release of the hormone. Although unusual in children, they can be life threatening and cause circulatory collapse. These "storms" are characterized by severe irritability and restlessness, vomiting, diarrhea, hyperthermia, hypertension, and prostration. They are precipitated by acute infection, surgical emergencies, and discontinuation of antithyroid therapy, especially after the use of iodine.

Diagnostic evaluation

Diagnosis is made on the basis of clinical observations and the presence of increased levels of protein-bound iodine, thyroxine, and free thyroxine. [131]I uptake by the thyroid gland is accelerated. Not infrequently the white count shows granulocytopenia.

Therapeutic management

The management of hyperthyroidism is controversial but most favor a trial of medical therapy before subtotal thyroidectomy is contemplated. Medical management involves administration of antithyroid drugs that interfere with the biosynthesis of thyroid hormone, primarily pro-

pylthiouracil (PTU) and methimazole (Tapazole). Symptomatic response to these drugs occurs in 1 or 2 weeks as evidenced by decreased nervousness, less fatigue, increased strength, a lowered pulse, and weight gain. In many children an initial treatment course of 1 to 3 years will be followed by a complete remission of the disorder. Those who relapse often benefit from a second course of therapy but may also be candidates for surgical intervention.

Subtotal thyroidectomy is a permanent form of therapy but it has a number of serious disadvantages, particularly the postoperative risks of hypothyroidism, hypoparathyroidism, and laryngeal nerve damage. Therefore, surgery is reserved for children who are hypersensitive to antithyroid drugs, who do not respond to or comply with the use of the drugs, or who are prone to recurrences.

Nursing considerations

Much of the child's care during diagnosis and initial medical therapy is related to the physical symptoms. He needs a quiet, unstimulated environment that is conducive to rest, and sometimes hospitalization is necessary during the immediate treatment phase to remove the child from a troubled home. A regular routine is beneficial with frequent rest periods, minimizing the stress of coping with unexpected demands, and meeting the child's needs promptly. Despite the excessive activity of these children, they tire easily, experience muscle weakness, and are unable to relax to recoup their strength.

Emotional lability is often manifest by sudden episodes of crying or elation. Such behavior, together with irritability, disrupts interpersonal relationships, creating difficulties within and outside the home. Heat intolerance may produce considerable family conflict. Since the child prefers a cooler environment than others, he is likely to open windows, complain about the heat, wear minimum clothing, and kick off blankets while sleeping.

Dietary requirements are regulated to meet the child's increased metabolic rate. Although his need for calories is increased, these should be provided in wholesome foods rather than "junk" foods. He may require vitamin supplements to meet his daily requirement. Rather than three large meals, the child's appetite may be better satisfied by five or six moderate meals throughout the day.

Once therapy is instituted, the nurse explains the drug regimen, emphasizing the importance of observing for side effects of antithyroid drugs. Untoward effects of propylthiouracil and related compounds include skin rash, drug fever, enlargement of the salivary and cervical lymph glands, diminished sense of taste, hepatitis, and edema of the lower extremities. Since sore throat and fever accompany the grave complication of leukopenia, these children should be seen by a physician if they occur. Parents should also be aware of the signs of hypothyroidism, which can occur from overdose of the drugs. The most common indications are lethargy and somnolence.

If surgery is anticipated, iodine (Lugol's solution or saturated potassium iodide solution [SSKI]) is usually administered for a few weeks prior to the procedure. Since oral iodine preparations are unpalatable, they should be mixed with a strong tasting fruit juice, such as grape or punch flavors, and given through a straw. Compliance with iodine therapy is essential to avoid the danger of thyroid crisis after sudden discontinuation.

Psychologic preparation of the child for thyroidectomy is similar to that for any other surgical procedure (p. 585). However, of special consideration is the site of the incision. The fear of cutting one's throat is very real and in older children is associated with death. The nurse explains that the throat is not cut, only the skin, to allow for removal of the gland. The child should be prepared for the dressing around the neck and the possibility of an endotracheal or "breathing" tube after surgery.

Postoperative care involves observation for bleeding into the operative site, which can rapidly lead to asphyxiation. The nurse inspects the dressing for bleeding and checks behind the neck for accumulation of draining blood and reports any signs of hemorrhage or respiratory distress. The child should be positioned with the neck slightly flexed to avoid strain on the sutures.

Another complication is damage to the recurrent laryngeal nerve. If damage is bilateral, airway obstruction will usually occur within a few hours. Any evidence of stridor is reported immediately, and a tracheostomy set is placed at the bedside. Unilateral injury to the nerve causes dysphonia. Although the hoarseness often improves in a few weeks, the child may have a permanent speech defect.

Since hypothyroidism and/or hypoparathyroidism may result, the nurse observes for signs of these conditions. The earliest indication of hypoparathyroidism may be anxiety and mental depression, followed by paresthesia and evidence of heightened neuromuscular excitability, such as the Chvostek sign (spasm of facial muscles elicited by light taps over the area of the facial nerve) and the Trousseau sign (carpal muscle spasm induced by pressure on the principal vessels and nerves of the upper arm) and carpopedal spasm (tetany). The behavioral manifestations, including those of hypothyroidism, must be differentiated from emotional depression as a reaction to the stress of surgery. Each of these conditions may require appropriate chemical replacement, which is discussed with the family prior to discharge.

PARATHYROID DYSFUNCTION

The parathyroid glands secrete parathormone (PTH), whose main function is to maintain homeostasis of blood calcium concentration. Parathormone exerts its effect by (1) increasing the release of calcium and phosphate from the bone (bone demineralization), (2) increasing the absorption of calcium and the excretion of phosphate by the kidneys, and (3) promoting calcium absorption in the gastrointestinal tract. The net result of these actions is to increase the plasma calcium concentration while lowering the plasma phosphate concentration.

HYPOPARATHYROIDISM

Two classic forms of primary hypoparathyroidism present during childhood: *idiopathic hypoparathyroidism,* in which there is a deficiency in the production of parathyroid hormone, and *pseudohypoparathyroidism,* in which there is adequate parathyroid hormone production but the end organ responsiveness to the hormone is deficient. Secondary hypoparathyroidism may also occur when the glands are removed during parathyroid or thyroid surgery or the short-lived disease in neonates born to mothers with hypoparathyroidism. Regardless of the cause, the clinical manifestations, treatment, and nursing considerations are essentially similar.

Clinical manifestations

The most common presenting sign is generalized convulsions. Other manifestations of neuromuscular excitability are evident, such as carpopedal spasms, muscle cramps and twitching, paresthesia, and laryngeal stridor. In addition, the child may exhibit abnormalities of the teeth, such as delayed dentition, premature loss of teeth, enamel hypoplasia, and caries; cracking and transverse ridging of the nails; alopecia; dry, scaly skin; and eye disorders, including blepharospasm, photophobia, keratoconjunctivitis, and cataracts. Digestive symptoms caused by irritability of the gastrointestinal tract include nausea and vomiting and diarrhea or constipation.

Since hypoparathyroidism results in decreased bone resorption and inactive osteoclastic activity, skeletal growth is retarded. Developmental abnormalities include short stature, round face, short neck, and stocky body build. Mental retardation is a prominent feature of pseudohypoparathyroidism but occurs less frequently in late onset disease. It is observed sometimes in idiopathic disease also. Papilledema may occur in idiopathic hypoparathyroidism but is rare in pseudohypoparathyroidism.

Diagnostic evaluation

Physical assessment may yield clues to the diagnosis, such as positive Trousseau and Chvostek signs. Laboratory tests include serum assays of calcium, phosphate, and parathormone. Kidney function tests are included in the differential diagnosis to rule out renal insufficiency. Although bone radiographs are usually normal, they may demonstrate increased bone density and suppressed growth.

Therapeutic management

The treatment of hypoparathyroidism includes the administration of oral calcium supplements and vitamin D to facilitate absorption of the mineral. For acute hypocalcemia, intravenous calcium gluconate is administered for relief of symptoms.

Nursing considerations

The initial nursing objective is recognition of hypocalcemia. Unexplained convulsions, irritability, especially to external stimuli, gastrointestinal symptoms, and positive signs of tetany should lead the nurse to suspect this disorder. Initial nursing care is related to these physical manifestations and includes (1) institution of seizure and safety precautions, (2) reduction of environmental stimuli, such as minimum holding of the infant, dim lights, and decreased noise, and (3) observation for signs of laryngospasm, such as stridor, hoarseness, and a feeling of tightness in the throat. A tracheostomy set and injectable calcium gluconate should be placed near the bedside for emergency use. If a low-phosphorus diet is recommended, the parents are advised to eliminate foods such as milk, cheese, and eggs. Restriction of dairy products may necessitate formula substitutions in infants.

When emergency administration of intravenous calcium gluconate is instituted the nurse is responsible for monitoring the infusion and exerting the needed care in preparation of the drug, such as understanding the substances with which it is incompatible.

HYPERPARATHYROIDISM

Hyperparathyroidism may be either primary or secondary. *Primary* hyperparathyroidism is primarily a disease of adults but is being recognized more often in childhood and may result from idiopathic hyperplasia of the parathyroid gland or a tumor (adenoma). *Secondary* hyperparathyroidism is caused by a variety of conditions (transplacental, intestinal, hepatic, or renal), which decrease the serum calcium ion concentration, resulting in a compensating parathyroid hyperplasia. The most common cause of secondary hyperparathyroidism is chronic renal failure.

Clinical manifestations

Increased parathyroid hormone causes retention of calcium; therefore, the clinical manifestations are those of hypercalcemia, including (1) bone resorption with signs of rickets, skeletal pain, and pathologic fractures; (2) hypercalciuria and associated deposition of calcium in the kidney, which produce renal calculi; (3) decreased neuromuscular irritability, such as muscular weakness, constipation, bradycardia, and cardiac irregularities; and (4) central nervous system disturbances, especially lethargy, stupor, and sometimes psychosis. The most common symptoms are caused by renal involvement, particularly polyuria, polydipsia, dysuria, nocturia, and renal colic. Advanced renal destruction may cause kidney failure.

Diagnostic evaluation

Blood studies reveal elevated calcium and lowered phosphorus levels. Measurement of parathormone, as well as several tests to isolate the cause of the hypercalcemia, such as renal function studies, are included. Other procedures employed to evaluate the physiologic consequences of the disorder include electrocardiography and radiographic bone surveys.

Therapeutic management

Treatment is directly related to the etiology of hyperparathyroidism. The treatment of primary hyperparathyroidism is surgical removal of the hyperplastic tissue. Whenever possible the underlying cause contributing to secondary hyperparathyroidism is treated, which consequently restores the serum calcium balance. However, in some instances the underlying disorder is irreversible, such as in chronic renal failure. In this instance treatment is the same as that discussed for renal osteodystrophy (p. 796).

Nursing considerations

Much of the initial nursing care is related to the physical symptoms and prevention of complications. To minimize renal calculi formation, hydration is essential. Fruit juices that maintain a low urinary pH, such as cranberry or apple juice, are encouraged, since acidity of body fluids promotes calcium resorption. All urine should be strained for evidence of renal casts.

Safety precautions, such as side rails in place at all times and assistance with ambulation, are instituted because of the tendency toward fractures and muscular weakness. Children with renal rickets (osteodystrophy) may wear braces to correct skeletal deformities. These are worn as prescribed. If the child is confined to bed, the physical therapist is consulted regarding proper use of orthopedic appliances.

Vital signs are taken frequently, and the pulse is counted for 1 full minute to detect irregularities. A decrease in pulse rate is reported, since it may signal severe bradycardia and cardiac arrest. The diet needs supervision to ensure compliance with low-phosphate foods, particularly dairy products. The nurse instructs parents regarding foods that need to be avoided and the necessity of administering calcium and vitamin D.

If surgery is anticipated the care is similar to that discussed for the child with hyperthyroidism. Since hypocalcemia is a potential complication, the nurse observes for signs of tetany, institutes seizure precautions, and has calcium gluconate available for emergency use.

ADRENAL CORTEX DYSFUNCTION

The adrenal cortex secretes three main groups of hormones collectively called steroids and classified according to their biologic activity: (1) glucocorticoids (cortisol, corticosterone), (2) mineralocorticoids (aldosterone), and (3) sex steroids (androgens, estrogens, and progestins). Alterations in the levels of these hormones produce significant dysfunction in a variety of body tissues and organs. Most are rare in children.

Disorders of adrenocortical hypofunction include adrenal hypoplasia, Addison disease, and adrenal crisis. The disorders of adrenocortical hyperfunction may be related to an excessive production of any of the hormones, such as cortisol (Cushing syndrome), androgens (adrenogenital syndrome), aldosterone (primary hyperaldosteronism), and estrogens (adrenal feminization syndrome). Since the adrenocortical cells are capable of producing any of the steroids, pathologic conditions may result in a deficiency or an excess of more than one type of hormone.

ADRENOCORTICAL INSUFFICIENCY

Deficient cortisol and/or aldosterone secretion can be caused by numerous disorders of the hypothalamus, pituitary gland, or adrenal cortex. They can be acute or chronic, mild or severe, transient or permanent, congenital or acquired, and present at any time during infancy and childhood. Some of the more common etiologic factors include hemorrhage into the gland from trauma, including a prolonged, difficult labor; fulminating infections, such as meningococcemia, which result in hemorrhage and necrosis (Waterhouse-Friderichsen syndrome); abrupt withdrawal of exogenous sources of cortisone or failure to increase exogenous supplies during stress; and destructive lesions of the adrenal cortex, which cause the most common disorder in older children, *Addison disease*.

Clinical manifestations

The age of onset and clinical manifestations depend upon the etiology of the disorder:

Adrenal hypoplasia. Signs of primary adrenal aplasia or hypoplasia are evident shortly after birth and are primarily those of salt loss—failure to thrive, lethargy, poor feeding, vomiting, and dehydration.

Addison disease. In older children the signs and symptoms of Addison disease, or chronic adrenocortical insufficiency, are muscular weakness, lassitude, mental fatigue, weight loss and general wasting, anorexia, and low blood pressure. There may be recurrent unexplained convulsions, an intense craving for salt, and acute abdominal pain.

Pigmentary changes of the skin, first noticeable on the face and hands and over pressure points (elbows, knees, or waist) should alert the observer to the possibility of adrenocortical insufficiency. Hyperpigmentation of freckles and scars is especially pronounced.

Adrenal crisis. Adrenal crisis, or acute adrenal insufficiency, may occur if the condition is not recognized, usually in the child with undiagnosed Addison disease, withdrawal of corticosteroid therapy, and during complications in Addison disease. The child is in a shocklike state with a weak, rapid pulse, decreased blood pressure, shallow and rapid respirations, cold clammy skin, and cyanosis. Without immediate therapy the condition progresses rapidly to circulatory collapse and death.

Adrenal crisis in the newborn is accompanied by extreme hyperpyrexia, tachypnea, cyanosis, and convulsions. Usually there is no evidence of infection or purpura. However, hemorrhage into the adrenal gland may be evident as a palpable retroperitoneal mass.

Diagnostic evaluation

There is no rapid, definitive test for confirmation of acute adrenocortical insufficiency. Diagnosis is usually made on clinical presentation, especially when a fulminating sepsis is accompanied by hemorrhagic manifestations and signs of circulatory collapse despite adequate antibiotic therapy.

Diagnosis of Addison disease is based on measurements of functional cortisol reserve. The cortisol and urinary 17-hydroxycorticosterone levels are low and fail to rise while plasma ACTH levels are elevated with corticotropin (ACTH) stimulation, the definitive test for the disease.

Therapeutic management

Treatment of acute adrenal insufficiency must be immediate and vigorous. It consists of intravenous replacement of cortisol, fluid replacement, administration of glucose solutions to correct hypoglycemia, and specific antibiotic therapy in the presence of infection. Salt-retaining hormones may be needed initially to restore serum sodium and potassium to normal levels rapidly.

For the treatment of Addison disease, most children are maintained on oral supplements of cortisol (cortisone or hydrocortisone preparations) with a liberal intake of salt. A salt-retaining hormone is administered only to those children with aldosterone deficiency. In the event of surgery, complicating bacterial infections, or other severe stresses parenteral steroid therapy may be needed to sustain the child through the stressful period.

Nursing considerations

Infants or children with adrenal crisis require intensive nursing care. Once the disorder is diagnosed and the crisis period is over, parents need guidance concerning drug therapy. For the child with Addison disease they must be aware of the continuous need for cortisol replacement. Sudden termination of the drug because of inadequate supplies or inability to ingest the oral form because of vomiting places the child in danger of an acute adrenal crisis. Therefore, parents should always have a spare supply of the medication in the home. Ideally they should have a prefilled syringe of hydrocortisone in the home and be instructed in proper technique for intramuscular administration of the drug in case of a crisis. Unnecessary administration of cortisone will not harm the child but, if needed, may be lifesaving. Any evidence of adrenal crisis is reported to the physician immediately.

Parents also need to be aware of side effects of the drugs. Undesirable side effects of cortisone include gastric irritation (which is minimized by ingestion with food or the use of an antacid), increased excitability and sleeplessness, weight gain that may require dietary management to prevent obesity, and, rarely, behavioral changes, including depression or euphoria.

Since the body cannot supply endogenous sources of cortical hormones during times of stress, the home environment should be stable and relatively unstressful. The child should wear a Medic Alert tag to permit medical personnel to adjust his requirements during emergency care.

CUSHING SYNDROME

Cushing syndrome is a characteristic pattern of obesity, often with hypertension, and short stature. The disorder is the result of maintaining abnormally high levels of glucocorticoids over a period of time. The source of the hormones can be in the pituitary gland, the adrenal gland, or exogenous. It can be caused by tumors, primary hyperplasia of the adrenals, or administration of steroids. Cushing syndrome is rare in children and when seen is often caused by excessive or prolonged steroid therapy that produces a cushingoid appearance.

Clinical manifestations

The physical features of Cushing syndrome are truncal obesity, with thin extremities, pendulous abdomen with purple striae, fat pads on the neck and back ("buffalo hump"), and rounded or "moon" face. Masculinization is often evident. There is weakness, plethora ("red cheeks"), easy bruisability, poor wound healing, growth retardation, and increased susceptibility to infection.

Diagnostic evaluation

Excess cortisol levels can be measured in blood and urine, especially 24-hour collections. Blood sugar levels are usually elevated and osteoporosis may be evident on roentgenographs. Special studies are needed to differentiate between adrenal hyperplasia and tumors, one of which is the dexamethasone (cortisone) suppression test. Administration of an exogenous supply of cortisone normally suppresses adrenocorticotropic hormone production. However, in individuals with Cushing syndrome, cortisol levels remain elevated. This test is also helpful in differentiating between children who are obese and those who have Cushing syndrome.

Therapeutic management

Treatment depends on the cause. Tumors are removed surgically. If the entire gland is removed hormone replacement therapy is implemented and may be continued indefinitely. The condition is reversible when cushingoid features are caused by steroid therapy, once the steroids are discontinued. Gradual withdrawal of exogenous supplies is necessary to allow the anterior pituitary an opportunity to secrete increasing amounts of adrenocorticotropic hormone to stimulate the adrenals to produce cortisol. Abrupt withdrawal will precipitate acute adrenal insufficiency.

Nursing considerations

Nursing care is related to the cause and treatment regime. If the cushingoid features are the result of steroid therapy, the main intervention is to ensure that parents know and realize the importance of correct drug administration.

When cushingoid features are caused by steroid therapy, the effects may be lessened with administration of the drug early in the morning and on an alternate-day basis. Giving the drug early in the day maintains the normal diurnal pattern of cortisol secretion. An alternate-day schedule allows the anterior pituitary an opportunity to maintain more normal hypothalamic-pituitary-adrenal control mechanisms.

If surgery is contemplated, parents need to be adequately informed of the operative benefits and disadvantages. They will also require education regarding drug administration following surgery and the signs and symptoms of complications.

ADRENOGENITAL SYNDROME (AGS)

Adrenogenital syndrome, also known as *adrenocortical hyperplasia* and *congenital adrenocortical hyperplasia*, is the result of excessive secretion of androgens by the adrenal cortex. Although hyperfunction of the adrenal gland can occur from a number of causes, such as a virilizing adrenal tumor and maternal ingestion of steroids during pregnancy, in children the most common is congenital adrenogenital hyperplasia (CAH), an inborn deficiency of any of several enzymes necessary for the biosynthesis of cortisol. Congenital adrenogenital hyperplasia is inherited as an autosomal-recessive disorder.

Pathophysiology

Interference with the biosynthesis of cortisol during fetal life results in an increased production of adrenocorticotropic hormone, which stimulates hyperplasia of the adrenal gland. This causes an increased secretion of hormones not dependent on cortisol precursors, primarily the adrenal androgens. The amount of cortisol and aldosterone secreted depends on the enzyme involved and the extent of its deficiency.

Clinical manifestations

Excessive secretion of androgens cause masculinization of the urogenital system during fetal development. The most pronounced abnormalities occur in the female, who is born with varying degrees of ambiguous genitalia (pseudohermaphroditism). The enlarged clitoris appears to be a small phallus and labial fusion produces a saclike structure resembling the scrotum without testes. However, no abnormal changes occur in the internal sexual organs, although the vaginal orifice is usually closed by the fused labia.

In the male enlargement of the genitals (macrogenitosomia precox) and frequent erections are the principal signs. When androgen production is not excessive, virilizing effects in the female may be minimal or absent and the male may have evidence of pseudohermaphroditism, such as microphallus, hypospadias, and incompletely fused scrotum.

Untreated congenital adrenogenital hyperplasia results in early sexual maturation, with enlargement of the external sexual organs; axillary, pubic, and facial hair; deepening of the voice; acne; and marked increase in musculature with changes toward an adult male physique. However, in contrast to precocious puberty, breasts do not develop in the female, and she remains amenorrheic and infertile. In the boy the testes remain small and spermatogenesis does not occur. In both sexes linear growth is accelerated and epiphyseal closure is premature, resulting in short stature by the end of puberty.

Diagnostic evaluation

Clinical diagnosis is initially based on congenital abnormalities that lead to difficulty in assigning sex to the newborn and on signs and symptoms of adrenal insufficiency or hypertension. Definitive diagnosis is confirmed by evidence of increased 17-ketosteroid levels in most types of congenital adrenogenital hyperplasia. Blood electrolytes demonstrate loss of sodium and chloride and elevation of potassium. In older children bone age is advanced and linear growth is increased. A buccal smear for positive sex determination should always be done in any case of ambiguous genitalia.

Visualizing the presence of pelvic structures by ultrasonography is especially useful in congenital adrenogenital hyperplasia because it readily identifies the absence or presence of female reproductive organs in a newborn or child with ambiguous genitalia.

Therapeutic management

The initial medical objective is to confirm the diagnosis and assign a sex to the child, usually in accordance with the genotype (see also p. 807). In both sexes cortisone is administered to suppress the abnormally high secretions of adrenocorticotropic hormone. As a result the signs and symptoms of masculinization in the female gradually disappear and excessive early linear growth is slowed. Puberty occurs normally at the appropriate age. In those children with the salt-losing type of congenital adrenogenital hyperplasia, the replacement of aldosterone as is outlined under chronic adrenal insufficiency is instituted. Because these children, particularly infants, are prone to adrenal crises during periods of stress, they may require the same emergency treatment as discussed for adrenal crisis.

Depending on the degree of masculinization in the female, reconstructive surgery may be required to reduce the size of the clitoris, separate the labia, and create a vaginal orifice. This should be done after the infant is physically able to withstand the procedure and before she is old enough to be aware of the abnormal genitalia. Plastic reconstruction is generally performed in stages and yields excellent cosmetic results. Reports concerning sexual satisfaction after partial clitoridectomy indicate that the capacity for orgasm and sexual gratification is not necessarily impaired.

Unfortunately all children with congenital adrenogenital hyperplasia are not diagnosed at birth and are raised

SUMMARY OF NURSING CARE OF THE CHILD WITH ADRENOGENITAL SYNDROME

GOALS	RESPONSIBILITIES
Recognize adrenogenital syndrome early	Assess newborn infants for signs of virilization, especially infants with ambiguous genitalia Suspect possibility in older children 　　Female: Masculinized external genitalia 　　Male: Early sexual maturation
Assist with diagnosis	Collect urine specimen for routine examination and 24-hour specimen for steroids Take buccal smear for sex chromatin tests Collect or order blood for analysis Assist with ultrasonography and radiographic examinations
Replace adrenal hormone	Administer cortisone preparation as prescribed
Prevent complications	Be alert for signs of impending adrenal crisis Be alert to evidence of salt loss
Assign correct gender	Assess genitalia carefully Assist with or perform diagnostic tests for gender
Assist in preparation for surgical correction	Prepare child and family for surgical procedure in manner appropriate to age of child and type of surgery anticipated
Support parents	Explain and clarify explanations of disorder and tests being performed Use correct vocabulary when discussing sex organs Allow for expression of feelings Help parents to cope with a delay in infant's sex determination Provide parents with information and support in explaining disorder to others Instruct parents regarding administration of medication and observing for signs of crisis Secure psychiatric consultation if indicated Refer to supportive agencies as appropriate Refer for genetic counseling

according to their assigned sex rather than their genetic sex. This usually occurs in affected females when masculinization of the external genitalia may have led to sex assignment as a male. Because of the psychologic trauma in these situations it is advisable to continue rearing the child as a male in accordance with his assigned sex and phenotype. Hormonal replacement is required to permit linear growth and to initiate male pubertal changes. Surgery is usually indicated to remove the female organs and reconstruct the phallus for satisfactory sexual relations. Obviously these individuals are not fertile.

Nursing considerations

Of major importance is recognition of ambiguous genitalia in newborns. If there is any question regarding assignment of sex, the parents need to be told immediately to prevent the embarrassing situation of informing family members of the child's sex and then having to change the pronouncement. As with any congenital defect, the parents require an adequate explanation of the condition and a period of time to grieve for the loss of perfection.

Parents need an explanation regarding this disorder that facilitates their explaining it to others. Prior to confirmation of the diagnosis and sex, the nurse should refer to the infant as "child" or "baby" rather than by the pronouns "he" or "she" and definitely not "it." When referring to the external genitalia, it is preferable to refer to them as sex organs and to emphasize the similarity between the penis/clitoris and scrotum/labia during fetal development. In this way one can explain that the sex organs were overdeveloped because of secretion of too much male hormone. Using a correct vocabulary allows parents to explain the abnormalities to others in a straightforward manner as they would if the defect involved the heart or an extremity.

The nurse also stresses that sex assignment and rearing depend on psychosocial influences, not on genetic sex or hormonal influences during fetal life. Parents often fear that the infant will retain "male behavioral characteristics'' because of prenatal masculinization and will not be able to develop "feminism." Using the word "hermaphrodite" is erroneous and often confuses parents because they interpret this term to mean that the child is "half male–half female." It is also beneficial to mention that ambiguous genitalia have no relationship with homosexual or bisexual activity later in life.

In the unfortunate situation in which sex is erroneously assigned and later diagnosed, parents need a great deal of help in understanding the reason for the incorrect sex identity and the options for sex reassignment and/or medical/surgical intervention. Since children become aware of their sexual identity by 18 months to 2 years of age, it is believed that any reassignment after this period can cause tremendous psychologic conflicts in the child. Therefore, sex rearing should be continued as previously established with medical/surgical intervention as required. (See the discussion of ambiguous genitalia in Chapter 24.)

Since congenital adrenogenital hyperplasia is an autosomal-recessive disorder, parents are referred for genetic counseling prior to conceiving another child (see p. 57). Advice regarding cortisol and aldosterone replacement is the same as that discussed under chronic adrenocortical insufficiency.

ADRENAL MEDULLA DYSFUNCTION

The adrenal medulla secretes the catecholamines epinephrine and norepinephrine. Both hormones have essentially the same effects on various organs as those caused by direct sympathetic stimulation, except that the hormonal effects last several times longer. Catecholamine-secreting tumors are the primary cause of adrenal medullary hyperfunction. In children the most common neoplasms of this type are pheochromocytoma, neuroblastoma, and ganglioneuroma.

PHEOCHROMOCYTOMA

Pheochromocytomas in children are frequently bilateral or multiple and are generally benign. Often there is a familial transmission of the condition as an autosomal-dominant trait that tends to favor males.

The clinical manifestations of pheochromocytoma are caused by an increased production of the catecholamines, causing hypertension, tachycardia, headache, decreased gastrointestinal activity evidenced by constipation, and increased metabolism with anorexia, weight loss, hyperglycemia, polyuria, polydipsia, hyperventilation, nervousness, and diaphoresis. In severe cases signs of congestive

heart failure are evident. Definitive treatment consists of surgical removal of the tumor.

Nursing considerations

Prior to surgical removal vital signs are monitored frequently. The nurse observes for evidence of hypertensive attacks, congestive heart failure, and hyperglycemia, including daily urine tests for sugar and acetone.

The environment should be conducive to rest and free from emotional stress. Adequate preparation for and during hospital admission and prior to surgery is essential. Parents should be encouraged to room-in with their child and to participate in his care. Play activities are tailored to the child's energy level but are not overly strenuous or challenging, since these can increase the metabolic rate and create frustration and anxiety.

After surgery the child is observed for signs of shock and removal of excess catecholamines. If a bilateral adrenalectomy is performed, the nursing interventions are the same as those discussed for adrenal insufficiency.

PANCREATIC HORMONE DYSFUNCTION

The islets of Langerhans of the pancreas have three major functioning cells:

1. The alpha cells produce glucagon, which increases the blood glucose levels by stimulating the liver and other cells to release stored glucose (glycogenolysis).
2. The beta cells produce insulin, which lowers blood glucose levels by facilitating the entrance of glucose into the cells for metabolism.
3. The delta cells produce somatostatin, which is believed to regulate the release of insulin and glucagon.

The discussion of disorders of pancreatic hormone secretion is limited to diabetes mellitus.

DIABETES MELLITUS

Diabetes mellitus is a disorder involving primarily carbohydrate metabolism that is characterized by a deficiency or diminished effectiveness of the hormone insulin. Without insulin, except for a very few specialized cells, the body is unable to metabolize carbohydrates adequately. It is the most frequent endocrine disorder of childhood.

Classification

To reduce confusion and facilitate communication among health professionals, a revised classification of the disease has been issued by the National Diabetes Data Group. This incorporates newer concepts into the terminology. The terms with which nurses should become familiar relative to children are:

Diabetes mellitus—previously qualified with the term "overt." The disease is further delineated as:

Insulin dependent (IDDM), or **type I**—formerly called "juvenile-onset diabetes," "juvenile onset–type diabetes," "ketosis-prone diabetes," and "brittle diabetes." It is characterized by catabolism and the development of ketosis in the absence of insulin replacement therapy. Onset is typically in childhood and adolescence but can be at any age. The disease has distinctive associations with inheritance of histocompatibility antigens and organ-specific autoimmunity, although there is much evidence for heterogeneity within this subclass.

Noninsulin dependent (NIDDM), or **type II**—previously known as "adult-onset diabetes," "maturity-onset diabetes," "maturity onset–type diabetes," "nonketosis-prone diabetes," or "stable diabetes." Adolescents with this type are obese. When the condition occurs in nonobese young people, it tends to be strongly familial and apparently autosomal dominant and thus referred to as maturity-onset diabetes of the young. There appears to be considerable heterogeneity within this clinical category, as well as in IDDM.

Other types (including diabetes associated with certain conditions and syndromes)—this category includes secondary diabetes, such as steroid-induced diabetes as well as primary diabetes associated with genetic syndromes, drug- or chemical-induced diabetes, and diabetes resulting from pancreatectomy for hypoglycemia. Syndromes with insulin receptor abnormality are classified in this group.

Etiology

Heredity is unquestioned as a prominent factor in the etiology of diabetes mellitus, although the mechanism of inheritance is unknown. A variety of genetic mechanisms have been proposed, but most favor a multifactorial inheritance or a recessive gene somehow linked to the tissue-typing antigens, the human leukocyte–A (HL-A) system. However, the inheritance of type I and type II diabetes appears to be different. Nearly 100% of offspring of parents who both have type II diabetes develop that type of diabetes, but only 45% to 60% of the offspring of both parents who have type I will develop the disease.

An autoimmune response to viruses has been proposed as an etiologic factor in development of diabetes. Tumors of the pancreas, pancreatitis, stress drugs such as steroids, stress diseases that involve other endocrine organs, and viral diseases are now believed to play a part in causing diabetes. There is also an increased risk of diabetes with obesity.

Pathophysiology

Insulin deficiency brings about metabolic adjustments or physiologic changes in almost all areas of the body. In type II diabetes disturbed carbohydrate metabolism may be a result of a sluggish or insensitive secretory response in the pancreas or a defect in body tissues that requires unusual amounts of insulin, or the insulin secreted may be rapidly destroyed, inhibited, or inactivated in affected persons. A lack of insulin because of reduction in islet cell mass or destruction of the islets is the hallmark of the person with type I diabetes.

Insulin is needed for the entry of glucose into the muscle and fat cells, for the prevention of mobilization of fats from fat cells, and for storage of glucose as glycogen in the cells of liver and muscle. (Insulin is not needed for the entry of glucose into nerve cells or vascular tissue.) When insulin is unable to enter the cell its concentration in the bloodstream increases, producing an osmotic gradient that causes the movement of body fluid from the intracellular space to the extracellular space and into the glomerular filtrate in order to "dilute" the hyperosmolar filtrate. Normally the renal tubular capacity to transport glucose is adequate to reabsorb all the glucose in the glomerular filtrate. When the glucose concentration in the glomerular filtrate exceeds the threshold (180 mg/100 ml), glucose "spills" into the urine (glycosuria) along with water causing *polyuria,* one of the cardinal signs of diabetes. The urinary fluid losses are the cause of the excessive thirst *(polydipsia)* observed in diabetes. As might be expected, this water washout results in a depletion of other essential chemicals from the body.

The child may be *hyperglycemic,* with elevated blood glucose levels and glucose in the urine; may be in *diabetic ketosis,* with ketones as well as glucose in the urine but not noticeably dehydrated; or may be in *diabetic ketoacidosis,* with dehydration, electrolyte imbalance, and acidosis.

Ketoacidosis. When insulin is deficient, glucose is unavailable for cellular metabolism and the body chooses alternate sources of fuel. Consequently fats break down into fatty acids and glycerol in the fat cells and in the liver and are converted to ketone bodies (β-hydroxybutyric acid, acetoacetic acid, and acetone), which are used as the alternative to glucose as a source of fuel but are utilized in the cells at a limited rate. Ketones are organic acids that readily produce excessive quantities of free hydrogen ions, causing acidosis. The respiratory buffering system attempts to eliminate the excess carbon dioxide by increased depth and rate—*Kussmaul respirations,* the hyperventilation characteristic of metabolic acidosis. Excess ketones are excreted by the urine and lungs, producing acetone in the urine *(ketonuria)* and the characteristic acetone odor to the breath.

Protein is also wasted during insulin deficiency. Since glucose is unable to enter the cells, protein is broken down and converted to glucose by the liver *(glucogenesis)*. This new glucose contributes further to the hyperglycemia.

If these conditions are not reversed by insulin therapy in combination with correction of the fluid deficiency and electrolyte imbalance, progressive deterioration occurs with dehydration, electrolyte imbalance, acidosis, coma, and death.

Clinical manifestations

The child may start wetting the bed, become grouchy and "not himself," or act overly tired. Abdominal discomfort is common. Weight loss, though quite observable on the charts, may be a less frequent presenting complaint because of the fact that the family might not have noticed the change. Another outstanding sign of overt diabetes is thirst. At a certain point in the illness the child may actually refuse fluid and food, adding to the increasing state of dehydration and malnutrition.

The sequence of chemical events described previously results in hyperglycemia and acidosis, which in turn produce the three "polys" of diabetes—polyphagia, or frequent eating associated with weight loss; polydipsia, or frequent water drinking; and polyuria, or frequent urination—the cardinal symptoms of the disease. Other symptoms are dry skin, blurred vision, and sores that are slow to heal. More commonly in children, tiredness and bedwetting are the chief complaints that prompt parents to take their child to the physician.

Diagnostic evaluation

The urine test will show positive glucose only when the disease is actually manifest. A negative urine test does not necessarily rule out early diabetes, nor does a positive test necessarily indicate diabetes. For example, renal glycosuria, unrelated to diabetes, can result in glucose in the urine. The fasting blood glucose test may miss the diagnosis of early diabetes and has been known to miss as many as 85% of children who had an abnormal glucose tolerance test with asymptomatic disease. The 4-hour glucose tolerance test has been found to be the most useful test for the diagnosis of early or chemical diabetes, whereas the 6-hour glucose tolerance test is most helpful for the diagnosis of hypoglycemia. To make the information more meaningful, insulin values should also be obtained during glucose tolerance testing.

Therapeutic management

The management program for any child with diabetes mellitus should be flexible with 24-hour insulin coverage and designed to accommodate the child's life-style. The insulin treatment is based on the understanding that the effective duration of action of insulin in children may be somewhat different from that in adults. In children the duration of effective action for intermediate-acting insulin has been found to be 12 to 14 hours. Lente insulin is the longest acting of the intermediate-acting insulins, but even it lasts only 14 to 16 hours (Table 26-2).

The most commonly used insulins are the intermediate-acting insulins, principally NPH, which are usually given in a single early morning dose combined with a small amount of short-acting insulin (usually regular). Both are available in either purified animal insulin, obtained from beef or pork pancreata, or human insulin (Humulin), derived from modified bacterial sources. Only regular insulin can be administered intravenously.

The diabetic child may be admitted to the hospital under several circumstances. The newly diagnosed child is usually admitted for definitive diagnosis and regulation of insulin dosage. During nondiabetes-related illnesses, such as an acute infection or surgery, the child frequently requires adjustment of insulin. The reaction that may be the initial manifestation of the disease or a severe response to physical or emotional stress is diabetic ketoacidosis. The other serious response that affects diabetic persons is hypoglycemia.

Diabetic ketoacidosis (DKA).   Diabetic ketoacidosis, the most complete state of insulin deficiency, is a life-threatening situation that was once synonymous with death. Management with adequate insulin, along with fluids and appropriate electrolytes, can reverse the ketoacidosis within a few hours. The insulin is administered in one of two ways:

1. The initial dose of regular insulin is administered intravenously as a bolus—some give half the dose as a bolus and half subcutaneously. This initial dose is followed by subcutaneous administration in 3 to 4 hours, again in 3 to 4 hours, and then every 6 hours until ketoacidosis is relieved.
2. Regular insulin is infused intravenously and the dose is controlled at a rate to lower the blood glucose about 100 mg/100 ml/hour until a blood glucose level of about 200 mg/100 ml is reached. Subcutaneous insulin is then instituted.

Vital signs, hourly blood sugar determinations, and cardiac monitoring are other parameters to observe. The cardiac monitor is employed to determine changes in the potassium levels of the child (a U wave after the T wave will indicate hypokalemia; an elevated and spreading T wave indicates increasingly abnormal hyperkalemia). Blood sugar measurements are made with a glucose monitor, which gives a digital readout of blood glucose. If a glucose monitor is not available, reagent strips (such as Dextrostix, Chemstrip bG, or Visidex) can be used. However, these are best read in the specially designed reflectance meters following the manufacturer's directions to en-

TABLE 26-2. ONSET, PEAK, AND DURATION OF ACTION FOR VARIOUS INSULIN PREPARATIONS IN CHILDREN

TYPE OF INSULIN	ONSET (hours after administration)	PEAK (hours)	EFFECTIVE DURATION OF ACTION (hours)
Short acting			
Crystalline zinc (regular insulin)*	½-1	2-4	6-8
Semilente (prompt insulin zinc suspension)	½-1	2-4	8-10
Intermediate acting			
Globin zinc (globulin zinc insulin)	1-2	6-8	12-14
Isophane (neutral protamine Hagedorn [NPH])*	1-2	6-8 +	12-14
Lente (insulin zinc suspension; 30% Semilente and 70% Ultralente)	1-2 +	8-12	14-16
Longer acting			
Ultralente (extended insulin zinc suspension)	4-6	8-12	24-36
Protamine zinc (protamine zinc insulin suspension [PZI])	4-6	18 +	36-72

*Available as human insulin as well as animal insulin.

sure accuracy of the test. Urine examinations for sugar and acetone are performed periodically.

Plasma expanders may be administered during the initial phase of treatment of diabetic ketoacidosis in order to establish renal blood flow. The fluids may then be changed to balanced solutions with dextrose as soon as plasma expansion is accomplished. Potassium is added as soon as renal output is established. Bicarbonate is added if the pH and/or serum bicarbonate levels are quite low.

Once the child has recovered from the most acute state, regular insulin is administered on a proportional basis. As oral feedings are tolerated, clear liquids are advanced to soft foods and then to a regular diet, in a three-meal, bedtime snack pattern. Blood glucose measurements (by glucose monitor) are made before meals and at bedtime.

If a glucose monitor is unavailable, urine samples are obtained in either of two methods—double-voided specimens or collected as fractional or block specimens:

1. Double-voided specimens are obtained by having the child void one half hour before the measurement is needed. This specimen is measured and discarded. A second voiding one half hour later is collected and measured for glucose and acetone. Specimens are tested before meals and at bedtime.
2. Measurements are made on fractional specimens of all urine voided, from before breakfast to before lunch, from before lunch to before supper, from before supper to about 11 PM, and from 11 PM to before breakfast. A Clinitest, Acetest, and total urine volume are recorded for each fraction.

Insulin dosages are adjusted according to the previous day's tests. U100 insulin is used but can be diluted for

readability and accuracy to U50, U25, or U10, as necessary. Once the child is stabilized on regular insulin, the total amount of insulin is gradually decreased. A split-dose insulin schedule and a three-meal, three-snack feeding pattern are begun. NPH and regular insulin are given together. Two thirds of the total daily dose of insulin is given about ½ hour before breakfast, and one third is given ½ hour before supper. Hypoglycemia should be avoided at this time.

Hypoglycemia. Low blood glucose levels can be equally as life threatening as elevated blood glucose levels. Just as administering insulin to the individual with diabetic ketoacidosis is an emergency, so is administering glucose to the individual with hypoglycemia. The brain depends on glucose, therefore, lack of this essential nutrient can cause coma and even permanent brain damage. Neurologic signs and symptoms appear when the blood glucose drops below about 30 mg/100 ml.

The causes of hypoglycemia are opposite of those for diabetic ketoacidosis. They include the ingestion of too little food, the increase in exercise without adequate food support, or the increase in insulin, whether accidental or on purpose, without adequate support by additional food. Gastroenteritis, in which there is a gastric stasis, may impede the absorption of food, resulting in hypoglycemia, and is probably the most threatening cause of hypoglycemia.

A mild insulin reaction is one that is described as the body's response to a falling blood sugar level. Epinephrine is released, causing the feelings of hunger, increased pulse rate, hyperactivity, increased respiratory rate, and weakness. Epinephrine triggers a glycogenolysis, which will raise the blood glucose level. If the blood glucose level

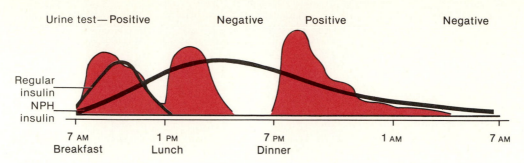

Fig. 26-1

Relationships between insulin levels, blood glucose levels, and meals. Red areas indicate blood sugar levels. (Adapted from Travis, L.B.: An instructional aid on juvenile diabetes mellitus, ed. 6, Galveston, Tex., Univ. of Texas Medical Branch, 1980.)

falls further, cerebral function may be affected. Symptoms include yawning, lethargy, and increasing difficulty in the thought process, along with irritability and belligerence. Food taken when the initial symptoms appear in their mildest form reverses the lowered blood glucose level. Milk is a very good food to use in children.

Moderate insulin reactions result from more severe lowering of the blood glucose level with a decline in cerebral activity and a more profound sympathetic response. Sweating, if not generalized, becomes noticeable on the extremities, the back of the neck, and the axilla area. Extreme nervousness and tremors may be noted. Stomachache and headache are common complaints. Vomiting may shortly follow. The pulse rate will usually increase and become stronger. Blood pressure may become lower, leading to faintness or dizziness. Blurring of vision may be noted at this state. Treatment must be with a simple sugar, preferably in the form of concentrated sugar. The simpler the sugar, the more rapidly it is absorbed. The treatment may be repeated in 10 to 15 minutes if the initial response is not satisfactory. With good response to the simple sugar, the pulse rate should show a noticeable change in 2 to 3 minutes. Rest and the addition of food should be part of the plan.

The severe insulin reaction is often the most feared aspect of having diabetes, since severe brain symptoms may develop. The signs of hypoglycemia include (in order of appearance): increased drowsiness, perspiration, tachycardia, loss of consciousness, seizure activity, deeper coma, and decreasing reflexes. The treatment of choice is 50% glucose administered intravenously.

Glucagon is sometimes prescribed for home treatment of hypoglycemia. It is available as a tablet to be mixed with diluting fluid from its accompanying bottle and is administered intramuscularly or subcutaneously. It requires about 15 to 20 minutes to elevate the blood glucose level by releasing the stored glucose from the liver. Once the child is responsive, the lost glycogen stores are replaced

by small amounts of sugar-containing fluid administered frequently until the child feels comfortable about trying solid foods.

With few exceptions hypoglycemia is preventable and efforts are made to modify management to avoid this complication. For example, more food is needed for more activity, and less food is needed for less activity. The extra food for activity is given preferably before the activity and repeated for increased activity every 45 to 60 minutes if activity continues. The only "excuse" for a severe insulin reaction is the development of unknown gastroenteritis.

Somogyi reflex should be recognized as a separate response, although not actually an acute emergency. This phenomenon is a physiologic reflex that occurs when the blood glucose level decreases to the point where stress hormones (epinephrine, growth hormone, and corticosteroids) are released causing the blood glucose level to rise. Instead of the expected decrease in blood glucose level with exercise, the blood glucose level is raised. The treatment is to increase the food and/or decrease the insulin.

Chronic care. Chronic care consists of a flexible, individualized program of day-to-day management, usually supervised on an outpatient basis. The more frequent use of short-acting insulin adds more flexibility to the individual's program, and the intermediate-acting insulins administered with an adequate overlap give satisfactory 24-hour insulinization. The split-dose insulin schedule, using mixtures of regular and intermediate-acting insulins twice daily, is the closest approximation of a four-dose schedule of regular insulin without giving four shots per day (Fig. 26-1).

A three-meal, three-snack feeding pattern is the most common pattern used for young children, and the distribution of calories can be altered to fit the activity pattern of any individual child. For example, the child who is more active in the afternoon will need the larger snack at that time. This larger snack might also be split to allow some food at school and some food after school. Alterations in food intake should be made so that food, insulin, and exercise are balanced. Extra food is needed for extra activity.

The food intake may be planned in a variety of ways. The family may follow the more conventional exchange system approved by the American Diabetes Association (ADA) or the approach called the point system, which is based on 75 kcal equaling 1 point. Concentrated sweets are eliminated, and foods are chosen from food groups similar to the basic four. Since the carbohydrate content of the diet does not have, in the majority of instances, a specific effect on blood glucose elevation, carbohydrates are not restricted except for simple sugars.

Exercise should be encouraged and never restricted unless other health conditions necessitate it. Insulin in children should not be reduced for increased activity unless the needed increase in food cannot be tolerated.

Blood glucose or urine records should be reviewed by the family weekly. At these times they look for frequent, even if insignificant, insulin reactions and plan to increase food or decrease the insulin. If urine testing is used instead of blood glucose monitoring, the tests are sometimes based on first-voided urine specimens, as it is difficult to obtain a second-voided specimen from a child. The first-voided urine test provides information about how the food is being handled by the insulin in relation to the exercise over a period of time rather than at a point in time. Some authorities, however, prefer second-voided specimens. The type of specimen obtained is recorded with the results of the test. In general a urine glucose level of +1 is considered to indicate adequate control because it reflects a slight spillage of sugar, ruling out hypoglycemia, and insufficient glucose to produce hyperglycemia.

Nursing considerations: acute care

Diabetic children in the hospital are generally admitted at the time of their initial diagnosis, during illness or surgery, or for episodes of ketoacidosis, which may be precipitated by any of a variety of factors. Most diabetic children are able to keep the disease under control with periodic assessment and adjustment of insulin, diet, and activity as needed under the supervision of the physician. Except for unusual circumstances these children can be managed very well at home. However, there are a small number of diabetic children (''brittle'' diabetics) who exhibit a degree of metabolic lability and who have repeated episodes of diabetic ketoacidosis that require hospitalization, which interferes with education and social development.

It is often difficult to distinguish between ketoacidosis and a hypoglycemic reaction (Table 26-3). Since the symptoms are similar and usually begin with changes in behavior, the simplest way to differentiate between the two

TABLE 26-3. COMPARISON OF MANIFESTATIONS OF HYPOGLYCEMIA AND HYPERGLYCEMIA

	HYPOGLYCEMIA	HYPERGLYCEMIA
Onset	Rapid	Gradual
Cause	Too much insulin Increased exercise with no increase in food intake Diminished food intake Gastroenteritis	Too little insulin Improper diet Reduced exercise with no reduction in food intake Emotional stress Physical stress such as infection, injury Drugs such as thiazides or corticosteroids
Manifestations	Lability of mood Irritability Shaky feeling Headache Impaired vision Hunger Convulsions	Weakness Increased thirst Frequent urination Signs of dehydration such as dry mucous membranes or soft eyeballs Nausea and vomiting Abdominal pain Acetone breath Rapid, deep respirations
Ominous features	Shock—coma—death	Acidosis—coma—death
Urinary findings		
Glucose	Negative	Positive
Acetone	Usually negative	Positive
Diacetic acid	Negative	Positive
Blood findings		
Glucose	Decreased (60 mg/100 ml or less)	Increased (250 mg/100 ml or more)
Acetone	Negative	Usually positive
Bicarbonate (HCO$_3$)	Usually normal	Decreased (less than 20 mEq/liter); leukocytosis present

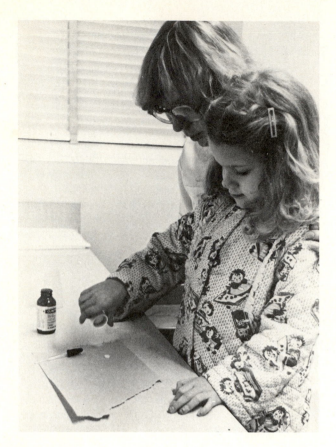

Fig. 26-2

School-age children are able to take responsibility for urine testing.

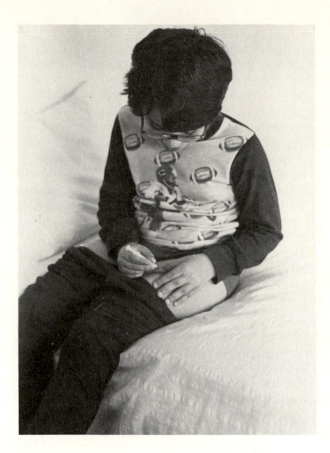

Fig. 26-3

School-age children are able to administer their own insulin.

is to check the blood glucose or obtain a urine sample and test for glucose content. The urine will be negative for glucose in hypoglycemia, or hyperinsulinism, whereas in hyperglycemia the glucose content will be excessive. The young child may not be able to void on command. However, urine output is diminished in hypoglycemia and there is increased urine formation in hyperglycemia. This should provide an additional clue to the alert observer. In doubtful situations and when a urine specimen cannot be obtained for analysis, it is safer to give the child some simple sugar. This will help alleviate the symptoms in the case of hypoglycemia but will do little harm if the child is hyperglycemic.

The child with diabetic ketoacidosis requires intensive nursing care. On admission to the hospital an intravenous infusion is started immediately to hydrate the child and to administer insulin either as a single bolus or as a continuous infusion (see medical management, p. 878). The blood glucose level is monitored at regular intervals and the insulin administered as ordered.

Sodium, potassium, and bicarbonate levels are monitored and replaced as indicated. Since potassium and sodium reenter the cells rapidly after administration of insu-

lin, depletion of these electrolytes can be a serious consequence. The child is generally attached to a cardiac monitor for continual assessment of cardiac status, especially when potassium levels are markedly altered.

Careful and accurate records are maintained, including vital signs (pulse, respiration, temperature, and blood pressure), intravenous fluids, electrolytes, insulin, blood glucose level, and intake and output. A urine collection device or retention catheter is used to obtain the urine measurements, which include volume, specific gravity, and glucose and acetone values. The volume relative to the glucose content is important, since 5% glucose in a 300 ml sample is a significantly greater amount than a similar reading from a 75 ml sample. A diabetic flow sheet maintained at the bedside provides an ongoing record of the vital signs, urine and blood tests, amount of insulin given, and intake and output of the patient. The level of consciousness is assessed and recorded at frequent intervals. The comatose child generally regains consciousness fairly soon after initiation of therapy but is managed as any unconscious child during that time.

When the critical period is over, the task of regulating insulin dosage to diet and activity is begun. The

SUMMARY OF NURSING CARE OF THE CHILD WITH DIABETIC KETOACIDOSIS

GOALS	RESPONSIBILITIES
Recognize diabetic ketoacidosis	Be alert to signs of acidosis, especially in children with known diabetes mellitus Observe for evidence of precipitating factors such as infection, stress, or not receiving insulin injections
Replace fluid and electrolyte losses	Monitor intravenous infusion Assess state of hydration Insert retention catheter or attach urine collection bag Monitor fluid intake and output Observe for signs of sodium, chloride, potassium, or bicarbonate ion imbalances and acidosis Monitor serum electrolytes
Correct hyperglycemia	Administer insulin intravenously and subcutaneously as prescribed Monitor blood glucose levels every 1 to 2 hours as ordered Monitor urine glucose and acetone every 1 to 2 hours as ordered
Correct acidosis	Administer sodium bicarbonate if prescribed Monitor serum pH and blood gases Assess for signs of altered serum pH

Detect alterations in status	Maintain meticulous records
	Assess vital signs frequently
	   Pulse quality and rate
	   Depth and rate of respirations
	   Blood pressure
	   Temperature
	Monitor mental status, level of consciousness
	Monitor serum electrolytes, pH, glucose, and blood gases
	Monitor urine glucose, acetone, specific gravity, and volume frequently
	Attach to cardiac monitor
	Assess degree of shock, if present, and implement therapeutic measures
	Observe for signs of complications such as cerebral edema, hyperkalemia, or hypokalemia

Treat associated problems	Carry out therapeutic regimen as prescribed for infection if present Implement appropriate care for the unconscious child
Support the child	Keep the child warm Orient the child to time and place, if indicated Explain equipment and procedures Answer questions and allow for expression of feelings Provide reassurance
Support the parents	Keep the family informed of the child's status and progress Answer questions and deal with parental concerns, fears, and feelings of guilt

same meticulous records of intake and output, blood or urine glucose and acetone levels, and insulin administration are maintained. The capable child is actively involved in his own care and is given responsibility for keeping the intake and output record, testing the urine, and, when appropriate, administering his own insulin—all under the supervision and guidance of the nurse (Figs. 26-2 and 26-3).

Nursing considerations: long-term care

Once the diabetic child is diagnosed and insulin therapy initiated, the major nursing responsibility is the education of the family and reinforcement of information.* The par-

---

*A book written for children and parents by Travis, L.B.: An instructional aid on juvenile diabetes mellitus, is available from the American Diabetes Association, P.O. Box 12946, Austin, TX 78711.

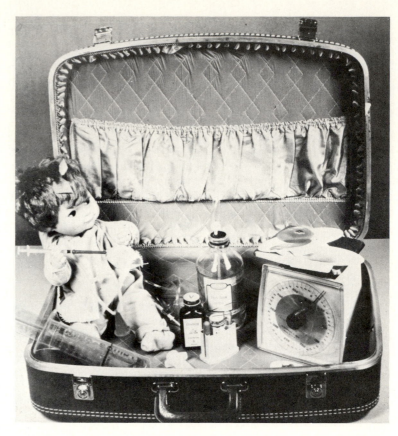

Fig. 26-4
Diabetic play equipment conveniently collected and stored in a small suitcase.

ents must supervise and manage the child's therapeutic program, but the child should assume responsibility for self-management as soon as he is capable. Children can begin to test their own urine at a relatively young age, and most should be able to check their blood glucose and administer their own insulin at about 9 years of age. In situations in which the parents are inconsistent and/or unreliable, the child is taught self-care at an earlier age.

A child learns best when sessions are kept short, no more than 15 to 20 minutes. The parents do best in periods of 45 to 60 minutes and, often, longer if they are inquisitive. Education should involve all the senses, and, although visual aids are valuable tools, participation is the most effective method for learning. For example, to teach urine testing, the technique is explained, the procedure is demonstrated, the learner is allowed to perform the procedure followed by a review of the material by visual aids, and the learning is validated by some testing method that includes a feedback. Varying the presentation with a variety of audiovisual materials including motion pictures, slide-tape programs, and books stimulates the senses and helps the individual to learn (Fig. 26-4). The American Diabetes Association, Inc.,* and the Juvenile Diabetes Foundation† are valuable resources for educational material.

The following information will allow the family to manage the daily aspects of care.

Nature of diabetes. The better the parents understand the pathophysiology of diabetes and the function and action of insulin and glucagon in relation to calorie intake, the better their understanding of the disease and its effect on the child. Parents have a number of questions (voiced or unvoiced) that give them an increased feeling of mental adjustment when answered.

Meal planning. Normal nutrition is a major aspect of information included in order that the family can learn how the meal plan relates to the requirements of normal development and the disease process. Diet instruction is usually conducted by the dietitian with reinforcement and guidance from the nurse. Learning about foods within specific food groups helps in choices. Weights and measures of foods, used as eye-training devices in defining food volumes, should be practiced for about 3 months with gradual conversion to estimating foods. Members of the family are also guided in reading labels for the nutritional value of foods and food contents.

Medication. Families need to understand the treatment method and to learn about the effective duration, onset, and peak action of the insulin prescribed. They should know the characteristics of the various types of insulins, the proper mixing and dilution of insulins, and how to substitute another type when their usual brand is not available.

---

*1 West 48th Street, New York, NY 10020.
†23 East 26th Street, Room 104, New York, NY 10010.

Injection procedure. Learning to give the insulin injections is a source of anxiety for the parents and the child. It is helpful for the learner to know that this important aspect of care will become as routine as brushing the teeth. First the basic injection technique is taught using an orange or similar item for practice. To gain the confidence of the child, the nurse demonstrates the technique by giving a skillful injection to the parent and then the parent returns the demonstration by giving the nurse an injection. Thus with practice the parents soon are able to give the insulin injection to the child and he will trust them. Both parents should participate, and as little time as possible should elapse between instruction and the actual injection, especially with parents and the teenage learner.

Insulin can be injected into any area in which there is skin over muscle with fatty tissue in between. The length and angle of the needle are altered according to the thickness of the skin. Usually the smaller the child, the thinner the skin. The pinch technique is the most effective method for obtaining skin tightness to allow easy entrance of the needle to subcutaneous tissues in children. The parents and child are helped to work out a rotation pattern. The site selected will sometimes depend on whether the child or parent administers the insulin. The arms, thighs, hips, and abdomen are usual injection sites for insulin. The child can reach the thighs, abdomen, and part of the hip and arm easily but may require help to inject other sites. For example, a parent can pinch a loose fold of skin of the arm while the child injects the insulin. Injections are rotated to various areas of the body to enhance absorption, since insulin absorption is slowed by the fat pads that develop in overused areas of injection. A rotation plan involves giving about four or five injections in one area (each injection about 1 inch from the previous injection) and then moving to another area. In this way injection sites for an entire month can be worked out in advance on a simple chart or illustration, such as an outline of a body. It is a good idea for the parent to give one or two shots each a week in the areas that are difficult to reach in order to keep in practice.

The teaching includes the proper way to equalize pressure in the bottle by injecting an amount of air equal to the amount of solution withdrawn and removal of air bubbles from the syringe. When insulin dosages are small, an air bubble in the syringe can displace a significant amount of medication. The parents and the child are taught always to remove insulin from the same bottle first so that only one bottle is apt to be adulterated by the contents of the other. The recommended procedure is to withdraw regular insulin first, then the modified insulin so that the regular insulin does not become modified, rendering it unsuited for emergency use. Some physicians advocate premixing the insulins in the bottle both for convenience and to reduce the chance for contamination of one insulin with the other. This option should not be taught unless the child's physician approves it and the person who mixes the insulins is

reliable. Insulin syringes should be compared for accuracy, comfort, and strength, and the family and/or child should be able to choose both "their" insulin and "their" syringe from a variety of samples. Use of the same syringe (even during hospitalization) is recommended to prevent errors in dosage due to varying amounts of dead space among syringes.

When a child is to use a portable insulin pump, both the child and the parents are taught to operate the device, including the mechanics of the pump, battery changes, and alarm systems. They learn how to dilute the insulin, load the syringe, insert the catheter, adjust the insulin flow for routine needs and for illnesses, and connect and disconnect the catheter. Nurses who work where the pumps are part of the therapeutic regimen should become familiar with the operation of the specific device being used and the protocol of the regimen.

Glucose monitoring. Nurses are also prepared to teach and supervise blood glucose monitoring, which is used in conjunction with the insulin pump and is rapidly replacing urine testing. The relatively inexpensive reagent strips are a satisfactory means for measuring blood glucose levels but the greatest accuracy is obtained from the more expensive mechanical monitors. Except for young children, these are well accepted by patients.

Urine testing. Urine testing is easily taught and should include all methods of urine testing, not just the test to be used for the particular child. Use of the copper reduction test (Clinitest) includes instruction of the 5-, 2-, and 1-drop methods. Instruction also includes the pass-through phenomenon, which occurs when there is more glucose in the specimen than the test can record. It responds by "going backward" on the color scale or "passes-through" the bright orange color at the top of the scale. This may occur during the "boiling" or during the 15-second waiting period. The likelihood for this pass-through to occur is much less with the 2-drop test, since it is able to show more glucose in the urine than the 5-drop test. More programs are using the 2- and 1-drop method when there is pass through on the 5-drop method. The copper reduction test may give false-positive results when certain antibiotics are being taken and with the introduction of sugars other than glucose. Shaking the test tube during the "boiling" will increase the addition of oxygen and cause an alteration in the test results; therefore, shaking of the test tube should not occur until after the 15-second wait. Families are cautioned about handling the tablet, which contains lye, and to keep the bottle out of reach of small children.

The glucose oxidase tests (Diastix, Clinistix, and Tes-Tape) are more sensitive tests and are responsive to glucose only. These tests are very useful for travel and for school but are a little too sensitive for daily control. Directions for interpreting the tests should be read carefully. The percentage readings are the same as those for the Clinitest, but there are differences in the plus values.

The tests for acetone are the Ketostix and the Acetest. The test is read after a 30-second wait. The acetone tests are not done daily, as the glucose tests are, but should be performed during times of illness or high sugar spills.

Moisture will cause changes to take place in the tablets. Families are instructed to discard tablets that are discolored, that have been open for a specified period of time, or after an expiration date.

Hyperglycemia and hypoglycemia. Severe hyperglycemia is most often caused by illness, growth, or emotional upset. Parents who are accustomed to seeing negative urine tests respond immediately when they see their child start to spill some sugar in the urine. The parents should understand how to adjust food, activity, and insulin at the time of illness and when the child is treated for an illness with a medication known to raise the blood glucose level.

Hypoglycemia is caused by imbalances of food intake, insulin, and activity. Ideally hypoglycemia should be prevented and parents need to be prepared to prevent, recognize, and treat the problem. They should be familiar with the signs of hypoglycemia and instructed in treatment, including care of the child with seizures (p. 848). Hypoglycemia can be managed effectively as follows:

> **Mild reaction** treat with food
> **Moderate reaction** treat with simple sugar followed by food
> **Severe reaction** treat with glucagon (or simple sugar administered rectally) followed by simple sugar in 15 to 20 minutes

All diabetic children should be provided with identification that explains their condition so that it will be noticed in times of emergency. This will bring aid to the child more quickly. Identification is noticed more readily if it is in the form of a bracelet rather than a necklace or dog tag.

Hygiene. All aspects of personal hygiene are emphasized for the child with diabetes. The child has not had time to develop the blood vessel disease that causes a decrease in peripheral circulation; therefore, foot care is not as important in the child as it is in the adult with diabetes. However, the correct method of nail and extremity care instituted for each particular child (with the guidance of a podiatrist) can begin health practices that last a lifetime. Eyes should be checked once a year unless the child wears glasses and then as directed by the ophthalmologist. Regular dental care is emphasized, and cuts and scratches should be treated with plain soap and water unless otherwise indicated.

Exercise. Exercise should be planned for the sedentary teenager, and observed in active children. If the child is more active at one time of the day than at another, food and/or insulin can be altered to meet the activity pat-

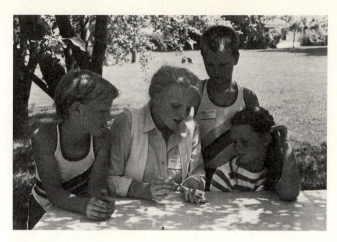

Fig. 26-5
Nurse demonstrates the withdrawal of insulin at a summer camp for diabetic children.

tern of the individual child. Food should be increased in the summer when children tend to be more active. The child who is active in team sports will need an increase in food intake on the days of activity, and races or other competition may call for a slightly higher food intake than practice times. Food will usually need to be repeated for prolonged activity periods, often as frequently as every 45 minutes to 1 hour. Families should be informed that if increased food is not tolerated, decreased insulin is the next course of action.

Record keeping. Keeping information about food, insulin, and glucosuria is useful to the physician as well as to the family. Insulin reactions are noted, including the time, severity, treatment, and response to treatment. Dietary variations are noted so that an increased blood glucose or urinary glucose spill can be analyzed in relation to insulin dose, food intake, and activity level.

Emotional support. In any educational program psychologic needs are just as important as the physical needs of the child. Adjustment to a chronic illness is difficult and follows the grief process (see Chapter 16). A noticeable adjustment cycle occurs during the week-long education course. First there is interest and perhaps some anger and doubt, followed by denial and accompanied by the overwhelming feeling of ''Why me?'' There are doubts regarding the ability to absorb so much essential information. Then there are the acceptance and synthesis of material as the learners realize that they are able to state and demonstrate their understanding of the material.

Camping and other special groups are very useful. In the camp for children with diabetes, these children learn that they are not alone (Fig. 26-5). As a result they become more independent and resourceful in the nondiabetic camp setting, especially if they have had experience in a

SUMMARY OF NURSING CARE OF THE CHILD WITH DIABETES MELLITUS

GOALS	RESPONSIBILITIES
Recognize diabetes mellitus	Be alert for signs and symptoms of diabetes
Assist with diagnosis	Obtain and check urine specimen for glucose, acetone, and specific gravity Collect 24-hour urine for glucose if ordered Order or obtain blood for analysis Assist with glucose tolerance testing

Replace insulin deficit	Understand action of insulin
	Understand differences in composition, time of onset, and duration of action for various insulin preparations
	Employ correct techniques when preparing and administering insulin
	    Subcutaneous injection
	    Rotation of sites

Assess status	Maintain bedside flow sheet including vital signs, intake, output, blood glucose, Clinitest, Acetest, and insulin administered (varies according to institutions)
Vital signs	Measure vital signs as ordered, usually every 4 hours

Urine	Measure intake and output
	Test for glucose, acetone, and specific gravity
	Time measurement as ordered, such as
	    Preprandial and bedtime
	    Double-voided specimens
	    Every 4 hours
	Perform Clinitest using method (1-, 2-, or 5-drop) and Acetest as ordered

Blood glucose	Check blood glucose as before meals and as ordered Order fasting blood sugar daily or as requested Withhold breakfast and insulin until after blood is drawn for test
Recognize signs of hypoglycemia early	Be particularly alert at times when blood glucose levels are lowest Observe for lability of mood, irritability, seizures, and indications of subjective symptoms such as shaky feeling, headache, hunger, and impaired vision Obtain blood glucose measurement Obtain urine specimen and test for glucose
Treat hypoglycemia	Offer readily absorbed carbohydrate such as milk, orange juice, or hard candy Administer glucagon, if ordered
Maintain nutrition	Provide balanced, nutritious diet as prescribed Consult with dietitian regarding diet Avoid concentrated sugars Offer three regular meals plus snacks as prescribed
Maintain general health status	Avoid exposure to infections
Provide for exercise and diversion	Provide activities in and around hospital unit Arrange for occupational therapy program that includes physical activity
Prepare for home care Educate the parents and child	Assess understanding and level of intelligence of learners Select methods, vocabulary, and content appropriate to level of learner Allow 3 or 4 days for the parents and child to begin to get over initial impact of diagnosis

Continued.

SUMMARY OF NURSING CARE OF THE CHILD WITH DIABETES MELLITUS—cont'd

GOALS	RESPONSIBILITIES

Educate the parents and child—cont'd	Select environment conducive to learning
	Allow ample time for education process
	Restrict length of teaching sessions
	    Child: 15 to 20 minutes
	    Parents: 45 to 60 minutes
	Involve all senses and employ a variety of teaching strategies
	Provide pamphlets or other supplementary materials

Nature of the disease	Provide information regarding pathophysiology of diabetes and function and actions of insulin and glucagon in relation to caloric intake Answer questions and clarify misconceptions Explain function and expected effect of procedures and tests
Meal planning	Enlist services of dietitian Emphasize relationship between normal nutritional needs and disease Become familiar with family's food preferences Teach or reinforce learners' understanding of basic food groups Assist the child and family to estimate food weights by volume Suggest low-carbohydrate snack items Guide the parents in assessing the labels of food products Teach or reinforce their understanding of concept of calories Relate caloric equivalents to familiar foods Retain cultural patterns and family preferences as much as possible
Medication	Teach the child and family characteristics of insulins prescribed for the child Teach proper mixing of insulins and acceptable substitutions (when familiar brand is unavailable)
Injection procedure	Impress on learners that procedure will be routine part of the child's life Involve both the parents and the child, if the child is old enough Teach basic techniques using an orange or similar item Use demonstration and return demonstration techniques on another person before injecting the child Help the parents and child work out a set rotation pattern Teach management, operation, and care of insulin infusion pump if prescribed Teach proper care of insulin and equipment
Glucose testing	Teach use of glucose monitor parents have selected and interpret results Teach care and maintenance of monitor
Urine testing	Teach all methods of urine testing and interpretation of results Teach proper care of test materials and equipment
Hygiene	Emphasize importance of personal hygiene Encourage regular dental care and yearly ophthalmologic examinations Teach proper care of cuts and scratches
Exercise	Help plan exercise program Reiterate physician instructions regarding adjustment of food and/or insulin to meet the child's activity pattern

SUMMARY OF NURSING CARE OF THE CHILD WITH DIABETES MELLITUS—cont'd

GOALS	RESPONSIBILITIES
Hyperglycemia and hypoglycemia	Instruct learners regarding prevention of hyper- or hypoglycemia Instruct them to recognize signs of hyperglycemia and hypoglycemia (especially hypoglycemia) (p. 881) Explain relationship of insulin needs to illness, activity, and emotional upset Teach how to adjust food, activity, and insulin at times of illness and other situations that alter blood sugar levels Suggest carrying source of carbohydrate Instruct the parents and child how to treat hypoglycemia with food, simple sugars, or glucagon Encourage acquisition of means of identification and explanation of the child's condition in case of emergency, such as an identification bracelet

Record keeping	Help the parents and child to design form for keeping records of
	   Insulin administered
	   Blood glucose
	   Urine tests
	   Food intake
	   Marked variation in exercise
	   Illness
	Encourage honesty in recording, such as eating a forbidden candy bar

Self-management	Encourage independence in applying concepts learned in teaching sessions Instruct when to seek assistance from medical personnel
Positive adjustment to disease	Assist child and parents to solve problems associated with each of the child's developmental stages Encourage the child to maintain normal activity pattern Encourage interpersonal relationships with peers Suggest involvement with special groups and facilities for diabetic children Be alert to signs that may indicate rebellion against disease, such as noncompliance or other forms of acting-out Be available for consultation when needed
Support parents	Allow for expression of feelings Encourage the parents in their efforts to adjust to the child's disease and its effect on the family life-style Assist the parents in problem-solving Assess interpersonal relationships within the family, especially behaviors that reflect parental attitudes toward affected child Intervene where behaviors indicate rejection or overprotection Refer parents to the American Diabetes Association and other agencies and services that help meet their special needs

diabetic camp. Useful information about such camps and organizations can be obtained from the American Diabetes Association. Many families find solace and comfort from their religious faith, and, where appropriate, a representative of the faith should be contacted to help provide for this very special need.

BIBLIOGRAPHY
General

Kreuger, J.A, and Ray, J.C.: Endocrine problems in nursing, St. Louis, 1976, The C.V. Mosby Co.

Hurwitz, L.S.: Nursing implications of selected pediatric endocrine problems, Nurs. Clin. North Am. **15**:525-536, 1980.

Lessick, M.L.: Genetic counseling of families with endocrine disorders, Issues Compr. Pediatr. Nurs. **4**(2):27-40, 1980.

Wong, D.L.: The significance of dead space in syringes, Am. J. Nurs. **82**:1237, 1982.

Disorders of pituitary function

Camuñas, C.: Transphenoidal hypophysectomy, Am. J. Nurs. **80**:1820-1823, 1980.

Hobdell, E.F.: Growing up without growing: the child with growth hormone deficiency, Am. J. Maternal Child Nurs. **2**:299-303, 1977.

Solomon, B.L.: The hypothalamus and the pituitary gland: an overview, Nurs. Clin. North Am. **15**:435-451, 1980.

Thyroid and parathyroid disorders

Arcangelo, V.P.: Simple goiter, Nursing 83, **13**(3):47, 1983.

Hoffmann, J.T.T, and Newby, T.B.: Hypercalcemia in primary hyperparathyroidism, Nurs. Clin. North Am. **15**:469-480, 1980.

Honigman, R.E.: Thyroid function tests, Nursing 82 **12**(4):68-71, 1982.

Sharkey, P.L., and Meyer, S.A.: Hyperthyroidism, Crit. Care Update **8**(5):12-24, 1981.

Wake, M.M., and Brensinger, J.F., III: The nurse's role in hypothyroidism, Nurs. Clin. North Am. **15**:453-467, 1980.

Adrenal disorders

Burnett, J.: A boy with CAH, Am. J. Nurs. **80**:1304-1305, 1980.

Burnett, J.: Congenital adrenocortical hyperplasia: the syndrome, Am. J. Nurs. **80**:1306-1308, 1980.

Camunas, C.: Pheochromocytoma, Am. J. Nurs. **83**:887-891, 1983.

Hill, S.: The child with ambiguous genitalia, Am. J. Nurs. **77**(5):810-814, 1977.

McFarlane, J.: Congenital adrenal hyperplasia, Am. J. Nurs. **76**(8):1290-1292, 1976.

McGann, M.: Cushing's syndrome: its complexities and care, RN **38**:40-43, Aug. 1975.

Sanford, S.J.: Dysfunction of the adrenal gland: physiologic considerations and nursing problems, Nurs. Clin. North Am. **15**:481-498, 1980.

Strobele, B.: How to counsel patients on cortisone, RN **38**:57-60, July 1975.

Diabetes mellitus

Ahlfield, J.E., Soler, N.G., and Marcus, S.D.: Adolescent diabetes mellitus: parent/child perspectives of the effect of the disease on family and social interactions, Diabetes Care **6**:393-398, 1983.

Burke, E.: Insulin injection; the site and the technique, Am. J. Nurs. **72**:2194-2196, 1976.

Cavalier, J.P.: Diabetes mellitus, Crit. Care Update **10**(9):39-45, 1983.

Childs, B.P.: Insulin infusion pumps, Nursing 83 **13**(11):55-54, 1983.

Dexter, D.M.: The new insulins, Am. J. Nurs. **81**:146-148, 1981.

Dillon, R.S.: Improved serum insulin profiles in diabetic individuals who massaged their insulin injection sites, Diabetes Care **6**:399-401, 1983.

Faro, B.: Maintaining good control in children with diabetes, Pediatr. Nurs. **9**:368-373, 1983.

Fendya, D.G., and Flynn, K.: Nursing care for children with hypoglycemia due to hyperinsulinism, Am. J. Maternal Child Nurs. **6**:100-105, 1981.

Fow, S.M.: Home blood glucose monitoring in children with insulin-dependent diabetes mellitus, Pediatr. Nurs. **9**:439-442, 1983.

Fredholm, N., Vignati, L., and Brown, S.: Insulin pumps: the patient's verdict, Am. J. Nurs. **84**:36-38, 1984.

Fredholm, N.Z.: The insulin pump: new method of insulin delivery, Am. J. Nurs. **81**:2024-2026, 1981.

Friedland, G.M.: Learning behaviors of a preadolescent with diabetes, Am. J. Nurs. **76**:59-61, 1976.

Guthrie, D.W.: Exercise, diets, and insulin for children with diabetes, Nursing 77 **7**(2):48-54, 1977.

Guthrie, D.W., and Guthrie, R.A.: Diabetes mellitus update! Crit. Care Update **5**(8):5-18, 1978.

Guthrie, D.W., and Guthrie, R.A., editors: Nursing management of diabetes mellitus, ed. 2, St. Louis, 1982, The C.V. Mosby Co.

Guthrie, D.W., and Guthrie, R.A.: The disease process of diabetes mellitus, Nurs. Clin. North Am. **18**:617-630, 1983.

Hardin, T., and Fischer, R.G.: Pediatric drug information, Pediatr. Nurs. **9**:457, 1983.

Heins, J.M.: Dietary management in diabetes mellitus, Nurs. Clin. North Am. **18**:631-643, 1983.

Hoette, S.J.: The adolescent with diabetes mellitus, Nurs. Clin. North Am. **18**:763-776, 1983.

Hopper, S.V.: Meeting the needs of the economically deprived diabetic, Nurs. Clin. North Am. **18**:813-825, 1983.

Jackson, R.L.: Insulin-dependent diabetes in children and young adults, Nutr. Today **14**(6):26-32, 1979.

Jackson, R.L.: Education of the parents of a child with diabetes, Nutr. Today **15**(3):30-35, 1980.

Jackson, R.L.: Management and treatment of the child with diabetes, Nutr. Today **15**(2):6-29, 1980.

Joyce, M.A., Kuzich, C.M., and Murphy, D.M.: Those new blood tests, RN **45**:46-52, April, 1983.

Kennell, C.: Outpatient management of the juvenile diabetic, Pediatr. Nurs. **2**(6):19-24, 1976.

Kiser, D.: The Somogyi effect, Am. J. Nurs. **80**:236-238, 1980.

Knott, S.P., and Herget, M.J.: Teaching self-injection to diabetics: an easier and more effective way, Nursing 84 **14**(1):57, 1984.

Krauser, K.L., and Madden, P.B.: The child with diabetes mellitus, Nurs. Clin. North Am. **18**:749-762, 1983.

Lavine, R.L.: How to recognize and what to do about hypoglycemia, Nursing 79 **9**(4):525-55, 1979.

Lillo, R.: Outpatient management of children with diabetic ketoacidosis, Pediatr. Nurs. **8**:383-385, 1982.

Lindsey, N.M.: Coping with diabetes, Nursing 83 **13**(3):48-49, 1983.

Lobo, M.L.: Nursing implications in camps for children with diabetes. In Chinn, P.L., and Leonard, K.B., editors: Current practice in pediatric nursing, vol. 3, St. Louis, 1980, The C.V. Mosby Co.

Loman, D., and Galgani, C.: Monitoring diabetic children's blood-glucose levels at home, Am. J. Maternal Child Nurs. **9**:192-196, 1984.

Managing diabetes properly, Horsham, Pa., 1977, Nursing Skillbooks, Intermed Communications.

Metzger, M.J.: A new test for blood sugar, Am. J. Nurs. **83**:763-764, 1983.

Miller, B.K., and White, N.E.: Diabetes assessment guide, Am. J. Nurs. **80**:1314-1316, 1980.

Miller, B.K., and White, N.E.: An assessment guide for diabetic patients, Crit. Care Update **9**(8):28-34, 1982.

Moorman, N.H.: Acute complications of hyperglycemia and hypoglycemia, Nurs. Clin. North Am. 18:707-719, 1983.

Nemchik, R.: Diabetes today: a startling new body of knowledge, RN **44**:31-37, 1982.

Nemchik, R.: The news about insulin, RN **44**:499-54, 1982.

Nemchik, R.: The new insulin pumps: tight control—at a price, RN **45**:52-59, 1983.

Ory, M.G., and Dronenfeld, J.J.: Living with juvenile diabetes mellitus, Pediatr. Nurs. **6**(5):47-50, 1980.

Pelczynski, L., and Reilly, A.: Helping your diabetic patients help themselves, Nursing 81 **11**(5):76-81, 1981.

Plasse, N.J.: Monitoring blood glucose at home: a comparison of three products, Am. J. Nurs. **81**:2028-2029, 1981.

Price, M.J.: Insulin and oral hypoglycemic agents, Nurs. Clin. North Am. **18**:687-706, 1983.

Resler, M.M.: Teaching strategies that promote adherence, Nurs. Clin. North Am. **18**:799-811, 1983.

Saucier, C.P.: Self concept and self-care management in school-age children with diabetes, Pediatr. Nurs. **10**:135-138, 1984.

Simpson, O.W., and Smith, M.A.: Lightening the load for parents of children with diabetes, Am. J. Maternal Child Nurs. **4**:293-296, 1979.

Stevens, A.D.: Monitoring blood glucose at home: who should do it, Am. J. Nurs. **81**:2026-2027, 1981.

Stock-Barkman, P.: Confusing concepts. Is it diabetic shock or diabetic coma? Nursing 83 **13**(6):33-41, 1983.

Surr, C.W.: Teaching patients to use the new blood-glucose monitoring products. Part I, Nursing 83 **13**(1):42-45, 1983.

Surr, C.W.: Teaching patients to use the new blood-glucose monitoring products. Part II, Nursing 83 **13**(2):58-62, 1983.

Tauer, K.M.: Physiologic mechanisms in childhood hypoglycemia, Pediatr. Nurs. **9**:341-344, 1983.

Valenta, C.L.: Urine testing and home blood-glucose monitoring, Nurs. Clin. North Am. **18**:645-659, 1983.

Welk, D.S.: Preventing insulin-induced lipodystrophies, Nursing 79 **9**(12):42-45, 1979.

Wolfe, L.: Insulin: paving the way to a new life, Nursing 77 **7**(11):38-41, 1977.

Traisman, H.: Management of juvenile diabetes mellitus, St. Louis, ed. 3, 1980, The C.V. Mosby Co.

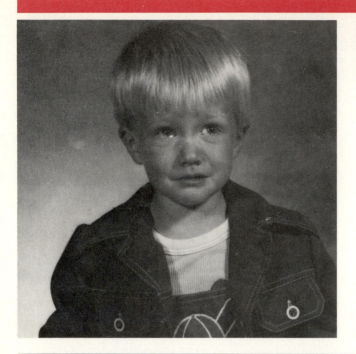

27

THE CHILD WITH INTEGUMENTARY DYSFUNCTION

OBJECTIVES

On completion of this chapter the reader will be able to:

- Describe the distribution and configuration of the various skin lesions

- Discuss the nursing care related to therapies for skin disorders

- Contrast the manifestations of and therapies for bacterial, viral, and fungal infections of the skin

- Compare the skin manifestations related to age in children

- Outline a plan of care for a child with eczema

- Formulate a teaching plan for an adolescent with acne

- Describe the methods for assessing a burn wound

- Discuss the physical and emotional care of a child with a severe burn wound

NURSING DIAGNOSES

Nursing diagnoses identified for the child with integumentary dysfunction include, but are not restricted to, the following:

Nutritional-metabolic pattern

- Fluid volume deficit related to excessive fluid losses

- Nutrition, alteration in: less than body requirements related to increased metabolic needs

- Skin integrity, impairment of: potential, related to (1) denuded skin; (2) presence of infective organisms; (3) nutritional deficit

Activity-exercise pattern

- Activity intolerance, related to increased metabolic demands

- Airway clearance, ineffective, related to (1) decreased energy; (2) pain

- Breathing pattern, ineffective, related to (1) fatigue; (2) immobility; (3) discomfort

- Diversional activity deficit related to (1) immobility; (2) schedule of therapies

- Mobility, impaired physical, related to (1) pain; (2) anxiety; (3) decreased activity tolerance

- Self-care deficit: feeding, bathing/hygiene, dressing/grooming, toileting, related to (1) developmental level; (2) discomfort; (3) immobility

Sleep-rest pattern

- Sleep pattern disturbance related to (1) physical discomfort; (2) schedule of therapies

Cognitive-perceptual pattern

- Comfort, alterations in: pain related to (1) tissue damage; (2) therapies; (3) position

- Sensory-perceptual alteration: visual, auditory, tactile, related to (1) application of topical therapy; (2) isolation; (3) discomfort

Self-perception—self-concept pattern

- Anxiety related to (1) strange environment; (2) perception of impending events; (3) separation; (4) anticipated discomfort; (5) knowledge deficit; (6) pain

- Self-concept, disturbance in: body image, self-esteem, related to perception of physical effects of integumentary disruption

Role-relationship pattern

- Family process, alteration in, related to situational crisis

- Grieving, anticipatory, related to expected change in appearance

- Parenting, alterations in, potential, related to (1) hospitalization; (2) skill deficit; (3) family stress

- Social isolation related to (1) impaired mobility; (2) self-concept disturbance; (3) physical isolation

Coping-stress tolerance pattern

- Coping, family: potential for growth

- Coping, ineffective family: compromised, related to (1) situational crisis; (2) temporary family disorganization

- Coping, ineffective individual, related to (1) situational crisis; (2) skill deficit

The skin, the largest organ in the body, is not merely a covering but is a complex structure that serves many functions, the most important of which are to protect the tissues that it encloses and to protect itself. This pliable sheath is a vital shield against the shifting physical and chemical stresses of the environment, and this role is fulfilled to the extent that outside changes are not transmitted inward to upset the body's internal equilibrium. The skin is primarily an insulator, not an organ of exchange.

DISEASES OF THE SKIN

Diseases of the skin focus sharply on the epidermis, which is the site of many distinctive patterns ranging from the vesiculation of contact dermatitis to common superficial tumors. Clearly visible, these morphologic changes produce the varied patterns on which a dermatologic diagnosis is made.

Lesions of the skin or disorders with skin manifestations can be a result of a wide variety of specific etiologic factors. In general, skin lesions originate from (1) contact with injurious agents such as infective organisms, toxic chemicals, and physical trauma, (2) hereditary factors, or (3) some external factor that produces a reaction in the skin, for example, allergens. In this situation the damage is caused by the body's response to the agent rather than by the agent itself. Such responses are highly individualized. An agent that may be harmless to one individual may be damaging to another, and a single agent may produce various types of responses in different individuals.

Among other factors involved in the etiology of skin manifestations is the age of the child. For example, infants are subject to "birthmark" malformations and atopic dermatitis that appear early in life, the school-age child is susceptible to ringworm of the scalp, and acne is a characteristic skin disorder of puberty. Contact dermatitis, such as poison ivy, is seen only where the noxious agent is a feature of the area. Similarly reactions to animal bites are associated with their life cycle and seasonal activities. Although less common in children, tension and anxiety may produce, modify, or prolong many skin conditions.

Skin of younger children

Several characteristics influence skin responses in infants and young children. Their skin is far more susceptible to superficial bacterial infection. They are more likely to have associated systemic symptoms with some infections and are more apt to react to a primary irritant than to a sensitizing allergen. In the infant and small child the epidermis is still loosely bound to the corium. Consequently the layers may easily separate during an inflammatory process to form blisters or during careless handling (such as removal of adhesive tape). The infant's skin is much more prone to develop a toxic erythema as a result of skin eruptions or drug reactions and is subject to maceration, infection, and the sweat retention associated with diaper rash.

The transitional zone between the epidermal layers, which allows fluid from lower layers to outer layers, is less effective in young children than in older children and adults. Consequently the small child's skin chaps more easily. Also, sebaceous glands are very active prenatally when they produce the protective *vernix caseosa*. The sebaceous activity slowly subsides after birth and continues to decrease throughout infancy. In the newborn period and early infancy, sebaceous secretions may cause minor problems such as "cradle cap" in some infants. The secretion gradually rises in childhood to increase markedly at puberty where it remains constant and contributes greatly to the disturbing skin problems of adolescence.

Diagnostic evaluation

One of the more advantageous aspects of skin disorders is that often the diagnosis is readily established after simple, careful inspection. Much can be determined by the distribution, size, morphology, and arrangement of the lesions. In addition, intrinsic causes must be distinguished from extrinsic causes. Extrinsic causes usually result from physical, chemical, or allergic irritants or from an infectious agent such as bacteria, fungi, viruses, or animal parasites. Skin manifestations can be produced by such intrinsic causes as a specific infection (such as measles or chickenpox), drug sensitization, or other allergic phenomena. Other diagnostic tools are subjective symptoms, history, and medical and laboratory studies.

Lesion. According to the nature of the pathologic process, lesions assume more or less distinct characteristics. A reddened area is usually caused by increased amounts of oxygenated blood in the dermal vasculature and is described as *erythema*. Hemorrhages into the skin produce localized red or purple discolorations such as *ecchymoses* (bruises), caused by extravasation of blood into dermis and subcutaneous tissues, and *petechiae*, pinpoint tiny and sharply circumscribed spots in the superficial layers of the epidermis. *Primary* lesions (Fig. 27-1) are skin changes produced by some causative factor; *secondary* lesions (Fig. 27-2) are changes that result from alteration in the primary lesions, such as those caused by rubbing, scratching, medication, or involution and healing. Nurses should become familiar with the more common terms used to describe skin lesions:

distribution pattern the pattern in which lesions are distributed over the body, whether local or generalized, and specific areas associated with the lesions.
configuration and arrangement the size, shape, and arrangement of a lesion or groups of lesions, such as discrete, clustered, diffuse, or confluent.

Fig. 27-1

Primary skin lesions.

Flat circumscribed area of color changes less than 1 cm in diameter, neither elevated nor depressed and with no alteration in skin texture

Example: Freckle, nevus, measles

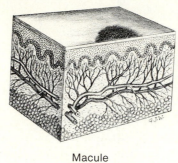

Macule

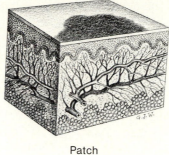

Patch

Flat circumscribed discoloration of skin greater than 1 cm in diameter

Example: Mongolian spot, vitiligo

Small, circumscribed solid elevation of the skin, less than 1 cm in diameter; exists mostly above the plane of the skin surface, and the more superficial it is, the more distinct are the borders

Example: Wart, ringworm

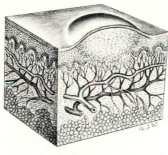

Papule

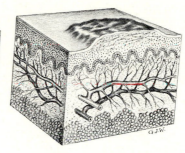

Plaque

Flattened, raised lesion in which the surface area involved is relatively large in relation to its height

Example: Psoriasis

Solid circumscribed elevation, round or ellipsoid, located deep in dermis or subcutaneous tissue

Example: Dermatofibroma

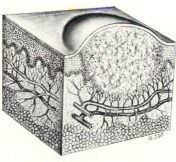

Nodule

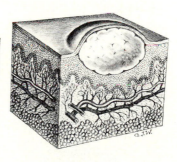

Tumor

Circumscribed infiltration of skin or subcutaneous tissue that is larger (greater than 1 cm in diameter) and deeper than nodule

Example: Cavernous hemangioma

Encapsulated semisolid or fluid-filled mass in dermis or subcutaneous tissue

Example: Epidermoid cyst

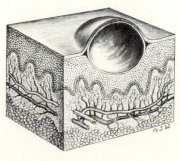

Cyst

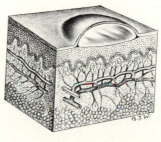

Vesicle

Small (less than 1 cm in diameter), superficial circumscribed elevation of the skin containing serous or blood-tinged fluid

Example: Chickenpox, herpes, poison ivy, dermatitis

Vesicle filled with pus that
may or may not be
caused by infection

Example: Acne, impetigo,
folliculitis

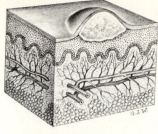

Pustule

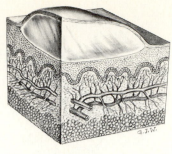

Bulla

Fluid-filled vesicle greater
than 1 cm in diameter; a
large vesicle; bleb;
blister

Example: Second-degree
burn

Round or flat-topped and
irregularly shaped,
evanescent lesions
resulting from acute
accumulation of edema
fluid in upper dermis

Example: Mosquito bites,
urticaria

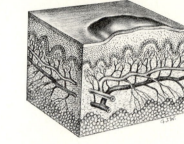

Wheal

Fig. 27-2

Secondary skin lesions.

Flakes of dead, cornified
tissue being shed from
skin

Example: Psoriasis,
ringworm

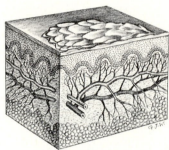

Scale

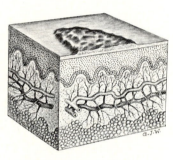

Crust

Dried masses of serum,
pus, dead skin, and
debris that can be found
surmounting any lesion

Example: Impetigo, other
infectious dermatitis

Ireegularly shaped
excavation caused by
loss of substance with
gradual disintegration
and necrosis of tissue

Example: Decubiti

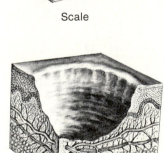

Ulcer

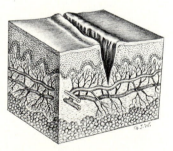

Fissure

Deep linear split through
epidermis into dermis

Example: Chapping

Permanent dermal changes
with production of
excess collagen
following damage to
corium

Example: Vaccination,
burns, deep scratches

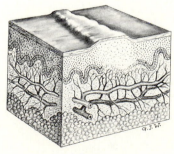

Scar

History and subjective symptoms. Many cutaneous lesions are associated with local symptoms, the most common of which is itching that varies in kind and intensity. Pain or tenderness often accompanies some skin lesions, and other sensations may be described as burning, prickling, stinging, or crawling. Alterations in local feeling or sensation include absence of sensation (anesthesia), excessive sensitiveness (hyperesthesia), or diminished or lessening of sensation (hypesthesia or hypoesthesia). These symptoms may remain localized or may migrate, may be constant or intermittent, and may be aggravated by a specific activity or circumstance, such as exposure to sunlight.

It is also important to determine whether the child has had an allergic condition such as asthma or hay fever or has had previous skin disease. Eczema, often associated with allergies, frequently begins in infancy. It should be determined when the lesion or symptom first became apparent as well as whether it is related to ingestion of a food or other substance, including any medication the child might be taking. It should be kept in mind that it may be related to an activity such as contact with plants, insects, or chemicals.

Laboratory studies. When it is suspected that a skin problem might be related to a systemic disease, such as one of the collagen diseases or immune deficiency disease, studies are needed to rule out these possibilities. Microscopic examination of a skin lesion may be essential in many chronic conditions and in pigmented nevi. Cultures in bacterial infections, scrapings for fungal infections, allergic skin testing, and various other laboratory tests (blood count, sedimentation rate) are employed when indicated.

General therapeutic management

The major aim of any treatment is to prevent further damage, eliminate the cause, prevent complications, and provide relief from discomfort while tissues undergo healing. Factors that contribute to the dermatitis and may prolong the course of the disease must be eliminated where possible. The most common offenders in pediatrics are environmental factors, such as soaps, bubble baths, shampoos, rough or tight clothing, blankets, and toys, and the natural elements, such as dirt, sand, heat, cold, moisture, and wind. Dermatitis can also be aggravated by home remedies and medications.

Topical therapy. A variety of agents and methods are available for treatment of dermatologic problems. In selecting a therapeutic program the practitioner considers (1) a choice of active ingredient, (2) a proper vehicle or base, (3) the cosmetic effect, (4) the cost, and (5) instructions for its use. In addition, several basic concepts are kept in mind. Overtreatment is avoided. For example, when the dermatitis is acute, the applications should be mild and bland to avoid further irritation. Broken or inflamed skin, especially in children, is more absorbent than intact skin, and chemicals that are nonirritating to intact skin may be quite irritating to inflamed skin.

Topical applications may be given to treat the disorder, reduce the itching associated with many diseases, decrease external stimuli, or apply external heat or cold. The emollient action of soaks, baths, and lotions provides a soothing film over the skin surface that reduces external stimuli. Application of heat tends to aggravate most conditions, and its use is usually reserved for reducing specific inflammatory processes, such as folliculitis and cellulitis. Ordinarily applications offer most relief when they are lukewarm, tepid, or cool. When more than one preparation is prescribed the nurse should clarify the correct order in which the substances are to be applied. This is especially important when providing directions to the person(s) who will be carrying out the therapy.

Wet dressings. Probably the mildest form of topical therapy, open wet dressings, cool the skin by evaporation, relieve itching and inflammation, and cleanse the area by loosening and removing crusts and debris. Any of a variety of ingredients can be applied on kerlix gauze, plain gauze, or (preferably) soft cotton cloths such as freshly laundered handkerchiefs or strips from diaper, sheeting, or pillowcase material. Dressings immersed in the desired solution are wrung out slightly and applied to the affected area wet but not dripping. They are applied flat and smooth and in such a way that motion is not totally restricted—fingers are wrapped separately and arms and legs are wrapped so that elbows and knees can bend. Dressings are kept in place by kerlix or other cotton wrap, tubular stockinette, mittens, and socks (two pair—one to hold the dressings in place, the other to take up movement) but are left uncovered. When evaporation begins to dry them, the dressings are removed, rewet in the solution, and reapplied to the area using aseptic technique. The solution is not poured or syringed directly over the dressings. The most commonly used solutions are normal saline and Burow's solution (aluminum sulfate and calcium acetate).

Fresh solution at room temperature is applied at 2-, 3-, or 4-hour intervals and is allowed to remain on anywhere from 30 minutes to 1½ hours. Wet dressings are seldom continued after about 48 hours. The child must be guarded against chilling during treatment, and no more than one third of the body should be covered at one time. After treatment the skin is dried thoroughly by patting with a towel. Application of lotion or other medication may be ordered at this time.

Occlusive dressings. Used primarily in association with topical steroids, occlusive dressings are usually restricted to treatment of chronic dermatoses. A thin application of ointment or cream is covered with a thin, transparent pliable plastic film that is anchored with adhesive. Occlusive dressings promote moisture retention, nonevaporation of the vehicle, and maceration of the epidermis, all of which increase the penetration of medications.

Soaks. When young children are uncooperative in the use of wet dressings, soaks are often employed for removal of crusts and for their mild astringent action, using the same solution employed for wet compresses. To gain young children's cooperation for hand or foot soaks is difficult unless the procedure is made attractive to them through play. Older infants and toddlers delight in playing with brightly colored marbles scattered over the bottom of the receptacle, and preschoolers can be challenged to hold a floating item beneath the water surface. These activities require supervision, because infants and small children will often place items in their mouths and children can easily lose control with water play. Washing dishes, cars, dolls, or doll clothes will occupy many children for quite some time. The older child is able to cooperate but may need something to do while confined during the procedure.

Lotions and shake solutions. Lotions are preparations of powder suspended in solution. As the liquid evaporates, it not only cools but a coating of soothing, lubricating, protective, and drying powder remains on the skin. Lotions are applied evenly over the skin with gauze or an ordinary paintbrush (children love this method), frequently after wet dressings or soaks.

Baths. Baths are especially useful in the treatment of widespread dermatitis by evenly distributing the soothing antipruritic and antiinflammatory effects of the solution. The solution is added to a tub well filled with lukewarm water. The duration of treatment is usually 15 to 30 minutes. Providing diversion such as reading a story, watching television, or providing floating toys helps obtain cooperation of the child with a short attention span or exaggerated time concept.

Creams and ointments. Creams and ointments are easily and evenly spread over the skin. Creams contain water with cold cream or oil emulsified in it; the main constituent of ointments is oil. Creams tend to disappear when rubbed into the skin and are less occlusive than ointments. If ointment is not absorbed but remains on the skin, too much is being applied.

Pastes. Pastes are powders mixed with an ointment base. More porous and less occlusive than ointments, they absorb moisture and produce a drying effect, and medications incorporated into pastes are released more slowly than from creams and ointments. Because they are difficult to apply and must be removed from the skin with mineral oil, pastes are used less frequently than other preparations. They are most easily applied with a tongue depressor and "buttered" on.

Powders. Powders have a controversial use in pediatrics. They are very effective for soothing, absorbing moisture, and protecting the skin by reducing friction. Chemically inert, their chief use is prophylactic when ap-

plied to intertriginous areas. However, powder must be applied in a fine film that does not cake or form lumps when wet, and care must be exerted to prevent the child from inhaling the powder, especially those that contain talc or kaolin. To reduce the risk of inhalation, powder is sprinkled in the palm of the hand and then applied to the skin surface. Powder is never sprinkled directly onto the patient's skin and the container is placed well out of the child's reach.

Soaps and shampoos. Germicidal soaps are useful adjunctive therapy for skin infections. Bactericidal agents incorporated in soaps include hexachlorophene and the halogenated salicylanilides and carbanilides, one or more of which are found in many of the well-known soaps. Another effective topical microbicide is povidone-iodine (Betadine) skin cleanser, which contains a detergent mixture with iodine and polyvinyl pyrrolidone that assists in disinfecting the skin and is effective in eliminating common pathogens including *Staphylococcus aureus*.

Shampoos that are used in dermatologic skin conditions include tar shampoos for resistant scalp seborrhea and psoriasis and antiparasitic shampoos such as lindane (Kwell) for pediculosis capitis. Soaps containing hexachlorophene are used with caution to reduce the risk of absorption, especially on broken or denuded areas. Large amounts of the drug when absorbed can cause central nervous system symptoms.

Sunscreening agents. Some chemicals have the capacity to absorb certain wavelengths of light and thus provide protection to the cutaneous surface when applied to the skin. They are especially useful in dermatoses in which light plays an important causative role. They are applied to light-exposed areas and provide protection for about 3 to 4 hours under ordinary circumstances.

Topical glucocorticoid therapy. The glucocorticoids are the therapeutic agents used most widely for skin disorders. Corticosteroids are applied directly to the affected area, and, because they are essentially nonsensitizing and have only minor side effects, they can be applied over prolonged periods with continuing effectiveness.

Other topical treatments. Other topical treatments include chemical cautery (especially useful for warts), cryosurgery, electrodesiccation (chiefly used for warts, granulomas, and nevi), ultraviolet therapy (primarily used in psoriasis and acne), and special acne therapies such as dermabrasion and acne "surgery."

Systemic therapy. Therapeutic agents are often used as an adjunct to topical therapy in dermatologic disorders, and those most frequently used therapeutically are the corticosteroids and the antibiotics. The corticosteroid hormones with their capacity to inhibit inflammatory and allergic reactions are valuable in the treatment of severe skin disorders. Dosage is carefully adjusted and gradually tapered to the minimum that is effective and tolerated and, in infants and children, is larger than is usually calculated from body-weight ratios. Protracted use may temporarily suppress growth, however.

Antibiotics, which interfere with the growth of micro-organisms, are used in severe or widespread skin infections. The danger inherent in the use of antibiotics is their tendency to produce a hypersensitivity in the patient; therefore, they are used with caution. Antifungal agents are the only means for treating systemic fungal infections.

Nursing considerations

Skin disorders present nurses with some of their most challenging problems. Nurses are involved in recognizing and describing deviations from normal skin character, determining the cause, carrying out a treatment plan, and dealing with the affected child and his family.

Identification of skin disorders. To assist in establishing a diagnosis, it is important for nurses to accurately describe any deviation in the character of the skin, using both inspection and palpation. The color, shape, and distribution of the lesions are noted, including absence of pigment (vitiligo). The individual lesions are described according to the accepted terminology and may involve more than one type, such as a maculopapular rash.

To confirm or amplify the findings made by inspection, the skin is gently palpated to detect characteristics such as temperature, moisture, texture, elasticity, and the presence of edema in the skin. It should be indicated whether the findings are restricted to the area of the lesion(s) or are generalized.

The child's subjective symptoms provide additional information. Older children are able to describe the condition as painful, itching, tingling, or so on. However, much can be determined by observation of the child's behavior and the parents' account of his reactions.

Nurse's role in therapy. Since only a few skin diseases are contagious, it is usually not necessary to isolate the affected child unless there is a danger that he may acquire a secondary infection. This is usually the child who is receiving large doses of corticosteroids or other immunosuppressant drugs or the child with an immunologic deficiency disorder. If the skin manifestation is caused by a viral exanthem, such as measles or chickenpox, the child should be prevented from exposing other susceptible children.

Autoinoculation is a constant hazard in some disorders such as impetigo, poison ivy, or (to a lesser extent) warts. The cooperation of older children can be obtained, although they may need reminding to stop scratching or rubbing, but smaller and uncooperative children require the implementation of techniques and devices such as mittens, restraints, or special coverings. These methods, along with general cleanliness and hygiene, also serve to reduce the

likelihood of secondary infection of a primary lesion.

Therapeutic programs are usually designed to provide general measures such as rest, protection, and relief of discomfort and specific treatments such as a definitive medication or physical technique. They usually involve some type of topical treatment, and the mode of application depends on the nature and location of the lesion being treated. Most of the therapeutic regimens are directed toward relief of pruritus, the most common subjective complaint. Cooling applications that reduce external stimuli to the part are highly beneficial along with maintenance of cleanliness and good aeration. Clothing and bed linen should be soft and lightweight to decrease the irritation from friction and stimulation. During any type of treatment, both affected and unaffected skin is protected from damage and secondary infection.

Child and parental support. Childhood dermatologic conditions always involve the parents. Since few situations require hospitalization and children who do require hospitalization will complete a therapy program at home, the parents are the persons who must carry out the treatment plan; therefore, their cooperation is essential. Child and parents are more apt to be motivated if they are told why something is being done in a certain way. Success of treatment depends on the correct interpretation of instructions, and it is often the nurse's responsibility to teach the parent how to carry out the physician's instructions and offer encouragement, support, and assistance with problem solving. Several additional suggestions for encouraging the child's cooperation with treatments are discussed in Chapter 19.

BACTERIAL INFECTIONS

Normally the skin harbors a variety of bacterial flora, including the major pathogenic varieties of staphylococci and streptococci. The degree of their pathogenicity depends on the specific organism's invasiveness and toxigenicity, the integrity of the skin, the barrier of the host, and the immune and cellular defenses of the host. Children with immune deficiency states are highly susceptible to bacterial invasion. This includes infants, children with congenital immune deficiency disorders, children in a debilitated condition, those on immunosuppressive therapy, and those with a generalized malignancy such as leukemia or lymphoma.

Because of the characteristic "walling off" process of the inflammatory reaction, that is, abscess formation, staphylococci are more difficult to attack and the local infected area is associated with an increase in numbers of bacteria all over the skin surface that serve as a source of continuing infection. Staphylococcal infections occur most often in children in the younger age-groups, and the inci-

SUMMARY OF NURSING CARE OF THE CHILD WITH A DISORDER OF THE SKIN

GOALS	RESPONSIBILITIES
Identify lesion and its cause	Describe skin lesion accurately; use descriptive terminology for type, configuration, and distribution of lesion(s)
	Describe any associated characteristics, such as temperature, moisture, texture, elasticity, and hardness of skin in general or in area of lesion(s)
	Obtain history of onset, possible precipitating events, and course of development
	Determine any symptoms associated with disorder, such as itching, pain, fever, and so on
	Participate in special tests, such as collection of specimens for laboratory examination, use of Wood's light, or elimination diet
Prevent secondary infection	Maintain careful handwashing before handling affected child; wear surgical gloves when handling or dressing affected parts if indicated by nature of lesion
	Teach the child and family hygienic care and medical asepsis
	Devise methods to prevent secondary infection of lesion in small or uncooperative children
Protect healthy skin surface	Teach and impress on child importance of keeping hands away from lesion(s)
	Assist the child to determine ways of preventing autoinoculation
	Devise means for keeping small or uncooperative children from spreading infection to other areas
	Protect healthy skin from maceration by keeping it dry
Prevent spread of infection to self and others	Isolate the affected child from susceptible individuals
	Maintain careful handwashing after caring for the child
	Avoid unnecessary close contact with the affected child during infective stage of disease
	Use correct technique for disposal of dressing, solutions, and other fomites in contact with lesion(s)
Prevent occurrence and/or recurrence	Avoid or reduce contact with agents or circumstances known to precipitate skin reaction
	Teach child to recognize agents or circumstances that produce reaction

TABLE 27-1. BACTERIAL INFECTIONS

DISORDER	ORGANISM	SKIN MANIFESTATIONS
Impetigo contagiosa (Fig. 27-3)	*Streptococcus* *Staphylococcus*	Begins as a reddish macule
		Becomes vesicular
		Ruptures easily, leaving a superficial, moist erosion
		Tends to spread peripherally in sharply marginated irregular outlines
		Exudate dries to form heavy, honey-colored crusts
		Pruritus common
Pyoderma	*Staphylococcus* *Streptococcus*	Deeper extension of infection into dermis
		Tissue reaction more severe
Folliculitis (pimple), furuncle (boil), carbuncle (multiple boils)	*Staphylococcus aureus*	Folliculitis: infection of hair follicle
		Furuncle is a larger lesion with more redness and swelling at a single follicle
		Carbuncle is a more extensive lesion with widespread inflammation and "pointing" at several follicular orifices
Cellulitis	*Streptococcus* *Hemophilus influenzae*	Inflammation of skin and subcutaneous tissues with intense redness, swelling, and firm infiltration
		Lymphangitis "streaking" frequently seen
		Involvement of regional lymph nodes common

GOALS	RESPONSIBILITIES
Promote healing	Carry out therapeutic regimen as prescribed or support and assist the parents to carry out treatment plan Prevent secondary infection and autoinoculation Encourage rest Reduce external stimuli that aggravate condition Encourage well-balanced diet
Relieve discomfort	Avoid or reduce external stimuli that aggravate discomfort, such as rough clothing and bed linen Apply soothing treatments and topical applications as ordered Administer medications to relieve discomfort and/or restlessness and irritability
Support the child	Teach self-care where appropriate Involve the child in planning treatment schedules Support and encourage the child in his efforts to deal with the multiple problems that may be associated with disorder, including discomfort, rejection, discouragement, and feelings of self-revulsion Encourage the child to maintain usual activities
Promote habits of hygiene	Teach and reinforce positive habits of hygienic care
Teach the parents	Teach the parents skills needed to carry out therapeutic program Inform the parents of expected and unexpected results of therapy and a course of action to follow Help devise special techniques to carry out therapy
Support the parents	Encourage the parents in their efforts to carry out plan of care Provide assistance when appropriate Refer to agencies and services that assist with social, financial, and medical problems

SYSTEMIC EFFECTS	TREATMENT	COMMENTS
Minimal or asymptomatic	Careful removal of undermined skin, crusts, and debris by softening with 1:20 Burow solution compresses Topical application of bacteriocidal ointment (Garamycin, Neo-Polycin, Neosporin) Systemic administration of oral or parenteral antibiotics (penicillin) in severe or extensive lesions	Tends to heal without scarring unless secondary infection Autoinoculable and contagious Very common in toddler, preschooler
Fever, lymphangitis	Soap and water cleansing Wet compresses (saline solution, Burow solution, or potassium permanganate solution)	Autoinoculable and contagious May heal with or without scarring
Malaise if severe	Skin cleanliness Local warm, moist compresses (Burow solution, saline solution, potassium permanganate) Topical application of antibiotic agents Systemic antibiotics in severe cases Incision and drainage of severe lesions, followed by wound irrigations with antibiotics or suitable drain implantation	Autoinoculable and contagious Furuncle and carbuncle tend to heal with scar formation
Fever, malaise	Oral or parenteral penicillin Rest and immobilization of both the affected area and the child	Hospitalization may be necessary for the child with systemic symptoms

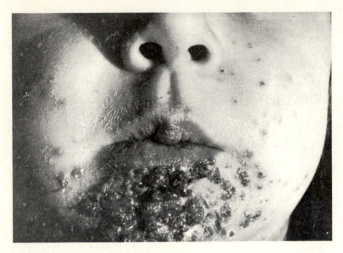

Fig. 27-3
Impetigo contagiosa. (From Stewart, W.D., Danto, J.L., and Maddin, S.: Dermatology: diagnosis and treatment of cutaneous disorders, ed. 4, St. Louis, 1978, The C.V. Mosby Co.)

dence decreases with advancing age. All of these factors emphasize the importance of careful handwashing and cleanliness when caring for infected children and their lesions to prevent spread of the infection and as an essential prophylactic measure when caring for infants and small children.

The most common bacterial infections are outlined in Table 27-1.

VIRAL INFECTIONS

Viruses are intracellular parasites that produce their effect by using the intracellular substances of the host cells. Composed of only a DNA or RNA core enclosed in an antigenic protein shell, viruses are unable to provide for their own metabolic needs or to reproduce themselves. After a virus penetrates a cell of the host organism, it sheds the outer shell and disappears within the cell where the nucleic acid core stimulates the host cell to form more vi-

TABLE 27-2. VIRAL INFECTIONS

DISEASE	MANIFESTATIONS	TREATMENT	COMMENTS
Verruca (warts)	Small, benign tumors Usually well-circumscribed, gray or brown, elevated firm papules with a roughened, finely papillomatous texture Occur anywhere but usually appear on exposed areas such as fingers, hands, face, and soles	Not uniformly successful Local destructive therapy, individualized according to location, type, and number—surgical removal, electrocautery, curettage, cryotherapy (liquid nitrogen), caustic solutions (bichloracetic acid, salicylic acid plasters), x-ray treatment Psychotherapy often effective	Common in children Tend to disappear spontaneously Course unpredictable Most destructive techniques tend to leave scars Autoinoculable Repeated irritation will cause to enlarge
Variants: Verruca vulgaris (common wart)	A skin-colored to brown, rough-surfaced epithelial growth May be single or multiple Asymptomatic Most frequent sites are dorsal and palmar surfaces of hands, fingers, and around nails		
Verruca plana juvenilis (juvenile wart)	Flat, skin-colored to brown, slightly raised, smooth lesion Asymptomatic Lesions multiple Commonly located on face and dorsum of hands		

rus material from its intracellular substance. In a viral infection the epidermal cells react with inflammation and vesiculation (as in herpes simplex) or by proliferating to form growths (warts).

The most common viral infections are outlined in Table 27-2.

FUNGAL INFECTIONS

Superficial infections caused by fungi live on, not in, the skin. They are confined to the dead keratin layers of the skin, hair, and nails but are unable to survive in the deeper layers. Superficial fungal infections are transmitted from one person to another or, more commonly, from infected animals to humans. Of the superficial fungal infections, ringworm is the most prevalent. Diseases in this category are the tineas with further designation related to the area of the body where they are found, for example, tinea capitis or ringworm of the scalp. (The most common fungal infections are outlined in Table 27-3.)

When teaching families regarding the care of the child with ringworm, it is important to emphasize good health and hygiene. Because of the infectious nature of the disease, several basic hygienic measures are particularly pertinent. The affected child should not exchange any groom-

TABLE 27-2. VIRAL INFECTIONS—cont'd			
DISEASE	**MANIFESTATIONS**	**TREATMENT**	**COMMENTS**
Verruca plantaris (plantar wart)	Located on plantar surface of feet and, because of pressure, are practically flat; may be surrounded by a collar of hyperkeratosis		
Herpes simplex* (cold sore, fever blister)	Grouped, burning, and itching vesicles on an inflammatory base, usually on or near mucocutaneous junctions (lips, nose, genitals, buttocks) Vesicles dry, forming a crust, followed by exfoliation and spontaneous healing in 8-10 days May be accompanied by regional lymphadenopathy	Avoidance of secondary infection Burow solution compresses during weeping stages Ointments (bacitracin or neomycin) when lesions are dry and crusted Aggravated by corticosteroids	Heal without scarring unless secondary infection
Herpes zoster (shingles)	Caused by same virus that causes varicella (chicken pox) Virus has affinity for posterior root ganglia, posterior horn of spinal cord, and skin; crops of vesicles usually confined to dermatome following along the course of the affected nerve Usually preceded by neuralgic pain, hyperesthesia, or itching May be accompanied by constitutional symptoms	Control of pain with analgesics Mild sedation sometimes helpful Local moist compresses three times daily soothing Drying lotions may be helpful Ophthalmic variety: systemic corticotropin (ACTH) and/or corticosteroids	Pain in children usually minimal Postherpetic pain does not occur in children Chickenpox may follow exposure to herpes zoster; thus affected child should be isolated from other children in a hospital May occur in children with depressed immunity; can be fatal
Molluscum contagiosum	Caused by a pox virus Flesh-colored papules with a central caseous plug Usually asymptomatic	Cases in well children resolve spontaneously in about 18 months Treatment reserved for troublesome cases	Common in school-age children Spread by person-to-person contact and by autoinoculation

*See p. 417 for genital herpes

TABLE 27-3. SUPERFICIAL MYCOSES CAUSED BY FUNGI

DISEASE/ORGANISM	MANIFESTATIONS	DIAGNOSIS	TREATMENT	COMMENTS
Dermatophytosis (ringworm) Tinea capitis— *Microsporum audouinii, M. canis* (see Fig. 27-4, *A*)	Lesions in the scalp but may extend to hairline or neck Scaly, circumscribed patches to patchy, scaling areas of alopecia Generally asymptomatic, but severe, deep inflammatory reaction may occur that manifests as boggy, encrusted lesions (kerions) Pruritic	Characteristic configuration Fluoresce green under Wood light Direct examination of scales and culture if doubtful Check at 2-week intervals with Wood's light	Oral griseofulvin (Gris-PEG, Fulvicin-U/F, Grifulvin V, Grisactin) Effectiveness of drug is enhanced by frequent shampoos and clipping hair Sometimes local application of strong antifungal ointment such as Whitfield ointment is advisable	Person-to-person transmission Animal-to-person transmission Rarely, permanent loss of hair *M. audouinii* transmitted from one human being to another; M. canis usually contracted from household pets
Tinea corporis— *Trichophyton, Microsporum* (see Fig. 27-4, *B*)	Generally round or oval, erythematous scaling patch that spreads peripherally and clears centrally; may involve nails (tinea unguium)	Direct microscopic examination of scales	Oral griseofulvin Local application of antifungal preparation such as Whitfield ointment, tolnaftate (Tinactin), haloprogin (Halotex), miconazole (Micatin), clotrimazole (Mycelex)	Usually of animal origin from infected pets Majority of infections in children caused by *M. canis* and *M. audouinii*

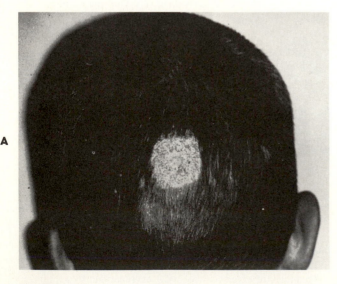

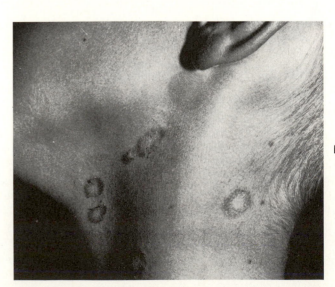

A

B

Fig. 27-4

A, *Tinea capitis.* **B,** *Tinea corporis. Both infections caused by* Microsporum canis, *the "kitten" or "puppy" fungus. (From Stewart, W.D., Danto, J.L., and Maddin, S.: Dermatology: diagnosis and treatment of cutaneous disorders, ed. 4, St. Louis, 1978, The C.V. Mosby Co.)*

TABLE 27-3. SUPERFICIAL MYCOSES CAUSED BY FUNGI—cont'd

DISEASE/ORGANISM	MANIFESTATIONS	DIAGNOSIS	TREATMENT	COMMENTS
Tinea cruris ("jock itch")—*Epidermophyton floccosum, T. rubrum*	Skin response similar to tinea corporis Localized to medial proximal aspect of thigh and crural fold; may involve scrotum in males Pruritic	Same as for tinea corporis	Local application of tolnaftate liquid Wet compresses or sitz baths may be soothing	Rare in preadolescent children Health education regarding personal hygiene
Tinea pedis *(athlete's foot)*—*E. floccosum, T. rubrum, T. interdigitale*	On intertriginous areas between toes or on plantar surface of feet Lesions vary: Maceration and fissuring between toes Patches with pinhead-sized vesicles on plantar surface Pruritic	Direct microscopic examination of scrapings	Oral griseofulvin Local applications of tolnaftate liquid and antifungal powder containing tolnaftate Acute infections: Compresses or soaks for 15 minutes twice daily followed by application of glucocorticoid cream Elimination of conditions of heat and perspiration by clean, light socks and well-ventilated shoes; avoidance of occlusive shoes	Most frequent in adolescents and adults; rare in children Transmission to other individuals is rare despite general opinion to the contrary Ointments not successful
Candidiasis (moniliasis)—*Candida albicans*	Grows in chronically moist areas Inflamed area with white exudate, peeling, and easy bleeding Pruritic	Characteristic appearance	Amphotericin B or nystatin ointment to affected areas	Common form of diaper dermatitis Oral form common in infants (p. 172)

ing items, headgear, scarves, or other articles of apparel that have been in proximity to the infected area. The affected child should have his own towel and wear a protective cap at night to avoid transmitting the fungus to bedding, especially if he sleeps with another person. Since the infection can be acquired by animal-to-human transmission, all household pets should be examined for the presence of the disorder.

Treatment with the drug griseofulvin frequently lasts for weeks or months, and because subjective symptoms subside the child or parent may be tempted to decrease or discontinue the drug. The nurse should impress on members of the family the importance of maintaining the prescribed dosage schedule. They are also instructed regarding the possibility of side effects from the drug such as headache, gastrointestinal upset, fatigue, insomnia, and photosensitivity. For children who take the drug over a period of many months, periodic testing is required to monitor leukopenia and assess liver and renal function.

Systemic or deep fungal infections (Table 27-4) have the capacity to invade the viscera as well as the skin. The best known of these are primarily lung diseases, which are usually acquired by inhalation. They produce a variable spectrum of disease, and some are quite common in certain geographic areas. They are not transmitted from person to person but appear to reside in the soil, from which their

TABLE 27-4. SYSTEMIC OR DEEP DISEASES CAUSED BY FUNGI

DISEASE/ORGANISM	SKIN MANIFESTATIONS	SYSTEMIC MANIFESTATIONS	TREATMENT	COMMENTS
Actinomycosis—*Actinomyces israelii*	Deep-seated granulomatous nodules and subcutaneous abscesses that drain as chronic fistulas, especially in jaw or neck	General health not affected	Penicillin or other antibiotics Incision and wide débridement of lesions	Access frequently through a carious tooth or mucous membranes of mouth Less prevalent in children Noninfectious
North American blastomycosis—*Blastomyces dermatitidis*	Chronic granulomatous lesions and microabscesses in any part of body Initial lesion is a papule; undergoes ulceration and peripheral spread	Pulmonary symptoms such as cough, chest pain, weakness, and weight loss May have skeletal involvement, with bone destruction and formation of cutaneous abscesses	Intravenous administration of amphotericin B (Fungizone)	Usual portal of entry is the lungs Source of infection unknown Noninfectious
Cryptococcosis—*Cryptococcus neoformans (Torula histolytica)*	Usually on face; acneiform, firm, nodular, painless eruption	Central nervous sytem (CNS) manifestations: headache, dizziness, stiff neck, and signs of increased intracranial pressure Low-grade fever, mild cough, lung infiltration	Intravenous amphotericin B may be administered intrathecally for CNS involvement 5-Fluorocytosine (Ancobon) Excision and drainage of local lesions	Acquired by inhalation of dust, but may enter through skin Prognosis serious Noninfectious
Histoplasmosis—*Histoplasma capsulatum*	Not distinctive or uniform but most appear as punched-out or granulomatous ulcers	General systemic symptoms may include pallor, diarrhea, vomiting, irregular spiking temperature, hepatosplenomegaly, and pulmonary symptoms Any tissue of the body may be involved with related symptoms	Intravenous amphotericin B for severe cases Triple sulfonamides Sulfadiazine	Organism cultured from soil, especially where contaminated with fowl droppings Fungus enters through skin or mucous membranes of mouth and respiratory tract Endemic in Mississippi and Ohio River valleys Disseminated diseases most common in infants and children
Coccidioidomycosis (valley fever)—*Coccidioides immitis*	Erythema nodosum	Primary lung disease usually asymptomatic May be sign of acute febrile illness Disseminated disease is very serious	Intravenous amphotericin B Intravenous miconazole (synthetic imidazole) Intrathecal administration of either drug for CNS involvement Surgical resection of persistent pulmonary cavities	Inhalation of aerospores from soil Endemic in southwestern United States Usually resolves spontaneously

TABLE 27-5. ERUPTIONS CAUSED BY RICKETTSIAE

DISEASE/RICKETTSIA	ORGANISM/HOST	MANIFESTATIONS	COMMENTS
Rocky mountain spotted fever—*R. rickettsii*	Arthropod: tick Transmission: tick bite Mammal source: wild rodents; dogs	Gradual onset: fever, malaise, anorexia, myalgia Abrupt onset: rapid temperature elevation, chills, vomiting, myalgia, severe headache Maculopapular or petechial rash primarily on extremities (ankles and wrists) but may spread to other areas	Usually self-limited in children Onset in children may resemble any infectious disease Severe disease rare in children See Table 27-6 for management of ticks
Epidemic typhus—*R. prowazekii*	Arthropod: body louse Transmission: infected feces into broken skin Mammal source: humans	Abrupt onset of chills, fever, diffuse myalgia, headache, malaise Maculopapular rash 4 to 5 days later spreading from trunk outward	Patient should be isolated until deloused See discussion on p. 911 for management of pediculosis
Rickettsialpox—*R. akari*	Arthropod: mouse mite Transmission: mite Mammal source: house mouse	Maculopapular rash following primary lesion at site of bite	Self-limited nonfatal disease Eliminate mice
Q fever—*Coxiella burnetti*	Arthropod: tick Transmission: inhalation of dried, infected material Mammal source: domestic farm animals (cattle, sheep, goats)	Abrupt onset of chills, fever, weakness, and nonspecific symptoms After 1 week—cough and chest pains	Milk should be pasteurized Persons who work around farm animals are at risk

spores are airborne. The cutaneous lesions are granulomatous and appear as ulcers, plaques, nodules, fungating mosses, and abscesses. The course of deep fungal diseases is chronic with slow progression that favors sensitization.

RICKETTSIAL INFECTIONS

Rickettsiae are intracellular parasites, similar in size to bacteria, that inhabit the alimentary tract of a wide range of natural hosts. With the exception of Q fever, mammals become infected only through the bites of infected insects (lice and fleas) or arachnids (ticks and mites), both of which serve as both infectors and reservoirs. Rickettsial diseases are more common in temperate and tropical climates and in areas where humans live in association with arthropods. Infection in humans is incidental (except epidemic typhus) and not necessary for the survival of the rickettsial species. However, once the organism invades a

human they cause a disease that varies in intensity from a benign, self-limiting illness to a fulminating and frequently fatal one. Some rickettsial infections are outlined in Table 27-5.

MISCELLANEOUS SKIN LESIONS

There are a number of skin lesions caused by extrinsic or intrinsic factors. Table 27-6 lists some of the common manifestations. In addition there are two common types of skin disorders that are encountered frequently by nurses in their practice.

Contact dermatitis

Contact dermatitis is an inflammatory reaction of the skin to chemical substances, natural or synthetic, that evoke a hypersensitivity response or to those agents that cause di-

TABLE 27-6. MISCELLANEOUS SKIN DISORDERS

DISEASE	CAUSATIVE AGENT	LOCAL MANIFESTATIONS	SYSTEMIC MANIFESTATIONS
Intertrigo	Mechanical trauma and aggravating factors of excessive heat, moisture, and sweat retention	Red, inflamed, moist, partially denuded, marginated areas, the shape of which is determined by location Appear where opposing skin surfaces rub together, that is, intergluteal folds, groin, neck, and axilla are common sites where chafing, warmth, and moisture enable microorganisms to produce dermatitis Hyperhidrosis and obesity are often factors	None unless severe secondary infection
Urticaria	Usually allergic response	Development of wheals Vary in size and configuration and tend to appear quickly, spread irregularly, and fade within a few hours May be constant or intermittent, sparse or profuse, small or large, discrete or confluent May be acute, chronic, or recurrent in acute attacks	May be accompanied by malaise, sometimes fever and lymphadenopathy Severe cases may involve mucous membranes, internal organs, and joints Obstruction to air passages constitutes medical emergency
Psoriasis	Unknown Hereditary predisposition	Round, thick, dry, reddish patches covered with coarse, silvery scales over trunk and extremities; first lesions commonly appear in scalp; facial lesions more common in children than adults Affected cells proliferate at a much more rapid rate than normal cells	Persons are otherwise healthy individuals

rect irritation. The initial reaction occurs in an exposed region, most commonly the face and neck, backs of the hands, forearms, male genitalia, and lower legs. Characteristically there is a sharp delineation between inflamed and normal skin early in the reaction that ranges from a faint, transient erythema to massive bullae on an erythematous swollen base. Itching is a constant symptom.

The major goal in treatment is to prevent further exposure of the skin to the offending substance. Providing there is not further irritation, the normal recuperative powers of the skin will produce satisfactory results without treatment.

The most frequent offenders are plant and animal irritants, the prototype of which is poison ivy. Contact with the dry or succulent portions of the plant produces localized, streaked or spotty, oozing and painful impetiginous lesions. The most effective management of the lesions includes administration of corticosteroids to reduce inflammation, cooling compresses, and a sedative such as diphenhydramine (Benadryl). Avoidance of contact by teaching the child to recognize the plant and its removal from the environment when feasible are prophylactic measures.

The most common contact dermatitis in infants occurs on the convex surfaces of the diaper area as a result of chemical irritation from ammonia, putrefactive enzymes acting on urinary amino acids, or, less often, laundry products. Other agents that frequently produce dermatologic responses from contact are animal irritants such as wool, feathers, and furs, vegetable irritants such as oleoresins, oils, and turpentine, and chemicals of all kinds, including synthetic fabrics, dyes, metals, cosmetics, perfumes, and soaps. The list is endless.

Several cosmetic products advertised as safe for children include a cream hair relaxer that contains lye and preparations to curl or straighten hair. These products are stronger than those intended for adults because children's hair is more resistant to these attempts. Frequent causes of genital irritation in girls are bubble baths and feminine hygiene products.

TREATMENT	COMMENTS
Affected areas are kept clean and dry Cool compresses of Burow solution provide relief Skin folds may be kept separated with a generous supply of nonmedicated powder Area is exposed to air and light Treat superimposed infections Remove excess clothing	A form of diaper irritation Prevent recurrence by keeping susceptible areas clean and dry Frequently associated with overheating from too much clothing
Local soothing and antipruritic applications Antihistamines Epinephrine or ephedrine Cortisone or ACTH in severe cases Severe upper respiratory involvement may require tracheostomy	Known etiologic agents should be avoided
Exposure to sunlight, ultraviolet light Children respond well to topical applications of coal tar ointments, which act synergistically with ultraviolet light Topical corticosteroid cream Systemic (used only in acute refractory cases): corticosteroids, methotrexate	Uncommon in children under age 6 years

Drug reactions

Adverse reactions to drugs are seen more often in the skin than in any other organ. Cutaneous manifestations can resemble almost any skin disease and can be seen in almost any degree of severity. With few exceptions, the distribution of a drug eruption is widespread since it results from a circulating agent, appears as an inflammatory response with itching, is sudden in onset, and may be associated with constitutional symptoms such as fever, malaise, gastrointestinal upsets, anemia, or liver and kidney damage.

The most frequent offenders in drug reactions are penicillin and sulfonamides. However, even commonplace drugs including aspirin, barbiturates, and chemical agents found in a number of foods, flavoring agents, and preservatives are capable of producing an undesired response.

Treatment for cutaneous reactions consists of discontinuation of the drug. Nurses who suspect that a rash is caused by a medication should withhold any further dose and report the eruption to the attending physician. In urticarial-type eruptions antihistamines may be ordered, and,

for widespread and severe lesions, corticosteroids are beneficial.

INFESTATIONS, BITES, AND STINGS

Young children are curious by nature and fascinated by the world around them. School children's social nature and proximity to other children render them highly susceptible to communicable diseases, including those caused by parasites. Because they spend a great deal of time outdoors and in fields and vacant lots, children often come in contact with insects. Consequently children are frequently the victims of insects that puncture the skin for the purpose of sucking blood, injecting venom, or laying their eggs. In the process of these activities, substances foreign to the victim may create an allergic sensitivity in that individual to produce pruritus, urticaria, or systemic reactions

TABLE 27-7. ERUPTIONS CAUSED BY INFESTATIONS

DISEASE	ORGANISM	MECHANISM	MANIFESTATIONS
Scabies (7-year itch)	*Sarcoptes scabiei*	Impregnated female burrows into superficial stratum corneum of epidermis, depositing eggs and fecal material; burrows form a minute linear, grayish-brown, threadlike lesion Transmitted by skin-to-skin contact	Characteristic minute linear lesion seen with difficulty Intense pruritus that leads to punctate discrete excoriations secondary to pruritus; maculopapular lesions characteristically distributed in intertriginous areas: interdigital surfaces, axillary-cubital area, popliteal folds, and inguinal region Alopecia in scalp involvement Diagnosis confirmed by demonstrating mite or ova from skin scrapings
Pediculosis capitis (head lice)	*Pediculus humanus capitis*	Saliva of louse on the skin produces itching	Pruritus of scalp Close examination of scalp reveals white eggs (nits) firmly attached to hair shafts near the scalp; adult lice are seldom found because of brief life span and mobility Excoriations are produced from itching and may become secondarily infected
Pediculosis corporis (body lice) including pediculosis pukis (''crabs'')	*Pediculus humanus corporis*	Lice present on the skin only when feeding Diagnosis established when lice and nits identified in seams of clothing	Pruritus Erythematous macules, wheals, and excoriated papules Most often found on upper back and pressure areas caused by tight clothing

of greater or lesser degree depending on the child's sensitivity.

INFESTATIONS

Infestations with insect parasites are relatively common, and those encountered most frequently in childhood are scabies and pediculosis capitis. Body lice infestations are seen less often, and pubic lice (pediculosis pubis, or ''crabs'') are rare in childhood. The major infestations are outlined in Table 27-7.

Scabies

Scabies is an endemic infestation that becomes pandemic at 15 year cyclic intervals with each incidence lasting approximately 15 years. The current pandemic is nearing completion. The lesions are created as the female scabies mite burrows into the stratum corneum (never into living tissue) to bury her eggs. The inflammatory response and itching occur after the host becomes sensitized to the mite, approximately 30 to 60 days following initial contact. After this time, anywhere the mite has traveled will begin to itch and develop the characteristic eruption. Consequently mites will not necessarily be located at all sites of eruption.

In children over 2 years of age the largest percentage of eruptions are found in the hands and wrists and, in children less than 2 years, on feet and ankles. The clinical picture is often confusing in infants who often develop an eczematous eruption; therefore, the observer must look for discrete papules, burrows, or vesicles. A mite is identified as a black dot at the end of a burrow.

The treatment of scabies is the application of a scabicide. Nurses instructing families in use of the scabicide should emphasize the importance of following the directions accurately. The lotion is applied to cool dry, skin—not following a hot bath—and left on for the recommended time, usually 4 hours for infants and 6 hours for older

TREATMENT	COMMENTS
Lindane (Kwell) in vanishing cream base	All infected members of a family should be treated at the same time
Benzyl benzoate emulsion	
Crotamiton (Eurax)	Previously worn clothing should be washed in very hot water and ironed
The prescribed drug is applied over entire cutaneous surface from the neck down; is left on for the prescribed length of time	Nurses caring for affected children in the hospital should wear gloves and reduce holding
Only fresh laundered bed linen and underclothing should be used	
Touch and holding contacts should be reduced until treatment is completed	
Soothing ointments for pruritus	
Lindane (Kwell) shampoo	Caregivers, including nurses, should protect themselves from infection during examination and treatment by wearing gloves
Pyrethrins with peperonyl butoxide (RID, A-200 Pyrinate) shampoo	
Malathion 0.5% (Prioderm) lotion	Launder or dry clean clothing, bed linen, and items that have been in contact with scalp in very hot water
Apply according to directions	
After treatment, remaining nits are removed with an extra-fine comb and/or between fingernails or tweezers	Soak all combs, brushes, curlers, barrettes, etc. in pediculocide solution for 10 minutes
Treatment is repeated in 8 to 10 days to exterminate hatched nits	Vacuum all carpets, upholstery, and mattresses thoroughly
	Treat all persons in household who have signs of infestation
	If lindane is used, observe for central nervous system toxicity (especially seizures)
All clothing should be thoroughly laundered and seams ironed	Associated with unhygienic environmental conditions

children and adults. Since it is a superficial skin disorder penetration need not be promoted. One liberal application is sufficient, but all persons in the family (including baby sitters, etc.) should be treated. Parents need to know that, although the mite will be killed, the rash and the itch will not be eliminated until the stratum corneum is replaced, which takes approximately 2 to 3 weeks.

Pediculosis capitis

Pediculosis capitis, head lice, or "cooties" are very common parasites, especially in school-age children. There are several things that nurses should be aware of in order to successfully manage or to assist parents in coping with the problem. It should be emphasized that *anyone* can get pediculosis. It has no respect for age, socioeconomic level, or cleanliness. The louse does not jump nor fly but it can be transmitted from one person to another on personal items. Therefore, children are cautioned against sharing combs, hats, caps, scarves, coats, and other items used on or near the hair. Also, lice are not carried nor transmitted by household pets.

Parents should carefully inspect the head of a child who scratches his head more than usual for bite marks, redness, and nits. The nits, or eggs, appear as tiny whitish oval specks adhering to the hair shaft about ¼ inch from the scalp. The adherent nature of the nits distinguish them from dandruff, which falls off readily. Empty nit cases, indicating hatched lice, are translucent rather than white and are located more than ¼ inch from the scalp.

It is also important to perform the treatment according to the directions described on the label of the pediculocide. For example, apply the shampoo to wet hair and leave on for a specified time before rinsing. The child should be made as comfortable as possible during the application process because the pediculocide must remain on the scalp and hair for several minutes. Playing "beauty parlor" is a useful strategy. The child lies supine with his head over a sink or or basin and covers his eyes with a dry towel or washcloth during the shampoo to protect them from splashing medication into the eyes, which can cause a chemical conjunctivitis. If eye irritation occurs, the operator must flush the eyes well with tepid water.

Nonwashable, noncleanable items should be placed in a tightly closed plastic bag that remains sealed for 35 days. Ova are able to lie dormant for this length of time. Families should also be advised that the pediculocide is relatively costly, especially when several members of the household require treatment.

BITES AND STINGS

Bites and stings account for a significant incidence of mild to moderate discomfort and, fortunately, a relatively small number of severe reactions in children. However, severe reactions can be life-threatening. The major offending ar-

thropods and animals, their manifestations, and management are outlined in Table 27-8.

Arthropod bites and stings

Mosquitos are probably the most common cause of insect bites in children. Children play in or near infested areas and their summer clothing leaves maximum skin surface exposed. Prevention by spraying the exposed areas with insect repellent is the most useful management. Sensitization follows repeated bites and, once sensitized, the child initially experiences a delayed reaction (24 to 48 hours) following exposure. Subsequently the wheals appear immediately after the child is bitten.

Fleas are probably the next most frequent source of bites in children. Fleas favor geographic areas with moderate temperatures and high humidity. They will live for

TABLE 27-8. ERUPTIONS CAUSED BY BITES AND STINGS

BITE OR STING	ORGANISM	MECHANISM	MANIFESTATIONS
Insect bites	Flies, gnats, mosquitoes, fleas, and flies	Hypersensitivity reaction Little or no reaction in nonsensitized person Foreign protein in insects' saliva introduced when skin penetrated for a bloodsucking meal	Papular urticaria termed lichen urticatus Firm papules; may be capped by vesicles or excoriated
Hymenoptera stings	Bees, wasps, hornets, yellow jackets, and ants	Injection of venom through stinging apparatus Venom contains histamine, allergenic proteins, and often a spreading factor, hyaluronidase Some proteins are species specific; others are common to a number of species, therefore cross-reactivity is common Severe reactions caused by hypersensitivity and/or multiple stings	Local reaction: small red area, wheal, itching, and heat Systemic reactions: may be mild to severe, including generalized edema, pain, nausea, and vomiting, confusion, respiratory embarrassment, and shock
Arachnid bites	Spiders	All produce venom via fangs; few are able to pierce skin or the venom is insufficiently toxic	Local tissue reaction
	Black widow spider	Venom injected through a clawlike appendage Has a neurotoxic action	Mild sting at time of bite Area becomes swollen, painful, and erythematous Dizziness, weakness, and abdominal pain May produce delirium, paralysis, convulsions, and (if large amount of venom absorbed) death

very long periods in carpeting, upholstery, mats, and debris collected in corners and floor cracks. However, because of their close proximity to household pets, children frequently acquire fleas from dogs or cats, which can harbor fleas in the winter months as well as the warmer seasons. Sensitization takes place in the same manner as with mosquitoes. Prevention involves eliminating fleas from pets and spraying carpets and furniture with environmental flea spray.

Persons who have become sensitized to the bites of certain hymenoptera such as bees may demonstrate a severe anaphylactic response that can be life threatening. Intramuscular administration of epinephrine provides immediate relief and must be available for emergency use. Hypersensitive children need a kit available that contains epinephrine, a hypodermic syringe, a tourniquet (to delay spread of venom from an extremity), and perhaps ephed-

rine and an antihistamine preparation. Ideally the person who reacts severely to hymenoptera stings should keep an automatic syringe loaded with epinephrine (EpiPen, Ana-Kit) with them at all times. A child with a history of generalized reactivity to an insect sting should undertake a program of skin testing and desensitization to prevent serious or fatal reactions.

Animal bites

Contrary to the popular conception, animal bites to children occur more often from animals belonging to the family or to neighbors than from strange animals. Boys are bitten more often by dogs; girls are bitten more often by cats. One third of dog bites and two thirds of cat bites or scratches occur to the upper extremities. However, children less than 4 years of age, because of their shorter stat-

TREATMENT	COMMENTS
Antipruritic agents and t176 baths Antihistamines Prevent secondary infection Painful bites: rub with cotton ball soaked with meat tenderizer for 15 min. If no meat tenderizer apply ammonia; apply ice cube to area	Avoidance of contact Removing focus such as treating furniture, mattresses, carpets, and so on, where insects may live Apply insect repellant to exposed areas before going outdoors or into wooded areas
Carefully scrape off stinger if present Cleanse with soap and water Apply cool compresses or ice packs Elevate involved extremity Apply cotton ball soaked with meat tenderizer Moisten skin and rub aspirin into it Apply a paste made of baking soda and water and keep in place with a bandaid Antihistamines Severe reactions: epinephrine, corticosteroids; treat for shock	Persons with known sensitivity to bites or stings should wear identifying tag to indicate allergy and therapy needed; parents should keep emergency medication and be taught its administration Child should be taught to wear shoes, to avoid wearing bright clothing or perfumed grooming products that might attract the insect, and to avoid places where the insect may be contacted Persons who develop anaphylaxis should keep an automatic syringe loaded with epinephrine
Local compresses	Most spiders are harmless, including tarantulas
Cleanse wound with antiseptic; application of ice packs Antivenin Muscle relaxant such as calcium gluconate Morphine sulfate for pain Phenobarbital	Spider is recognized by red or orange hourglass-shaped marking on underside Avoids light and bites in self-defense

Continued.

TABLE 27-8. ERUPTIONS CAUSED BY BITES AND STINGS—cont'd

BITE OR STING	ORGANISM	MECHANISM	MANIFESTATIONS
Arachnid bites— cont'd	Brown recluse spider	Venom contains powerful necrotoxic, hemolytic, and spreading factors	Mild sting at time of bite Transient erythema followed by bleb or blister; mild to severe pain in 2-8 hours; purple, star-shaped area in 3-4 days; necrotic ulceration in 7-14 days Heals with scar formation Systemic reactions may include fever, malaise, restlessness, nausea and vomiting, and joint pain Generalized petechial eruption
	Scorpions	Sting by means of a hooked caudal stinger that discharges venom Venom of more venomous species contains hemolysins, endotheliolysins, and neurotoxins	Some species produce only local tissue reaction with swelling at puncture site (distinctive) Intense local pain, erythema, numbness, and burning Ascending motor paralysis with convulsions, weakness, rapid pulse, excessive salivation, thirst, and dysuria
	Ticks	Feed on blood of mammals Significant in man because of pathologic organisms they carry In the process of sucking blood, the head and mouth parts are buried in the skin	Produce firm, discrete, intensely pruritic nodules at site of attachment May cause urticaria or persistent localized edema
Animal bites	Household pets (e.g., dogs, cats, mice, hamsters) Wild animals (e.g., mice, skunks, raccoon)	Puncture wounds and tears from direct penetration of skin with teeth (claws)	Puncture wound, laceration, bruise

ure, sustain almost two thirds of bites to the head, face, or neck. Small children are relatively defenseless and at greater risk.

Dog bites are primarily laceration or evulsion injuries but can be associated with considerable crush injury. Cat bites become infected more easily than dog bites but the incidence is no greater than lacerations from other causes. It is typical, however, that injuries to poorly vascularized areas such as the hands are more likely to become infected than the more vascularized areas such as the face; puncture wounds are more apt to become infected than lacerations.

The wound care involves rinsing with copious amounts of water or saline under pressure (syringe), washing surrounding skin with mild soap, elevation of the injured part, and application of a pressure dressing to control bleeding. Antibiotics are indicated in puncture wounds and wounds in areas that may prove to be cosmetically or functionally impaired if infected. Tetanus toxoid is administered according to standard guidelines and rabies protocol followed. Plastic surgery may be required for severe injury.

The most important aspect related to animal bites is prevention. Children should be taught the proper behavior around and toward animals both their own and those of

TREATMENT	COMMENTS
Local application of cool compresses Antibiotics Large doses of corticosteroids Relieve pain Some advocate early excision of necrotic area and surrounding tissue	Spider is fawn to dark brown and recognized by fiddle-shaded mark on head
Delay absorption of venom by application of tourniquets for 10-15 minutes and apply cold with ice packs or submersion in cold water Supportive measures Treat shock	Usual habitat is southwestern United States Symptoms subside in a few hours Deaths occur among children under 4 years of age
Remove tick, making every effort to avoid breaking off embedded head 　Grasp with tweezers as close as possible to the point of attachment and roll *forward* slowly and steadily to loosen grip; if tweezers are unavailable, use fingers protected with facial tissue; if head remains in skin, remove with a sterile needle Wash wound with soap and water If bare hands touch the tick during removal, wash thoroughly with soap and water	May be vectors of various infectious diseases such as Rocky Mountain spotted fever, Q fever, tularemia, and relapsing fever Immediately check children who have been hiking in tick-infested areas
Thorough rinsing with water or saline and washing surrounding area with soap Observe animal for rabies; if animal is positive for rabies, immunization series is begun immediately Tetanus immunization as indicated	May be vectors of bacterial infections and rabies Usual habitat is very wooded area

others. Small children should be supervised closely when around animals.

SKIN DISORDERS ASSOCIATED WITH SPECIFIC AGE-GROUPS

Several common and important dermatologic conditions are confined primarily, but not exclusively, to children in specific age-groups. This includes atopic, seborrheic, and diaper dermatitis and the acne of adolescence. The treatment modalities include those described in the previous segment. However, there are some special needs and therapies involved with these disorders.

ECZEMA (ATOPIC DERMATITIS)

Eczema is a common pruritic disease that usually appears in three phases: (1) the infantile form (infantile eczema) with distribution on the cheeks, trunk, and extremities; (2) the childhood form, which involves primarily the extensor, antecubital, and popliteal surfaces; and, (3) the preadolescent and adolescent form with distribution on the face, neck, flexor surfaces, hands, and feet. Because the disease appears predominantly in infancy this discussion is restricted to infantile eczema.

The manifestations appear first in children at about 2 to 4 months of age as an allergic response to foods, environmental inhalants, or pollens. During infancy foods such as cow's milk and egg albumin are the chief offenders. As the child grows older, environmental inhalants and pollen become stronger allergens. The majority of children with infantile eczema have a family history of atopic dermatitis, asthma, or hay fever, which strongly supports a genetic predetermined allergic disorder although a mode of inheritance has not been established. The disorder can be controlled but not cured.

Clinical manifestations

The disease appears on the face, scalp, and extensor aspects of the arms and legs. The eczematous lesions are characterized by erythema, vesicles, papules, weeping, oozing, and crusting accompanied by intense itching. The unaffected areas of the body tend to be dry and rough.

The child may be very irritable, fretful, and unable to sleep because of the persistent pruritus, and scratching the lesions contributes to a high frequency of secondary infection.

Therapeutic management

The major management modality is local therapy with wet, cool compresses that are soothing, antipruritic, and antiinflammatory. The compresses are applied loosely to allow for evaporation for 5 to 10 minutes for up to six times a day. Local steroids are sometimes helpful and, if secondary infection is suspected, the appropriate systemic antibiotic is administered. Since pruritus increases at night, a mild sedative may be needed. Tepid baths, with or without emollient substances, are beneficial as a comfort measure. Hot baths and soap are contraindicated. The processed oatmeal preparation, Aveeno, provides an excellent medium for a soothing bath.

The allergic nature of the disorder necessitates removal of the allergen if possible. The onset of eczema is frequently associated with the introduction of cow's milk to breast-fed infants or new foods, particularly egg white, to other infants. The child is placed on a hypoallergenic diet that restricts the following foods: milk or milk products, eggs, wheat, fish, citrus fruits, nuts, peanut butter, chocolate, strawberries, tomatoes, pork, and pineapple. It is now recommended that susceptible infants remain on breast-feedings with delayed introduction of solid foods until at least 6 months of age.

Nursing considerations

Long-term treatment of eczema is usually established on an outpatient basis. As a result the major burden of responsibility and physical care rests on the parents in the home. A vicious cycle of exacerbations–scratching–infection–irritability–frustration is the usual course unless the initial phase can be altered.

Probably the most difficult problem of caring for the child with eczema is controlling the intense pruritus. In order to prevent infection, the child must be restricted from scratching. Aside from the use of topical or systemic medications, other measures can be taken to minimize the scratching. Fingernails and toenails are cut short, kept clean, and filed frequently to prevent sharp edges. Gloves or cotton stockings may have to be placed over the hands and pinned to shirt-sleeves. To prevent any contact with the skin, elbow restraints are sometimes necessary. One-piece outfits with long sleeves and long pants also decrease direct contact with the skin. Whether gloves or restraints are used, the child needs time when he is free from such restrictions. An excellent time to remove any protective devices is during the bath or after receiving sedative or antipruritic medication. Restraints should not be removed during sleep, because the child will scratch in his sleep and can severely traumatize the skin.

The elimination of conditions that increase itching is another approach. Woolen clothes or blankets, rough fabrics, and furry stuffed animals are irritating to the skin and are removed. All (100%) cotton fabrics appear to be the least irritating. During cold months, synthetic—not wool—fabrics are used for overcoats, hats, gloves, and snowsuits. Heat and humidity cause perspiration, which intensifies itching; therefore, proper dress for climatic conditions is a prime consideration. Since sunlight has a beneficial drying effect on weeping lesions, exposure to ultraviolet light is encouraged but monitored carefully to prevent burning. Any topical beauty aid, such as perfumes, powder, or oils, is avoided. Clothes and sheets should be laundered in a mild detergent and rinsed thoroughly in clear water (without fabric softeners and antistatic chemicals). Putting the clothes through a second complete wash cycle without using detergent minimizes the amount of residue remaining in the fabric.

Preventing infection is usually secondary to preventing scratching. Personal hygiene is accomplished without the liberal use of soap. Baths are given infrequently (unless otherwise prescribed), the water is kept tepid, and bubble baths are avoided as well as the use of oils or powder. Skin folds and diaper areas need frequent cleansing with plain water and without the use of any antidiaper rash preparation. If antiseptic soaks are prescribed, they are applied as directed.

Since adequate rest is also important for these children, who are usually fretful and irritable, planning meals,

SUMMARY OF NURSING CARE OF THE CHILD WITH ECZEMA

GOALS	RESPONSIBILITIES

Prevent exacervations	Eliminate the precipitating allergen
	    Provide hypoallergenic diet as ordered
	    Avoid foods and other substances known to produce exacerbations
	Maintain health

Reduce irritation	Avoid substances that irritate the skin, such as soap, perfumed lotions, etc. Dress in loose-fitting, one-piece, long-sleeve and long-pants outfit (if appropriate for weather conditions) Avoid overheating, high humidity, and perspiration Encourage exposure to ultraviolet light, but avoid sunburn Eliminate any woolen or rough garment or furry stuffed toys; nylon garments promote sweating Launder all clothes or bedsheets in mild detergent and rinse very well in clear water
Prevent or minimize scratching	Provide bath with antipruritic solution Keep fingernails and toenails short and clean Wrap hands in soft cotton gloves or stockings; pin to shirt cuff Use elbow restraints when absolutely necessary, but allow supervised periods for unrestricted movement
Prevent infection	Administer good personal hygiene—baths with tepid water, little or no soap Demonstrate proper procedure for applying wet dressing; suggest quiet times of day for applying them to the child's skin Demonstrate carefully the proper dilution of soaks at home Schedule times for administering oral antibiotics that maintain continuous high blood levels of the drug
Promote rest	Plan meals, baths, medications, and treatments around nap or bedtime Make child as comfortable as possible before sleep to enhance restfulness (for example, give sedation and then give bath before bedtime) Carry out any distressing procedure when the child is well rested and after he has received medication for itching Administer analgesics, sedatives, and ataractics as prescribed
Promote nutrition	Feed the child when he is well rested Do not force foods or introduce a restricted food to encourage eating Stress need for vitamin and mineral supplements Allow the child to feed himself if that is usual routine
Encourage play activities that are suitable to skin condition and child's developmental age	Avoid any furry, hairy stuffed toys or dolls Provide kinesthetic, moving toys, large toys, which require less fine motor skills if hands are covered, and quiet musical or visual toys Remember that there is no substitution for the stimulation and comfort of human contact
Assist parents in avoiding causative allergens	Stress reason for hypoallergenic diet or removal of inhalants, especially that positive results are not immediate Give written list of foods restricted as well as those allowed Identify hidden sources of milk, wheat, and eggs Assess home environment before suggesting ways to eliminate inhalants
Provide emotional support for the child and parents	Provide consistent caregiver for the hospitalized child Encourage the parents to play with the child and to realize that the irritable behavior is directly related to physical discomfort Stress to the parents that the child still needs limit setting and discipline Be aware of overprotectiveness and restrictiveness, which can stifle the child's emotional growth Allow and encourage the parents, particularly the one who cares for the child most of the time, to express their negative feelings, such as anger, frustration, and perhaps guilt Stress that negative feelings are normal, acceptable, and expected but that they must have an outlet in order for parents and child to remain healthy Make public health referral for long-term home care follow-up

baths, medications, and treatments during awake periods is paramount. Sleepy, tired children are normally cranky, and such behavior only intensifies the urge to scratch. During periods of irritability, these children tend to be anorectic, which is made worse by restriction of many foods.

Diet modification is another source of frustration to parents. When a hypoallergenic diet is prescribed, parents need help in understanding the reason for the diet and guidelines for following it. A typical hypoallergenic diet for an infant includes a milk substitute such as soy formula, rice cereal, apples, apricots, carrots, string beans, beef, and aqueous multiple-vitamin supplements. The diet is followed for 10 days; if remission occurs, each food from the restricted list is added one at a time at weekly intervals to identify specific food allergens. Milk and then wheat are usually the first two foods added for suspected sensitivity. Even if all foods can be accepted, eggs are usually not permitted. If the response to the hypoallergenic diet is unsuccessful, environmental control is attempted to lessen the amount of inhalants.

Parents can be assured that the lesions will not produce scarring (unless secondarily infected) and that the disease is not contagious. However, the child will be subject to repeated exacerbations and remissions and, although spontaneous and permanent remission takes place at approximately 2 to 3 years of age in most children, a large number will develop asthma as children and hay fever as adults. A few children will progress to a chronic phase that persists throughout childhood.

SEBORRHEIC DERMATITIS (CRADLE CAP)

Seborrheic dermatitis is a chronic, recurrent, inflammatory reaction of the skin. It occurs most commonly in the scalp but may involve the eyelids (blepharitis), external ear canal (otitis externa), nasolabial folds, and inguinal region. The cause is unknown, although it is more common in early infancy when sebum production is increased. The lesions are characteristically thick, adherent, yellowish, scaly, oily patches. Occasionally areas of transient alopecia may be evident.

Although the appearance of cradle cap resembles eczematous eruptions, it differs from them in several important aspects. It is not necessarily associated with a positive family history for allergy, it is very common (approximately 50%) in infants shortly after birth, the lesions are greasy in appearance and more pink or yellow than red, and lichenification (induration and thickening of the skin from persistent irritation) does not occur. Probably the most significant distinguishing characteristic of seborrheic dermatitis is the absence of pruritus. The child's behavior is unchanged by the presence of the lesions. Diagnosis is made primarily on the appearance of the crusts and the absence of pruritus.

Nursing considerations

The initial objective is prevention of cradle cap through adequate scalp hygiene. Not infrequently parents omit shampooing the infant's hair from fear of damaging the "soft spots" or fontanels. It is important to discuss how to shampoo the infant's hair and emphasize that the fontanel is like skin anywhere else on the body. It does not puncture or tear with mild pressure.

When seborrheic lesions are present, parents are taught the appropriate procedure to clean the scalp thoroughly. At this point, a demonstration may be necessary to ensure that the parents can institute meticulous hygiene. Shampooing should be done three to four times a week, using a mild soap or commercial shampoo, such as the no-tear preparations. If an oil is applied, it is massaged into the scalp and allowed to penetrate the crusts for a few minutes and then thoroughly removed. Using a fine-toothed comb after shampooing helps remove the loosened crusts from the strands of hair.

The nurse stresses prevention of secondary bacterial or fungal infection through hygiene measures and frequent changing of bed linen and clothing that comes in contact with affected sites, such as hats or diapers. Since the lesions are not pruritic, measures to prevent scratching are not necessary. However, as a general precaution the infant's hands are kept clean to prevent infecting areas such as the eyelids.

If topical preparations are used, the nurse consults with the physician regarding specific procedures for use. For example, coal tar ointments such as Pragmatar may need to be diluted with a few drops of water for use in infants. They are sometimes applied overnight and then removed with a shampoo in the morning, or they may be left on indefinitely. Parents are cautioned to avoid the eyes when applying any preparation. Sometimes it is helpful to use a light cotton cap to cover the infant's head to avoid accidental rubbing of the medication in the eyes.

DIAPER DERMATITIS

Dermatitis in the diaper area is encountered frequently by nurses in all pediatric settings. It is caused by prolonged and repetitive contact with an irritant, principally urine, feces, soaps, detergents, ointments, and friction. The eruptions can be manifest primarily on convex surface or in the folds and the lesions can represent a variety of types and configurations.

Eruptions involving the skin in most intimate contact

with the diaper (that is, the convex surfaces of buttocks, inner thighs, mons pubis, and scrotum) but sparing the folds are likely to be caused by chemical irritants. The chemicals most often involved are ammonia and end-products of putrefactive enzymes. Other causes are detergents or soaps from inadequately rinsed cloth diapers.

Inflammatory processes involving primarily the areas in which skin surfaces are touching, such as the groin and gluteal folds, are caused by intertrigo or seborrheic dermatitis. When seborrheic dermatitis is complicated by secondary infection with *Candida albicans,* satellite lesions can be detected beyond the sharply demarcated reddened area.

Perianal involvement is usually the result of chemical irritation from feces, especially diarrheal stools. Perianal dermatitis is more common in bottle-fed than in breast-fed infants. *Candida albicans* infection produces perianal inflammation with satellite lesions.

Bands of reddened areas at the margins of the diaper, that is, around the waist and the thighs, are caused by plastic edges of diapers or plastic rubber pants. Small vesiculopustules in the diaper area, sometimes called ''heat rash'' or ''prickly heat,'' are the result of the hot, humid atmosphere created in the plastic-covered, wet, warm diaper.

Impetigo, manifested by the presence of large vesicles or bullae, may be observed in the diaper area, especially in the younger infant, and is frequently a part of a more generalized eruption.

Nursing considerations

The single most significant factor associated with diaper dermatitis is the hot, humid environment created in the diaper area. Consequently, airing and cooling the area are highly beneficial. This is accomplished by removing excess clothing and any occlusive diaper coverings to permit evaporation. Changing the diaper as soon as it becomes wet eliminates a large part of the problem, and removing the diaper entirely for extended periods to expose the area to light and air facilitates drying and healing.

After soiling the perianal area is cleansed. Wiping the area with a wet cloth is usually sufficient to remove urine. Parents should be advised that the use of disposable wet towels can aggravate the problem because the child may be sensitive to one or more agents in the product. After stooling, the area needs thorough cleansing and in some instances, especially with diarrheal stools, may require a sponge bath.

The selection and care of diapers are very important aspects in preventing inflammation or further irritation. Plastic or rubber diaper covers (especially those with elastic edges) should not be used except for brief social occa-

sions. Disposable diapers, which are preferable to cloth diapers with plastic overpants, have a plastic covering that inhibits evaporation but they do allow some air circulation. Soft, thoroughly laundered and sterilized cloth diapers are best. Licensed, commercial diaper laundries provide the least irritating diapers. If diapers are laundered at home they should be soaked in a quaternary ammonium compound (such as Diaparene), washed in hot water with a simple laundry soap (such as Ivory), and run through the rinse cycle twice. Using a dryer enhances diaper softness.

Topical glucocorticoid preparations are sometimes required for stubborn inflammations that do not respond to the simple measures just described. However, ointment applications to inflamed areas are avoided since they tend to be occlusive and contribute to sweat retention. *Candida* infections are treated with nystatin dusting powder, using precautions against the infant's inhaling the powder. Where *Candida* is the causative agent, oral administration of nystatin is advised also since the gastrointestinal tract is usually the source of infection. Occasionally prevention can be accomplished by zinc oxide applied to the noninflamed diaper area of highly sensitive infants.

ACNE

There is one skin disorder that, although not limited to the adolescent age-group, appears predominantly at this time—*acne vulgaris*. Acne is an almost universal occurrence during these years and involves anatomic, physiologic, biochemical, genetic, immunologic, and psychologic factors of significant import.

It is estimated that over 90% of all teenage boys and 80% of all teenage girls suffer from acne. The degree to which they are affected may range from nothing more than a few isolated comedones to a severe inflammatory reaction. The greatest incidence is in late adolescence, from about ages 16 to 20 years, after which it usually diminishes, but it may persist well into adulthood. Although the disease is self-limited and is not life threatening, its significance to the adolescent is great, and it is a mistake to underestimate the impact it can have on young persons.

The etiology of acne is still unclear, although a number of factors appear to be related to its development. Its distribution in families and a high degree of concordance in identical twins suggest that hereditary factors predispose to susceptibility to acne.

Pathophysiology

Acne is a disease that involves the pilosebaceous follicles (the hair follicle and sebaceous gland complex) of the face,

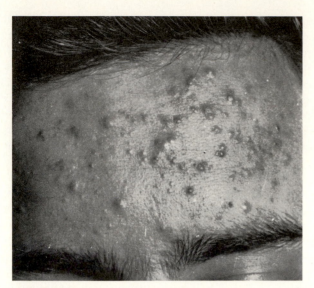
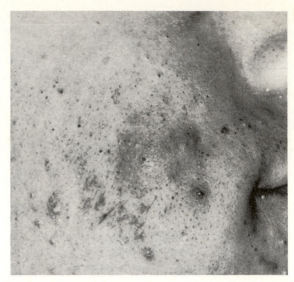

Fig. 27-5

Acne vulgaris. Papular pustules and comedones. (From Stewart, W.D., Danto, J.L., and Maddin, S.: Dermatology: diagnosis and treatment of cutaneous disorders, ed. 4, St. Louis, 1978, The C.V. Mosby Co.)

neck, shoulders, back, and upper chest—the so-called flush areas of the skin. There are two basic types of lesions seen in acne:

1. **noninflamed** lesions called *comedomes*, consisting of compact masses of keratin, lipids, fatty acids, and bacteria that dilate the follicular duct, which may be plugged (closed comedones, or whiteheads, with no visible opening) or open (blackheads, with visible dilated openings that are discolored as fatty acids are oxidated by air)
2. **inflamed** lesions that result when the follicular wall ruptures to produce papules, pustules, nodules, and cysts (Fig. 27-5). The inflammatory acne is responsible for the destructiveness and propensity for scarring.

Androgens are implicated and the disease seems to be aggravated by emotional stress, winter weather, some stimulant drugs, and the premenstrual period. There is no positive evidence that any specific foods are factors, except perhaps with individual youngsters.

Secondary invasion by *Staphylococcus albus* can complicate the acne lesion, and adolescents' concern about their appearance tempts them to pick, finger, squeeze, and otherwise manipulate the lesions, which plays an important role in the perpetuation of acne. In addition to the precipitating factors mentioned previously, the application of creams, oils, and some cosmetics that add to the plugging of the follicles may aggravate acne; therefore, cosmetic agents should be selected to avoid those with greasy or occlusive bases.

Therapeutic management

There is little evidence that treatment shortens the duration of the entire course of the disease. However, much can be done to control acne, reduce the inflammatory process and scarring, and improve the appearance. The management if acne is directed toward preventing comedo formation, removing the comedo, controlling excessive sebaceous gland activity, controlling infection, and preventing scar formation.

Improvement of the adolescent's overall health status is part of the general management. Adequate rest, moderate exercise, a well-balanced diet, reduction of emotional stress, elimination of any foci of infection, and correction of constipation (if it exists) are all part of general health promotion. There is no convincing evidence to implicate any single dietary item or combination of foods in the exacerbation of acne with the possible exception of iodides and bromide in therapeutic amounts. Occasionally a youngster will demonstrate an aggravation of symptoms after each ingestion of a given food. In such instances the food is eliminated for a period of time to assess its influence on the disease.

Noninflammatory acne is predominantly an obstructive disease characterized by open and closed comedones. Therefore, the treatment consists of the removal of these comedones and the prevention or reduction of the formation of new lesions. Open comedones, or blackheads, can be effectively expressed by direct pressure with a comedo extractor, a small metal scoop with a hole in the center.

The hole is placed directly over the blackhead and pressure applied against the skin with a slight sliding movement across the skin. Closed comedones, or whiteheads, cannot be removed easily with the extractor alone. The epidermal covering of the whitehead must be gently and superficially nicked with a Bard-Parker No. 11 blade before extrusion with the comedo extractor.

A number of therapeutic modalities that produce erythema and desquamation have proved effective in diminishing the development of new lesions and contributing to the loosening of the comedo for easy extraction. These agents include (1) cleansing agents such as soaps and detergents, (2) astringents containing substances such as alcohol or acetone, (3) creams, lotions, gels, etc., (4) cryoslush therapy that freezes the skin to produce erythema and desquamation, (5) ultraviolet light, and (6) topical applications of vitamin A acid. Not all dermatologists subscribe to all of these methods, but the majority prescribe some form of peeling agent either as a single agent or one or more of these in combination. Some dermatologists prescribe frequent shampooing.

The modalities employed in therapy of the pustular and cystic forms include (1) surgical techniques, such as incision and drainage of cystic or pustular lesions and intralesional injection of corticosteroids, (2) chemotherapy, including long-term administration of antibiotic agents, especially the tetracyclines, short-term therapy with corticosteroids, and estrogen-progestin therapy in a cyclic routine, and (3) dermabrasion (abrading the skin with a high-speed rotating wire brush or steel abrasive wheel after the skin has been hardened and anesthetized with a refrigerant) in selected individuals.

Nursing considerations

The adolescent should be encouraged to seek medical treatment for the skin lesions from a sympathetic and understanding dermatologist; however, the extent of physician involvement varies. Simple over-the-counter acne remedies are available, and most adolescents do not see a physician, but they need education regarding the many factors associated with the disorder and a supportive, caring individual to help them maintain the persistence required to deal with the disorder over such an extended period of time. It is essential that the youngster with inflammatory lesions obtain medical treatment in order to control the process and reduce the incidence of scarring.

The adolescent needs education regarding the disease process and instruction in the prescribed therapy. Instruction should be definite and as specific as practical for each individual youngster. A written instruction sheet that describes the etiology and therapeutic regimen is often helpful, and parents should be cautioned against nagging. Ad-

olescents should assume responsibility for following through on the instructions. They need to be cautioned against damaging the skin through too vigorous scrubbing. The importance of using only those preparations and appliances (such as the ultraviolet light) prescribed for their particular needs and carrying out associated directions such as hairstyling and shampooing, and for girls not leaving cosmetics on the face overnight, are emphasized. Nurses can help girls select proper cosmetic preparations. The nurse is often the person who teaches a family member in the use of a comedo extractor.

Initially the procedures are carried out in the physician's office by the physician or nurse, but a parent or other family member often can be taught to use the extractor. The face is washed with soap and water before and after extraction, and the instrument is cleaned and cared for in the manner directed by the individual physician, which usually consists of cleaning it with soap and water and then either storing it in alcohol or wiping it with alcohol and storing in a clean receptacle such as a clean, dry envelope. The parent is cautioned against excessive pressure that might bruise the skin. The blackhead that cannot be removed readily should be left until another time. Some dermatologists limit home treatment to removal of blackheads only.

During conversations with teenagers, the nurse can dispel the common myths often associated with acne and allow them to discuss any feelings related to the disorder, such as self-consciousness and anxieties regarding relationships with others, and, sometimes, help them explore job or other after-school interests. The acne lesions need not become an excuse to avoid social contacts and activities after school.

THERMAL INJURY

Thermal injuries are usually attributed to injury from extreme heat sources. Although thermal burns are the most frequent type of burns, harmful effects also occur from exposure to cold or hot environments.

BURNS

Minor burn injuries are experienced by everyone in day-to-day living and are relatively commonplace in nursing practice. Extensive burns, on the other hand, are relatively uncommon; however, they account for some of the most difficult nursing problems encountered in the pediatric age-group. As a cause of accidental death in childhood, burns

SUMMARY OF NURSING CARE OF THE ADOLESCENT WITH ACNE

GOALS	RESPONSIBILITIES
Obtain medical treatment	Be alert to cues that adolescent wants to discuss his problem Broach subject of therapy for adolescent with obvious skin lesions Suggest an understanding dermatologist who is sympathetic to the special needs of adolescents Discourage self-treatment with over-the-counter preparations
Educate the adolescent	Dispel myths regarding etiology of condition Reassure adolescent regarding unfounded fears Provide accurate information regarding disease process and therapy to be implemented
Promote general health	Encourage adequate rest and moderate exercise Help adolescent plan a well-balanced diet Help adolescent find mechanisms to reduce emotional stress Implement measures to correct constipation (if it exists) Assess for any foci of infection and initiate measures to eliminate them Eliminate any given food adolescent has found aggravates symptoms

Prevent inflammation and scarring	Periodic expression of comedones
	  Blackheads—by direct pressure with comedo extractor
	  Whiteheads—nick gently and superficially with No. 11 blade before extrusion
	Carefully cleanse skin with soap and water prior to expression
	Caution against using excessive pressure
	Express limited number of comedones each day
	Apply peeling agent(s) as prescribed
	Teach correct cleansing techniques and medical asepsis
	Caution against too vigorous scrubbing to prevent skin damage
	Impress importance of following instructions, such as using only prescribed preparations and appliances
	Instruct about shampooing, hairstyling, and selection and use of cosmetics
	Instruct in proper care of equipment used for therapy

Reduce number of lesions	Avoid oily applications to skin Shampoo hair and scalp frequently (if prescribed) Style hair off forehead
Prevent inflammation and infection	Administer antibiotics as prescribed Administer oral corticosteroids and assist with intralesion injections of drug Reemphasize importance of cleanliness and medical asepsis
Treat more resistant forms	Prepare the adolescent for surgical procedure(s) Assist with incision and drainage of cystic or pustular lesions Prepare the adolescent for and assist with x-ray therapy
Reduce androgenic effect	Administer estrogens (in selected female cases)
Encourage self-care	Provide written instructions, including cause of lesions and therapeutic regimen outlined Motivate the adolescent to assume responsibility for following through on instructions Instruct in technique of comedo extraction and other therapeutic and hygienic measures Discourage mirror gazing
Obtain cooperation and understanding of parents	Explain disorder and therapy prescribed Caution the parents against nagging about compliance Teach the parents technique of comedo extraction Explain nature of adolescent personality and effect disorder has on self-image and identity formation
Support the adolescent	Allow the adolescent to express feelings about disorder, its effect on appearance, and length of time required for therapy Provide positive reinforcement for compliance Encourage maintenance of normal activities and interaction with peers Explore job opportunities and after-school interests with adolescent Emphasize positive aspects, such as self-limited nature of disorder, efficacy of therapy, and improvement in appearance

are outranked only by automobile casualties and drownings. In addition, serious burn injury accounts for a very large number of children who must undergo prolonged, painful, and restrictive hospitalization.

Burns can be caused by thermal, chemical, electric, or radioactive agents. Most burn injuries are caused by thermal agents, principally flame and hot water (including steam), and to a lesser extent friction. Chemical burns can be caused by either acids or alkalis, radiation burns by either x-rays or ultraviolet radiation, and electrical burns by life wires, transformers, or lightning. The extent of tissue destruction is determined by the intensity of the heat source, the duration of contact or exposure, and the speed with which the heat energy is dissipated by the burned surface. For example, a brief exposure to high-intensity heat, such as a flame, or a longer exposure to a low-intensity heat, such as hot water, can produce similar burn injuries. Contact burns from heated metal or liquids (such as tar) at extreme temperatures, prolonged immersion in hot water, chemical burns without rinsing with water, and electric burns are all significant in the etiology of severe burn trauma. Chemical agents continue to cauterize the tissues until the injurious agent is chemically united with tissue elements, neutralized, or removed by washing with running water. Electric burns are especially deceptive, since they are characterized by more extensive thrombosis that is not evident until 24 to 36 hours after injury. Their extensive destruction has been described as resembling a crush injury.

Assessment of burn wound

The physiologic responses, therapy, prognosis, and disposition of the injured child are all directly related to the *amount of tissue destroyed;* therefore, the severity of the burn injury is assessed on the basis of the percentage of surface burned and the depth of the burn. Also important in determining the seriousness of the injury are the location of the burn(s), the age of the child, causative agent, the presence or absence of respiratory involvement, the general health of the child, and the presence of any associated injury or condition.

Percentage of body surface. The size of a burn is usually expressed as a percentage of total body surface area, which is most accurately estimated by using specially designed age-related charts (Fig. 27-6). Because of the

Fig. 27-6
Estimation of distribution of burns in children. **A,** *Children from birth to age 5 years.* **B,** *Older children.*

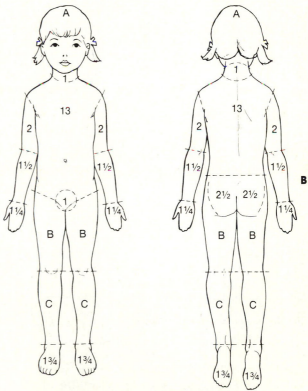

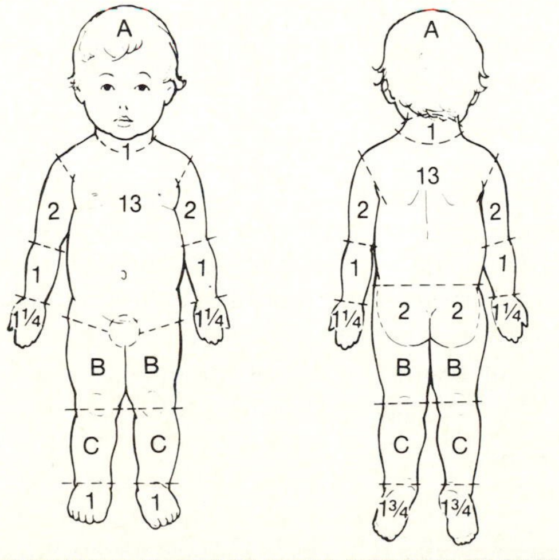

RELATIVE PERCENTAGES OF AREAS AFFECTED BY GROWTH

AREA	BIRTH	AGE 1 YR	AGE 5 YR
A = ½ of head	9½	8½	6½
B = ½ of one thigh	2¾	3¼	4
C = ½ of one leg	2½	2½	2¾

RELATIVE PERCENTAGES OF AREAS AFFECTED BY GROWTH

AREA	AGE 10 YR	AGE 15 YR	ADULT
A = ½ of head	5½	4½	3½
B = ½ of one thigh	4½	4½	4¾
C = ½ of one leg	3	3¼	3½

Fig. 27-7

Characteristics of burn wounds.

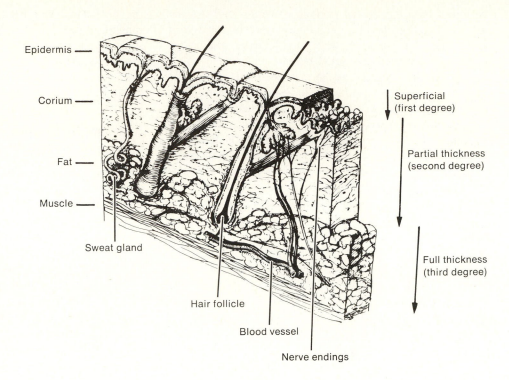

body proportions, especially the head and lower extremities, the standard "rule of nines" charts used for adults are not applicable to small children.

Depth of injury.   A thermal injury is a three-dimensional wound and therefore, is also assessed in relation to depth of injury. Traditionally the terms "first-," "second-," and "third-degree" have been used to describe the depth of tissue injury. However, with the current emphasis on burn healing, these are gradually being replaced by more descriptive terms based on the extent of destruction to the epithelializing elements of the skin (Fig. 27-7).

Erythema or **epidermal** (first-degree) burns are usually of minor significance. There is frequently a latent period followed by erythema. Tissue damage is minimal, protective functions remain intact, and systemic effects are rare. Pain is the predominant symptom.

Partial-thickness (second-degree) burns are deeper and involve not only the epithelium but a minimal to substantial portion of the corium. The severity of the injury and the rate of healing are directly related to the amount of undamaged corium from which new tissue can regenerate. Superficial partial-thickness burns are painful whereas deep, dermal burns are often anesthetic for the first 1 or 2 days after injury.

Full-thickness (third-degree) burns are serious injuries in which all layers of the skin are destroyed, may involve underlying tissues as well, and are usually combined with extensive partial-thickness damage. Systemic effects can be life threatening and involve every organ system in the body.

Other factors.   Burns involving the head, face, hands, feet, genitalia, and flexion creases are considered serious. Also serious, no matter how much tissue is destroyed, are instances where inhalation of heated air and/or toxic fumes is suspected, because there is risk of developing airway obstruction. Because infants' skin is so thin, it is readily destroyed by thermal agents. Children less than 2 years of age have a significantly higher mortality rate than older children with burns of similar magnitude. Acute or chronic illnesses or superimposed injuries complicate burn care and response to treatment.

Pathophysiology

Thermal injury produces both local and systemic effects that are directly related to the extent of tissue destruction. In superficial burns the tissue damage is minimal. The burning sensation and pain resolve in 48 to 72 hours and, in 5 to 10 days, the damaged epithelium peels off in small scales or sheets, leaving no scarring. In partial-thickness burns there is considerable edema and more severe capillary damage. In 3 to 5 days a crust of dried exudate and injured tissue covers the wound to form a protective seal while healing takes place from underneath. With reasonable care, superficial burns heal spontaneously. The crust separates in 10 to 14 days with minimal or no scarring.

Deep-dermal burns heal more slowly. A thin epithelial covering develops in 25 to 35 days, but this type of burn may require several months to heal. Scarring is common, and trauma or infection can easily convert a partial thickness burn to a full-thickness injury, especially in young children with their normally thinner skin. Fluid loss and metabolic effects may be considerable.

Along with and subsequent to the pathophysiologic response at the site of thermal injury, a number of systemic responses occur. Swelling takes place in and around the wound site as a result of increased capillary permeability and vasodilation. The edema can reach tremendous proportions and, in severe burns, loss of circulating fluid can precipitate shock. Loss of fluid, protein, and electrolytes at the wound surface further complicates the management of these patients.

Other systemic responses to severe burns include anemia caused by direct heat destruction of red blood cells, hemolysis of heat-damaged red blood cells, and depressed bone marrow; massive protein loss from the burn wound and from gluconeogenesis; and increased metabolism to maintain body heat and provide for the increased energy needs of the body.

Complications. Thermally injured persons are subject to a number of serious complications, both from the wound and from systemic alterations resulting from the wound. The immediate threat to life is asphyxia resulting from irritation and edema of the lungs and respiratory passages. In the first 48 to 72 hours the greatest hazard is unremitting shock, followed by possible renal shutdown and potassium excess during the first week. During healing, infection—both local and generalized sepsis—is the primary complication.

Pulmonary problems persist as the major cause of fatality in patients with thermal burns or a result of injury to or complications in the respiratory tract. A full range of respiratory insufficiency can occur, including inhalation injury, aspiration in unconscious patients, bacterial pneumonia, pulmonary edema, pulmonary embolus, and post-traumatic pulmonary insufficiency. The most common causative factor in respiratory failure in the pediatric age-group is bacterial pneumonia, which may be secondary to airway injury or contamination from a tracheostomy or acquired through hematogenous spread of bacteria, usually from the burn wound.

Sepsis is the most critical problem in treatment of burns and is an ever-present threat after the shock phase. Initially burns are relatively pathogen free, unless the wound is contaminated with potentially infectious material (dirt, polluted water, and so on). However, dead tissue and exudate provide a fertile field for bacterial growth. Early colonization of the wound surface by a preponderance of gram-positive organisms (primarily staphylococci) changes, on about the third postburn day, to predominantly gram-negative organisms, particularly *Pseudomonas aeruginosa* organisms. By the fifth postburn day the bacterial invasion is well underway beneath the surface of the wound.

Recurrent or intermittent bleeding resulting from Curling, or stress, ulceration is a major noninfectious complication of burns. Routine antacid administration has reduced the incidence of this complication in recent years, but these superficial erosive lesions still occur in a number of burn injuries.

Immediate treatment

The aims of immediate treatment of thermal injury are stopping the burning process, covering the burn, transporting the child to medical aid, and providing reassurance.

In flame burns the chief aim in rescue is to smother the fire, not to fan it. Children tend to panic and run, which only serves to fan the flames and make assistance more difficult. The victim should not run and should not remain standing. The injured child is placed in a horizontal position and rolled in a blanket, rug, or similar article, being careful not to cover the child's head and face because of the danger of the child's inhaling the toxic fumes. If no covering is available, he is made to lie down and roll over slowly. If the victim remains in a vertical position, the hair may be ignited or it may cause him to inhale flames, heat, or smoke. Spontaneous cooling of burns by slow immersion in cold water or any nonflammable liquid helps to relieve the pain, inhibit edema formation, and slow the process of heat damage. Ice water or ice packs are contraindicated because the resulting vasoconstriction interferes with capillary perfusion and carries the risk of further damage from cold burn. Unless there is nothing else available, no dirt or sand should be thrown on the burn. In chemical burns it is particularly important to wash the burn with copious amounts of cool running water for 10 to 15 minutes.

Burned clothing is removed to prevent further damage from smoldering fabric or hot beads of melted synthetic material. The wound is then covered with a clean cloth to prevent contamination and to alleviate pain by avoiding air contact. Application of topical ointments, oils, or other home remedies is avoided.

The child with an extensive burn is not given anything by mouth because of the risk of aspiration and water intoxication. The child is transported to the nearest place where medical aid is available. Providing reassurance and psychologic support to both the parents and the child helps immeasurably during postinjury crisis. Reducing anxiety helps to conserve energy needed to cope with the physiologic and emotional stress of a traumatic injury.

Therapeutic management of minor burns

Treatment of burns classified as minor usually can be managed adequately on an outpatient basis when it is determined that the parents can be relied on to carry out instructions for care and observation. The wound is cleansed and debrided (all foreign material and devitalized tissue removed) with a tepid or cool dilute, nonirritating soap solution and rinsed with sterile saline solution. Coolness reduces pain and probably reduces edema that can interfere with capillary flow in the area. Because they provide a sterile covering for the wound, intact blisters may or may not be debrided.

Most physicians favor covering the wound with a dry dressing or fine-mesh gauze lightly lubricated with water-soluble antiseptic or antimicrobial cream and then wrapping it with bulky dry gauze dressings. Some physicians prefer that an occlusive dressing be left in place for 7 to 10 days if the dressing remains clean and the child afebrile. The parents are instructed to cleanse the wound with mild soap and tepid water, change the dressings once or twice daily, and return to the office or clinic as directed for wound observation. If there is a high probability of infection or other complications or if there is doubt about their ability to carry out the directions, the parents may be directed to return daily for dressing change and inspection or a nurse may be assigned to make a home visit for that purpose. Soaking the dressing in tepid water prior to removal will help loosen the dressings and debris and reduce the discomfort. Burns about the face are usually treated by exposure, since a protective crust will form in 24 to 36 hours provided the atmosphere is cool and dry.

A tetanus history is obtained on admission and tetanus toxoid administered if indicated. Administration of antibiotics for minor burns is controversial.

Analgesics, such as aspirin or acetaminophen, are effective for relief of discomfort, and the antipyretic action of the drug alleviates the sensation of heat. Most mild burns heal with little difficulty, but if the wound margin becomes erythematous, gross purulence is noted, or the child develops evidence of systemic reaction, such as fever or tachycardia, hospitalization is indicated.

Therapeutic management of major burns

When a child with serious burns is admitted to the hospital for treatment, a variety of assessments are made and therapies initiated. Of these, the priority concerns are (1) to establish and maintain an adequate airway, (2) to establish a lifeline for fluid resuscitation, and (3) to care for the burn wound. Other needs and therapies, including nutritional support, splinting to prevent contractures, treatment of anemia and hypoproteinemia, and the rehabilitative aspects of burn management, are initiated as appropriate throughout the course of treatment.

Establishment of adequate airway. The first priority of care is airway maintenance. If there is evidence of respiratory involvement, oxygen is administered and blood gases, including carbon monoxide, are quickly determined. If the child exhibits air hunger or otherwise appears in critical condition, an endotracheal tube is inserted to maintain the airway. Since early edema subsides within 24 to 48 hours and many have been managed successfully for longer periods of time without significant damage, nasotracheal intubation is safer and preferred to a tracheostomy.

Frequently, placing the child in a Croupette or under an oxygen hood with a high flow of oxygen and maximum humidity is sufficient to reduce reflex bronchospasm produced by trauma to the bronchial mucosa.

Fluid replacement therapy. The objectives of fluid therapy are to (1) compensate for water and sodium lost to traumatized areas and interstitial spaces, (2) replenish sodium deficits, (3) restore plasma volume, (4) obtain adequate perfusion, (5) correct acidosis, and (6) improve renal function.

The predominant therapy at the present time is the use of crystalloid rather than colloid solutions in resuscitation of burn shock. The composition of the fluid selected varies with the philosophy of the physician and may consist of isotonic saline solution, a near-isotonic solution (such as Ringer's lactate), or even a hypertonic saline solution.

After diuresis, in 48 to 72 hours, when capillary permeability is restored, colloid solutions such as albumin or plasma are useful in maintaining plasma volume. Oral fluids are usually withheld in the early resuscitative phase but may be administered in 24 to 48 hours.

Fluid balance may continue to be a problem throughout the course of treatment, especially during the periods in which there may be considerable evaporative loss from the wound.

Nutrition. The high metabolic requirements and catabolism in severe burns make nutritional needs of paramount importance and often difficult to provide. The diet must provide sufficient protein to avoid protein breakdown and extra calories to utilize the proteins, sustain the adaptive hypermetabolism, and spare protein breakdown. Extra calories should be derived from carbohydrates, since fat, although higher in total calories, will not spare protein.

Most burn patients are able to eat, and the child is given oral feedings as soon as possible. The caloric requirements of burned children may be as much as two to three times their usual requirements for size and age; therefore, the diet is high in calories and protein, supplemented with high doses of vitamins B and C and iron. Burned children are often anorexic. Consequently, nasogastric feedings may be needed to supplement oral intake, and intravenous hyperalimentation has been used to provide a large amount of concentrated glucose and amino acids, especially in infants.

Care of burn wound. After the initial period of shock and restoration of fluid balance, the primary concern is the burn wound. The objectives of management for epidermal and superficial burns is to prevent infection by providing as aseptic an environment as possible, prevent mechanical trauma, and relieve pain. Occlusive dressings

TABLE 27-9. METHODS OF BURN CARE

METHOD	DESCRIPTION	ADVANTAGES	DISADVANTAGES
Exposure therapy	After cleansing, wound remains exposed to air and allowed to dry Natural protective barrier formed by hard coagulum from exudate of partial-thickness burns and dry eschar of full-thickness burns	Patient not immobilized with bulky dressings Allows frequent inspection Dry crust is poor culture medium Fluid loss less in initial phases Less odor	Risk of cross contamination greater Requires strict isolation technique Requires maintenance of optimum environmental temperature Often requires restraints on extremities to prevent picking at crust Presents unsightly appearance
Occlusive dressings	Wound surface covered with non-adherent, water-permeable fine-mesh gauze Inner layer covered with even layer of absorptive, resilient, fluffed gauze held in place by nonconstricting stretch gauze bandages	Protection from cross contamination Protection from injury Better immobilization, if desired Aids in positioning and putting injured part at rest Less pain initially	Requires skilled nursing care Higher incidence of hyperpyrexia Warm, moist environment more conducive to bacterial growth Often requires pain medication for uncomfortable dressing changes
Primary excision	Immediate surgical excision of devitalized tissue and grafting	Immediate removal of necrotic eschar Permanent coverage of damaged skin Reduces exposure to infection	Difficult to distinguish between full-thickness and deep partial-thickness injury Associated with significant blood loss

protect the wound from injury and help to reduce pain by minimizing exposure to air. The objectives for management of full-thickness wounds are prevention of invasive infection, removal of dead tissue, and closure of the wound.

There are essentially three methods of therapy for the burn wound, each of which has its place in the treatment of children. All meet the objectives of preparation for permanent wound coverage (Table 27-9). The occlusive dressings are used more frequently, although primary excision is gaining popularity as a major modality of burn care. Both the exposure and the occlusive methods employ topical antibacterial applications and daily hydrotherapy or tubbing to remove loose tissue and debris and to allow inspection of the wound.

Soaking in the Hubbard tank for 20 to 30 minutes once or twice daily facilitates the loosening and removal of sloughing tissue, eschar, exudate, and topical medications. The mesh gauze serves to entrap exudative slough and is readily removed during the tubbing procedure (Fig. 27-8). Any loose tissue or eschar is carefully trimmed away before redressing. Debridement is painful and usually requires premedication with an adequate dose of an appropriate narcotic.

A number of topical agents are employed, but those

Fig. 27-8

An analgesic is administered prior to removal of dressings and débridement. In this instance the analgesic is injected directly into the intravenous line at the time of tubbing.

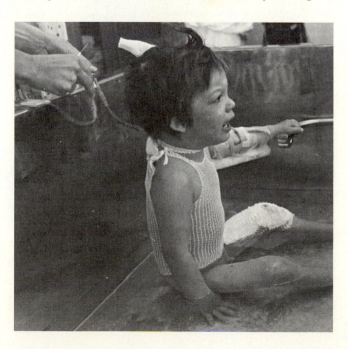

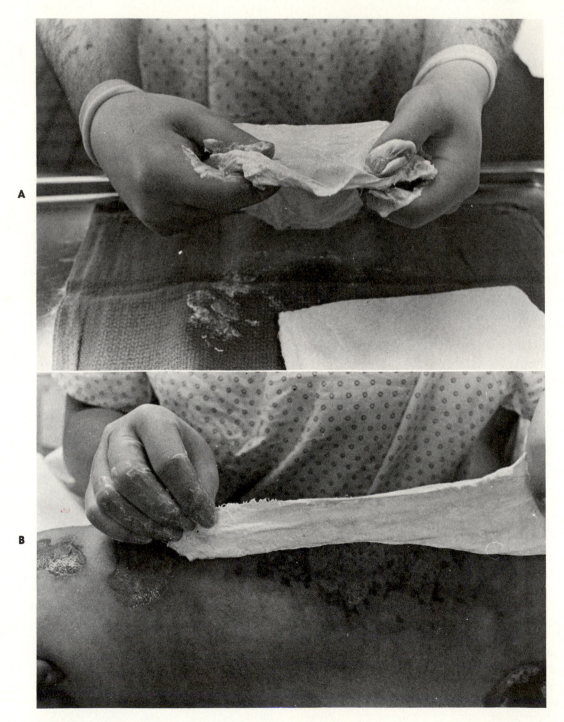

Fig. 27-9

Application of burn dressing. **A,** *Gauze impregnated with ointment.* **B,** *Ointment and gauze applied to burn wound.*

used most frequently are 0.5% silver nitrate solution, 10% mafenide acetate (Sulfamylon), and 1% silver sulfadiazine (Silvadene). All three are effective bacteriostatic agents, but each has advantages and disadvantages. Less frequently used are 0.1% gentamycin sulfate (Garamycin) and povidone-iodine (Betadine) ointment.

Ointments are applied directly to the burn wound surface with sterile tongue blades or the hand with a sterile glove. The layer of cream or ointment should be applied thick enough so that the wound cannot be seen. It can be left uncovered or covered with a layer of fine-mesh gauze and secured with stretch gauze or elastic tubular netting. For areas that are small or difficult to cover, strips of fine-mesh gauze are impregnated with the medication and then applied to the wound (Fig. 27-9).

Temporary or permanent coverage of full-thickness wounds is accomplished with grafts. Temporary grafts are those that provide biologic dressings during the acute phase of therapy to protect the wound from bacterial invasion and to minimize fluid loss. Permanent grafting is part of the rehabilitative stage to restore cosmetic appearance and to achieve maximum functional capacity. In recent years the early application of temporary biologic dressings to partial-thickness burns, especially in children, has significantly improved burn management and is gaining in popularity.

Grafts are derived from several sources. Permanent grafts are obtained from only two sources:

autografts tissues obtained from undamaged areas of the patient's own body.
isografts histocompatible tissue obtained from genetically identical individuals, that is, the patient's identical twin.

Temporary grafts include:

allografts (homografts) tissues obtained from genetically different members of the same species, living or dead— usually cadavers—that are free from disease.
xenografts (heterografts) tissues obtained from members of a different species. At present most xenografts are derived primarily from pigskin, either fresh or frozen.

Biologic (pigskin, amnion, cadaver skin) and biosynthetic (Biobrane, Biobrin) dressings (Fig. 27-10) are frequently employed as temporary covering until the wound bed has developed sufficient granulation for permanent grafts. Permanent grafting of full-thickness burns is usually accomplished with a split-thickness skin graft. This consists of the epidermis and part of the dermis being removed from an undamaged area by a special instrument, the dermatome, which is designed to excise split-thickness skin. The priority areas for coverage are the face, neck, and areas around joints, especially the hands.

The donor site is dressed with either a xenograft or fine-mesh gauze and left exposed until the graft falls off in

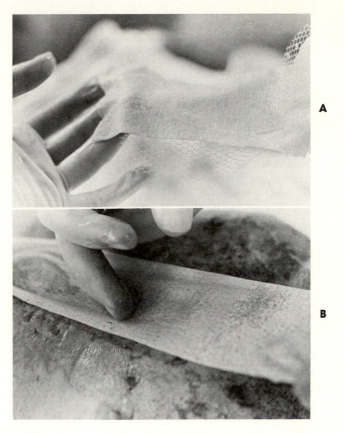

Fig. 27-10
Porcine dressing. **A,** *Removed from net backing.* **B,** *Applied to wound.*

about 10 to 14 days. Dressings are not changed on donor sites to prevent tearing the new, delicate epithelium.

Nursing considerations

Nursing care is the most important aspect of burn therapy. The care of the severely burned child encompasses a broad range of skills and foci. The primary emphasis during the initial phases of burn care is prevention of burn shock. Checking vital signs, monitoring the intravenous infusion, and measuring urinary output are ongoing nursing activities in the hours immediately after injury. The intravenous infusion is started immediately by intracatheter or cutdown and is regulated according to urine output and specific gravity, laboratory data, and objective signs of adequate hydration. Urine volume, measured at least every hour, should be:

20 to 30 ml/hour in a child over 2 years of age
10 to 20 ml/hour in a child less than 2 years of age

The child requires constant observation and assessment with special attention to signs of complications. Respiratory, cardiac, and renal complications may appear early in the postburn period.

The burn wound is treated according to the protocol of the specific burn facility. Extensive wounds may require the use of special beds and other equipment, such as CircOelectric beds, flotation beds, alternating pressure mattresses, and many other devices, depending on the extent and location of the wound.

Throughout the acute phase of care the child's emotional needs should not be overlooked. The child is frightened, uncomfortable, and often confused. He is isolated from familiar persons and surroundings, and the often overwhelming physical needs at this time are the primary focus of staff and parents. The child needs to be reassured that he is all right and that he will get better.

Pain management. The severe pain of the wound and the therapies, the anxiety generated by these experiences, and the conscious and unconscious interpretations of traumatic events contribute to the psychologic reactions frequently observed in burned children. Much of the difficulty encountered in managing burned children is related to these factors. Soon after hospitalization many burned children become irritable, depressed, hostile, and aggressive toward the members of the health team. In his helplessness, the child often resorts to angry outbursts against anything and anybody.

The burn pain is overwhelming, engulfing, and irrepressible. Consequently the pain causes anxiety and a feeling of profound helplessness in the child and can produce reactions of confusion, fear, and panic. Compounding the pain is the child's interpretation of it and of the procedures; this is closely related to the developmental level of the child. Many burned children believe their pain is punishment for past misdeeds and therefore deserved. There are often feelings of anger, guilt, and depression, and, as in all illness, regressive behavior. When a child appears to accept his pain and shows little or no aggressive behavior, psychologic consultation is usually in order.

It is always difficult to deal with a child in pain, and to inflict pain on a helpless child is contrary to the empathetic nature of nursing. Although inflicting pain is unavoidable, adequate management of pain can greatly reduce the discomfort. When administering drugs for adequate pain control during procedures the nurse must consider the following factors: (1) selection of appropriate analgesic—mild analgesics (such as acetaminophen) are sufficient to relieve mild discomfort whereas narcotics are needed for severe pain; (2) adequate dosage of the drug—a sufficient amount is given to achieve the desired effect; and (3) timing of administration—the peak effect occurs at the time the procedure is performed. (See Chapter 18 for additional suggestions for nursing management of pain.)

Wound care. After the patient's condition is stabilized, the long management phase begins. The nurse has the major responsibility for cleansing, debriding, and applying topical medication and dressings to the burn wound. Because dressing removal is a painful procedure, the child should receive adequate analgesia before the scheduled tubbing. Both nurse and child must recognize it for exactly what it is—a dreadful but absolutely necessary procedure. Because it is painful, the child should know that it is all right to cry when the treatment hurts, but only *when it hurts*. Since it is easy for the child to give way to emotional excesses he cannot control, he needs the firm control of a caring adult. This includes both actual and anticipated hurt. The child needs help to gain and maintain control of his emotions. He benefits from knowing why things are being done to him, how they will help him get better, and how he can contribute. New procedures or changes in routine need to be explained. Children feel comfortable with the known, the routine.

Outer dressings (if any) are removed before placing the child in the tub, but adherent dressings are more easily removed after soaking in the water. It is helpful to involve the child in the process. Whereas a child will cry and protest vigorously when others remove the dressings, he will remove adherent gauze with a minimum of fuss. In this way he maintains some control of the situation. Loose or easily detached tissue is also removed during hydrotherapy, and the child is encouraged to move about as much as possible to exercise muscles and reduce contracture formation. Providing something constructive for the child to do during dressing application, such as holding a package of dressings or a roll of kerlix or simply holding someone's hand, helps him to focus on something other than the procedure. In dressing the wound, it is important that all areas are clean, that medication is amply applied, and that no two burned surfaces touch, such as fingers or toes. Application of the medication can be a painful experience also, especially when mafenide (Sulfamylon) cream is the agent employed. Both nurse and child must understand that there is a painful sensation often described as "burning" that may have special significance for burned children. They must be reassured that the medication is not inflicting further injury and that the sensation is only a transient discomfort.

When occlusive dressings are applied, elastic bandages are worn over dressings to prevent epithelial breakdown, stimulate circulation, and make mobility easier. This is especially important when the child is ambulatory.

Nutrition. After the initial phase of care, children are usually allowed oral feedings (unless paralytic ileus persists). Because children are frequently anorexic and their caloric needs and protein needs are markedly increased, a great deal of encouragement, help, and patience are required on the part of the nursing staff. Consultation with the parents and the dietitian is arranged to determine the best way to provide needed nutrients in foods the child will be more likely to eat. Children who are old enough to participate should be included in the planning. Nourishing snacks are provided between regularly scheduled mealtimes, and, if a child eats better at a time other than a scheduled mealtime, that is the time he should be fed. Most importantly, meals should not be scheduled immediately after a dressing change. Most children are too physically exhausted and too emotionally upset to eat at this time. If they will not eat, tube feeding is necessary, but every effort should be made to encourage oral intake. (See Chapter 19 for suggestions for feeding the anorexic child.)

To reduce caloric expenditure as much as possible, the ambient temperature in the environment is usually maintained at a temperature above the temperature of the burn surface to reduce evaporative loss. The heat is often provided by means of a heat cradle over the child, but, if employed, the heat source should be situated well away from the child's body. Other methods include electric heaters, which if used should be situated 4 to 5 feet away to avoid overheating.

Prevention of complications. The chief danger in this phase of burn care is infection—wound infection, generalized sepsis, and bacterial pneumonia. It is important to make accurate ongoing assessments. Wound cultures are obtained at least three times weekly and antacids are usually administered prophylactically to prevent or minimize the effect of Curling ulcer.

Because the child is reluctant to move and doing so causes pain or discomfort, stiffness and joint contracture develop easily. In an effort to prevent this complication, he is encouraged to move whenever feasible and active physiotherapy is included as an essential aspect of burn care. When the child is resting or sleeping, contracture is prevented by proper splinting. The child's natural tendency is to be active, and he will usually move spontaneously unless the pain is severe.

Care of skin graft. Effort in the care of children with skin grafts is directed toward facilitating a "take." Trauma, infection, and bleeding must be avoided for a successful transplantation to occur. When the grafted area is left exposed, the child must be immobilized to prevent the graft from becoming dislodged. Flat surfaces usually pose few problems, but grafts over irregular or mobile areas may require special techniques such as splints or skeletal traction. Small children may need to be restrained. Sedation might be needed for very restless and/or uncooperative children for the first 2 or 3 days after surgery.

The grafted areas can be left exposed (which allows for easy inspection of the grafts), dressed with occlusive pressure dressings, or secured with sutures attached to normal surrounding skin and tied over the grafted skin to hold it in place. Wet dressings are occasionally applied over lace grafts and kept moist with antimicrobial agents, silver nitrate, or normal saline and covered with dry absorbent gauze.

Wound contraction and scar tissue formation are nor-

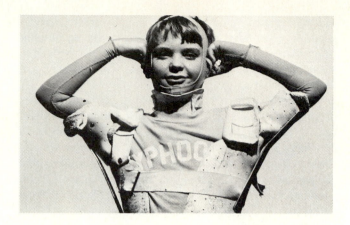

Fig. 27-11
Child in elasticized garment (Jobst) and "airplane" splints.

mal parts of wound healing. Scar tissue is metabolically active tissue that continually rearranges itself; as a result disabling contractures, deformity, and disfigurement are ever-present possibilities. Physical therapy, splints, and other methods are employed to minimize these long-term effects. Pressure splints and elastic bandages or elasticized (Jobst) garments help reduce scar hypertrophy and are sometimes worn for months after hospitalization (Fig. 27-11). Often severely burned children must return to the hospital periodically for additional skin grafts and scar revisions, especially to release contractures over joint spaces and for cosmetic considerations. Achievement of optimum results frequently requires years. In the meantime, burn scars are unsightly and, although improvements can be made, hope should not be extended to the parents and child for total cosmetic and functional repair.

Emotional support. The child should be encouraged to participate in as many aspects of his care as possible. With illness, children always regress to the developmental level that allows them to deal with the stress. As their condition permits, children can be expected to do things that they were capable of doing for themselves before they were burned, such as oral hygiene, face washing, feeding themselves, and playing. Allowing the child to make choices and to help make decisions about the time of his care and recreational activities makes him feel a part of the team and provides him a measure of control. The child will probably require assistance; however, as the child sees himself contributing to his care, he gains confidence and self-esteem.

The psychologic pain and sequelae of severe burn trauma are as intense as the physical trauma. Each burned child goes through a tremendous amount of pain, often continuous for varying periods, and separation from families for extended periods. In addition, there is a continual barrage of painful therapeutic and diagnostic procedures that are inflicted by others. He wonders why this has happened to *him*—what he has done that he should be punished so. Past experiences cannot serve him in this crisis. He does not understand the "ugliness" and disfigurement he sees as his body.

The impact of such severe injury taxes the capabilities of children at all ages, but the young child, who suffers acutely from separation anxiety, and the adolescent, who is developing an identity, are probably most affected psychologically. The toddler cannot begin to comprehend why the parents whom he loves and who have protected him from hurt can leave him in such a dreadful place and allow others to inflict such painful indignities on him.

The adolescent, in the process of achieving independence from his family and seeking to find out who he is in the world, finds himself in a dependent position with a damaged body. Being different from others at a time when conformity and being like his peers are so important is difficult to accept. These children need understanding adults to help them deal with the struggles concerning resentment and other feelings generated by such a catastrophe.

Members of the family as well as the child feel the impact of severe burn injury. They are concerned about the child's survival, recovery, and future appearance. Nurses are in the most opportune position to assist parents to cope with the stresses of the child's illness and their feelings of guilt and helplessness. The parents need to be informed of the child's progress and helped in their efforts to cope with their feelings while providing support to the child. The nurse is the person who can help them understand that it is not selfish to look after themselves and their own needs in order that they can better meet the needs of the child. For parents whose response to the illness is too severe or whose response to stress is manifest in destructive behavior, professional help may be needed.

SUNBURN

Sunburn is a very common skin injury caused by ultraviolet light waves. The sun emits a continuous spectrum of visible and nonvisible light rays that range in length from very short to very long. The shorter higher frequency waves are more damaging than longer wavelengths, but much of the light is filtered out as it travels through the atmosphere. Of the light that does filter through, ultraviolet A (UVA) waves are the longest and cause only minimum burning but play a significant role in photosensitive and photoallergic reactions. Ultraviolet B (UVB) waves are shorter and responsible for tanning, burning, and most of the harmful effects attributed to sunlight.

Numerous factors influence the amount of UVB ex-

posure. Maximum exposure occurs at midday (11 AM to 3 PM) when the distance from the sun to a given spot on the earth is shortest. There is more exposure at higher altitudes, less when the sky is hazy (although its effect is easily underestimated), and window glass effectively screens out UVB but not UVA. Fresh snow and water reflect ultraviolet rays, especially when the sun is directly overhead; some is reflected by sand.

Protection from sunburn is the major goal of medical and nursing management, and the harmful effects of the sun on the delicate skin of infants and children is receiving increased attention. The safest time to sunbathe is when the sun is nearest the horizon (before 9 or 10 AM and after 3 or 4 PM) when rays must travel the greatest distance. When skin is exposed to the sun for more extended periods a protective covering is advised.

Two types of products are available for sun protection: topical sunscreens, which partially absorb ultraviolet light, and sun blockers, which block out ultraviolet rays by reflecting sunlight. The most frequently recommended sun blockers are zinc oxide and titanium dioxide ointments. Sunscreens are products containing a sun protective factor (SPF) based on evaluation of effectiveness against ultraviolet rays. The SPF is indicated by number with an SPF of 15 providing the maximum protection. The most effective sunscreens are para-aminobenzoic acid (PABA) and para-aminobenzoic acid esters (PABA-esters). PABA is more effective but may stain clothing; PABA-esters are less likely to stain clothing but are less effective than PABA.

Sunburn is usually an epidermal burn, although severe sunburn can be partial thickness with blister formation. Treatment involves stopping the burning process, decreasing the inflammatory response, and rehydrating the skin. Local application of cool tap water soaks or emersion in a tepid water bath for 20 minutes or until the skin is cool limits tissue destruction and relieves the discomfort. An oil-in-water moisturizing lotion is then applied. Oil-based products should be avoided because they can trap irradiant heat in the tissues (Anders, 1982). Partial thickness burns are treated the same as those from any heat source.

COLD INJURY

Cold injuries are most commonly seen in very cold regions. The nature of the heat regulating mechanisms of the body are such that the inner portion of the body, or core, produces heat, and the periphery, or outer area, conserves or dissipates the heat. When the body attempts to conserve heat the the outer tissues are subjected to low temperatures, and local trauma may result.

Chilblain occurs when extremities, usually the hands, are exposed intermittently to temperatures 30° to 60° F.

SUMMARY OF NURSING CARE OF THE CHILD WITH BURNS

GOALS	RESPONSIBILITIES
Immediate care	
Implement care	Have respiratory resuscitation equipment ready
	Remove all clothing, jewelry, and so on
	Evaluate level of consciousness
	Give analgesic if ordered
	Insert Foley catheter
	Insert nasogastric tube
	Administer tetanus prophylaxis
Obtain baseline information	Take vital signs
	Weigh the child
	Help evaluate extent and depth of burn wound
	Help assess condition
	Request laboratory studies as ordered—hematocrit, sodium, chloride, potassium, carbon dioxide, blood urea nitrogen, creatinine, and serum protein levels
Prevent shock	Help establish intravenous line
	Administer fluids as ordered
	Monitor vital signs (including central venous pressure, if employed)
	Monitor intravenous infusion closely
	Monitor urinary output, specific gravity, and pH (sometimes protein) every ½ to 1 hour
	Obtain needed specimens for examination or perform needed studies
Prevent complications	
Acute respiratory distress	Administer humidified oxygen
	Observe for signs of respiratory distress
	Obtain blood for blood gas determination, if indicated
	Have respiratory resuscitation equipment available
	Have tracheostomy tray available
	Check for constricting eschar of chest
	Observe nasopharynx for edema or redness
	Obtain chest x-ray film
Fluid overload	Monitor vital signs frequently
	Observe for signs of impending overhydration
	Be alert for altered behavior or sensorium
	Perform or request laboratory studies
Abdominal distention, nausea and vomiting	Insert nasogastric tube and attach to low Gomco suction
	Administer nothing by mouth
Impaired circulation in extremities	Check circulation in extremities or other areas peripheral to burns—color, capillary filling, pulses, sensation
	Check for constricting eschar
Cardiac failure	Check vital signs
	Order electrocardiogram if indicated
Renal failure	Check hourly urine for amount, color
Ongoing care	
Prevent heat loss	Adjust ambient temperature according to child's temperature
	Use direct-probe thermometer when feasible
	Avoid drafts

Continued.

SUMMARY OF NURSING CARE OF THE CHILD WITH BURNS—cont'd

GOALS	RESPONSIBILITIES
Relieve pain	Administer analgesics as indicated
Control bacterial growth on wound	Maintain clean environment Maintain careful handwashing Wear sterile gown, mask, and gloves when handling burn wound Carefully cleanse wound and remove devitalized tissue and eschar Apply prescribed topical antimicrobial preparation and dressings (if ordered) to wound Administer good oral hygiene Avoid injury to crusts and eschar Avoid contact with infected persons Obtain wound cultures three times per week to ascertain any increase in wound flora
Facilitate wound healing	Keep the child from scratching and picking at wound Maintain care in handling wound to avoid damaging epithelializing and granulating tissues Administer supplementary vitamins and minerals—vitamins A, B, and C and zinc sulfate Offer high-calorie, high-protein meals and snacks Prevent infection Protect graft from trauma Protect from infection Position for minimum disturbance of graft site Restrain if necessary

Maintain adequate nutrition and prevent nitrogen loss	Provide high-calorie, high-protein meals and snacks
	Encourage oral feeding by
	    Providing foods the child likes
	    Allowing self-help
	    Providing meals when the child is most apt to eat well
	    Providing attractive meals and surroundings
	    Providing companionship at meals
	    Employing ''contract'' with older children

Recognize signs of complications	Take vital signs (temperature, pulse, respirations, blood pressure) as ordered Observe, record, and report deviations from expected vital signs Record intake and output
Wound infection	Assess wound for signs of invasive infection, including redness, purulent drainage, unpleasant odor

Generalized sepsis	Recognize signs of septicemia
	    Marked temperature elevation (40.0°–41.6° C [104°–107° F], rectally)
	    Chills
	    Rapid, irregular pulse
	    Hypotension
	    Diminished urine output
	    Paralytic ileus (distention, vomiting, absent bowel sounds)
	    Alterations in sensorium
	Obtain blood culture of the child with temperature of 39.5° C or over

Curling ulcer	Assess for abdominal discomfort Check for recurrent or intermittent bleeding Determine hematocrit Administer antacids as ordered
Fecal impaction	Record regular bowel movements Administer enema or remove impacted feces

SUMMARY OF NURSING CARE OF THE CHILD WITH BURNS—cont'd

GOALS	RESPONSIBILITIES
Hypertension	Check blood pressure regularly
Pneumonia	Observe for signs of respiratory distress, elevated temperature, presence of rales, lethargy
Renal	Observe amount, color, specific gravity, and reaction of urine daily or as ordered Send specimens for laboratory examination periodically

Cerebral disorders	Observe for seizures
	    Alterations in sensorium
	    Behavioral changes

Prevent pressure necrosis	Turn frequently Stimulate circulation
Preserve body function	Encourage mobility Carry out range of motion exercises if child is unable to move extremities Splint joints to prevent contracture deformity Position for minimum deformity and optimum function Ambulate as soon as feasible Encourage and promote self-help activities
Minimize scar formation	Position in functional attitude Apply splints as ordered and designed Wrap healing tissue with elastic bandage or dress in elastic garments as ordered Carry out physical therapy
Support the child psychologically	Reassure the child and parents Allow the parents to visit the child Facilitate parent-child interaction Do not allow isolation technique to unduly separate parent and child Allow the child to express anger and distress Answer questions as honestly as possible

Support the parents	Reinforce factual information
	Answer questions regarding therapy
	Allow for expression of feelings
	    Help alleviate feelings of guilt
	Instruct in techniques required for visiting the child
	    Isolation procedures
	Help to devise means for providing tactile contact with the child
	Help the parents deal with anxiety regarding pain to the child

Prepare the child for discharge	Begin early in hospitalization to discuss ''going home'' Accept regressive behavior where appropriate Help the child develop independence and self-help capabilities Explore feelings about returning to home and family, school, and friends Explore feelings concerning physical appearance Provide reinforcement of positive aspects of appearance and capabilities Discuss aids that camouflage disfigurement, e.g., wigs, clothing (for example, turtleneck sweaters), makeup Help the parents set realistic goals for themselves, the child, and other family members Help the parents acquire needed equipment and supplies

The response may vary but is characterized by intense vasodilation that increases the temperature of involved tissues above unaffected tissue and produces edematous, reddish-blue patches that itch and burn (DeLapp, 1980). As warming takes place the sensations become more intense but ordinarily subside in a few days.

Frostbite results from sufficient exposure to cool the tissues to the point that small ice crystals form in interstitial spaces of superficial and deep structures, resulting in variable degrees of tissue loss and function. The frostbitten part appears white or blanched, feels solid, and is without sensation. Rapid rewarming produces a flush (sometimes deep purple) and a return of sensation, which is extremely painful. Large blisters appear in 24 to 48 hours after rewarming, which begin to reabsorb within 5 to 10 days followed by formation of a hard black eschar. Superficial injury often heals without incident. Rewarming in accomplished by immersing the part in well-agitated water at 100° to 108° F. Discomfort is managed with analgesics and sedatives. Care of blistered skin is similar to that described for burns. It is seldom possible to estimate the extent of tissue loss until new skin layers are revealed after the eschar layer separates.

REFERENCES

Anders, J.E., and Moeller, P.J.: Topicals: a welter of options calls for refined application techniques, RN **44**(9):33-42, 1982.

DeLapp, T.D.: Taking the bite out of frostbite and other cold-weather injuries, Am. J. Nurs. **80**:56-60, 1980.

BIBLIOGRAPHY
General

Burson, I.J.: Drug reactions, insect bites, and fungal infections, Issues Compr. Pediatr. Nurs., pp. 12-21, 1976.

Fisher, A.A., and Maibach, H.: Cooling poison-plant dermatitis, Patient Care **10**(11):60-65, 1976.

Fleming, J.W.: Common dermatologic conditions in children, Am. J. Maternal Child Nurs. **6**:346-354, 1981.

Forbes, M., and Scipien, G.: Communicable diseases and some infections of the skin, Issues Compr. Pediatr. Nurs., pp. 1-11, 1976.

Hawkins, K.: Wet dressings: putting the damper on dermatitis, Nursing 78 **8**(2)64-67, 1978.

Hawkins, K.: Wet dressings, Crit. Care Update **6**(11):25-28, 1979.

Krugman, S., and Katz, S.L.: Infectious diseases of children, ed. 7, St. Louis, 1981, The C.V. Mosby Co.

Matus, N.R.: Topical therapy: choosing and using the proper vehicle, Nursing 77 **7**(11):8-10, 1977.

Infections

Nortarangelo, P.R., and Dixon, D.M.: Opportunistic systemic mycoses and the critical care patient, Crit. Care Update **10**(5):7-11, 1983.

North, C., and Weinstein, G.D.: Treatment of psoriasis, Am. J. Nurs. **76**:410-412, 1976.

Rees, P.L., and Dixon, D.M.: Opportunistic mycoses, Am. J. Nurs. **81**:1160-1163, 1981.

Infestations

Clore, E.R.: Lice: ancient pest with new resistance, Pediatr. Nurs. **9**:347-350, 1983.

Hall, V.A., Shaw, P.K., and Smith, E.B.: Could that itching be scabies? Nurs. Update **7**(8):1, 13-16, 1976.

Hall, V.A., Shaw, P.K., and Smith, E.B.: Exterminating the scabies mite, Patient Care **10**(9):102, 1976.

McLaury, P.: Head lice. Pediatric social disease, Am. J. Nurs. **83**:1300-1303, 1983.

Minster, J.: Nursing management of patients with scabies and lice, Nurs. Clin. North Am. **15**:747-756, 1980.

Bites and stings

Derbes, V.J., and others: Treating severe reaction to bee sting, Patient Care **10**(11):66-77, 1976.

Frazier, C.A.: Severe toxic and allergic reactions to insect bites and stings, Crit. Care Update **8**(9):17-24, 1981.

Huchinson, R.: What to do and what to worry about when treating stings and bites, Nursing 77 **7**(6):69-71, 1977.

King. R.C., and Giles, J.: Dealing with insect bites, RN **46**(5):53-55, 1984.

Thompson, S.: Summertime and ticks, Am. J. Nurs. **83**:758, 1983.

Acne

Evans, J.C., and Singleton, C.E.: Acne: the scourge of adolescence, Issues Compr. Pediatr. Nurs., pp. 60-68, 1976.

Fischer, R.G.: Acne vulgaris: a common disease, Pediatr. Nurs. **4**(2):9-14, 1978.

Lawlis, G.F., and Achterberg, J.: Acne: the disease and stress, Top. Clin. Nurs. **5**(2):23-31, 1983.

Rasmussen, J.E.: A new look at old acne, Pediatr. Clin. North Am. **25**:263-284, 1978.

Stone, A.C.: Facing up to acne, Pediatr. Nurs. **8**:229-234, 1983.

Burns

Bell, J.G.: Bitsy was so little . . . and her problems so big, Nursing 77 **7**(6):35-37, 1977.

Campbell, L.: Special behavioral problems of the burned child, Am. J. Nurs. **76**:220-224, 1976.

Conrad, F.L.: Tips for treating corrosive burns, Nursing 83 **13**(2):55-57, 1983.

Fonger, L.: Emergency! First aid for burns, Nursing 82 **12**(9):70-77, 1982.

Frye, S., and Lander, J.: The initial management of the acutely burned child, Issues Compr. Pediatr. Nurs, pp. 39-59, 1976.

Gaston, S.F., and Pathak, M.A: Burn wound management, Crit. Care Update **7**(10):5-17, 1980.

Gentry, W.C., and Pathak, M.A.: Help for your sunburn-prone patients, Patient Care **10**(11):40-45, 1976.

Jacoby, F.G.: Individualized burn wound dressings, Nursing 77 **7**(6):62-63, 1977.

Jones, C.A., and Feller, I.: Burns, what to do during the first crucial hours, Nursing 77 **7**(3):23-31, 1977.

Kavanagh, C.: A portrait of need and of giving, Am. J. Maternal Child Nurs. **2**(4):229, 1977.

Kavanagh, C.: Should children participate in burn care? Am. J. Nurs. **84**:601, 1984.

Kenner, C., and Manning, S.: Emergency care of the burn patient, Crit. Care Update **7**(10):24-33, 1980.

Kneut, C.: Acute stress ulcers in childhood, Issues Compr. Pediatr. Nurs. **3**(4):41-50, 1978.

Marvin, J.A.: Burn nursing as a specialty, Heart Lung **8**:913-917, 1979.

Marvin, J.A.: Planning home care for burn patients, Nursing 83 **13**(8):65-67, 1983.

McHugh, M.L., Dimitroff, K., and Davis, N.D.: Family support group in a burn unit, Am. J. Nurs. **79**:2148-2150, 1979.

Savedra, M.K.: The child and his family at home: what then? Am. J. Maternal Child Nurs. **2**(4):224-227, 1977.

Savedra, M.K.: Moving from hospital to home, Am. J. Maternal Child Nurs. **2**(4):220-222, 1977.

Siner, E., and Allyn, P.: Emergency burn care, Crit. Care Update **4**(3):24-27, 1977.

Smith, E.C., and others: Reestablishing a child's body image, Am. J. Nurs. **77**:445-447, 1977.

Surveyer, J.A., and Clougherty, D.M.: Burn scars: fighting the effects, Am. J. Nurs. **83**:746-751, 1983.

Surveyer, J.A., and Halpern, J.: Age-related burn injuries and their prevention, Pediatr. Nurs. **7**(5):29-34, 1981.

Talabere, L., and Graves, P.: A tool for assessing families of burned children, Am. J. Nurs. **76**:225-227, 1976.

Van Oss, S.: Emergency burn care: Those crucial first minutes, RN **44**:45-49, 1982.

Wagner, M.M.: Emergency care of the burned patient, Am. J. Nurs. **77**:1788-1795, 1977.

Wingate, E.: Emergent burn care: a time for life-saving measures, Crit. Care Update **10**(8):49-54, 1983.

Wooldridge, M., and Surveyer, J.A.: Skin grafting for full-thickness burn injury, Am. J. Nurs. **80**:2000-2004, 1980.

Zitomer, M.M.: Protecting children from the tragedy of burns, Am. J. Maternal Child Nurs. **2**:129-130, 1977.

Sunburn and frostbite

Anders, J.E., and Leach, E.E.: Sun versus skin, Am. J. Nurs. **83**:1015-1020, 1983.

Boyd, L.T., Shurett, P.H., and Coburn, C.: Heat and heat-related illnesses, Am. J. Nurs. **81**:1298-1302, 1981.

Gedrose, J.: When cold can be a killer, Nursing 80 **10**(2):334-36, 1980.

Robinson, L.A.: Sun exposure and sun protection, Pediatr. Nurs. **8**:272-273, 1982.

Wingate, E.: A nursing perspective on frostbite, Crit. Care Update **10**(1):8-15, 1983.

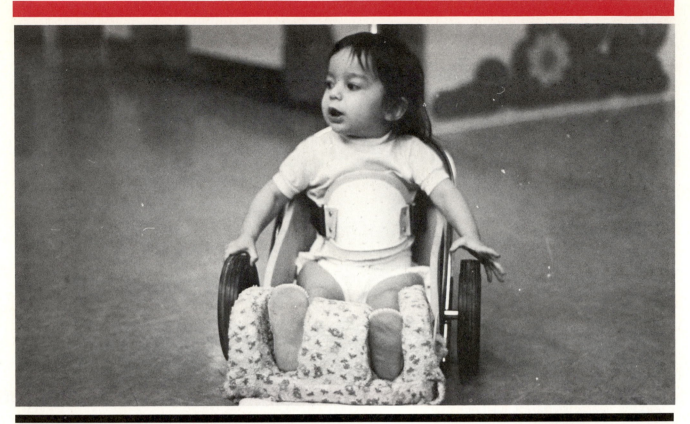

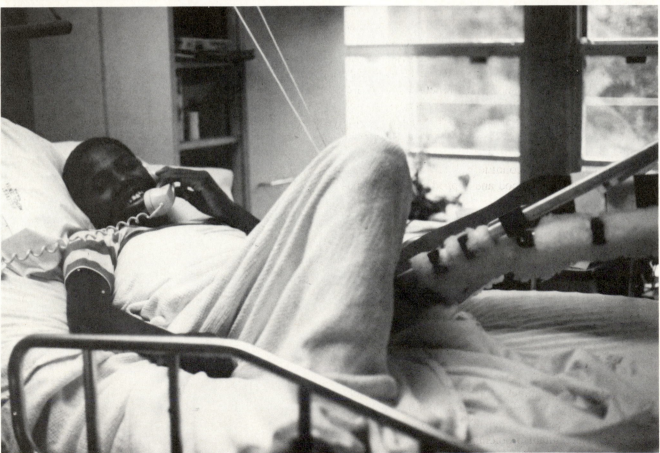

UNIT 12

THE CHILD WITH A PROBLEM THAT INTERFERES WITH LOCOMOTION

Childhood is the age of onset for a variety of physically disabling conditions with hereditary, infectious, or traumatic etiologies. Many disorders that interfere with locomotion are present at birth; others appear later in childhood. Defects in locomotion can be associated with diseases or deficits in the supporting structures (the skeleton), the movement-producing structures (muscle or their innervation), or the articulating structures (joints) of the body. Some of these defects occur at any age, such as fractures, and others make their appearance at ages characteristic for the specific condition, such as muscular dystrophy during early childhood and slipped epiphysis at puberty.

Some locomotor disabilities are acquired in an instant (such as amputation or spinal cord injury); others develop over an extended period (such as tuberculosis or progressive muscular atrophy). Some need only short-term therapy (such as fractures); others require long-term therapy and a longer term of adjustment and involve all aspects of daily living (such as spinal cord injuries and cerebral palsy).

The physical limitations may involve only temporary inconvenience, or they may be permanent with the need to substitute an alternative form of locomotion. Some are helped by specific treatments; for others therapy is merely supportive. A large number of these disabilities require a health team approach with contributions from a variety of specialists. Concomitant problems associated with perma-

nent disabilities, particularly those acquired in later childhood, are emotional adjustment and alterations in self-image.

Chapter 28, *The Child with Skeletal or Articular Dysfunction,* is concerned with disorders that involve the skeleton and articular systems. Also included in this discussion is the collagen disease, systemic lupus erythematosus. Chapter 29, *The Child with Neuromuscular Dysfunction,* deals with disorders that involve muscle dysfunction of either muscular or neurologic origin.

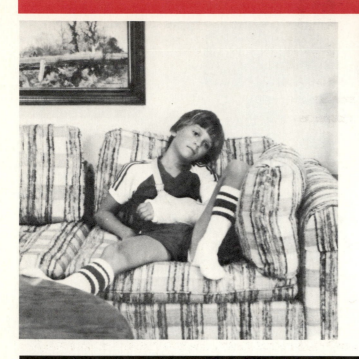

28

THE CHILD WITH SKELETAL OR ARTICULAR DYSFUNCTION

OBJECTIVES

On completion of this chapter the reader will be able to:

■ Formulate a teaching plan for the parents of a child in a cast

■ Explain the functions of the various types of traction

■ Devise a nursing care plan for a child in traction

■ Differentiate between the various congenital skeletal defects

■ Design a teaching plan for the parents of a child with a congenital skeletal deformity

■ Describe the therapies and nursing care of the child with scoliosis

■ Outline a plan of care for the child with osteomyelitis

■ Differentiate between osteosarcoma and Ewing sarcoma

■ Describe the nursing care of a child with juvenile rheumatoid arthritis

■ Demonstrate an understanding of the management of systemic lupus erythematosis

NURSING DIAGNOSES

Nursing diagnoses identified for the child with skeletal or articular dysfunction include, but are not restricted to, the following:

Health perception-health management pattern

■ Injury, potential for, related to use of unaccustomed appliances

Nutritional-metabolic pattern

■ Nutrition, alteration in: potential for more than body requirements related to immobility

■ Skin integrity, impairment of: potential related to (1) immobility; (2) pressure from corrective devices

Elimination pattern

■ Bowel elimination, alteration in: constipation related to immobility

Activity-exercise pattern

- Activity intolerance related to fatigue

- Diversional activity deficit related to (1) immobility; (2) corrective devices

- Mobility, impaired physical, related to (1) injury (specify); (2) corrective device(s); (3) absence of limb

- Self-care deficit: feeding, bathing/hygiene, dressing/grooming, toileting related to (1) developmental level; (2) discomfort; (3) immobility

Sleep-rest pattern

- Sleep pattern disturbance related to (1) effects of injury; (2) schedule of therapies; (3) orthopedic appliances

Cognitive-perceptual pattern

- Comfort, alterations in: pain related to (1) effects of injury or disease; (2) position

Self-perception—self-concept pattern

- Anxiety related to (1) strange environment; (2) perception of impending events; (3) separation; (4) anticipated discomfort; (5) knowledge deficit; (6) discomfort

- Powerlessness related to application of corrective devices

- Self-concept, disturbance in: body image, self-esteem, related to (1) perception of disability; (2) nonintegration of change in body function or limitations

Role-relationship pattern

- Family process, alteration in, related to situational crisis

- Grieving, anticipatory related to (1) expected loss; (2) expected change

- Parenting, alterations in: potential, related to (1) skill deficit; (2) family stress

- Social isolation related to (1) impaired mobility; (2) self-concept disturbance

Coping-stress tolerance pattern

- Coping, family: potential for growth

- Coping, ineffective family: compromised related to (1) situational crisis; (2) temporary family disorganization

Disorders that affect the skeletal and associated structures are of congenital, traumatic, infectious, neoplastic, or idiopathic origin. Some appear at any age, such as fractures, whereas others have a predilection for a particular stage of childhood. For example, there are those disorders detected at birth or shortly thereafter, such as congenital deformities and defects; Legg-Calvé-Perthes disease affects children in middle childhood; and slipped femoral capital epiphysis and scoliosis are characteristic of late childhood and adolescence.

TRAUMATIC INJURY

Children, with their natural tendency toward active mobility and their limited gross motor coordination, are highly susceptible to physical injury. Cuts, bruises, and contusions are a part of growing up, and fractures occur frequently in the pediatric age-groups.

FRACTURES

Bones fracture when the resistance of bone against the stress being exerted yields to the stress force. Fractures are a common injury at any age but are more likely to occur in children and elderly persons. Because of the characteristics of the child's skeleton, there are some differences in the pattern of fractures, problems of diagnosis, and methods of treatment.

Etiology

Fracture injuries in children are the result of traumatic incidents at home, at school, in a motor vehicle, or in association with recreational activities. Children's everyday activities include vigorous play that predispose them to injury—climbing, falling down, running into immovable objects, and receiving blows to any part of their bodies.

Aside from automobile accidents, true accidents that cause fractures rarely occur in infancy; therefore, bone injury in children of that age-group warrants further investigation. In any small child radiographic evidence of fractures at various stages of healing are, with few exceptions, the result of physical abuse. Fractures in school-age children are often the result of bicycle-automobile or skateboard accidents. Adolescents are vulnerable to multiple and severe trauma because they are mobile on bikes and motorcycles and active in sports. Speed and congested surroundings often intensify the impact. Young children and teenagers usually do not calculate risks as they learn to manipulate their environment and achieve developmental

goals. Therefore, accidents are a part of most childhood experience.

The fracture wound

A fractured bone consists of fragments—the fragment closer to the midline, or the proximal fragment, and the fragment farther from the midline, or the distal fragment. When fracture fragments are separated, the fracture is *complete;* when fragments remain attached the fracture is *incomplete.* The fracture line can be:

transverse crosswise, at right angles to the long axis of the bone
oblique slanting but straight, between a horizontal and a perpendicular direction
spiral slanting and circular, twisting around the bone shaft

The twisting of an extremity while the bone is breaking results in a spiral break. If the fracture does not produce a break in the skin, it is a *simple,* or *closed,* fracture. *Open,* or *compound,* fractures are those with an open wound through which the bone is or has protruded. If the bone fragments cause damage to other organs or tissues (such as the lung or bladder), the injury is said to be *complicated.* When small fragments of bone are broken from the fractured shaft and lie in the surrounding tissue, the fracture is called *comminuted.* This type of fracture is rare in children. The types of fractures seen most often in children are shown in Fig. 28-1.

bends a child's flexible bone can be bent 45 degrees or more before breaking. However, if bent, the bone will straighten slowly, but not completely, to produce some deformity but without the angulation seen when the bone breaks. Bends occur more commonly in the ulna and fibula, often associated with fractures of the radius and tibia.
buckle fracture compression of the porous bone produces a *buckle,* or *torus,* fracture. This appears as a raised or bulging projection at the fracture site. Torus fractures occur in the most porous portion of the bone near the metaphysis (the portion of the bone shaft adjacent to the epiphysis) and are more common in young children.
green-stick fracture a green-stick fracture occurs when a bone is angulated beyond the limits of bending. The compressed side bends and the tension side fails, causing an incomplete fracture similar to the break observed when a green stick is broken.
complete fracture complete fractures are those that divide the bone fragments. They often remain attached by a periosteal hinge, which can aid or hinder reduction.

Immediately after a fracture occurs the muscles contract and physiologically splint the injured area. This phenomenon accounts for the muscle tightness observed over a fracture site and the deformity that is produced as the muscles pull the bone ends out of alignment. This muscle

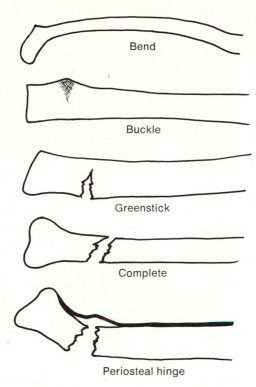

Fig. 28-1

Types of fractures in children.

response must be overcome by traction or complete muscle relaxation, that is, anesthesia, in order to realign the distal bone fragment to the proximal bone fragment.

Bone healing and remodeling. Bone healing is characteristically rapid in children because of the thickened periosteum and generous blood supply. When there is a break in the continuity of bone, the osteoblasts are in some way stimulated to maximum activity. New bone cells are formed in immense numbers almost immediately after the injury and, in time, are evidenced by a bulging growth of new bone tissue between the fractured bone fragments. This is followed by deposition of calcium salts to form a *callus*.

Fractures heal in less time in children than in adults. The approximate healing times for a femoral shaft are:

Neonatal period—2 to 3 weeks
Early childhood—4 weeks
Later childhood—6 weeks
Adolescence—8 to 10 weeks

Clinical manifestations

Children demonstrate the usual signs of injury—generalized swelling, pain or tenderness, and diminished functional use of the affected part. There may be bruising, severe muscular rigidity, and crepitus (a grating sensation at the fracture site), which are also frequent signs in adults. More often the fracture is remarkably stable because of the frequently intact periosteum. The child may even be able to use an affected arm or walk on a fractured leg. However, a fracture should be strongly suspected in a small child who refuses to walk.

Diagnostic evaluation

A history is often lacking in childhood injuries. Infants are unable to communicate, and older children are unreliable informants and seldom volunteer information (even under direct questioning) when the injury occurred during forbidden activities. Unless they are witnesses to the injury, parents may misinterpret what the child is trying to say. In cases of child abuse parents may give false information deliberately in order to protect themselves.

Radiographic examination is the most useful diagnostic tool for assessing skeletal trauma. The calcium deposits in bone make the entire structure radiopaque. Radiographic films are taken after fracture reduction and, in some cases, may be taken during the healing process to determine satisfactory progress.

Therapeutic management

The majority of children's fractures heal well, and nonunion is rare. Most are readily reduced by simple traction and immobilization until healing takes place. However, the position of the bone fragments in relation to one another influences the rapidity of healing and the residual deformity. Healing is prompt and complete with end-to-end apposition, but a gap between fragments delays (or prevents) healing. The goals of fracture management are:

1. To regain alignment and length of the bony fragments (reduction)
2. To retain alignment and length (immobilization)
3. To restore function to the injured parts

In children the bone fragments are usually realigned and immobilized by traction or by closed manipulation and casting until adequate callus is formed. Weight bearing on lower extremity fractures and active movement for the purpose of regaining function can begin after the fracture site is stable. The child's natural tendency to be active is usually sufficient to restore normal mobility, and physical therapy is rarely needed. In most cases children's fractures can be managed by closed reduction and plaster immobilization, which is most often provided on an outpatient basis with reevaluation in 7 to 10 days. Open reduction is seldom required and is limited to alignment that cannot be maintained by conservative methods and when there is interposed tissue or injury to arteries or nerves.

Children are most frequently hospitalized for fractures

of the femur and the supracondylar area of the distal humerus. If simple reductions cannot be achieved or if a neurovascular problem is detected after injury, observation in a hospital is indicated. Severe contusions with profound swelling cannot be treated with a cast, which would act as a tourniquet on the extremity. A badly malaligned fracture requires traction for a period of time before a cast is applied.

The major methods for immobilizing a fracture, casting and traction, are described in the following section in relation to the nursing care involved.

The child in a cast: application and nursing considerations

Nurses are frequently the persons who make the initial assessment of a child with a suspected fracture. The child and his parents are frightened and upset, the child is in pain, and since most fractures are obvious, the parents and (frequently) the child are already convinced of the diagnosis. Therefore, if the child is alert and if there is no evidence of hemorrhage, the initial nursing interventions are directed toward calming and reassuring the child and his parents so that a more extensive assessment can be more easily accomplished.

While maintaining a calm manner and speaking in a quiet voice, the nurse can ask the parents to describe what happened and how they feel about it. Since the child usually arrives with the limb supported in some manner, this time does not delay or endanger the treatment. Initially it is best not to touch the child but to ask him to point to the painful area and to wiggle his fingers or toes. By this time he usually feels relatively safe and will allow someone to gently touch him just enough to feel the pulse and test for sensation. A child's anxiety is greatly influenced by previous experiences with injury and health personnel. However, the child needs to be told what will happen and what he can do to help. The affected limb need not be palpated, and it should not be moved unless properly splinted. If the child is at home or if the physician is not present to examine the child, some type of splint is applied carefully for transport to the hospital and to the radiology department and cast room.

Cast application. The completeness of the fracture, the type of bone involved, and the amount of weight bearing influence how much of the extremity must be included in the cast to immobilize the fracture site completely. In most cases the joints above and below the fracture are immobilized to eliminate the possibility of movement that might cause displacement at the fracture site. The types of casts used for the more common fractures are illustrated in Fig. 28-2. If possible, the small child should be allowed to play with a doll that has a cast so that he understands what will be done.

While a cast is applied, it is often the nurse's role to set up the cast materials and to hold the extremity in alignment. In most instances only the cast material is required; however, special cast tables that hold the child's body are used for applying large hip spica casts.

Plaster casts. A tube of stockinette is first stretched over the area to be casted, and bony prominences are padded with soft cotton sheeting. Dry rolls of gauze impregnated with plaster of Paris are immersed in a pail of tepid water with the open end of the roll downward to allow soaking of the bandage. The wet plaster rolls are put on in a bandage fashion and molded to the extremity. A heat-producing chemical reaction occurs between the plaster and water as the plaster becomes a crystalline gypsum. During application of the cast the underlying stockinette is pulled over the raw edges of the cast and secured with a layer of wet plaster ½ to 1 inch below the rim to form a smooth padded edge to protect the skin.

Synthetic casts. Fiberglass, plastic, and resin materials are also used as casting materials. They are lightweight, dry quickly, can tolerate more contact with water, and can be lightly sponged when they become soiled. Preparation and application of these materials are similar to the application of plaster casts. The temperature of the water varies with the type of material, however.

Cast care. The complete evaporation of the water from a hip spica cast can take 24 to 48 hours when older types of plaster materials are used. Drying occurs within minutes with new quick-drying substances. The cast must remain uncovered to allow the cast to dry from the inside out. Turning the child in a plaster cast at least every 2 hours will help to dry a body cast evenly as well as prevent complications related to immobility. A regular fan to circulate air may be helpful during high-humidity weather. Heated fans or dryers should not be used, since they cause the cast to dry on the outside and remain wet beneath or cause burns from heat conduction by way of the cast to the underlying tissue.

A wet cast should be supported by a pillow that is covered with plastic and handled by the palms of the hands to prevent indenting the cast, which can create pressure areas. A dry plaster of Paris cast produces a hollow sound when it is tapped with the finger. If ''hot spots'' are felt on the cast surface, they are reported because this usually indicates an infection beneath the area. The cast may need to be removed or a window made in the cast so that the site can be observed.

If a protective edge is not provided at the time of casting, the raw edges of the dried cast can be protected by a ''petaled'' edge. Small pieces approximately 2 to 3 inches long are cut from 1- or 1½-inch wide adhesive tape. The edges are rounded with scissors, and each of these ''petals'' is placed over the edge of the cast, each petal slightly overlapping the previous petal to form a smooth, neat

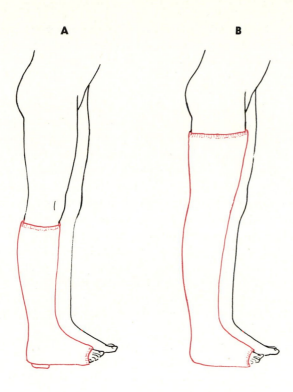

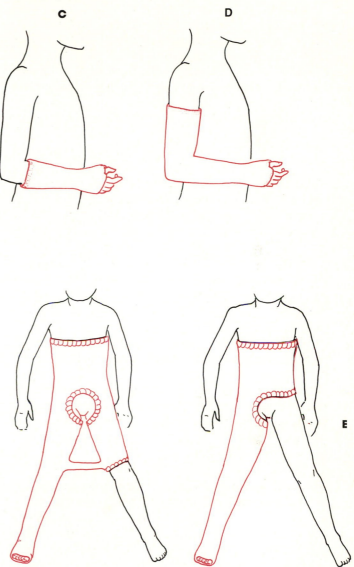

Fig. 28-2
Types of casts. **A,** *Short leg cast with walking attachment.*
B, *Long leg cast.* **C,** *Short arm cast.* **D,** *Long arm cast.*
E, *Hip spica casts.*

edge. A simple but more expensive alternative is to use appropriate size Band-Aids. It is easier to apply the petal to the underside of the cast first and then bring the other edge to the front, pressing firmly so that the edges remain securely attached.

During the first few hours after a cast is applied, the chief concern is that the extremity may continue to swell to the extent that the cast becomes a tourniquet, shutting off circulation and producing neurovascular complications. The casted extremity is observed at frequent intervals for any signs of pain, swelling, discoloration (pallor or cyanosis) of the exposed parts, lack of pulsation and warmth, and/or the inability to move the exposed part(s). A measure for reducing the likelihood of this potential problem is to elevate the body part, thereby increasing venous return. If edema is excessive, casts are bivalved, that is, cut to make an anterior and a posterior half that are held together with an elastic bandage.

When more extensive damage has occurred, variations of reduction and casting are employed. An extremity that has sustained an open fracture is often casted with a window over the wound area to allow for observation and dressing of the wound. A surgical reduction is usually casted as for a closed fracture. However, for the first few hours after surgery there may be substantial bleeding that will soak through the cast. Periodically the circumscribed blood-stained area is outlined with a ball-point pen or pencil and the time indicated to provide a guide for assessing the amount of bleeding.

Frequently the child will be discharged to home care after a cast is applied in the emergency room or clinic. Parents need instructions on care of the cast and symptoms that indicate that the cast is too tight. They are also instructed to bring the child for attention if the cast becomes too loose, since a loose cast no longer serves to maintain its purpose. Plaster casts cannot be submersed in water, which softens the plaster and alters its shape when dried; therefore, the cast requires protection during the child's bath. Plaster casts become soiled easily, but the surface can be wiped gently with a damp (not wet) cloth. Synthetic casts are immersible but must be rinsed and dried following bathing, showering, or swimming. The cast is first blotted with a towel then thoroughly dried with a blow drier on the cool or warm setting.

Cast removal. Cutting the cast to remove it or to relieve tightness is frequently a frightening experience for a child. He fears the sound of the cast cutter and is terrified that his flesh as well as the cast will be cut. Since it works by vibration, a cast cutter cuts only the hard surface of the cast. This can be demonstrated on the nurse or person removing the cast. However, the vibration generates heat that may be felt by the child, and this should be explained to him. Preparing the child for the procedure will help reduce his anxiety, especially if a trusting relationship has been established between the child and his nurse. Many young children come to regard the cast as a part of them-

selves, which intensifies their fear of its removal. Using the analogy of having fingernails or hair cut sometimes helps reduce their anxiety. They need continual reassurance that all is going well and that their behavior is accepted.

After the cast is removed the skin surface will be caked with desquamated skin and sebaceous secretions. Soaking the area in a bathtub usually removes this material, but it may take several days to eliminate the accumulation completely. Application of olive oil or lotion may provide comfort. The parents and child are instructed not to pull or forcibly remove this material with vigorous scrubbing, which may cause excoriation and bleeding.

SUMMARY OF NURSING CARE OF THE CHILD WITH A CAST

GOALS	RESPONSIBILITIES
Assist with diagnosis	Recognize deviation from normal alignment Assist with radiographs
Prepare the child for procedures	Maintain a calm, reassuring manner Explain procedures and equipment at the child's level of understanding

Assist with fracture reduction	Gather equipment as needed
	Help maintain extremity in alignment as needed
	Provide support to the child during the procedure
	   Explain what is happening
	   Remain with the child throughout the procedure

Prevent circulatory impairment	Elevate cast extremity
	   Place leg cast on pillows, making certain that leg is well supported and that there is no pressure on heel
	   Elevate arm on pillows or support in stockinette sling suspended from intravenous infusion pole—either in bed or during ambulation; triangular arm sling is adequate for lesser elevation and support

Monitor neurovascular status	Monitor peripheral pulses frequently Blanch skin on extremity distal to fracture to ascertain adequate circulation to the part Feel cast for tightness; cast should allow insertion of fingers between skin and cast after it has dried Assess for increase in pain, swelling, coldness, cyanosis Assess finger or toe movement and sensation Request the child to move his fingers or toes Report signs of impending circulatory impairment immediately Instruct the child to report any feelings of numbness or tingling
Detect signs of infection	Smell cast for foul odor Be alert to increased temperature, lethargy, and discomfort
Detect respiratory impairment	Assess the child's chest expansion Observe respiratory rate Observe color and behavior

GOALS	RESPONSIBILITIES
Prevent skin irritation	Make certain that all edges are smooth and free from irritating projections; trim and/or pad as necessary; petal cast edges if needed Keep crumbs and other items from getting between cast and skin Inspect skin for irritation or pressure areas In small children, inspect beneath cast for items that the child may place there In older children, caution not to place items under cast Keep exposed skin clean and free of irritants

Maintain optimum temperature	Check temperature; imbalance can be produced by
	    Chemical reaction in cast drying process, which generates heat
	    Water evaporation, which causes heat loss

Maintain cast integrity	Do not allow weight bearing until cast is completely dry—even if weight-bearing device is attached Caution against activities that might cause physical damage to cast
Hip spica cast	Change position periodically; small children can be managed easily; adolescents may require one or two persons; eventually children become very adept at moving themselves Do *not* use abduction stabilizer bar between legs of hip spica as handle for turning Position the child with buttocks lower than shoulders during toileting to prevent urine from flowing under cast at the back; body can be supported on pillows Protect rim of cast around perineal area of body cast with plastic film, or Saran wrap to prevent soiling during toileting For infants and small children who are not toilet trained or who are prone to "accidents," use plastic-backed disposable diaper with edges tucked underneath rim of cast; a sanitary napkin can also be used if waterproof material is placed between pad and cast Place the small child on Bradford frame
Maintain muscle use of unaffected areas	Encourage the child to ambulate as soon as possible Support casted arm in sling Teach use of mobilizing devices such as crutches for casted leg (walking device is applied when weight bearing allowed) With newer devices, encourage the child to ambulate as soon as general condition allows Provide and encourage use of muscles in play activities and diversions If unaffected limbs are paralyzed, carry out range of motion exercises
Provide comfort	Position for comfort; use pillows to support dependent areas Alleviate itching underneath cast with alcohol swabs, cool air blown from Asepto syringe or fan Avoid using powder or lotion under cast, since these substances have tendency to "ball" and produce irritation Place a piece of tape lengthwise beneath stockinette prior to cast application so that it can be moved up and down to "scratch" skin Remove soiled areas from plaster cast with damp cloth and small amount of white, low-abrasive cleanser Dry synthetic casts thoroughly after immersion
Educate the parents	Teach cast care and support of casted part Make certain that the parents understand signs of circulatory impairment and infection Help the parents plan suitable activities Help the parents in problem solving to modify clothing to fit over casted area Help the parents devise supportive devices and modification of furniture for positioning (such as pillows, pads and so on) Help the parents in problem solving of means of transporting the child
Support the child during cast removal	Explain procedure Demonstrate safety of equipment Provide reassurance

The child in traction: application and nursing considerations

Bone fragments that cannot be aligned initially by simple traction and stabilization with a cast require the extended pulling force provided by continuous traction. Traction may be used for purposes other than fracture alignment and immobilization. Some additional uses of traction are: to provide rest for an extremity, to help correct or prevent contracture deformity, or, rarely, to reduce muscle spasms. In these cases the traction may be applied at night and intermittently during the day. Muscle relaxants may be administered for muscle spasms.

The three essential components of traction management are traction, countertraction, and friction (Fig. 28-3). To reduce or realign a fracture site, traction is provided by weights applied to the distal bone fragment; body weight provides countertraction; and the patient's contact with the bed constitutes the frictional force. By adjusting the line of pull upward or downward or by adducting or abducting the extremity, the operator uses these forces to align the distal and proximal bone fragments.

Equilibrium is attained and maintained in two ways: (1) the amount of forward force is adjusted by adding weight to or subtracting weight from the traction, and/or (2) countertraction is increased by elevating the foot of the bed to create a greater gravitational pull to the backward force. A bed board placed under the mattress of heavy children prevents sagging, which can change the direction of the forces applied to the fracture.

The three primary purposes of traction are:

1. To fatigue the involved muscle and reduce muscle spasm so that bones can be realigned
2. To position the distal and proximal bone ends in desired realignment to promote satisfactory bone healing
3. To immobilize the fracture site until realignment has been achieved and sufficient healing has taken place to permit casting or splinting

The all-or-none law, characteristic of muscle contractibility, is used to attain complete relaxation. When muscle is stretched, muscle spasm ceases, permitting the realignment of the bone ends. The continuous maintenance of traction is essential during this phase because release of the traction allows the normal muscle contraction to again malposition the bone ends. The realignment of the fragments is a gradual process that is achieved more rapidly in infants, because of their limited muscle tone, than in muscular teenagers.

The traction pull serves to immobilize the fracture site; however, adjunctive immobilizing devices such as splints or casts are sometimes used with skeletal traction. In injuries with severe soft tissue swelling or vascular and nerve damage, it is customary to use traction until these complications have been resolved and it is safe to apply a cast. A cast can act as a tourniquet if swelling occurs beneath it. The desired line of pull and callus formation are assessed periodically by radiographic examination. Immobilization with traction will be maintained until the bone ends are in satisfactory realignment, after which a less-confining type of immobilization, usually a cast, will be applied.

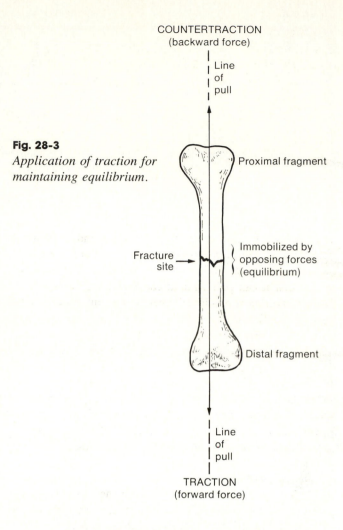

Fig. 28-3
Application of traction for maintaining equilibrium.

COUNTERTRACTION
(backward force)

Line of pull

Proximal fragment

Fracture site

Immobilized by opposing forces (equilibrium)

Distal fragment

Line of pull

TRACTION
(forward force)

Types of traction (general). The pull needed for traction can be applied to the distal bone fragment in several ways:

manual traction traction applied to the body part by the hand placed distally to the fracture site. Nurses frequently provide manual traction during cast application.

skin traction traction applied directly to the skin surface and indirectly to the skeletal structures. The pulling mechanism is attached to the skin with adhesive material or an elastic bandage.

skeletal traction traction applied directly to the skeletal structure by a pin, wire, or tongs inserted into or through the diameter of the bone distal to the fracture.

Manual traction is used to realign bone fragments for immediate cast application in uncomplicated arm or leg fractures in which there is little overriding of the bones and minimum muscle pull to overcome. Skin traction is ap-

Fig. 28-4

Upper extremity traction. (Redrawn from Hilt, N.E., and Schmitt, E.W.: Pediatric orthopedic nursing, St. Louis, 1975, The C.V. Mosby Co.)

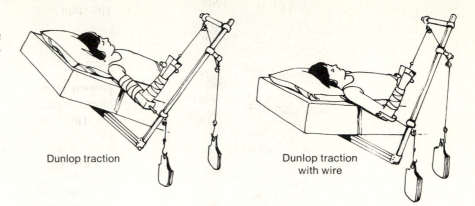

Dunlop traction

Dunlop traction
with wire

plied when there is minimum displacement and little muscle spasticity but is contraindicated when there is associated skin damage. Skin traction has specific limits of weight that it can pull without causing tissue breakdown. Skeletal traction is employed when significant traction pull must be applied in order to achieve realignment and immobilization. By inserting a pin or wire into the bone, the stress is placed on the bone and not on the surrounding tissue.

The type of traction applied is determined primarily by the age of the child, the condition of the soft tissues, and the type and degree of displacement of the fracture. The fractures most commonly treated by application of traction are those involving the humerus, femur, and vertebrae.

Upper extremity traction.   Treatment of fractures of the humerus by traction is accomplished by: (1) overhead suspension, in which the arm (bent at the elbow) is suspended vertically by skin or skeletal attachment and traction applied to the distal end of the humerus; or (2) Dunlop traction.

Dunlop traction.   With Dunlop traction (Fig. 28-4) the arm is suspended horizontally, using either skin or skeletal attachment. When skin traction is used, straps are placed on the lower and upper arm with the arm flexed to accomplish pull in two directions: one along the longitudinal direction of the upper arm and one to maintain alignment of the lower arm.

Fractures of the humerus, which usually result from a fall with the arm in extension, frequently involve the supracondylar portion. These fractures are especially at risk for nerve damage and angulation deformities and, therefore, must be reduced carefully. Because of the danger of complications, children with closed reduction of supracondylar fractures are frequently hospitalized for observation. Severely malaligned fractures are reduced under anesthesia and followed by application of skeletal traction for 2 to 3 weeks, after which a long arm cast is applied for an additional 2 to 3 weeks.

Lower extremity traction.   The force direction of muscle pull and bone displacement varies with the location of the fracture. A fracture in the middle third of the shaft

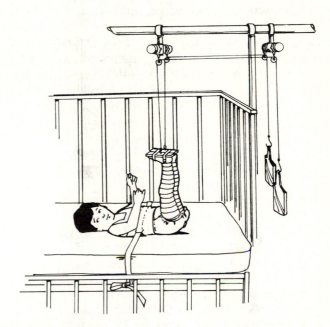

Fig. 28-5

Lower extremity traction used in treatment and care of children (Bryant traction). (Redrawn from Hilt, N.E., and Schmitt, E.W.: Pediatric orthopedic nursing, St. Louis, 1975, The C.V. Mosby Co.)

results in significant overriding but minimum displacement. In a fracture in the lower third of the shaft, the pull of the gastrocnemius muscle causes the distal fragment to become downwardly displaced.

Fractures of the femur can often be reduced with immediate application of a hip spica cast in young children. When traction is required several types may be employed, based on the initial assessment.

Bryant traction.   When a traction pulls in only one direction it is called running traction. Bryant traction is this type of traction (Fig. 28-5). Adhesive traction strips are applied to the child's legs and secured with elastic bandages wrapped from the foot to the groin. Both of the child's hips are flexed at a 90-degree angle with the knees

Fig. 28-6

Buck extension. (Redrawn from Hilt, N.E., and Schmitt, E.W.: Pediatric orthopedic nursing, St. Louis, 1975, The C.V. Mosby Co.)

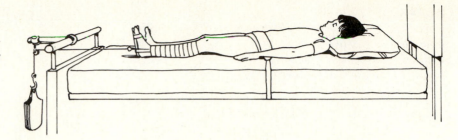

extended and the legs suspended by pulleys and weights. The child's weight supplies the countertraction; therefore, the buttocks are elevated slightly off the bed. Applying the same amount of traction to both legs and restraining the torso, prevents the pelvis and hips from rotating and places equal stress on the growing extremities. The ankle bones are protected with stockinette or cotton wadding.

This type of traction is employed for children younger than 2 years of age whose weight is not sufficient to provide adequate countertraction without the additional gravitational force. Both legs are suspended, even though only one may be involved. Bryant traction is unsuited to older children and is usually limited to children who weigh less than 12 to 14 kg (26 to 30 pounds) because of the risk of postural hypertension and to those without spasticity or contractures of the hamstring muscles.

Sufficient room is maintained between the child's foot and the traction foot plate to permit foot movement and thereby prevent ankle problems. The legs must be maintained perpendicular to the trunk, and the buttocks are not allowed to rest on the mattress. Sometimes the child, especially the very active child, is placed in a jacket restraint or on a Bradford frame to prevent his turning and twisting out of alignment.

The child's position is monitored, and the alignment of the fracture is checked periodically by radiographic examination with traction adjustments made as needed. Remodeling and callus formation occur rapidly, within 2 to 3 weeks, after which the child is placed in a hip spica cast for an additional 3 to 9 weeks.

Buck extension traction.   Buck extension (Fig. 28-6) is also skin traction with the legs extended, but it differs from Bryant's traction in that the hips are not flexed. This traction allows for greater mobility and prevents the postural hypertension that might develop as a result of Bryant traction. Turning from side to side is permitted with care to maintain the involved leg in alignment. Buck extension is used primarily for short-term immobilization or, frequently, for correcting contracture or bone deformities such as Legg-Calvé-Perthes disease.

Russell traction.   Russell traction (Fig. 28-7) uses skin traction on the lower leg and a padded sling under the knee. Two lines of pull are produced—one along the longitudinal line of the lower leg and one perpendicular to the

leg. This combination allows realignment of the lower extremity and immobilizes the hip and knee in a flexed position. The hip flexion must be kept at the prescribed angle to prevent fracture malalignment since there is no direct support beneath the fracture and the skin traction may slip. Special nursing measures include careful assessment to assure that the amount of desired hip flexion is maintained and that damage to the common peroneal nerve under the knee does not produce footdrop.

Ninety-degree–90-degree traction.   The most commonly used skeletal traction is 90-degree–90-degree traction (Fig. 28-8), in which the lower leg is encased in a boot cast and a skeletal Steinmann pin or Kirschner wire is placed in the distal fragment of the femur. From a nursing standpoint this traction facilitates position changes, toileting, and hygienic care and prevents traction complications.

Balance suspension traction.   Balance suspension traction (Fig. 28-9) may be used with or without skin or skeletal traction. Unless combined with another type of traction, the balanced suspension merely suspends the leg in a desired flexed position to relax the hip and hamstring muscles without exerting traction on a body part directly. A Thomas splint that extends from the groin to midair above the foot and a Pearson attachment support the lower leg with ropes attached to create a balanced traction. Towels or pieces of felt that are covered with stockinette, clipped or pinned to the splints provide leg support. When the child is lifted from the bed, the traction lifts with him without loss of alignment. This is especially useful for moving an older and heavier child. Splints and ropes are assessed regularly to detect any signs of slippage or fraying.

Cervical traction.   The cervical area is vulnerable to flexion or extension injuries to muscle, vertebrae, and/or spinal cord. Cervical muscle trauma without complications is treated with a cervical soft or hard collar to relieve the weight of the head from the fracture site. Intermittent cervical skin traction is often employed with a chin halter and weight to decrease muscle spasms.

Cervical traction is usually accomplished by the insertion of Crutchfield or Cone-Barton tongs through burr holes in the skull and weights attached to the hyperextended head. As the neck muscles fatigue as a result of continual traction pull, the vertebral bodies gradually sep-

Fig. 28-7

Russell traction. (Redrawn from Hilt, N.E., and Schmitt, E.W.: Pediatric orthopedic nursing, St. Louis, 1975, The C.V. Mosby Co.)

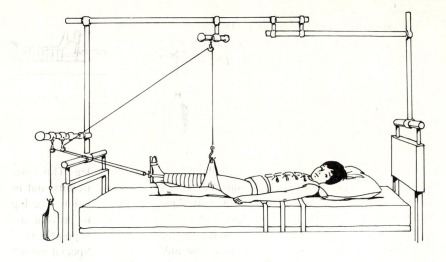

Fig. 28-8

Ninety-degree–90° traction. (Redrawn from Hilt, N.E., and Schmitt, E.W.: Pediatric orthopedic nursing, St. Louis, 1975, The C.V. Mosby Co.)

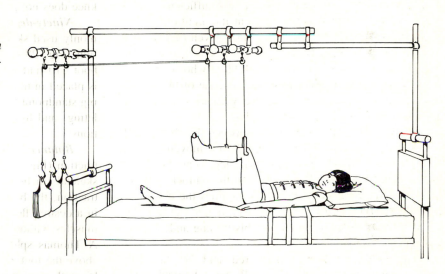

Fig. 28-9

Balanced suspension with Thomas ring splint and Pearson attachment. (Redrawn from Hilt, N.E., and Schmitt, E.W.: Pediatric orthopedic nursing, St. Louis, 1975. The C.V. Mosby Co.)

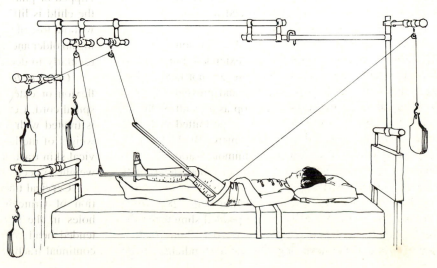

arate so that the cord is no longer pinched between. Immobilization until fracture healing can occur is a second goal of cervical traction. If the injury has been limited to a vertebral fracture without neurologic deficit, a halo cast is applied to permit earlier ambulation.

Traction care. Generally the child in traction is hospitalized under the direct care of nurses who develop individualized nursing care plans based on an understanding of correct traction management. There are a number of physical needs that require attention and vigilance. It is essential that nurses understand the basic principles of traction, the specific type of traction employed, and their role in its maintenance. Skeletal traction is never released by the nurse, but, under certain circumstances, such as the child with Legg-Calvé-Perthes disease or scoliosis, nurses may remove nonadhesive skin traction. In these cases intermittent traction is periodically released and reapplied as ordered. When skin traction must be constantly maintained, such as in fractures, nurses may occasionally remove and reapply the Ace bandage if this is approved by the attending physician, provided that *someone maintains the traction manually during the rewrapping process*. It is not uncommon for a child to have several types of traction at one time, and each traction must be assessed separately to avoid problems.

When the child is first placed in traction he may have increased discomfort as a result of the traction pull fatiguing the muscle. Analgesics and muscle relaxants will help during this phase of care, but helping the child to cope with the confinement and the new experience requires more than medications. The child needs an explanation, at his level of understanding, of what is happening and why he is confined in the device. He needs to be reassured that someone will be present to aid him in adjusting to the traction and coping with the problems of immobilization.

SUMMARY OF NURSING CARE OF THE CHILD IN TRACTION

GOALS	RESPONSIBILITIES
Decrease anxiety and gain cooperation	Explain traction apparatus to the child Explain to the child what his nursing care will involve Determine with the child how he can participate in his care Make certain that the child knows how to call for help Assure the child that he will not be left totally helpless

Maintain traction	Understand purpose of traction
	Understand function of traction in each specific situation
	Check desired line of pull and relationship of distal fragment to proximal fragment—directed upward, adducted, or abducted
	Check function of each component part
	  Position of bandages, frames, splints
	  Ropes—in center track of pulley, taut, no fraying, knots tied securely
	  Pulleys—in original position on attachment bar, have not moved from original site, wheels freely movable
	  Weights—correct amount of weight, hanging freely, in safe location
	Assess bed position—head or foot elevated as directed for desired amount of pull and countertraction
	Do not remove skeletal traction or adhesive traction straps on skin traction

Skin traction	Replace nonadhesive strips and/or Ace bandage on skin traction when permitted and/or absolutely necessary; make certain that traction on limb is maintained by someone during procedure Assess bandages to ascertain correct application (diagonal or spiral), not too loose or too tight (which could cause slippage and malalignment of traction)
Skeletal traction	Assess pin sites frequently for signs of bleeding, inflammation, or infection Clean and dress pin sites as ordered Apply topical antiseptic or antibiotic daily as ordered Cover ends of pins with protective cord or padding to prevent the child's being scratched by pin Note pull of traction on pin (pull should be even) Check pin screws to be certain that screws are tight in metal clamp that attaches traction apparatus to pin

GOALS	RESPONSIBILITIES

Maintain alignment	Observe for correct body alignment with emphasis on alignment of shoulders, hips, and leg(s)
	Reassess after the child has moved
	Apply restraints when indicated
	Maintain correct angles at joints, for example:
	    Bryant traction—90-degree angle at hip
	    Russell traction—20-degree angle at hip

Prevent complications	Assess the child's behavior to determine if traction causes pain or discomfort
Pressure areas	Change position at least every 2 hours to relieve pressure Stimulate circulation with gentle massage over pressure areas Provide sheepskin, egg carton, or alternating pressure mattress underneath hips and back Make total body skin checks for redness or breakdown, especially over areas that receive greatest pressure Wash and dry skin at least twice daily

Circulation	Note any neurovascular changes, such as
	    Color in skin and nail beds
	    Alterations in sensation
	    Alterations in motor ability
	Take immediate action to correct problem or report to the physician if neurovascular change is detected
	Record neurovascular assessments
	Assess circular dressings for excessive tightness
	Assess restraining devices
	    Make certain that they are not too loose or too tight
	    Remove periodically and check for pressure areas

Disuse atrophy and contractures	Carry out passive, active, or active-with-resistance exercises as prescribed Note if any tightness, weakness, or contractures are developing in uninvolved joints and muscles Take measures to correct or prevent further development, such as applying foot plate to prevent footdrop Move uninvolved joint or muscle frequently to avoid contractures Encourage the child in activities that provide exercise for uninvolved muscles and joints
Respiratory	Encourage deep breathing frequently with maximum inspiratory chest expansion
Provide adequate nutrition and hydration	Encourage fluid intake so the child stays well hydrated Provide nourishing, nonconstipating diet with preferred foods when possible and foods that the child can manage unassisted Make certain that the child ingests sufficient amount of calcium-rich foods
Promote elimination	Check frequency and consistency of bowel movements Adjust fluid and food intake according to stools, for example, increase fluids, fruits, grains, for constipation Administer stool softeners as indicated Administer rectal suppository or mild laxative if indicated Use fracture pan for bowel movements Assure adequate renal output by increasing fluids when indicated
Relieve pain and discomfort	Administer pain medication as needed during first 2 or 3 days after fracture Use pads, pillows, and rolls to position for comfort
Support family	Explain treatments Reinforce information Provide opportunity to discuss feelings and concerns

Surgical intervention

When surgical intervention is required to realign a fracture, the child needs physical and psychologic preparation. The preoperative teaching is the same as for any other surgical procedure, except that orthopedic surgery uses a variety of rods, screws, and plates. The child needs to know about these unfamiliar things and how they will appear when he returns from the operation. Usually rods are driven down the shaft of the long bones; screws and plates are attached to the surface of the bone shaft.

Postoperatively bone healing proceeds the same as a new fracture with the callus formation and remodeling. Generally the child with an internal fixation device is able to mobilize in a chair and to a walker or crutches within a few hours or days. The most common postoperative complications are infection and slippage of the fixation device. The nurse's responsibility includes close monitoring of neurovascular changes in the involved extremity, prevention of postanesthesia problems, and observation for early evidence of complications.

AMPUTATION

The child may be a victim of a traumatic loss of an extremity or he may need a surgical amputation for a pathologic condition such as osteosarcoma. With today's surgical technology and the rapid action of a bystander who saves a traumatically amputated body part, some children have had fingers and arms replaced with variable degrees of functional use regained. A severed part should be wrapped in a clean cloth moistened with saline if possible and placed in a plastic bag, which is sealed and placed on ice. It is taken to the hospital with the victim.

Operative amputation or the surgical repair of a permanently severed limb focuses on constructing an adequately nourished stump. A smooth, healthy, padded stump that is free of nerve endings is important in prosthesis fitting and subsequent ambulation. In situations where there is no vascular or neurologic deficit, a cast is applied to the stump at the time of surgery and a pylon with metal extension and artificial foot is attached. The patient is able to walk on this temporary prosthesis within a few hours.

Stump elevation may be prescribed during the first 24 hours, but after this time the extremity should not remain in a position that contributes to joint contractures. For example, contractures in the proximal joint of a lower extremity can develop and seriously hamper ambulation. Monitoring proper body alignment will further decrease the risk of flexion contractures.

Stump shaping begins postoperatively. It is accomplished by means of an elastic figure-8 bandage, which applies and maintains pressure in a cone-shaped fashion. This technique decreases stump edema, controls hemorrhage, and aids in developing desired contours that facili-

tate prosthesis attachment. The shaping allows the child with a lower extremity amputation to bear weight on the posterior aspect of the skin flap rather than on the end of the stump.

For older children and adolescents, arm exercises, bed push-ups, and parallel bars, which are used in prosthesis training programs, help to build up the arm muscles necessary for walking with crutches. Full range of motion of joints above the amputation must be performed several times daily, using active and isotonic exercises. Young children are spontaneously active and require little encouragement.

Depending on the child's age, he or his parents are taught stump hygiene, which includes careful cleansing with soap and water and observation for skin irritation, breakdown, or infection. A tube of stockinette or some type of powder is used to slide the prosthesis on more easily. A careful skin check is carried out each time the prosthesis is removed, and the time the prosthesis is worn (tolerance time) is adjusted to prevent skin breakdown.

The child who has had an amputation can expect to experience phantom limb pain, because the nerve-brain connections are still present. These sensations fade gradually. Preoperative discussion of this phenomenon will aid the child in understanding these ''unusual feelings'' so that he will not hide such sensations from others. Limb pain, especially pain that increases with ambulation, should be evaluated for the possibility of a neuroma at the free nerve endings in the stump. Psychogenic phantom limb pain is a complex problem involving the child's response to the altered body image and the coping mechanisms he uses to handle the new experience. The problem of amputation, particularly the psychologic aspects, is discussed further on p. 975.

INJURY TO JOINTS AND SOFT TISSUE

A variety of injuries can result when an external force exerts severe stress on tissue, muscle, and skeletal structures. The body structures attempt to accommodate the force, but, when unable to do so, they are subjected to a variety of injuries (Fig. 28-10).

Contusion

A contusion consists of damage to the soft tissues (subcutaneous structures and muscle) without breaking the skin and is characterized by swelling, discoloration, and pain. The escape of blood into the tissues is observed as *ecchymosis,* a black and blue discoloration.

Early application of cold to the damaged area decreases pain and triggers local vasoconstriction that reduces hemorrhage and edema. Local cold therapy has the additional advantage of lessening muscle spasm, probably

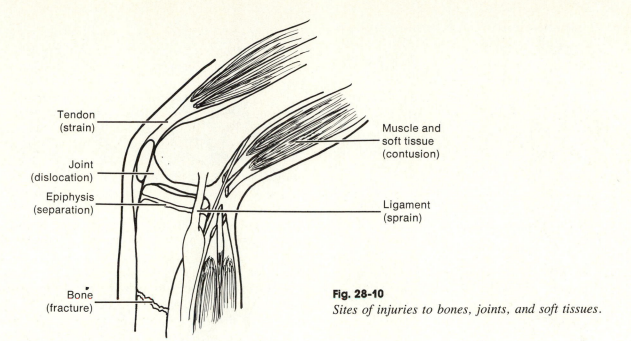

Tendon
(strain)

Joint
(dislocation)

Epiphysis
(separation)

Bone
(fracture)

Muscle and
soft tissue
(contusion)

Ligament
(sprain)

Fig. 28-10
Sites of injuries to bones, joints, and soft tissues.

by decreasing muscle irritability and the responsiveness of muscle spindles to stretch. Adjunctive therapies that promote venous return include compression bandaging and elevation of the extremity.

Strains and sprains

A *strain* consists of damage to any portion of the musculature, caused by overstretching or overexertion, that results in pain and swelling. Application of cold, immobilization with elastic bandage, and elevation of the extremity will help alleviate these symptoms.

A *sprain* is a traumatic injury that occurs when a ligament is partially or completely torn or stretched when a joint is twisted or wrenched. They are often accompanied by damage to associated blood vessels, muscles, tendons, and nerves. Generally sprains require only support, heat, and muscle relaxants with occasional use of intermittent traction. Major sprains or tears to the ligamentous tissue rarely occur in growing children. Ligaments are stronger than bone, and the epiphysis and growth plate are the weakest areas of the bone; therefore, the more usual sites of injury are at the growth plate.

Therapy for a sprained joint consists of elevating and immobilizing the injured joint, applying an ice pack as soon as possible to relieve pain and swelling, and wrapping the injured region with an elastic bandage to control swelling. The ice is applied for 20 to 30 minutes intermittently for 24 to 48 hours, according to the instructions of practitioners. The cold cellular temperature reduces metabolic demand and cellular activity and constricts the capillaries. No weight-bearing is allowed for 5 to 7 days or until there is no edema and no pain on weight-bearing.

Torn ligaments, especially those in the knee, are usually treated by immobilization with a cast for 3 to 4 weeks or strapping of the joint with adhesive or Elastoplast bandage. Passive leg exercises, gradually increased to active ones, are begun as soon as sufficient healing has taken place.

Dislocations

Long bones are maintained in approximation at the joint by ligaments. A dislocation occurs when the force of stress on the ligament is so great that there is displacement of the normal position of the opposing bone ends or the bone end to its socket. The predominant symptom is pain that increases with attempted passive or active movement of the extremity. There may be an obvious deformity and inability to move the joint.

Dislocations are less common in children than in older persons. Before final closure of the epiphyses, injuries to the joints are more likely to cause epiphyseal separation than dislocation. For example, shoulder dislocation is seen only in older adolescents, and dislocation unaccompanied by fracture is rare.

Dislocation of the hip is probably the most common dislocation and, in children younger than 5 years of age, is usually caused by a fall. However, trauma is minimum because of general joint laxity and the largely cartilaginous nature of the acetabulum. The cause of dislocation between 6 and 10 years of age is more often an athletic injury. Thereafter, automobile accidents are the most frequent cause.

Dislocation of the patella is a recurrent episode in some children; in others it is the result of injury. It is quite common in adolescent girls. The patella is always dislocated laterally. Most dislocations are reduced either spontaneously or by a companion before the child is seen by a health professional. Surgery may be required for recurrent dislocations.

The most common dislocation injury, often managed in a pediatrician's office, is subluxation of the head of the radius. This occurs when a child between ages 1 and 4 years is pulled along or stumbles while holding onto the hand of an adult causing the arm to be jerked upward while in a position of extension. The child complains of pain in the elbow and wrist, refuses to move the arm, and holds it slightly flexed and pronated. The dislocation is reduced by application of firm finger pressure to the head of the radius while supinating and flexing the forearm returning the bone structures to normal alignment.

Dislocations are reduced by manipulation to replace the bones in anatomic alignment, often under anesthesia. Temporary joint restriction, such as the application of a sling or bandage that secures the arm to the chest in a shoulder dislocation, provides sufficient comfort and immobilization until the child can receive medical help. Following reduction, immobilization for 3 weeks or more is necessary for healing of any torn ligaments followed by gentle, graduated exercises without stretching, usually performed by the child himself.

CONGENITAL DEFECTS

There are numerous skeletal defects that can be diagnosed at or shortly after birth. The alert nurse is frequently the person who detects the defect and refers the family for correction of the condition. The deviation is often difficult to detect without careful inspection. Therefore, it is imperative that nurses become acquainted with signs of these defects and understand the principles of therapy in order to direct others in the care and management of these children.

CONGENITAL HIP DYSPLASIA

The broad term *congenital hip dysplasia* and the more common term *congenital dislocated hip (CDH)* are applied to malformations of the hip with various degrees of deformity that are present at birth. Three degrees of congenital dysplasia can be identified (Fig. 28-11):

acetabular dysplasia (or preluxation) the mildest form, in which there is neither subluxation nor dislocation. The dysplasia reflects an apparent delay in acetabular development evidenced by osseous hypoplasia of the acetabular roof that is oblique and shallow, although the cartilaginous roof is comparatively intact. The femoral head remains in the acetabulum.

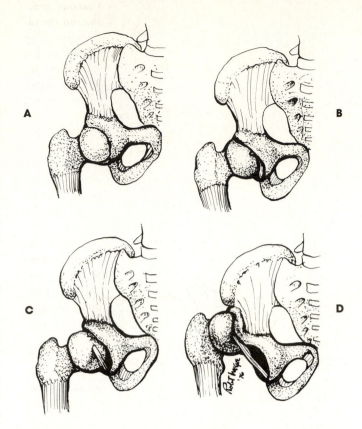

Fig. 28-11
Configuration and relationship of structure in congenital hip deformities. **A,** *Normal;* **B,** *acetabular dysplasia;* **C,** *subluxation;* **D,** *dislocation.*

subluxation accounts for the largest percentage of congenital hip dysplasias. Subluxation implies incomplete dislocation or dislocatable hip and is sometimes regarded as an intermediate state in the development from primary dysplasia to complete dislocation. The femoral head remains in contact with the acetabulum, but a stretched capsule and ligamentum teres cause the head of the femur to be partially displaced. Pressure on the cartilaginous roof inhibits ossification and produces a flattening of the socket.

dislocation in which the femoral head loses contact with the acetabulum and is displaced posteriorly and superiorly over the fibrocartilaginous rim. The ligamentum teres is elongated and taut.

Although it is one of the most common congenital defects, the cause of hip dysplasia is unknown. The incidence is about one in 500 to 1000 births, and it occurs more frequently in females than in males (7:1). The disorder occurs 25 to 30 times more often in first-degree relatives than in the general population, which suggests that genetic factors play a role in the causation. One fourth of all cases involve both hips, and when only one hip is involved the left hip is affected three times more often than the right. Congenital hip dysplasia is frequently associated with other conditions, such as spina bifida, breech presen-

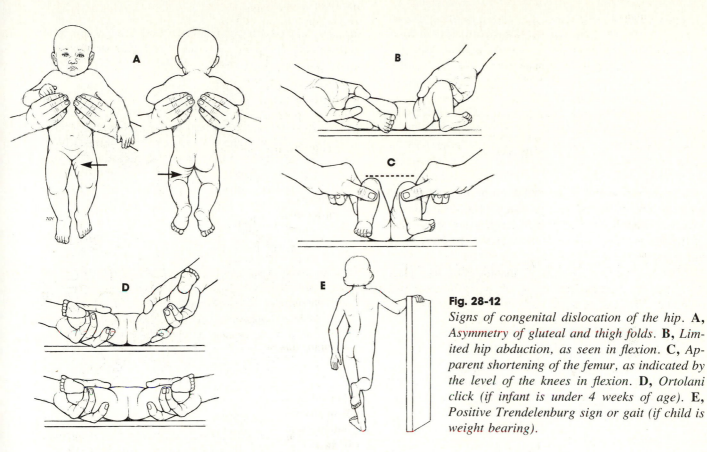

Fig. 28-12

Signs of congenital dislocation of the hip. **A,** *Asymmetry of gluteal and thigh folds.* **B,** *Limited hip abduction, as seen in flexion.* **C,** *Apparent shortening of the femur, as indicated by the level of the knees in flexion.* **D,** *Ortolani click (if infant is under 4 weeks of age).* **E,** *Positive Trendelenburg sign or gait (if child is weight bearing).*

tations, and cesarean section (often necessary because of abnormal intrauterine position). Legs in frank breech position, that is, with the hips acutely flexed and knees extended, is an important factor in the development of hip dislocation.

The disorder is virtually unknown in the Far East and relatively common among Navajo Indians and Canadian Eskimos. There appears to be a striking relationship between the development of dislocation and methods of handling infants. Among the cultures with the highest incidence of dislocation, newly born infants are tightly wrapped in blankets or other swaddling material or are strapped to cradle boards. In cultures where mothers traditionally carry infants on their backs or hips in the widely abducted straddle position, the incidence is lowest.

Clinical manifestations

In the newborn period dysplasia usually appears as hip joint laxity rather than as outright dislocation. The infant with hip dislocation manifests physical signs such as restricted abduction of the affected hip, shortening of the limb on the affected side (Allis sign), asymmetric thigh and gluteal folds, and broadening of the perineum (in bilateral dislocation) (Fig. 28-12). Sometimes weight bearing will precipitate a transition from subluxation to dislo-

cation in unrecognized cases; the disorder is not always apparent at birth.

In the older infant and child the affected leg will be shorter than the other with telescoping or piston mobility, that is, the head of the femur can be felt to move up and down in the buttock when the extended thigh is pushed first toward the child's head and then pulled distally. Instability of the hip on weight bearing delays walking and produces a characteristic limp. When the child stands first on one foot and then on the other (holding onto a chair, rail, or someone's hands) bearing weight on the affected hip, the pelvis tilts downward on the normal side instead of upward as it would with normal stability (Trendelenburg sign). In both unilateral and bilateral dislocations the greater trochanter is prominent and appears above a line from the anterior superior iliac spine to the tuberosity of the ischium. The child with bilateral dislocations has marked lordosis and a peculiar waddling gait.

Diagnostic evaluation

The diagnosis of congenital hip dysplasia should be made in the newborn period if possible since treatment initiated before 2 months of age achieves the highest rate of success. Subluxation and the tendency to dislocate can be demonstrated by the Ortolani manipulation (Fig. 28-12) or the Barlow modification of the maneuver performed by persons skilled in the techniques. There are cases in which dislocation is not diagnosed by these standard tests. It is recommended that hip examination be included as part of the well-baby visits until the child begins to walk and the gait is obviously normal.

In older infants and children radiographic examination is useful in confirming the diagnosis. An upward slope in the roof of the acetabulum (the acetabular angle) greater than 40 degrees with upward and outward displacement of the femoral head is a frequent finding in older children. Radiographic examination in early infancy is not reliable because the bones are largely cartilaginous and difficult to visualize. However, sonographic images show the unossified head of the femur and its relationship to the acetabulum; therefore, this test is being used with increased frequency.

Therapeutic management

Treatment is begun as soon as the condition is recognized, since early intervention is more favorable to the restoration of normal bony architecture and function. The longer treat-

ment is delayed, the more severe the deformity, the more difficult the treatment, and the less favorable the prognosis. The treatment varies with the age of the child and the extent of the dysplasia.

Infant.   In the child less than 1 year of age a dislocated hip securely held in abduction is usually sufficient to produce a stable joint. In many instances where the defect is recognized within the first week of life, simple abduction by way of double diapering is recommended by some authorities to create secure positioning that will produce a stable joint and prevent dislocation. For infants beyond the neonatal period an abduction device, which may be constructed from plastic, metal, leather, or a soft pillow (Frejka pillow splint), is worn that can be removed for bathing (Fig. 28-13). A lightweight harness (Pavlik harness) is the device preferred by most authorities. When adduction contracture is present, the hips are slowly and gently stretched to abduction and maintained with a device until stability is attained. This is accomplished by devices that can be adjusted as the amount of abduction is gradually increased. The device is worn for variable periods of time from days (in the newborn) to several weeks.

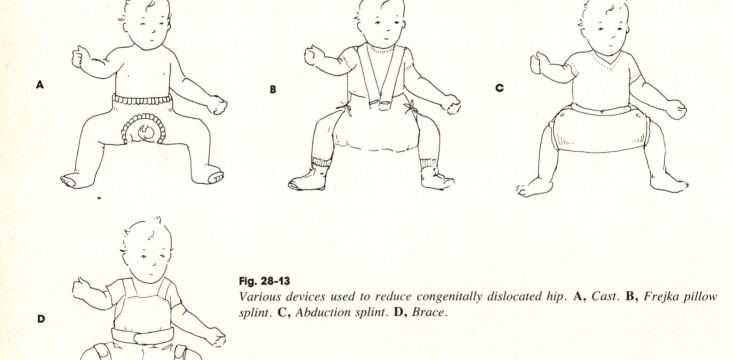

Fig. 28-13
Various devices used to reduce congenitally dislocated hip. **A,** *Cast.* **B,** *Frejka pillow splint.* **C,** *Abduction splint.* **D,** *Brace.*

When there is difficulty in maintaining stable reduction, a plaster hip spica cast is applied and changed periodically to accommodate the child's growth. After 3 to 6 months, sufficient stability is acquired to allow transfer to a removable protective abduction brace. The duration of treatment depends on development of the acetabulum but is usually accomplished within the first year.

Toddler. In this age-group the dislocation is not recognized until the child begins to walk, when attendant shortening of the limb and contractures of hip adductor and flexor muscles become apparent. Gradual reduction by traction is followed by plaster cast immobilization, which is maintained until radiographic examination confirms a stable joint. Often soft tissue may obstruct and complicate reduction and subsequent joint development. In this case open reduction is performed to remove the obstruction with postoperative spica cast immobilization and, after 4 to 6 months, replacement with an abduction splint.

Older child. Correction of the hip deformity in the older child is inherently more difficult than in the preceding age-groups since secondary adaptive changes complicate the condition. Operative reduction, which may involve preoperative traction, tenotomy of contracted muscles, and any one of several innominate osteotomy procedures designed to construct an acetabular roof, is usually required. After cast removal and before weight bearing is permitted, range of motion exercises help restore movement. Next, rehabilitative measures are instituted. Successful reduction and reconstruction become increasingly difficult after the age of 4 years and are usually impossible or inadvisable over 6 years of age because of severe shortening and contracture of muscles and deformity of the femoral and acetabular structures.

Nursing considerations

Nurses are in a unique position to detect congenital dislocation of the hip in the newborn. During the infant assessment process and routine nurturing activities the hips and extremities are inspected for any deviations from the normal. Usually only nurses specially trained in the technique are permitted to perform Barlow's maneuver, but any nurse can be alert to other signs such as leg shortening, gluteal folds, and limited abduction. Diapering, for example, provides an excellent opportunity to observe for limited movement and a wide perineum. These observations are reported to the attending physician, and the ambulatory child who displays a limp or an unusual gait should be referred for evaluation. This may indicate an orthopedic or neurologic problem.

Care of the child in a reduction device. The major nursing problems in the care of an infant or child in a cast or other device are related to maintenance of the device and adapting nurturing activities to meet the needs of the infant or child. Generally treatment and follow-up care of these children are carried out in a clinic, physician's office, or outpatient unit. However, hospitalization may be necessary for cast application or brace fitting but seldom exceeds 24 to 48 hours. Longer hospitalization is required for open reduction procedures or if the child is hospitalized for a concurrent illness.

The simplest devices to care for are multiple diapers and the Frejka pillow splint. With diapers, two or more are applied in the routine manner and maintained in position to achieve the desired abduction. They should fit snugly but not tightly. The pillow splint, a firm, rectangular pillow held in place by a romperlike outer garment, must be removed and reapplied with each diaper change. Although plastic pants worn over the diaper reduces the chance of soiling, it is necessary to have a second cover for the pillow to permit removal for laundering. These devices allow for easy handling of the infant and usually produce less apprehension in the parent. The Pavlik harness is removed during the child's bath and/or for cleaning.

Casts and braces offer more challenging nursing problems since they cannot be removed for routine care, although sometimes a brace may be removed for bathing. Care of an infant or small child with a cast requires nursing innovation to reduce irritation and to maintain cleanliness of both the child and the cast, particularly in the diaper area. (See p. 944 for care of the child in a cast.)

Parents are taught the proper care of the cast (or brace) and are helped to devise means for maintaining cleanliness. Plastic film or other waterproof material is applied around the edges of the cast in the perineal area to protect the cast from becoming wet and soiled. This material is removed, washed, dried, and replaced at least once a day. The skin is kept clean and dry around and under the cast and is checked frequently for evidence of irritation or pressure. Foam rubber can be used to provide extra protection if needed. Since older infants and small children may stuff bits of food, small toys, or other items under the cast, parents are alerted to this possibility and suitable preventive measures implemented.

Feeding the infant in a hip spica cast or brace offers problems of positioning. Very young infants can be fed in the supine position with head elevated, and (with the infant's hips and legs supported on a pillow at her side) the mother can cuddle the infant in her arms during feeding. A somewhat similar position can be used for breast-feeding, that is, with the infant supported on pillows or held in a "football" hold facing the mother and with the legs behind her. An alternate position is to hold the infant upright on the mother's lap. When the infant is able to sit up, he can be fed in a feeding table or a modified high chair. The parents may be able to fashion a tilt board with a padded seat or an adjustable chair.

It is important for nurses, parents, and other caregiv-

SUMMARY OF NURSING CARE OF THE CHILD WITH CONGENITAL DISLOCATION OF THE HIP (CDH)

GOALS	RESPONSIBILITIES
Recognize congenital dislocation of the hip	Inspect and assess the infant Repeat hip inspection at every postnatal well-baby check for undetected or overlooked signs
Maintain corrective positioning of hip	Apply reduction device correctly Maintain care of reduction device Assist with application of cast
Prevent complications	Observe for tightness of cast or apparatus, which indicates need for change or adjustment Check for evidence of impaired circulation Check for skin irritation and carry out appropriate skin care
Maintain care of corrective device	Maintain care of cast to prevent soiling or damage Administer correct care of braces or splints Position with suitable arrangement of pillows
Maintain nutrition	Feed in upright position whenever possible (appetite is seldom affected by the disorder or treatment) Avoid soiling cast or appliance with food Allow self-help as the child is able
Provide comfort	Encourage the parents to fondle and hold the infant or child Maintain accustomed routine at home and, when possible, if hospitalized
Facilitate developmental progress	Provide appropriate stimulation and activities for stage of development
Support parents	Provide ongoing and follow-up care Refer to public health agency and Special Child Health Services Teach the parents care of cast or appliance Help devise modifications for routine activities

ers to understand that these children need to be involved in all the activities of any child in the same age-group. Confinement in a cast should not exclude children from family (or unit) activities. They can be held astride a lap for comfort and transported to areas of activity, for example. The child may be allowed to walk in the cast. An excellent means for providing mobility is a low plastic or wooden platform (available at many toy and orthopedic supply stores) with rollers on which the child can propel himself. This device also helps develop the upper extremities.

CONGENITAL CLUBFOOT

"Clubfoot" is a general term used to describe a common deformity in which the foot is misshapen or malpositioned. Any foot deformity involving the ankle is called *talipes*, derived from *talus*, meaning ankle, and *pes*, meaning foot. Deformities of foot and ankle are conveniently described according to the position of the ankle and foot. The more common positions involve the variations:

talipes varus an inversion or a bending inward

talipes valgus an eversion or bending outward

talipes equinus plantar flexion in which the toes are lower than the heel

talipes calcaneus or dorsiflexion in which the toes are higher than the heel

Most clubfeet are a combination of these positions. Approximately 95% of the cases consist of the composite deformity *talipes equinovarus*, in which the foot is pointed downward and inward in varying degrees of severity (Fig. 28-14). Unilateral clubfoot is somewhat more common than bilateral clubfoot and may occur as an isolated defect or in association with other disorders or syndromes such as chromosomal aberrations, arthrogryposis (a generalized immobility of the joints), cerebral palsy, or spina bifida.

The frequency of clubfoot in the general population is one in every 700 to 1000 live births, and boys are affected twice as often as girls. The precise cause is unknown. There is an increased incidence in some families, which suggests a hereditary component. There are those who attribute the defect to abnormal positioning and restricted movement in utero, although the evidence is not conclu-

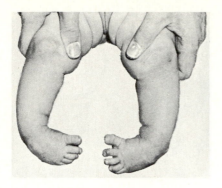

Fig. 28-14

Bilateral congenital talipes equinovarus (congenital club-foot) in 2-month-old infant. (From Brashear, H.R., Jr., and Raney, R.B.: Shands' handbook of orthopaedic surgery, ed. 9, St. Louis, 1978, The C.V. Mosby Co.)

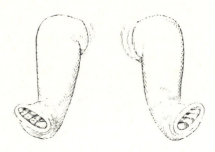

Fig. 28-15

Feet casted for correction of bilateral congenital talipes equinovarus. (From Brashear, H.R., Jr., and Raney, R.B.: Shands' handbook of orthopaedic surgery, ed. 9, St. Louis, 1978, The C.V. Mosby Co.)

sive. Others implicate arrested or anomalous embryonic development.

Diagnostic evaluation

The deformity is readily apparent and easily detected at birth. However, it must be differentiated from some positional deformities that can be corrected passively or over-corrected. The true clubfoot is fixed. Paralytic changes in the lower extremity of children with neuromuscular involvement often produce equinovarus deformity.

Therapeutic management

Treatment, which is begun as soon as the deformity is recognized, involves three stages: first, correction of the deformity; second, maintenance of the correction until normal muscle balance is regained; and third, follow-up observation to avert possible recurrence of the deformity. Some feet respond to treatment readily; some respond only to prolonged, vigorous, and sustained efforts; and the improvement in others remains disappointing even with maximum effort on the part of all concerned.

Correction of talipes equinovarus is most reliably accomplished by the application of a series of casts begun immediately or shortly after birth and continued until marked overcorrection is reached (Fig. 28-15). Successive casts allow for gradual stretching of tight structures on the medial side and gradual contraction of lax structures on the lateral side of the foot. The adduction deformity is corrected first, the inversion deformity next, and the plantar flexion deformity last. Weekly manipulations and cast changes are needed in the beginning to accommodate the rapid growth of early infancy.

Some authorities favor the use of gentle but firm manipulations for 1 or 2 weeks prior to casting a newborn in order to take advantage of the pliability of the infant's foot

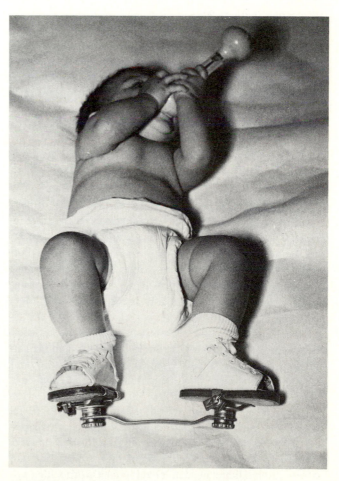

Fig. 28-16

Child in Denis Browne splint.

at this early age. Much of the correction can be obtained during this period, but the success of treatment is based on its early initiation and consistent application. Manipulations are carried out on a regular basis (at least five to six times per day) by the nursery staff and the mother according to detailed instruction.

An alternative method is use of the Denis Browne splint, a device that consists of two padded metal plates to which the infant's feet are securely fastened with adhesive tape and connected to a metal crossbar. Another device uses shoes affixed to the metal crossbar. The foot plates are adjusted to achieve the desired positioning. This device makes use of the infant's natural kicking movements to accelerate the correction process (Fig. 28-16).

Maintaining the correction is accomplished by use of special clubfoot shoes designed to maintain the correction (Fig. 28-17). The lateral side of the shoe is raised to maintain correction of the varus deformity and the front portion of the shoe turns outward to maintain forefoot abduction. Sometimes corrective shoes or splints are worn at night, and walking is encouraged to help strengthen the muscles. It is important for the feet to be observed throughout childhood since there is frequently a tendency for recurrence, which demands prompt attention.

Surgical intervention is sometimes required for children with recurrent deformity or in cases that are resistant to more conservative measures. Surgery may be performed to correct bony deformity, to release tight ligaments, or to lengthen or transplant tendons. Again the extremity or extremities are casted until the desired result is achieved.

Nursing considerations

Nursing care of the child with nonsurgical correction of clubfoot is the same as it is for any child who has limited mobility and whose limbs are confined with casts or braces. The child will spend considerable time in a corrective device; therefore, nursing care plans include both long-term and short-term goals. Conscientious observation of skin and circulation is particularly important in young infants because of their normally rapid growth rate. Since treatment and follow-up care are carried out in the orthopedist's office, clinic, or outpatient department, parent education and support are important aspects in nursing care of these children. Parents need to understand the overall treatment program, the importance of regular cast changes, and the role they play in the long-term effectiveness of the therapy. Reinforcing and clarifying the orthopedist's explanations and instructions, teaching parents about care of a cast or appliance, including vigilant observation for potential problems, and encouraging parents to facilitate normal development within the limitations imposed by the deformity or therapy are all part of nursing responsibilities.

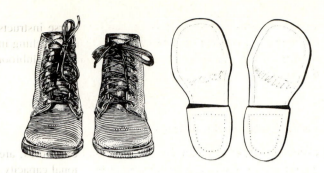

Fig. 28-17
Clubfoot shoes. The lateral side of the sole and heel of each shoe is raised to maintain correction of varus deformity, and the front half of each shoe is turned outward to maintain correction of forefoot adduction. (From Brashear, H.R., Jr., and Raney, R.B.: Shands' handbook of orthopaedic surgery, ed. 9, St. Louis, 1978, The C.V. Mosby Co.)

METATARSUS ADDUCTUS (VARUS)

Metatarsus adductus, or metatarsus varus, is probably the most common congenital foot deformity. In most instances it is the result of abnormal intrauterine positioning, and it is usually detected at birth. The deformity is characterized by medial adduction of the toes and forefoot, it is frequently associated with inversion, and there is a convexity of the lateral border of the foot. Unlike talipes equinovarus, with which it is often confused, the angulation occurs at the tarsometatarsal joint while the heel and ankle remain in a neutral position. This deformity is often responsible for a pigeon-toed gait in the young child.

The management depends on the rigidity of the deformity. Correction can usually be accomplished by gentle manipulation and passive stretching of the foot, which the parents are taught to perform. Repeated and consistent stretching is continued for the first 6 weeks, after which the treatment is based on the flexibility of the foot. Those feet that do not respond to the manipulation require orthopedic therapy. If the child is able to overcorrect the deformity voluntarily on stimulation, continued stretching is generally sufficient. If the foot cannot be overcorrected actively or passively, some type of passive corrective device is indicated. The device selected depends on the orthopedist and may involve reverse-shoes, a Denis Browne splint, or a series of casts followed by corrective shoes.

Nursing considerations

The primary nursing role is early identification of the defect and parent teaching. The nurse teaches the parents how to hold the heel firmly and to stretch only the forefoot. Otherwise, undue force on the heel may produce a valgus deformity. If casting is needed, the nurse instructs the parents in cast care and observation. Parent teaching in the use of other devices is the same as that for clubfoot deformities.

SKELETAL LIMB DEFICIENCY

Congenital limb deficiencies, or reduction deformities, are manifest by variable degrees of loss in functional capacity. They are characterized by underdevelopment of skeletal elements of the extremities. The range of defects can extend from minor defects of the digits to serious abnormalities such as *amelia,* absence of an entire extremity, or *meromelia,* partial absence of an extremity, including *phocomelia* (seal limbs), an intercalary deficiency of long bones with relatively good development of hands and feet attached at or near the shoulders or hips.

In rare instances prenatal destruction of limbs has been reported, but most reduction deformities are primary defects of development (agenesis, aplasia). Therefore, congenital amputations, in the literal sense, are not amputations since nonexistent limbs cannot be amputated.

Limb deficiencies are attributed to both heredity and environment and can originate at any stage of limb development. Formation of limbs may be suppressed at the time of limb bud formation, or there might be interference in later stages of differentiation and growth. Heredity appears to play a prominent role, and prenatal environmental insults have been implicated in a number of cases. The well-publicized thalidomide tragedy is a dramatic illustration of the effects of environmental interference with limb development. Children damaged by maternal ingestion of the drug displayed a variety of serious limb anomalies that demonstrated a clear relationship between the time of exposure and the presence and type of limb deformity.

Therapeutic management

It is generally agreed that children with congenital limb deficiencies should be fitted with prosthetic devices whenever possible and that such a functional replacement should be applied at the earliest possible stage of development in an attempt to match the motor readiness of the infant. This favors natural progression of prosthetic use. For example, an infant with an upper extremity deficiency is fitted with a simple passive device, such as a mitten prosthesis, between 3 and 6 months of age when limb exploration is active, sitting begins (with the extremities needed for support), and bilateral hand activities are encouraged.

Lower limb prostheses are applied when the infant is ready to pull himself to a standing position. Preparation for prosthetic devices often involves surgical modification

to assure the most favorable use of the device, especially if the deformity is severe. Phocomelic digits are preserved for controlling switches of externally powered appliances in upper extremities. Digits (in both upper and lower extremities) provide the child with surfaces for tactile exploration and stimulation. Prostheses are replaced to accommodate growth and increasing capabilities of the child.

Nursing considerations

Prosthetic application training and habilitation involve a team of health professionals including the parents, who must encourage the child in making age-commensurate adjustments to the environment. Although these children need assistance, excessive overprotection may produce overdependency with later maladjustment to school and other situations.

As in the case of any other congenital anomaly, parents need emotional support in their grieving process for the loss of the perfect child. Because of the visibility of a lost limb, these parents may have greater difficulty accepting the child. Psychologic care for these families is discussed in Chapter 16.

OSTEOGENESIS IMPERFECTA (OI)

Osteogenesis imperfecta is a rare hereditary disorder characterized by fractures, osteoporosis, and skeletal deformities. The disease may be apparent at birth or appear at variable ages, and it appears to be manifest in four different forms.

Osteogenesis imperfecta Type I. Type I, the most common variety, is inherited as an autosomal-dominant trait. The tendency to fracture appears at variable ages with a marked reduction in frequency of fractures after puberty. During childhood the shafts of the long bones are slender with reduced cortical thickness resulting from defective periosteal bone formation. Features associated with the disease are blue sclerae, thin skin, hyperextensibility of ligaments, and hypoplastic and deformed teeth; these children are prone to develop otosclerosis with hearing loss in adolescence and adulthood. Tendency to recurrent epistaxis, excess diaphoresis, easy bruising, and mild hyperpyrexia are also common manifestations. The disease shows variable expressivity, that is, the number and extent of pathologic features present in any individual range from severe to minimum involvement.

Osteogenesis imperfecta Type II. Type II is a rare and severe form of the disease believed to be the result of an autosomal-recessive gene. The disorder is apparent at birth and is characterized by multiple intrauterine or perinatal fractures with considerable deformity and early death. Approximately 50% of these children are stillborn.

Osteogenesis imperfecta Type III. Type III is manifest at birth or in early infancy with severe bone fragility and multiple fractures that produce progressive skeletal deformity. Sclerae may be blue at birth but become less so with age. The inheritance pattern is autosomal-recessive.

Osteogenesis imperfecta Type IV. Type IV is an autosomal-dominant disorder with variable age of onset from birth to adulthood. It is characterized by osteoporosis that leads to bone fragility, blue sclerae that become less blue with age, and spontaneous improvement with puberty.

Therapeutic management

The treatment for osteogenesis imperfecta is primarily supportive. Fractures are reduced and immobilized as any fracture, and internal fixation with metal rods and pins has proved effective in many instances. Medical therapies have been uniformly disappointing.

Nursing considerations

Infants and children with this disorder require careful handling to avoid fractures. Even activities such as feeding, bathing, changing a diaper, or taking vital signs may cause a fracture in severely affected infants. Turning by means of a blanket placed beneath the entire length of the child provides needed support without undue pressure or stretching. Diapers are changed by lifting the buttocks with a hand firmly supporting the pelvis, and feeding is accomplished easily with the infant in an infant seat (Guerrein, 1982).

Parental anxiety regarding handling such a fragile child creates numerous problems. They need guidance and support to overcome the fear of touching, holding, and providing other means for meeting both the parents' and child's need for close body contact. Nurses participate with parents in devising ways to protect the child with the use of pillows, blankets, and other devices as well as providing encouragement for their efforts to provide all types of sensory stimulation.

Both parents and the affected child need education regarding the child's limitations and guidelines in planning suitable activities that promote optimum development and socialization as well as protect him from harm. Realistic occupational planning and genetic counseling are part of the long-term goals of care. The Osteogenesis Imperfecta Foundation, Inc.* and The American Brittle Bone Society† provide information and support to families who have a child with this disorder.

---

*P.O. Box 838, Manchester, NH 03105.
†1256 Merrill Drive, Marshallton, West Chester, PA 19380.

ACQUIRED DEFECTS

There are a number of skeletal defects that are acquired during the childhood years. Most of these defects are age-related. Nurses caring for children in an ambulatory setting should be aware of the possibility of these correctable conditions and be alert to signs that indicate their presence so that corrective therapy can be implemented early.

COXA PLANA (LEGG-CALVÉ-PERTHES DISEASE)

Coxa plana or *osteochondritis deformans juvenilis*, more commonly known as Legg-Perthes or Legg-Calvé-Perthes disease, is a self-limited disorder in which aseptic necrosis of the femoral head produces hip deformation and dysfunction of varying degrees. The disease affects children 3 to 12 years of age, and most cases occur in males between 4 and 8 years of age as an isolated event. In approximately 10% to 15% of all cases the involvement is bilateral, and most of the affected children have a skeletal age significantly below their chronologic age. The male to female ratio is 4:1 or 5:1, and white children are affected 10 times more frequently than black children.

Pathophysiology

The cause of the disease is unknown, but there is a disturbance of the circulation to the femoral capital epiphysis that produces an ischemic aseptic necrosis of the femoral head. This circulatory impairment seems to extend to the epiphysis and acetabulum as well.

The pathologic events appear to take place in three stages, each usually consisting of 9 months to 1 year:

Initial or **avascular stage** there is aseptic necrosis of the femoral capital epiphysis with degenerative changes producing flattening of the upper surface of the femoral head

Fragmentation or **revascularization stage** revascularization takes place with fragmentation (vascular resorption of the epiphysis) that gives a mottled appearance on radiographs

Reparative or **regeneration stage** new bone forms with gradual reformation of the femoral head

The entire process may encompass as little as 18 months or it may continue for several years. The reformed femoral head may be severely altered or appear entirely normal.

Clinical manifestations

The child usually complains of persistent pain that may be accompanied by joint dysfunction with limp and limitation of motion and may or may not have been preceded by trauma. The diagnosis is established by radiographic examination.

Therapeutic management

Since deformity occurs early in the disease process, the aim of treatment is to keep the head of the femur in the acetabulum and maintain a full range of motion. This can be accomplished by non–weight-bearing devices such as an abduction brace, leg casts, or a leather harness sling that prevents weight bearing on the affected limb; use of abduction-ambulation braces or casts after a period of bed rest and traction; or surgical reconstructive and containment procedures. Conservative therapy must be continued for 2 to 4 years, whereas surgical correction, although a

---

SUMMARY OF NURSING CARE OF THE CHILD WITH LEGG-CALVÉ-PERTHES DISEASE (coxa plana)

GOALS	RESPONSIBILITIES
Assist with diagnosis	Recognize signs and symptoms of disorder Refer suspected cases for medical evaluation Assist with radiographic examination
Avoid weight-bearing on affected hip	Instruct the child and parents regarding what constitutes non–weight-bearing, for example, no standing or kneeling on affected leg Supervise application and/or use of 　Non–weight-bearing devices 　Abduction brace 　Cast (see p. 944 for cast care) 　Harness sling 　Abduction-ambulation braces or casts
Maintain alignment of head of femur in acetabulum	Supervise use of above mechanisms Provide proper care of the child in traction (p. 952) Educate the child and parents regarding correct use of appliances and other elements of therapy
Maintain full range of motion in affected hip	Supervise active exercises as prescribed Carry out passive exercises as prescribed
Gain cooperation in therapy	Allow the child as much autonomy as possible in planning activities Help the child assume as much responsibility as feasible for orthopedic device Encourage the child to become involved in therapy Provide positive reinforcement for compliance
Assist with surgical correction of deformity	Prepare the child for surgical experience Provide postoperative care commensurate with the child's age
Facilitate growth and development	Encourage age-appropriate activities within limitations imposed by therapeutic measures Assist the child and family in selecting activities according to the child's age, interests, and physical limitations, for example 　Quiet games 　Hobby such as collections, model building, crafts, indoor gardening, etc. Encourage peer interaction Involve the child in planning activities and therapy
Maintain therapy	Assist the parents in coping with the child and his therapy Refer to appropriate health agencies as indicated by the parents' needs Enlist cooperation of school personnel
Maintain peer associations	Encourage interaction with peers Help the child to determine alternatives to weight-bearing activity, such as score keeping, sideline ''coach'' Help the child devise explanations for appliances and inability to participate actively with peers

relatively recent advance and subject to additional risks (such as anesthesia, infection, and blood transfusion), returns the child to normal activities in 3 to 4 months.

The disease is self-limited, but the ultimate outcome of therapy depends on early and efficient treatment and the age of onset of the disorder—the younger the child, the more complete the recovery appears to be. In most cases the prognosis is excellent.

Nursing considerations

Nursing care of the child with coxa plana depends on the therapy implemented. Care of the child in traction or in a cast is discussed elsewhere and the reader is referred to these for more definitive nursing interventions. Nurses are often the first health professionals to identify affected children and to refer them for medical evaluation. They are also persons on whom the child and his family can rely to help them to understand and adjust to the therapeutic measures.

One of the most difficult aspects associated with the disorder is coping with a normally active child who feels well but must remain relatively inactive. Suitable activities must be devised to meet the needs of the child in the process of developing a sense of initiative or industry. Activities that meet his creative urges are well received, and this is an opportune time to encourage the child to begin a hobby such as collections, model building, or crafts. It is especially important that relationships with peers are maintained and encouraged.

SLIPPED FEMORAL CAPITAL EPIPHYSIS

Slipped femoral capital epiphysis, or *coxa vara*, refers to the spontaneous displacement of the proximal femoral epiphysis in a posterior and inferior direction. It develops most frequently shortly before or during accelerated growth and the onset of puberty (children between the ages of 10 and 16 years—median age, 13 years for boys, 11 years for girls) and occurs most often in ''overlarge'' youngsters or very tall, thin, rapidly growing children. Bilateral involvement has been reported variously as 16% to 40%. The cause is unknown.

Pathophysiology

The pathologic processes as seen on radiographs involves first a rarefication of bone on the lower femoral side of the epiphysis with widening of the growth plate. After trauma or slight injury the femoral portion of the epiphysis slides upward. As slipping increases, the epiphyseal displacement becomes posterior and inferior.

The following different varieties of clinical behavior have been observed: (1) an episode of trauma in which the epiphysis is acutely displaced in a previously functional joint; (2) gradual displacement without definite injury with progressively increased hip disability; (3) intermittent bouts of displacement alternating with periods of well-being with gradual appearance of symptoms associated with ambulation (such as external rotation); and (4) a combined gradual and traumatic displacement, in which there is gradual slippage with further displacement caused by injury.

Clinical manifestations

Slipped femoral epiphysis is suspected when an adolescent or preadolescent youngster, especially one who is obese or tall and lanky, begins to limp and complains of pain in the hip continuously or intermittently. The pain is frequently referred to the groin, anteromedial aspect of the thigh, or knee. Physical examination reveals early restriction of internal rotation on adduction and external rotation deformity with loss of abduction and internal rotation as the severity increases. The diagnosis is confirmed by radiographic examination.

Therapeutic management

The treatment varies with the degree of displacement but involves surgical stabilization and correction of deformity. In mild cases simple pin fixation is sufficient. More extensive displacement requires skeletal traction followed by pin fixation or osteotomy. Weight bearing is prohibited and traction may be necessary before surgery to relieve muscle spasms and correct any external rotation contractures that have developed. The prognosis depends on the degree of deformity and on whether or not complications, such as avascular necrosis and cartilaginous necrosis, affect the progress. As in other disorders, early diagnosis and implementation of therapy increase the likelihood of a satisfactory cure.

Nursing considerations

Nursing care is the same as that for a child in a cast or a child in traction.

KYPHOSIS AND LORDOSIS

The spine, consisting of numerous segments, can acquire deformation curves of three types: kyphosis, lordosis, and scoliosis (Fig. 28-18). Kyphosis is an abnormally increased convex angulation in the curvature of the thoracic spine (Fig. 28-18, *B*). The most common form is ''postural'' kyphosis. Children are prone to exaggeration of a

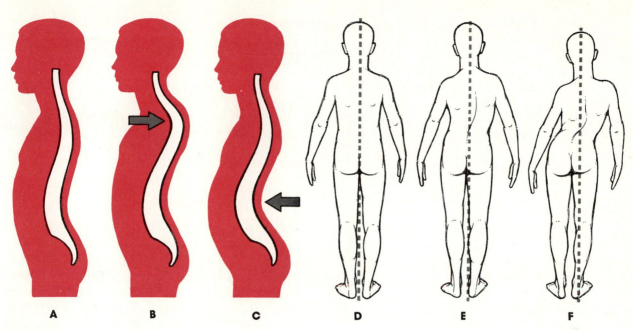

Fig. 28-18

Defects of the spinal column. **A,** *Normal spine.* **B,** *Kyphosis.* **C,** *Lordosis.* **D,** *Normal spine in balance.* **E,** *Mild scoliosis in balance.* **F,** *Severe scoliosis, not in balance.* **G,** *Rib hump and flank asymmetry seen in flexion due to rotary component. (Redrawn from Hilt, N.E., and Schmitt, E.W.: Pediatric orthopedic nursing, St. Louis, 1975, The C.V. Mosby Co.)*

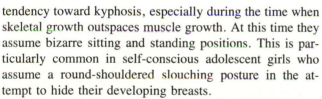

tendency toward kyphosis, especially during the time when skeletal growth outspaces muscle growth. At this time they assume bizarre sitting and standing positions. This is particularly common in self-conscious adolescent girls who assume a round-shouldered slouching posture in the attempt to hide their developing breasts.

Postural kyphosis is almost always accompanied by a compensatory postural lordosis, an abnormally exaggerated concave lumbar curvature (Fig. 28-18, *C*). Treatment consists of postural exercises to strengthen shoulder and abdominal muscles and bracing for more marked deformity. Unfortunately treatment is difficult because of the normal rebellious tendencies of the adolescent together with continual parental nagging to "stand up straight," which often interferes with compliance to a therapeutic regimen. The best approach is to emphasize the cosmetic value of corrective therapy and to place the responsibility on the adolescent for carrying out an exercise program at home with regular visits to and assessments by a therapist.

Most adolescents respond well to selected sports as a supplement to regular exercise. Boys prefer weight lifting (preferably performed from a prone or supine position on a bench) and track sports. Girls respond well to dance classes (ballet or modern dancing). Swimming is excellent for these children and has the added advantages of exercising for all muscles, eliminating gravity, and teaching breath control.

SCOLIOSIS

Scoliosis is a lateral curvature of the spine usually associated with a rotary deformity that eventually causes cosmetic and physiologic alterations in the spine, chest, and pelvis. Although it can appear at any age, it is seen most frequently in adolescent girls.

Scoliosis can be caused by a number of etiologic agents, and it may occur spontaneously or in association with other diseases or deformities. When the curve is flexible and corrects by bending, it is called a "nonstructural" curve. When the curve fails to straighten on side-bending, it is termed a "structural" curve and is characterized by changes in the spine and its supporting structures.

Nonstructural scoliosis may be postural with a slight curve that disappears when the child lies down, or a curve that maintains balance when there is a leg-length discrepancy. A transient scoliosis may be produced by pressure on a nerve root or inflammation. Structural scoliosis, on the other hand, is characterized by loss of flexibility and noncorrectable deformity. The cause in 70% of cases is "idiopathic" (without apparent cause); however, evidence indicates that it is probably genetic (transmitted as an autosomal-dominant trait with incomplete penetrance). Early

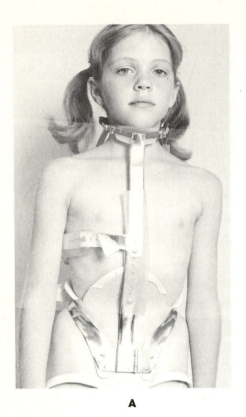
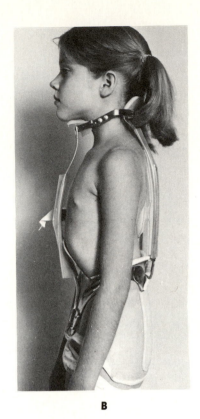
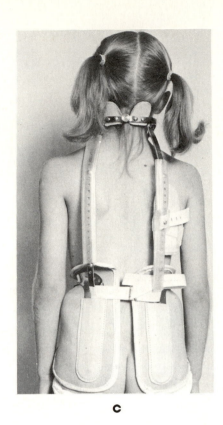

A   B   C

Fig. 28-19
Milwaukee brace. **A,** *Front view.* **B,** *Side view.* **C,** *Rear view. (From the clinical material of Dr. Walter P. Blount, Milwaukee, Wis.)*

detection and treatment are essential to successful management.

Clinical manifestations and diagnosis

There is rarely discomfort with scoliosis, and there are few outward signs until the deformity is well established. Viewing the undressed child from the posterior side will often reveal primary curvature and a compensatory curvature that places the head in alignment with the gluteal fold (Fig. 28-18, *E*). In uncompensated scoliosis the head and hips are not in alignment (Fig. 28-18, *F*). In advanced cases with rotary deformity, rib hump and flank asymmetry are observed when the child bends from the waist unsupported with the arms (Fig. 28-18, *G*). Radiographic films taken in the standing position establish the state of deformity.

Therapeutic management

A thorough examination, history, and assessment of the child are carried out in order to evaluate the status of the deformity, factors contributing to the defect, and factors that may influence the outcome of therapy. Treatment is best undertaken in a center in which a team is available that specializes in management of scoliosis. Cur-

rent management involves straightening and realignment of the vertebrae by either external or internal fixation techniques.

Bracing and exercise. Exercises can often help postural scoliosis but are rarely of value with structural defects. Nonoperative treatment by application of a properly constructed and well-fitted external bracing device and close supervision are successful in halting the progression of most curvatures. The most commonly used device is the Milwaukee brace, an individually adapted steel and leather brace that extends from a chin cup and neck pads to the pelvis, where lumbar pads rest on the hips (Fig. 28-19). The brace is used for minimum curvatures and is worn 23 hours a day and offers little interference with normal activity. Supplemental exercises are employed daily both in and out of the brace. The brace is adjusted at regular trimonthly intervals and, when radiographic examinations reveal bone maturity, the child is gradually weaned from the brace over a 1- to 2-year period. The brace is then worn only at night until the spine is absolutely mature.

Electrical stimulation. A newer approach to nonsurgical correction is surface electrical stimulation, which uses the child's muscle contractions to alter spinal configuration. It involves a pulse generator that evokes muscle contractions, approximately 5 per hour, in much the same manner as a cardiac or phrenic nerve pacemaker. Used primarily during sleep, this method is expected to replace the need for 24-hour bracing.

Surgery. For many curvatures surgical intervention is needed. Spinal fusion techniques followed by casting for a period of 6 months to a year produce satisfactory results. The surgical techniques for internal vertebral fixation are: (1) implantation of metal (Harrington) rods by way of clips to hold the vertebrae and bone fragments for permanent fusion; (2) a titanium cable through cannulated screws transfixed to each vertebra (Dwyer instrumentation); or (3) a flexible metal rod fixed by wires to the bases of the spinous processes (Luque segmental instrumentation).

For the most severe scoliotic curvatures, traction devices are employed for a time prior to spinal fusion. The traction is applied to the spine by way of a metal ring, or halo, attached to the skull and pins inserted into either the distal femur or the iliac wings of the pelvis. With halo-femoral traction and following Harrington rod instrumentation, the child is placed on a special Stryker frame and traction is applied by weight. Halo-pelvic traction is applied by means of turnbuckles, and the child can remain ambulatory. After traction a spinal fusion is performed and an immobilizing plaster jacket is applied from occiput to pelvis, which is worn for 8 months to 1 year.

Nursing considerations

Treatment for scoliosis extends over a significant portion of the affected child's period of growth. In adolescents this period is the one in which their physical and psychologic identity is formed. For some youngsters much of this time is spent in the hospital sitting immobilized in complex, unattractive appliances. For those treated on an outpatient basis it means a modified life-style and being "different" from their peers, even though they are usually able to engage in many activities enjoyed by other youngsters.

When the child first faces the prospect of a prolonged period in a brace, cast, or other device, the therapy program and the nature of the device must be explained thoroughly to the child and parents so that they will have an understanding of the anticipated results, how the appliance corrects the defect, the freedoms and constraints imposed by the device, and what they can do to help achieve the desired goal. The management involves the skills and services of a team of specialists, including the orthopedist, physical therapist, orthotist (a specialist in fitting orthopedic braces), nurse, social worker, and sometimes pulmonary specialists. The services of two organizations are available that provide information and education for families and health professionals: The National Scoliosis Foundation* and The Scoliosis Research Society.† The latter publishes a useful booklet for patients and families, "Sco-

liosis: A Handbook for Patients," which can be obtained by sending $1.00 to the organization. The Scoliosis Association,* a national self-help group, has a number of chapters throughout the country.

It is difficult for a child to be restricted at any phase of development, but especially for the teenager who needs continual positive reinforcement, encouragement, and as much independence as can be safely assumed during this time. Socialization with peers is encouraged, and every effort is expended to help the adolescent feel attractive and worthwhile.

Nursing care following surgical procedures involves preparing the child and family for the postoperative period on the Stryker frame. Postoperative discomfort, urinary retention, and the hazards of immobility are the major physical problems encountered. A Foley catheter is usually inserted for a day or two after surgery, appropriate analgesics are prescribed for pain, and the patient is placed on a Stryker frame to allow for frequent turning, which maintains spinal stability and reduces the discomfort associated with position changes. Special attention is directed toward skin care, especially the bony prominences. The patient is removed from the Stryker frame in 7 to 10 days, placed in a body cast, and then discharged.

INFECTIONS OF BONES AND JOINTS

Like other body tissues, bones, joints, and accessory structures are subject to infection and, because of their inaccessibility, are often difficult to treat. Because they are rigid structures, the inflammatory process is extremely painful. Early detection and therapy significantly shorten the term of treatment and reduce the degree of deformity and disability that often results from infections of these tissues.

OSTEOMYELITIS

Osteomyelitis is an infectious process of bone that can occur at any age but that occurs most frequently between 5 and 14 years of age. It is twice as common in boys as in girls.

Pathophysiology

Osteomyelitis can be acquired from *exogenous* or *hematogenous* sources. Exogenous osteomyelitis is acquired by direct invasion of the bone by direct extension from the outside as a result of a penetrating wound, open fracture, contamination during surgery, or secondary extension from

---

*48 Stone Road, Belmont, MA 02178.
†444 North Michigan Avenue, Chicago, IL 60611.

*1 Penn Plaza, New York, NY 10119.

SUMMARY OF NURSING CARE OF THE ADOLESCENT WITH MILD STRUCTURAL SCOLIOSIS

GOALS	RESPONSIBILITIES

Recognize deformity	Check spine alignment as part of the child's assessment
	Be alert to comments by the child or parent that indicate possible problems such as
	    Clothes do not fit right
	    Skirt hems are uneven
	    One hip seems higher than other
	Recommend screening for other family members

Assist in medical evaluation	Encourage the child and parents to seek medical evaluation Refer to the family physician and/or specialized services Determine if referrals were used

Prepare for application of brace	Reinforce and clarify explanations provided by orthopedist—explanations of
	    Appliance
	    Plan of care
	    Activities allowed/restricted
	    The child's and parents' responsibilities in therapy

Provide for supportive services	Refer to social services and/or Special Child Health Services for financial assistance, transportation, and so on, if needed
Assist in physical adjustment to appliance	Assess brace and its fit Attempt to determine source of any discomfort Refer to orthotist for needed adjustment and service Examine skin surfaces in contact with braces for signs of irritation; implement corrective action to treat or prevent skin breakdown Assist with plan for personal hygiene Help in selection of appropriate wearing apparel to wear over brace and footwear to maintain proper balance Reinforce teaching regarding removal and reapplication of appliance Investigate any complaints of discomfort
Help the child adjust to restricted movement	Demonstrate alternative modes of accomplishing tasks such as getting in and out of bed, dressing Help devise alternatives for restricted activities and coping with awkwardness
Prevent injury	Assess environment for hazards Teach safety precautions such as using hand rail on stairways, avoiding slippery surfaces, and so on Help develop safe methods of mobilization
Encourage compliance to regimen	Establish communication with the child and family Assess understanding of plan of care Instruct the child and family in various aspects of therapy and care as needed Provide feedback and praise for positive behavior Provide assistance and encouragement when needed Arrange appointments Assist family with transportation to appointments Identify goals with achievable outcomes Include family in setting goals Allow child and family to express discouragement at what appears to be slow progress and interference with activities
Support normal growth and development	Encourage independence where appropriate Allow for dependence when needed Involve in scheduling appointments and other aspects of care Encourage school attendance and socialization with peers Encourage involvement in activities compatible with limitations
Help the child develop positive self-image	Accentuate positive aspects of appearance Motivate to good habits of personal hygiene Encourage the child to wear attractive clothes and hairstyle Emphasize positive long-term outcome Help devise positive ways to deal with reactions of others

an overlying abscess or burn. Hematogenous spread of organisms from a preexisting focus is the most common source of infection. Frequent infectious foci include furuncles, skin abrasions, impetigo, upper respiratory tract infections, acute otitis media, tonsillitis, abscessed teeth, pyelonephritis, or infected burns.

Any organism can cause osteomyelitis, and there is some relationship between the age of the child and the type of organism responsible. In older children staphylococci are the most common organisms, approximately 80% of which are *Staphylococcus aureus;* in younger children other organisms predominate, especially *Haemophilus influenzae*. In children with sickle cell anemia, *Salmonella* organisms are frequently the responsible agents. Other factors that predispose to development of osteomyelitis are poor physical condition, inadequate nutrition, and surroundings that are not hygienic.

Infective emboli from the focus of infection travel to the small end arteries in the bone metaphysis, where they set up an infectious process that leads to local bone destruction and abscess formation.

Clinical manifestations

The signs and symptoms of *acute* hematogenous osteomyelitis begin abruptly and build to a maximum intensity during the first few days of the disease, usually in less than 1 week. There is frequently a history of trauma to the affected bone.

The child with acute osteomyelitis appears very ill. He is irritable and restless with elevated temperature, rapid pulse, and dehydration. There is usually localized tenderness, increased warmth, and diffuse swelling over the involved bone. The extremity is painful, especially on movement. The child holds it in semiflexion, and the surrounding muscles are tense and resist passive movement. Most cases involve the femur or tibia and to a lesser extent the humerus and hip. In infants the diagnosis is more difficult because of lack of systemic symptoms and may involve multiple bones or joints because of the difficulty in confining an infectious process in children in this age-group.

In *subacute* hematogenous osteomyelitis, symptoms have been present for a longer period of time, and the child sometimes has been treated with antibiotics, often for another infection, which modifies the clinical symptoms. In some instances the infection may produce a walled-off abscess rather than a spreading infection.

Diagnostic evaluation

In acute osteomyelitis there is marked leukocytosis and an elevated erythrocyte sedimentation rate. Blood culture is usually positive during the early stage, and radiographic findings are often negative or show only soft tissue swelling for 10 to 14 days. After this time the radiographic findings reveal new bone formation. Tomography may reveal bone changes at an early stage.

Similar symptoms are observed in rheumatic fever, rheumatoid arthritis, leukemia and other malignant lesions, cellulitis, erysipelas, and scurvy. Osteomyelitis may be unrecognized if it occurs as a complication of a severe toxic and debilitating illness.

Therapeutic management

As soon as blood cultures have been drawn, prompt and vigorous intravenous antibiotic therapy is initiated. The choice of antibiotic is influenced by age, and the dosage determined is sufficient to ensure high blood and tissue levels. Since most cases of osteomyelitis in the pediatric age group are caused by staphylococci, large doses of penicillin G are administered and supplemented by other antibiotics. In children younger than 3 years of age, the infectious agents are more likely to be penicillin-resistant staphylococci or gram-negative organisms; therefore, the agents of choice are usually methicillin, nafcillin, or clindamycin in conjunction with ampicillin. Neonates in whom coliform organisms are likely to be involved are given kanamycin or gentamicin, either intramuscularly or *slowly* by the intravenous route in addition to intravenously administered ampicillin.

Antibiotic therapy is accompanied by local treatment. The child is placed on complete bed rest. Immobilization of the affected extremity with a splint or bivalved cast is continued throughout therapy to limit the spread of infection and, when it is a complication of a fracture, to maintain alignment of bone fragments.

Opinions differ regarding surgical intervention, but many advocate sequestrectomy (removal of dead bone) and surgical drainage to prevent abscess formation. When surgical drainage is carried out, polyethylene tubes are placed in the wound—one tube instills an antibiotic solution directly into the infected area by gravity, and the other, connected to a suction apparatus, provides drainage.

Nursing considerations

During the acute phase of illness any movement of the affected limb will cause discomfort to the child; therefore, he should be positioned comfortably with the affected limb supported. Moving and turning are carried out carefully and gently to minimize discomfort. The child may require pain medication or sedation. Vital signs are taken and recorded frequently, and measures are implemented to reduce a significant temperature elevation.

Antibiotic therapy requires careful observation and monitoring of the intravenous equipment and site. Since more than one antibiotic is usually administered, the compatibility of the drugs is determined and care is taken to

SUMMARY OF NURSING CARE OF THE CHILD WITH OSTEOMYELITIS

GOALS	RESPONSIBILITIES
Assist with diagnosis	Recognize symptoms that could indicate osteomyelitis Obtain specimens as needed Order radiographs

Facilitate wound healing	Administer antibiotics as prescribed
	Care for wound
	    Assess area for swelling, heat, tenderness
	    Note and record amount and type of drainage, if any
	    Maintain asepsis
	    Clean area as ordered including irrigation if prescribed
	    Apply appropriate medication, wound packing, etc., as ordered
	    Dress wound according to instructions
	Maintain immobilization with positioning, devices such as casts, splints, traction
	Perform wound irrigations as prescribed

Prepare for surgical procedure (if prescribed)	See preparation for surgery (p. 585)

Maintain intravenous infusion	Monitor rate, amount, and type of intravenous solution
	Assess integrity of infusion site
	Ascertain compatibility of drugs administered (if more than one)
	    Use appropriate method to prevent mixing of incompatible drugs, such as piggyback set-up, adequate rinsing of tubing
	If heparin-lock mechanism used, maintain integrity and sterility
	    Secure properly

Relieve discomfort	Position for comfort Assess immobilization for fit and application Administer analgesics as appropriate
Reduce temperature	Apply appropriate temperature-reducing techniques for disseminating heat Administer antipyretic drugs as ordered
Facilitate growth and development	Provide diversional activities appropriate to the child's condition, physical limitations, and developmental level Involve the child in planning his care to the extent of his capabilities Arrange for and encourage interaction with others as feasible
Prepare for discharge	Instruct the parents regarding administration of oral medications Instruct the parents how to change dressings as indicated
Arrange for follow-up care	Make clinic appointment Refer to public health nurse

avoid mixing noncompatible drugs. A double, or piggy-back, setup is safest because there is less opportunity for the two drugs to come in contact with each other. The stability of the drugs, especially ampicillin, is also considered when determining the rate of administration.

The child with an opened wound is placed on complete or wound isolation precautions, depending on the policies of the institution. The wound is managed as prescribed. Antibiotic solution administered directly into the wound is most efficiently accomplished with a regular intravenous infusion setup that is prepared and regulated as any other. The drainage tubes are connected to low Gomco or wall suction for continuous removal. Intake and output are measured and recorded, and the character of the wound drainage is noted. The amount and character of drainage on the wound dressing are also noted.

Casts are sometimes employed for immobilization, and, if so, routine cast care is carried out. The extremity is examined for sensation, circulation, and pain, and the area over the inflammation is usually left open for observation. The affected area, casted or uncasted, is assessed for color, swelling, heat, and tenderness.

The child usually has a poor appetite at first, and he may be subject to vomiting. Nourishment in the form of high-calorie liquids such as fruit juices, gelatin, and juice bars should be encouraged until the child begins to feel better. The appetite returns as the acute symptoms subside. During convalescence adequate nutrition must be maintained to aid healing and reconstitution of new bone.

When the acute stage subsides, the child begins to feel better, his appetite improves, and he becomes interested in his surroundings and relationships. He wishes to move about in bed and is allowed to do so. However, weight bearing on the affected limb is not permitted until healing is well under way in order to avoid pathologic fractures. Diversional and constructive activities become important nursing interventions. The child is usually confined to bed for some time after the acute phase but may be allowed about the unit on a gurney or in a wheelchair when isolation and bed rest are no longer necessary. At this stage the continuous intravenous infusion may be replaced by a heparin lock to allow greater freedom.

As the infection subsides, physical therapy is instituted to ensure restoration of optimum function. The child is usually discharged with oral antibiotics, and his progress is followed closely for some time.

SEPTIC (SUPPURATIVE, PYOGENIC, PURULENT) ARTHRITIS

The source of infection of the joints, like infection of bone, is usually by hematogenous dissemination and spread from another focus. Occasionally it results from direct extension of a soft tissue infection. The infection occurs predominantly in males, especially in the adolescent age-group. In infancy the age distribution is more nearly equal. Any joint may be involved, but the hip, knee, shoulder, and other large joints are more commonly affected. It usually affects only one joint.

The signs and symptoms of suppurative arthritis, unlike osteomyelitis, are usually characteristic. The presence of a warm and tender joint that is painful on even gentle pressure is sufficient to differentiate it from osteomyelitis, in which gentle passive motion is tolerated. When superficial joints are involved they are exquisitely painful and swollen; deep-seated joints show little superficial evidence. In most instances there is history of a traumatic injury to the affected joint. Fever, leukocytosis, and increased erythrocyte sedimentation rate are present but may not be demonstrated in affected infants.

The most common pathogens are *Staphylococcus aureus,* group A streptococci, and *Haemophilus influenzae.* Diagnosis is made from blood culture, joint fluid aspirate, and radiographs.

Treatment consists of open surgical drainage of hip and shoulder joint disease and repeated needle aspirations of the joint space in other joints. The goals are (1) to clean the joint to avoid destruction of articular cartilage, (2) to decompress the joint to avoid interference with the blood supply to the epiphysis, (3) to eradicate the infection with adequate antibiotic therapy, and (4) to prevent secondary bone infection and hematogenous spread. Therapy is similar to that for osteomyelitis: intravenous antibiotic therapy, relief of pain, immobilization of the joint, and prohibition of weight bearing until healing is complete. Nursing care is the same as that for osteomyelitis.

TUBERCULOSIS

Tubercular infection of the bones is acquired by hematogenous dissemination from a primary tubercular focus. The most common sites in infants and small children are the carpals and phalanges and the corresponding bones of the feet. A single bone or several bones may be involved with spindle-shaped swelling and tenderness as soft tissues are affected. The process, relatively painless, persists with intermittent symptoms for several months and may leave a permanent deformity. The affected areas are immobilized with a splint or cast.

Tuberculosis of spine (Pott disease)

In older children the infection attacks the body of one or more vertebrae, destroying the bone, and spreads to all the articular tissues, producing a kyphotic deformity. The lower thoracic spine is most frequently affected. Symptoms are insidious. The child will be irritable and complain of persistent or intermittent pain over the areas innervated by spinal nerves that arise adjacent to the affected vertebrae. There is muscle splinting and pain when there is increased pressure on his head. The child assumes a position that best eases the weight on the diseased vertebrae, such as avoiding bending, walking stiffly and carefully on the toes, and resting on the abdomen or across a chair or a lap.

Treatment consists of immobilization with extension on a Bradford frame until there is no evidence of active infection followed by spinal fusion. Antimicrobial therapy and drainage of tubercular abscess are standard therapies.

The reparative process is slow, but, in most instances, recovery takes place with little or no deformity.

Tuberculosis of hip

The hip is the most common joint affected by tuberculosis, but the process usually begins in the epiphysis of the femoral head and then erupts into the joint capsule. The initial manifestation is a limp that occurs intermittently, most often on arising in the morning or after exercise. There is progressive destruction of the femoral head with symptoms of pain, and the thigh gradually becomes fixed and adducted with internal rotation. There may be swelling around the hip and abscess formation.

Treatment involves bed rest, traction to reduce muscle spasm, and appropriate drug therapy. Hip fusion may be necessary in severe cases.

BONE TUMORS

Malignant bone tumors represent less than 1% of all malignant neoplasms but are more frequent in children than adults. The peak ages during childhood are 15 to 19 years. The sexes are affected equally until puberty, at which time the ratio approaches 2:1 in favor of males.

Neoplastic disease can arise from any tissues involved in bone growth, such as osteoid matrix, bone marrow elements, fat, blood and lymph vessels, nerve sheath, and cartilage. The basic classifications are spindle-cell sarcoma (osteosarcoma or osteogenic sarcoma) and small-cell sarcoma (Ewing sarcoma). In children these two types account for 85% of all primary malignant bone tumors and the manifestations and diagnosis are similar in both.

Clinical manifestations

Most malignant bone tumors produce severe or dull localized pain in the affected site. In most cases this pain is attributed to trauma or to the vague complaint of ''growing pains.'' The pain is often relieved by a flexed position, which relaxes the muscles overlying the stretched periosteum. The condition is brought to the attention of others when the child limps, curtails his own physical activity, or is unable to hold heavy objects.

Diagnostic evaluation

Diagnosis begins with a thorough history and physical examination in order to rule out causes such as trauma or infection. Careful questioning regarding pain is essential in attempting to determine the duration and rate of tumor growth. Physical assessment focuses on functional status of the affected area, signs of inflammation, size of the mass, involvement of regional lymph nodes, and any systemic indication of generalized malignancy, such as anemia, weight loss, and frequent infection.

A definitive diagnosis is established by radiographic or tomographic studies that determine the extent of the lesion, radioisotope bone scans that evaluate metastasis, and a bone biopsy that determines the type of tumor. Bone marrow aspiration is helpful in diagnosing Ewing sarcoma. Radiographic findings are also characteristic for each type of tumor.

Several tests may be performed for differential diagnosis of secondary bone metastasis from Wilms tumor, neuroblastoma, retinoblastoma, rhabdomyosarcoma, lymphoma, or leukemia. Lung tomography is usually a standard procedure, since pulmonary metastasis is the most common complication of primary bone tumors.

Prognosis

Children with nonmetastastic Ewing sarcoma who are given intensive radiotherapy and chemotherapy have an 80% chance of cure. Those with osteosarcoma arising from the small bones of the hands and feet, where radical amputation is most easily accomplished, have a better than 50% chance of 5-year survival. However, tumors closer to the trunk carry poorer prognoses, especially if metastasis occurs.

OSTEOSARCOMA

Osteosarcoma is the most frequently encountered malignant bone cancer in children; its peak incidence is between 10 and 25 years of age. Most primary tumor sites are in the diaphysis (shaft) of long bones, especially in the lower extremities. Over half occur in the femur, particularly in the distal portion; the remainder involve the humerus, tibia, pelvis, jaw, and phalanges.

Therapeutic management

Aggressive treatment is mandatory and consists of radical surgical ablation followed by intensive chemotherapy. Depending on the tumor site, surgery involves amputation of the affected extremity at least 7.5 cm (3 inches) above the proximal tumor margin or above the joint proximal to the involved bone. With tumors of the distal femur, preservation of the hip joint may be possible. Other procedures include an above-the-knee amputation for tumors of the tibia or fibula, a hemipelvectomy for tumors of the innominate (hip) bone, and a forequarter amputation (removal of arm, scapula, and portion of the clavicle on the affected side) for tumors of the upper humerus.

Chemotherapy is implemented following surgery and, although the period of treatment varies according to institutions, many centers advocate adjuvant chemotherapy for 2 years in nonmetastatic osteosarcoma and for 3 years when metastasis is present.

An alternative approach is intensive preoperative chemotherapy followed by an en bloc resection of the primary tumor with prosthetic replacement of the involved bone. For example, osteosarcoma of the distal femur requires total femur and joint replacement. After surgery adjuvant chemotherapy is continued for approximately 1 year. At present, long-term survival rates to determine limb function and disease-free status are encouraging.

Nursing considerations

The main nursing consideration is preparation of the child and family for an amputation. Straightforward honesty is essential in gaining the cooperation and trust of the child. The diagnosis of cancer should not be disguised with falsehoods such as "infection." For the child to gradually accept the need for an amputation, he must be aware that there is no alternative treatment. Conservative surgery offers virtually no hope for a cure. He should also know if the operation will follow the biopsy procedure immediately. Informing him that just a biopsy will be performed in the hope of sparing him anxiety over the operation only serves to weaken his trust once he becomes aware of the deception.

The physician has the responsibility of telling the child about the surgery. Ideally the nurse should be present at the discussion or be made aware of precisely what is told to the child. The child should be told a few days before surgery to allow him time to adjust to the diagnosis, to think about the consequent treatment, and to ask questions.

Sometimes children have many questions about the prosthesis, limitations on physical ability, and prognosis in terms of cure. At other times they react with silence or impassivity that belies their concern and fear. Either response is accepted as a part of the grieving process that follows any loss. For those who wish information, it may be helpful to introduce them to another amputee prior to surgery or to show them pictures of the prosthesis. However, the nurse must be careful not to overwhelm them with information.

A sound approach involves answering their questions without offering additional information. For those who do not pursue the discussion, the nurse expresses a willingness to pursue the topic with such expressions as, "Anytime you would like to talk or ask questions about the surgery, tell me." The subject should not be broached unless the child initiates the conversation. Si-

lence does not always mean nonacceptance.

The child is also informed of the need for chemotherapy. Although it is well to introduce this subject prior to surgery, since treatment begins as soon as possible postoperatively, caution is exercised to avoid offering too much information at one time. A discussion of hair loss should emphasize the positive aspects, such as wearing a wig. Since bone tumors affect adolescents and young adults, it is not unusual for them to become angry over all the radical body changes that drastically alter their developing sense of identity.

In most instances the child is fitted with a temporary prosthesis immediately after surgery. For a leg amputation the prosthesis consists of a rigid dressing pylon with a foot-ankle assembly, which permits early ambulation and helps to foster psychologic adjustment to a lost limb. A permanent prosthesis is usually fitted within 6 to 8 weeks. During hospitalization the child begins physical therapy to develop proficiency in the use and care of the device.

Discharge planning must begin early during the postoperative period. Once the child has begun physical therapy, the nurse consults with the therapist and physician to evaluate the child's physical and emotional readiness to reenter school. It is an opportune time to involve a community nurse in the home care of the child. Every effort is made to promote a normal and gradual resumption of realistic preamputation activities.

EWING SARCOMA

Ewing sarcoma arises in the marrow spaces of the bone rather than from osseous tissue. The principal sites of origin are the shafts of long bones and trunk bones. Most often affected are the femur, tibia, fibula, humerus, ulna, vertebra, scapula, ribs, pelvic bones, and skull. The tumor occurs almost exclusively in individuals under age 30 years—the majority between 4 and 25 years of age.

Therapeutic management

Surgical tumor excision and/or amputation have not demonstrated improved survival rates. The treatment of choice is intensive irradiation of the involved bone, usually for a period of 6 to 8 weeks, combined with chemotherapy for a period of 2 years. A widely used drug regimen includes vincristine, actinomycin D, and cyclophosphamide (this regimen is often referred to as VAC).

Investigational therapeutic approaches include totalbody irradiation to destroy widespread foci of disease and immunotherapy to control and/or prevent metastasis. However, at the present time these techniques represent ancillary, not primary, modes of therapy.

SUMMARY OF NURSING CARE OF THE CHILD WITH A BONE TUMOR

GOALS	RESPONSIBILITIES

General
Recognize bone tumor early
	Be alert to signs and symptoms that might indicate bone tumor
	Obtain thorough history
	Carry out thorough physical assessment, especially regarding affected area, including
	    Functional status
	    Signs of inflammation
	    Size of mass
	    Regional lymph node involvement
	Assist with diagnostic tests such as
	    Radiographs
	    Tomography of bone and lungs
	    Bone scan
	    Bone marrow aspiration
	Order and/or collect blood for analysis
	Prepare the child and family for surgical biopsy

Osteogenic sarcoma Prepare the child and family for probable amputation	Employ straightforward honesty Avoid disguising diagnosis with terms such as "infection" Emphasize lack of alternatives Answer questions regarding information presented by the surgeon and clarify any misconceptions Avoid overwhelming the child or parents with too much information Be available and willing to listen and to talk to the child and parents about their concerns Allow for and encourage expression of feelings
Begin preparation for supplemental therapies	Introduce, but do not elaborate on, information regarding need for chemotherapy Reserve extensive discussion of chemotherapy and rehabilitation until after surgery
Give postoperative care	Employ appropriate stump care according to limb involved Assist with early ambulation and use of temporary prosthesis Arrange for, carry out, or supervise physical therapy as prescribed Arrange for preparation of permanent prosthesis Teach use of auxiliary appliances such as wheelchair or crutches
Prepare for discharge	Arrange for and emphasize importance of maintaining physical therapy regimen Arrange for acquisition of needed supplies such as dressing, crutches, wheelchair in addition to prosthesis Teach stump care to the parents and child, if the child is old enough to assume some responsibility Assess home for environmental handicaps (such as stairs), accessibility of school, and so on Refer to agencies for aid and assist family to prepare environment
Prepare for effects of chemotherapy	Impress on the child importance of therapy Explain probable side effects of antimetabolites, such as nausea and hair loss

Nursing considerations

The psychologic adjustment to Ewing sarcoma is typically less traumatic than to osteosarcoma because the affected limb can be preserved. Many families accept the diagnosis with a sense of relief knowing that this type of bone cancer does not require amputation. However, they still need preparation for the various diagnostic tests, including bone marrow aspiration and surgical biopsy, and adequate explanation of the treatment regimen. High-dose radiotherapy often causes dry or moist skin desquamation followed by hyperpigmentation. Therefore, the child is advised to wear loose-fitting clothes over the irradiated area to decrease additional skin irritation. Because of increased sen-

SUMMARY OF NURSING CARE OF THE CHILD WITH A BONE TUMOR—cont'd

GOALS	RESPONSIBILITIES
Osteogenic sarcoma—cont'd	
Assist the child to adjust to disability	Encourage visits from friends before discharge to help prepare the child for reactions and questions of others
	Encourage early and consistent interaction with peers
	Assist the child to become adept in use of appliances
	Assist the child to select clothing to camouflage prosthesis
	Encourage good hygiene, grooming, and sex-appropriate items to enhance appearance, such as wig (for hair loss from antimetabolites), makeup, and attractive, sex-appropriate clothing
	Allow the child time and opportunity to go through grief process
	Allow for expression of feelings regarding the loss and the undesirable effects of chemotherapy
	Assist the child to cope with side effects
	Encourage independence
Support the parents	Allow the parents to express their feelings and concerns
	Interpret the child's emotional reactions, such as depression, expressions of anger, and hostility
	Answer questions regarding posthospital care
	Teach the parents skills and give information necessary for home care
	Encourage the parents to allow the child to live as normal a life as possible
	Refer to appropriate agencies and groups to facilitate care and adjustment such as the American Cancer Society, parent groups
	Maintain contact with the family
Ewing sarcoma	
Prepare the child and family for chemotherapy	Inform the parents and child of the side effects of antimetabolites and immunosuppressant drugs
	Suggest and/or implement measures to reduce physical and emotional impact
Prepare the child and family for radiotherapy	Explain procedure
	Remain with the child during the procedure
	Explain undesirable side effects of radiotherapy
	Suggest and/or implement measures to reduce physical effects of radiotherapy
	Select loose-fitting clothing over irradiated area to decrease additional irritation
	Protect area from sunlight and sudden changes in temperature (avoid ice packs, heating pads)
Support the child and family during therapy	Allow for expression of feelings
	Clarify misconceptions and provide technical information as needed
	Impress on both the child and family the need for continuing normal activities, interactions, and behaviors
	Refer to appropriate agencies and individuals as indicated by assessed needs of the child and family

sitivity, the area is protected from sunlight and sudden changes in temperature, such as from heating pads or ice packs. The child is encouraged to use the extremity as tolerated. An active exercise program may be planned by the physical therapist to preserve maximum function.

The child requires the same preparation for and support in adjusting to the effects of chemotherapy as any other cancer patient. The regimen usually causes hair loss, severe nausea and vomiting, peripheral neuropathy, and possibly cardiotoxicity. Every effort should be made to outline a treatment plan that allows the child maximum resumption of a normal life-style and activities.

DISORDERS OF THE JOINTS

Many disorders involving the joints have been discussed in relation to other problems of locomotion, for example sprains, dislocations, congenital hip dysplasia, and septic arthritis. This segment is primarily concerned with the inflammatory joint disease, juvenile rheumatoid arthritis, and one of the diseases with joint pain as a manifestation, lupus erythematosis.

JUVENILE RHEUMATOID ARTHRITIS (JRA)

Clinically and pathologically, juvenile rheumatoid arthritis is an inflammatory disease for which the inciting agent is not known. There are two peak ages of onset: between 2 and 5 years of age and between 9 and 12 years of age. Females are affected somewhat more frequently than males, and the incidence has been estimated variously as 1 in 1000, 1 in 5000, and 3 in 100,000. In many instances the disease remains undiagnosed for years.

Pathophysiology

The rheumatic process is characterized by a chronic inflammation of the synovium with joint effusion and eventual erosion, destruction, and fibrosis of the articular cartilage. Adhesions between joint surfaces and ankylosis of joints occur if the process persists long enough.

Clinical manifestations

Whether single or multiple joints are involved, stiffness, swelling, and loss of motion develop in the affected joints. They are swollen and warm to the touch but seldom red. The swelling results from edema, joint effusion, and synovial thickening. The affected joints may be tender and painful to the touch or relatively painless. The limited motion that occurs early in the disease is the result of muscle spasm and joint inflammation; it is later caused by ankylosis or soft tissue contracture. Morning stiffness or "gelling" of the joint(s) is characteristic and is seen when the child rises in the morning or after inactivity. Infections, injuries, or operations often precipitate a flare-up of the arthritis; therefore, prompt recognition and treatment of infections are necessary.

The onset of juvenile rheumatoid arthritis may be acute or gradual. In very small children there is frequently acute febrile onset, widespread systemic changes, and little joint involvement. In small children the onset tends to be severe and is more likely to involve many joints. In older children joint involvement is more often restricted to one or two large joints without significant systemic manifesta-

tions, and the course tends to be quiet and abates in the early teen years.

Juvenile rheumatoid arthritis is a variable disease and is now recognized to pursue at least three distinct disease courses: (1) systemic onset, (2) polyarticular onset, and (3) pauciarticular onset.

Systemic onset. General systemic involvement resembles the symptomatology seen in most childhood illness—low-grade fever frequently accompanied by a rash, anorexia, failure to gain weight, anemia, lymphadenopathy, myalgia, and generalized fatigue. Any joint may be involved, but arthritis may not be present initially. There are two ages of onset—1 to 3 years and 8 to 10 years.

Polyarticular onset. Polyarticular juvenile rheumatoid arthritis is characterized by multiple joint involvement, which may be accompanied by minimum systemic involvement. Any joint may be affected. Involvement is usually symmetric and frequently begins in large joints such as the knees, ankles, wrists, and elbows. Joints of fingers and toes become swollen and inflamed and assume a spindle, or fusiform, shape. Hip, cervical, and temporomandibular joint involvement is common. The onset of painful joint symptoms can be acute or gradual. A small number of children gradually develop a painless arthritis, usually morning stiffness, over a period of months or years without definable systemic manifestations.

Pauciarticular onset. Isolated arthritis is most commonly seen in the knee, ankle, hip, and eventually, the sacroiliac joint; sometimes the elbow is involved. Early onset disease appears in early childhood (under age 3 years), occurs predominantly in girls, and is frequently accompanied by chronic iridocyclitis (inflammation of the iris and ciliary body) and mucocutaneous lesions. A later onset disease (over 13 years) occurs predominantly in males and has a high incidence of spondylitis as a long-term complication, especially in boys positive for HLA-B27 (see p. 55).

Diagnostic evaluation

Radiographic findings are variable, but the earliest manifestations are widening joint spaces followed by gradual evidence of fusion and articular destruction.

There are no specific diagnostic tests for juvenile rheumatoid arthritis. The erythrocyte sedimentation rate may or may not be elevated, depending on the degree of inflammation present. Leukocytosis is generally present in the early stages of classic systemic disease. Latex fixation test, the most common test used to detect the presence of "rheumatoid factor" in adults, is seldom positive in juvenile rheumatoid arthritis. Antinuclear antibodies are present in many children with pauciarticular disease and may be present in those with polyarticular disease.

Therapeutic management

There is no specific cure for juvenile rheumatoid arthritis. The major goals of therapy are to preserve joint function, prevent physical deformities, and relieve symptoms without therapeutic harm. Whenever possible the child is treated at home under the supervision of the health team and intermittent treatment by qualified professionals is administered. Hospitalization may be needed during severe exacerbations or when intercurrent illness warrants. Iridocyclitis requires the attention of an ophthalmologist.

Drugs. Several drugs, including salicylates, corticosteroids, and gold salts, are effective in suppressing the inflammatory process and relieving pain. Acetylsalicylic acid (aspirin) is administered with each meal and at 10:00 or 11:00 PM. To avoid the acute gastritis and bleeding associated with large amounts of aspirin, especially when administered with daily corticosteroids, it may be given in an enteric-coated form or accompanied by an antacid.

Corticosteroids are administered in the lowest effective dose, given on alternate days rather than daily, and used for the shortest period of time possible. Indications for daily corticosteroid (prednisone) therapy are life-threatening disease (such as pericarditis), incapacitating systemic disease unresponsive to other antiinflammatory therapy, and iridocyclitis.

Gold salts, such as gold sodium thiomalate, are often useful in severe forms of the disease and indomethacin, approved for use in patients over 14 years of age, appears to be effective in those with lower limb ankylosing spondylitis. Although the action is unknown, antimalarial drugs such as hydroxychloroquine (Plaquenil) and chloroquine (Aralen) are also proving to be effective in relieving symptoms of arthritis.

Physical management. Programs of physical management are individualized for each child and designed to reach the ultimate goal—the preservation of function. Physical therapy is directed toward (1) specific joints, focusing on strengthening muscles, mobilizing restricted joint motion, and preventing or correcting deformities, and (2) generalized mobility and performance of activities of daily living. Normal activities of daily living and the child's natural tendencies to be active are usually sufficient to maintain muscle strength and joint mobility.

Exercising in a pool is excellent therapy, since it allows freedom of movement with support and minimum gravitational pull. When joints are inflamed, heavy resistance aggravates the pain, and, at these times, simple isometric or tensing exercises that do not involve joint movement are generally tolerated and should be encouraged. Range of motion exercises are an important aspect of therapy and are continued after evidence of disease has disappeared in order to detect any signs of recurrence.

Use of splints for these children is controversial, but most therapists recommend splinting and positioning dur-

ing rest to help minimize pain and prevent or reduce flexion deformity. Joints most frequently splinted are the knees, wrists, and hands. Positioning during rest is also important. The children rest on a firm mattress with no pillow or a very low one and have no support under the knee. Loss of extension in the knee, hip, and wrist causes special problems and requires vigilance to detect the earliest signs of involvement and vigorous attention to prevent deformity with specialized passive stretching, positioning, and resting splints.

Nursing considerations

The effects of this chronic illness are felt in every aspect of the child's life—in physical activities, social experiences, and personality development. Much of the child's adjustment to the stresses and demands of the disease and level of functioning he achieves is directly related to the reaction and support he receives from his family and the health professionals concerned with his care and management.

General health promotion. The general health of the child must be considered and is frequently overlooked as parents and health personnel concentrate on the disease. A well-balanced diet and assessment of nutritional status are integral parts of health supervision. Excessive fatigue and overexertion should be avoided with regular periods of rest, especially during acute flare-ups of arthritis. The child is susceptible to frequent upper respiratory infection, which should receive prompt treatment.

Posture and body mechanics are important for the child with juvenile rheumatoid arthritis, both when he is at rest and when he is active. He must have a firm mattress to maintain good alignment of spine, hips, and knees and no pillow or a very thin one. The child who is confined to bed either at home or in the hospital may require sandbags, splints, or other types of support to maintain positioning. Lying in the prone position is encouraged to straighten hips and knees, such as during rest periods or television viewing.

Heat and exercise. Heat has proved beneficial to children with arthritis. Moist heat is best for relieving pain and stiffness, and the most efficient and practical method for accomplishing this is to place the child in the bathtub. A daily whirlpool bath, paraffin bath, or hot packs may be used as needed for temporary relief of acute swelling and pain. Painful hands or feet can be immersed in a pan of water for 10 minutes two or three times daily in addition to tub baths.

Pool therapy is the easiest method for exercising a large number of joints. Swimming activities strengthen muscles and maintain mobility in larger joints. Most children have access to a therapy pool, although transportation may be a problem for some families. Very small children

SUMMARY OF NURSING CARE OF THE CHILD WITH JUVENILE RHEUMATOID ARTHRITIS

GOALS	RESPONSIBILITIES
Assist with diagnosis	Recognize signs and symptoms Assist with laboratory tests such as erythrocyte sedimentation rate, latex fixation test Assist with radiographic tests, joint aspiration
Reduce inflammation	Administer antiinflammatory drugs

Preserve joint function	Carry out or supervise physical therapy regimen
	   Muscle strengthening exercises
	   Joint mobilization exercises
	Incorporate therapeutic exercises in play activities, such as swimming, throwing a ball, hanging from a monkey bar, riding tricycle or bicycle
	Supervise and encourage activities of daily living
	Encourage the child's natural tendency to be active
	Apply splints or sandbags, if needed, to maintain position and reduce flexion deformity
	Maintain good body alignment during periods of rest
	   Lie flat in bed with joints extended
	   Use prone position frequently
	   Use no pillow or a very thin one

Promote general health	Assure well-balanced diet that does not produce excessive weight gain Avoid exposure to infections Schedule regular exercise program appropriate to the child's age, interests, and capabilities but avoid overexertion or fatigue Schedule regular periods for sleep and rest, especially during acute flareups Stress importance of regular ophthalmologic examination for early detection of possible eye complications Carry out frequent assessments for evidence of improvement, exacerbation, or complications, especially iridocyclitis (blurred vision, pain and/or redness in eye) Seek medical treatment promptly for upper respiratory (or other) infections
Reduce discomfort	Provide heat to painful joints by way of tub baths, including whirlpool, paraffin baths, warm moist packs, soaks Maintain schedule of drug administration Avoid overexercising painful, swollen joints

Carry out activities of daily living	Encourage maximum independence
	Provide and/or help devise methods to facilitate independent functioning
	   Select clothes for convenience in putting on and fastening
	   Modify utensils (such as spoons, toothbrush, comb) for easier grasp
	   Elevate toilet seat, if needed
	   Install handrails for convenience and safety (as in hallways, bathroom)
	Teach application of splints (when able) and encourage responsibility for their use

Help the child adjust to chronic illness	Plan schedule of activities that includes exercise and rest
	Promote independence
	Encourage regular school attendance
	   Enlist aid of school nurse regarding medication schedule and rest periods
	Discourage activities that increase isolation from others
	Explore the child's feelings regarding disability
	   Limitations
	   Stress of being "different"
	   Difficulty in competing
	   Relationships with peers
	   Self-image
	Help the child to learn about his disease and its therapies

SUMMARY OF NURSING CARE OF THE CHILD WITH JUVENILE RHEUMATOID ARTHRITIS—cont'd

GOALS	RESPONSIBILITIES
Provide parental education	Reinforce explanation of disease Instruct in administration of prescribed medications 　Assist to plan regular schedule of administration 　Instruct regarding special precautions of administration 　Instruct regarding signs of toxicity Educate regarding carrying out physical therapies Impress importance of compliance in medication and exercise
Support the parents	Explore attitude toward the child and his disease Allow for expression of feelings Be alert for cues that signal undue anxiety and guilt, such as 　Preoccupation with causative factors 　Constant analysis of effect of therapies 　Experimentation with diets and folk remedies 　Seeking magical cures Be alert for overprotective behaviors, such as 　Assuming self-care activities for the child 　Restricting the child's activities and interaction with peers Refer to parent support groups Refer to agencies that provide special services, such as Arthritis Foundation, Special Child Health Services

who are frightened of the water can carry out their exercises in the bathtub.

Activities of daily living provide satisfactory exercise for older children to maintain maximum mobility with minimum pain. They should be encouraged in their efforts and patiently allowed to dress and groom themselves, to assume daily tasks, and to care for their belongings. It is often difficult for stiff fingers to manipulate buttons, comb or brush hair, and turn faucets, but parents and other caregivers should refrain from assisting them. Also, the child should learn and understand why others do not help him. Many helpful devices, such as Velcro fasteners, tongs for manipulating difficult items, and grab bars installed in bathrooms for safety, can be employed to facilitate tasks. A raised toilet seat often makes the difference between dependent and independent toileting, since weak quadriceps muscles and sore knees inhibit the ability to raise the body form a low sitting position.

The child's natural affinity for play offers many opportunities for incorporating therapeutic exercises. Throwing or kicking a ball, hanging from monkey bars, and riding a tricycle (with the seat raised to achieve maximum leg extension) are excellent moving and stretching exercises for preschool children. These are especially important for the very young child whose activities of daily living are physically limited. Parents are instructed in exercises that are designed to fit the needs of the individual child.

The parents are instructed regarding administration of medications as well as the value of a regular schedule of

administration to maintain a satisfactory drug level in the body. They need to know that aspirin should not be given on an empty stomach and to be alert for signs of aspirin toxicity, which include hyperventilation as a sign of acidosis, bleeding from decreased clotting capacity, tinnitus (ringing in the ears) as a sign of cranial nerve VIII involvement, and undue drowsiness that may indicate central nervous system depression.

The Arthritis Foundation* provides services for both parents and professionals, and nurses should refer families to this agency as an added resource. Health professionals can obtain up-to-date information regarding materials and programs from the Arthritis Information Clearinghouse.†

The child. Rheumatoid arthritis affects every aspect of the child's daily life. The physical pain and limitations interfere with performance of normal tasks and provision of self-care. There may be school difficulties related to transportation to and from school, stairs, and loss of time as a result of exacerbations and hospitalization. Physical limitations interfere with participation in many activities, both curricular and extracurricular, which limits peer contacts and interaction and increases social isolation.

Changes in personality usually accompany juvenile rheumatoid arthritis as they do in any child with a chronic illness. They may be temporary, such as demanding, irritable behavior, or they may be manifest in a more perma-

---
*1314 Spring Street, N.W. Atlanta, GA 30309.
†P.O. Box 9782, Arlington, VA 22209.

nent way, such as passive hostility, uncommunicativeness, and manipulativeness. Efforts should be made to break through the child's defenses and to identify his anxieties, concerns, and conflicts in order to intervene early to prevent the development of permanent personality problems (see Chapter 16 for problems of the child with chronic illness).

SYSTEMIC LUPUS ERYTHEMATOSUS (SLE)

Systemic lupus erythematosus, which literally means "red wolf" because of the characteristic butterfly rash on the face of some affected individuals, is a chronic inflammatory disease of the collagen or supporting tissues of the body and, because connective tissue is found extensively throughout the body, almost any organ or structure can be affected. Characteristically SLE follows an unpredicatable course of remissions and exacerbations and may remit spontaneously, continue for many years, or become progressively fatal. SLE in children is generally more acute and severe than SLE in adults.

Although considered predominantly a disease of early adulthood, a significant number of cases (20%) is diagnosed in childhood, usually in children over 8 years of age. Like many rheumatic disorders, SLE occurs 8 to 10 times more frequently in females than in males and is more common in the dark-skinned races such as blacks, Hispanics, and American Indians. The tendency for the disease to affect several members of the same family supports a polygenic mode of inheritance.

Pathophysiology

Systemic lupus erythematosus is a multisystem disorder characterized by the presence of autoantibodies responsible for immune-mediated tissue injury. An inciting event (such as infection, drugs, and ultraviolet light) causes fibroid deposition in connective tissue and blood vessels of affected organs. There is an accompanying inflammation and, if untreated, eventual degeneration of the involved connective tissue.

Clinical manifestations

Because SLE can involve almost any tissue, the clinical manifestations are highly variable. The onset is usually insidious, with vague signs such as low-grade fever, chills, weakness, generalized aching, and malaise. However, rapid involvement of vital organs, primarily the kidney, can herald an accelerated course with minimum or absent involvement of other sites.

The most common symptom is generalized weakness, usually accompanied by arthritis, myalgia, joint swelling, and stiffness. Usually the joint manifestations are not severe enough to cause deformity, although it may result in temporary disability because of pain. Evidence of neurologic involvement varies from forgetfulness, excitability, and headache to seizures, frank psychosis, and paralysis from spinal cord involvement. The serous linings of the lungs and heart may become inflamed, resulting in pleurisy or pericarditis, respectively. The glomerulus is the usual site of kidney destruction with signs and symptoms of progressive renal failure. Anemia from decreased erythrocytes is common, and sometimes the spleen and often the cervical, axillary, and inguinal lymph nodes are enlarged. Nausea and vomiting, diarrhea, and abdominal pain may be present and, at times, falsely suggest conditions such as appendicitis.

The most typical skin involvement, although seen in only a few patients, is the symmetrical "butterfly rash" over the bridge of the nose and extending to each cheek. It is described as "fleeting, faint to pink, pink to red, flat to slightly raised, and mild to severe." These same types of lesions can occur anywhere on the body, have a tendency to scar, and are aggravated by exposure to ultraviolet rays.

Diagnostic evaluation

Systemic lupus erythematosus has been called the "great imitator," since its clinical manifestations may point to a variety of unrelated conditions. Definitive diagnosis is essential, particularly to distinguish it from the other collagen diseases, because treatment and prognosis vary.

Numerous laboratory tests are employed in the diagnosis of SLE. Antinuclear antibodies are always present, but not necessarily diagnostic, and antibodies to DNA are diagnostic of SLE but are present only in severe or widespread disease. Other helpful tests findings include diminished serum hemolytic complement, hypergammaglobulinemia, positive Coombs test, and false-positive tests for syphilis, anemia, leukopenia or thrombocytopenia, and evidence of nephritis. LE cells are not always demonstrated.

Therapeutic management

The objectives of medical treatment are (1) to reverse the autoimmune and inflammatory process and (2) to prevent exacerbations and complications. Therapy involves the use of specific and supportive medications and regulation of activity and diet.

Medications. Corticosteroids, salicylates, and other nonsteroid agents offer relief of symptoms and adjunctive use of antimalarials and, in severe cases, anticancer drugs are the usual drugs employed. Because of the high incidence of serious renal disease and central nervous system involvement, careful follow-up care is essential.

Regulation of activity and diet. The goal of restricted activity is to prevent a recurrence of the disease. Although the exact relationship is unclear, fatigue, stress, or sudden exertion brings about a relapse of symptoms. An effective schedule must provide for gradual resumption of pre–lupus erythematosus activity and maximum rest periods.

Diet may be restricted depending on weight gain and/or fluid retention from steroids and renal damage. The most frequently prescribed diet modification is moderate or low salt. Low-protein diets may be necessary to prevent elevated nitrogen levels. Weight reduction may help preserve maximum joint function and conserve energy.

Prognosis. Since many children with mild disease are being recognized, the prognosis has improved but prolonged spontaneous remission is uncommon in children. A significant number succumb from nephritis, central nervous system complications, infections, pulmonary lupus, and possible myocardial infarction.

Nursing considerations

The principal nursing goal is to help the child and family adjust to the limitations and treatments of the disease and to prevent exacerbations and complications. Since older female adolescents are the most likely group to be affected, the nurse be aware of their special needs, such as body image changes, present and future vocational activities, and social relationships. See the principles of adjusting to a chronic illness in Chapter 16.

Family members need an understanding of the disease process to gain an appreciation of the need for regular, uninterrupted drug administration, moderate activity, and any diet modifications that may be imposed. Usually diagnostic tests are performed during hospitalization, which allows the nurse an opportunity to help the child and parents learn about the disease. Several booklets are available, and local lupus erythematosus organizations* have been formed to help sufferers learn about and adjust to the disease. The nurse should be aware of what information the family is receiving since learning about joint deformity, sudden bouts of pain and disability, a disfiguring rash, and the possibility of renal failure can be overwhelming. Nurses should also be aware of advertised nonmedical approaches to treatment because quackery abounds when no known cure exists.

To prevent exacerbations and complications the list of ''don'ts'' for these individuals is long. The importance of

---

*Addresses of local lupus erythematosus societies are available from the National Lupus Foundation, 5430 Van Nuys Ave., Van Nuys, CA 91401.

adequate rest and the need to adhere to the medication schedule are stressed. Individuals who are sensitive to the sun must avoid exposure. It is important to emphasize that sun filtered through clouds or reflected from snow, water, or white surfaces (such as cement) can cause a severe reaction. Although clothes can protect most areas of the body, special sunscreening agents are needed on exposed areas such as the face. An ingredient that effectively blocks ultraviolet rays is paraaminobenzoic acid (PABA), which is available in over-the-counter creams, lotions, and lip balms. The family is advised to read labels carefully and purchase those products with the greatest amount of screening capability. A large-brimmed hat helps in partially shading the face.

Affected persons are advised to maintain regular medical supervision and additional attention during periods of stress, illness, or prior to elective surgical procedures, such as dental extraction, because the body may require larger amounts of a drug. They should carry an identification card or Medic Alert tag emphasizing their dependence on steroids.

REFERENCES

Guerrein, A.T.: Osteogenesis imperfecta: a disorder that breaks more than our hearts, Am. J. Maternal Child Nurs. **7**:315-318, 1982.

BIBLIOGRAPHY
General

Diamond, L.: Triaging pediatric emergencies, Crit. Care Update **7**(2):28-32, 1980.

Hinkhouse, A.: Physical assessment: multiple trauma, Crit. Care Update **3**(12):15-19, 1976.

Hogan, K., and Sawyer, J.: Fracture dislocation of the elbow, Am. J. Nurs. **76**:1266-1268, 1976.

Larson, C.B., and Gould, M.: Orthopedic nursing, ed. 9, St. Louis, 1978, The C.V. Mosby Co.

O'Boyle, C.M.: Sports injuries in adolescents: emergency care, Am. J. Nurs. **75**:1732-1739, 1975.

Fractures

Alt, P.: Nursing care of a child in traction, Orthop. Nurs. Assoc. J. **3**:40, 1976.

Bailey, M.: Emergency! First aid for fractures, Nursing 82 **12**(11):72-79, 1982.

Cassels, C.J.: Fundamentals of long bone traction. Part I, Crit. Care Update **10**(3):36-39, 1983.

Cassels, C.J.: Fundamentals of long bone traction. Part II, Crit. Care Update **10**(4):26-31, 1983.

Cassels, C.J.: Fundamentals of long bone traction. Part III, Crit. Care Update **10**(5):38-39, 1983.

Deyerle, W.M., and Crossland, S.A.: Broken legs are to be walked on, Am. J. Nurs. **77**:1927-1930, 1977.

Kryschyshen, P.L., and Fischer, D.A.: External fixation for complicated fractures, Am. J. Nurs. **80**:156-159, 1980.

Lane, P.L., and Lee, M.M.: Special care for special casts, Nursing 83 **13**(7):50, 1983.

Programmed instruction: Nursing care of a patient in traction. Am. J. Nurs. **79:**1771-1798, 1979.

Richards, H.: A child with a fractured femur, Nurs. Times **78:**59-62, 1982.

Siner, E.: Emergency care update: skeletal trauma, Crit. Care Update **4**(2):20-23, 1977.

Siner, E.: Skeletal trauma, Crit. Care Update **4**(1):32-33, 1977.

Stout, J.A., and Gibbs, K.R.: The child undergoing a leg-lengthening procedure, Am. J. Nurs. **81:**1152-1155, 1981.

Swanson, V.M.: The school-age traction patient: toward better behavior patterns, J. Assoc. Care Child. Hosp. **9**(1):12-14, 1980.

Wassel, A.: Nursing assessment of injuries to the lower extremity, Nurs. Clin. North Am. **16:**739-748, 1981.

Congenital defects

Bunch, W.H.: Common deformities of the lower limb, Pediatr. Nurs. **5**(4):18-22, 1979.

Cantrell, D.: Osteogenesis imperfecta, Orthop. Nurs. Assoc. J. **3:**163, 1976.

Dubowski, F.M.: Children with osteogenesis imperfecta, Nurs. Clin. North Am. **11:**709-715, 1976.

Holland, S.H.: Up-to-date home care of a baby in a hip spica cast, Pediatr. Nurs. **9:**114-115, 1983.

McLaughlin, S.: Brittle bones or osteogenesis imperfecta, Can. Nurs. **78**(2):23, 1983.

Mercer, R.T.: Crisis: a baby is born with a defect, Nursing 77 **7**(11):45-47, 1977.

Meservey, P.M.: Congenital musculoskeletal abnormalities, Issues Compr. Pediatr. Nurs. **2**(4):15-22, 1977.

Mital, M.A.: Limb deficiencies: classification and treatment, Orthop. Clin. North Am. **7:**457-464, 1976.

Twoney, M.R.: Nursing care study: osteogenesis imperfecta, Nurs. Times **73:**123-129, 1977.

Scoliosis

Allard, J.L., and Dibble, S.L.: Scoliosis surgery: a look at Luque rods, Am. J. Nurs. **84:**609-611, 1984.

Anderson, B.: The patient with scoliosis: Carole, a girl treated with bracing, Am. J. Nurs. **79:**1592-1598, 1979.

Anderson, B., and D'Ambra, P.: The adolescent patient with scoliosis, Nurs. Clin. North Am. **11:**699-708, 1976.

Barrett, M.J.: Surviving adolescence in a back brace: Laura's experience, Am. J. Maternal Child Nurs. **2:**160-163, 1977.

Bowring, V.N.: Electro-spinal instrumentation: a new look at pediatric scoliosis, Orthop. Nurs. Assoc. J. **3:**172, 1976.

Brier, L., and Seligson, D.: Care of the patient in the halo, Crit. Care Update **9**(8):38-41, 1982.

Davis, S.E., and Lewis, S.A.: Managing scoliosis: fashions for the body and mind, Am. J. Maternal Child Nurs. **9:**186-187, 1984.

de Toledo, C.H.: The patient with scoliosis: the defect: classification and detection, Am. J. Nurs. **79:**1588-1591, 1979.

Hill, P.M., and Romm, L.S.: Screening for scoliosis in adolescents, Am. J. Maternal Child Nurs. **2**:156-159, May/June 1977.

Micheli, L.J., Magin, M.A., and Rouvales, R.: The patient with scoliosis: surgical management and nursing care, Am. J. Nurs. **79**:1599-1607, 1979.

Schatzinger, L.H., Brower, E.M., and Nash, C.L.: The patient with scoliosis: spinal fusion: emotional stress and adjustment, Am. J. Nurs. **79**:1608-1612, 1979.

Seigil, C.: Current concepts in the management of scoliosis, Nurs. Clin North Am. **11**:691-698, 1976.

Strong, C., and Gavaghan, M.: Scoliosis and its implications, Issues Compr. Pediatr. Nurs. **2**(4):33-45, 1977.

Wilson, R.: The MUD bed and its implications for nursing care, Nurs. Clin. North Am. **11**:725-730, 1976.

Miscellaneous skeletal disorders

Hussey, C.G.: Surviving a handicap in everyday life: how to help, Am. J. Maternal Child Nurs. **4**:46-50, 1979.

Rang, M.C., Rogers, L.F., and Zimmerman, R.C.: Growth plate injuries: treat or refer? Patient Care **10**(9):60-94, 1976.

Bone tumors

Ritchie, J.A.: Nursing the child undergoing limb amputation, Am. J. Maternal Child Nurs. **5**:114-120, 1980.

Staudt, A.R.: Femur replacement in osteogenic sarcoma, Am. J. Nurs. **75**(8):1346-1348, 1975.

Juvenile rheumatoid arthritis

Brown-Skeers, V.: How the nurse practitioner manages the rheumatoid arthritis patient, Nursing 79 **9**(6):26-35, 1979.

Dickinson, G.B.: A home care program for patients with rheumatoid arthritis, Nurs. Clin. North Am. **15**:403-418, 1980.

Lindsley, C.B.: The child with arthritis, Issues Compr. Pediatr. Nurs. **2**(4):23-32, 1977.

Spruck, M.: Gold therapy for rheumatoid arthritis, Am. J. Nurs. **79**:1246-1248, 1979.

Systemic lupus erythematosus

Ascheim, J.H.: The adolescent and systemic lupus erythematosus: a developmental and educational approach, Issues Compr. Pediatr. Nurs. **5**:293-307, 1981.

Torbett, M.P., and Ervin, J.C.: The patient with systemic lupus erythematosus, Am. J. Nurs. **77**(8):1299-1302, 1977.

White, J.F., and Ziegler, G.L.: Patient management of systemic lupus erythematosus, Crit. Care Update **7**(8):5-15, 1980.

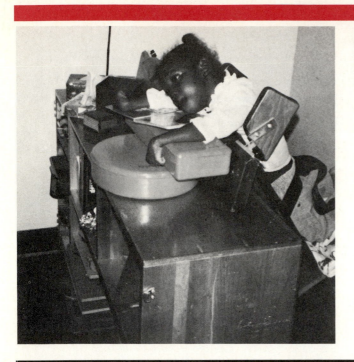

29

THE CHILD WITH NEUROMUSCULAR DYSFUNCTION

OBJECTIVES

On completion of this chapter the reader will be able to:

■ Discuss the nursing role in assisting the parents to cope with a child with cerebral palsy

■ Formulate a nursing care plan for the preoperative and postoperative care of a child with meningomyelocele

■ Discuss the prevention and treatment of tetanus

■ Differentiate between the various types of muscular dystrophy

■ Outline a plan of care for the child with Guillain-Barré syndrome

NURSING DIAGNOSES

Nursing diagnoses identified for the child with skeletal or articular dysfunction include, but are not restricted to, the following:

Health perception-health management pattern

■ Injury, potential for, related to (1) impaired coordination; (2) immobility

Nutritional-metabolic pattern

■ Nutrition, alteration in: potential for more than body requirements related to immobility

■ Skin integrity, impairment of: potential related to (1) immobility; (2) presence of incontinent secretions

Elimination pattern

■ Bowel elimination, alteration in: constipation related to immobility

■ Bowel elimination, alteration in: incontinence related to ineffective anal sphincter

■ Urinary elimination, alteration in patterns related to ineffective urinary sphincters

Activity-exercise pattern

■ Airway clearance, ineffective, related to (1) retention of secretions; (2) weak respiratory muscles

■ Diversional activity deficit related to (1) immobility; (2) difficulty coordinating movements; (3) muscular weakness

■ Mobility, impaired physical, related to muscle weakness

■ Self-care deficit: feeding, bathing/hygiene, dressing/grooming, toileting, related to (1) developmental level; (2) muscular weakness; (3) immobility

Sleep-rest pattern

■ Sleep pattern disturbance related to (1) discomfort; (2) schedule of therapies

Cognitive-perceptual pattern

■ Comfort, alteration in: pain related to movement

Self-perception—self-concept pattern

■ Anxiety related to (1) strange environment; (2) perception of impending events; (3) separation; (4) predicted outcome of injury and/or therapy; (5) knowledge deficit; (6) perceived powerlessness

■ Powerlessness related to immobility

■ Self-concept, disturbance in: body image, self-esteem, related to (1) perception of physical impairment; (2) nonintegration of change in body function or limitations

Role-relationship pattern

■ Family process, alteration in, related to situational crisis

■ Grieving, anticipatory, related to expected change(s)

■ Parenting, alterations in: potential related to (1) skill deficit; (2) family stress

■ Social isolation related to (1) impaired mobility; (2) self-concept disturbance

Coping-stress tolerance pattern

■ Coping, family: potential for growth

■ Coping, ineffective family: compromised related to (1) situational crisis; (2) temporary family disorganization

Abnormal muscle performance may result from (1) defects within the muscle itself, (2) defective transmission of nerve impulses to muscles, (3) dysfunction of peripheral motor or sensory nerves, or (4) damage to the central nervous system.

CEREBRAL PALSY (CP)

Cerebral palsy is a nonspecific term that is applied to impaired neuromuscular control that results from a nonprogressive abnormality in the pyramidal motor system (motor cortex, basal ganglia, and cerebellum). The etiology, clinical features, and course are variable, and abnormal muscle tone and coordination are the primary disturbances. It is the most frequently occurring permanent physical disability of childhood, and, although the incidence is not known, various studies suggest that it varies from 1.5 to 5 per 1000 live births.

Various prenatal, perinatal, and postnatal factors contribute to the etiology of cerebral palsy singly or in combination, such as developmental anomalies, infections, cerebral trauma, hypoxia, metabolic disturbances, and toxicoses. Cerebral anoxia, which has long been associated with cerebral damage, is an important cause during the prenatal and perinatal periods.

Pathophysiology

It is difficult to establish a precise location of neurologic lesions based on etiology or clinical signs because there is no characteristic pathologic picture. In some cases there are gross malformations of the brain. In others there may be evidence of vascular occlusion, atrophy, loss of neurons, and degeneration. Anoxia plays the most significant role in the pathology of brain damage, although trauma, neonatal diseases (such as hypoglycemia and kernicterus), trauma, cerebrovascular accident, and prematurity are important factors.

Clinical manifestations

The alert observer may be suspicious when a child demonstrates some of the following groups of manifestations.

Delayed gross motor development is a universal manifestation of cerebral palsy. The child shows delay in all motor accomplishments, and the discrepancy between motor ability and expected achievement tends to increase with successive developmental milestones as growth advances.

Abnormal motor performance is evidence of neuromuscular dysfunction. This includes very early preferential unilateral hand use, abnormal and asymmetric crawl using the unaffected arm and leg to propel the child on either the buttocks or the abdomen, standing or walking on the toes, and uncoordinated or involuntary movements. Other significant signs of motor dysfunction are poor sucking and feeding difficulties with persistent tongue thrust.

Alterations of muscle tone are displayed by increased or decreased resistance to passive movements. The child may exhibit opisthotonic postures (exaggerated arching of the back), he may feel stiff on handling or dressing, and there is difficulty in diapering him because of spasticity of hip adductor muscles and lower extremities. When the child is pulled to a sitting position, he may extend the entire body, rigid and unbending at the hip and knee joints. This is an early sign of spasticity.

Abnormal postures may be assumed by children at rest or when their position is changed. From an early age a child lying in a prone position will maintain the hips higher than the trunk with the legs and arms flexed or drawn under the body. In the supine position spasticity is demonstrated by scissoring and extension of legs and with the feet plantar flexed. This posture is exaggerated when the child is suspended vertically or when others try to make him bear weight. A persistent infantile resting and sleeping posture—that is, arms abducted at shoulders, elbows flexed, and hands fisted—is a sign of spasticity when it remains constant after 4 to 5 months of age.

Reflex abnormalities, including persistence of primitive infantile reflexes, are some of the earliest clues to cerebral palsy, for example, obligatory tonic neck reflex at any age or nonobligatory persistence beyond 6 months of age and the persistence or even hyperactivity of the Moro, plantar, and palmar grasp reflexes. Hyperreflexia, ankle clonus, and stretch reflexes can be elicited on many muscle groups on fast passive movements, for example, resistance to passive abduction when hips are suddenly separated (adductor catch).

Clinical classification. Cerebral palsy has been classified in several ways. The most useful classification is based on the nature and distribution of neuromuscular dysfunction.

Spastic. This is the most common clinical type; it is characterized by hypertonicity with poor control of posture, balance, and coordinated motion and impairment of fine and gross motor skills. Active attempts at motion increase abnormal postures and are accompanied by an overflow of movement to other parts of the body.

Dyskinetic. Dyskinesia implies abnormal involuntary movement. The major manifestation of dyskinetic cerebral palsy is athetosis, which is characterized by slow, wormlike, writhing movements that usually involve all extremities, the trunk, neck, facial muscles, and tongue. Involvement of the pharyngeal, laryngeal, and oral muscles causes drooling and dysarthria (imperfect speech articulation), which makes it difficult to understand what the child is saying. Involuntary movements may take on choreoid (involuntary, irregular, jerking movements) and dystonic (disordered muscle tone) manifestations that increase in intensity under emotional stress and around adolescence.

Ataxic. The least common type of cerebral palsy is ataxia. Affected children have a wide-based gait and perform rapid repetitive movements poorly. There is disintegration of movements of the upper extremities when the child reaches for objects.

Mixed-type. A combination of spasticity and athetosis is described as mixed-type cerebral palsy. Many affected children are severely disabled.

Rigid, tremor, and atonic. These types of cerebral palsy are uncommon. Both rigid and atonic types have a poor prognosis, with deformities and lack of active movement.

Associated disabilities. Some of the disabilities associated with cerebral palsy are subnormal learning and reasoning capacity (mental retardation), impaired behavioral and interpersonal relationships (attention deficit disorder), seizures, and impairment of special senses.

Diagnostic evaluation

The neurologic examination and history are the primary modalities for diagnosis. A thorough knowledge of normal variations of motor development is required for detecting abnormal progress, and a careful history is elicited to detect possible etiologic factors. The child's spontaneous movements and behavior are observed, including posture, attitude, and muscle size, function, and tone.

Supplemental diagnostic tests may be employed, such as electroencephalography, tomography, screening for metabolic defects, and serum electrolyte values. The possibility that the manifestations are those of slowly progressive degenerative disease or early onset, slowly growing brain tumors must be ruled out.

Therapeutic management

The goals of therapy for children with cerebral palsy are early recognition and promotion of an optimum developmental course in order that the child may realize his potential within the limits of his brain dysfunction. The disorder is permanent, and therapy is chiefly symptomatic and preventive.

The broad aims of therapy are (1) to establish locomotion, communication, and self-help; (2) to gain optimum appearance and integration of motor functions; (3) to correct associated defects as effectively as possible; and (4) to provide educational opportunities adapted to the individual child's needs and capabilities. Each child is evaluated and managed on an individual basis. The plan of therapy may involve a variety of settings, facilities, and specially trained persons, including the parents.

Braces are often used to help prevent or reduce deformity, and orthopedic surgery may be required to decrease or abolish spastic muscle imbalance. Surgical intervention is usually reserved for the child who does not respond to the more conservative measures, but it is also indicated for the child whose spasticity causes progressive deformities. Surgery is primarily used to improve function and is followed by physical therapy. Surgery is not performed for cosmetic purposes.

Drugs that decrease spasticity have little usefulness in improving function in cerebral palsy. Antianxiety agents have been used to some extent to relieve excessive motion and tension, particularly in the athetoid child. Skeletal muscle relaxants, such as dantrolene (Dantrium) and diazepam (Valium), which has a direct influence on spastic hypertonicity, have been tried with encouraging results in decreasing stiffness and thus facilitating ease of motion. Local nerve block to motor points of a muscle with a neurolytic agent such as phenol solution reduces spasticity temporarily.

Children with seizures should receive anticonvulsant medications, and hyperactive, dyskinetic children perform better when given dextroamphetamine or other drugs used for the child with attention deficit disorder. Care of visual and auditory deficits requires the attention of appropriate specialists, and speech therapy involves the services of a speech therapist.

Physical therapy is one of the most frequently employed conservative treatment modalities. It requires the specialized skills of a qualified therapist with an extensive repertoire of exercise methods who can design a program to stimulate each child to achieve his functional goals. In general, physical therapy is directed toward good skeletal alignment for the spastic child; training in purposeful acts, even in the face of involuntary motion, for the athetoid child; and maximum development of proprioceptive sense for the ataxic child.

Nursing considerations

Early recognition of cerebral palsy is often a result of alert observation by the nurse. Detection begins at birth, and the nurse should be especially observant for signs in an infant who has a history that includes any of the prenatal and perinatal conditions that predispose to brain damage. An infant in the nursery who displays any sign that may indicate that all is not well, for example, poor feeding, rigidity, tenseness, or hypotonia, merits closer scrutiny and evaluation.

Delayed attainment of developmental milestones is one of the most valuable clues to recognizing cerebral palsy; therefore, slow development in a child is cause for concern. Nurses working with children need to be well acquainted with normal child growth and development and with the tools of assessment. The earlier any deviation

SUMMARY OF NURSING CARE OF THE CHILD WITH CEREBRAL PALSY

GOALS	RESPONSIBILITIES
Recognize disorder early	Take careful history of prenatal factors and circumstances surrounding birth that predispose to fetal anoxia Be alert for evidence of cerebral palsy
Promote general health	Assure balanced diet Provide extra calories to meet extra energy demands of increased muscle activity Monitor weight gain Provide vitamin, mineral, and/or protein supplements if eating habits are poor Protect from exposure to infections Assure regular routine health maintenance including physical assessment, dental care, immunizations
Establish locomotion	Encourage sitting, crawling, and walking at appropriate ages Carry out therapies that strengthen and improve control Assist the child to use reciprocal leg motion when learning to walk Provide incentives to locomote Assure adequate rest before attempting locomotion activities Incorporate play that encourages desired behavior Employ aids that facilitate locomotion, such as parallel bars and crutches Prepare the child and family for surgical procedures if indicated
Facilitate communication	Enlist services of speech therapist early Talk to the child slowly Use articles and pictures to reinforce speech Employ feeding techniques that help facilitate speech, such as using lips, teeth, and various tongue movements Teach and use nonverbal communication methods to dysarthric child who would benefit
Prevent deformity	Apply and correctly use braces Carry out and teach the family to perform stretching exercises Employ appropriate range of motion exercises Provide preoperative and postoperative care to children who require corrective surgery

Prevent injury	Implement measures that provide safe physical environment, such as
	    Furniture padded
	    Side rails on bed
	    Study furniture that does not slip
	    Avoidance of scatter rugs and polished floors
	Select toys appropriate to age and physical limitations
	Encourage sufficient rest
	Use restraints when the child is in chair or vehicle
	Provide the child who is prone to falls with protective helmet and enforce its use
	Institute seizure precautions for susceptible children

Encourage self-help	Encourage the child to assist in his care as his age and capabilities permit Select toys and activities that allow maximum participation by the child and that improve motor function and sensory input Avoid undue persistence to accomplish a goal Encourage activities that require both unimanual and bimanual activities Adapt utensils, foods, and clothing to facilitate self-help; for example, large bowled spoon with padded handle, finger foods and foods that adhere rather than slip from utensil, and clothing that opens from front with Velcro closings rather than buttons Assist the parents in toilet training the child

SUMMARY OF NURSING CARE OF THE CHILD WITH CEREBRAL PALSY—cont'd

GOALS	RESPONSIBILITIES
Promote relaxation	Maintain a well-regulated schedule that allows for adequate rest and sleep periods
	Be alert to evidence of fatigue, which tends to aggravate symptoms
Promote positive self-image	Capitalize on the child's assets and compensate for his liabilities
	Praise the child for accomplishments and "near" accomplishments such as partial completion of a task
	Set realistic goals for the child
	Encourage appealing physical appearance
	Good body hygiene, clean straight teeth, and good grooming
	Stylish clothing
	Makeup for teenage girls
	Encourage recreational outlets and after-school activities appropriate to the child's capabilities
	Allow the child to discuss himself, his disorder, and how he thinks others feel about him
	Encourage the child to become involved with children who have similar problems
	Encourage attendance at schools with facilities that meet his special needs
	Talk to the child at his mental level
Treat and/or correct associated defects	Administer anticonvulsant drugs
	Prepare the child and family for needed surgical procedures
	Arrange for hearing and visual tests and assist the parents to acquire corrective devices
Support the parents	Allow for expression of feelings regarding the child, their own guilt regarding disease, and the impact that disorder has on the family
	Help them explore their frustations and concerns
	Assist the parents in problem solving
	Assist the parents in carrying out the prescribed treatment regimen and in assuming the responsibility at their own pace and readiness
	Encourage early and consistent participation in treatment programs
	Provide praise and encouragement for compliance and innovation
	Help the parents to achieve realistic view of the child's capabilities and outlook for future
	Help the parents to view the child rather than the defects
	Support siblings and help them to understand the affected child, his special needs, and the impact this has on their lives
	Refer to counseling services as appropriate, parent groups, and organization with special services, such as the United Cerebral Palsy Association
	Maintain contact with the family

from the normal is detected, the better the outlook for therapeutic intervention.

Nurses in a community setting, especially those in public health, in physicians' offices and clinics, and in schools, are more likely to become involved with a family in which there is a child with cerebral palsy. Both the child and the family need the help, support, and encouragement that nurses are prepared to offer, and nurses are involved in all aspects of the child's management. Nurses who know the family and their special needs and problems are in the best position to provide guidance and support to that family.

Parents can also find help and solace from parent groups with whom they can share problems and concerns and from whom they can derive comfort and practical information. The national organization, United Cerebral Palsy Association,* has branches in most communities that are listed in the telephone directory, and the address of the nearest branch can be obtained from a local agency directory or a local health department or by writing to the national headquarters. The association provides a variety of services for children and families. There are also a number of excellent books available to serve as guides for parents and nurses who work with the child with cerebral palsy.†

Hospitalized child. Cerebral palsy is not a disorder that requires hospitalization; therefore, when children with cerebral palsy are hospitalized they are usually admitted for another reason or for corrective surgery. Consequently

---

*66 E. 34th St., New York, NY 10016

†Especially recommended is Levy, J.: The baby exercise book, New York, 1975, Random House, Inc.

many nurses are not accustomed to handling these children. Nurses who have never been associated with a child with cerebral palsy may react in a variety of ways, including fear, revulsion, or overwhelming pity. The basic concept to keep in mind when caring for these children is that they are, first of all, children, who happen to be afflicted with a disorder that limits their capacities in performing some activities of daily living and, for some, communicating with others. They should be approached and treated the same as any child in the hospital. The nurse's actions should convey acceptance, affection, and friendliness and promote a feeling of trust and dependability in the child. This is especially true with older children who have normal intelligence but who may have communication problems. All too frequently nurses tend to ''talk down'' to these children and do things for them that they are perfectly capable of doing for themseslves, although not as adeptly. This is especially humiliating to a teenager who values his independence and self-esteem.

To facilitate the care and management of the child, the therapy program should be continued, insofar as his condition allows, during the time he is hospitalized. This should be incorporated into his nursing care plan and every effort expended to make certain that the ground that has been so laboriously gained is not lost. Encouraging the parent to room-in and actively participate in the child's care facilitates a continuation of the home therapy program and helps the child adjust to an unfamiliar environment.

SPINA BIFIDA

Abnormalities along the neural axis constitute a significant portion of congenital malformations. The defects may extend the entire length of the neural tube or they may be restricted to a small area. The amount of deformity and disability depends on the degree of neural involvement. *Myelodysplasia* is an all-inclusive term that refers to defective development of any part of the spinal cord. It is usually used to describe abnormalities without gross superficial defects, especially those of the lower segment. The more severe defects are *rachischisis,* a fissure in the spinal column that leaves the meninges and spinal cord exposed, and *anencephaly* (absence of the brain), which consists of only an exposed vascular mass and no bony covering.

The majority of neural tube malformations consist of defects in closure of the vertebral column with varying degrees of tissue protrusion through the bony cleft called *spinal dysraphism,* or *spina bifida.* If the anomaly is not visible externally, it is termed *spina bifida occulta;* if there is an external saccular protrusion, the defect is termed *spina bifida cystica* and is further classified as *meningocele* or *meningomyelocele,* according to the extent of neural involvement (Fig. 29-1). A herniation of brain and meninges through a defect in the skull that produces a fluid-filled sac in the occipital region is termed *encephalocele*.

The cause of neural tube malformations is unknown, although the increased incidence in families lends support to a genetic influence. There is some speculation regarding a viral cause of spina bifida since there appears to be an increased incidence of the defect in infants conceived during the early winter months. Radiation and other environmental influences have also been implicated, based on animal experiments.

Pathophysiology

The primary defect in neural tube malformations is believed by most authorities to be a failure of neural tube closure during early development of the embryo. However, there is evidence to indicate that the defects are a result of splitting of the already closed neural tube as a result of an abnormal increase in cerebrospinal fluid pressure during the first trimester of pregnancy. The degree of neurologic dysfunction is directly related to the anatomic level of the defect and thus the nerves involved.

Clinical manifestations

The cystic defect affects 0.2 to 4.2:1000 live births and appears most commonly as a saclike structure that may be located at any point along the spinal column. The sac is usually encased in a fine membrane that is prone to tears through which cerebrospinal fluid leaks. In other instances the sac may be covered by dura, meninges, or skin, in which instances there is rapid and spontaneous epithelialization. The largest number of meningomyeloceles are found in the lumbar or lumbosacral area (Fig. 29-2). When the defect is located below the second lumbar vertebra, the nerves of the cauda equina are involved, giving rise to symptoms such as flaccid, areflexic partial paralysis of the lower extremities and varying degrees of sensory deficit. Sensory disturbances usually parallel motor dysfunction.

Defective nerve supply to the bladder affects both sphincter and detrusor tone to produce overflow incontinence with constant dribbling of urine. Often there is poor anal sphincter tone and poor anal skin reflex, which result in lack of bowel control and, sometimes, rectal prolapse. If the defect is located below the third sacral vertebra, there is no motor impairment but there may be saddle anesthesia with bladder and anal sphincter paralysis.

Sometimes the denervation to the muscles of the lower extremities will produce joint deformities in utero. These are primarily flexion or extension contractures, talipes valgus or varus contractures, kyphosis, lumbosacral scoliosis, and hip dislocations. The extent and severity of these associated deformities depend on the degree of nerve involvement.

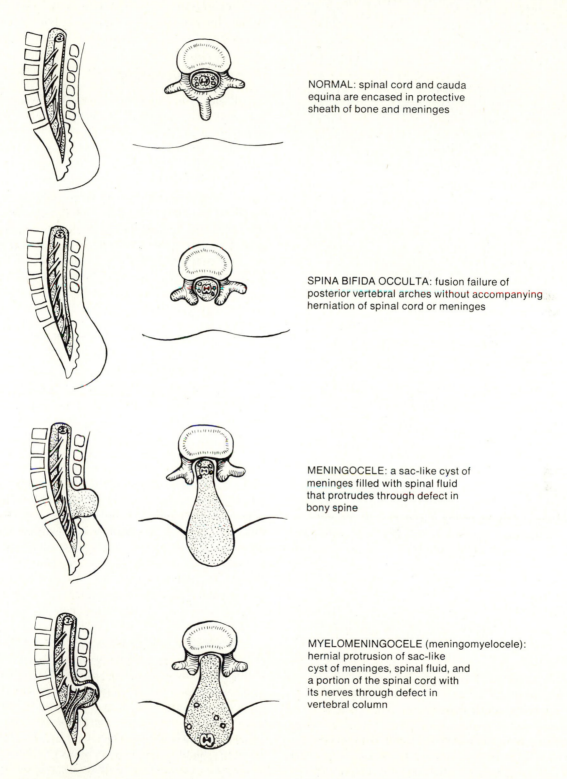

NORMAL: spinal cord and cauda equina are encased in protective sheath of bone and meninges

SPINA BIFIDA OCCULTA: fusion failure of posterior vertebral arches without accompanying herniation of spinal cord or meninges

MENINGOCELE: a sac-like cyst of meninges filled with spinal fluid that protrudes through defect in bony spine

MYELOMENINGOCELE (meningomyelocele): hernial protrusion of sac-like cyst of meninges, spinal fluid, and a portion of the spinal cord with its nerves through defect in vertebral column

Fig. 29-1

Midline defects of the osseous spine with varying degrees of neural herniations.

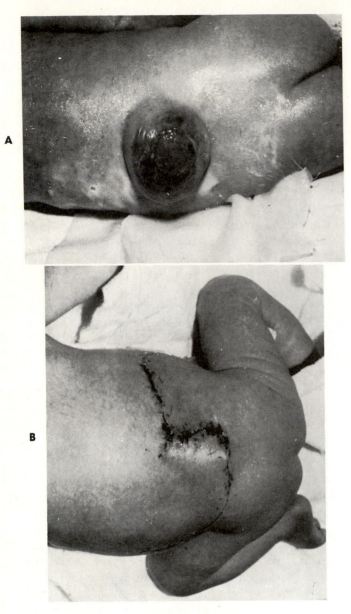

Fig. 29-2

A, *Meningomyelocele before surgery. (An antibacterial dressing was used.)* **B,** *Same patient after surgery. (Courtesy M.C. Gleason, M.D., San Diego, Calif. From Ingalls, A.J., and Salerno, M.C.: Maternal and child health nursing, ed. 4, St. Louis, 1979, The C.V. Mosby Co.)*

Noncystic spina bifida is failure of the spinous processes to join posteriorly in the lumbosacral area. Routine radiographic examinations indicate that the disorder is quite common, but it may not be apparent unless there are associated cutaneous manifestations or neuromuscular disturbances. Superficial indications include a skin depression or dimple (which may also mark the outlet of a dermal

sinus tract that extends to the subarachnoid space), port-wine angiomatous nevi, dark tufts of hair, or soft, subcutaneous lipomas. These signs may be absent, appear singly, or be present in combination.

Diagnostic evaluation

The diagnosis is made on the basis of clinical manifestations and examination of the meningeal sac. Supplementary diagnostic measures include plain radiographic films to disclose the precise bony defect in symptomatic lesions and to establish the diagnosis in the suspected, nonsymptomatic occult variety. Occasionally spinal tomograms and myelography are employed to differentiate between spina bifida occulta and other spinal pathology. Skull tomography helps to establish the presence or absence of hydrocephalus (a frequent complication) in spina bifida cystica.

Prenatal detection. It is possible to determine the presence of some major open neural tube defects prenatally. Ultrasonic scanning of the uterus and elevated concentrations of α-fetoprotein (AFP), a fetal-specific α-1 globulin, in amniotic fluid can indicate the presence of anencephaly or meningomyelocele. The optimum time for these diagnostic tests to be carried out is between the fourteenth and sixteenth weeks of gestation before AFP concentrations normally diminish and in sufficient time to permit a therapeutic abortion.

Therapeutic management

Care and management of the child who has spina bifida with meningomyelocele require a multidisciplinary approach involving the specialties of neurology, neurosurgery, pediatrics, urology, orthopedics, and rehabilitation and physical therapy, as well as intensive nursing care in a variety of specialty areas. The collaborative efforts of these specialists are directed toward the five major problems associated with this serious defect—meningomyelocele, hydrocephalus, urinary tract paralysis, locomotion, and rehabilitation and education of both the child and family.

Surgical treatment. Initial care involves prevention of infection, neurologic assessment, including observation for associated anomalies, and dealing with the impact of the anomaly on the parents. Although meningoceles are repaired early, especially if there is danger of rupture of the sac, the philosophy regarding skin closure of meningomyeloceles varies radically among authorities. At the present time, however, most authorities believe that early closure, within the first 24 to 48 hours, offers the most favorable outcome, especially in regard to morbidity and mortality from serious infection.

The preferred method of surgical repair of the lesion employs skin grafts of Z closure without disturbing the neural elements or removal of any portion of the sac (see Fig. 29-2, *B*). Wide excision of the large membranous covering may damage functioning neural tissue. Where the skin over the defect is intact, as often occurs with meningocele, surgical intervention may be performed for cosmetic reasons.

Recently some experimentation has been carried out using small, individual oxygen chambers that fit over the lesion. There is evidence to indicate that this relatively simple procedure hastens healing and prevents spread of infection in infants already infected or in those who are otherwise unable to undergo immediate surgery.

Orthopedic considerations. According to most orthopedists, musculoskeletal problems that will affect later locomotion should be evaluated early, and treatment, where indicated, should be instituted without delay. Casting, bracing, traction, and surgical techniques for correction of hip, knee, and foot deformities are employed when they may aid later ambulation. Corrective procedures, when indicated, are best initiated at an early age in order that the infant will not lag significantly behind age-mates in developmental progress. Where there is little hope for lower extremity functioning, surgery is seldom recommended.

Management of excretory function. Meningomyelocele is one of the most common causes of neurogenic bladder dysfunction in childhood. Since the majority of these children suffer from incontinence and are subject to recurrent or persistent pyuria, prevention and treatment of renal complications are a constant goal. Treatment of renal disorders includes (1) lifetime administration of urinary tract antiseptic drugs, (2) reduction of urinary stasis with suprapubic manual expression of urine (Credé maneuver) or self-catheterization, and (3) a system for bladder drainage, such as an indwelling catheter or collecting device, to reduce vesicoureteral reflux and hydronephrosis. Drugs such as bethanechol (Urecholine), propantheline (Pro-Banthine), phenoxybenzamine (Dibenzyline), and ephedrine prove useful in some cases, and in many institutions the surgically implanted artificial urinary sphincter and bladder pacemaker are being used with increasing frequency. In cases of intractable severe hydronephrosis or incontinence, urinary diversion such as a ureteroileostomy, ureterostomy, or cystostomy may be necessary.

Fecal incontinence can usually be controlled with diet modification and bowel training. Colostomy may prove more convenient for social reasons in children who are otherwise able to function.

Nursing considerations

Care of the infant and child with defective development of the spinal cord requires both immediate and long-term nursing and medical supervision. At the time of delivery an examination is performed to assess the intactness of the membranous cyst, and every effort is made to prevent trauma to this protective covering. It is inspected for possible spinal fluid leaks through tears in the membrane, and a moist saline dressing is applied. In the newborn period nursing responsibilities are directed toward preventing infection of and trauma to the fragile cyst, observation for complications, and providing support for and education of the parents. Long-term management is directed toward preventing complications and improving the quality of life for the child and family.

Care of meningomyelocele sac. The infant is usually placed in an Isolette or beneath a warmer so that his temperature can be maintained without clothing or covers that might irritate the delicate lesion. When an overhead warmer is used, the dressings over the defect require more frequent moistening because of the dehydrating effect of the dry heat.

Before surgical closure, a sterile, moist gauze dressing that is applied over the defect prevents the meningomyelocele from drying. The moistening solution is usually sterile normal saline, although soaks with antibacterial solutions such as silver nitrate or bacitracin are also advocated. Soaks are changed frequently (every 2 to 4 hours), and the sac is closely inspected for leaks, abrasions, irritation, or any signs of infection. Any opening in the sac greatly increases the risk of infection to the central nervous system. The area must be carefully cleaned with hydrogen peroxide solution if it becomes soiled or contaminated. If surgical closure is to be delayed, measures are directed toward facilitating the drying and epithelialization of the sac. In this instance the sac is usually left exposed to the air or covered with a dry gauze or nonadherent dressing.

Special measures may be indicated to toughen the skin or membrane, such as application of benzoin tincture, but care must be taken to prevent a dressing from adhering to and damaging the sac. Prolonged use of ointments or moist dressings is usually contraindicated to avoid maceration and breakdown of the tissues. A large doughnut-shaped piece of foam rubber or other spongy material can be fashioned to provide a protective shield for the sac. The edges should be left sufficiently wide to allow for adequate anchoring with strips of bandage or paper tape. A sterile drape or gauze cover can form a roof over the opening but should not come in contact with the sac.

Positioning. One of the most difficult, important, and challenging aspects in the early care of the infant with meningomyelocele is positioning. Before surgery the infant is kept in the prone position to minimize tension on the sac and the risk of trauma. The prone position allows for optimum positioning of legs, especially in cases of associated hip dysplasia. Ideally the infant is placed in a low Trendelenburg's position to reduce spinal fluid pressure in the defect, with the hips only slightly flexed to reduce tension on the defect. The legs are maintained in abduction with a pad between the knees to counteract hip subluxation, and a small roll is placed under the ankles to maintain a neutral foot position. Sometimes, however, positioning with the head of the bed elevated is desirable and preferred by the neurosurgeon, especially after closure of the defect and where there is increased intracranial pressure from impending hydrocephalus. A variety of aids, including diaper rolls, pads, small sandbags, or specially designed frames and appliances, can be used to maintain the desired position.

The prone position affects other aspects of the infant's care. For example, in this position the infant is more difficult to keep clean, pressure areas are a constant threat, and feeding becomes a problem. The infant's head is turned to one side and tilted upward for bottle-feeding. Until the child is able to lift the head and shoulders from the bed, solid foods are best mixed with formula and fed through a nipple with an enlarged hole. Fortunately most defects are repaired early and the infant can be held for feeding as soon as the surgical site is sufficiently healed to permit handling.

The prone position is maintained after operative closure, although many neurosurgeons allow a side-lying or partial side-lying position unless it aggravates a coexisting hip dysplasia or permits undesirable hip flexion. This offers an opportunity for position changes, which reduces the risk of pressure sores and facilitates feeding. If permitted by the physician, the infant can be held upright against the body as one would normally do with care to avoid pressure on the operative site.

General care. Diapering the infant is contraindicated until the defect has been repaired and until healing is well advanced or epithelialization has taken place. The padding beneath the diaper area is changed as needed to keep the skin dry and free of irritation. When urinary retention is present, gentle pressure applied to the suprapubic area will facilitate emptying of the bladder, which is still an abdominal organ in early infancy.

Since the bowel sphincter is frequently affected, there is continual passage of stool, often misinterpreted as diarrhea, which is a constant irritant to the skin and a source of infection to the spinal lesion. This provides another rationale for closure before the infant's first feeding since the meconium is still free of organisms.

Areas of sensory and motor impairment are subject to skin breakdown and therefore require meticulous care. Placing the infant on a soft foam or fleece pad reduces pressure on the knees and ankles. Periodic cleansing with application of lotion and gentle massage aid circulation. Changing linen is best accomplished by two persons—one changes the linen while the other holds the infant, assuring that the spine is maintained in good alignment without tension in the area of the defect.

Gentle range of motion exercises are sometimes car-

ried out to prevent contractures, and stretching of contractures is done when indicated. However, these exercises may be restricted to the foot, ankle, and knee joint. Where the hip joints are unstable, stretching against tight hip flexors or adductor muscles, which act much like bowstrings, may aggravate a tendency toward subluxation. In addition, the bones of these infants tend to be fragile and subject to fractures.

Since infants with meningomyelocele cannot be held in the arms and cuddled for some time as unaffected infants are, their need for tactile stimulation is met by fondling, stroking, and other comfort measures. Bright mobiles or other objects can be placed within the infant's view, and other stimulating activities usually provided for infants are appropriate. All infants respond to pleasant sounds.

Observation. The nurse is in a position to aid the physician in determining the extent of neuromuscular involvement. Movement of the extremities or skin response, especially an anal reflex, that might provide cues to the degree of motor or sensory status is noted. The head circumference is measured daily (see p. 90), and the fontanels are examined for signs of tension or bulging. The nurse is also alert to early signs of infection, such as an elevated temperature (axillary), irritability, lethargy, and nuchal rigidity, and to signs of increased intracranial pressure.

Parent education and long-term supervision. As soon as the parents are emotionally able to cope with the infant's condition, they should become actively involved in his care. They need to learn how to continue at home the care that has been initiated in the hospital—positioning, feeding, skin care, manual expression of urine, and range of motion exercises when appropriate. In cases in which the defect has not been repaired, they are taught to care for the lesion and to observe for signs of complications.

The long-range planning with and support of the parents and child begin in the hospital and extend throughout childhood and beyond. Long-term care of these children is of uncertain length. The child will need numerous hospitalizations over the years, and each one will be a source of stress to which the younger child is especially vulnerable. The multiple aspects in care of the child include bowel and bladder control, orthopedic appliances, and the observation and management of complications, especially urinary tract infections and pressure necrosis.

The Spina Bifida Association of America* has a network of chapters throughout the country where health professionals and families can obtain information, education, and a list of resources providing financial and other types of support.

---

*343 S. Dearborn Street, Chicago, IL 60604.

SUMMARY OF NURSING CARE OF THE INFANT WITH MENINGOMYELOCELE

GOALS	RESPONSIBILITIES
Prevent local infection	Cleanse meningomyelocele carefully with sterile saline or hydrogen peroxide solution as ordered
	Inspect meningomyelocele for any changes in appearance, for example, abrasions, tears, signs of infection
	Apply sterile dressings (moisten with sterile solution as ordered—saline, silver nitrate, antibiotic)
	Report any change in appearance
	Position the infant to prevent contamination from urine and stool
	Administer antibiotics as ordered
	Administer similar care of operative site postoperatively
Prevent local trauma	Handle the infant carefully
	Place the infant in prone position or side-lying position, if permitted
	Apply protective devices
	Modify routine nursing activities, for example, feeding, making bed, comforting activities
Prevent complications	Observe for signs of hydrocephalus
	Measure head circumference daily
	Check fontanels for tenseness or bulging
	Note irritability, lethargy, difficulty in feeding, high-pitched cry
	Observe for signs of meningeal irritation and inflammation, for example, fever, nuchal rigidity, irritability (take vital signs every 2 to 4 hours as ordered)
Prevent urinary tract infection	Avoid contamination with stool
	Empty bladder periodically (apply gentle, downward pressure to bladder—Credé's manuever)
Prevent skin breakdown	Change position frequently
	Place soft foam or fleece pad under the infant
	Rub skin periodically to stimulate circulation
	Maintain meticulous skin cleanliness
	Apply protective substance to areas where excoriation is most likely—anal and perineal areas, knees, elbows, ankles, and chin
Prevent or minimize hip and lower extremity deformity	Carry out passive range of motion exercises
	Carry out muscle stretching when indicated
	Carry out exercises with care to avoid fracturing fragile bones
	Maintain hips in slight to moderate abduction to prevent dislocation
Maintain hydration and electrolyte balance	Measure intake and output
	Administer fluids as ordered
	Observe for signs of dehydration
Maintain warmth	Place the infant in Isolette or use an overhead warmer
Provide nutrition	Provide diet for age
	Devise feeding techniques to assure adequate intake
Provide tender, loving care	Fondle and caress
	Speak to the child
	Encourage the parents to visit and fondle the infant
	Use an *en face* position as often as possible
Deal with parental anxiety about recurrence in future children	Refer the parents to genetic counseling service

Continued.

SUMMARY OF NURSING CARE OF THE INFANT WITH MENINGOMYELOCELE—cont'd

GOALS	RESPONSIBILITIES

Prepare the parents for discharge of the child	Assess ability of the parents to care for the infant
	Teach the parents essential aspects of the infant's physical care
	    Allow ample time for preparation
	    Encourage questions and expression of feelings
	    Allow for supervised practice in care
	Refer for evaluation of foster-care placement when the parents are unable or unwilling to care for the child
	
	Give anticipatory guidance regarding development expectations
	Teach the parents to observe for signs of complications
	    Signs of infection
	    Signs of possible shunt failure (when shunt procedure has been performed for hydrocephalus)

Facilitate developmental progress	Help the parents plan activities appropriate to developmental level Assist with nursery school and educational placement
Support the parents	Provide or arrange for ongoing contact with the family Refer to parent groups
Coordinate services	Plan for home visits where needed Maintain contact with the family Make appointments for follow-up care Make referrals to special agencies as needed Act as liaison between inpatient and outpatient services

SPINAL MUSCULAR ATROPHY

The disorders designated as the spinal muscular atrophies are characterized by progressive weakness and wasting of skeletal muscles caused by progressive degeneration of anterior horn cells. These diseases are inherited as autosomal-recessive traits and appear primarily in infancy.

Progressive spinal muscular atrophy of infants (Werdnig-Hoffmann paralysis)

The most severe form of neurogenic atrophy and the most common paralytic form of the "floppy infant syndrome" is Werdnig-Hoffmann paralysis. The site of the pathologic condition is the anterior horn cells of the spinal cord and the motor nuclei of the brainstem. The primary effect is atrophy of skeletal muscles.

This disorder is manifest early, usually at birth, frequently in utero, and almost always before age 2 years. Inactivity of the infant is the most prominent feature. The child lies with his legs in the frog position; breathing is diaphragmatic with sternal retractions caused by intercostal muscle paralysis; and there are weakness and limited movements of the shoulder and arm muscles. The child's cry and cough are weak, and secretions tend to pool in the pharynx. The facies are alert, and sensation and intellect are normal.

The diagnosis is established from electromyography, which demonstrates a denervation pattern, and is confirmed by muscle biopsy. Early death from respiratory failure or infection is usual. The most common complication is pneumonia. Few children with this type of paralysis live beyond 4 or 5 years of age.

Juvenile spinal muscular atrophy (Kugelberg-Welander disease)

Juvenile spinal muscular atrophy is also characterized by anterior horn cell and motor nerve degeneration. The onset of proximal muscle weakness (especially of the pelvic girdle) appears later, in early childhood or adolescence, and the progression is slower. Muscles of the lower arms and legs are involved relatively late, and muscles of the trunk and those supplied by the cranial nerves are usually unaffected. Many affected persons have a normal life expectancy.

Nursing considerations

The infant and small child with extensive paralysis requires frequent change of position to prevent complications, especially pneumonia. The pharynx requires frequent suctioning to remove secretions, and feeding must be carried out slowly and carefully to prevent aspiration. Since these children are intellectually normal, verbal, tactile, and auditory stimulation are important aspects of care. Supporting them so that they can see the activities around them and transporting them in a buggy to provide them with a change of environment provide stimulation and a broader scope of contacts.

Parents of a chronically ill or potentially fatally ill child require a great deal of support and encouragement (see Chapter 16). The parents of a child with a genetically transmitted disorder also need to be encouraged to seek genetic counseling.

PROGRESSIVE NEUROPATHIC (PERONEAL) MUSCULAR ATROPHY (CHARCOT-MARIE-TOOTH DISEASE)

Progressive neuropathic (peroneal) muscular atrophy is a slowly progressive disorder characterized by gradual wasting of distal limb musculature. The disease is usually inherited by autosomal-dominant transmission, although exceptions have been reported. The age of onset is late childhood or adolescence, and muscle wasting involving first the intrinsic foot muscles and those of the anterolateral aspect of the lower leg is seen. In time the wasting extends proximally to include the entire lower leg and sometimes the lower thigh. This distal wasting gives the "stork leg" appearance to the lower extremities, and the footdrop leads to the high-stepping, foot-slapping gait. No specific treatment is available. The disease is slowly progressive but has no effect on the life span. With orthopedic assistance it usually causes little disability.

MYOTONIAS

The myotonias are a group of muscle disorders characterized by increased irritability and contractility of skeletal muscles with decreased power of relaxation and either wasting or hypertrophy of the affected muscles. All are aggravated by cold. Myotonia is also a symptom of other disorders, such as familial hyperkalemia periodic paralysis and McArdle's disease, a glycogen storage disease caused by deficiency of muscle phosphorylase.

MUSCULAR DYSTROPHIES

The muscular dystrophies constitute the largest and most important single group of muscle diseases of childhood. They all have a genetic origin in which there is gradual degeneration of muscle fibers and are characterized by progressive weakness and wasting of symmetric groups of skeletal muscles with increasing disability and deformity. In all forms of muscular dystrophy there is insidious loss of strength, but each differs in regard to muscle groups affected, age of onset, rate of progression, and inheritance patterns (Fig. 29-3). The most common form, *Duchenne muscular dystrophy,* is considered separately in the next section.

Fascioscapulohumeral (Landouzy-Déjérine) muscular dystrophy is inherited as an autosomal dominant disorder with onset in early adolescence. It is characterized by difficulty raising the arms over the head, lack of facial mobility, and a forward slope of the shoulders. The progression is slow.

Limb-girdle muscular dystrophy is an autosomal-recessive disease of later childhood or adolescence with variable, but usually slow, progression and characterized by weakness of proximal muscles of both pelvic and shoulder girdles.

Treatment of the muscular dystrophies consists mainly of supportive measures. This includes physical therapy to improve mobility, orthopedic procedures to minimize deformity, and assistance for the affected child in meeting the demands of daily living.

Pseudohypertrophic (Duchenne) Muscular Dystrophy

The most severe and the most common muscular dystrophy seen in childhood is pseudohypertrophic muscular dystrophy. The incidence is approximately 0.14:1000 children, and an X-linked inheritance pattern is identified in 50% of cases; the remainder appear as sporadic cases and probably represent fresh mutations. As in all X-linked disorders, males are affected almost exclusively. The basic defect in muscular dystrophy is unknown.

Clinical manifestations. Evidence of muscle weakness usually appears during the third year, although there may have been a history of delay in motor development, particularly walking. Difficulty in running, riding a bicycle, and climbing stairs are usually the first symptoms noted. Later abnormal gait on a level surface becomes apparent. In the early years rapid developmental gains may mask the progression of the disease. Questioning the parents may reveal difficulty in rising from a sitting or supine position. Occasionally enlarged calves may be noticed by parents.

Typically the affected male has a waddling gait and

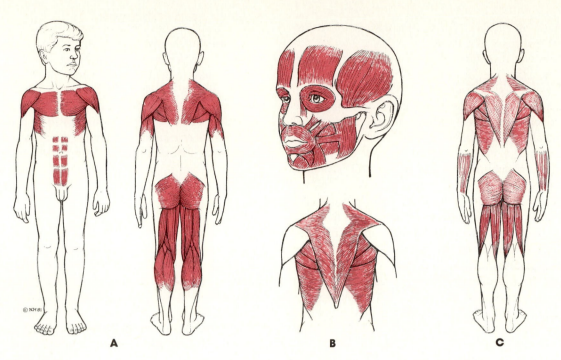

Fig. 29-3

Initial muscle groups involved in the muscular dystrophies. **A,** *Pseudohypertrophic.* **B,** *Facioscapulohumerol.* **C,** *Limb-girdle.*

lordosis, falls frequently, and develops a characteristic manner of rising from a squatting or sitting position on the floor (Gower sign)—he turns onto his side or abdomen, flexes his knees to assume a kneeling position, then with knees extended gradually pushes his torso to an upright position by "walking" his hands up his legs. The muscles, especially those of the thighs and upper arms, become enlarged from fatty infiltration and feel unusually firm or woody on palpation.

The name "pseudohypertrophy" is derived from this muscular enlargement. Profound muscular atrophy occurs in later stages, and as the disease progresses, contractures and deformities involving large and small joints are common. Ambulation usually becomes impossible by 12 years of age. Facial, oropharyngeal, and respiratory muscles are spared until the terminal stages of the disease. Ultimately the disease process involves the diaphragm and auxiliary muscles of respiration, and cardiomegaly is common.

Diagnostic evaluation

The disease is confirmed by serum enzyme measurement, muscle biopsy, and electromyography. The serum creatine phosphokinase, aldolase, and serum glutamic-oxaloacetic transaminase levels are extremely high in the first 2 years of life before onset of clinical weakness. They diminish with muscle deterioration but do not reach normal levels until severe muscle wasting and incapacitation have oc-

curred. Muscle biopsy reveals degeneration of muscle fibers with fibrosis and fatty tissue replacement. Electromyography shows decrease in amplitude and duration of motor unit potentials. Ultrasound imaging is assuming a more prominant place in the diagnosis of muscle disease.

Therapeutic management

There is no effective treatment for childhood muscular dystrophy. Maintaining function in unaffected muscles for as long as possible is the primary goal. It has been found that children who remain as active as possible are able to avoid wheelchair confinement for a longer period of time. Early recourse to a wheelchair accelerates deconditioning and promotes the development of lower extremity contractures. Maintenance of function often includes range of motion exercises, surgery to release contracture deformities, bracing, and performance of activities of daily living (ADL).

The major complications of muscular dystrophy (contractures, disuse atrophy, infection, obesity, and cardiopulmonary problems) are managed with appropriate therapies. The cause of death is usually respiratory tract infection or cardiac failure.

Genetic counseling is recommended for parents, female siblings, and maternal aunts and their female offspring.

Nursing considerations

The major emphasis of nursing care is to assist the child and his family to cope with the progressive, incapacitating, and fatal nature of the disease, to help design a program that will afford a greater degree of independence and reduce the predictable and preventable disabilities associated with the disorder, and to assist them to deal constructively with the limitations the disease imposes on their daily lives.

Working closely with other team members, nurses help the family in developing the child's self-help skills to give the child the satisfaction of being as independent as possible for as long as possible. This requires continual evaluation of the child's capabilities, which are often difficult to assess. It is not always possible to know when the child seeks parental assistance because he wants a little extra attention or because his muscles are overtired. Fortunately most children with muscular dystrophy instinctually recognize this need to be as independent as possible and strive to do so.

Practical difficulties faced by families are physical limitations of housing and mobility. Parents also need help in buying and modifying clothing for their disabled child. It is difficult to find clothing and footwear to wear comfortably in a wheelchair, to fit over contracted limbs, and to fit the obese child. Parent's social activities are also restricted, and the family's activities must be continually modified to the needs of the affected child.

The concentrated efforts and full-time commitment to the care of these children in the later stages of the disease is frequently cause for their placement in a skilled nursing facility. Helping the parents with this decision and supporting them through their guilt and distress are important nursing functions.

No matter how successful the program and how well the family adapts to the disorder, superimposed on the physical and emotional problems associated with a child with a long-term disability is the constant presence of the ultimate outcome of the disease. All of the manifestations seen in the child with a fatal illness are encountered in these families (see Chapter 16). The guilt feelings of the mother may be particularly pronounced in this disorder because of the mother-to-son transmission of the defective gene.

Nurses can be alert to problems and needs of the families and make necessary referrals when supplementary services are indicated. The Muscular Dystrophy Association of America, Inc.* has branches in most communities to provide assistance to families in which there is a member with muscular dystrophy.

---

*810 Seventh Avenue, New York, NY 10019

ACQUIRED NEUROMUSCULAR DISORDERS

Neuromuscular disorders can be acquired. Most are caused by either trauma or infectious agents. Botulism and tetanus are discussed later in this chapter. Rhabdomyosarcoma, a tumor involving muscle tissue, is not a neuromuscular disorder, but it is considered here for convenience.

INFECTIOUS POLYNEURITIS (GUILLAIN-BARRÉ SYNDROME)

Infectious polyneuritis, also known as infectious neuronitis and Landry's or Guillain-Barré syndrome, is probably the most common form of polyneuritis and may occur at any age. Although children are less often affected than adults, the incidence in the pediatric age-group appears to be increasing, with higher susceptibility in children between ages 4 and 10 years. Both sexes are affected with equal frequency.

Pathophysiology

The precise etiologic agent is unknown. Since the disease has been associated with a number of viral infections or the administration of vaccines, it has been suggested that it may be a toxic sequela of an original infection, an activated latent virus, or a manifestation of an acute infection. It is an acute polyneuropathy in which motor dysfunction predominates over sensory disturbance and in which there is bilateral facial paresis or paralysis and, occasionally, weakness of the bulbar and respiratory musculature. Some believe that it may represent a cell-mediated immunologic response directed at the peripheral nerves. Pathologic changes show inflammation and segmented demyelination of peripheral nerves.

Clinical manifestations

The paralytic manifestations are usually preceded by a mild influenza-like illness or sore throat. In 3 to 12 days neurologic symptoms appear, initially involving muscle tenderness and sometimes accompanied by paresthesia and cramps. Symmetric muscle weakness, which progresses to paralysis, starts in the periphery and rapidly ascends from the lower extremities, frequently involving the muscles of the trunk, upper extremities, and those supplied by cranial nerves. Paralysis is flaccid with loss of reflexes and may include variable degrees of sensory impairment. Paralysis of facial, extraocular, labial, lingual, pharyngeal, and laryngeal muscles may be affected. Evidence of intercostal and phrenic nerve involvement includes breathlessness in vocalizations and shallow, irregular respirations. Most patients complain of muscle tenderness or sensitivity to slight pressure. Urinary incontinence or retention and constipation are frequently present.

Course. The general health of the child and the extent of paralysis influence the outcome of the illness. Almost all deaths are caused by respiratory failure; therefore, early diagnosis and access to respiratory support are especially important. Muscle function begins to return 2 days to 2 weeks after the onset of symptoms, and recovery is complete in most cases. The rate of recovery is usually related to the degree of involvement, which may extend from a few weeks to months. The greater the degree of paralysis, the longer the recovery phase.

Diagnostic evaluation

Cerebrospinal fluid analysis reveals an increased protein concentration, but other laboratory studies are noncontributory. The symmetric nature of the paralysis helps differentiate this disorder from spinal paralytic poliomyelitis, which usually affects sporadic muscles.

Therapeutic management

Treatment of Guillain-Barré syndrome is symptomatic. Corticosteroid therapy has been of benefit in the early stages. Respiratory and pharyngeal involvement require assisted ventilation, frequently with tracheostomy.

Nursing considerations

Nursing care is essentially supportive and is the same as that required for quadriplegia from any cause. The emphasis of care is on close observation to assess the extent of paralysis and on prevention of complications.

During the acute phase of the disease the child's condition should be carefully observed for possible difficulty in swallowing and respiratory involvement. A respirator with a cardiac monitor attached is kept on standby, and suction apparatus, tracheostomy tray, and vasoconstrictor drugs are kept available at the bedside. Vital signs and level of consciousness are monitored frequently. The child who develops respiratory dysfunction requires the same care as any child who requires mechanical ventilation and who suffers paralysis.

Physical therapy is limited to passive range of motion exercises during the evolving phase of the disease. Later, as the disease stabilizes and as recovery begins, an active physical therapy program is implemented to prevent contracture deformities and facilitate muscle recovery. This may include active exercise, gait training, and bracing.

Throughout the course of the illness child and parent support is paramount. The rapidity of the paralysis and the long period of recovery greatly tax the emotional reserves of all family members. The parents and child benefit from repeated reassurance that recovery is occurring and from realistic information regarding the possibility of permanent disabililty. In the event of a residual handicap, the family needs assistance in accepting and adjusting to the loss of function (see Chapter 16).

RHABDOMYOSARCOMA

Soft-tissue sarcomas are malignant neoplasms that originate from undifferentiated mesenchymal cells in muscle, tendons, bursae, and fascia or fibrous, connective, lymphatic, or vascular tissue. They derive their name from the specific tissue(s) of origin, such as myosarcoma (*myo,* muscle). Rhabdomyosarcoma (*rhabdo,* striated) is the most common soft-tissue sarcoma in children. Because striated (skeletal) muscle is found almost anywhere in the body, these tumors occur in many sites, the most common of which are the head and neck, especially the orbit.

Rhabdomyosarcoma occurs in children of all age-groups, but is seen most commonly in children younger than 5 years of age. Males are affected more frequently than females.

Clinical manifestations

The initial signs and symptoms are related to the site of the tumor and compression of adjacent organs. Some tumor locations, particularly the orbit, produce symptoms early in the course of the illness and contribute to rapid diagnosis and improved prognosis. Such symptoms include unilateral proptosis (protrusion of the eyeball), ecchymosis of the conjunctiva, and strabismus. Other tumors, such as those of the retroperitoneal area, produce no symptoms until they become large, invasive, and widely metastasized. At this point, an abdominal mass, pain, and signs of intestinal or genitourinary obstruction are seen. In some instances a primary tumor site is never identified.

Diagnostic evaluation

Diagnosis begins with a careful examination of the head and neck area, particularly palpation of a nontender, firm, hard mass. This is especially important because the signs and symptoms of the disorder are vague and frequently suggest a common childhood illness. The nasopharynx and oropharynx are inspected for any evidence of visible mass.

Radiographic studies are performed to isolate a tumor site. Chest radiographic examinations, lung tomograms, bone surveys, and bone marrow aspiration are also carried out to rule out metastasis. Other tests that are used include a lumbar puncture for head and neck tumors, and a lymphangiogram for tumors of lower extremities and genital regions. An excisional biopsy confirms the histologic type.

Therapeutic management

Since the tumor is highly malignant, with metastasis at the time of diagnosis, aggressive multimodal therapy is recommended. Complete removal of the primary tumor is advocated whenever possible. However, biopsy only is required in certain tumor locations, such as those of the orbit when followed by radiation and chemotherapy. This is a fortunate change because it avoids the devastating effects of enucleation, amputation, or pelvic exenteration.

High-dose radiation to the primary tumor is recommended in combination with chemotherapy. Chemotherapy is indicated in all stages of the disease and discontinued after 1 to 2 years.

Nursing considerations

The nursing responsibilities for children with rhabdomyosarcoma are similar to those for other types of cancer, especially the solid tumors when surgery is employed. Specific objectives include (1) careful assessment for signs of the tumor, particularly during routine physical examinations; (2) preparation of the child and family for the multiple diagnostic tests; and (3) supportive care during each stage of multimodal therapy (see Chapter 16).

SPINAL CORD INJURIES

Spinal cord injuries with major neurologic involvement are not a common cause of physical handicap in childhood. However, there are a sufficient number of children with these injuries admitted to major medical centers and, because of the increased survival rate as the result of improved management, nurses are more likely to become involved with such children.

Mechanisms of injury

In automobile accidents, most spinal cord injuries in children are the result of indirect trauma caused by sudden hyperflexion or hyperextension of the neck, often combined with a rotational force. Trauma to the spinal cord without evidence of vertebral fracture or dislocation is particularly likely to occur in a motor vehicle accident when proper restraints are not used. An unrestrained child becomes a projectile during sudden deceleration and is subject to injury from contact with a variety of objects inside and outside the vehicle.

Falling from heights takes place less often in children than in adults, but vertebral compression from blows to the head or buttocks can occur in water sports (diving and surfing), falls from horses, or other athletic injuries. Birth injuries may occur in breech deliveries from traction force on the cord during delivery of the head and shoulders. A number of teenagers receive cord injuries when they are accidentally shot or stabbed in the back.

The injury sustained can affect any of the spinal nerves, and the higher the injury, the more extensive the damage. The child can be left with complete or partial paralysis of the lower extremities (paraplegia) or sustain damage at a higher level, which leaves him without functional use of all four extremities (quadraplegia). A high cervical cord injury that affects the phrenic nerve paralyzes the diaphragm and leaves the child dependent on a respirator.

Therapeutic management

In any situation in which spinal cord injury is suspected or a possibility, the child is calmed, reassured, and advised not to move, and no person should be allowed to move him unless they are able to do so carefully. He must be lifted gently and without undue haste (preferably by a coordinated team) to avoid twisting or bending the spine. If the child is conscious, he is placed supine on a rigid surface to prevent sagging. Because of the complexity and relative infrequency of these injuries, it is usually recommended that the injured person be transferred to a spinal injury center for care by a team of specially trained professionals.

Nursing considerations

The nursing care of the paraplegic or quadriplegic child is complex and challenging. As a member of the acute care and rehabilitation teams, the nurse is invovled in all aspects of care. Ideally initial care takes place in a special intensive care unit with personnel trained to handle spinal cord injuries. Nursing management is concerned primarily with prevention of complications and maintenance of function.

Once the acute period is over, the lesion is usually static and nonprogressive, regardless of whether the paralysis is secondary to trauma, congenital defects, infection, treated tumor, or surgery. In the treatment of children with spinal cord injuries, nurses are members of a team that consists of specialists, including physicians from a number of specialty areas, physical and occupational therapists, psychologists, social workers, teachers, and vocational counselors. Each member has a unique contribution to make, and mutual agreement for specific areas of responsibility is determined during regularly scheduled team conferences.

The complexity of the care and the extensive knowledge required are beyond the scope of this volume. The reader who is interested in the multiple problems of spinal cord rehabilitation is directed to the more extensive coverage in Whaley and Wong (1983) or to books that deal exclusively with the problem.

DISEASES OF THE NEUROMUSCULAR JUNCTION

Several diseases are responsible for muscle weakness or paralysis as a result of a defect in transmission of nerve impulses at the myoneural junction. Normally nerve impulses are transmitted to skeletal muscles across the neuromuscular junction by acetylcholine. Any interference with this physiologic function will block transmission of nerve impulses and prevent muscular contraction. Several toxic substances act at the myoneural junction to inhibit nerve impulses to the skeletal muscles. Examples of toxins that prevent release of acetylcholine are those that produce the paralysis of botulism and tick paralysis. Action at receptor sites is blocked by the drug tubocurarine (Curare). Paralysis caused by the inhibition of cholinesterase release can be caused by poisoning with organic phosphate insecticides.

TETANUS

Tetanus, or lockjaw, is an acute, preventable, and often fatal disease caused by the exotoxin produced by the anaerobic spore-forming, gram-positive bacillus *Clostridium tetani*. It is characterized by painful muscular rigidity primarily involving the masseter and neck muscles. There are four requirements for the development of tetanus: (1) presence of tetanus spores or vegetative forms of the bacillus, (2) injury to the tissues, (3) wound conditions that encourage multiplication of the organism, and (4) a susceptible host.

Tetanus spores are found in the soil and dust and in the intestinal tracts of humans and animals, especially herbivorous animals. The organisms are more prevalent in rural areas but are readily carried to urban areas by the wind. The organisms are not invasive but enter the body by way of wounds, particularly a puncture wound, burn, or crushed area. They may enter through a very minor, unnoticed break in the skin such as a thorn or needle prick, bee sting, or scratch. In the newborn, infection may occur through the umbilical cord, usually in situations in which infants are delivered in contaminated surroundings. The disease has the greatest incidence in months when persons are more involved in outdoor activities. Drug addicts are especially susceptible because of poor injection technique and the use of street heroin, which is often mixed with quinine, a protoplasmic poison that favors the growth of the organism.

Pathophysiology

When conditions are favorable, the organisms proliferate and elaborate an exotoxin that acts at the myoneural junc-

tion to produce the muscular stiffness and lower the threshold for reflex excitability. The ideal conditions for growth of the organisms are devitalized tissues without access to air, such as wounds that have not been washed or kept clean and those that have crusted over, trapping pus beneath.

Clinical manifestations

The incubation period for tetanus varies from 1 to 54 days but is generally less than 14 days. The more extensive the injury, the shorter the incubation period and the more severe the symptoms.

There are several forms of the disease, but the generalized form is the most common and dangerous. The manner of onset varies, but the initial symptoms are usually a progressive stiffness and tenderness of the muscles in the neck and jaw. The characteristic difficulty in opening the mouth (*trismus*), which is caused by sustained contraction of the jaw-closing muscles, is evident early and gives the disease its common name, lockjaw. Spasm of facial muscles produces the so-called sardonic smile (*risus sardonicus*).

Progressive involvement of the trunk muscles causes opisthotonos and a boardlike rigidity of abdominal and limb muscles. There is difficulty in swallowing, and the patient is highly sensitive to external stimuli. The slightest noise, a gentle touch, or bright light will trigger convulsive muscular contractions that last from a few seconds to minutes. The paroxysmal contractions recur with increased frequency until they become almost continuous. The patient's mentation is unaffected; therefore, he remains alert and reflects his pain and distress with rapid pulse, sweating, and an anxious expression.

Laryngospasm and tetany of respiratory muscles and accumulated secretions predispose to respiratory arrest, atelectasis, and pneumonia. Fever is usually absent or only mild; presence of fever generally indicates a poor prognosis. As the child recovers from the disease, the paroxysms become less and less frequent and gradually subside. Survival beyond 4 days usually indicates recovery, but complete recovery may require weeks.

Therapeutic management: prevention

Preventive measures are based on the immune status of the affected child and the nature of the injury. Specific prophylactic therapy after trauma is administration of either tetanus toxoid or tetanus antitoxin. Children who have completed the immunization series (see p. 241) are given a tetanus toxoid booster prophylactically if none has been given in the prior 10 years for a clean minor wound or, if there is a heavily contaminated wound, if none has been given in the previous 5 years. Protective levels of antibody are maintained for at least 10 years; therefore, antitoxin is not indicated for the fully immunized child. (See also Tables 8-4 and 8-5.)

The unprotected or inadequately immunized child who sustains a "tetanus-prone" wound (contaminated soil, crush injury, burn, compound fracture, retained foreign body, or a wound unattended for 24 hours, for example) should receive human tetanus immune globulin (TIG). Human tetanus immune globulin is preferred to bovine or horse tetanus antitoxin (TAT) because of its absence of sensitivity reactions and longer half-life. Concurrent administration of both human tetanus immune globulin and (when indicated) toxoid at separate sites is recommended both to provide protection and to initiate the active immune process. Completion of active immunization is carried out according to the usual pattern.

Therapeutic management: treatment

The affected child is best treated in an intensive care facility where close and constant observation and equipment for monitoring and respiratory support are readily available. A quiet environment is preferred to reduce external stimuli. Neonates are placed in an open unit or Isolette to maintain a constant environmental temperature and oxygen supply.

General supportive care is provided, including maintenance of adequate fluid and electrolyte balance and caloric intake. Indwelling oral or nasogastric feedings are used whenever possible, but severe laryngospasm may be an indication for intravenous alimentation or gastrostomy feeding. Recurrent laryngospasm or excessive accumulation of secretions may require endotracheal intubation.

Antitoxin therapy to neutralize toxins not yet bound to nervous tissue is the most specific therapy for tetanus. Human tetanus immune globulin is preferred, but, if unavailable, bovine or horse tetanus antitoxin is given. Antibiotics are administered to control the proliferation of the vegetative forms of the organism at the site of infection. When the child recovers, active immunization should take place since the disease does not confer a permanent immunity.

Local care of the wound by surgical débridement and cleansing helps reduce the numbers of proliferating organisms at the site of injury. An antibacterial agent such as povidone-iodine (Betadine) followed by a dilute solution of hydrogen peroxide has proved effective. The cleansing should be repeated several times during the first 48 hours, and deep infected lacerations are usually exposed and débrided.

Sedatives or muscle relaxants are administered to help reduce muscle spasm and prevent convulsions. The most widely used is diazepam (Valium), but phenobarbital, chloral hydrate, the phenothiazines, and paraldehyde may be employed. Patients with severe tetanus and those who do not respond to other sedatives may require the administration of a neuromuscular blocking agent, such as tubocurarine (Curare) or pancuronium bromide (Pavulon). Because of their paralytic effect on respiratory muscles, use of these drugs requires mechanical ventilation and constant attendance by trained personnel until muscle spasms are controlled.

Tracheostomy is often indicated and should be performed before severe respiratory distress develops. Administration of corticosteroid preparations has met with success in some instances.

Nursing considerations

In caring for the child with tetanus, every effort is made to control or eliminate stimulation from sound, light, and touch. Although a darkened room is ideal, sufficient light is essential in order that the child can be carefully observed; light appears to be less irritating than vibratory or auditory stimuli. The infant or child is handled as little as possible, and extra effort is expended to avoid any sudden and/or loud noise.

Medications are administered as prescribed, and vital signs are observed and recorded at frequent intervals. The location and extent of muscle spasms and assessment of their severity are important nursing observations. Respiratory status is carefully evaluated for any signs of embarrassment, and appropriate emergency equipment is kept available at all times. Muscle relaxants and sedatives that may be prescribed can also cause respiratory depression; therefore, the child must be assessed for excessive central nervous system depression. Blood gases are obtained frequently to evaluate the respiratory status. Attention to hydration and nutrition may involve monitoring an intravenous infusion, monitoring nasogastric or gastrostomy feedings, and suctioning oropharyngeal secretions when indictated.

If a potent muscle relaxant, such as pancuronium bromide or tubocurarine, is used, the total paralysis makes oral communication impossible. Therefore, the child's needs must be anticipated and all procedures are carefully explained beforehand. As the dose of medication is decreased, the child regains movement of the eyelids and facial muscles, giving him some opportunity to express emotions and indicate choices through a signal system, for example, blinking the lids to indicate "yes" or "no."

Although most affected children are neonates and receive the nursing care and assessment of any high-risk infant (Chapter 7), the older child may acquire a tetanus infection. Since the child's mental status is clear, he is aware of what is happening to him and is often in a state of terror. He should not be left alone, and all efforts are made to reduce his anxiety, which can contribute to muscular spasms. A calm and reassuring manner and sympathetic understanding can help immeasurably in getting the child and his parents through this crisis situation. Emotional support of parents is an essential part of comprehensive care as it is in all high anxiety situations.

BOTULISM

Botulism is a serious food poisoning that results from ingestion of the preformed toxin produced by the anaerobic bacillus *Clostridium botulinum*. The most common source of the toxin is improperly sterilized home-canned foods. Nervous system symptoms appear abruptly about 12 to 36 hours after ingestion of contaminated food and may or may not have been preceded by acute digestive disturbance. There is weakness, dizziness, headache, difficulty in talking and speaking, diplopia, and vomiting. Progressive respiratory paralysis is life threatening.

Infant botulism (unlike the disease in older persons) is caused by the ingestion of spores or vegetative cells of *C. botulinum* which colonize the gastrointestinal tract and release a powerful toxin. There appears to be no common food or drug source of the organisms; however, the *C. botulinum* organisms have been found in honey fed to affected infants. Characteristic symptoms include constipation, lethargy, and poor feeding in a previously well infant. Neurologic examination reveals general weakness, hypotonia, and cranial nerve involvement.

Treatment consists of intravenous administration of botulism antitoxin (this is controversial for infants) and general supportive measures, including respiratory support and nutrition. Since the toxin has a relatively short half-life and does not bind to tissues firmly, therapy is continued until paralysis abates.

Nursing responsibilities include observing for and reporting signs of muscle impairment and providing intensive nursing care when the infant is hospitalized. Parental support and reassurance is important. Most infants recover when the disorder is recognized and therapy implemented. Home supervision of the outpatient and education regarding prevention of infection (such as using properly canned foods and avoiding use of honey as formula sweetener) are nursing responsibilities.

TICK PARALYSIS

Saliva from certain ticks contains a neurotoxin that inhibits the release of acetylcholine, producing a rapidly ascending paralysis that is often accompanied by pain and hypersensitivity. Diagnosis is established on discovery of the imbedded tick. Total removal of the tick is followed by rapid improvement and recovery; otherwise death may result from respiratory paralysis (see Table 27-8).

MYASTHENIA GRAVIS

Myasthenia gravis is relatively uncommon in childhood but may appear in two forms: neonatal and juvenile. The precise mechanism has not been determined, although the abnormality is associated with altered function of cholinesterase on the acetylcholine released at the neuromuscular junction. An autoimmune response has also been implicated.

Neonatal myasthenia gravis

A *transient* form of myasthenia gravis occurs in infants born to mothers with myasthenia gravis who may not be aware that they have the disease. These infants display generalized weakness and hypotonia at birth with a depressed Moro reflex, ptosis, ineffective sucking and swallowing reflexes, and weak cry. There is no evidence of neurologic damage. In this form the symptoms usually disappear within 2 to 4 weeks.

Persistent neonatal myasthenia gravis appears indistinguishable from the transient form, but the mother usually does not have the disease. The disease persists throughout life, and more than one sibling may be affected, which suggests a genetic etiology. Sex distribution is equal. The disorder is relatively resistant to drug therapy, and the eyelid and extraocular muscles are usually the muscles most severely affected.

Juvenile myasthenia gravis

Juvenile myasthenia gravis appears to be identical to that seen in adults and usually has its onset after age 10 years but may appear as early as age 2 years. Girls are affected six times as often as boys. The most common symptoms are general paralysis of the optic muscles with ptosis and diplopia. Difficulty in swallowing, chewing, and speaking are also prominent, accompanied by weakness and paralysis of all skeletal muscles. The signs and symptoms are more pronounced in the late afternoon and evening. They are relieved by rest and made worse by exercise.

The diagnosis is made on the basis of the characteristic distribution of muscle weakness and the progressive weakness on repeated or sustained muscular contraction. The diagnosis is established by observation of the response to the anticholinesterase drugs. Intravenous administration of a small test dose of edrophonium (Tensilon) or neostigmine (Prostigmin) produces a beneficial effect in 1 minute but lasts for less than 5 minutes. Electromyography is helpful in diagnosis and reveals high amplitude muscle responses followed by contractions of rapidly diminishing amplitude.

Treatment consists of the oral administration of anticholinesterase drugs, the least toxic of which is pyridostigmine (Mestinon). An initial small dose is given and the dosage is gradually increased until a satisfactory result is obtained. The child must be observed for signs of parasympathetic stimulation from overmedication. These include lacrimation, salivation, abdominal cramps, sweating, diarrhea, vomiting, bradycardia, and weakness of respiratory muscles.

These children need continuous medical and nursing supervision. The parents are taught the importance of accurate administration of medications, with special emphasis on recognizing side effects with the dangers of choking, aspiration, and respiratory distress.

Parents are counseled regarding promoting a life-style that minimizes stress and maximizes relaxation. Strenuous activity is discouraged. They are also warned of the possibility of a sudden exacerbation of symptoms during times of physical or emotional stress (myasthenia crisis) that requires immediate medical attention. They should receive instruction in providing respiratory assistance until help arrives or the child can be transported to medical aid.

The prognosis in persistent congenital myasthenia gravis is usually good. Although there is gradual worsening of symptoms with age, the life span is not affected significantly. A high percentage of persons with childhood-onset (juvenile) myasthenia gravis become resistant or unresponsive to medication, with the danger of exacerbation and respiratory failure. Spontaneous remissions are infrequent.

REFERENCE

Whaley, L.F., and Wong, D.L.: Nursing care of infants and children, ed. 2, St. Louis, 1983, The C.V. Mosby Co.

BIBLIOGRAPHY

Beall, M.S., Jr.: Evaluation of the musculoskeletal system in the pediatric patient, Issues Compr. Pediatr. Nurs. **2**(4):1-13, 1977.
Conway, B.L.: Pediatric neurologic nursing, St. Louis, 1977, The C.V. Mosby Co.
Conway-Rutkowski, B.L.: Carini and Owens' neurological and neurosurgical nursing, ed. 8, St. Louis, 1982, The C.V. Mosby Co.

Cerebral palsy

Brown, M.S.: How to tell if a baby has cerebral palsy and what to tell his parents when he does, Nursing 79 **9**(5):88-91, 1979.
Lepler, M.: Having a handicapped child, Am. J. Maternal Child Nurs. **3**(1):32-33, 1978.

Spina bifida

Henderson, M.L., and Synhorst, D.M.: Bladder and bowel management in the child with myelomeningocele, Pediatr. Nurs. **3**(5):24-31, 1977.
Hill, M.L.: Meningomyelocele: the child and the family, Issues Compr. Pediatr. Nurs. **2**(5):51, 1978.

Jackson, P.L.: Ventriculo-peritoneal shunt, Am. J. Nurs. **80**:1104-1109, 1980.
Jeffries, J.S., Killam, P.E., and Varni, J.W.: Behavioral management of fecal incontinence in a child with myelomeningocele, Pediatr. Nurs. **8**:267-270, 1982.
Killam, P.E., and others: Behavioral pediatric weight rehabilitation for children with myelomeningocele, Am. J. Maternal Child Nurs. **8**:280-286, 1983.
Meservey, P.M.: Congenital musculoskeletal abnormalities, Issues Compr. Pediatr. Nurs. **2**(4):15-22, 1977.
Owen, L.V.: Orthopedic management of a child with a spinal cord disorder, Pediatr. Nurs. **3**(4):37-40, 1977.
Vigliarolo, D.: Managing bowel incontinence in children with meningomyelocele, Am. J. Nurs. **80**:105-107, 1980.

Muscular dystrophies

Brady, M.H.: Lifelong care of the child with Duchenne muscular dystrophy, Am. J. Maternal Child Nurs. **4**:227-230, 1979.
Nursing Grand Rounds: Muscular dystrophy: a nursing point of view, Nursing 80 **10**(1):45-49, 1980.
Pope-Gratten, M.M., and others: Human figure drawings by children with Duchenne's muscular dystrophy, Phys. Ther. **56**:168-176, 1976.

Guillain-Barré syndrome

Jemison-Smith, P., and Hubbell, H.: Guillain-Barré syndrome, Crit. Care Update **10**(6):12-16, 1983.
Kealy, S.: Respiratory care in Guillain-Barré syndrome, Am. J. Nurs. **77**:58-60, 1977.
Kealy, S.L.: The patient with Guillain-Barré syndrome, Crit. Care Update **5**(1):5-12, 1978.
Mills, N., and Plasterer, H.H.: Guillain-Barré syndrome: a framework for nursing care, Nurs. Clin. North Am. **15**:257-264, 1980.
Samonds, R.J.: Guillain-Barré syndrome: helping the patient in the acute stage, Nursing '80 **10**(8):35-41, 1980.
Samonds, R.J.: Guillain-Barraé syndrome: the acute stage, Crit. Care Update **8**(11):38-44, 1981.

Spinal cord injury

Andberg, M.M., Rudolph, A., and Anderson, T.P.: Improving skin care through patient and family training, Topics Clin. Nurs. **5**(2):45-54, 1983.
Buchanan, L.E.: Emergency! First aid for spinal cord injury, Nursing 82 **12**(8):68-75, 1982.
Coffey, H., and Koch, C.R.: Psycho-social care of the paralyzed child, Pediatr. Nurs. **1**(1):21, 1975.
D'Agnostino, J.: Nursing rehabilitation of the quadriplegic adolescent, J. Assoc. Care Child. Health, **9**(3):87-91, 1981.
Ford, J.R., and Duckworth, B.: Moving a dependent patient safely, comfortably. Part 1. Positioning, Nursing 76 **6**(1):27-36, 1976.
Ford, J.R., and Duckworth, B.: Moving a dependent patient safely, comfortably. Part 2. Transferring, Nursing 76 **6**(2):58-65, 1976.
Ginnity, S.W.: Assessment of cervical cord trauma by the nurse practitioner, J. Neurosurg. Nurs. **10**:193-197, 1978.
King, R.B., and Dudas, S.: Rehabilitation of the patient with a spinal cord injury, Nurs. Clin. North Am. **15**:225-243, 1980.
Larrabee, J.: The person with a spinal cord injury, physical care during early recovery, Am. J. Nurs. **77**:1320-1329, 1977.
Martinez, J.W.: Merry Christmas, David, Am. J. Nurs. **77**:1931, 1977.
Pepper, G.A.: The person with a spinal cord injury; psychological care, Am. J. Nurs. **77**:1330-1336, 1977.
Shearer, J.D.: The adolescent wheelchair athlete, Pediatr. Nurs. **3**(5):20-22, 1977.

Tetanus and botulism

Miller, D.K.: The challenge of infant botulism, Am. J. Maternal Child
  Nurs. **7:**180-183, 1982.
Polin, R.A., and Brown, L.W.: Infant botulism, Pediatr. Clin. North
  Am. **26:**345-354, 1979.
Research review: Tetanus: controlled, but still hazardous, Immunol. Up-
  date **2**(1):2-4, 1980.
Roderick, M.A.: Tetanus, Nursing 82 **12**(7):63, 1982.

Myasthenia gravis

Barry, L.: The patient with myasthenia gravis really needs you, Nursing
  82 **12**7:50-53, 1982.

APPENDIXES

TABLES OF NORMAL
LABORATORY VALUES

TABLE A-1. COMMON LABORATORY TESTS

TEST	SPECIMEN	AGE/SEX	NORMAL VALUE	
Ammonia nitrogen	Plasma or serum	Newborn	90-150 µg/dL	
		0-2 weeks	79-129 µ/dL	
		>1 month	29-70 µ/dL	
		Thereafter	15-45 µ/dL	
	Urine, 24 hr		1.3-7.0 mg/d	
Amylase (Amylochrome, 37° C)	Serum	Newborn	5-65 U/L	
	Urine, 24 hour	>1 yr	25-125 U/L	
		1-17	1-17 U/L	
Antistreptolysin O titer (ASO)	Serum			
Normal			<166 Todd units	
Recent streptococcal infection			200-2500 Todd units	
Base excess	Whole blood	Newborn	$(-10)-(-2)$ mmol/L	
		Infant	$(-7)-(-1)$ mmol/L	
		Child	$(-4)-(+2)$ mmol/L	
		Thereafter	$(-3)-(+3)$ mmol/L	
Bicarbonate (HCO_3)	Serum	Arterial	21-28 mmol/L	
		Venous	22-29 mmol/L	
			Premature (mg/dL)	*Full-term (mg/dL)*
Bilirubin, total	Serum	Cord	<2.0	<2.0
		0-1 day	<8.0	<6.0
		1-2 days	<12.0	<8.0
		2-5 days	<16.0	<12.0
		Thereafter	<2	0.2-1.0
Bilirubin, direct (conjugated)			0.0-0.2 mg/dL	
Bleeding time (Ivy)	Skin puncture	Normal:	2-7 min	
		Borderline:	7-11 min	
(Simplate)			2.75-8 min	
Blood volume	Whole blood	Male	52-83 mL/kg	
		Female	50-75 mL/kg	
C-reactive protein (CRP)	Serum	Cord	10-350 ng/mL	
		Adult	68-8200 ng/mL	
Calcium, ionized	Serum, plasma, or whole blood	Cord	5.5 ± 0.3 mg/dL	
		Newborn	4.3-5.1 mg/dL	
		24-48 hr	4.0-4.7 mg/dL	
		Thereafter	4.48-4.92 mg/dL or 2.24-2.46 mEq/L	

Modified from Behrman, R.E., and Vaughan, V.C., III: Nelson Textbook of pediatrics, ed. 12, Philadelphia, 1983, W.B. Saunders Co.

Continued.

TABLE A-1. COMMON LABORATORY TESTS—cont'd

TEST	SPECIMEN	AGE/SEX	NORMAL VALUE
Calcium, total	Serum	Cord	9.0-11.5 mg/dL
		Newborn, 3-24 hr	9.0-10.6 mg/dL
		24-48 hr	7.0-12.0 mg/dL
		4-7 d	9.0-10.9 mg/dL
		Child	8.8-10.8 mg/dL
		Thereafter	8.4-10.2 mg/dL
	Urine (24 hr)	Ca free diet:	5-40 mg/d
		Low to average Ca in diet:	50-150 mg/d
		Average:	100-300 mg/d
	CSF		4.2-5.4 mg/dL
			or
			2.1-2.7 mEq/L
	Feces	Average:	0.64 g/d
Carbon dioxide, partial pressure (Pco_2)	Whole blood, arterial	Newborn	27-40 mm Hg
		Infant	27-41 mm Hg
		Thereafter: Male	35-48 mm Hg
		Female	32-45 mm Hg
Carbon dioxide (total CO_2)	Serum or plasma	Cord	14-22 mmol/L
		Premature (1 week)	14-27 mmol/L
		Newborn	13-22 mmol/L
		Infant	20-28 mmol/L
		Child	20-28 mmol/L
		Thereafter	23-30 mmol/L
Cerebrospinal fluid pressure	CSF		70-180 mm water
Cerebrospinal fluid volume	CSF	Child	60-100 mL
		Adult	100-160 mL
Chloride	Serum or plasma	Cord	96-104 mmol/L
		Newborn	97-110 mmol/L
		Thereafter	98-106 mmol/L
	CSF		118-132 mmol/L
	Urine, 24 hr	Infant	2-10 mmol/d (diet-dependent)
		Child	15-40 mmol/d
		Thereafter	110-250 mmol/d
	Sweat	Normal homozygote	0-35 mmol/L
		Marginal (e.g., asthma, Addison disease, malnutrition)	30-60 mmol/L
		Cystic fibrosis	60-200 mmol/L
Cholesterol, total	Serum or plasma	Cord	45-100 mg/dL
		Newborn	53-135 mg/dL
		Infant	70-175 mg/dL
		Child	120-200 mg/dL
		Adolescent	120-210 mg/dL
		Thereafter	140-310 mg/dL

TABLE A-1. COMMON LABORATORY TESTS—cont'd

TEST	SPECIMEN	AGE/SEX	NORMAL VALUE
Clotting time (Lee-White)	Whole blood		5-8 minutes (glass tubes)
			5-15 minutes (room temp)
Copper	Serum	Birth-6 mo	20-70 μg/dL
		6 yr	90-190 μg/dL
		12 yr	80-160 μg/dL
		Adult: Male	70-140 μg/dL
		Female	80-155 μg/dL
Creatine kinase (CK, CPK)	Serum	Newborn	68-580 U/L
		Adult: Male	12-70 U/L
		Female	10-55 U/L
		Ambulatory: Male	25-90 U/L
		Female	10-70 U/L
		Higher after exercise	
Creatinine	Serum	Cord	0.6-1.2 mg/dL
		Newborn	0.3-1.0 mg/dL
		Infant	0.2-0.4 mg/dL
		Child	0.3-0.7 mg/dL
		Adolescent	0.5-1.0 mg/dL
		Adult: Male	0.6-1.2 mg/dL
		Female	0.5-1.1 mg/dL
	Urine, 24 hr	Infant	8-20 mg/kg/d
		Child	8-22 mg/kg/d
		Adolescent	8-30 mg/kg/d
		Adult	14-26 mg/kg/d
Creatinine clearance (endogenous)	Serum or plasma and urine	Newborn	40-65 ml/min/1.73m^2
		<40 yr: Male	97-137 ml/min/1.73m^2
		Female	88-128 ml/min/1.73 m^2
Eosinophil count	Whole blood, capillary blood		50-350 cells/mm^3 (μL)
Erythrocyte (RBC) count	Whole blood	cord	3.9-5.5 million/mm^3
		1-3 d	4.0-6.6 million/mm^3
		1 wk	3.9-6.3 million/mm^3
		2 wk	3.0-5.4 million/mm^3
		2 mo	2.7-4.9 million/mm^3
		3-6 mo	3.1-4.5 million/mm^3
		0.5-2 yr	3.7-5.3 million/mm^3
		2-6 yr	3.9-5.3 million/mm^3
		6-12 yr	4.0-5.2 million/mm^3
		12-18 yr: Male	4.5-5.3 million/mm^3
		Female	4.1-5.1 million/mm^3
Erythrocyte sedimentation rate (ESR)	Whole blood		
Westergren (modified)		Child	0-10 mm/hr
		<50 yr: Male	0-15 mm/hr
		Female	0-20 mm/hr
Wintrobe		Child	0-13 mm/hr
		Adult: Male	0-9 mm/hr
		Female	0-20 mm/hr

Continued.

TABLE A-1. COMMON LABORATORY TESTS—cont'd

TEST	SPECIMEN	AGE/SEX	NORMAL VALUE
ZETA			41-54%
Fat, fecal	Feces (72 hr)	Infant, breast-fed	<1 g/d
		0-6 yr	<2 g/d
		Adult	<7 g/d
Fatty acids, free	Serum or plasma	Adults	8-25 mg/dL
		Children and obese adults	<31 mg/dL
Fetal hemoglobin	Whole blood	1 d	77.0 ± 7.3% HbF
		5 d	76.8 ± 5.8% HbF
		3 wk	70.0 ± 7.3% HbF
		6-9 wk	52.9 ± 11.0% HbF
		3-4 mo	23.2 ± 16.0% HbF
		6 mo	4.7 ± 2.2% HbF
		Adult	<2.0 % HbF
Fibrinogen	Plasma	Newborn	125-300 mg/dL
		Thereafter	200-400 mg/dL
Galactose	Serum	Newborn	0-20 mg/dL
		Thereafter	<5 mg/dL
	Urine	Newborn	≤60 mg/dL
		Thereafter	<14 mg/dL
Glucose	Serum	Cord	45-96 mg/dL
		Premature	20-60 mg/dL
		Neonate	30-60 mg/dL
		Newborn, 1 d	40-60 mg/dL
		Newborn, > 1 d	50-90 mg/dL
		Child	60-100 mg/dL
		Thereafter	70-105 mg/dL
	Blood	Thereafter	65-95 mg/dL
	CSF	Adult	40-70 mg/dL
	Urine (quantitative)		<0.5 g/d
	(Qualitative)		negative
Glucose tolerance test (GTT)	Serum	Dosages	
		Adult: 75 g	
		Child: 1.75 g/kg of ideal weight up to maximum of 75 g	

	Time	Normal	Diabetic
	Fasting	70-105	>115
	60 min	120-170	≥200
	90 min	100-140	≥200
	120 mmin	70-120	≥140

TEST	SPECIMEN	AGE/SEX	NORMAL VALUE
Growth hormone (hGH, Somatotropin)	Plasma Fasting, at rest	Cord	10-50 ng/mL
		Newborn	10-40 ng/mL
		Child	<5 ng/mL
		Adult: Male	<5 ng/mL
		Female	<8 ng/mL

TABLE A-1. COMMON LABORATORY TESTS—cont'd

TEST	SPECIMEN	AGE/SEX	NORMAL VALUE
Hematocrit (HCT, Hct)	Whole blood	1 d (cap)	48-69%
		2 d	48-75%
		3 d	44-72%
		2 mo	28-42%
		6-12 yr	35-45%
		12-18 yr: Male	37-49%
		Female	36-46%
Hemoglobin (Hb)	Whole blood	1-3 d (cap)	14.5-22.5 g/dL
		2 mo	9.0-14.0 g/dL
		6-12 yr	11.5-15.5 g/dL
		12-18 yr: Male	13.0-16.0 g/dL
		Female	12.0-16.0 g/dL
Hemoglobin A	Whole blood		>95% of total
Hemoglobin F	Whole blood	1 d	77.0 ± 7.3% of total
		6 mo	4.7 ± 2.2% of total
		Adult	<2.0 % of total

TEST	SPECIMEN	AGE/SEX	IgA (mg/dL)	IgG (mg/dL)	IgM (mg/dL)
Immunoglobulin levels	Serum	Cord	0-5	760-1700	4-24
		Newborn	0-2.2	700-1480	5-30
		1/2-6 mo	3-82	300-1000	15-109
		6 mo-2 yr	14-108	500-1200	43-239
		2-6 yr	23-190	500-1300	50-199
		6-12 yr	29-270	700-1650	50-260
		12-16 yr	81-232	700-1550	45-240
		Thereafter	60-380	600-1600 (higher in Blacks)	40-345

TEST	SPECIMEN	AGE/SEX	NORMAL VALUE
Iron	Serum	Newborn	100-250 μg/dL
		Infant	40-100 μg/dL
		Child	50-120 μm/dL
		Thereafter, Male	50-160 μg/dL
		Female	40-150 μg/dL
		Intoxicated child	280-2550 μg/dL
		Fatally poisoned child:	>1800
Iron-binding capacity, total (TIBC)	Serum	Infant	100-400 μg/dL
		Thereafter	250-400 μg/dL
Lead	Whole blood	Child	<30 μg/dL
		Adult	<40 μg/dL
		Acceptable for industrial exposure	<60
		Toxic	≥100
	Urine, 24 hr		<80 μg/L
Leukocyte count (WBC count)	Whole blood		×1000 cells/mm³ (μL)
		Birth	9.0-30.0
		24 h	9.4-34.0
		1 mo	5.0-19.5
		1-3 yr	6.0-17.5
		4-7 yr	5.5-15.5
		8-13 yr	4.5-13.5
		Adult	4.5-11.0

Continued.

TABLE A-1. COMMON LABORATORY TESTS—cont'd

TEST	SPECIMEN	AGE/SEX	NORMAL VALUE
Leukocyte—cont'd	CSF		***×1000 cells/mm³ (μL)***
		Premature	0-25 mononuclear
			0-100 polymorphonuclear
			0-1000 RBC
		Newborn	0-20 mononuclear
			0-70 polymorphonuclear
			0-800 RBC
		Neonate	0-5 mononuclear
			0-25 polymorphonuclear
			0-50 RBC
		Thereafter	0-5 mononuclear
Leukocyte differential count	Whole blood	Myelocytes 0%	0 Cells/mm³ (μL)
		Neutrophils—"bands" 3-5%	150-400 Cells/mm³ (μL)
		Neutrophils—"segs" 54-62%	3000-5800 Cells/mm³ (μL)
		Lymphocytes 25-33%	1500-3000 Cells/mm³ (μL)
		Monocytes 3-7%	285-500 Cells/mm³ (μL)
		Eosinophils 1-3%	50-250 Cells/mm³ (μL)
		Basophils 0.075%	15-50 Cells/mm³ (μL)
Mean corpuscular hemoglobin (MCH)	Whole blood	Birth	31-37 pg/cell
		1-3 d (cap)	31-37 pg/cell
		1 wk-1 mo	28-40 pg/cell
		2 mo	26-34 pg/cell
		3-6 mo	25-35 pg/cell
		0.5-2 yr	23-31 pg/cell
		2-6 yr	24-30 pg/cell
		6-12 yr	25-33 pg/cell
		12-18 yr	25-35 pg/cell
		18-49 yr	26-34 pg/cell
Mean corpuscular hemoglobin concentration (MCHC)	Whole blood	Birth	30-36% Hb/cell or g Hb/dL RBC
		1-3 d (cap)	29-37% Hb/cell or g Hb/dL RBC
		1-2 wk	28-38% Hb/cell or g Hb/dL RBC
		1-2 mo	29-37% Hb/cell or g Hb/dL RBC
		3 mo-2 yr	30-36% Hb/cell or g Hb/dL RBC
		2-18 yr	31-37% Hb/cell or g Hb/dL RBC
		>18 yr	31-37% Hb/cell or g Hb/dL RBC
Mean corpuscular volume (MCV)	Whole blood	1-3 d (cap)	95-121 μm³
		0.5-2 yr	70-86 μm³
		6-12 yr	77-95 μm³
		12-18 yr: Male	78-98 μm³
		Female	78-102 μm³
Osmolality	Serum	Child, Adult:	275-295 mOsmol/kg H_2O
	Urine, random		50-1400 mOsmol/kg H_2O, depending on fluid intake. After 12 hr fluid restriction: >850 mOsmol/kg H_2O
	Urine, 24 hr		≈300-900 mOsmol/kg H_2O

TABLE A-1. COMMON LABORATORY TESTS—cont'd

TEST	SPECIMEN	AGE/SEX	NORMAL VALUE
Oxygen, partial pressure (pO_2)	Whole blood, arterial	Birth	8-24 mm Hg
		5-10 min	33-75 mm Hg
		30 min	31-85 mm Hg
		>1 hr	55-80 mm Hg
		1 d	54-95 mm Hg
		Thereafter	83-108 mm Hg
		(Decreased with age)	
Oxygen saturation	Whole blood, arterial	Newborn	40-90%
		Thereafter	95-99%
Partial thromboplastin time (PTT)	Whole blood (Na citrate)		
Nonactivated			60-85 s (Platelin)
Activated			25-35 s (differs with method)
pH	Whole blood, arterial	Premature (48 hr)	7.35-7.50
		Birth, full term	7.11-7.36
		5-10 min	7.09-7.30
		30 min	7.21-7.38
		>1 hr	7.26-7.49
		1 d	7.29-7.45
		Thereafter	7.35-7.45
		Must be corrected for body temperature	
	Urine, random	Newborn/neonate	5-7
		Thereafter	4.5-8
		(average ≃6)	
	Stool		7.0-7.5
Phenylalanine	Serum	Premature	2.0-7.5 mg/dL
		Newborn	1.2-3.4 mg/dL
		Thereafter	0.8-1.8 mg/dL
	Urine, 24 hr	10 d-2 wk	1-2 mg/d
		3-12 yr	4-18 mg/d
		Thereafter	trace-17 mg/d
			or: 6 ± 2 mg/g creatinine
Plasma volume	Plasma	Male	25-43 mL/kg
		Female	28-45 mL/kg
Platelet count (thrombocyte count)	Whole blood (EDTA)	Newborn	84-478 × 10^3/mm^3 (μL)
		(After 1 wk, same as adult)	
		Adult	150-400 × 10^3/mm^3 (μL)
Potassium	Serum	Newborn	3.9-5.9 mmol/L
		Infant	4.1-5.3 mmol/L
		Child	3.4-4.7 mmol/L
		Thereafter	3.5-5.1 mmol/L
	Plasma (heparin)		3.5-4.5 mmol/L
	Urine, 24 hr		2.5-125 mmol/d varies with diet

Continued.

TABLE A-1. COMMON LABORATORY TESTS—cont'd

TEST	SPECIMEN	AGE/SEX	NORMAL VALUE
Protein			
Total	Serum	Premature	4.3-7.6 g/dL
		Newborn	4.6-7.4 g/dL
		Child	6.2-8.0 g/dL
		Adults, recumbent	6.0-7.8 g/dL
			~0.5 g higher in ambulatory patients

Electrophoresis		*g/dL*				
		Albumin	*α_1-Globulin*	*α_2-Globulin*	*β-Globulin*	*γ-Globulin*
	Premature	3.0-4.2	0.1-0.5	0.3-0.7	0.3-1.2	0.3-1.4
	Newborn	3.6-5.4	0.1-0.3	0.3-0.5	0.2-0.6	0.2-1.0
	Infant	4.0-5.0	0.2-0.4	0.5-0.8	0.5-0.8	0.3-1.2
	Thereafter	3.5-5.0	0.2-0.3	0.4-1.0	0.5-1.1	0.7-1.2
						Higher in Blacks

TEST	SPECIMEN	AGE/SEX	NORMAL VALUE
Total	Urine, 24 hr		1-14 mg/dL
			50-80 mg/d (at rest)
			<250 mg/d after intense exercise
Total	CSF		Lumbar: 8-32 mg/dL
Prothrombin time (PT)			
One-stage (Quick)	Whole blood (Na citrate)	In general	11-15 s (varies with type of thromboplastin)
		Newborn	Prolonged by 2-3 sec
Two-stage modified (Ware and Seegers)	Whole blood (Na citrate)		18-22 sec
RBC count, see erythrocyte count			
Red cell volume	Whole blood	Male	20-36 mL/kg
		Female	19-31 mL/kg
Reticulocyte count	Whole blood	Adults	0.5-1.5% of erythrocytes or 25,000-75,000/mm^3 (μL)
	Capillary	1 d	3.2 ± 1.4%
		7 d	0.5 ± 0.4%
		1-4 wk	0.6 ± 0.3%
		5-6 wk	1.0 ± 0.7%
		7-8 wk	1.5 ± 0.7%
		9-10 wk	1.2 ± 0.7%
		11-12 wk	0.7 ± 0.3%
Salicylates	Serum, plasma		Therap. conc.: 15-30 mg/dL
			Toxic conc.: >30
Sedimentation rate, see erythrocyte sedimentation rate			

TABLE A-1. COMMON LABORATORY TESTS—cont'd

TEST	SPECIMEN	AGE/SEX	NORMAL VALUE	
Sodium	Serum or plasma	Newborn	136-146 mmol/L	
		Infant	139-146 mmol/L	
		Child	138-145 mmol/L	
		Thereafter	136-146 mmol/L	
			40-220 mmol/L (diet dependent)	
	Urine, 24 hr		10-40 mmol/L	
	Sweat	Cystic fibrosis	>70	
Specific gravity	Urine, random	Adult	1.002-1.030	
		After 12 hr fluid restriction	>1.025	
	Urine, 24 h		1.015-1.025	
Thrombin time	Whole blood (Na citrate)		Control time ± 2 sec when control is 9-13 sec	
Thyroxine, total (T_4)	Serum	Cord	8-13 µg/dL	
		Newborn	11.5-24 (lower in low birth weight infants)	
		Neonate	9-18 µg/dL	
		Infant	7-15 µm/dL	
		1-5 yr	7.3-15 µg/dL	
		5-10 yr	6.4-13.3 µg/dL	
		Thereafter	5-12 µg/dL	
		Newborn screen (filter paper)	6.2-22 µg/dL	
Tourniquet test (capillary fragility)			<5-10 petechiae in 2.5 cm circle on forearm (halfway between systolic and diastolic pressure for 5 min); 0-8 petechiae in 6 cm circle (50 torr for 15 min); 10-20 petechiae in 5 cm circle (80 mm Hg)	
Triglycerides (TG)	Serum, after ≥ 12 hr fast		*mg/dL*	
			M	F
		Cord blood	10-98	10-98
		0-5 yr	30-86	32-99
		6-11 yr	31-108	35-114
		12-15 yr	36-138	41-138
		16-19 yr	40-163	40-128
Triiodothyronine, free	Serum	Cord	130 ± 10(SE) mean pg/dL	
		1-3 d	410 ± 20	
		6 wk	400 ± 20	
		Adults (20-50 yr)	230-660 pg/dL	
Triiodothyronine, total (T_3-RIA)	Serum	Cord	30-70 ng/dL	
		Newborn	75-260 ng/dL	
		1-5 yr	100-260 ng/dL	
		5-10 yr	90-240 ng/dL	
		10-15 yr	80-210 ng/dL	
		Thereafter	115-190 ng/dL	

Continued.

TABLE A-1. COMMON LABORATORY TESTS—cont'd

TEST	SPECIMEN	AGE/SEX	NORMAL VALUE
Urea nitrogen	Serum or plasma	Cord	21-40 mg/dL
		Premature (1 wk)	3-25 mg/dL
		Newborn	3-12 mg/dL
		Infant/Child	5-18 mg/dL
		Thereafter	7-18 mg/dL
Uric acid	Serum		
Phosphotungstate		Newborn	2.0-6.2 mg/dL
		Adult: Male	4.5-8.2 mg/dL
		Female	3.0-6.5 mg/dL
Uricase		Child	2.0-5.5 mg/dL
		Adults: Male	3.5-7.2 mg/dL
		Female	2.6-6.0 mg/dL
Urine volume	Urine, 24 hr	Newborn	50-300 mL/d
		Infant	350-550 mL/d
		Child	500-1000 mL/d
		Adolescent	700-1400 mL/d
		Thereafter: Male	800-1800 mL/d
		Female	600-1600 mL/d
			(varies with intake and other factors)
WBC, see Leukocyte			

GROWTH MEASUREMENTS

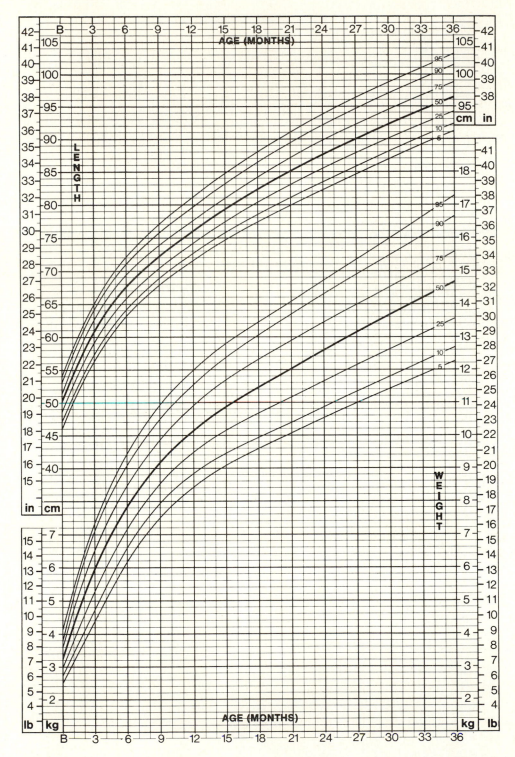

Fig. B-1

*Boys: birth to age 36 months—physical growth (length, weight), NCHS percentiles. (Adapted from Hamill, P.V.V., and others: Physical growth: National Center for Health Statistics percentiles, Am. J. Clin. Nutr. **32**:607-629, 1979. Data from the Fels Research Institute, Wright State University School of Medicine, Yellow Springs, Ohio. Provided as a service of Ross Laboratories, 1980.)*

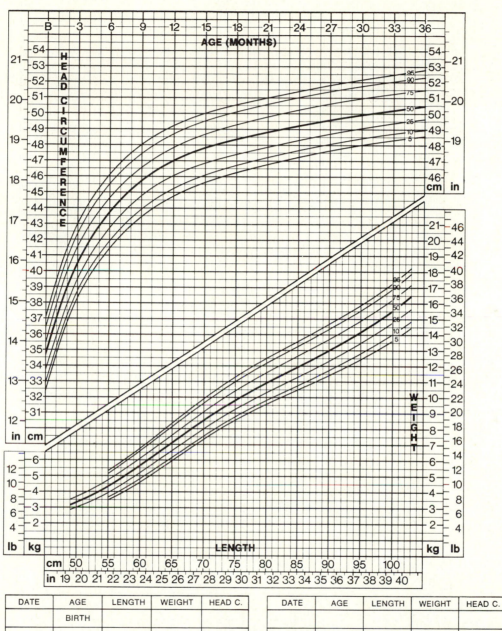

Fig. B-2

*Boys: birth to age 36 months—physical growth (head circumference, length, weight), NCHS percentiles. (Adapted from Hamill, P.V.V., and others: Physical growth: National Center for Health Statistics percentiles, Am. J. Clin. Nutr. **32**:607-629, 1979. Data from the Fels Research Institute, Wright State University School of Medicine, Yellow Springs, Ohio. Provided as a service of Ross Laboratories, 1980.)*

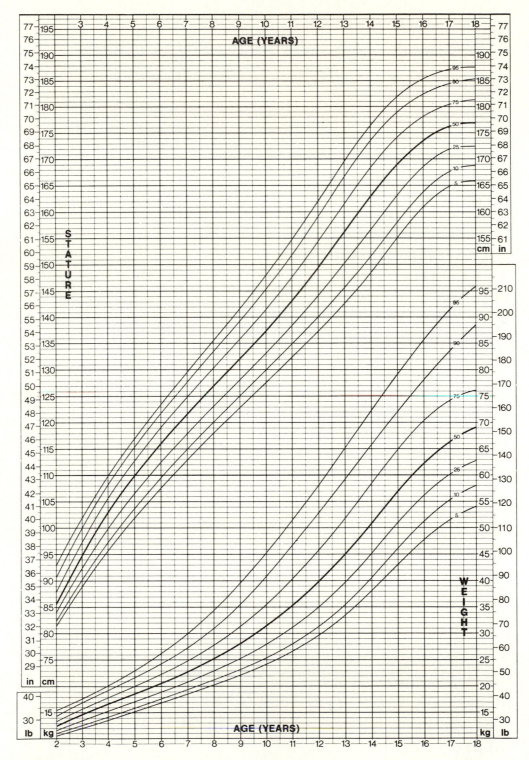

Fig. B-3

*Boys: ages 2 to 18 years—physical growth (stature, weight), NCHS percentiles. (Adapted from Hamill, P.V.V., and others: Physical growth: National Center for Health Statistics percentiles, Am. J. Clin. Nutr. **32:**607-629, 1979. Data from the National Center for Health Statistics [NCHS], Hyattsville, Md. Provided as a service of Ross Laboratories, 1980.)*

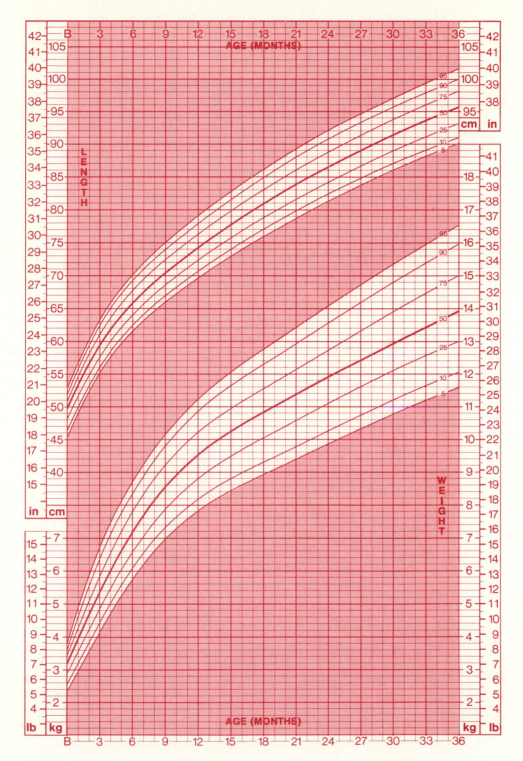

Fig. B-4

*Girls: birth to age 36 months—physical growth (length, weight), NCHS percentiles. (Adapted from Hamill, P.V.V., and others: Physical growth: National Center for Health Statistics percentiles, Am. J. Clin. Nutr. **32:**607-629, 1979. Data from the Fels Research Institute, Wright State University School of Medicine, Yellow Springs, Ohio. Provided as a service of Ross Laboratories, 1980.)*

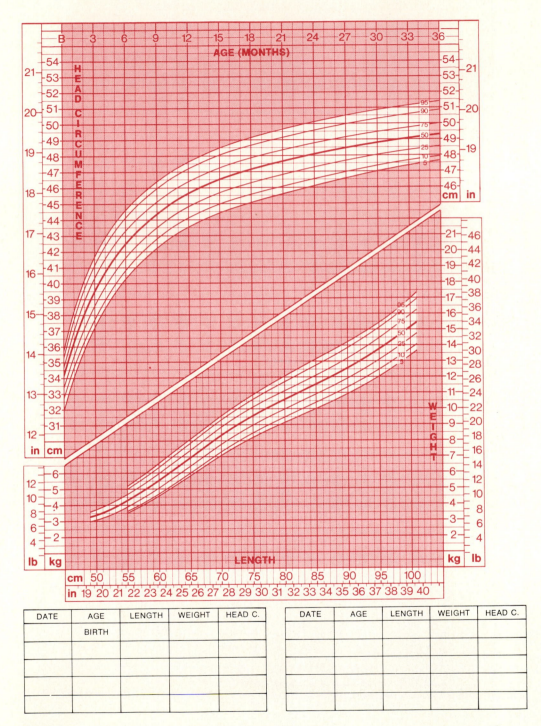

DATE	AGE	LENGTH	WEIGHT	HEAD C.
	BIRTH			

DATE	AGE	LENGTH	WEIGHT	HEAD C.

Fig. B-5

*Girls: birth to age 36 months—physical growth (head circumference, length, weight), NCHS percentiles. (Adapted from Hamill, P.V.V., and others: Physical growth: National Center for Health Statistics percentiles, Am. J. Clin. Nutr. **32**:607-629, 1979. Data from the Fels Research Institute, Wright State University School of Medicine, Yellow Springs, Ohio. Provided as a service of Ross Laboratories, 1980.)*

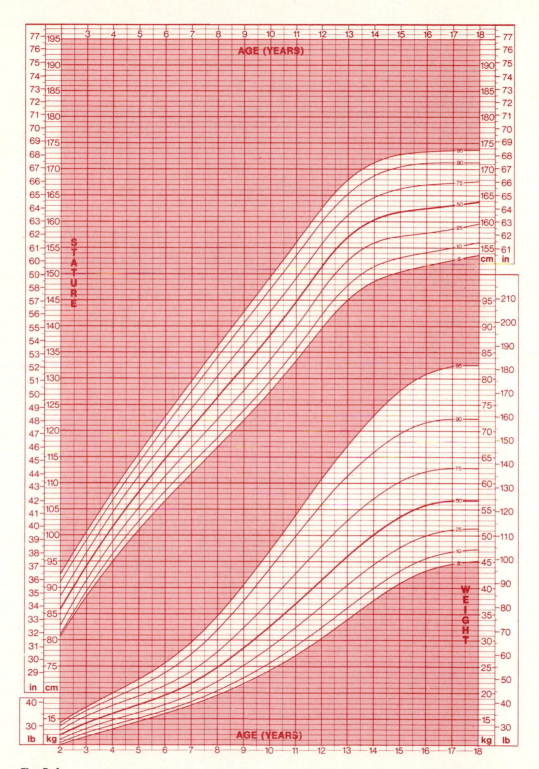

Fig. B-6

*Girls: ages 2 to 18 years—physical growth (stature, weight), NCHS percentiles. (Adapted from Hamill, P.V.V., and others: Physical growth: National Center for Health Statistics percentiles, Am. J. Clin. Nutr. **32**:607-629, 1979. Data from the National Center for Health Statistics [NCHS], Hyattsville, Md. Provided as a service of Ross Laboratories, 1980.)*

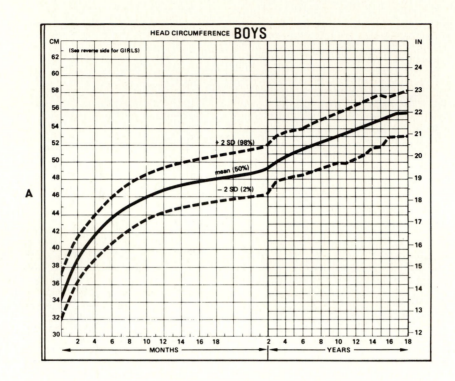

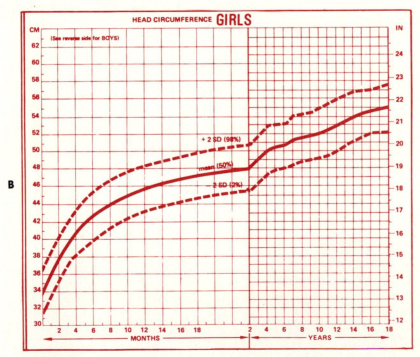

Fig. B-7

*Head circumference charts. **A,** Boys; **B,** girls. (From Nellhaus, G.: Composite international and interracial graphs, Pediatrics **41:**106, 1968. Reprinted by permission. Copyright American Academy of Pediatrics, 1968.)*

TABLE B-1 GROWTH STANDARDS OF HEALTHY CHINESE CHILDREN AND ADOLESCENTS (urban)*

AGE (months or years)	BOYS					GIRLS				
	WEIGHT (kg)	HEIGHT (cm)	TRUNK (cm)	HEAD CIRCUMFERENCE (cm)	CHEST CIRCUMFERENCE (cm)	WEIGHT (kg)	HEIGHT (cm)	TRUNK (cm)	HEAD CIRCUMFERENCE (cm)	CHEST CIRCUMFERENCE (cm)
Birth	3.27	50.6	33.7	34.3	32.8	3.17	50.0	33.4	33.7	32.6
1 mo	4.97	56.5	37.7	38.1	37.9	4.64	55.5	36.9	37.3	36.9
2 mo	5.95	59.6	39.7	39.7	40.0	5.49	58.4	38.7	38.7	38.9
3 mo	6.73	62.3	41.2	41.0	41.3	6.23	60.9	40.1	40.0	40.3
4 mo	7.32	64.4	42.3	42.0	42.3	6.69	62.9	41.2	41.0	41.1
5 mo	7.70	65.9	43.1	42.9	42.9	7.19	64.5	42.1	41.9	41.9
6 mo	8.22	68.1	44.1	43.9	43.8	7.62	66.7	43.2	42.8	42.7
8 mo	8.71	70.6	45.2	44.9	44.7	8.14	69.0	44.1	43.7	43.4
10 mo	9.14	72.9	46.3	45.7	45.4	8.57	71.4	45.4	44.5	44.2
12 mo	9.66	75.6	47.8	46.3	46.1	9.04	74.1	46.6	45.2	45.0
15 mo	10.15	78.3	49.0	46.8	46.8	9.54	76.9	48.0	45.6	45.8
18 mo	10.67	80.7	50.1	47.3	47.6	10.08	79.4	49.4	46.2	46.6
21 mo	11.18	83.0	51.2	47.8	48.3	10.56	81.7	50.4	46.7	47.3
24 mo	11.95	86.5	52.7	48.2	49.2	11.37	85.3	51.9	47.1	48.2
2½ yr	12.84	90.4	54.4	48.8	50.2	12.28	89.3	53.6	47.7	49.0
3 yr	13.63	93.8	55.5	49.1	50.8	13.1	92.8	54.7	48.1	49.8
3½ yr	14.45	97.2	56.9	49.4	51.5	14.00	96.3	56.1	48.5	50.5
4 yr	15.26	100.8	58.3	49.7	52.2	14.89	100.1	57.8	48.9	51.2
4½ yr	16.07	103.9	59.7	50.0	53.0	15.63	103.1	59.1	49.1	51.8
5 yr	16.88	107.2	61.1	50.2	53.6	16.46	106.5	60.4	49.4	52.5
5½ yr	17.65	110.1	62.2	50.5	54.4	17.18	109.2	61.8	49.6	53.0
6 yr	19.25	114.7	64.5	50.8	55.6	18.67	113.9	63.8	50.0	54.2
7 yr	21.01	120.6	66.6	51.1	57.1	20.35	119.3	65.8	50.2	55.5
8 yr	23.08	125.3	68.7	51.4	58.8	22.43	124.6	68.2	50.6	57.1
9 yr	25.33	130.6	70.7	51.7	60.8	24.57	129.5	70.2	50.9	58.6
10 yr	27.15	134.4	72.3	51.9	62.0	27.05	134.8	72.5	51.3	60.7
11 yr	30.13	139.2	74.4	52.3	64.3	30.51	140.6	75.3	51.7	63.5
12 yr	33.05	144.2	76.7	52.7	66.5	34.82	146.6	78.4	52.3	67.2
13 yr	36.90	149.3	79.5	53.0	68.9	38.52	150.7	80.7	52.8	70.3
14 yr	42.03	156.5	83.0	53.5	72.4	42.26	153.7	82.6	53.1	73.3
15 yr	46.91	162.0	86.3	54.3	76.0	45.37	155.5	84.1	53.4	75.6
16 yr	50.90	165.6	88.8	54.9	78.8	47.43	156.8	85.0	53.8	76.6
17 yr	53.11	167.7	90.3	55.2	80.8	48.57	157.4	85.5	53.9	77.9

Adapted from Practical Pediatrics, edited by Peking Children Hospital, 1979.

*Measurements of rural Chinese children are slightly lower.

NOTE: A comparison of the average growth of American and Chinese children demonstrates that on the standard NCHS growth charts the mean height and weight for Chinese children falls on the 10th percentile, as compared to the mean growth measurements for American children, which comprise the 50th percentile.

DEVELOPMENTAL ASSESSMENT

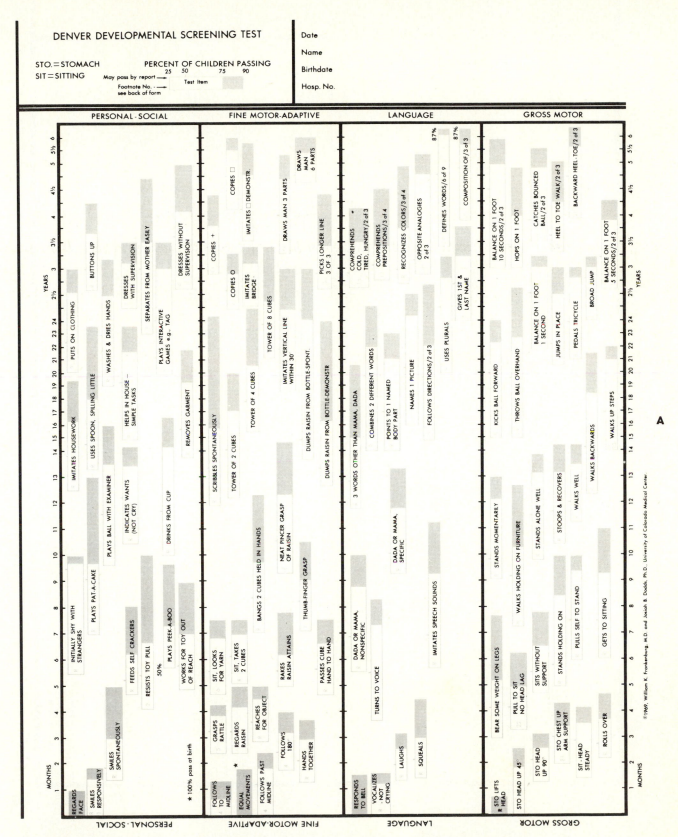

Fig. C-1

A, *Denver Developmental Screening Test. (From W.K. Frankenburg and J.B. Dodds, University of Colorado Medical Center, 1969.)*

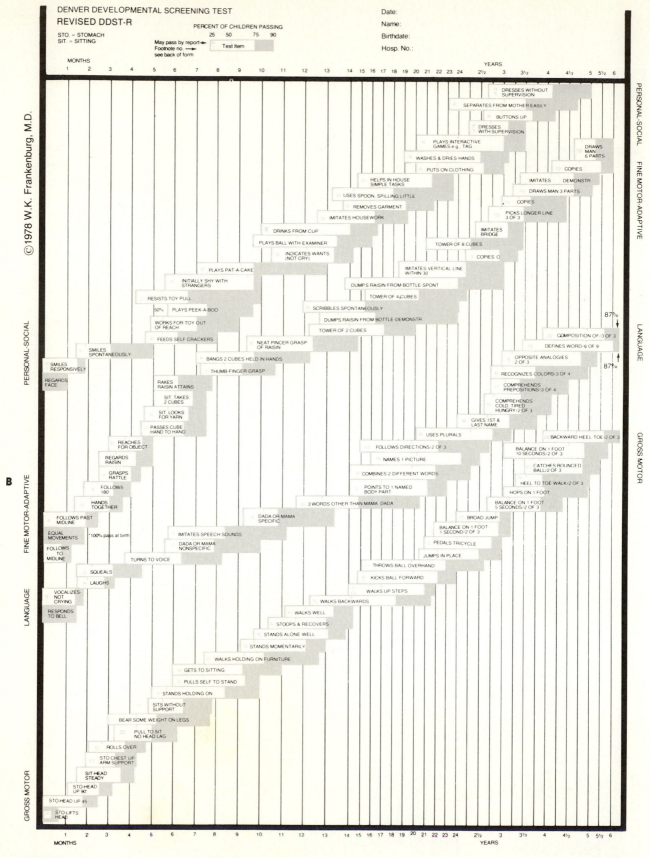

Fig. C-1 cont'd

B, *DDST revised (DDST-R). Resembling a growth curve, this form places items at lowest age level starting at bottom left and progresses upward to right with increasing age. (B from Frankenburg, W.K., Sciarillo, W., and Burgess, D.: The newly abbreviated and revised Denver Developmental Screening Test, J. Pediatr. 99(6):995-999, 1981.)*

DATE:

NAME:

DIRECTIONS BIRTHDATE:

HOSP. NO.:

1. Try to get child to smile by smiling, talking or waving to him. Do not touch him.
2. When child is playing with toy, pull it away from him. Pass if he resists.
3. Child does not have to be able to tie shoes or button in the back.
4. Move yarn slowly in an arc from one side to the other, about 6" above child's face.
    Pass if eyes follow 90° to midline. (Past midline; 180°)
5. Pass if child grasps rattle when it is touched to the backs or tips of fingers.
6. Pass if child continues to look where yarn disappeared or tries to see where it went. Yarn
    should be dropped quickly from sight from tester's hand without arm movement.
7. Pass if child picks up raisin with any part of thumb and a finger.
8. Pass if child picks up raisin with the ends of thumb and index finger using an over hand
    approach.

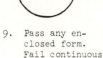

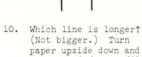

9. Pass any en-   10. Which line is longer?   11. Pass any   12. Have child copy
    closed form.   (Not bigger.) Turn   crossing   first. If failed,
    Fail continuous   paper upside down and   lines.   demonstrate
    round motions.   repeat. (3/3 or 5/6)

    When giving items 9, 11 and 12, do not name the forms. Do not demonstrate 9 and 11.

13. When scoring, each pair (2 arms, 2 legs, etc.) counts as one part.
14. Point to picture and have child name it. (No credit is given for sounds only.)

  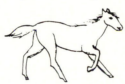 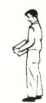

15. Tell child to: Give block to Mommie; put block on table; put block on floor. Pass 2 of 3.
    (Do not help child by pointing, moving head or eyes.)
16. Ask child: What do you do when you are cold? ..hungry? ..tired? Pass 2 of 3.
17. Tell child to: Put block on table; under table; in front of chair, behind chair.
    Pass 3 of 4. (Do not help child by pointing, moving head or eyes.)
18. Ask child: If fire is hot, ice is ?; Mother is a woman, Dad is a ?; a horse is big, a
    mouse is ?. Pass 2 of 3.
19. Ask child: What is a ball? ..lake? ..desk? ..house? ..banana? ..curtain? ..ceiling?
    ..hedge? ..pavement? Pass if defined in terms of use, shape, what it is made of or general
    category (such as banana is fruit, not just yellow). Pass 6 of 9.
20. Ask child: What is a spoon made of? ..a shoe made of? ..a door made of? (No other objects
    may be substituted.) Pass 3 of 3.
21. When placed on stomach, child lifts chest off table with support of forearms and/or hands.
22. When child is on back, grasp his hands and pull him to sitting. Pass if head does not hang back.
23. Child may use wall or rail only, not person. May not crawl.
24. Child must throw ball overhand 3 feet to within arm's reach of tester.
25. Child must perform standing broad jump over width of test sheet. (8-1/2 inches)
26. Tell child to walk forward, ⌒⌒⌒⌒➤ heel within 1 inch of toe.
    Tester may demonstrate. Child must walk 4 consecutive steps, 2 out of 3 trials.
27. Bounce ball to child who should stand 3 feet away from tester. Child must catch ball with
    hands, not arms, 2 out of 3 trials.
28. Tell child to walk backward, ◀⌒⌒⌒⌒ toe within 1 inch of heel.
    Tester may demonstrate. Child must walk 4 consecutive steps, 2 out of 3 trials.

DATE AND BEHAVIORAL OBSERVATIONS (how child feels at time of test, relation to tester, attention
span, verbal behavior, self-confidence, etc,):

Fig. C-1, cont'd

C, *Directions for numbered items of testing form. (From W.K. Frankenburg and J.B.
Dodds, University of Colorado Medical Center, 1969.)*

DENVER ARTICULATION SCREENING EXAM
for children 2 1/2 to 6 years of age

Instructions: Have child repeat each word after you. Circle the underlined sounds that he pronounces correctly. Total correct sounds is the Raw Score. Use charts on reverse side to score results.

NAME

HOSP. NO.

ADDRESS

Date: _____ Child's Age: _____ Examiner: _____ Raw Score: _____
Percentile: _____ Intelligibility: _____ Result: _____

1. table   6. zipper   11. sock   16. wagon   21. leaf
2. shirt   7. grapes   12. vacuum   17. gum   22. carrot
3. door   8. flag   13. yarn   18. house
4. trunk   9. thumb   14. mother   19. pencil
5. jumping   10. toothbrush 15. twinkle   20. fish

Intelligibility: (circle one)   1. Easy to understand   3. Not understandable
                                 2. Understandable 1/2   4. Can't evaluate
                                       the time.

Comments:

A

Date: _____ Child's Age: _____ Examiner: _____ Raw Score _____
Percentile: _____ Intelligibility: _____ Result: _____

1. table   6. zipper   11. sock   16. wagon   21. leaf
2. shirt   7. grapes   12. vacuum   17. gum   22. carrot
3. door   8. flag   13. yarn   18. house
4. trunk   9. thumb   14. mother   19. pencil
5. jumping   10. toothbrush 15. twinkle   20. fish

Intelligibility: (circle one)   1. Easy to understand   3. Not understandable
                                 2. Understandable 1/2   4. Can't evaluate
                                       the time.

Comments:

Date: _____ Child's Age: _____ Examiner: _____ Raw Score _____
Percentile: _____ Intelligibility: _____ Result: _____

1. table   6. zipper   11. sock   16. wagon   21. leaf
2. shirt   7. grapes   12. vacuum   17. gum   22. carrot
3. door   8. flag   13. yarn   18. house
4. trunk   9. thumb   14. mother   19. pencil
5. jumping   10. toothbrush 15. twinkle   20. fish

Intelligibility: (circle one)   1. Easy to understand   3. Not understandable
                                 2. Understandable 1/2   4. Can't evaluate
                                       the time.

Fig. C-2

A, *Denver Articulation Screening Examination for children 2½ to 6 years of age. (From A.F. Drumwright, University of Colorado Medical Center, 1971.)*

To score DASE words: Note Raw Score for child's performance. Match raw score line (extreme left of chart) with column representing child's age (to the closest <u>previous</u> age group). Where raw score line and age column meet number in that square denotes percentile rank of child's performance when compared to other children that age. Percentiles above heavy line are ABNORMAL percentiles, below heavy line are NORMAL.

<u>PERCENTILE RANK</u>

Raw Score	2.5 yr.	3.0	3.5	4.0	4.5	5.0	5.5	6 years
2	1							
3	2							
4	5							
5	9							
6	16							
7	23							
8	31	2						
9	37	4	1					
10	42	6	2					
11	48	7	4					
12	54	9	6	1	1			
13	58	12	9	2	3	1	1	
14	62	17	11	5	4	2	2	
15	68	23	15	9	5	3	2	
16	75	31	19	12	5	4	3	
17	79	38	25	15	6	6	4	
18	83	46	31	19	8	7	4	
19	86	51	38	24	10	9	5	1
20	89	58	45	30	12	11	7	3
21	92	65	52	36	15	15	9	4
22	94	72	58	43	18	19	12	5
23	96	77	63	50	22	24	15	7
24	97	82	70	58	29	29	20	15
25	99	87	78	66	36	34	26	17
26	99	91	84	75	46	43	34	24
27		94	89	82	57	54	44	34
28		96	94	88	70	68	59	47
29		98	98	94	84	84	77	68
30		100	100	100	100	100	100	100

To Score intelligibility:

	NORMAL	ABNORMAL
2 1/2 years	Understandable 1/2 the time, or, "easy"	Not Understandable
3 years and older	Easy to understand	Understandable 1/2 time Not understandable

Test Result: 1. NORMAL on Dase and Intelligibility = NORMAL

2. ABNORMAL on Dase and/or Intelligibility = ABNORMAL

* If abnormal on initial screening rescreen within 2 weeks. If abnormal again child should be referred for complete speech evaluation.

Fig. C-2, cont'd

B, *Percentile rank. (From A.F. Drumwright, University of Colorado Medical Center, 1971.)*

DIRECTIONS FOR SNELLEN SCREENING*
Preparation

1. Hang the Snellen chart on a light-colored wall so that the 20- to 30-foot lines are at eye level when children 6 to 12 years old are tested in the standing position.
2. Secure the chart to the wall with double-stick tape on the back side at all four corners. If the chart must be reversed for use of the letter or E chart, secure it at the top and bottom with tacks. Make sure that the chart does not swing when in place.
3. The illumination intensity on the chart should be 10 to 30 footcandles, without any glare from windows or light fixtures. The illumination should be checked with a light meter.
4. Mark an exact 20-foot distance from the chart. Mark the floor with a piece of tape or ''footprints'' positioned so that the heels touch the 20-foot line.

Procedure

1. Place the child at the 20-foot mark, with the heel edging the line if the child is standing or with the back of the chair placed at the marker if the child is seated.
2. If the E chart is used, accustom the child to identifying which direction the ''legs of the E'' are pointing. Use a demonstration E card for this purpose.
3. Teach the child to use the occluder to cover one eye. Instruct him to keep both eyes open during the test. Provide a clean cover care for each child and then discard after use.
4. If the child wears glasses, test only with glasses on.
5. Test both eyes together, then right eye, then left eye.
6. Begin with the 40- or 30-foot line and proceed with test to include the 20-foot line.
7. With the child suspected of low vision, begin with the 200-foot line and proceed until the child can no longer correctly read three out of four or four out of six symbols on a line.
8. Use covers on the Snellen chart to expose only one symbol or one line at a time. When screening kindergarten or older children, expose one line but use a pointer to point to one symbol at a time.

*Adapted from recommendations in National Society to Prevent Blindness: Children's eye health guide, 1982, New York, The Society.

Recording and referral

1. Record the last line the child read correctly (three out of four or four out of six symbols).
2. Record visual acuity as a fraction. The numerator represents the distance from the chart, and the denominator represents the last line read correctly. For example, 20/30 means that the child read the 30-foot line at a 20-foot distance.
3. Observe the child's eyes during testing and record any evidence of squinting, head tilting, thrusting the head forward, excessive blinking, tearing, or redness.
4. Only make referrals after a second screening has been made on children who are potential candidates for referral.
5. The following children should be referred for a complete eye examination:
   a. All children who consistently present any of the signs of possible visual disturbance, regardless of visual acuity.
   b. Any child with a one-line difference between each eye.
   c. Three-year-old children with visual acuity of 20/50 or less (inability to read the 40-foot line).
   d. Four-year-old children and above with visual acuity of 20/40 or less (inability to read the 30-foot line).

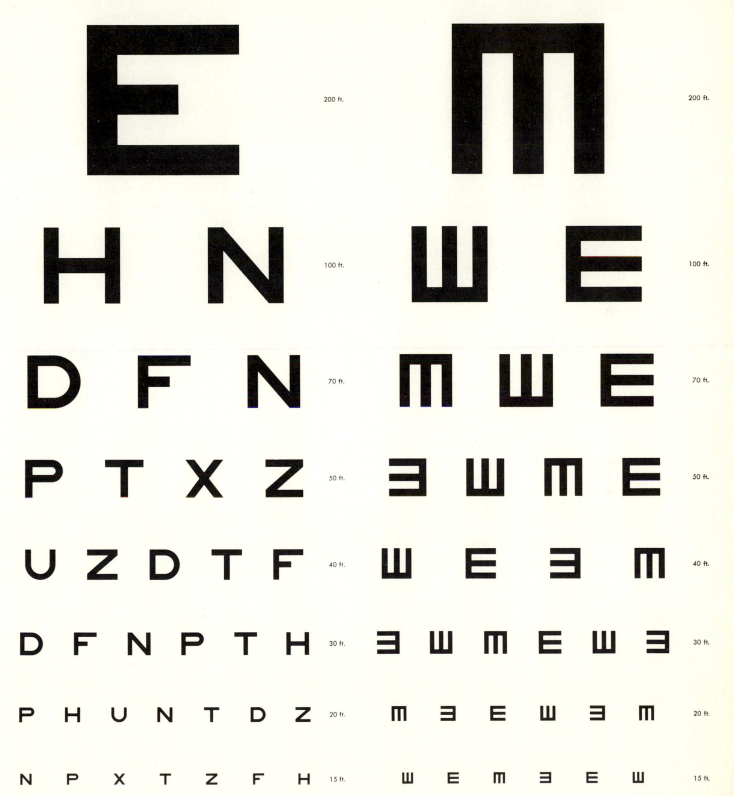

Fig. C-3

Snellen Chart. (From National Society to Prevent Blindness, New York. Member of National Health Council.)

Lit. 217

DENVER EYE SCREENING TEST

Name:
Hospital No.:
Ward:
Address:

	1ST SCREENING: DATE:						RESCREENING: DATE:					
	Right Eye			Left Eye			Right Eye			Left Eye		
Vision Tests	Normal	Abnormal	Untestable	Normal	Abnormal	Untestable	Normal	Abnormal	Untestable	Normal	Abnormal	Untestable
1. "E" (3 years and above—3 to 5 trials)	3P	3F	U	3P	3F	U	3P	3F	U	3P	3F	U
2. Picture card (2 1/2 - 2 11/12 yrs.—3 to 5 trials)	3P	3F	U	3P	3F	U	3P	3F	U	3P	3F	U
3. Fixation (6 months - 2 5/12 years)	P	F	U	P	F	U	P	F	U	P	F	U
4. Squinting	yes			yes			yes			yes		

Tests for Non-Straight Eyes	Normal	Abnormal	Untestable	Normal	Abnormal	Untestable
1. Do your child's eyes turn in or out, or are they ever not straight?	NO	YES		NO	YES	
2. Cover Test	P	F	U	P	F	U
3. Pupillary Light Reflex	P	F	U	P	F	U

Total Test Rating (Both Eyes)

Normal (passed vision test plus no squint, plus passed 2/3 tests for non-straight eyes) — Normal

Abnormal (abnormal on any vision test, squinting or 2 of 3 procedures for non-straight eyes) — Abnormal

Untestable (untestable on any vision test or untestable on 2/3 tests for non-straight eyes) — Untestable

Future Rescreening Appointment for Total Test Rating (Abnormal or Untestable)

Date: Date:

Fig. C-4

Denver Eye Screening Test. (From W.K. Frankenburg and J.B. Dobbs, University of Colorado Medical Center, 1969.)

NUTRITION

TABLE D-1. RECOMMENDED DAILY DIETARY ALLOWANCES (designed for the maintenance of good nutrition of

	AGE (years)	WEIGHT KG	WEIGHT LB	HEIGHT CM	HEIGHT IN	PROTEIN (g)	FAT-SOLUBLE VITAMINS VITAMIN A (μg RE)[a]	FAT-SOLUBLE VITAMINS VITAMIN D (μg)[b]	FAT-SOLUBLE VITAMINS VITAMIN E (mg α TE)[c]
Infants	0.0-0.5	6	13	60	24	kg × 2.2	420	10	3
	0.5-1.0	9	20	71	28	kg × 2.0	400	10	4
Children	1-3	13	29	90	35	23	400	10	5
	4-6	20	44	112	44	30	500	10	6
	7-10	28	62	132	52	34	700	10	7
Males	11-14	45	99	157	62	45	1000	10	8
	15-18	66	145	176	69	56	1000	10	10
	19-22	70	154	177	70	56	1000	7.5	10
	23-50	70	154	178	70	56	1000	5	10
	51 +	70	154	178	70	56	1000	5	10
Females	11-14	46	101	157	62	46	800	10	8
	15-18	55	120	163	64	46	800	10	8
	19-22	55	120	163	64	44	800	7.5	8
	23-50	55	120	163	64	44	800	5	8
	51 +	55	120	163	64	44	800	5	8
Pregnant						+30	+200	+5	+2
Lactating						+20	+400	+5	+3

From Food and Nutrition Board, National Academy of Sciences—National Research Council, Washington, D.C., 1980.

*The allowances are intended to provide for individual variations among most normal persons as they live in the United States under usual environmental stresses. Diets should be based on a variety of common foods in order to provide other nutrients for which human requirements have been less well defined.

[a]Retinol equivalents. 1 Retinol equivalent = 1 μg retinol or 6 μg β carotene.

[b]As cholecalciferol. 10 μg cholecalciferol = 400 IU vitamin D.

[c]α tocopherol equivalents. 1 mg d-α-tocopherol = 1 α TE.

[d]1 NE (niacin equivalent) is equal to 1 mg of niacin or 60 mg of dietary tryptophan.

[e]The folacin allowances refer to dietary sources as determined by *Lactobacillus casei* assay after treatment with enzymes ("conjugates") to make polyglutamyl forms of the vitamin available for the test organism.

[f]The RDA for vitamin B_{12} in infants based on average concentration of the vitamin in human milk. The allowances after weaning are based on energy intake (as recommended by the American Academy of Pediatrics) and consideration of other factors such as intestinal absorption.

[g]The increased requirement during pregnancy cannot be met by the iron content of habitual American diets nor by the existing iron stores of many women; therefore the use of 30-60 mg of supplemental iron is recommended. Iron needs during lactation are not substantially different from those of nonpregnant women, but continued supplementation of the mother for 2 to 3 months after parturition is advisable in order to replenish stores depleted by pregnancy.

TABLE D-2. ESTIMATED SAFE AND ADEQUATE DAILY DIETARY INTAKES OF ADDITIONAL SELECTED VITAMINS

	AGE (years)	VITAMINS VITAMIN K (μg)	VITAMINS BIOTIN (μg)	VITAMINS PANTOTHENIC ACID (mg)	COPPER (mg)	MANGANESE (mg)
Infants	0.0-0.5	12	35	2	0.5-0.7	0.5-0.7
	0.5-1.0	10-20	50	3	0.7-1.0	0.7-1.0
Children	1-3	15-30	65	3	1.0-1.5	1.0-1.5
	4-6	20-40	85	3-4	1.5-2.0	1.5-2.0
	7-10	30-60	120	4-5	2.0-2.5	2.0-3.0
Adolescents	11 +	50-100	100-200	4-7	2.0-3.0	2.5-5.0
Adults		70-140	100-200	4-7	2.0-3.0	2.5-5.0

From Recommended dietary allowances, Food and Nutrition Board, National Academy of Sciences—National Research Council, Washington, D.C., 1980.

*Because there is less information on which to base allowances, these figures are not given in the main tables of the RDA and are provided here in the form of ranges of recommended intakes.

†Since the toxic levels for many trace elements may be only several times usual intakes, the upper levels for the trace elements given in this table should not be habitually exceeded.

practically all healthy people in the United States)*

WATER-SOLUBLE VITAMINS							MINERALS					
VITAMIN C (mg)	THIAMIN (mg)	RIBOFLAVIN (mg)	NIACIN (mg NE)d	VITAMIN B6 (mg)	FOLACINe (µg)	VITAMIN B12 (µg)	CALCIUM (mg)	PHOSPHORUS (mg)	MAGNESIUM (mg)	IRON (mg)	ZINC (mg)	IODINE (µg)
35	0.3	0.4	6	0.3	30	0.5f	360	240	50	10	3	40
35	0.5	0.6	8	0.6	45	1.5	540	360	70	15	5	50
45	0.7	0.8	9	0.9	100	2.0	800	800	150	15	10	70
45	0.9	1.0	11	1.3	200	2.5	800	800	200	10	10	90
45	1.2	1.4	16	1.6	300	3.0	800	800	250	10	10	120
50	1.4	1.6	18	1.8	400	3.0	1200	1200	350	18	15	150
60	1.4	1.7	18	2.0	400	3.0	1200	1200	400	18	15	150
60	1.5	1.7	19	2.2	400	3.0	800	800	350	10	15	150
60	1.4	1.6	18	2.2	400	3.0	800	800	350	10	15	150
60	1.2	1.4	16	2.2	400	3.0	800	800	350	10	15	150
50	1.1	1.3	15	1.8	400	3.0	1200	1200	300	18	15	150
60	1.1	1.3	14	2.0	400	3.0	1200	1200	300	18	15	150
60	1.1	1.3	14	2.0	400	3.0	800	800	300	18	15	150
60	1.0	1.2	13	2.0	400	3.0	800	800	300	18	15	150
60	1.0	1.2	13	2.0	400	3.0	800	800	300	10	15	150
+20	+0.4	+0.3	+2	+0.6	+400	+1.0	+400	+400	+150	g	+5	+25
+40	+0.5	+0.5	+5	+0.5	+100	+1.0	+400	+400	+150	g	+10	+50

AND MINERALS*

TRACE ELEMENTS†				ELECTROLYTES		
FLUORIDE (mg)	CHROMIUM (mg)	SELENIUM (mg)	MOLYBDENUM (mg)	SODIUM (mg)	POTASSIUM (mg)	CHLORIDE (mg)
0.1-0.5	0.01-0.04	0.01-0.04	0.03-0.06	115-350	350-925	295-700
0.2-1.0	0.02-0.06	0.02-0.06	0.04-0.08	250-750	425-1275	400-1200
0.5-1.5	0.02-0.08	0.02-0.08	0.05-0.1	325-975	550-1650	500-1500
1.0-2.5	0.03-0.12	0.03-0.12	0.06-0.15	450-1350	775-2325	700-2100
1.5-2.5	0.05-0.92	0.05-0.2	0.1-0.3	600-1800	1000-3000	925-2775
1.5-2.5	0.05-0.2	0.05-0.2	0.15-0.5	900-2700	1525-4575	1400-4200
1.5-4.0	0.05-0.2	0.05-0.2	0.15-0.5	1100-3300	1875-5625	1700-5100

INDEX

1043

P

P$_{CO^2}$; *see* Partial pressure of carbon dioxide
PABA; *see* Para-aminobenzoic acid
PABA esters; *see* Para-aminobenzoic acid esters
Pacifiers, aspiration of, 248
Packed red blood cells, 796
Pain
    abdominal; *see* Abdominal pain
    and adolescent, 507-508
    assessment of, 512-513
    burns and, 930
    coxa plana and, 964
    dislocations and, 955
    fractures and, 943
    infant reactions to, 500
    juvenile rheumatoid arthritis and, 979
    in leukemia, 760
    management of, 513-515
    nurse's role in, 511-515
    osteomyelitis and, 971
    phantom limb, 954
    and preschooler, 504-505
    psychosomatic, 505
    rating scale for, 512-513
    and school-age child, 506-507
    skin disorders and, 897
    slipped femoral capital epiphysis and, 966
    and toddler, 504
Pain flow chart, 514
Pain management, 513-515
Pain rating scale, 512-513
Painful stimuli in newborn, 139
Palate
    cleft; *see* Cleft lip and/or cleft palate
    hard, 109
    soft, 109
Palatine tonsils, 109, 341
Palmar crease, single, 95
Palmar grasp, 233
Palpation
    of abdomen, 118
    in blood pressure measurement, 43
    of heart, 114
    of lungs, 111
Palpebral conjunctiva, 97
Palpebral fissures, 97
Palsy; *see also* Paralysis
    brachial, 170-172
    Erb, 170
    Klumpke, 170-171
    lower plexus, 170-171
    upper plexus, 170
Pancreas, 876
    cystic fibrosis and, 624
Pancrease; *see* Pancrelipase
Pancreatic amylase deficiency, 137
Pancreatic ducts, obstruction of, 625, 626
Pancreatic enzymes, 221
    cystic fibrosis and, 626
Pancreatic hormone dysfunction, 876-890
Pancreatic lipase deficiency, 137
Pancreatin, 626
Pancrelipase, 626
Pancuronium
    in Reye syndrome, 843
    tetanus and, 1005
Panendoscopy, 687
Panteric; *see* Pancreatin
Pantothenic acid, 260-261
    daily allowances for, 1040
Pap smear; *see* Papanicolaou smear
Papanicolaou smear, 419

Paper-doll technique of examination, 85-86
Papilledema
    in brain tumors, 830
    in cerebral dysfunction, 814
    in increased intracranial pressure, 812
Papule, 895
Para-aminobenzoic acid
    sunburn and, 932
    systemic lupus erythematosus and, 983
Para-aminobenzoic acid esters, 932
Parachute reflex, 220
    rolling over and, 225
Paradoxical pulse pressure, 728
Parainfluenza viruses, 606, 607
Paralanguage, 64
Paraldehyde
    in neonatal seizures, 202
    tetanus and, 1005
    and unconscious child, 817
Parallel play, 42
    in toddler, 291
Paralysis
    diaphragmatic, 172
    Erb-Duchenne, 170-172
    facial, 170
    infectious polyneuritis and, 1001-1002
    in neonate, 170-172
    phrenic nerve, 172
    tick, 1004, 1006
    Werdnig-Hoffmann, 998
Paraplegia, 1003
Parasites, 413
Parasympathetic ganglion cell absence, 650
Parathormone, 39, 863, 870
Parathyroid dysfunction, 39, 870-872
Paregoric, 208
Parent groups, exceptional problems and, 458; *see also* Parents
Parent-child attachment deprivation syndrome, 270
Parent-child bonding, 159-163, 235-236, 237; *see also* Parents, attachment and
Parenteral alimentation, 684
Parenteral fluids; *see* Fluid therapy; Intravenous fluids
Parents; *see also* Families; Father; Mother
    adolescents and, 72, 400-401, 406
    anticipatory guidance for, 254
        adolescence and, 406
        preschool child and, 325
    attachment and, 159-163, 235-236, 237
        deprivation syndrome and, 270
        high-risk infant and, 177
        needs and, 14-15
        visual impairment and, 489
    bonding and; *see* Parents, attachment and
    bureaucratic, 21
    casts and, 945, 949
    and child abuse, 360-361, 362, 363
    communication with, 65-69
        heart disease in, 715-716
    Down syndrome and, 475
    drug administration and, 557, 567-568
    exceptional problems and, 442-450, 453-456; *see also* Families, exceptional problems and
    expectations of, 67
    failure of child to thrive and, 271
    foreign body aspiration and, 612-613
    hydrocephalus and, 855-856
    infants and, 235-236, 237, 253-254
        high-risk, 177-178
    informed consent of, 532
        negligence and, 533

Parents—cont'd
    informed consent of—cont'd
        treatment without, 533
    interpersonal relationships and, 40-41
        adolescents and, 72
        nurses and, 520
        school-age child and, 377-378
    pain assessment and, 512
    plumbism and, 356
    rape victim and, 420
    reactions of, to ill child, 521
    rooming-in, 508-510
    skin disorders and, 899
    of toddler, 306-308
    ulcerative colitis and, 685
    and unconscious child, 820
Paroxysmal abdominal pain, 269-270
Paroxysmal contractions of tetanus, 1004
Parrot speech, 277
Partial pressure
    of carbon dioxide, 1012
    of oxygen, 1017
Partial seizures, 845-846
Partial thromboplastin time, 1017
Partially seeing, 483
Partial-thickness burns, 924
Participation in care, 456
Parties, adolescents and, 399
Passive immunity, 138
Passive inhalation injury, 615
Passivity, 444
Past history, 77-79
Pastes for skin care, 898
Patau syndrome, 52
Patch, 895
Patching of eye, 484
Patellar dislocations, 955-956
Patent airway of newborn, 150
Patent ductus arteriosus, 709, 710
Paternal engrossment, 162; *see also* Parents, attachment and
Patient profile, 82
Patterns
    of development, 28-29; *see also* Growth and development
    of sleep of newborn, 149
Pauses, nonverbal communication and, 64
Pavlik harness, 958
Pavulon; *see* Pancuronium
PBI; *see* Protein-bound iodine
PCM; *see* Protein and calorie malnutrition
PDA; *see* Patent ductus arteriosus
PDQ; *see* Denver Prescreening Developmental Questionnaire
PE tubes; *see* Pressure-equalizer tubes
Pearson attachment, 950
Pedestrian traffic accidents, 301
Pedialyte, 646
Pediatric nursing, 2-17
    child in, 14-16
    evolution of health care in, 7-9
    health during childhood and, 3-7
    nurse in, 9-12
    process of, 12-14
Pediculosis, 910, 911-912
    as sexually transmitted disease, 416, 418
Pediculosis capitis, 910, 911-912
Pediculosis corporis, 910
Pediculus humanus capitis, 910
Pediculus humanus corporis, 910
PEEP; *see* Positive and expiratory pressure
Peers, 40-41
    adolescence and, 72, 401-402

CONVERSION OF POUNDS TO KILOGRAMS FOR PEDIATRIC WEIGHTS

POUNDS→ ↓	0	1	2	3	4	5	6	7	8	9
0	0.00	0.45	0.90	1.36	1.81	2.26	2.72	3.17	3.62	4.08
10	4.53	4.98	5.44	5.89	6.35	6.80	7.35	7.71	8.16	8.61
20	9.07	9.52	9.97	10.43	10.88	11.34	11.79	12.24	12.70	13.15
30	13.60	14.06	14.51	14.96	15.42	15.87	16.32	16.78	17.23	17.69
40	18.14	18.59	19.05	19.50	19.95	20.41	20.86	21.31	21.77	22.22
50	22.68	23.13	23.58	24.04	24.49	24.94	25.40	25.85	26.30	26.76
60	27.21	27.66	28.22	28.57	29.03	29.48	29.93	30.39	30.84	31.29
70	31.75	32.20	32.65	33.11	33.56	34.02	34.47	34.92	35.38	35.83
80	36.28	36.74	37.19	37.64	38.10	38.55	39.00	39.46	39.93	40.37
90	40.82	41.27	41.73	42.18	42.63	43.09	43.54	43.99	44.45	44.90
100	45.36	45.81	46.26	46.72	47.17	47.62	48.08	48.53	48.98	49.44
110	49.89	50.34	50.80	51.25	51.71	52.16	52.61	53.07	53.52	53.97
120	54.43	54.88	55.33	55.79	56.24	56.70	57.15	57.60	58.06	58.51
130	58.96	59.42	59.87	60.32	60.78	61.23	61.68	62.14	62.59	63.05
140	63.50	63.95	64.41	64.86	65.31	65.77	66.22	66.67	67.13	67.58
150	68.04	68.49	68.94	69.40	69.85	70.30	70.76	71.21	71.66	72.12
160	72.57	73.02	73.48	73.93	74.39	74.84	75.29	75.75	76.20	76.65
170	77.11	77.56	78.01	78.47	78.92	79.38	79.83	80.28	80.74	81.19
180	81.64	82.10	82.55	83.00	83.46	83.91	84.36	84.82	85.27	85.73
190	86.18	86.68	87.09	87.54	87.99	88.45	88.90	89.35	89.81	90.26
200	90.72	91.17	91.62	92.08	92.53	92.98	93.44	93.89	94.34	94.80

CONVERSION OF POUNDS AND OUNCES TO KILOGRAMS FOR PEDIATRIC WEIGHTS

Pounds	Kilograms	Pounds	Kilograms	Ounces	Kilograms	Ounces	Kilograms
1	0.454	9	4.082	1	0.028	9	0.255
2	0.907	10	4.536	2	0.057	10	0.283
3	1.361	11	4.990	3	0.085	11	0.312
4	1.814	12	5.443	4	0.113	12	0.340
5	2.268	13	5.897	5	0.142	13	0.369
6	2.722			6	0.170	14	0.397
7	3.175			7	0.198	15	0.425
8	3.629			8	0.227		

CONVERSION FACTORS FOR TEMPERATURE*

Celsius	Fahrenheit	Celsius	Fahrenheit	Celsius	Fahrenheit	Celsius	Fahrenheit
34.0	93.2	36.4	97.5	38.6	101.5	41.0	105.9
34.2	93.6	36.6	97.9	38.8	101.8	41.2	106.1
34.4	93.9	36.8	98.2	39.0	102.2	41.4	106.5
34.6	94.3	37.0	98.6	39.2	102.6	41.6	106.8
34.8	94.6	37.2	99.0	39.4	102.9	41.8	107.2
35.0	95.0	37.4	99.3	39.6	103.3	42.0	107.6
35.2	95.4	37.6	99.7	39.8	103.6	42.2	108.0
35.4	95.7	37.8	100.0	40.0	104.0	42.4	108.3
35.6	96.1	38.0	100.4	40.2	104.4	42.6	108.7
35.8	96.4	38.2	100.8	40.4	104.7	42.8	109.0
36.0	96.8	38.4	101.1	40.6	105.2	43.0	109.4
36.2	97.2			40.8	105.4		

*(°C) × (9/5) + 32 = °F
(°F − 32) × (5/9) = °C
°C = temperature in Celsius (centigrade) degrees
°F = temperature in Fahrenheit degrees